AF779009

Chinese Materia Medica
Combinations and Applications

Biographical details

Xu Li graduated from Tianjin College of Traditional Chinese Medicine in 1985 with a bachelor's degree in medicine, having studied both Western and traditional Chinese medicine. He was a teacher in the college's Department of Acupuncture from 1985 to 1993, since when he has taught in the International School of Tianjin College of TCM. He is now Vice-Professor and Dean of the International School. Dr. Xu has extensive clinical and teaching experience and has lectured and practised abroad in several countries including the UK. He has been involved in the writing or compilation of a number of TCM books including *Chinese Materia Medica, A Teaching Guide to Commonly-Used Chinese Materia Medica, Traditional Chinese Medicine Formulae* (a textbook in English for overseas students), *A Compendium of Diagnosis and Treatment in Integrated Chinese and Western Medicine* and *A Complete Manual of Modern Acupuncture, Channels and Points* (English edition).

Wang Wei graduated from Tianjin College of Traditional Chinese Medicine in 1985 with a bachelor's degree in medicine, having studied both Western and traditional Chinese medicine. She then became a teacher in the college's Department of Acupuncture and is now Vice-Professor and Director of the Acupuncture Treatment Division of this department. She has extensive clinical and teaching experience and has lectured and practised abroad in several countries including the UK. Dr. Wang has published a number of articles and has been involved as deputy editor-in-chief in the writing of several books including *Chinese Materia Medica, Traditional Chinese Medicine, Acupuncture Therapy* (English edition), *Collected Explanations of TCM Formulae* (a commentary on the classic work) and *Essential Readings from the Medical Tradition.*

Simon Fielding practises acupuncture and Chinese herbal medicine in Leicester. He trained first in acupuncture, graduating from the London School of Acupuncture in 1991, and later in herbs, graduating from the London Academy of Oriental Medicine in 1995. He teaches at the London College of Traditional Acupuncture and Oriental Medicine and works on the editorial board of The European Journal of Oriental Medicine. He is a member of the British Acupuncture Council and the Register of Chinese Herbal Medicine.

Chinese Materia Medica
Combinations and Applications

Compiled and translated by

Xu Li

Vice-Professor and Dean,
International School of Tianjin College of TCM

Wang Wei

Vice-Professor and Director of the Acupuncture Treatment Division,
Department of Acupuncture, Tianjin College of TCM

Foreword by

Giovanni Maciocia

CAc (Nanjing)

Subject editor

Simon Fielding

MBAcC MRCHM

Donica Publishing Ltd

Note

Medical knowledge is constantly changing. As new information becomes available, changes in treatment, procedures, equipment and the use of drugs and/or materia medica become necessary. The editors/authors/contributors and the publishers have, as far as it is possible, taken care to ensure that the information given in this text is accurate and up to date. However, readers are strongly advised to confirm that the information, especially with regard to the permitted usage of materia medica, complies with the latest legislation and standards of practice.

Although every effort has been made to indicate appropriate precautions with regard to the legal status and usage of materia medica, neither the publishers nor the authors can accept responsibility for any treatment advice or information offered, neither will they be liable for any loss or damage of any nature occasioned to or suffered by any person acting or refraining from acting as a result of reliance on the material contained in this publication.

Copyright © 2002 by Donica Publishing Ltd

All rights reserved. No part of this book may be reprinted or reproduced or utilized in any form or by any electronic, mechanical or other means, now known or hereafter invented, including photocopying and recording, or in any information storage or retrieval system (including the Internet), without prior permission in writing from the publishers. For information, please contact Donica Publishing Ltd, 2 Waddington Road, St. Albans, Herts AL3 5EX.

First published 2002

ISBN 1 901149 02 1

British Library Cataloguing in Publication Data
A catalogue record for this book is available from the British Library

Commissioning editor Yanping Li
Managing editor Rodger Watts
Cover design Phill Butterworth

Typeset by Aarontype Ltd.
Printed in the UK by CPI.
The publisher's policy is to use paper manufactured from sustainable forests.

Contributors

Li Zhidao

Zhang Liancheng
Li Chengli
Diao Xi
Li Lanyuan
Li Lixiang
Ma Zuoying
Li Ling
Yang Xuemei

Acknowledgements

This book could not have been written without the constant help and encouragement of our teachers, colleagues and friends.

We are deeply indebted to our mentors Professor Shi Xuemin, Academician of the Chinese Academy of Engineering, Member of the Council of the China Acupuncture Association and President of the First Hospital Affiliated to Tianjin College of TCM and Professor Li Zhidao of Tianjin College of TCM.

We are also very grateful to Mr. Giovanni Maciocia for kindly agreeing to write a foreword to this volume.

In addition, this book could not have been compiled without the assistance of our fellow editors and translators Zhang Liancheng, Li Chengli, Diao Xi, Li Lanyuan, Li Lixiang, Ma Zuoying, Li Ling and Yang Xuemei.

Further help in the translation of English terminology was provided by Anna-Katharina Lehr, Stephanie Sommer and Adi Gerlitz.

Without the unflagging assistance and support of Yanping Li at Donica Publishing, this book could never have been completed.

To all of them, we express our heartfelt gratitude.

SUMMARY OF CONTENTS

DETAILED LIST OF CONTENTS

Chapter 4

Chapter 5

Chapter 6

Chapter 7

Chapter 12

Chapter 13

Foreword

Chinese medicine was introduced in the West primarily with acupuncture but Chinese herbal medicine is becoming more and more popular in many countries. Compared to acupuncture, Chinese herbal medicine allows us to treat a broader spectrum of diseases and often serious diseases such as hepatitis, cancer and leukaemia. To practise Chinese herbal medicine safely and effectively, the student needs to pass a series of hurdles: the most important of these are making a correct diagnosis and following a correct treatment principle. If we have a clear idea of the diagnosis, a clear idea of the full or empty character of the condition and a clear idea of the treatment principle, the choice of herbal prescription follows almost automatically.

However, the art of Chinese herbal medicine consists also in adapting the chosen formula to the patient, carefully adjusting it to treat the patient's unique pattern configuration. Apart from the empty or full and hot or cold character of the condition, the practitioner needs to take into account many other factors such as the nature (hot or cold), taste and directional tendencies of the formula as a whole and of the individual herbs. Learning and memorizing single herbs and formulae is a daunting prospect for all students of Chinese herbal medicine. No matter how many herbs we learn, we always seem to come across a new formula that contains a herb we have not studied.

The harmonization of herbs within a formula is comparable to a balanced composition in a beautiful painting: it is this composition which makes beautiful art in the same way as the balanced mixture of herbs according to their nature, taste and directional tendencies makes an effective formula with the maximum therapeutic effect and minimum strain on the digestive system.

Adapting a formula to a patient's particular disharmony of course requires a profound knowledge of single herbs and of the differences and peculiarities of herbs in the same categories with similar effects. The book *Chinese Materia Medica: Combinations and Applications* is an invaluable help to students and practitioners precisely for such a task. This book fills a gap in the existing literature on Chinese herbal medicine by presenting the herbs in a very clear, easily memorized way. Furthermore, a real strength of the book is the presentation of much of the information in tabular form for easy reference. Other details make the book extremely useful to students such as the reference to herbs with similar functions within each monograph. Another important feature of the book is the inclusion of the legal status of certain herbs in the UK, an important consideration in the current regulatory climate. Thus, rather than a textbook, this book places itself squarely in the market as an excellent clinical reference text.

A particularly welcome feature of the book is the comprehensive system of indexes: apart from the usual indexes of names (by pinyin, Chinese characters, Latin name and English name), there are also very useful cross-references of functions to individual herbs, of individual herbs to combinations and of symptoms to relevant combinations as well as an index of patterns with applicable herbs.

The authors of this work are teachers in the International School of Tianjin College of TCM. They have extensive clinical practice and experience in teaching foreign students. The chief author, Xu Li, is Vice-Professor and Dean of the School and has lectured abroad in several countries including Britain. The book has been translated paying particular attention to terminology and style and avoids the often heavy prose of Chinese books in English.

In conclusion, this book represents a welcome addition to the literature on Chinese herbal medicine and one that can be highly recommended to students and practitioners alike.

Giovanni Maciocia
Amersham 2001

Preface

The growing interest around the world in complementary and alternative medicines in general and traditional Chinese medicine in particular makes the publication of a handy reference book on the combination and application of Chinese materia medica particularly apposite. The science of Chinese materia medica involves the study of the basic theories, sources, methods of collection and processing, properties, functions, combinations and applications of various Chinese medicinal materials. Much of this has been handed down from generation to generation throughout the long history of Chinese culture, but the greater awareness of the effectiveness of these materia medica in the treatment of a wide variety of conditions and the growing desire both in China and the West to identify the scientific basis governing their functions have resulted in an increased level of research and in greater application of these substances in the treatment of certain of the 'modern' diseases afflicting society all over the world at the start of the 21st century.

PRINCIPLES GOVERNING THE SELECTION OF MATERIAL

There are more than 2,200 materia medica listed in the *National Collection of Chinese Herbs*, a two-volume encyclopaedia whose second edition was published in 1996.[1] We have selected more than 350 of the most commonly-used materia medica for inclusion in this book. We have generally followed the traditional chapter denominations and classifications of Chinese books through the ages, although this does allow a certain amount of scope in classifying some herbs with two functions of similar importance. Some of the combinations may be familiar to Western readers, others may give a fresh insight into the use of the materia medica included in the book. Whatever the case, we hope that the combinations and applications listed will be of use to those working in the TCM field in achieving a better understanding of these commonly-used herbs and raising the overall effectiveness of the treatment given.

The herbs chosen and the functions, combinations and applications associated with them are based on the teaching material that we have prepared for the Chinese materia medica degree course at the International School of the Tianjin College of TCM. This material in turn was based on the standard TCM classics, the recently-published *Zhong Yao Xue* [Chinese Materia Medica] by Gao Xuemei,[2] and the TCM teaching syllabus for specialist TCM colleges and universities. This book was written by combining traditional Chinese medicine theories with the authors' practical clinical and teaching experience.

COMPILATION PRINCIPLES

The focus of this book is on the combination and application of Chinese materia medica. A knowledge of the basics of traditional Chinese medicine has been assumed. The book has been written primarily for practitioners, although it is hoped that study of the functions, combinations and applications detailed will also prove invaluable to intermediate and advanced students.

The text relating to combinations and applications has essentially been laid out in tabular form to facilitate the process of reference and consultation. It is our intention that this volume should serve as a reference book in clinical practice. Each chapter and many chapter sections begin with a summary of the herbs covered by that particular chapter or section. The clear arrangement of the tabular format and the comprehensive indexing is designed to make it easy for practitioners to find the reference or assistance they require in a matter of seconds, allowing them to focus their attention on treating the patient.

Throughout this book, the term 'herbs' can be taken to mean materia medica. In those instances where the materia medica referred to consist entirely of mineral or animal substances, other designations may also be employed. Although materia medica is technically the more correct term, we have essentially adopted the use of the term 'herbs', as this appears to be in more general use among practitioners.

Herbs are referred to throughout by their Chinese names in pinyin and their pharmaceutical names in Latin. Within each individual herb monograph, the Latin name of the main herb is generally not repeated (the only exception to this rule can be found in the comparison of functions subsection). Each monograph title also includes the Chinese characters for the herb and an English name. As many herbs have several English names, it is not practical to refer to them in the text with these names, which is one of the reasons why we have opted for the pinyin-Latin designation. All main herbs (and those that only appear in combinations rather than having a monograph to themselves) are listed in Appendices 1 and 2 by pinyin name, Chinese characters, English name and pharmaceutical name to aid cross-reference.

Ideally, the designation, ordering and prescription of Chinese herbs would be carried out using characters in order to reduce the risk of errors to a minimum. However, we recognize that this is not a practical proposition for many Western practitioners, which is another reason for the pinyin-Latin approach. The Latin designations of herbs are based primarily on the *Pharmacopoeia of the People's Republic of China (English Edition) 2000.*[3] Where necessary, we have increased the precision of these designations to conform to general practice in the West (for example, when only one plant is used for a particular herb). We hope that this will not lead to confusion.

The plants or other substances used for any particular herb have essentially been taken from the *Pharmacopoeia*[3] or the *National Collection of Chinese Herbs.*[1] More than one plant may sometimes be used for a particular herb; this has been indicated where appropriate.

It is important at this point to draw readers' attention to the legal status of certain of the herbs included in this book. Although they are all available in China, a few herbs are subject to export restrictions and others are considered too toxic for use in some Western countries. Readers are advised to consult the section at the end of the introduction for more details; this section should be read before prescribing any of the herbs. The situation regarding restrictions and bans tends to change over time and from country to country. The position described in this book is to the best of our knowledge and belief that existing in the United Kingdom at the time of publication. Readers should consult the appropriate authorities in their own countries for the latest developments. Inclusion of a herb in this book does not imply that its use is permitted in all countries and in all circumstances.

Research into the active ingredients of herbs continues, but knowledge about the constituents of each individual herb varies from herb to herb. Some herbs have been identified as having a large number of major ingredients, others have been subject to little research. It is not the aim of this book to give an exhaustive listing of all the ingredients of every herb, but to provide some background understanding as a guide to usage. In addition, there is not always agreement on what actually constitutes the main ingredients of particular herbs; we have tried to provide a synthesis of the current situation in China.

Unless indicated otherwise, the common dosage of each herb given in the book refers to the dosage (in grams) suitable for an adult to drink in a decoction. It should be borne in mind that Chinese patients are often more tolerant of large dosages than their Western counterparts. Exact dosages of herbs for external use are not given; they should be decided according to such factors as the size of area affected, the constitution of the patient, and the severity and nature of the disease.

Further details relating to properties, channels entered, functions and indications, precautions and contraindications, and combinations and applications are given in the introduction. It should be pointed out here that the combinations and applications chosen are just a small cross-section of the huge number included in the books on Chinese herbal medicine. In addition, some herbs can be used on their own or as subsidiary herbs in other combinations for particular indications, with the result that there may be some instances where some indications do not have corresponding combinations.

Many herbs have similar functions and we consider it important that practitioners are in a position to understand how to differentiate between these herbs and decide which herb is most appropriate in a given situation. We have therefore included direct comparisons of herbs in a number of monographs with the aim of offering a greater insight into their actions. The *Remarks* subsection gives additional information on usage and differentiation.

In recent years, a considerable amount of research has been carried out in China into Chinese herbs and their functions. Much of this research remains inaccessible to many Western practitioners since it has not been published in English or other Western languages. We have aimed to provide a brief indication of some of the main research on herbs by listing the sources in which it can be found. This is a first step towards the huge task of making it more generally available. Readers should be aware of the ongoing debate on the rigour with which this research, especially less recent research, has been carried out. It should also be noted that, unless otherwise indicated, the modern research results noted refer to laboratory experiments conducted on animals. Much less research has been carried out into the effect of herbs on humans; readers should be aware that the results of animal tests may not necessarily be replicated in humans. A detailed description of the experiments conducted is not within the scope of this book, as it would expand its size considerably as well as diverting attention away from the main focus. Nevertheless, we consider that the indication of possible benefits as identified by modern research will be of interest to readers.

A significant element of the research that has been carried out has focused on the toxicity of certain herbs. Where such work has been undertaken, we have summarized the results in the *Toxicity* subsection. Again, most of the experiments have been performed on animals, but the results give an indication of the likely effect on humans. The most widely used measure of toxicity is the dosage that will lead to the death of 50 percent of the animals used in the experiments concerned – this is commonly referred to as LD_{50}. In addition, clinical reports on symptoms appearing after toxic overdoses (generally far in excess of normal dosages for humans) provide useful guidelines. Clearly, overdosage and erroneous use of materia medica can lead to unwanted side-effects, and practitioners must always bear this in mind when prescribing.

TERMINOLOGY AND TRANSLATION

The issue of terminology and translation always excites passionate debate in TCM circles. Even in China, renowned and experienced doctors still argue about the exact interpretation of the ancient texts. The problem of finding precise equivalents for TCM terms in a foreign language is even more challenging. There are a number of bilingual (Chinese-English) TCM dictionaries available in China compiled by Chinese authors. However, these all generally suffer from the drawback that the compilers have preferred to find a Western medical equivalent for TCM terms, even where there is no direct correlation. The only comprehensive glossary of TCM terminology in English compiled by a Westerner available in China is the *English-Chinese Chinese-English Dictionary of Chinese Medicine* by Nigel Wiseman.[4] The translation of many of the terms used in this book (especially the less common ones) is therefore based on this dictionary.

However, certain of the terms used in the dictionary still seem to be the subject of much debate in the West and there are a few instances where the terminology adopted to date in Western TCM books seems to us to be more appropriate. We have therefore employed as our standard the 'middle way' adopted in the UK between the longer-standing translations employed by respected authors such as Giovanni Maciocia[5] and the move towards a more literal approach used by Wiseman. One major example recently of what can be achieved with this approach is *A Manual of Acupuncture* by Peter Deadman, Mazin al-Khafaji and Kevin Baker.[6]

We have included two appendices relating to terminology at the end of the book – one to indicate the terminology utilized in translating the functions of herbs and the other to highlight the meaning of some of the terms used in the book. It is hoped that this will clarify the situation where there are differences from the translations employed in other books.

We have opted to translate most Chinese terms into English, but there are a few exceptions. As most people now accept that Yin, Yang and Qi are untranslatable terms, we have left them in the original Chinese. We have also preferred to leave Jiao untranslated (rather than the Energizer favoured by Chinese translators or the Burner of Western texts). In addition, we prefer Bi syndrome, Lin syndrome and Wei syndrome for painful obstruction syndrome, painful urinary syndrome (or dysfunction) and atrophy syndrome respectively and Shan disorders for hernial disorders, as we consider that the meaning of these terms is sufficiently well-known not to require translation.

Where there is the possibility of confusion in relation to body organs or functions, we have opted to indicate the TCM term with a capital letter and the Western understanding of the term with a small letter (thus, Kidney deficiency, but kidney stones).

Although most applications have been translated in TCM terms, Western medical terms have occasionally been used for more 'modern' disorders or disorders not recognized as such in classical works (for example, hypertension). In a few other instances, notably skin diseases, we have included both a literal translation of the original Chinese and the generally accepted Western medical equivalent. As far as gynaecological conditions are concerned, we have not used Western medical terminology, preferring to go back to a literal translation of the original Chinese, as this makes the nature of the condition clear.

It is our sincere hope that debates on terminology will take second place to consideration of the treatment principles underlying the combinations and applications of the herbs discussed in this book.

Xu Li, Wang Wei
Tianjin, October 2001

References

1. Xie Zongwan et al., *Quan Guo Zhong Cao Yao Hui Bian* [National Collection of Chinese Herbs], 2nd edition (Beijing: People's Medical Publishing House, 1996).
2. Gao Xuemei et al., *Zhong Yao Xue* [Chinese Materia Medica] (Beijing: People's Medical Publishing House, 2000).
3. Pharmacopoeia Commission of the PRC, *Pharmacopoeia of the People's Republic of China (English Edition 2000)* (Beijing: Chemical Industry Press, 2000).
4. Nigel Wiseman, *English-Chinese Chinese-English Dictionary of Chinese Medicine* (Changsha: Hubei Science and Technology Publishing House, 1996).
5. Giovanni Maciocia, *The Foundations of Chinese Medicine* (Edinburgh: Churchill Livingstone, 1989).
6. Peter Deadman, Mazin al-Khafaji and Kevin Baker, *Manual of Acupuncture* (Hove: Journal of Chinese Medicine Publications, 1998).

General introduction

CHARACTERISTICS AND FUNCTIONS OF HERBS USED IN TRADITIONAL CHINESE MEDICINE

Traditional Chinese medicine (TCM) attributes certain characteristics to each herb, classifying them for example as cold or hot, upward-bearing or downward-bearing, drying or moistening. Herbs are used according to their intrinsic characteristics to treat diseases, regulate Yin and Yang and help the body re-establish its normal physiological functions by curing disorders and restoring health. The classification of traditional Chinese herbs according to their characteristics and functions forms the basis for treating diseases with Chinese herbs.

Nature and taste

Herbs are classified in traditional Chinese medicine according to the four natures (*sì qì*) and five tastes (*wŭ wèi*). Each herb possesses these two characteristics – one of the four natures and at least one of the five tastes. The functions of each herb have a very close relationship with the taste and nature of that herb. Thus, *sì qì* and *wŭ wèi*, as the basic method of describing the nature and taste of traditional Chinese herbs, function as important guidelines in clinical practice.

Sì qì describes the four different natures of herbs as cold, hot, warm and cool. As a general rule, herbs used for treating heat patterns are characterized as being cold or cool, whereas those for treating cold patterns are designated as hot or warm. So the nature of a herb, i.e. cold, hot, warm or cool, can be considered as antagonistic to the nature of the disease.

The nature of herbs can essentially be divided into two categories – cool and cold on the one hand, and warm and hot on the other; within the two categories, differences are only a matter of degree. Cool is less conspicuous than cold and warm is less apparent than hot. In some texts, the characteristics of slightly cold and slightly warm are attributed to certain herbs. In this context, 'slightly cold' is similar to or slightly less cold than 'cool' and 'slightly warm' is not as hot as 'warm'.

Cool or cold herbs perform such functions as clearing heat or fire, relieving toxicity and enriching Yin and can therefore be used to treat heat patterns. Warm or hot herbs act against cold patterns by dispelling cold, warming the interior, supplementing Yang and treating collapse.

In addition to the four natures mentioned above, some herbs are described as 'neutral'. As they are neither obviously hot or warm, nor cold or cool, they are considered as having moderating functions. They can be combined with other herbs for the treatment of both cold and heat patterns.

Wŭ wèi refers to the five different tastes – acrid, sweet, sour, bitter and salty. Additionally, the terms bland and astringent are sometimes mentioned in the ancient texts, resulting in the term *qì wèi*, or seven tastes, being coined. As taste is not always easy to determine rigorously, people a long time ago did not discriminate between bland and sweet, simply classifying some herbs as having both tastes. In addition, as astringent is similar to sour, further distinction was not always made between them.

Herbs with different tastes vary in their pharmacologically-active substances and functions, whereas herbs with similar tastes have similar functions and ingredients. The functions of the various types of herbs are described below:

1. **Acrid herbs** have a dissipating function and promote the movement of Qi and Blood. As a general rule, most of the herbs for inducing sweating and moving or regulating Qi are acrid. They are used mainly to treat exterior patterns and disorders due to Qi stagnation and Blood stasis. For example, *Ma Huang* (Herba Ephedrae) induces sweating, *Xiang Fu* (Rhizoma Cyperi Rotundi) regulates Qi, and *Hong Hua* (Flos Carthami Tinctorii) quickens the Blood and dispels Blood stasis.

2. **Sweet herbs** have a supplementing, harmonizing and adjusting function and can alleviate spasms and convulsions. They are commonly used to treat deficiency patterns, harmonize the properties of herbs and alleviate pain. Examples include *Ren Shen* (Radix Ginseng), which strongly supplements original Qi, *Shu Di Huang* (Radix Rehmanniae Glutinosae Conquita), which nourishes the Blood, and *Gan Cao* (Radix Glycyrrhizae) which adjusts and harmonizes the properties of other herbs and relaxes tension to alleviate pain.
3. **Sour herbs** have an astringent function and secure the Essence. Most of the sour herbs are used to treat sweating due to deficiency, enduring diarrhoea, seminal emission and vaginal discharge. For example, *Wu Wei Zi* (Fructus Schisandrae) constrains sweating, *Wu Bei Zi* (Galla Rhois Chinensis) stops diarrhoea and *Shan Zhu Yu* (Fructus Corni Officinalis) has a securing and containing function.
4. **Bitter herbs**: Most of the herbs which clear heat and fire, free the bowels, dry dampness and bear counterflow Qi downwards are bitter. They are commonly used to treat heat patterns, constipation, fullness in the stomach and abdomen due to obstruction of dampness, and coughing and vomiting due to ascending counterflow Qi. For example *Huang Lian* (Rhizoma Coptidis) clears heat and drains fire, *Da Huang* (Radix et Rhizoma Rhei) drains downwards to treat constipation, *Xing Ren* (Semen Pruni Armeniacae) stops coughing by bearing counterflow Qi downwards, *Cang Zhu* (Rhizoma Atractylodis) dries dampness and fortifies the Spleen, and *Zhi Mu* (Rhizoma Anemarrhenae Asphodeloidis) clears heat by purgation in order to preserve body fluids.
5. **Salty herbs** dissipate lumps and free the bowels. They are commonly used to treat scrofula, abdominal masses and constipation. Examples include *Mang Xiao* (Mirabilitum), which guides out stagnation to treat constipation, and *Mu Li* (Concha Ostreae), which treats scrofula and Phlegm nodes by softening hardness and dissipating lumps.
6. **Bland herbs**: Herbs with a bland taste perform the functions of percolating dampness and promoting urination. They are mostly used to treat disorders due to obstruction of dampness and inhibited urination. Examples include *Fu Ling* (Sclerotium Poriae Cocos) and *Tong Cao* (Medulla Tetrapanacis Papyriferi).
7. **Astringent herbs** have similar functions to sour herbs.

Herbs with different tastes also vary in their functions as a result of the chemical constituents they contain. For example, most sour herbs contain tannins and organic acids; bitter herbs contain alkaloids, glycosides and amaroids; sweet herbs contain carbohydrates; and acrid herbs contain volatile oils.

As clinical practice has developed, the classification of herbs according to their taste has changed. Accordingly, herbs with astringent functions have been classified as sour herbs and herbs that dissipate lumps as salty herbs. Thus, the description of the taste of different herbs does not necessarily coincide with their actual taste. In the early days of Chinese medicine, herbs were classified by their perceivable tastes; later on, the system was reorganized to classify them according to their therapeutic functions.

Nature and taste are the two main characteristics of herbs. Generally speaking, herbs with a similar nature and taste have similar functions. For instance, most acrid and warm herbs have the function of diffusing and dissipating cold to treat exterior patterns. Nevertheless, each herb still possesses its own special characteristics. For example, both *Zi Su Ye* (Folium Perillae Frutescentis) and *Sheng Jiang* (Rhizoma Zingiberis Officinalis Recens) are acrid and warm and have the function of dissipating cold by inducing sweating, but *Zi Su Ye* is more effective than *Sheng Jiang* in this respect. *Zi Su Ye* has the additional function of moving Qi, whereas *Sheng Jiang* is also able to warm the Middle Jiao to stop vomiting.

The functions of herbs which differ in nature and taste are obviously different. For instance, both *Huang Lian* (Rhizoma Coptidis) and *Fu Ping* (Herba Spirodelae Polyrrhizae) are cold, but as *Huang Lian* is bitter and cold, it clears heat and dries dampness, whereas *Fu Ping* is acrid and cold, thus having the function of diffusing and dispersing wind-heat. *Huang Qi* (Radix Astragali seu Hedysari) and *Shi Hu* (Herba Dendrobii) are both sweet, but *Huang Qi* is sweet and slightly warm, thus warming Yang Qi, whereas *Shi Hu*, being sweet and slightly cold, enriches Yin and abates fever.

Many herbs are recognized as having several kinds of taste, so they exhibit a larger functional range than herbs with only one taste. This implies that the use of herbs in clinical practice should not only be guided by the basic theories of *sì qì* and *wǔ wèi,* but also by the special characteristics and curative functions attributed to each herb.

Directional tendencies

The directional tendencies of the functions of herbs are usually classified as upward-bearing, downward-bearing, floating and sinking. In this context, the function of a herb shows a certain tendency towards upward, downward, outward or inward movement in relation to the body. 'Upward-bearing' signifies rising or sending up while 'downward-bearing' means falling or sending down. 'Floating' indicates going outwards or sending to the surface, whereas 'sinking' signifies going inwards or purging to eliminate.

Upward-bearing and floating herbs which have upward and outward tendencies are used for bearing Yang upwards, releasing the exterior by means of artificially-induced sweating, dissipating external wind and cold, inducing vomiting and bringing about resuscitation. Downward-bearing and sinking herbs exhibit downward and inward actions and are thus used for clearing heat, purging, promoting urination, percolating dampness and subduing Yang. Additionally, they bear ascending counterflow Qi downwards in order to stop coughing and calm wheezing, stop vomiting, disperse food accumulation and quiet the Spirit.

The actions of upward-bearing, downward-bearing, floating and sinking correspond to the location of a disease, but oppose the tendency of the development of the disease. As a general rule, for diseases located in the upper or exterior part of the body, such as an exterior pattern caused by wind-cold, it is appropriate to use upward-bearing and floating herbs. For diseases located in the lower or interior part of the body, such as Intestinal dryness with constipation, it is appropriate to use downward-bearing and sinking herbs. For diseases which have an upward tendency, such as headache, dizziness and red eyes due to ascendant hyperactivity of Liver Yang, downward-bearing and sinking herbs should be used. For diseases which have downward tendencies, such as enduring diarrhoea or prolapse of the rectum or uterus, upward-bearing and floating herbs should be selected.

The characteristics of upward-bearing, downward-bearing, floating and sinking have a certain relationship to the nature, taste and consistency of herbs. Most hot or warm herbs with an acrid or sweet taste have upward-bearing and floating actions; herbs with a bitter, sour or salty taste, which are cool or cold, also possess downward-bearing and sinking actions. Most substances with a low physical density have lifting and floating actions. By contrast, most heavy materials have the actions of downward-bearing and sinking. However, there are some exceptions. *Man Jing Zi* (Fructus Viticis) and *Cang Er Zi* (Fructus Xanthii Sibirici) are comparatively heavy, as they are seeds, but they have floating properties; on the other hand, *Xuan Fu Hua* (Flos Inulae) and *Fan Xie Ye* (Folium Sennae) are flower and leaf respectively, but they perform downward-bearing actions.

Although the actions of herbs are based on their nature and taste, they can also be influenced by pharmacological processing and combination with other herbs. Downward-bearing and sinking herbs can have upward-bearing and floating actions after being processed with alcohol or when used together with a large quantity of floating and upward-bearing herbs. Upward-bearing and floating herbs can have downward-bearing and sinking actions after being processed with salt or when used together with large amounts of sinking and downward-bearing herbs.

Channels entered

The expression 'channels entered' refers to the fact that a certain kind of herb performs its major therapeutic function in a certain part of the body by acting along one or more channels and exercising its effect on the corresponding organ. For example, some herbs for clearing heat are used mainly for clearing Lung-heat, whereas others are used mainly for clearing Liver-heat; some supplementing herbs act on the Lungs, others on the Spleen.

Hence, TCM ascribes each herb to one or more of the twelve channels used to explain the curative effect according to Zang-Fu and channel theory. For instance, *Bai Jie Zi* (Semen Sinapis Albae) and *Zi Wan* (Radix Asteris Tatarici) can be used to stop coughing and calm wheezing and they are consequently said to enter the Lung channel; *Quan Xie* (Buthus Martensi) and *Tian Ma* (Rhizoma Gastrodiae Elatae) extinguish wind and alleviate tetany, so they are considered as entering the Liver channel. Some herbs enter several channels, which means that they are effective in different parts of the body represented by these channels. For example, the Lung and Stomach channels are attributed to *Shi Gao* (Gypsum Fibrosum), which can clear heat in both the Lungs and the Stomach; the Spleen and Lung channels are attributed to *Dang Shen* (Radix Codonopsitis Pilosulae), which can boost both Spleen and Lung Qi.

The theory of channels entered describes the effect of herbs and is widely used in the clinic. But, as disorders of different Zang-Fu organs and channels are often complex and can affect each other, it is not normally sufficient to select herbs which only enter one channel. For instance, herbs for the Lungs and the Spleen should be combined when treating a disease consisting of a disorder of the Lungs and deficiency of the Spleen.

Supplementation and draining functions of herbs

Although the pathology of diseases is complicated, traditional Chinese medicine classifies diseases into two groups: deficiency patterns caused by insufficiency of Qi, Blood, Yin or Yang; and full patterns due to functional hyperactivity. The supplementation and draining functions of herbs are characteristics which describe their antagonistic effect on deficiency or full patterns in the human body. In this context, supplementation refers to the ability of herbs to supplement original Qi and nourish Yin and Blood as well as supplementing Yang and boosting Qi. Thus, herbs that have a supplementing function counteract functional disorders, strengthen the body and prevent illness. Herbs that have a draining function are able to disperse pathogenic factors, regulate hyperactivity and stop or inhibit the further development of a disease.

The supplementation and draining functions of herbs have a close connection to their nature and taste. As herbs with antagonistic functions are used to treat deficiency and full patterns, it is indispensable to distinguish properly between these two kinds of patterns. A thorough diagnosis must precede the selection of supplementing herbs to treat deficiency patterns and draining herbs to treat full patterns. For instance, most herbs which dispel cold are acrid and sweet in taste and warm or hot in nature; herbs for clearing heat are generally acrid, sweet or salty in taste and cold in nature; and herbs which supplement Yin are mostly acrid, bitter and salty in taste and cold in nature. On the other hand, herbs that supplement Qi and the Blood are sweet and warm, and herbs for treating fever due to Blood deficiency are sweet and cool.

In addition, there is a close relationship between the Zang-Fu organs, as the state of one organ affects that of others. This is also very important in applying supplementing and draining herbs correctly in treatment.

Toxicity of herbs

The term 'toxicity' implies that an overdosage of certain herbs may lead to toxic reactions, or that application of the therapeutic dosage of the herb may actually cause severe side-effects. In Chinese texts on herbal medicine, the degree of toxicity is expressed as 'slightly toxic', 'toxic', 'extremely toxic' or 'deadly toxic'.

In order to ensure safety while using herbs for treatment, it is advisable to adjust the dosage according to the toxicity and side-effects of herbs, the patient's constitution and age, and the severity and location of the disease. The dosage of herbs, especially that of extremely toxic herbs, must be strictly controlled and the medication should be stopped as soon as the condition of the patient has improved. In addition, the toxicity of some poisonous herbs can be eliminated or reduced by certain processing techniques.

PROCESSING OF HERBS

The processing of herbs refers to the methods used to process herbs in their natural state so as to adapt them to meet the requirements for dispensing and preparation before they can be used for treatment. The term 'processing' includes the general treatment of all natural herbs and the special treatment of certain types. Since most traditional Chinese herbs are of natural origin, they can be contaminated while being gathered. Some cannot be stored for a long time because they deteriorate easily, some cannot be used directly because of their toxicity or potency and others need to be treated in a special way in order to meet therapeutic requirements. In short, all herbs must be processed prior to application. Only after processing can herbs exert their full range of therapeutic effects and only then can safe usage be guaranteed.

Purposes of processing

The main purposes of the processing of herbs are:

1. to eliminate or reduce the toxicity, moderate the potency and diminish the side-effects of certain herbs;
2. to increase the curative effects of herbs;
3. to modify the characteristics and functions of herbs to fulfil therapeutic requirements;
4. to enhance the quality of herbs;
5. to facilitate the decoction and preparation of remedies;
6. to facilitate the storage of herbs.

Processing methods

Different processing methods and procedures can increase the therapeutic effect, reduce the toxicity, alter the functions and facilitate the preservation of herbs.

Processing methods can be divided into the following categories:

1. *Processing with water*

   Processing with water is undertaken to remove foreign substances from the herbs, soften and clean them, reduce the toxic content of certain herbs, and purify mineral substances. The most commonly-used methods are:

   (1) washing (*xǐ*): using water to wash off clay, sand and other impurities from the surface of the herbs;

   (2) rinsing (*piǎo*): soaking herbs in clean standing or running water to rid them of salt, fishy odours and other smells, and poisonous components so as to facilitate preparation and administration;

   (3) moistening (*rùn*): sprinkling clean water on herbs repeatedly, and then covering them with a wet cloth to soften them so that they can easily be cut into pieces;

   (4) grinding into a powder with water (*shuǐ fēi*): insoluble minerals can be ground with water into a fine powder. This is accomplished by the following procedure. Crushed, coarse particles of a mineral are put into a container and ground with water. The suspension is then decanted. The procedure is repeated several times with water being added and the mineral ground again until no sediment of coarse particles is left. After the superfluous water is discarded, the precipitate is dried to

obtain a fine powder. The powder obtained is very fine and loss of the drug is minimized.

2. *Processing with heat*

This method processes herbs by exposing them directly or indirectly to fire. The most common methods include:

(1) stir-frying (*chǎo*): this involves heating the raw herbs in a pan while stirring constantly. The duration and temperature of stir-frying varies according to the substance. Different herbs are stir-fried until they change colour to yellow or brown, or until they are charred.

In addition, there are other methods of stir-frying, such as stir-frying with sand. Here, the sand is stir-fried in a pan until it is hot; the materia medica are then mixed with the heated sand to make them light and crispy. This method is mainly used for crustaceans.

(2) mix-frying with auxiliary substances (*zhì*): this method involves frying the herbs with liquids such as honey, vinegar, alcohol, ginger juice or salt water to allow the liquid to penetrate into or attach itself to the surface of the herbs. The liquids themselves have some therapeutic effect, thus enhancing the overall therapeutic effect of the materia medica they are processed with;

(3) calcining (*duàn*): this involves placing herbs directly or indirectly in the flames to make them light, crispy and easy to crush so as to release all their therapeutic effects. Minerals or shellfish are usually calcined directly until they glow red. Indirect calcining means roasting the materia medica in a tightly-sealed fireproof container;

(4) wet-coated roasting in cinders (*wēi*): this method involves wrapping the herbs in wet paper or dough and roasting them in fresh cinders until the wrapping turns black. This procedure reduces the fat content of the herbs and moderates the potency of some of them;

(5) high-temperature frying (*páo*): this method is basically similar to mix-frying with auxiliary substances, but frying is performed quickly at a high temperature until the herbs turn dark brown and puff up. The purpose is to reduce toxicity or change the nature of the materia medica while avoiding charring;

(6) baking (*hōng*): with this method, dry herbs are heated slowly in front of a weak fire to achieve dehydration, thus permitting longer storage and easier grinding.

3. *Processing with both water and heat*

Some herbs are processed with heat and water or other liquids. Common methods include:

(1) steaming (*zhēng*): this method involves steaming the herbs with other substances over a low fire until cooked, thus altering their properties;

(2) boiling (*zhǔ*): the herbs are boiled in water or other liquids to enhance their power or reduce their toxicity;

(3) scalding (*dàn*): a herb is dipped in boiling water until the water comes to the boil again, thus facilitating the drying of the herb or the removal of the non-medicinal part.

COMPATIBILITY, DOSAGE, ADMINISTRATION AND CONTRAINDICATIONS OF HERBS

As most diseases are complex, the use of a single herb is not normally sufficient to obtain a good curative effect. Herbs must therefore be combined for application, with the result that consideration should be given to their compatibility before they are administered. To ensure safe usage and a satisfactory curative effect, attention must be paid to the contraindications, dosage and administration of single herbs and complex prescriptions.

Compatibility of herbs

Using two or more herbs in conjunction to treat a disease according to the clinical requirements and theoretical principles of the application of herbs exploits their combined effect. This effect is used to modify, enhance or decrease the therapeutic effects and reduce the side-effects of herbs. Seven features are used to describe the effects of combination:

1. going alone (*dān xíng*): one herb is used on its own to treat a disorder;
2. mutual need (*xiāng xū*): two or more herbs with similar characteristics and functions are used in combination to strengthen their therapeutic effect;
3. mutual enhancement (*xiāng shǐ*): two or more herbs with different characteristics and functions are used together in a combination within which one herb enhances the effect of the other(s);
4. mutual counteraction (*xiāng wèi*): when two or more herbs are used together, one herb can reduce or eliminate the toxicity and side-effects of the other(s);
5. mutual antagonism (*xiāng wù*): when two herbs are used together, their original therapeutic effect is diminished or cancelled out by their interaction;
6. mutual suppression (*xiāng shā*): the combination of two herbs can reduce or eliminate the toxic effects or side-effects of one (or both) of the herbs;
7. mutual incompatibility (*xiāng fǎn*): when two herbs are used together, their combination causes toxicity or severe side-effects that do not occur when used alone.

With the exception of herbs used alone, each of these expressions illustrates a different aspect of the possible interaction of herbs. Mutual need and mutual enhancement apply to situations where herbs work together to enhance their effects; as a result, they are commonly used in combination. Mutual counteraction and mutual suppression refer to the reduction and elimination of toxicity and side-effects, so these herbs can be combined when using toxic herbs. Herb combinations which can be described by mutual antagonism or mutual incompatibility result in the therapeutic effect of the herbs being decreased or eliminated, or may even give rise to toxic symptoms and side-effects. Consequently, such combinations should be avoided in the clinic.

The compatibility of herbs is the basis of prescriptions and is of crucial significance for the application of herbs and prescriptions.

Dosage of herbs

The dosage of herbs refers to the quantity of herbs to be prescribed for a certain medication. It indicates the daily amount of each herb for an adult, as well as the relative amount of the different ingredients of prescription herbs in a recipe. The dosage of each herb given in this book, unless otherwise indicated, refers to the amount of dried herb to be taken in decoction per day by an adult person.

When treating diseases with herbs, attention should be paid to the dosage, as it has a direct influence on the therapeutic effect. If the dosage is too small to treat a serious case effectively, the desired result will not be achieved, while a dosage which is too large for a mild case will frequently damage vital Qi as well as being a waste of the medical substance. Therefore, proper dosage is of great importance for satisfactory therapeutic results.

Usually, dosage is calculated by weight, although sometimes it is determined by quantity or volume. Since most of the materia medica in this book are raw herbs, the range of safe dosage is comparatively wide and dosage is not as strict as that for chemical substances. Some herbs, however, potentially have very serious side-effects or are extremely toxic, so their dosage should be strictly controlled to prevent poisoning.

In general, the following aspects should be considered when deciding the dosage of a herb:

1. the nature of the herb: for herbs with a mild nature, the dosage can be large, whereas for toxic and potent herbs, it should be small; for herbs that are light in weight, it should be small, whereas for heavy, non-toxic materia medica, such as minerals and shells, it should be large. In addition, for effective but very expensive herbs, the dosage should be small in order

not to impose an unnecessary financial burden on the patient. For fresh medicinal herbs, which usually contain some water, the dosage should be approximately twice as much as that for the dried herb.

2. combinations and preparations: for a single-herb prescription, the dosage is usually large. In compound prescriptions, the dosage is decided according to the number of ingredients in the prescription. In formulae with many herbs, each of them will have a relatively small dosage, whereas in prescriptions with fewer ingredients, each herb can be present in larger dosages. The dosage of the herb with the main function is generally larger than that of auxiliary ingredients. The dosage of one herb may vary in different preparations. The dosage of a herb in a decoction should be larger than that for pills and powders.
3. the condition, constitution and age of the patient: as a general rule, the dosage for severe and acute cases should be large, for mild and chronic cases small; the dosage for patients with a weak constitution should be small, although it can be larger for those with a strong constitution. Dosage for children and elderly patients should be small. Generally, the dosage for a child over six will be half the dosage for an adult, and the dosage for children under five a quarter of the adult dosage (even smaller for infants). Special attention should always be paid to the dosage of toxic herbs.

Administration of herbs

Decoction is a very common form of preparation for Chinese herbs. This section describes the method of decoction and indicates what precautions should be taken.

1. *Decoctions*

   The term decoction is used to describe a type of liquid preparation made by boiling herbs in water or other liquids (such as alcohol or vinegar). As a general rule, herbs are placed in a vessel, which should be made of a chemically inert material such as earthenware or enamel; pots made of iron or copper should never be used. The herbs should be soaked for 30-60 minutes in an amount of water which just covers them. They should then be boiled, initially over a strong heat, subsequently over a gentle heat. Depending on requirements, herbs can be decocted repeatedly after being drained from the decoction. Herbs can normally be decocted two or three times. The liquid obtained by successive decoctions should be mixed and split into several draughts to be taken orally. The quantity of water, the temperature and the boiling time are adjusted according to the herbs used. Herbs which release the exterior and clear heat are boiled quickly in a comparatively small amount of water for 5-10 minutes; supplementing herbs are simmered in a comparatively large quantity of water for 30-40 minutes.

   Some herbs need to be decocted separately to guarantee the quality of the decoction or increase their curative effect. The methods employed are indicated below:

   (1) decoct first (*xiān jiān*): this method is suitable for minerals and shells as their texture is hard and it is difficult to extract their effective ingredients. They should be crushed into small pieces and decocted first for 15 minutes before adding the other ingredients of a prescription. Substances requiring this method include *Shi Gao* (Gypsum Fibrosum), *Mu Li* (Concha Ostreae), *Shi Jue Ming* (Concha Haliotidis) and *Gui Ban* (Plastrum Testudinis);

   (2) add at the end (*hòu xià*): this method is suitable for aromatic herbs or herbs whose effective ingredients would be destroyed easily if boiled for too long. These herbs should be put in after the other herbs have been boiled for 5-10 minutes and should only be boiled themselves for about 5-10 minutes. These herbs include *Bo He* (Herba Menthae Haplocalycis), *Sha Ren* (Fructus Amomi), *Da*

Huang (Radix et Rhizoma Rhei) and *Fan Xie Ye* (Folium Sennae);

(3) decoct in wrapping (*bāo jiān*): this method is suitable for some powder-like or sticky substances and hairy herbs which are wrapped in gauze in order to prevent the decoction from becoming turbid, irritating to the throat or burning at the bottom of the pot. These herbs include *Xuan Fu Hua* (Flos Inulae) and *Che Qian Zi* (Semen Plantaginis);

(4) decoct separately (*lìng jiān*): this method is particularly suitable for expensive substances such as *Ren Shen* (Radix Ginseng), *Xi Yang Shen* (Radix Panacis Quinquefolii) and *Ling Yang Jiao* (Cornu Antelopis). The decoction obtained can be taken separately or mixed with a decoction of other herbs in order to avoid wasting anything of these precious medicinals;

(5) melt in boiled decoction (*yáng huà*): some viscous or very sticky substances such as *E Jiao* (Gelatinum Corii Asini) should be melted or dissolved in a boiled decoction that has already been prepared. This method can prevent these substances from sticking to other herbs or to the pot;

(6) direct oral application with warm water or a prepared decoction (*chōng fú*): some herbs such as *Hu Po* (Succinum) cannot be used for a decoction. They should be ground into a fine powder and mixed with warm water or a prepared decoction for administration. Liquid herbs such as *Zhu Li* (Succus Bambusae) and *Sheng Jiang Zhi* (Succus Rhizomatis Zingiberis Officinalis Recens) should also be taken this way.

2. *Directions for use*

As a general rule, one dose should be taken twice a day (two decoctions). For acute, severe or emergency cases, two doses (four decoctions) or more may be given per day at an interval of four hours. For chronic cases, one dose can be taken over two days (i.e. one decoction per day).

With regard to the time of administration, supplementing substances should be taken before meals, whereas those irritant to the stomach and intestines should be ingested after meals. Herbs for killing worms should be taken on an empty stomach, while herbs for quieting the Spirit should be taken before sleep. Herbs which stop vomiting can be taken repeatedly in small doses. For unconscious patients and those with lockjaw, the decoction can be administered nasally. The application of herbs for inducing sweating and of downward-draining herbs should be stopped as soon as the patient begins to sweat or have bowel movements so as to avoid causing excessive sweating or purgation which might damage vital Qi. Powders should be taken with warm water that has been boiled. Herbs prescribed in a large dosage, herbs with a strong, unpleasant smell or those which cause choking can be taken with honey.

Decoctions are usually taken while still warm. Decoctions of cold herbs for the treatment of heat patterns are taken cold, while decoctions of hot herbs which treat cold patterns are taken hot. In the case of cold patterns with pseudo-heat symptoms ('true cold, false heat'), it is better to take the medicine cold even though the nature of the herbs is hot; on the other hand, in the case of heat patterns with pseudo-cold symptoms ('true heat, false cold'), a hot decoction of cold drugs can be taken.

Contraindications of herbs

Besides their preventive and curative effects, some Chinese herbs can also cause harmful side-effects. Therefore, it is not only necessary to acquire a clear understanding of their positive effects in prevention and treatment, but also of their side-effects.

1. *Contraindications for certain patterns*

Each herb or class of herbs has a certain indication. For diseases or patterns which are not included, the herb is contraindicated.

For example, *Ma Huang* (Herba Ephedrae) induces sweating and calms wheezing; it is indicated for lack of sweating due to full-type exterior patterns and for cough due to the obstruction of Lung Qi caused by external wind-cold; however, it is contraindicated in cases with spontaneous sweating due to an exterior pattern of the deficiency type or cough due to deficiency of Kidney Qi.

Cold and cool herbs drain heat, yet they may also damage Yang Qi. Hot herbs eliminate cold, but may also consume Yin. Herbs with a powerful purgative action eliminate pathogenic factors, but can impair vital Qi as well. Supplementing herbs boost vital Qi, yet may also influence pathogenic Qi and prolong the duration of the disease. If herbs with upward-bearing and floating actions are used in cases of Yang hyperactivity, they may make the situation even worse. If herbs for suppressing ascending counterflow Qi are applied in cases of prolapse, they may cause aggravation of the condition.

2. *Contraindications in writing prescriptions*

In ancient Chinese literature about herbal medicine, it is recorded that some herbs are incompatible with others and may never be used in combination, otherwise toxic reactions, harmful side-effects or a diminished therapeutic effect may result. The most important are the 'eighteen incompatible herbs' and the 'nineteen antagonistic herbs'.

(i) The Eighteen Incompatible Herbs *(Shi Ba Fan)* are:

Wu Tou (Radix Aconiti), which is incompatible with *Ban Xia* (Rhizoma Pinelliae Ternatae), *Gua Lou* (Fructus Trichosanthis), *Bei Mu* (Bulbus Fritillariae), *Bai Lian* (Radix Ampelopsis Japonicae) and *Bai Ji* (Rhizoma Bletillae Striatae); *Gan Cao* (Radix Glycyrrhizae), which is incompatible with *Hai Zao* (Herba Sargassi), *Jing Da Ji* (Radix Euphorbiae Pekinensis), *Gan Sui* (Radix Euphorbiae Kansui) and *Yuan Hua* (Flos Daphnes Genkwa); and *Li Lu* (Radix et Rhizoma Veratri), which is incompatible with *Ren Shen* (Radix Ginseng), *Sha Shen* (Radix Glehniae seu Adenophorae), *Dan Shen* (Radix Salviae Miltiorrhizae), *Xuan Shen* (Radix Scrophulariae Ningpoensis), *Xi Xin* (Herba cum Radice Asari) and *Bai Shao* (Radix Paeoniae Lactiflorae).

(ii) The Nineteen Antagonistic Herbs *(Shi Jiu Wei)* are:

Liu Huang (Sulphur), which antagonizes *Po Xiao* (Mirabilitum Non-Purum); *Shui Yin* (Hydrargyrum), which antagonizes *Pi Shuang* (Arsenicum); *Lang Du* (Radix Euphorbiae Fischerianae), which antagonizes *Mi Tuo Seng* (Lithargyrum); *Ba Dou* (Semen Crotonis Tiglii), which antagonizes *Qian Niu Zi* (Semen Pharbitidis); *Ding Xiang* (Flos Caryophylli), which antagonizes *Yu Jin* (Radix Curcumae); *Chuan Wu* (Radix Aconiti Carmichaeli) and *Cao Wu* (Radix Aconiti Kusnezoffii), both of which antagonize *Xi Jiao* (Cornu Rhinoceri); *Ya Xiao* (Mirabilitum Equidens), which antagonizes *San Leng* (Rhizoma Sparganii Stoloniferi); *Guan Gui* (Cortex Tubiformis Cinnamomi Cassiae), which antagonizes *Chi Shi Zhi* (Halloysitum Rubrum); and *Ren Shen* (Radix Ginseng), which antagonizes *Wu Ling Zhi* (Excrementum Trogopteri).

However, there have been differences of opinion in both ancient and modern times as to the incompatibility of some of the herbs listed above. Experiments have indicated that some are toxic if combined, whereas others do not give rise to any negative side-effects. As yet, no consensus of opinion has been reached and further research remains to be done. However, until final results are available, it is advisable to follow the traditional doctrine.

3. *Contraindications during pregnancy*

As some herbs harm the vital Qi of the foetus and may lead to threatened or actual miscarriage, attention must be paid to those herbs that are contraindicated during pregnancy. Extremely toxic or purgative herbs, and aromatic herbs which quicken the Blood and dissipate Blood stasis or generally have a dispersive action should not be prescribed at all or only with great caution. Substances in this category include *Ba Dou* (Semen Crotonis Tiglii), *Ban Mao* (Mylabris), *Qian Niu Zi* (Semen Pharbitidis), *Jing Da Ji* (Radix Euphorbiae Pekinensis), *Gan Sui* (Radix Euphorbiae Kansui), *Yuan Hua* (Flos Daphnes Genkwa), *Shang Lu* (Radix Phytolaccae), *San Leng* (Rhizoma Sparganii Stoloniferi), *E Zhu* (Rhizoma Curcumae), *Shui Zhi* (Hirudo seu Whitmania), *Meng Chong* (Tabanus), *Tao Ren* (Semen Persicae), *Hong Hua* (Flos Carthami Tinctorii), *Da Huang* (Radix et Rhizoma Rhei), *Zhi Shi* (Fructus Immaturus Citri Aurantii), *Fu Zi* (Radix Lateralis Aconiti Carmichaeli Praeparata), *Gan Jiang* (Rhizoma Zingiberis Officinalis) and *Rou Gui* (Cortex Cinnamomi Cassiae). However, if a pregnant woman is seriously ill and cannot be treated without one or more of the above-mentioned herbs, they may be prescribed with great care depending on the condition of the patient.

4. *Contraindications relating to diet*
In general, uncooked, cold, greasy, fishy and fatty, indigestible, and irritating food should not be taken at all or only in small amounts during treatment with the materia medica described in this book. In detail, this means that uncooked or cold food should be avoided in cases of cold patterns; hot, pungent, and greasy food in cases of heat patterns; peppers, chilli peppers, alcohol and garlic in cases of dizziness, insomnia and mental disorders; fried, greasy and sticky food is not suitable for patients suffering from indigestion due to deficiency of the Spleen and Stomach; and fish, shrimps, crabs, and other fishy or irritating food should not be eaten by patients suffering from a suppurative infection or pruritus.

SPECIAL NOTE ON LEGAL RESTRICTIONS AFFECTING CHINESE MATERIA MEDICA IN THE UNITED KINGDOM AND THE USA

Laws affecting the importation and prescription of Chinese materia medica vary from country to country. In the United Kingdom, the legal status of substances included in the Chinese pharmacopoeia changes continually to reflect factors such as toxicity and the endangerment of species. The legal situation in the United Kingdom at the time of publication and as described in this book is based on information provided by the Medicines Control Agency (www.mca.gov.uk) and the Register of Chinese Herbal Medicine (www.rchm.co.uk).

There are two categories of restricted substances covered by the Convention on International Trade in Endangered Species of Wild Fauna and Flora (CITES), listed as Appendices I and II:

1. Appendix I: All trade in these substances is currently banned.
   The following materia medica referred to in this book are listed in CITES Appendix I: *She Xiang* (Secretio Moschi); *Bie Jia* (Carapax Amydae Sinensis); *Dai Mao* (Carapax Eretmochelydis); *Mu Xiang* (Radix Aucklandiae Lappae); and *Xi Jiao* (Cornu Rhinoceri), although the latter substance is only included for information purposes in relation to antagonisms between herbs.
2. Appendix II: Trade allowed with the appropriate trade permits.
   The following materials referred to in this book are listed in CITES Appendix II: *Chuan Shan Jia* (Squama Manitis Pentadactylae); *Ling Yang Jiao* (Cornu Antelopis); *Shi Hu* (Herba Dendrobii); *Bai Ji* (Rhizoma Bletillae Striatae); *Tian Ma* (Rhizoma Gastrodiae Elatae); *Gou Ji* (Rhizoma Cibotii Barometz); *Xi Yang Shen* (Radix Panacis Quinquefolii), in whole root form only; *Lu Hui* (Herba Aloes); and *Gui Ban* (Plastrum Testudinis) and its derivatives.

The following materia medica referred to in this book are restricted by law because of their toxic nature:

1. Completely illegal: *Guang Fang Ji* (Radix Aristolochiae Fangchi), *Ma Dou Ling* (Fructus Aristolochiae), *Guan Mu Tong* (Caulis Aristolochiae Manshuriensis) and all other species of aristolochia; *Han Fang Ji* (Radix Stephaniae Tetrandrae); *Mu Tong* (Caulis Mutong); *Guan Zhong* (Rhizoma Dryopteris Crassirhizomae) and all other species of dryopteris; *Zhu Sha* (Cinnabaris); *Qing Fen* (Calomelas); *Xiong Huang* (Realgar); *Mi Tuo Seng* (Lithargyrum); and *Ying Su Ke* (Pericarpium Papaveris Somniferi). *Pi Shuang* (Arsenicum) and *Shui Yin* (Hydrargyrum), which are also banned, are mentioned in this introduction only, as they are traditionally included among the Nineteen Antagonistic Herbs.
2. Illegal for internal use: *Fu Zi* (Radix Lateralis Aconiti Carmichaeli Praeparata), *Chuan Wu* (Radix Aconiti Carmichaeli), *Cao Wu* (Radix Aconiti Kusnezoffii) and *Wu Tou* (Radix Aconiti).
3. Dosage restricted: *Ma Huang* (Herba Ephedrae); maximum permitted dosage of 0.6g thrice daily.

There are several reasons for keeping the above-mentioned substances in this book. Firstly, in most cases, it is not possible to suggest a simple substitute for a herb; only by understanding its properties and actions will the practitioner be able to decide what to use in its place in a given situation. Secondly, the legal status of herbs changes over time: a substance which is illegal or restricted now may be available for use in the future. Thirdly, as has been mentioned already, legal status varies from country to country, and the use of substances that are illegal in the United Kingdom may be permitted in other countries. Practitioners are advised to check with their local regulatory agency in case of doubt.

In addition, the Medicines Control Agency (MCA) issued a document in September 2001 entitled *Traditional Ethnic Medicines: Public Health and Compliance with Medicines Law*, which restricted the use of non-herbal ingredients in unlicensed herbal remedies. The document stated that 'unlicensed herbal remedies are not permitted to contain as active ingredients non-herbal ingredients, such as animal parts or minerals. A medicine containing such ingredients would need a product licence.'

In another document issued in the same month and entitled *A Review of Restricted Herbal Ingredients*, the MCA went further down the road towards the possible imposition of tighter controls on the use of Chinese herbs, focusing essentially on ingredients where specific safety concerns had been identified independently of the review and on ingredients identified from lists supplied by trade associations and others relating to products which are or may be on the UK market and where the MCA has provisional concerns on public health grounds (some of these ingredients are already classified as restricted in Hong Kong). Practitioners will be able to judge just how legitimate these concerns are from the reasons given for any possible restrictions on use.

The MCA is therefore looking critically at the potential need for regulatory action where the inherent toxicity of an ingredient is a safety issue and/or the safe use of an ingredient is critically dependent on such factors as the competence of the practitioner, the patient being given precise instructions on usage, and quality control in manufacture.

This book includes the following herbs listed in the MCA review: *Bai Fu Zi* (Rhizoma Typhonii Gigantei), *Bai Guo* (Semen Ginkgo Bilobae), *Ban Xia* (Rhizoma Pinelliae Ternatae), *Bu Gu Zhi* (Fructus Psoraleae Corylifoliae), *Cang Er Zi* (Fructus Xanthii Sibirici), *Gan Sui* (Radix Euphorbiae Kansui), *Gua Lou* (Fructus Trichosanthis), *Jing Da Ji* (Radix Euphorbiae Pekinensis), *Nan Gua Zi* (Semen Cucurbitae Moschatae), *Sang Ji Sheng* (Ramulus Loranthi), *Shan Dou Gen* (Radix Sophorae Tonkinensis), *Tian Hua Fen* (Radix Trichosanthis), *Tian Nan Xing* (Rhizoma Arisaematis), *Wu Bei Zi* (Galla Rhois Chinensis), *Xi Xin* (Herba cum Radice Asari), *Yang Jin Hua* (Flos Daturae) and *Yin Chai Hu* (Radix Stellariae Dichotomae). Practitioners should be aware that restrictions may be imposed on the use of these herbs at some time in the future in the UK.

In the USA, the Food and Drug Administration (FDA) has been moving since May 2000 towards banning several Chinese herbs. The FDA is concerned with overseas incidences of nephropathy linked to aristolochic acid in Chinese herbal products and with reports that two patients in the United States had been diagnosed with end-stage renal disease in association with the use of botanical preparations containing aristolochic acids. The FDA therefore decided to take regulatory action against herbs that may contain aristolochic acids, may be mistakenly substituted by an aristolochic acid-containing herb or may have been adulterated by aristolochic acids. In a letter in April 2001, it asked herbal manufacturers and suppliers to recall on a voluntarily basis several different herbs classified under these categories as well as various formulae in which these herbs were included as ingredients.

The letter contained two attachments listing botanicals known or suspected to contain aristolochic acid (Attachment A) or botanicals which may be adulterated with aristolochic acid (Attachment B). The following herbs in this book are covered by the regulatory action set in motion by the FDA:

- Attachment A: *Guan Mu Tong* (Caulis Aristolochiae Manshuriensis), *Ma Dou Ling* (Fructus Aristolochiae), *Guang Fang Ji* (Radix Aristolochiae Fangchi);
- Attachment B: *Mu Tong* (Caulis Mutong), *Xi Xin* (Herba cum Radice Asari), *Wei Ling Xian* (Radix Clematidis), *Han Fang Ji* (Radix Stephaniae Tetrandrae).

Chapter 1

Herbs for releasing the exterior

解表药

Herbs for releasing the exterior

Herbs for releasing the exterior are herbs that can dispel external pathogenic factors to release patterns affecting the exterior.

Most of these herbs are acrid; they mainly enter the Lung channel. They can dispel external pathogenic factors from the surface of body through sweating. In so doing, they prevent internal transmission of these pathogenic factors and bring about a cure of the disease. Herbs for releasing the exterior are mainly used for chills, fever, headache and generalized pain, soreness of the limbs, sweating or absence of sweating, and a floating pulse, where these symptoms are caused by external pathogenic factors penetrating the body surface. These herbs can also be applied where there is disharmony between the Ying and Wei levels. Some herbs for releasing the exterior also stop coughing and calm wheezing, alleviate pain, vent papules and promote urination; they are therefore used to treat externally-contracted coughing and wheezing, wind-damp Bi syndrome, wind papules, urticaria (dormant papules), measles and oedema.

If the usage of herbs for releasing the exterior is incorrect or the dosage too high, Yang Qi may be consumed and body fluids may be damaged; it is even possible that collapse of Yin or Yang might occur due to profuse sweating. In clinical practice, attention should therefore be paid to the following aspects:

1. Herbs for releasing the exterior should be used with caution or not at all in cases of profuse sweating, spontaneous sweating due to Qi deficiency, night sweating due to Yin deficiency, damage to body fluids, loss of blood, chills due to Yang deficiency, and fever due to Yin deficiency.
2. The herbs used and their dosage should be adjusted according to the season and climate.
3. Most of these herbs contain volatile ingredients, so they should not be decocted for a lengthy period.
4. Herbs for releasing the exterior should be used in combination with herbs for clearing summerheat, herbs for transforming dampness, and herbs for supplementing Yin, Yang or Qi. The combination will depend on the complexity of the patterns and the strength or weakness of the patient's constitution. The dosage of herbs for releasing the exterior is reduced in these combinations.
5. Decoctions for releasing the exterior should be taken warm or combined with hot liquids in order to strengthen their curative effect.

Herbs for releasing the exterior can be divided, according to their characteristics, into herbs for dissipating wind-cold (acrid, warm herbs for releasing the exterior) and herbs for dissipating wind-heat (acrid, cool herbs for releasing the exterior).

ACRID, WARM HERBS FOR RELEASING THE EXTERIOR

Acrid, warm herbs for releasing the exterior possess the common feature of a strong sweat-inducing effect; they function very effectively in dispelling external pathogenic factors lodged between the muscles and the skin. They are used mainly for wind-cold-type exterior patterns manifesting as slight fever, severe chills, an absence of sweating, headache, generalized pain, nasal congestion and an absence of thirst, accompanied by a floating and tight pulse and a thin tongue with white fur.

In addition, some of these herbs can warm the channels, dissipate wind-cold, dispel external wind-damp pathogenic factors, adjust the Ying and Wei levels, and alleviate pain. They are commonly used for headache, generalized pain and wind-cold-damp Bi syndrome. Certain of these herbs can promote the dispersing function of the Lungs and bear counterflow Lung Qi downwards in order to stop coughing and calm wheezing; they can therefore be used for coughing and wheezing caused by external pathogenic factors invading the Lungs. As a result of their strong diaphoretic effect, these herbs can be used to treat oedema by inducing sweating. Some of them have the functions of regulating the passage of body fluids and warming Yang to promote urination. They can therefore be used for oedema and painful urination combined with an exterior pattern, or for oedema in the upper part of the body.

Tab. 1.1 Acrid, warm herbs for releasing the exterior

Herb	Functions	Indications
Ma Huang (Herba Ephedrae)	Inducing sweating and dissipating cold to release the exterior, diffusing Lung Qi to stop coughing and calm wheezing, promoting urination and dispersing swelling	Full type of wind-cold exterior patterns, coughing and wheezing due to external wind-cold invading the Lungs, oedema combined with exterior patterns, Yin abscesses
Gui Zhi (Ramulus Cinnamomi Cassiae)	Inducing sweating and releasing the exterior, adjusting and harmonizing the Ying and Wei levels, warming the channels and dissipating cold, quickening the Blood, freeing Yang and transforming Qi, warming and transforming water-fluids	Full- and deficiency-type exterior patterns due to wind-cold, wind-cold-damp Bi syndrome pain, soreness of the shoulders, back and joints, obstruction of Qi in the chest due to Heart Yang deficiency, Phlegm-fluids due to damp obstruction
Xi Xin (Herba cum Radice Asari)	Dissipating wind-cold or dispelling wind to alleviate pain, warming the Lungs and transforming fluids, freeing obstructions and opening the orifices	Headache due to wind-cold, nasal congestion, deep-source nasal congestion, toothache, deafness, cough due to Phlegm-fluids, wind-cold-damp Bi syndrome
Zi Su Ye (Folium Perillae Frutescentis)	Dissipating cold and releasing the exterior, moving Qi and loosening the Middle Jiao, treating seafood poisoning by relieving toxicity	Full type of wind-cold exterior patterns, oppression in the chest and vomiting due to Qi stagnation in the Spleen and Stomach; pain in the abdomen, vomiting and diarrhoea caused by seafood poisoning

Jing Jie (Herba Schizonepetae Tenuifoliae)	Dispelling wind and releasing the exterior, venting papules and alleviating itching, regulating the Blood and stopping bleeding	Full type of wind-cold exterior patterns, the initial stage of measles and sores combined with exterior patterns, nosebleed and uterine bleeding
Fang Feng (Radix Ledebouriellae Divaricatae)	Dispelling wind and releasing the exterior, overcoming dampness and alleviating pain, expelling wind to relieve tetany, stopping bleeding and stopping diarrhoea	Wind-cold type of exterior patterns, Bi syndrome due to wind, cold or damp, headache and generalized pain, itchy skin, tetanus, blood in the stool, uterine bleeding, and diarrhoea due to Spleen deficiency
Qiang Huo (Rhizoma et Radix Notopterygii)	Dispelling wind and releasing the exterior, overcoming dampness and alleviating pain	Wind-cold type of common cold, headache without sweating, wind-cold-damp Bi syndrome pain, stiffness of the neck, aching and painful joints, dizziness, red eyes
Bai Zhi (Radix Angelicae Dahuricae)	Dissipating cold and releasing the exterior, dispelling wind and drying dampness, freeing the orifices and alleviating pain, dispersing swelling and expelling pus	Headache due to common colds, pain in the supra-orbital region, nasal congestion and toothache, red and white vaginal discharge, sores, itchy skin
Gao Ben (Rhizoma et Radix Ligustici)	Dissipating wind, dispelling dampness and alleviating pain	Headache due to wind-cold, parietal headache, toothache, pain due to wind-damp, pain in the abdomen due to damp-cold, diarrhoea, scabies and abscesses
Cang Er Zi (Fructus Xanthii Sibirici)	Dispelling wind-damp, freeing the orifices to alleviate pain	Headache due to wind-cold, deep-source nasal congestion, toothache, sore eyes, wind-cold-damp Bi syndrome, spasms of the limbs, itchy skin
Xin Yi Hua (Flos Magnoliae)	Dispelling wind-cold, freeing the orifices to alleviate pain	Headache due to wind-cold, deep-source nasal congestion, allergic rhinitis, stuffy nose, toothache
Sheng Jiang (Rhizoma Zingiberis Officinalis Recens)	Inducing sweating and releasing the exterior, warming the Stomach and stopping vomiting, warming the Lungs and stopping coughing, relieving toxicity	Wind-cold type of common cold, cough, vomiting due to Stomach-cold; also reduces the toxicity of *Ban Xia* (Rhizoma Pinelliae Ternatae) and *Dan Nan Xing* (Pulvis Arisaematis cum Felle Bovis) and treats seafood poisoning
Xiang Ru (Herba Elsholtziae seu Moslae)	Inducing sweating and releasing the exterior, clearing summerheat and transforming dampness, promoting the movement of water and dispersing swelling	Summerheat type of common cold, headache and fever, chills with an absence of sweating, oppression in the chest, pain in the abdomen, vomiting, diarrhoea, oedema
Cong Bai (Bulbus Allii Fistulosi)	Inducing sweating and releasing the exterior, dissipating cold and freeing Yang, relieving toxicity and dissipating lumps	Wind-cold type of common cold, pain in the abdomen, diarrhoea, and cold limbs due to Yin cold

Ma Huang 麻黄 (Ephedra, Herba Ephedrae)

Ma Huang is the herbaceous stem of *Ephedra sinica* Stapf., *E. intermedia* Schrenk et C. A. Mey. or *E. equisetina* Bge., family Ephedraceae.

Legal status *Ma Huang* is listed in the UK in Schedule III of The Medicines (Retail Sale or Supply of Herbal Remedies) Order 1977 and may only be supplied to the public in restricted circumstances, in particular where there has been a one-to-one consultation; in addition the dosage of *Ma Huang* is restricted to 0.6g three times a day.

Main ingredients *Ma Huang* contains many kinds of alkaloids (including ephedrine, pseudoephedrine, norephedrine, norpseudoephedrine, methylephedrine and methylpseudoephedrine), ephedine and volatile oils (including terpineols, myrcene and tricin).

Properties Taste: acrid and slightly bitter; nature: warm.

Channels entered Lung and Bladder.

Functions and indications Induces sweating and dissipates cold to release the exterior, diffuses Lung Qi to stop coughing and calm wheezing, promotes urination and disperses swelling. It is mainly indicated for the full type of wind-cold exterior patterns, coughing and wheezing due to external wind-cold invading the Lungs, oedema combined with exterior patterns, and Yin abscesses.

Common dosage 3-10g, or about 20g for a large dosage (see legal status above for dosage restrictions in the UK).

Precautions and contraindications

1. *Ma Huang* strongly promotes perspiration in exterior deficiency-type patterns with sweating or night sweating due to Yin deficiency or coughing and wheezing due to deficiency of Kidney Qi. Overdosage may result in profuse sweating, which weakens the body.
2. For the treatment of oedema, 25-45g of *Shi Gao* (Gypsum Fibrosum) should be used together with 15-20g of *Ma Huang* to reduce the latter's diaphoretic function and diffuse Lung Qi to promote urination (see legal status above for dosage restrictions in the UK).

Remarks Raw *Ma Huang* has a strong diaphoretic effect. After stir-frying with honey (*Zhi Ma Huang*), this effect is reduced and its function in stopping coughing and calming wheezing is strengthened. *Ma Huang Gen* (Radix Ephedrae) can be used to stop sweating due to Qi deficiency (see Chapter 18).

Comparison of functions See *Xi Xin* (Herba cum Radice Asari), *Xiang Ru* (Herba Elsholtziae seu Moslae), *Fu Ping* (Herba Spirodelae Polyrrhizae) and *Xing Ren* (Semen Pruni Armeniacae).

Toxicity The LD_{50} for subcutaneous injection of ephedrine in rats is 650mg/kg, whereas for intraperitoneal injection in mice of a 10% emulsion solution of the volatile oils contained in *Ma Huang*, it is 1.35mg/kg. Oral administration of 5-10 times the normal therapeutic amount of ephedrine can cause toxic side-effects, with such symptoms as headache, dizziness, tinnitus, facial flushes, sweating, nausea and vomiting, vexation and agitation, palpitations, an increase in blood pressure, precordial pain, dilated pupils and blurred vision, and difficult urination. Ingestion by patients of 15ml of a 1% ephedrine solution resulted in profuse sweating, body temperature rising to 39°C, pain in the upper abdomen, nausea and vomiting, and difficulty in swallowing. As overdosage is the main cause of the appearance of toxic symptoms, dosage limits must be strictly adhered to (see *Legal status* above).

Modern research

1. An aqueous extract of *Ma Huang* had a diaphoretic effect in animals.[1]
2. Stimulates spasm of the bronchial smooth muscle to calm wheezing.[2-4]

3. The volatile oils contained in *Ma Huang* can inhibit group A streptococci and Streptococcus pneumoniae,[5] and influenza viruses.[6]
4. Ephedrine can raise blood pressure by contracting the blood vessels and can also stimulate the central nervous system.[2]

Combinations and applications

Functions	Combinations	Applications
Inducing sweating and dissipating cold to release the exterior	*Gui Zhi* (Ramulus Cinnamomi Cassiae) *Xing Ren* (Semen Pruni Armeniacae) *Gan Cao* (Radix Glycyrrhizae)	Full type of wind-cold exterior patterns, manifesting as chills, fever without sweating, absence of thirst, headache and generalized pain, with a floating and tight pulse
	Gui Zhi (Ramulus Cinnamomi Cassiae) *Qiang Huo* (Rhizoma et Radix Notopterygii) *Wu Tou* (Radix Aconiti) (see notes on legal status)	Wind-cold-damp Bi syndrome
Diffusing Lung Qi to stop coughing and calm wheezing	*Xing Ren* (Semen Pruni Armeniacae) *Ban Xia* (Rhizoma Pinelliae Ternatae) *Qian Hu* (Radix Peucedani)	Cough due to wind-cold, manifesting as cough with an itchy throat, oppression in the chest and thin sputum
	Shi Gao (Gypsum Fibrosum) *Xing Ren* (Semen Pruni Armeniacae) *Gan Cao* (Radix Glycyrrhizae) *Huang Qin* (Radix Scutellariae Baicalensis)	Cough due to Lung-heat, manifesting as cough with thick, yellow sputum, a dry throat, yellow tongue fur and a rapid pulse
	Gan Jiang (Rhizoma Zingiberis Officinalis) *Xi Xin* (Herba cum Radice Asari) *Ban Xia* (Rhizoma Pinelliae Ternatae)	Cough with thin sputum, rasping and rapid breathing, and oppression in the chest due to cold fluids collecting internally
Promoting urination and dispersing swelling	*Lian Qiao* (Fructus Forsythiae Suspensae) *Bai Mao Gen* (Rhizoma Imperatae Cylindricae) *Che Qian Zi* (Semen Plantaginis) *Shi Gao* (Gypsum Fibrosum)	Oedema of the face, head and upper part of the body, scant urine, fever and chills, and cough with a floating pulse
	Sheng Jiang (Rhizoma Zingiberis Officinalis Recens) *Shi Gao* (Gypsum Fibrosum) *Gan Cao* (Radix Glycyrrhizae) *Bai Zhu* (Rhizoma Atractylodis Macrocephalae)	Loss of control of the water passages, skin water swellings, generalized oedema, fever, aversion to wind and inhibited urination due to Qi deficiency of the Lungs and Spleen
	Fu Zi (Radix Lateralis Aconiti Carmichaeli Praeparata) (see notes on legal status) *Rou Gui* (Cortex Cinnamomi Cassiae) *Bai Zhu* (Rhizoma Atractylodis Macrocephalae) *Ze Xie* (Rhizoma Alismatis Orientalis)	Oedema due to Yang deficiency, manifesting with a bright white facial complexion, scant urine, loose stool, a pale tongue with white fur, and a sunken and fine pulse

Shu Di Huang (Radix Rehmanniae Glutinosae Conquita) *Rou Gui* (Cortex Cinnamomi Cassiae) *Bai Jie Zi* (Semen Sinapis Albae) *Lu Jiao Jiao* (Gelatinum Cornu Cervi)	Yin abscesses (manifesting as swelling with no local change of colour) or Phlegm nodes due to congealing and stagnation of Qi and Blood associated with Yang deficiency cold binding

Gui Zhi 桂枝 (Cinnamon twig, Ramulus Cinnamomi Cassiae)

Gui Zhi is the tender branch of *Cinnamomum cassia* Presl., family Lauraceae.

Main ingredients *Gui Zhi* contains 0.2-0.9% of volatile oils (mainly cinnamic aldehyde), as well as transcinnamic acid, coumarin, β-sitosterol and protocatechuic acid.

Properties Taste: acrid and sweet; nature: warm.

Channels entered Heart, Lung and Bladder.

Functions and indications Induces sweating and releases the exterior, adjusts and harmonizes the Ying and Wei levels, warms the channels and dissipates cold, quickens the Blood, frees Yang and transforms Qi, and warms and transforms water-fluids. It is indicated for exterior patterns due to wind-cold, including both the full type (without sweating) and the deficiency type (with sweating); it is also indicated for wind-cold-damp Bi syndrome pain, soreness of the shoulders, back and joints, obstruction of Qi in the chest due to Heart Yang deficiency, and Phlegm-fluids due to damp obstruction.

Common dosage 3-10g, or 30g for large dosages.

Precautions and contraindications

1. As *Gui Zhi* is warm, it can supplement Yang, damage Yin and stir the Blood; it is therefore contraindicated in cases of effulgent Yin deficiency-fire, for bleeding due to heat in the Blood, and in febrile diseases.
2. *Gui Zhi* should be used with caution during pregnancy and for patients with profuse menstruation.

Remarks The tip of *Gui Zhi* has a strong effect in freeing the vessels and can be used for pain in the upper limbs; it is therefore a guiding herb for disorders of the upper limbs. Fried *Gui Zhi* has a strong effect in warming the channels and can be used for limb joint pain due to wind-cold-damp.

Comparison of functions See *Xi Xin* (Herba cum Radice Asari), *Sang Zhi* (Ramulus Mori Albae) and *Rou Gui* (Cortex Cinnamomi Cassiae).

Toxicity The LD_{50} for intravenous injection of cinnamic aldehyde in mice is 132mg/kg, that for oral administration is 2225mg/kg. In experiments on mice, *Gui Zhi* was more toxic and caused more deaths during the day than at night.

Modern research

1. Has a diaphoretic effect.[7]
2. Has a strong inhibitory effect on Staphylococcus aureus and Salmonella typhi.[8]
3. Has an obvious pain-relieving effect.[9]

Combinations and applications

Functions	Combinations	Applications
Inducing sweating and releasing the exterior, adjusting and harmonizing the Ying and Wei levels	*Ma Huang* (Herba Ephedrae) (see notes on legal status) *Jing Jie* (Herba Schizonepetae Tenuifoliae) *Fang Feng* (Radix Ledebouriellae Divaricatae)	Full type of wind-cold exterior patterns, manifesting as fever and chills, lack of sweating, headache and generalized pain, with a floating and tight pulse
	Bai Shao (Radix Paeoniae Lactiflorae) *Da Zao* (Fructus Ziziphi Jujubae) *Sheng Jiang* (Rhizoma Zingiberis Officinalis Recens)	Deficiency type of wind-cold exterior patterns, manifesting as fever and chills and spontaneous sweating, with a floating and moderate pulse
Warming the channels and dissipating cold, quickening the Blood	*Jiang Huang* (Rhizoma Curcumae Longae) *Fang Feng* (Radix Ledebouriellae Divaricatae)	Pain in the shoulder and upper limbs due to obstruction of Qi and Blood in the channels resulting from an invasion of wind-cold
	Fu Zi (Radix Lateralis Aconiti Carmichaeli Praeparata) (see notes on legal status) *Dang Gui* (Radix Angelicae Sinensis) *Du Huo* (Radix Angelicae Pubescentis) *Wei Ling Xian* (Radix Clematidis)	Joint pain, hypertonicity of the limbs, difficulty in bending and stretching and Bi syndrome of the joints due to wind, cold and damp pathogenic factors
	Shen Jin Cao (Herba Lycopodii Japonici) *Chi Shao* (Radix Paeoniae Rubra) *Du Zhong* (Cortex Eucommiae Ulmoidis) *Hong Hua* (Flos Carthami Tinctorii)	Spasms, pain and inhibited bending and stretching due to damp-cold
	Ai Ye (Folium Artemisiae Argyi) *Wu Zhu Yu* (Fructus Evodiae Rutaecarpae) *Chuan Xiong* (Rhizoma Ligustici Chuanxiong) *Xiang Fu* (Rhizoma Cyperi Rotundi)	Painful menstruation due to cold or insufficiency of Yang Qi
	Dang Gui (Radix Angelicae Sinensis) *Chuan Xiong* (Rhizoma Ligustici Chuanxiong) *Tao Ren* (Semen Persicae) *Hong Hua* (Flos Carthami Tinctorii)	Menstrual block and abdominal masses due to Blood stasis (e.g. fibroids)
	Gan Jiang (Rhizoma Zingiberis Officinalis) *Wu Zhu Yu* (Fructus Evodiae Rutaecarpae) *Bai Shao* (Radix Paeoniae Lactiflorae) *Gan Cao* (Radix Glycyrrhizae)	Cold and pain in the abdomen due to Yang deficiency of the Spleen and Stomach or intake of too much raw and cold food
	Chuan Lian Zi (Fructus Meliae Toosendan) *Xiao Hui Xiang* (Fructus Foeniculi Vulgaris)	Cold and pain in the testicles due to insufficiency of Yang Qi or externally-contracted cold

Freeing Yang and transforming Qi, warming and transforming water-fluids	*Fu Ling* (Sclerotium Poriae Cocos) *Zhu Ling* (Sclerotium Polypori Umbellati) *Ze Xie* (Rhizoma Alismatis Orientalis) *Bai Zhu* (Rhizoma Atractylodis Macrocephalae) *Zhi Gan Cao* (Radix Glycyrrhizae Praeparata)	Palpitations, oedema and scant urine due to water-fluids invading the Heart
	Zhi Shi (Fructus Immaturus Citri Aurantii) *Xie Bai* (Bulbus Allii Macrostemi) *Hou Po* (Cortex Magnoliae Officinalis)	Congestion and obstruction of Phlegm turbidity, obstruction of the Heart vessels, and chest Bi syndrome pain due to failure to rouse chest Yang
	Bai Zhu (Rhizoma Atractylodis Macrocephalae) *Fu Ling* (Sclerotium Poriae Cocos)	Coughing and wheezing, dizziness and oedema due to Phlegm-fluids
	Bai Zhu (Rhizoma Atractylodis Macrocephalae) *Bai Jie Zi* (Semen Sinapis Albae) *Zi Su Ye* (Folium Perillae Frutescentis) *Hou Po* (Cortex Magnoliae Officinalis)	Cold fluids lying latent internally, coughing and wheezing with spitting of sputum, alternating chills and fever, aching in the lumbar region, twitching of the body

Xi Xin 细辛 (Chinese wild ginger, Herba cum Radice Asari)

Xi Xin is the dried herb of *Asarum heterotropoides* Fr. Schmidt var. *mandshuricum* (Maxim.) Kitag., *A. sieboldii* Miq. or *A. sieboldii* Miq. var. *seoulense* Nakai, family Aristolochiaceae.

Legal status *Xi Xin* was listed in a document entitled *A Review of Restricted Herbal Ingredients* issued by the Medicines Control Agency (MCA) in the UK in September 2001 with a view to the possible imposition of restrictions on its use at a future date. The MCA is concerned that this herb contains small quantities of aristolochic acid, which is considered by medical supervisory authorities as nephrotoxic and potentially carcinogenic.

Main ingredients *Xi Xin* contains 3% of volatile oils (including methyleugenol, safrole, α-pinene, β-pinene, myrcene, limonene, estragole, eucarvone, camphene and asarylketone) and various trace elements.

Properties Taste: acrid; nature: warm.

Channels entered Lung and Kidney.

Functions and indications Dissipates wind-cold or dispels wind to alleviate pain, warms the Lungs and transforms fluids, frees obstructions and opens the orifices. It is indicated for headache due to wind-cold, nasal congestion, deep-source nasal congestion, toothache, deafness, cough due to Phlegm-fluids, and wind-cold-damp Bi syndrome.

Common dosage 1-3g, or 10g for large dosages; appropriate dosage of the herb in powder form for nasal insufflation therapy.

Precautions and contraindications

1. As *Xi Xin* has a strong taste and a powerful warming and dissipating effect, it is easy for it to consume Qi and damage Yin. It is therefore contraindicated in cases of profuse sweating due to Qi deficiency, headache due to Blood deficiency, or cough due to Yin deficiency.
2. *Xi Xin* is incompatible with *Li Lu* (Radix et Rhizoma Veratri).

Remarks Traditional sources such as *Ben Cao Bie Shuo* [Discussions on Materia Medica] indicate that '*Xi Xin* cannot be used in dosages higher than 3g'. The herb is frequently decocted with *Gan Cao* (Radix Glycyrrhizae) to decrease the drastic nature of its effect. *Xi Xin* can also be processed with honey to diminish its toxicity and reduce its warming and dissipating characteristics.

Comparison of functions *Xi Xin* (Herba cum Radice Asari), *Ma Huang* (Herba Ephedrae) and *Gui Zhi* (Ramulus Cinnamomi Cassiae), all of which are acrid in taste and warm in nature, are commonly used in the clinic for releasing the exterior and dissipating wind-cold to treat common colds or other exterior patterns due to wind-cold. *Ma Huang* and *Gui Zhi* are key herbs for inducing sweating and releasing the exterior and are often used in combination to enhance each other's effect in the treatment of exterior patterns due to wind-cold.

Ma Huang, which opens with acridity and discharges with bitterness, mainly diffuses and dissipates defensive Qi, opens the interstices (*cou li*), induces sweating and releases the exterior, and dissipates wind-cold in the Lung and Bladder channels. It has a comparatively strong effect in inducing sweating and dissipating cold to release the exterior, and in diffusing Lung Qi; it is therefore mainly used for wind-cold fettering the exterior, full-type Lung Qi congestion, blockage of the orifices, and severe common colds due to full-type wind-cold exterior patterns without sweating.

Gui Zhi reinforces Heart Yang, adjusts and harmonizes the Ying and Wei levels, releases flesh and induces sweating, and releases the exterior and dispels wind. It functions well in dissipating wind-cold in the Lung and Bladder channels, but its effect in inducing sweating is less powerful than that of *Ma Huang*. *Gui Zhi* is good for both full-type and deficiency-type exterior patterns as it can warm the channels and dissipate cold, free Yang and transform Qi. It can be used for common colds due to wind-cold irrespective of whether these manifest as exterior full patterns without sweating or exterior deficiency patterns with sweating.

Xi Xin penetrates the exterior and passes into the interior. It can disperse wind-cold in the Lung and Kidney channels. Its ability to induce sweating is inferior to that of *Ma Huang* and *Gui Zhi*, but it is effective in dissipating cold. It can be used for common colds due to wind-cold, as well as for cold invading in the Shaoyin stage, for an absence of sweating and an aversion to cold, and for cold with Yang deficiency accompanied by fever and a sunken pulse.

Toxicity The minimum lethal dosage for intraperitoneal injection in mice of the volatile oils contained in *Xi Xin* is 200mg/kg, with the LD_{50} being 247mg/kg. Extracts of the herb have higher toxicity than decoctions. The volatile oils in *Xi Xin* initially stimulated activity in animals before inhibiting it, resulting in a slowing down of voluntary movement and respiration before eventual death due to respiratory paralysis. *Xi Xin* directly inhibits the cardiac muscle and there have been reports that overdosage has caused arrhythmia. Toxic side-effects mainly arise through oral administration of large dosages of a powder of *Xi Xin* on its own or large dosages of the herbal decoction cooked for a very short time.

Modern research

1. The volatile oils contained in *Xi Xin* possess a tranquillizing function and can inhibit convulsions.[10]
2. Blood pressure can be raised by the volatile oils contained in *Xi Xin*, but lowered by decoctions of the herb.[11]
3. Decoctions of *Xi Xin* can abate fever[10] and alleviate pain.[12]
4. Calms wheezing.[13]
5. The safrole contained in *Xi Xin* has an inhibitory effect on Shigella shigae and Salmonella typhi.[14]

Combinations and applications

Functions	Combinations	Applications
Dissipating wind-cold and alleviating pain	*Fang Feng* (Radix Ledebouriellae Divaricatae) *Bai Zhi* (Radix Angelicae Dahuricae) *Chuan Xiong* (Rhizoma Ligustici Chuanxiong)	Wind-cold type of common cold, fever and chills; used especially for heavy nasal congestion and headache
Dispelling wind and alleviating pain	*Fang Feng* (Radix Ledebouriellae Divaricatae) *Fang Ji* (Radix Stephaniae Tetrandrae) (see notes on legal status) *Gui Zhi* (Ramulus Cinnamomi Cassiae) *Wu Tou* (Radix Aconiti) (see notes on legal status)	Limb joint pain due to wind-cold Bi syndrome, with worsening of pain when cold
	Du Huo (Radix Angelicae Pubescentis) *Sang Ji Sheng* (Ramulus Loranthi) *Xu Duan* (Radix Dipsaci) *Wu Yao* (Radix Linderae Strychnifoliae)	Pain in the lumbar region, knees and abdomen due to externally-contracted cold
Warming the Lungs and transforming fluids	*Gan Jiang* (Rhizoma Zingiberis Officinalis) *Ban Xia* (Rhizoma Pinelliae Ternatae) *Rou Gui* (Cortex Cinnamomi Cassiae)	Cough and rapid breathing with copious thin sputum due to Lung-cold
	Gui Zhi (Ramulus Cinnamomi Cassiae) *Fu Zi* (Radix Lateralis Aconiti Carmichaeli Praeparata) (see notes on legal status) *Ting Li Zi* (Semen Lepidii seu Descurainiae) *Wu Jia Pi* (Cortex Acanthopanacis Gracilistyli Radicis)	Coughing and wheezing with copious thin sputum, cold limbs, oedema and scant urine due to water Qi intimidating the Heart and containing the Lungs
Freeing obstructions and opening the orifices	*Xin Yi Hua* (Flos Magnoliae) *Bai Zhi* (Radix Angelicae Dahuricae) *Huang Qin* (Radix Scutellariae Baicalensis)	Nasal congestion, deep-source nasal congestion, headache
	Xie Bai (Bulbus Allii Macrostemi) *Dan Shen* (Radix Salviae Miltiorrhizae) *Gui Zhi* (Ramulus Cinnamomi Cassiae)	Chest Bi syndrome due to Yang deficiency
	Chi Shao (Radix Paeoniae Rubra) *Hong Hua* (Flos Carthami Tinctorii) *Chuan Xiong* (Rhizoma Ligustici Chuanxiong)	Distension of the breasts with pain, menstrual block

Zi Su Ye 紫苏叶 (Perilla leaf, Folium Perillae Frutescentis)

Zi Su Ye is the leaf of *Perilla frutescens* (L.) Britt. var. *acuta* (Thunb.) Kudo, family Labiatae.

Main ingredients The whole plant contains 0.5% of volatile oils, of which 55% is perillaldehyde and 20-30% l-limonene. Other ingredients include β-pinene, l-linalool, camphene, menthol, menthone, perilla alcohol, eugenol and perilla ketone.

Properties Taste: acrid; nature: warm.

Channels entered Lung and Spleen.

Functions and indications Dissipates cold and releases the exterior, moves Qi and loosens the Middle Jiao, and treats seafood poisoning by relieving toxicity. It is indicated for the full type of wind-cold exterior patterns, oppression in the chest and vomiting due to Qi stagnation in the Spleen and Stomach; and for pain in the abdomen, vomiting and diarrhoea caused by seafood poisoning.

Common dosage 3-10g, or 30g for large dosages. Lengthy decoction is not appropriate.

Precautions and contraindications *Zi Su Ye* should be used with caution in cases of spontaneous sweating due to exterior deficiency.

Remarks To release the exterior, use *Zi Su Ye* (Folium Perillae Frutescentis); to move Qi and loosen the Middle Jiao, use *Su Geng* (Caulis Perillae Frutescentis); to harmonize the Stomach and stop vomiting, use *Zi Su Ye* and *Su Geng* together; to bear counterflow Qi downwards and disperse Phlegm, use *Su Zi* (Fructus Perillae Frutescentis) (see Chapter 13).

Comparison of functions See *Huo Xiang* (Herba Agastaches seu Pogostemi).

Toxicity The LD_{50} for oral administration to mice of the eugenol contained in *Zi Su Ye* is 1.95mg/kg. Intravenous injection of 10mg/kg of perilla ketone in nanny goats can cause death; 30mg/kg injected intravenously in calves can have the same result. Perilla alcohol is the most toxic constituent of *Zi Su Ye*; it has a stimulatory effect and can cause an allergic reaction. Perilla ketone caused extensive pulmonary oedema in mice with a large quantity of peritoneal exudate.

Modern research

1. Stops bleeding by causing contraction of the blood vessels.[15]
2. Stops coughing and calms wheezing.[16]
3. Decoctions of *Zi Su Ye* can inhibit Staphylococcus aureus and epiphytes.[17]
4. Inhibits carcinoma.[18]

Combinations and applications

Functions	Combinations	Applications
Dissipating cold and releasing the exterior	*Xiang Fu* (Rhizoma Cyperi Rotundi) *Chen Pi* (Pericarpium Citri Reticulatae)	Fever and chills, headache without sweating and oppression in the chest due to externally-contracted wind-cold with internal Qi stagnation
	Xing Ren (Semen Pruni Armeniacae) *Qian Hu* (Radix Peucedani) *Jie Geng* (Radix Platycodi Grandiflori)	Fever without sweating, cough and oppression in the chest due to externally-contracted wind-cold

	Huo Xiang (Herba Agastaches seu Pogostemi) *Chen Pi* (Pericarpium Citri Reticulatae) *Sheng Jiang* (Rhizoma Zingiberis Officinalis Recens) *Shen Qu* (Massa Fermentata)	Wind-cold type of common cold with oppression in the chest, nausea, vomiting, pain in the stomach or diarrhoea
Moving Qi and loosening the Middle Jiao	*Chen Pi* (Pericarpium Citri Reticulatae) *Ban Xia* (Rhizoma Pinelliae Ternatae) *Dai Zhe Shi* (Haematitum)	Oppression in the chest, belching, nausea and vomiting due to Qi stagnation in the Spleen and Stomach
	Ban Xia (Rhizoma Pinelliae Ternatae) *Hou Po* (Cortex Magnoliae Officinalis)	Oppression in the chest, nausea and vomiting due to Qi stagnation and binding of Phlegm
	Chen Pi (Pericarpium Citri Reticulatae) *Sha Ren* (Fructus Amomi) *Bai Shao* (Radix Paeoniae Lactiflorae)	Vomiting during pregnancy, and stirring foetus due to inhibited Qi dynamic
Treating seafood poisoning by relieving toxicity	*Huang Lian* (Rhizoma Coptidis) *Huo Xiang* (Herba Agastaches seu Pogostemi) *Ban Xia* (Rhizoma Pinelliae Ternatae) *Sheng Jiang* (Rhizoma Zingiberis Officinalis Recens)	Pain in the abdomen, vomiting and diarrhoea due to seafood poisoning

Appendix

***Su Geng* 苏梗 (Perilla stem, Caulis Perillae Frutescentis)**

Su Geng is the stem of *Perilla frutescens* (L.) Britt. var. *acuta* (Thunb.) Kudo, family Labiatae. It is acrid and sweet in taste and slightly warm in nature and enters the Lung, Spleen and Stomach channels. Its main functions are regulating Qi to quiet the foetus, and loosening the chest and benefiting the diaphragm. It is used to treat vomiting during pregnancy and distension in the abdomen due to Qi stagnation during pregnancy.

Jing Jie 荆芥
(Schizonepeta herb, Herba Schizonepetae Tenuifoliae)

Jing Jie is the dried aerial parts of *Schizonepeta tenuifolia* Briq., family Labiatae.

Main ingredients The whole plant contains 1.8% of volatile oils; the spike contains 4% of volatile oils. The main volatile oils include d-menthone and racemin-menthone, together with small quantities of α- and β-pinene, d-limonene, camphene and 3-octanone.

Properties Taste: acrid; nature: slightly warm.

Channels entered Lung and Liver.

Functions and indications Dispels wind and releases the exterior, vents papules and alleviates itching, regulates the Blood and stops bleeding. It is indicated for the full type of wind-cold exterior patterns, the initial stage of measles and sores combined with exterior patterns, nosebleed and uterine bleeding.

Common dosage 3-10g; or appropriate dosage for external use in crushed or powder form or as a wash. Lengthy decoction is not advisable.

Precautions and contraindications *Jing Jie* is contraindicated in cases of spontaneous sweating due to exterior deficiency, and headache due to Yin deficiency.

Remarks Raw *Jing Jie* has a strong diaphoretic effect, fried *Jing Jie* has a mild function in releasing the exterior, and the charred herb, *Jing Jie Tan* (Herba Schizonepetae Tenuifoliae Carbonisata), is mainly used to stop bleeding, being particularly useful for nosebleed, blood in the stool, haemorrhoids and uterine bleeding. The spike of the plant, *Jing Jie Sui* (Spica Schizonepetae Tenuifoliae), is more effective than the whole plant.

Comparison of functions See *Fang Feng* (Radix Ledebouriellae Divaricatae) and *Bo He* (Herba Menthae Haplocalycis).

Toxicity The LD_{50} for intraperitoneal injection in mice of a decoction of *Jing Jie* was 30.05g/kg after seven days.

Modern research

1. A decoction of *Jing Jie* reduced fever considerably when injected intravenously into the ears of rabbits and brought slight relief through stomach perfusion.[19]
2. Has a tranquillizing function and alleviates pain.[19]
3. Inhibits inflammation.[20-22]
4. In its charred form, it can stop bleeding.[23]
5. Decoctions of *Jing Jie* can inhibit Staphylococcus aureus and Corynebacterium diphtheriae.[24]

Combinations and applications

Functions	Combinations	Applications
Dispelling wind and releasing the exterior	*Qiang Huo* (Rhizoma et Radix Notopterygii) *Fang Feng* (Radix Ledebouriellae Divaricatae) *Chai Hu* (Radix Bupleuri)	Wind-cold type of common cold, manifesting as fever and chills, headache and generalized pain
	Ju Hua (Flos Chrysanthemi Morifolii) *Bo He* (Herba Menthae Haplocalycis) *Da Qing Ye* (Folium Isatidis seu Baphicacanthi)	Wind-heat type of common cold, manifesting as high fever and slight chill, cough and swollen throat
	Jin Yin Hua (Flos Lonicerae) *Chi Shao* (Radix Paeoniae Rubra) *Mu Dan Pi* (Cortex Moutan Radicis) *Fang Feng* (Radix Ledebouriellae Divaricatae)	Swelling and toxins of sores at the initial stage, with local warmth, pain and redness, combined with fever and chills
Venting papules and alleviating itching	*Bo He* (Herba Menthae Haplocalycis) *Chan Tui* (Periostracum Cicadae)	Initial stage of measles before development of a rash
	Ku Shen (Radix Sophorae Flavescentis) *Huang Bai* (Cortex Phellodendri) *She Chuang Zi* (Fructus Cnidii Monnieri)	Itchy skin, eczema
Regulating the Blood and stopping bleeding	*Huang Qi* (Radix Astragali seu Hedysari) *Mu Dan Pi* (Cortex Moutan Radicis) *Da Huang Tan* (Radix et Rhizoma Rhei Carbonisatae) *Sheng Di Huang* (Radix Rehmanniae Glutinosae)	Red and profuse advanced menstruation, feverishness, a red tongue with a thin body and yellow fur, and a rapid pulse

Huai Hua (Flos Sophorae Japonicae)	Blood in the stool
Di Yu (Radix Sanguisorbae Officinalis) *Huai Jiao* (Fructus Sophorae Japonicae) *Hu Huang Lian* (Rhizoma Picrorhizae Scrophulariiflorae) *E Jiao* (Gelatinum Corii Asini)	Haemorrhoidal bleeding

Note: In addition, a powder of *Jing Jie Sui* (Spica Schizonepetae Tenuifoliae) can be taken orally to treat profuse sweating and uterine bleeding after childbirth.

Fang Feng 防风 (Ledebouriella root, Radix Ledebouriellae Divaricatae)

Fang Feng is the root of *Ledebouriella divaricata* (Turcz.) Hiroe, family Umbelliferae. This herb is also known as *Saposhnikovia divaricata* (Turcz.) Schischk. (Radix Saposhnikoviae Divaricatae).

Main ingredients *Fang Feng* contains 0.1% of volatile oils (including pentanal, hexanal, octanal and α-pinene), naphthalene, cimifugin, psoralen, bergapten, β-sitosterol, daucosterol and mannitol.

Properties Taste: acrid and sweet; nature: slightly warm.

Channels entered Bladder, Liver and Spleen.

Functions and indications Dispels wind and releases the exterior, overcomes dampness and alleviates pain, expels wind to relieve tetany, stops bleeding and stops diarrhoea. It is indicated for the wind-cold type of exterior patterns, Bi syndrome due to wind, cold or damp, headache and generalized pain, itchy skin, tetanus, blood in the stool, uterine bleeding, and diarrhoea due to Spleen deficiency.

Common dosage 3-10g, or 20g for large dosages.

Precautions and contraindications *Fang Feng* is contraindicated in cases of effulgent Yin deficiency-fire, and spasms due to Blood deficiency where there is an absence of wind pathogenic factors.

Remarks Raw *Fang Feng* is used to induce sweating; baked *Fang Feng* can strengthen the effect of drying dampness and warming the channels; charred *Fang Feng* is good for stopping bleeding. Large dosages (above 20g) of *Fang Feng* are indicated for bleeding and diarrhoea.

Comparison of functions *Fang Feng* (Radix Ledebouriellae Divaricatae) and *Jing Jie* (Herba Schizonepetae Tenuifoliae) are commonly used in the clinic for dispelling wind, releasing the exterior and venting papules, but they have a less drastic action than *Ma Huang* (Herba Ephedrae) and *Gui Zhi* (Ramulus Cinnamomi Cassiae). They can treat common colds due to wind-cold and wind-heat and can also alleviate itching. The two herbs are often used together to dispel wind and release the exterior.

The acrid property of *Jing Jie* means that it has a stronger function in dispelling wind and venting papules as well as in treating the initial stage of sores combined with an exterior pattern. *Fang Feng* can overcome dampness and alleviate pain and is therefore used for wind, cold or damp Bi syndrome and limb joint pain; it can also dispel external wind and extinguish internal wind to treat tetanus due to external wind stirring internal wind, opisthotonos, convulsions and spasms.

Toxicity The LD_{50} for aqueous extracts of *Guan Fang Feng* (the variety of *Fang Feng* found in Northeast China) administered to mice is 37.18 ± 8.36g/kg.

Modern research

1. Decoctions of *Fang Feng* can abate fever.[25]
2. Inhibits inflammation.[26]
3. Alleviates pain[27] and inhibits convulsions.[28]
4. Juice from the fresh herb has a certain inhibitory effect on Staphylococcus aureus and Pseudomonas pyocyanea.[29]

Combinations and applications

Functions	Combinations	Applications
Dispelling wind and releasing the exterior	*Jing Jie* (Herba Schizonepetae Tenuifoliae) *Qiang Huo* (Rhizoma et Radix Notopterygii)	Headache, generalized pain and lack of sweating due to externally-contracted wind-cold pathogenic factors
	Bo He (Herba Menthae Haplocalycis) *Lian Qiao* (Fructus Forsythiae Suspensae)	Fever, sore throat and red eyes due to externally-contracted wind-heat
	Chan Tui (Periostracum Cicadae) *Sheng Ma* (Rhizoma Cimicifugae) *Ze Xie* (Rhizoma Alismatis Orientalis)	Red, sore and swollen eyes due to wind-fire attacking upwards
	Ku Shen (Radix Sophorae Flavescentis) *Jing Jie* (Herba Schizonepetae Tenuifoliae) *Bai Xian Pi* (Cortex Dictamni Dasycarpi Radicis)	Itchy skin due to urticaria (dormant papules) or other dermatological diseases
Overcoming dampness and alleviating pain	*Du Huo* (Radix Angelicae Pubescentis) *Qin Jiao* (Radix Gentianae Macrophyllae) *Wei Ling Xian* (Radix Clematidis)	Bi syndrome due to an invasion of wind, with wandering pain
	Gui Zhi (Ramulus Cinnamomi Cassiae) *Wu Tou* (Radix Aconiti) (see notes on legal status) *Xi Xin* (Herba cum Radice Asari)	Bi syndrome due to externally-contracted cold, with worsening of pain when cold
	Cang Zhu (Rhizoma Atractylodis) *Fen Bi Xie* (Rhizoma Dioscoreae Hypoglaucae) *Fang Ji* (Radix Stephaniae Tetrandrae) (see notes on legal status)	Bi syndrome due to an invasion of damp, with pain in a fixed location
	Du Huo (Radix Angelicae Pubescentis) *Niu Xi* (Radix Achyranthis Bidentatae) *Sang Ji Sheng* (Ramulus Loranthi)	Pain in the lumbar region and inhibited bending and stretching due to insufficiency of the Liver and Kidneys leading to enduring Bi syndrome
Expelling wind to relieve tetany	*Tian Nan Xing* (Rhizoma Arisaematis) *Bai Fu Zi* (Rhizoma Typhonii Gigantei) *Tian Ma* (Rhizoma Gastrodiae Elatae) (see notes on legal status) *Bai Zhi* (Radix Angelicae Dahuricae)	Tetanus manifesting as opisthotonos and clenched jaw

Stopping bleeding and stopping diarrhoea	*Bai Shao* (Radix Paeoniae Lactiflorae) *Bai Zhu* (Rhizoma Atractylodis Macrocephalae) *Chen Pi* (Pericarpium Citri Reticulatae)	Pain in the abdomen and diarrhoea due to stagnated Liver Qi invading the Spleen
	Jing Jie Tan (Herba Schizonepetae Tenuifoliae Carbonisata) *Di Yu Tan* (Radix Sanguisorbae Officinalis Carbonisata) *Chao Huai Hua* (Flos Sophorae Japonicae, stir-fried)	Uterine bleeding and blood in the stool due to the Spleen failing to control the Blood

Qiang Huo 羌活
(Notopterygium root, Rhizoma et Radix Notopterygii)

Qiang Huo is the rhizome and root of *Notopterygium incisum* Ting ex H. T. Chang or *N. forbesii* Boiss., family Umbelliferae.

Main ingredients *Qiang Huo* contains 2.7% of volatile oils (including α-thujene, α- and β- pinene, β-ocimene, limonene, bornyl acetate and sabinene), coumaric acids, lysine, arginine, fructose, glucose and sucrose.

Properties Taste: acrid and bitter; nature: warm.

Channels entered Bladder and Kidney.

Functions and indications Dispels wind and releases the exterior, overcomes dampness and alleviates pain. It is indicated for the wind-cold type of common cold, headache without sweating, wind-cold-damp Bi syndrome pain, stiffness of the neck, aching and painful joints, dizziness, and red eyes.

Common dosage 3-10g.

Precautions and contraindications *Qiang Huo* is acrid, warm and extremely dry; it should therefore be used with caution for headaches due to Blood deficiency and in cases of lack of strength.

Remarks A large dosage of this herb may result in vomiting because of the strong smell.

Comparison of functions According to classical texts: '*Du Huo* can treat latent wind, *Qiang Huo* can treat wandering wind.' Both *Qiang Huo* (Rhizoma et Radix Notopterygii) and *Du Huo* (Radix Angelicae Pubescentis) can be used for dispelling wind, overcoming dampness and alleviating pain. *Qiang Huo* is drier and harsher in nature and is better at dissipating exterior pathogenic factors to alleviate pain occurring in the upper part of the body and wind-cold-damp Bi syndrome pain. *Du Huo* is milder and its dissipating effect is weaker than that of *Qiang Huo*. It is more effective in dispelling wind and damp in the sinews and bones and is commonly used for wind-cold-damp Bi syndrome in the lower part of the body. When the two herbs are used together for limb joint pain, the pain-alleviating effect is increased.

For an additional comparison, see *Gao Ben* (Rhizoma et Radix Ligustici).

Toxicity The LD_{50} for the volatile oils contained in *Qiang Huo* administered to mice is 6.64 ± 0.87ml/kg. No abnormal reactions were observed after a single intravenous injection in mice of 10ml/kg of a 2% solution of *Qiang Huo*.

Modern research

1. The volatile oils contained in *Qiang Huo* can relieve myocardial ischaemia.[30]
2. Decoctions of *Qiang Huo* can inhibit the formation of embolisms.[31]
3. Can inhibit arrhythmia.[31]

Combinations and applications

Functions	Combinations	Applications
Dispelling wind and releasing the exterior	*Jing Jie Tan* (Herba Schizonepetae Tenuifoliae Carbonisata) *Fang Feng* (Radix Ledebouriellae Divaricatae)	Wind-cold type of common cold, headache without sweating; used especially for occipital headache
	Ju Hua (Flos Chrysanthemi Morifolii) *Man Jing Zi* (Fructus Viticis)	Red eyes due to wind-heat
	Niu Bang Zi (Fructus Arctii Lappae) *Bo He* (Herba Menthae Haplocalycis) *Pu Gong Ying* (Herba Taraxaci cum Radice)	Wind-heat type of influenza
Overcoming dampness and alleviating pain	*Du Huo* (Radix Angelicae Pubescentis) *Fang Feng* (Radix Ledebouriellae Divaricatae) *Chuan Xiong* (Rhizoma Ligustici Chuanxiong)	Wind-cold-damp Bi syndrome pain, especially with pain in the upper part of the body
	Du Huo (Radix Angelicae Pubescentis) *Fang Feng* (Radix Ledebouriellae Divaricatae) *Gao Ben* (Rhizoma et Radix Ligustici) *Man Jing Zi* (Fructus Viticis)	Wind-damp in the exterior, headache and painful stiff neck, aching in the lumbar region and back, and generalized pain
	Jiang Huang (Rhizoma Curcumae Longae) *Gui Zhi* (Ramulus Cinnamomi Cassiae)	Pain in the upper limbs and fingers
	Cang Zhu (Rhizoma Atractylodis) *Fang Feng* (Radix Ledebouriellae Divaricatae) *Cang Er Zi* (Fructus Xanthii Sibirici)	Headache due to wind-damp

Note: In addition, *Qiang Huo* can also bear Yang Qi upwards in the Taiyang channel and Du vessel and is indicated for disorders of the Du vessel manifesting as stiffness of the back and convulsions.

Bai Zhi 白芷 (White angelica root, Radix Angelicae Dahuricae)

Bai Zhi is the root of *Angelica dahurica* (Fisch. ex Hoffm.) Benth. et Hook. f. and *A. dahurica* (Fisch. ex Hoffm.) Benth. et Hook. f. var. *formosana* (Boiss.) Shan et Yuan, family Umbelliferae.

Main ingredients *Bai Zhi* contains imperatorin, alloimperatorin, bergaptene, phellopterin, byak-angelicin, oxypeucedanin, byak-angelicol, xanthotoxin, scopoletin, xanthotoxol and anomalin.

Properties Taste: acrid; nature: warm.

Channels entered Lung and Stomach.

Functions and indications Dissipates cold and releases the exterior, dispels wind and dries dampness, frees the orifices and alleviates pain, disperses swelling and expels pus. It is indicated for headache due to common colds, pain in the supra-orbital region, nasal congestion and toothache, red and white vaginal discharge, sores, and itchy skin.

Common dosage 3-10g; or appropriate dosage for external application when ground into a powder.

Precautions and contraindications *Bai Zhi* should be used with caution in cases of effulgent Yin deficiency-fire.

Comparison of functions See *Cang Er Zi* (Fructus Xanthii Sibirici).

Toxicity The LD_{50} for oral administration to mice of the coumarins contained in the species of *Bai Zhi* grown in Yunnan is 2110mg/kg. The LD_{50} for oral administration to mice of the imperatorin contained in the herb is 100g/kg. It is rare for internal use of *Bai Zhi* or external application of the dried herb to provoke allergic reactions, but contact with the fresh herb may lead to contact dermatitis.

Modern research

1. An aqueous extract of *Bai Zhi* can contract the blood vessels, whereas an acetic extract of the herb can dilate them.[32]
2. Too large a dosage can result in convulsions.[33]
3. Can alleviate pain[34] and abate fever.[35]

Combinations and applications

Functions	Combinations	Applications
Dissipating cold and releasing the exterior	*Qiang Huo* (Rhizoma et Radix Notopterygii) *Fang Feng* (Radix Ledebouriellae Divaricatae) *Man Jing Zi* (Fructus Viticis)	Wind-cold type of common cold with severe headache and nasal congestion
	Qiang Huo (Rhizoma et Radix Notopterygii) *Chuan Xiong* (Rhizoma Ligustici Chuanxiong)	Headache due to wind-cold
Dispelling wind and drying dampness	*Cang Zhu* (Rhizoma Atractylodis) *Hai Piao Xiao* (Os Sepiae seu Sepiellae) *Qian Shi* (Semen Euryales Ferocis)	Vaginal discharge due to cold-damp, aching in the lumbar region, limp and cold limbs, cold and pain in the lower abdomen
	Huang Bai (Cortex Phellodendri) *Che Qian Zi* (Semen Plantaginis)	Vaginal discharge due to damp-heat
	Jing Jie (Herba Schizonepetae Tenuifoliae) *Ku Shen* (Radix Sophorae Flavescentis) *Chan Tui* (Periostracum Cicadae)	Eczema, itchy skin
	He Zi (Fructus Terminaliae Chebulae) *Rou Dou Kou* (Semen Myristicae Fragrantis) *Fu Ling* (Sclerotium Poriae Cocos) *Qian Shi* (Semen Euryales Ferocis)	Diarrhoea due to Spleen deficiency with dampness
Freeing the orifices and alleviating pain	*Xi Xin* (Herba cum Radice Asari) *Chuan Xiong* (Rhizoma Ligustici Chuanxiong)	Frontal headache due to wind-cold
	Cang Er Zi (Fructus Xanthii Sibirici) *Xin Yi Hua* (Flos Magnoliae) *Bo He* (Herba Menthae Haplocalycis)	Nasal disorders such as nasal congestion or deep-source nasal congestion

Dispersing swelling and expelling pus	*Gua Lou* (Fructus Trichosanthis)	Breast abscess
	Mu Dan Pi (Cortex Moutan Radicis) *Bai Jiang Cao* (Herba Patriniae cum Radice) *Da Huang* (Radix et Rhizoma Rhei) *Hong Teng* (Caulis Sargentodoxae Cuneatae)	Intestinal abscess
	Jin Yin Hua (Flos Lonicerae) *Mu Dan Pi* (Cortex Moutan Radicis) *Chuan Shan Jia* (Squama Manitis Pentadactylae) (see notes on legal status) *Dang Gui* (Radix Angelicae Sinensis)	Swelling and toxins of sores, regardless of whether they have ulcerated or not

Gao Ben 藁本 (Chinese lovage root, Rhizoma et Radix Ligustici)

Gao Ben is the rhizome and root of *Ligusticum sinense* Oliv. or *L. jeholense* Nakai et Kitag., family Umbelliferae.

Main ingredients *Gao Ben* contains volatile oils, mainly 3-butylphthalide, cnidilide and methyl eugenol, with smaller amounts of α- and β-pinene, camphene, sabinene, myrcene, α-phellandrene, α-terpinene and terpine-4-ol.

Properties Taste: acrid; nature: warm.

Channel entered Bladder.

Functions and indications Dissipates wind, dispels dampness and alleviates pain. It is indicated for headache due to wind-cold, parietal headache, toothache, pain due to wind-damp, pain in the abdomen due to damp-cold, diarrhoea, scabies and abscesses.

Common dosage 3-10g.

Precautions and contraindications *Gao Ben* is contraindicated for heat patterns and headache due to Blood deficiency.

Comparison of functions Both *Gao Ben* (Rhizoma et Radix Ligustici) and *Qiang Huo* (Rhizoma et Radix Notopterygii) are acrid and warm and are effective in dispelling pathogenic wind in the Bladder channel to dissipate cold and release the exterior, as well as in overcoming dampness and alleviating pain. They are often combined to strengthen their function.

Qiang Huo, which is bitter and dry, has a stronger function in drying dampness than *Gao Ben*. It is good at treating stiffness and pain in the neck and the back of the head caused by pathogenic wind, cold and damp invading the Taiyang channel. *Gao Ben* is warm and upward-bearing and functions better in reaching the vertex to treat Taiyang patterns due to an invasion of wind and cold manifesting as pain at the vertex.

For an additional comparison, see *Man Jing Zi* (Fructus Viticis).

Toxicity The LD_{50} of the volatile oils contained in *Gao Ben* given to mice via intragastric administration is 70.17 ± 4.95g/kg (calculated on the basis of the raw herb).

Modern research

1. Has a tranquillizing effect.[36]
2. Alleviates pain, inhibits inflammation, abates fever and lowers body temperature.[37]

Combinations and applications

Functions	Combinations	Applications
Dissipating wind, dispelling dampness and alleviating pain	*Bai Zhi* (Radix Angelicae Dahuricae) *Chuan Xiong* (Rhizoma Ligustici Chuanxiong)	Headache due to externally-contracted wind-cold
	Qiang Huo (Rhizoma et Radix Notopterygii) *Fang Feng* (Radix Ledebouriellae Divaricatae) *Ma Huang* (Herba Ephedrae)	Head-wind headache in the Taiyang channel with fever, aversion to cold and absence of sweating
	Dang Gui (Radix Angelicae Sinensis) *Chuan Xiong* (Rhizoma Ligustici Chuanxiong) *Qiang Huo* (Rhizoma et Radix Notopterygii)	Headache occurring at the vertex accompanied by chills
	Chuan Xiong (Rhizoma Ligustici Chuanxiong) *Xi Xin* (Herba cum Radice Asari) *Bai Zhi* (Radix Angelicae Dahuricae) *Gan Cao* (Radix Glycyrrhizae)	Migraine, numbness of the hands and feet
	Cang Zhu (Rhizoma Atractylodis)	Pain in the stomach
	Qiang Huo (Rhizoma et Radix Notopterygii) *Du Huo* (Radix Angelicae Pubescentis) *Fang Feng* (Radix Ledebouriellae Divaricatae) *Man Jing Zi* (Fructus Viticis)	Cold and pain in the back and lumbar region due to external wind-cold-damp

Cang Er Zi 苍耳子 (Cocklebur fruit, Fructus Xanthii Sibirici)

Cang Er Zi is the fruit of *Xanthium sibiricum* Patr., family Compositae.

Legal status *Cang Er Zi* was listed in a document entitled *A Review of Restricted Herbal Ingredients* issued by the Medicines Control Agency (MCA) in the UK in September 2001 with a view to the possible imposition of restrictions on its use at a future date. The MCA is considering introducing a requirement for medical supervision in use as a result of reported side-effects of seizures in one UK patient.

Main ingredients *Cang Er Zi* contains xanthostrumarin, xanthanol, xanthumin, fatty oils, resins, vitamin C and alkaloids.

Properties Taste: acrid and bitter; nature: warm; slightly toxic.

Channel entered Lung.

Functions and indications Dispels wind-damp, and frees the orifices to alleviate pain. It is indicated for headache due to wind-cold, deep-source nasal congestion, toothache, sore eyes, wind-cold-damp Bi syndrome, spasms of the limbs, and itchy skin.

Common dosage 3-10g.

Precautions and contraindications

1. *Cang Er Zi* is contraindicated for headache or Bi syndrome due to Blood deficiency.
2. Overdosage can cause toxic reaction manifesting as vomiting, pain in the abdomen or diarrhoea.

Comparison of functions Both *Cang Er Zi* (Fructus Xanthii Sibirici) and *Bai Zhi* (Radix Angelicae Dahuricae) are aromatic herbs with dissipating properties. They are effective in dispelling wind and dissipating pathogenic factors and in freeing the orifices and alleviating pain.

Bai Zhi can concurrently dry dampness and stop discharge, disperse swelling and expel pus. It is a key herb for pain in the face or frontal headache due to wind-cold invading the Yangming channel. *Cang Er Zi* is bitter in taste and is especially good for unblocking the nasal passages. It also has the functions of dispelling dampness and freeing the network vessels and is consequently used for wind-damp Bi syndrome, although it has a comparatively weak effect and is only used as an auxiliary herb for this purpose.

For an additional comparison, see *Xin Yi Hua* (Flos Magnoliae).

Toxicity The LD_{50} for intraperitoneal injection in mice of an infusion of *Cang Er Zi* is 0.93g/kg. The oils and proteins contained in *Cang Er Zi* have a low level of toxicity; the most toxic constituent is the yellow crystal glycoside AA_2, which has an LD_{50} of 46mg/kg and 10mg/kg for intraperitoneal injection in rats and mice respectively. Toxic overdose damages the kidneys and liver and can lead to encephaloedema. Initial toxic symptoms include headache and dizziness, general malaise, nausea and vomiting, slight distension in the abdomen, diarrhoea or constipation, fatigue and somnolence, progressing to shock, loss of consciousness, major haemorrhaging and hepatomegaly. To avoid toxic reactions, the maximum dosage must not be exceeded and the herb must be fully decocted.

Modern research

1. The glycosides contained in *Cang Er Zi* can lower the blood sugar level.[38]
2. Decoctions of *Cang Er Zi* can stop coughing.[38]
3. A 50% concentration of decoctions of *Cang Er Zi* can inhibit Staphylococcus aureus and epiphytes.[39]

Combinations and applications

Functions	Combinations	Applications
Dispelling wind-damp, freeing the orifices to alleviate pain	*Qiang Huo* (Rhizoma et Radix Notopterygii) *Fang Feng* (Radix Ledebouriellae Divaricatae)	Muscular spasm and Bi syndrome due to wind-damp
	Bai Zhi (Radix Angelicae Dahuricae) *Xi Xin* (Herba cum Radice Asari)	Headache due to wind-cold, deep-source nasal congestion
	Xin Yi Hua (Flos Magnoliae) *Bai Zhi* (Radix Angelicae Dahuricae) *Bo He* (Herba Menthae Haplocalycis)	Nasal congestion, deep-source nasal congestion, inability to distinguish smells, and fishy-smelling turbid and sticky nasal discharge due to pathogenic wind attacking upwards
	Qin Jiao (Radix Gentianae Macrophyllae) *Wei Ling Xian* (Radix Clematidis) *Fang Feng* (Radix Ledebouriellae Divaricatae)	Limb joint pain and numbness of the limbs due to wind-damp
	Tian Ma (Rhizoma Gastrodiae Elatae) (see notes on legal status) *Ju Hua* (Flos Chrysanthemi Morifolii)	Dizziness and distending headache
	Ku Shen (Radix Sophorae Flavescentis) *She Chuang Zi* (Fructus Cnidii Monnieri)	Itchy skin and eczema

Xin Yi Hua 辛夷花 (Magnolia flower, Flos Magnoliae)

Xin Yi Hua is the flower bud of *Magnolia biondii* Pamp., *M. denudata* Desr. or *M. liliflora* Desr., family Magnoliaceae.

Main ingredients *Xin Yi Hua* contains volatile oils (including α- and β-pinene, camphene, sabinene, myrcene, limonene, cineole, γ-terpinene, camphor and bornyl acetate) and alkaloids (including magnocurarine, salicifoline and magnosprengerine).

Properties Taste: acrid; nature: warm.

Channels entered Lung and Stomach.

Functions and indications Dispels wind-cold, and frees the orifices to alleviate pain. It is indicated for headache due to wind-cold, deep-source nasal congestion, allergic rhinitis, stuffy nose, and toothache.

Common dosage 3-10g in decoctions, pills or powders; appropriate dosage for external application. *Xin Yi Hua* should be decocted in a wrap for internal use because its trichome hairs may irritate the throat.

Precautions and contraindications *Xin Yi Hua* is contraindicated in cases of effulgent Yin deficiency-fire.

Comparison of functions Both *Xin Yi Hua* (Flos Magnoliae) and *Cang Er Zi* (Fructus Xanthii Sibirici) are acrid and warm, have diffusing and dissipating properties and are effective in freeing the orifices to alleviate pain. *Xin Yi Hua* is aromatic in smell and taste and tends to open the orifices specifically to treat headaches caused by deep-source nasal congestion due to pathogenic wind-cold or wind-heat invading upwards. *Cang Er Zi* dispels dampness and frees the network vessels and is especially good for unblocking the nasal passages.

Toxicity The LD_{50} for intraperitoneal injection in rats of a tincture of *Xin Yi Hua* is 22.5g/kg. Clinical reports of overdosage are extremely rare.

Modern research

1. The volatile oils contained in *Xin Yi Hua* have a local astringent function and can be used to treat nasal inflammation.[40]
2. Inhibits Staphylococcus aureus, group B streptococci, Corynebacterium diphtheriae and Shigella shigae.[41]

Combinations and applications

Functions	Combinations	Applications
Dispelling wind-cold, freeing the orifices to alleviate pain	*Bai Zhi* (Radix Angelicae Dahuricae) *Xi Xin* (Herba cum Radice Asari)	Deep-source nasal congestion due to wind-cold
	Huang Qin (Radix Scutellariae Baicalensis) *Ju Hua* (Flos Chrysanthemi Morifolii)	Deep-source nasal congestion due to wind-heat
	Sang Ye (Folium Mori Albae) *Jin Yin Hua* (Flos Lonicerae)	Wind-heat-type headache
	Bai Zhi (Radix Angelicae Dahuricae) *Bo He* (Herba Menthae Haplocalycis) *Sheng Ma* (Rhizoma Cimicifugae)	Fever and red, sore and swollen head and face due to wind-heat attacking upwards

Note: In addition to its internal use in a decoction, *Xin Yi Hua* is also prepared as an oil, cream or powder for external application topically to treat conditions in the nasal cavity.

Sheng Jiang 生姜 (Fresh ginger, Rhizoma Zingiberis Officinalis Recens)

Sheng Jiang is the fresh rhizome of *Zingiber officinale* (Willd.) Rosc., family Zingiberaceae.

Main ingredients *Sheng Jiang* contains volatile oils (including zingiberol, zingiberene, tricyclene, α- and β-pinene, β-fenchene, citral, methyl eugenol, acetaldehyde, camphene and perillal), gingerdione and gingerol.

Properties Taste: acrid; nature: slightly warm.

Channels entered Lung, Spleen and Stomach.

Functions and indications Induces sweating and releases the exterior, warms the Stomach and stops vomiting, warms the Lungs and stops coughing, and relieves toxicity. It is indicated for the wind-cold type of common cold, cough, vomiting due to Stomach-cold, and for reducing the toxicity of *Ban Xia* (Rhizoma Pinelliae Ternatae) and *Dan Nan Xing* (Pulvis Arisaematis cum Felle Bovis) and treating seafood poisoning.

Common dosage 3-10g in decoctions or as a juice.

Precautions and contraindications *Sheng Jiang* is contraindicated for dry cough due to Lung-heat, and in cases of deficiency-fire or full-heat.

Comparison of functions Ginger can perform a variety of functions depending on its preparation. *Sheng Jiang* (Rhizoma Zingiberis Officinalis Recens) is moderate in nature and taste and is good at dissipating exterior pathogenic factors and warming the Stomach to stop vomiting. *Gan Jiang* (dried ginger, Rhizoma Zingiberis Officinalis) warms the Middle Jiao and dissipates cold to dispel pathogenic cold in the interior; it also warms and returns Yang Qi verging on desertion (see Chapter 7). *Pao Jiang* (quick-fried dried ginger, Rhizoma Zingiberis Officinalis Praeparata) warms the channels and stops bleeding (see Chapter 11). Since it is not as dry as *Gan Jiang*, *Wei Jiang* (roasted ginger, Rhizoma Zingiberis Officinalis Usta) warms and harmonizes the Stomach to stop vomiting. *Sheng Jiang Pi* (ginger rhizome skin, Cortex Zingiberis Officinalis Recens) is used for promoting urination and reducing swelling.

Toxicity Amounts of up to 625 times the normal clinical dosage of fresh ginger juice were safely injected intravenously into mice. The LD_{50} for intraperitoneal injection in male mice of three types of zingiberol is more than 100mg/kg.

Modern research

1. Decoctions of *Sheng Jiang* can promote the secretion of gastric juices.[42]
2. Has an anti-emetic function.[42]
3. Can stimulate the respiratory and cardiac systems.[43]
4. Inhibits and kills pathogenic bacteria including Vibrio cholerae and Trichomonas.[43]

Combinations and applications

Functions	Combinations	Applications
Inducing sweating and releasing the exterior	*Jing Jie* (Herba Schizonepetae Tenuifoliae) *Fang Feng* (Radix Ledebouriellae Divaricatae)	Common cold due to an invasion of wind-cold
	Hong Tang (brown sugar)	Mild wind-cold-type exterior patterns
Warming the Stomach and stopping vomiting	*Ban Xia* (Rhizoma Pinelliae Ternatae) *Wu Zhu Yu* (Fructus Evodiae Rutaecarpae)	Vomiting due to Stomach-cold

	Huang Lian (Rhizoma Coptidis) *Zhu Ru* (Caulis Bambusae in Taeniis)	Vomiting due to Stomach-heat
	Huang Lian (Rhizoma Coptidis) *Huang Qin* (Radix Scutellariae Baicalensis) *Dang Shen* (Radix Codonopsitis Pilosulae)	Water-fluids in the Stomach
	Shi Chang Pu (Rhizoma Acori Graminei) *Gao Liang Jiang* (Rhizoma Alpiniae Officinari)	Cold and pain in the stomach due to wind-cold directly attacking the interior
Warming the Lungs and stopping coughing	*Zi Su Ye* (Folium Perillae Frutescentis) *Qian Hu* (Radix Peucedani) *Xing Ren* (Semen Pruni Armeniacae)	Cough with copious sputum and oppression in the chest due to cold invading the Lungs
	Wu Wei Zi (Fructus Schisandrae) *Kuan Dong Hua* (Flos Tussilaginis Farfarae) *Ban Xia* (Rhizoma Pinelliae Ternatae)	Enduring cough
Relieving toxicity	*Huo Xiang* (Herba Agastaches seu Pogostemi) *Pei Lan* (Herba Eupatorii Fortunei) *Huang Lian* (Rhizoma Coptidis)	Diarrhoea and vomiting due to fish toxins

Note: The juice of *Sheng Jiang* can also reduce the toxicity of *Ban Xia* (Rhizoma Pinelliae Ternatae) and *Dan Nan Xing* (Pulvis Arisaematis cum Felle Bovis).

Xiang Ru 香薷 (Aromatic madder, Herba Elsholtziae seu Moslae)

Xiang Ru is the dried aerial parts of *Elsholtzia splendens* Nakai ex F. Maekawa or *Mosla chinensis* Maxim., family Labiatae.

Main ingredients *Xiang Ru* contains volatile oils (including elsholtziaketone and acetophenone) and sesquiterpenes.

Properties Taste: acrid; nature: slightly warm.

Channels entered Lung and Stomach.

Functions and indications Induces sweating and releases the exterior, clears summerheat and transforms dampness, promotes the movement of water and disperses swelling. It is indicated for the summerheat type of common cold, headache and fever, chills with an absence of sweating, oppression in the chest, pain in the abdomen, vomiting, diarrhoea, and oedema.

Common dosage 3-10g. Decoct for a short time (5-10 minutes) for transforming dampness and releasing the exterior, decoct for longer (30 minutes) for promoting the movement of water and dispersing swelling.

Precautions and contraindications

1. As *Xiang Ru* has a powerful action in inducing sweating, it is contraindicated for exterior deficiency patterns with sweating.
2. Taking a decoction of *Xiang Ru* hot may induce vomiting because of its particular fragrance; it should therefore be cooled or mixed with *Huang Lian* (Rhizoma Coptidis) or *Huang Bai* (Cortex Phellodendri).

Comparison of functions Both *Xiang Ru* (Herba Elsholtziae seu Moslae) and *Ma Huang*

(Herba Ephedrae) can induce sweating and release the exterior, and promote urination and disperse swelling. They are often used in treating exterior wind-cold patterns.

Xiang Ru has a weaker effect in inducing sweating and is frequently selected in the summer to transform dampness and harmonize the Middle Jiao for the treatment of wind-cold-type common colds. It is said that using *Xiang Ru* to release the exterior in the summer is like using *Ma Huang* in the winter. *Ma Huang* has a strong function in inducing sweating and also diffuses Lung Qi; it is commonly used for wind-cold-type common colds in winter.

Xiang Ru is good at eliminating dampness in the Spleen to promote the movement of water and disperse swelling, whereas *Ma Huang* promotes urination and disperses swelling by diffusing Lung Qi. As a result, *Xiang Ru* is used for oedema due to dampness which causes the Spleen to fail in its transportation function, whereas *Ma Huang* is used for oedema due to inhibition of Lung Qi.

For an additional comparison, see *Pei Lan* (Herba Eupatorii Fortunei).

Modern research

1. The volatile oils contained in *Xiang Ru* can promote urination.[44]
2. Stops coughing.[44]
3. Inhibits inflammation.[45]
4. Decoctions of *Xiang Ru* had an inhibitory effect *in vitro* on Bacterium coli and Staphylococcus aureus, as did the volatile oils contained in the herb.[46]

Combinations and applications

Functions	Combinations	Applications
Inducing sweating and releasing the exterior	*Huo Xiang* (Herba Agastaches seu Pogostemi) *Pei Lan* (Herba Eupatorii Fortunei)	Summer cold manifesting as fever and chills, vomiting and oppression in the chest
	Jing Jie (Herba Schizonepetae Tenuifoliae) *Fang Feng* (Radix Ledebouriellae Divaricatae)	Wind-cold type of common cold
Clearing summerheat and transforming dampness	*Bai Bian Dou* (Semen Dolichoris Lablab) *Hou Po* (Cortex Magnoliae Officinalis)	Aversion to cold, nausea, headache with an absence of sweating, oppression in the chest, fatigued limbs, pain in the abdomen and vomiting and diarrhoea caused by excessive consumption of raw and cold food in summer accompanied by exterior cold and interior dampness
Promoting the movement of water and dispersing swelling	*Bai Mao Gen* (Rhizoma Imperatae Cylindricae) *Yi Mu Cao* (Herba Leonuri Heterophylli)	Oedema and painful urination due to obstruction of Yang Qi
	Bai Zhu (Rhizoma Atractylodis Macrocephalae)	Oedema, fatigue and lack of strength due to Spleen deficiency

Cong Bai 葱白 (Chinese green onion, Bulbus Allii Fistulosi)

Cong Bai is the white stalk of *Allium fistulosum* L., family Liliaceae.

Main ingredients *Cong Bai* contains allicin, vitamins A, B_1, B_2 and C, and palmitic, stearic, arachidic, oleic and linoleic acids.

Properties Taste: acrid; nature: warm.

Channels entered Lung and Stomach.

Functions and indications Induces sweating and releases the exterior, dissipates cold and frees Yang, relieves toxicity and dissipates lumps. It is indicated for the wind-cold type of common cold, pain in the abdomen, diarrhoea, and cold limbs due to Yin cold.

Common dosage 3-10g, or appropriate dosage for external application.

Precautions and contraindications *Cong Bai* cannot be used internally with *Feng Mi* (Mel) and is contraindicated in cases of spontaneous sweating due to exterior deficiency.

Modern research

1. The volatile ingredients of *Cong Bai* can inhibit such bacteria as Shigella shigae and Corynebacterium diphtheriae, and dermatophytes.[47]
2. Induces sweating, expels sputum and promotes urination.[48]
3. The mucus of *Cong Bai* can protect the mucous membrane and skin.[48]

Combinations and applications

Functions	Combinations	Applications
Inducing sweating and releasing the exterior	*Sheng Jiang* (Rhizoma Zingiberis Officinalis Recens) *Dan Dou Chi* (Semen Sojae Praeparatum)	Mild wind-cold exterior patterns
Dissipating cold and freeing Yang	*Fu Zi* (Radix Lateralis Aconiti Carmichaeli Praeparata) (see notes on legal status) *Gan Jiang* (Rhizoma Zingiberis Officinalis)	Pain in the abdomen and cold limbs due to Yin cold
	Zhi Zi (Fructus Gardeniae Jasminoidis) *Lian Qiao* (Fructus Forsythiae Suspensae) *Bo He* (Herba Menthae Haplocalycis)	Exterior cold patterns with interior heat in febrile diseases caused by cold or in the initial stage of warm-febrile diseases

Note: For external use, *Cong Bai* can relieve toxicity and dissipate the accumulation of pathogenic factors or lumps. For example, after pounding the herb into a paste and mixing it with *Feng Mi* (Mel), it can relieve the pain caused by abscesses and sores arising from the accumulation of toxins; in addition, a paste of *Cong Bai* and *Ru Xiang* (Gummi Olibanum) can be used to treat a swollen and painful scrotum.

ACRID, COOL HERBS FOR RELEASING THE EXTERIOR

Acrid, cool herbs for releasing the exterior have a mild diaphoretic effect. They can dissipate wind-heat pathogenic factors and release exterior heat patterns. These herbs can be used for high fever, mild chills, thirst, sweating or absence of sweating, sore throat, runny nose with concentrated discharge, a rapid and floating pulse, and a thin tongue with white or yellow fur, where these symptoms are caused by wind-heat or warm and dry pathogenic factors invading the Lungs.

In addition, some of these herbs can clear heat in the Liver to brighten the eyes, clear heat from the Lungs to stop coughing, benefit the throat, and vent papules. They are indicated for red, sore and swollen eyes, indistinct rashes, cough and sore throat. In cases of full-heat, they should be used together with herbs for clearing heat.

Tab. 1.2 Acrid, cool herbs for releasing the exterior

Herb	Functions	Indications
Bo He (Herba Menthae Haplocalycis)	Dissipating wind-heat, clearing the Liver and brightening the eyes, benefiting the throat and venting papules, allowing constrained Liver Qi to flow freely and relieving depression	Wind-heat type of common cold, headache, red eyes, sore throat, mouth and tongue sores, itchy skin, and distension and oppression in the chest and hypochondrium due to Liver depression and Qi stagnation
Niu Bang Zi (Fructus Arctii Lappae)	Dissipating wind-heat, diffusing Lung Qi and venting papules, clearing heat and benefiting the throat, transforming Phlegm and stopping coughing, relieving toxicity and dispersing swelling, moistening the Intestines and freeing the bowels	Wind-heat type of common cold, cough, sore and swollen throat, indistinct rashes, sores
Sang Ye (Folium Mori Albae)	Dissipating wind-heat, clearing the Lungs and moistening dryness, clearing the Liver and brightening the eyes	Wind-heat type of common cold, cough, dryness of the throat due to damage to the Lungs by dry-heat, and red, sore and swollen eyes due to Liver-fire flaming upwards
Ju Hua (Flos Chrysanthemi Morifolii)	Dissipating wind-heat, calming the Liver and brightening the eyes, clearing heat and relieving toxicity	Wind-heat type of common cold, red, sore and swollen eyes due to wind-heat, headache and dizziness due to ascendant hyperactivity of Liver Yang, clove sores
Chai Hu (Radix Bupleuri)	Harmonizing Shaoyang and abating fever, allowing constrained Liver Qi to flow freely and relieving depression, uplifting Yang Qi to restore prolapsed organs	Alternating chills and fever, bitter fullness in the chest and hypochondrium due to cold pathogenic factors in the Shaoyang channel, externally-contracted fever, malaria, menstrual irregularities and other gynaecological diseases due to heat entering the Blood chamber or Liver depression and Qi stagnation, prolapse of the rectum or other organs due to Qi deficiency fall

Ge Gen (Radix Puerariae)	Releasing flesh and abating fever, venting macules and papules, generating body fluids and allaying thirst, bearing Yang upwards and stopping diarrhoea	Externally-contracted wind-cold or wind-heat patterns, the initial stage of measles, damage to body fluids in febrile diseases, wasting and thirsting, diarrhoea due to Spleen deficiency
Dan Dou Chi (Semen Sojae Praeparatum)	Releasing the exterior, eliminating vexation, relieving toxicity	Febrile diseases caused by cold damage, headache, vexation and agitation, oppression in the chest
Chan Tui (Periostracum Cicadae)	Dissipating wind-heat, venting papules and alleviating itching, removing eye screen and brightening the eyes, extinguishing wind and relieving tetany	Exterior patterns due to wind-heat or seasonal febrile diseases, fever, headache, sore throat and hoarse voice, the initial stage of measles and non-eruption of measles, itching due to wind papules, red eyes and eye screen, child fright epilepsy, tetanus
Man Jing Zi (Fructus Viticis)	Dissipating wind-heat, clearing and benefiting the head and eyes, dispelling wind and overcoming dampness	Wind-heat type of common cold, headache and dizziness, red, sore and swollen eyes, pain and swelling of the gums, Bi syndrome due to pathogenic wind-damp
Sheng Ma (Rhizoma Cimicifugae)	Releasing the exterior and venting papules, clearing heat and relieving toxicity, uplifting Yang Qi	Headache due to wind-heat, non-eruption of measles, mouth sores and toothache, sore throat, prolapse of the organs (especially the rectum and uterus) due to Qi deficiency, enduring diarrhoea
Fu Ping (Herba Spirodelae Polyrrhizae)	Dispelling wind and releasing the exterior, venting papules and alleviating itching, promoting the movement of water and dispersing swelling	Externally-contracted pathogenic wind-heat, fever without sweating, non-eruption of measles, wind-heat-type urticaria (dormant papules), itchy skin, oedema, difficult urination
Mu Zei (Herba Equiseti Hiemalis)	Dissipating wind-heat and removing eye screen	Blurred vision and red eyes, profuse lacrimation induced by wind-heat, blood in the stool, haemorrhoids, pain in the hypochondrium

Bo He 薄荷 (Peppermint, Herba Menthae Haplocalycis)

Bo He is the branch and leaf of *Mentha haplocalyx* Briq., family Labiatae.

Main ingredients *Bo He* contains 0.8-1.0% of volatile oils (principally menthol, with smaller quantities of menthone, menthyl acetate, camphene, limonene, isomenthone, pinene and menthenone), isoraifolin, menthoside and rosmarinic acid.

Properties Taste: acrid; nature: cool.

Channels entered Liver and Lung.

Functions and indications Dissipates wind-heat, clears the Liver and brightens the eyes, benefits the throat and vents papules, allows constrained Liver Qi to flow freely and relieves depression. It is indicated for the wind-heat type of common cold, headache, red eyes, sore throat, mouth and tongue sores, itchy skin, and distension in the chest and hypochondrium due to Liver depression and Qi stagnation.

Common dosage 3-10g; *Bo He* should not be overcooked, and therefore should be added at the end of the decoction process.

Precautions and contraindications As *Bo He* is an acrid and dissipating aromatic herb that induces sweating and consumes Qi, it is contraindicated in cases of profuse sweating due to general deficiency, dryness of the Blood due to Yin deficiency, and hyperactivity of Liver Yang.

Remarks The leaves of *Bo He* should be selected for dissipating wind-heat, while the stem should be used for allowing constrained Liver Qi to flow freely.

Comparison of functions Both *Bo He* (Herba Menthae Haplocalycis) and *Jing Jie* (Herba Schizonepetae Tenuifoliae) enter the Lung and Liver channels and have the functions of dissipating or dispelling wind and releasing the exterior, venting papules and alleviating itching. They can be used for exterior patterns due to wind-heat, for fever and headache, and for swollen and painful throat. They are also often combined to treat the initial stage of measles before development of a rash and to alleviate itching due to wind papules.

Bo He is acrid and cool and is mainly used for exterior patterns due to wind-heat as well as for headache and red eyes due to wind-heat attacking upwards. In addition, it has the functions of dissipating constrained Liver Qi due to Liver depression and Qi stagnation, and stopping diarrhoea due to summerheat-damp. *Jing Jie* is acrid and slightly warm and can be used for exterior patterns due both to wind-heat and wind-cold. It also has the functions of dispelling wind and stopping bleeding.

For additional comparisons, see *Niu Bang Zi* (Fructus Arctii Lappae) and *Chan Tui* (Periostracum Cicadae).

Toxicity The LD_{50} for subcutaneous injection in mice and rats of natural menthol is 5000-6000mg/kg and 1000mg/kg respectively. Reports of toxic side-effects caused by *Bo He* are very rare. There was one report that erroneous administration of 20ml of *Bo He* oil to treat distension in the abdomen led to dizziness, nausea, vomiting, numbness of the hands and feet, fainting and a reduction in blood pressure. The patient recovered the following day after treatment by intravenous infusion.

Modern research

1. Menthol can stimulate the skin to regulate its vascular function.[49]
2. Can be used locally to inhibit inflammation and alleviate pain.[50]
3. A small intake can excite the central nervous system and dilate the blood vessels in the skin to induce sweating and abate fever.[51]
4. Decoctions of *Bo He* can inhibit such bacteria as Staphylococcus aureus, Bacterium coli, Pseudomonas aeruginosa and Corynebacterium diphtheriae.[52]

Combinations and applications

Functions	Combinations	Applications
Dissipating wind-heat	*Jin Yin Hua* (Flos Lonicerae) *Lian Qiao* (Fructus Forsythiae Suspensae) *Jing Jie* (Herba Schizonepetae Tenuifoliae)	Wind-heat type of common cold and the initial stage of seasonal febrile diseases, manifesting as headache, fever and mild chill
	Niu Bang Zi (Fructus Arctii Lappae) *Huang Qin* (Radix Scutellariae Baicalensis) *Ju Hua* (Flos Chrysanthemi Morifolii)	Headache and red eyes due to wind-heat invading the Upper Jiao
Clearing the Liver and brightening the eyes	*Chai Hu* (Radix Bupleuri) *Long Dan Cao* (Radix Gentianae Scabrae) *Jue Ming Zi* (Semen Cassiae)	Red, sore and swollen eyes, dizziness and blurred vision due to Liver depression transforming into fire
Benefiting the throat and venting papules	*Jie Geng* (Radix Platycodi Grandiflori) *Ban Lan Gen* (Radix Isatidis seu Baphicacanthi)	Sore throat due to wind-heat
	Niu Bang Zi (Fructus Arctii Lappae) *Ge Gen* (Radix Puerariae) *Jing Jie* (Herba Schizonepetae Tenuifoliae)	Initial stage of measles combined with the wind-heat type of exterior pattern
	Ku Shen (Radix Sophorae Flavescentis) *Chan Tui* (Periostracum Cicadae) *Bai Xian Pi* (Cortex Dictamni Dasycarpi Radicis)	Itching and a feeling of heat on the skin due to wind papules
Allowing constrained Liver Qi to flow freely and relieving depression	*Yu Jin* (Radix Curcumae) *Mei Gui Hua* (Flos Rosae Rugosae) *Chai Hu* (Radix Bupleuri)	Distension and fullness in the chest and hypochondrium due to constrained Liver Qi
	Chai Hu (Radix Bupleuri) *Bai Shao* (Radix Paeoniae Lactiflorae) *Dang Gui* (Radix Angelicae Sinensis) *Fu Ling* (Sclerotium Poriae Cocos)	Fullness and pain in the hypochondrium, fatigue, poor appetite or menstrual irregularities due to constrained Liver Qi and Blood deficiency, and Spleen-Stomach disharmony

Note: *Bo He* can also disperse food accumulation, bear counterflow Qi downwards and disperse distension. It can be used together with *Mu Xiang* (Radix Aucklandiae Lappae), *Jiao San Xian* (scorch-fried Fructus Crataegi, Massa Fermentata and Fructus Hordei Vulgaris Germinatus) and *Zhi Ke* (Fructus Citri Aurantii) to treat indigestion, cholera, diarrhoea and vomiting (for *Mu Xiang*, see notes on legal status).

Niu Bang Zi 牛蒡子 (Great burdock fruit, Fructus Arctii Lappae)

Niu Bang Zi is the fruit of *Arctium lappa* L., family Compositae.

Main ingredients *Niu Bang Zi* contains arctiin, arctigenin, isoarctigenin, arachidic acid, fatty oils, alkaloids, and vitamins A and B_1.

Properties Taste: acrid and bitter; nature: cold.
Channels entered Lung and Stomach.
Functions and indications Dissipates wind-heat, diffuses Lung Qi and vents papules, clears heat and benefits the throat, transforms Phlegm and stops coughing, relieves toxicity and disperses swelling, moistens the Intestines and frees the bowels. It is indicated for the wind-heat type of common cold, cough, sore and swollen throat, indistinct rashes, and sores.
Common dosage 3-10g; pound into pieces for decocting.
Precautions and contraindications The purgative function of *Niu Bang Zi* means that it should be used with caution in cases of loose stool due to Spleen and Stomach deficiency.
Comparison of functions Both *Niu Bang Zi* (Fructus Arctii Lappae) and *Bo He* (Herba Menthae Haplocalycis) can release the exterior. They have the functions of dissipating wind-heat, benefiting the throat and venting papules and are often used for exterior patterns due to externally-contracted wind-heat, non-eruption of measles, itching due to wind papules, and sore and swollen throat. The two herbs are often used together or in combination with *Chan Tui* (Periostracum Cicadae) to enhance their effect.

Niu Bang Zi has both upward-bearing and downward-bearing properties; it is bitter and cold and enters the Lung and Stomach channels. It is very effective in clearing heat and relieving toxicity and can be used for congestion of heat toxins in the head, face and neck. *Bo He* is acrid and cool and has upward-bearing, floating and dispersing functions. It enters the Lung and Liver channels and can dissipate wind-heat in both channels. It is used for headache and red eyes due to wind-heat in the Liver channel attacking upwards. It is also effective in allowing constrained Liver Qi to flow freely.

For an additional comparison, see *Sheng Ma* (Rhizoma Cimicifugae).

Toxicity There have been no clinical reports of overdose, but one case of allergic reaction has been reported involving oppression in the chest and rapid breathing 30 minutes after intake of the herb, followed by dizziness, vomiting, papular eruption, unbearable itching and a reduction in blood pressure.

Modern research

1. Inhibited pathogenic fungi *in vitro*.[53]
2. Preparations of *Niu Bang Zi* can lower the blood sugar level.[53]
3. Has a slight purgative and diuretic effect.[54]

Combinations and applications

Functions	Combinations	Applications
Dissipating wind-heat	*Bo He* (Herba Menthae Haplocalycis) *Jin Yin Hua* (Flos Lonicerae) *Lian Qiao* (Fructus Forsythiae Suspensae)	Wind-heat type of common cold combined with cough and an itchy throat
Diffusing Lung Qi and venting papules	*Bo He* (Herba Menthae Haplocalycis) *Chan Tui* (Periostracum Cicadae) *Lu Gen* (Rhizoma Phragmitis Communis)	Measles with non-eruption of rash accompanied by cough and a sore and swollen throat
Clearing heat and benefiting the throat	*Shan Dou Gen* (Radix Sophorae Tonkinensis) *Lian Qiao* (Fructus Forsythiae Suspensae) *Jie Geng* (Radix Platycodi Grandiflori)	Sore and swollen throat due to wind-heat or heat toxins

	Ban Lan Gen (Radix Isatidis seu Baphicacanthi) *Jie Geng* (Radix Platycodi Grandiflori) *Da Huang* (Radix et Rhizoma Rhei)	Tonsillitis
Transforming Phlegm and stopping coughing	*Jin Yin Hua* (Flos Lonicerae) *Bai Qian* (Radix et Rhizoma Cynanchi Stauntonii) *Bei Mu* (Bulbus Fritillariae)	Unproductive cough due to externally-contracted wind-heat
	Ma Huang (Herba Ephedrae) *Shi Gao* (Gypsum Fibrosum) *Xing Ren* (Semen Pruni Armeniacae) *Huang Qin* (Radix Scutellariae Baicalensis)	Coughing and wheezing due to Lung-heat
Relieving toxicity and dispersing swelling	*Jin Yin Hua* (Flos Lonicerae) *Lian Qiao* (Fructus Forsythiae Suspensae) *Mu Dan Pi* (Cortex Moutan Radicis) *Chi Shao* (Radix Paeoniae Rubra)	Swelling and toxins of sores, erysipelas with local redness, swelling, pain and heat, and Phlegm nodes
Moistening the Intestines and freeing the bowels	*Huo Ma Ren* (Semen Cannabis Sativae) *Xing Ren* (Semen Pruni Armeniacae)	Intestinal dryness with constipation

Sang Ye 桑叶 (White mulberry leaf, Folium Mori Albae)

Sang Ye is the leaf of *Morus alba* L., family Moraceae.
Main ingredients *Sang Ye* contains ecdysterone, rutin, quercetin, isoquercetin, moracetin, astragalin, sitosterols, campesterol, betulinic acid, vitamins B_1, B_2 and C, and small quantities of volatile oils, proteins, tannins, copper and zinc.
Properties Taste: bitter and sweet; nature: cold.
Channels entered Lung and Liver.
Functions and indications Dissipates wind-heat, clears the Lungs and moistens dryness, clears the Liver and brightens the eyes. It is indicated for the wind-heat type of common cold, cough, dryness of the throat due to damage to the Lungs by dry-heat, and red, sore and swollen eyes due to Liver-fire flaming upwards.
Common dosage 5-10g, or 30g for large dosages. A decoction of the herb can be used as an external wash for the eyes.
Remarks Processing *Sang Ye* with honey can strengthen the effect of moistening dryness and stopping coughing; in this form, it is therefore indicated for cough due to dryness in the Lungs.
Comparison of functions See *Ju Hua* (Flos Chrysanthemi Morifolii) and *Sang Bai Pi* (Cortex Mori Albae Radicis).
Toxicity Sub-acute toxicity tests indicated no injury to the internal organs of mice after intraperitoneal injection for 21 days of a 10% *Sang Ye* solution at 60 times the normal human dosage. When the amount was increased to more than 250 times the human dosage, there was damage to the lungs, liver and kidneys (including degeneration and haemorrhage). Intramuscular injection of *Sang Ye* has caused cold, fever or dizziness in some patients; others have suffered general malaise and pain in the lumbar region, back and lower limbs. Recovery normally takes place after lying down for one or two days.

Modern research

1. Decoctions of *Sang Ye* can inhibit such organisms as Staphylococcus aureus, β-haemolytic streptococci, Corynebacterium diphtheriae and Bacillus anthracis.[55]
2. Decoctions of *Sang Ye* can inhibit leptospirosis.[56]
3. Can lower the blood sugar level, thus benefiting insulin secretion.[57, 58]

Combinations and applications

Functions	Combinations	Applications
Dissipating wind-heat	*Jin Yin Hua* (Flos Lonicerae) *Gua Lou* (Fructus Trichosanthis) *Ju Hua* (Flos Chrysanthemi Morifolii)	Wind-heat type of common cold, cough with yellow sputum
Clearing the Lungs and moistening dryness	*Sha Shen* (Radix Glehniae seu Adenophorae) *Shi Gao* (Gypsum Fibrosum) *Bai Bu* (Radix Stemonae) *Ban Lan Gen* (Radix Isatidis seu Baphicacanthi) *Shan Dou Gen* (Radix Sophorae Tonkinensis)	Dry cough without sputum, dry mouth, and dry and sore throat due to dry-heat damaging the Lungs
	Sang Bai Pi (Cortex Mori Albae Radicis) *Mu Dan Pi* (Cortex Moutan Radicis) *Di Gu Pi* (Cortex Lycii Radicis) *Chuan Bei Mu* (Bulbus Fritillariae Cirrhosae)	Dry cough with scant sputum, cough-induced pain in the hypochondrium and coughing of blood or blood-streaked sputum due to Liver-fire scorching the Lungs
Clearing the Liver and brightening the eyes	*Jue Ming Zi* (Semen Cassiae) *Zhi Zi* (Fructus Gardeniae Jasminoidis) *Qing Xiang Zi* (Semen Celosiae Argenteae)	Red, sore and swollen eyes due to Liver-fire flaming upwards
	Hei Zhi Ma (Semen Sesami Indici) *Gou Qi Zi* (Fructus Lycii) *Nü Zhen Zi* (Fructus Ligustri Lucidi)	Blurred vision due to insufficiency of Liver Yin
	Ju Hua (Flos Chrysanthemi Morifolii) *Gou Teng* (Ramulus Uncariae cum Uncis) *Xia Ku Cao* (Spica Prunellae Vulgaris)	Headache, dizziness and blurred vision due to ascendant hyperactivity of Liver Yang

Ju Hua 菊花 (Chrysanthemum flower, Flos Chrysanthemi Morifolii)

Ju Hua is the flower of *Chrysanthemum morifolium* Ramat., family Compositae.

Main ingredients *Ju Hua* contains chrysanthemin, adenine, choline, stachydrine, acacetin, amino acids, flavones and a little vitamin B_1. The whole plant contains volatile oils.

Properties Taste: acrid, sweet and bitter; nature: slightly cold.

Channels entered Liver and Lung.

Functions and indications Dissipates wind-heat, calms the Liver and brightens the eyes, clears heat and relieves toxicity. It is indicated for the wind-heat type of common cold, red, sore and swollen eyes due to wind-heat, headache and dizziness due to ascendant hyperactivity of Liver Yang, and clove sores.

Common dosage 10-15g as a decoction or infusion; or appropriate dosage for external application.

Precautions and contraindications According to *Ben Cao Hui Yao* [Treasury of Words on the Materia Medica], *Ju Hua* should be used with caution in cases of Stomach-cold due to Qi deficiency or for patients with reduced appetite and diarrhoea.

Remarks Yellow chrysanthemum, or *Huang Ju Hua* (Flos Aureus Chrysanthemi Morifolii), is best for dissipating wind-heat, whereas white chrysanthemum, or *Bai Ju Hua* (Flos Albus Chrysanthemi Morifolii), is good for calming the Liver and brightening the eyes; *Ye Ju Hua* (Flos Chrysanthemi Indici) has the functions of clearing heat and relieving toxicity (see Chapter 2).

Comparison of functions Both *Ju Hua* (Flos Chrysanthemi Morifolii) and *Sang Ye* (Folium Mori Albae) can dissipate wind-heat and calm or clear the Liver to brighten the eyes. They are often used together to treat exterior patterns due to externally-contracted wind-heat, or in the initial stage of warm diseases, or for dizziness and red eyes due to ascendant hyperactivity of Liver Yang. The dissipating effect of *Sang Ye* is stronger than that of *Ju Hua*; as a result, it is extremely effective for exterior patterns due to wind-heat accompanied by cough and headache. *Ju Hua* has a stronger effect than *Sang Ye* in calming the Liver and brightening the eyes and can also relieve toxicity.

For additional comparisons, see *Qin Pi* (Cortex Fraxini), *Ye Ju Hua* (Flos Chrysanthemi Indici) and *Gou Teng* (Ramulus Uncariae cum Uncis).

Toxicity Although *Ju Hua* has a very low level of toxicity, its concentrated decoction or pills of its extract can cause pain in the upper abdomen and diarrhoea in some patients. Persistent use of large amounts of *Ju Hua* can affect gastrointestinal functions. Cases have been reported of *Hang Ju Hua* (the variety of *Ju Hua* grown in Hangzhou) causing contact dermatitis.

Modern research

1. Decoctions of *Ju Hua* can enlarge the coronary arteries and increase the volume of blood flow.[59]
2. Preparations of *Ju Hua* have a tranquillizing function and can improve the oxygen supply.[59, 60]
3. Decoctions of *Ju Hua* can inhibit such bacteria as Staphylococcus aureus, β-haemolytic streptococcus, Corynebacterium diphtheriae and Shigella shigae, as can its volatile oils.[61]

Combinations and applications

Functions	Combinations	Applications
Dissipating wind-heat	*Sang Ye* (Folium Mori Albae) *Chuan Xiong* (Rhizoma Ligustici Chuanxiong) *Shi Gao* (Gypsum Fibrosum)	Fever and headache in the initial stage of seasonal febrile diseases or due to externally-contracted wind-heat
Calming the Liver and brightening the eyes	*Sang Ye* (Folium Mori Albae) *Bai Ji Li* (Fructus Tribuli Terrestris) *Xia Ku Cao* (Spica Prunellae Vulgaris)	Red, sore and swollen eyes due to wind-heat in the Liver channel
	Shi Jue Ming (Concha Haliotidis) *Sheng Di Huang* (Radix Rehmanniae Glutinosae) *Bai Shao* (Radix Paeoniae Lactiflorae)	Headache and dizziness due to ascendant hyperactivity of Liver Yang

	Shu Di Huang (Radix Rehmanniae Glutinosae Conquita) *Gou Qi Zi* (Fructus Lycii)	Blurred vision due to Yin deficiency of the Liver and Kidneys
Clearing heat and relieving toxicity	*Pu Gong Ying* (Herba Taraxaci cum Radice) *Mu Dan Pi* (Cortex Moutan Radicis) *Zi Hua Di Ding* (Herba Violae Yedoensitis)	Swelling and toxins of clove sores

Chai Hu 柴胡 (Chinese thorowax root, Radix Bupleuri)

Chai Hu is the root of *Bupleurum chinense* D. C. or *B. scorzonerifolium* Willd., family Umbelliferae.

Main ingredients *Chai Hu* contains volatile oils (including bupleurumol, limonene and myrcene), oleic, linolenic, palmitic and stearic acids, plant sterols and saponins (including saikosaponins, saikogenin and longispinogenin). The stalk and leaves of the plant contain rutin.

Properties Taste: bitter and acrid; nature: slightly cold.

Channels entered Pericardium, Liver, San Jiao and Gallbladder.

Functions and indications Harmonizes Shaoyang and abates fever, allows constrained Liver Qi to flow freely and relieves depression, and uplifts Yang Qi to restore prolapsed organs. It is indicated for alternating chills and fever, bitter fullness in the chest and hypochondrium due to cold pathogenic factors in the Shaoyang channel, externally-contracted fever, malaria, menstrual irregularities and other gynaecological diseases due to heat entering the Blood chamber or Liver depression and Qi stagnation, and prolapse of the rectum or other organs due to Qi deficiency fall.

Common dosage 3-10g, or 30g for large dosages.

Precautions and contraindications The upward-bearing characteristic of *Chai Hu* means that this herb is contraindicated in cases of disorders due to effulgent Yin deficiency-fire or ascendant hyperactivity of Liver Yang.

Remarks *Bei Chai Hu* (*Bupleurum chinense*), or northern thorowax root, is mainly used for abating fever by harmonizing Shaoyang; *Nan Chai Hu* (*Bupleurum scorzonerifolium*), or southern thorowax root, is mild and is used mostly for allowing constrained Liver Qi to flow freely. Raw *Chai Hu* can abate fever, *Chai Hu* processed with vinegar can quicken the Blood to alleviate pain, and *Chai Hu* processed with alcohol can uplift vital Qi to stop diarrhoea. Smaller dosages should be employed for allowing constrained Liver Qi to flow freely and uplifting Yang Qi; a larger dosage is more suitable for abating fever.

Comparison of functions See *Ge Gen* (Radix Puerariae), *Qing Hao* (Herba Artemisiae Chinghao), *Yin Chai Hu* (Radix Stellariae Dichotomae) and *Qian Hu* (Radix Peucedani).

Toxicity Acute toxicity tests indicated that *Chai Hu* has a very low level of toxicity. The minimum lethal dosage for subcutaneous injection in moles of a 10% aqueous extract of *Chai Hu* is 100mg/kg. The LD_{50} for oral administration to mice of the saikosaponins contained in *Chai Hu* is 4.7g/kg. There has been a report of an injection of *Chai Hu* causing allergic shock in one case.

Modern research

1. In animal experiments, decoctions of *Chai Hu* and injections of the herb and the volatile oils it contains had an obvious effect in abating fever.[62, 63]
2. Has a tranquillizing function,[64] alleviates pain[65] and stops coughing.[66]
3. Inhibits streptococci, Mycobacterium tuberculosis and influenza viruses.[67, 68]
4. Inhibits inflammation.[69]
5. Strengthens the immune function.[70]

Combinations and applications

Functions	Combinations	Applications
Harmonizing Shaoyang and abating fever	*Jing Jie* (Herba Schizonepetae Tenuifoliae) *Fang Feng* (Radix Ledebouriellae Divaricatae) *Qiang Huo* (Rhizoma et Radix Notopterygii)	Severe chill and slight fever in the wind-cold type of common cold
	Lian Qiao (Fructus Forsythiae Suspensae) *Niu Bang Zi* (Fructus Arctii Lappae) *Jin Yin Hua* (Flos Lonicerae) *Ge Gen* (Radix Puerariae)	High fever, slight chill and sore throat in the wind-heat type of common cold
	Huang Qin (Radix Scutellariae Baicalensis) *Ban Xia* (Rhizoma Pinelliae Ternatae) *Gan Cao* (Radix Glycyrrhizae)	Alternating chills and fever, bitter fullness in the chest and hypochondrium, a bitter taste in the mouth, dry throat, agitation and nausea, and a tight pulse due to heat in Shaoyang diseases
	Chang Shan (Radix Dichroae Febrifugae) *Cao Guo* (Fructus Amomi Tsaoko)	Malaria
	Mu Dan Pi (Cortex Moutan Radicis) *Sheng Di Huang* (Radix Rehmanniae Glutinosae)	Alternating chills and fever due to external heat invading the Blood chamber during menstruation or postpartum
Allowing constrained Liver Qi to flow freely and relieving depression	*Dang Gui* (Radix Angelicae Sinensis) *Bai Shao* (Radix Paeoniae Lactiflorae) *Bai Zhu* (Rhizoma Atractylodis Macrocephalae)	Pain in the hypochondrium, menstrual irregularities and poor appetite due to Liver depression and Blood deficiency
	Chuan Lian Zi (Fructus Meliae Toosendan) *Xiang Fu* (Rhizoma Cyperi Rotundi) *Yu Jin* (Radix Curcumae)	Distension and pain in the abdomen, dizziness, distension and pain in the hypochondrium, painful menstruation, and distension of the breasts due to constrained Liver Qi
Uplifting Yang Qi to restore prolapsed organs	*Ren Shen* (Radix Ginseng) *Huang Qi* (Radix Astragali seu Hedysari) *Bai Zhu* (Rhizoma Atractylodis Macrocephalae) *Sheng Ma* (Rhizoma Cimicifugae)	Prolapse of the rectum and other organs due to Qi deficiency fall
	Huang Qi (Radix Astragali seu Hedysari) *Bai Zhu* (Rhizoma Atractylodis Macrocephalae) *Fu Ling* (Sclerotium Poriae Cocos) *Zhu Ling* (Sclerotium Polypori Umbellati)	Diarrhoea due to Spleen deficiency accompanied by generalized fever due to exterior patterns

Ge Gen 葛根 (Kudzu vine root, Radix Puerariae)

Ge Gen is the root of *Pueraria lobata* (Willd.) Ohwi. or *P. thomsonii* Benth., family Leguminosae.

Main ingredients *Ge Gen* contains up to 12% of flavones, including daidzin, daidzein, pueroside and puerarin, as well as arachidic acid, daucosterol and allantoin.

Properties Taste: acrid and sweet; nature: cool.

Channels entered Spleen and Stomach.

Functions and indications Releases flesh and abates fever, vents macules and papules, generates body fluids and allays thirst, bears Yang upwards and stops diarrhoea. It is indicated for externally-contracted wind-cold or wind-heat patterns, the initial stage of measles, damage to body fluids in febrile diseases, wasting and thirsting, and diarrhoea due to Spleen deficiency.

Common dosage 10-20g, or 30g for large dosages.

Precautions and contraindications *Ge Gen* is contraindicated in cases of profuse sweating due to exterior deficiency or in cases of vented maculopapular eruptions.

Remarks Raw *Ge Gen* should be used for clearing heat and generating body fluids, whereas roasted *Ge Gen* is suitable for stopping diarrhoea by bearing Yang upwards. The flower of the plant, *Ge Hua* (Flos Puerariae), is sweet and neutral, and thus relieves inebriation and fortifies the Spleen. It is mainly used for vomiting, vexation, and dizziness due to excessive drinking.

Comparison of functions *Ge Gen* (Radix Puerariae), *Chai Hu* (Radix Bupleuri) and *Sheng Ma* (Rhizoma Cimicifugae) are all acrid and cool and have the functions of releasing the exterior and bearing Yang upwards. They can be used for externally-contracted exterior patterns and for diarrhoea due to clear Yang in the Spleen and Stomach failing to bear upwards.

Chai Hu is effective in harmonizing Shaoyang and dispersing half-interior, half-exterior pathogenic factors from the Shaoyang channel. Since it also enters the Liver channel, it is very effective for allowing constrained Liver Qi to flow freely and for abating fever.

Ge Gen clears heat in the Yangming channel and is good at releasing flesh and abating fever, venting papules and generating body fluids. It is a key herb for treating fever caused by exterior patterns without sweating and accompanied by headache or stiffness and pain in the neck and back. Its function of uplifting Yang is reflected in the use of the roasted herb for bearing clear Yang upwards to stop diarrhoea. *Ge Gen* is only used rarely for prolapse of the rectum due to middle Qi fall.

Sheng Ma enters the Lung and Stomach channels and is good at venting papules, especially measles, and at bearing clear Yang upwards. Its upward-bearing effect is stronger than that of *Chai Hu*. It is not used frequently for exterior patterns due to wind-heat.

Toxicity *Ge Gen* generally has a very low level of toxicity, which varies depending on the plant involved. *Ge Gen* from Yunnan is more toxic than *Ge Gen* from E Mei (Sichuan) or wild *Ge Gen*; the powdered herb is the least toxic.

Modern research

1. Aqueous extracts of *Ge Gen* possess a strong fever-abating function.[71]
2. Decoctions of *Ge Gen* can lower blood pressure.[72]
3. Enlarges the coronary arteries and improves coronary circulation to relieve angina.[73]

Combinations and applications

Functions	Combinations	Applications
Releasing flesh and abating fever	*Ma Huang* (Herba Ephedrae) (see notes on legal status) *Gui Zhi* (Ramulus Cinnamomi Cassiae) *Bai Shao* (Radix Paeoniae Lactiflorae)	Exterior patterns due to wind-cold, chills without sweating, stiffness and pain in the back
	Shi Gao (Gypsum Fibrosum) *Chai Hu* (Radix Bupleuri) *Da Qing Ye* (Folium Isatidis seu Baphicacanthi)	High fever, slight chill, headache and dryness of the nose due to transformation of heat from the wind-cold type of common cold
	Cong Bai (Bulbus Allii Fistulosi) *Dan Dou Chi* (Semen Sojae Praeparatum) *Sheng Jiang* (Rhizoma Zingiberis Officinalis Recens)	Externally-contracted wind-heat or the initial stage of warm diseases, manifesting as vigorous generalized fever, headache, stiffness of the back and spine, slight cold of the mouth, nose, hands and feet, and reddish-yellow urine
Venting macules and papules	*Jie Geng* (Radix Platycodi Grandiflori) *Sheng Ma* (Rhizoma Cimicifugae) *Chan Tui* (Periostracum Cicadae)	Initial stage of measles, indistinct rashes with thirst or diarrhoea
Generating body fluids and allaying thirst	*Lu Gen* (Rhizoma Phragmitis Communis) *Tian Hua Fen* (Radix Trichosanthis)	Thirst during febrile diseases, wasting and thirsting due to damage to body fluids
Bearing Yang upwards and stopping diarrhoea	*Fu Ling* (Sclerotium Poriae Cocos) *Ren Shen* (Radix Ginseng)	Diarrhoea due to Spleen deficiency
	Huang Qin (Radix Scutellariae Baicalensis) *Huang Lian* (Rhizoma Coptidis) *Gan Cao* (Radix Glycyrrhizae)	Dysentery and diarrhoea due to damp-heat, combined with vexation and thirst

Dan Dou Chi 淡豆豉 (Prepared soybean, Semen Sojae Praeparatum)

Dan Dou Chi is the fermented seed of *Glycine max* (L.) Merr., family Leguminosae.

Main ingredients *Dan Dou Chi* contains large quantities of fats, proteins and enzymes, as well as chrysanthemin, daidzin, genistin, vitamins B_1 and B_2, and soyasaponins.

Properties Taste: acrid, sweet and slightly bitter; nature: cool, when fermented with *Qing Hao* (Herba Artemisiae Chinghao) and *Sang Ye* (Folium Mori Albae), or slightly warm, when fermented with *Ma Huang* (Herba Ephedrae) and *Zi Su Ye* (Folium Perillae Frutescentis).

Channels entered Lung and Stomach.

Functions and indications Releases the exterior, eliminates vexation, and relieves toxicity. It is indicated for febrile diseases caused by cold damage, headache, vexation and agitation, and oppression in the chest.

Common dosage 10-15g; or appropriate dosage for external application.

Precautions and contraindications Since *Dan Dou Chi* can restrict lactation, it is contraindicated for nursing mothers.

Remarks When fermented with *Qing Hao* (Herba Artemisiae Chinghao) and *Sang Ye* (Folium Mori Albae), *Dan Dou Chi* is mainly used for externally-contracted wind-heat, and for vexation and oppression in the chest in febrile diseases; when fermented with *Ma Huang* (Herba Ephedrae) and *Zi Su Ye* (Folium Perillae Frutescentis), *Dan Dou Chi* is mostly used for headache due to externally-contracted wind-cold.

Modern research

1. The soyasaponins contained in *Dan Dou Chi* can cause a significant reduction in the level of blood lipids.[74]
2. The soya flavones contained in *Dan Dou Chi* can relieve spasm of the intestinal muscle, abate fever, promote digestion and inhibit inflammation.[75]

Combinations and applications

Functions	Combinations	Applications
Releasing the exterior	*Cong Bai* (Bulbus Allii Fistulosi)	Common cold due to wind-cold
	Lian Qiao (Fructus Forsythiae Suspensae) *Jin Yin Hua* (Flos Lonicerae)	Common cold due to wind-heat, with headache and sore throat
Eliminating vexation	*Zhi Zi* (Fructus Gardeniae Jasminoidis)	Vexation and insomnia during febrile diseases
Relieving toxicity	Fried, made into powder and mixed with oil for use as a topical application	Infantile erysipelas with yellow discharge

Chan Tui 蝉蜕 (Cicada slough, Periostracum Cicadae)

Chan Tui is the slough shed by the nymph of the cicada *Cryptotympana pustulata* Fabr., family Cicadidae.

Main ingredients *Chan Tui* contains chitin, amino acids, proteins and trace elements.

Properties Taste: sweet; nature: cold.

Channels entered Lung and Liver.

Functions and indications Dissipates wind-heat, vents papules and alleviates itching, removes eye screen and brightens the eyes, extinguishes wind and relieves tetany. It is indicated for exterior patterns due to wind-heat or seasonal febrile diseases, fever, headache, sore throat and hoarse voice, the initial stage of measles and non-eruption of measles, itching due to wind papules, red eyes and eye screen, child fright epilepsy, and tetanus.

Common dosage 3-10g.

Precautions and contraindications

1. *Chan Tui* should be used with caution during pregnancy.
2. It is not advisable to take large dosages of *Chan Tui* in cases of Stomach Qi deficiency-cold, or in cases of reduced appetite and diarrhoea.

Comparison of functions Both *Chan Tui* (Periostracum Cicadae) and *Bo He* (Herba Menthae Haplocalycis) can dissipate wind-heat, clear heat to benefit the throat, and vent papules. They can treat exterior patterns due to wind-heat, non-eruption of measles, and itching due to wind papules. However, *Bo He* has the stronger effect in releasing the exterior and is better at dissipating wind-heat from the head and eyes as well as functioning effectively in allowing constrained Liver Qi to flow freely. *Chan Tui* is also good for brightening the eyes and removing eye screen, extinguishing wind and relieving tetany. It is thus used to treat all types of eye disorders, tetanus and child fright epilepsy.

Toxicity The LD_{50} for intraperitoneal injection in mice of the alcoholic extract of *Chan Tui* is 8000mg/kg. No deaths occurred after intravenous injection in the tail of the aqueous extract of *Chan Tui*. There are reports of abdominal pain when using *Chan Tui* to treat externally-contracted wind-heat. Symptoms included persistent pain in the upper abdomen accompanied by abdominal distension and rumbling intestines. These symptoms disappeared when intake of the medicinal was halted. There was also a report of an allergic reaction after drinking powdered *Chan Tui* mixed with yellow wine. The symptoms, which included generalized sweating, facial flushes and skin rash, disappeared once intake ceased.

Modern research

1. Has a tranquillizing function and inhibits convulsions.[76]
2. Decoctions of *Chan Tui* can abate fever and inhibit skin allergies.[77]

Combinations and applications

Functions	Combinations	Applications
Dissipating wind-heat	*Bo He* (Herba Menthae Haplocalycis) *Lian Qiao* (Fructus Forsythiae Suspensae)	Common cold due to wind-heat with fever and headache
	Niu Bang Zi (Fructus Arctii Lappae) *Jie Geng* (Radix Platycodi Grandiflori)	Sore throat and hoarse voice
Venting papules and alleviating itching	*Bo He* (Herba Menthae Haplocalycis) *Ge Gen* (Radix Puerariae)	Inhibited eruptions in the initial stage of measles and itchy skin due to wind-heat
	Jing Jie (Herba Schizonepetae Tenuifoliae) *Bai Ji Li* (Fructus Tribuli Terrestris)	Itching due to wind papules
Removing eye screen and brightening the eyes	*Ju Hua* (Flos Chrysanthemi Morifolii) *Mu Zei* (Herba Equiseti Hiemalis)	Red, sore and swollen eyes and eye screen due to wind-heat in the Liver channel or Liver-fire flaming upwards
Extinguishing wind and relieving tetany	*Gou Teng* (Ramulus Uncariae cum Uncis) *Jiang Can* (Bombyx Batryticatus)	Child fright epilepsy
	Dan Nan Xing (Pulvis Arisaematis cum Felle Bovis) *Quan Xie* (Buthus Martensi) *Fang Feng* (Radix Ledebouriellae Divaricatae)	Infantile tetanus
	Gou Teng (Ramulus Uncariae cum Uncis) *Dan Zhu Ye* (Herba Lophatheri Gracilis)	Night crying in infants due to wind-heat in the Liver channel

Man Jing Zi 蔓荆子
(Chaste-tree fruit, Fructus Viticis)

Man Jing Zi is the dried fruit of *Vitex trifolia* L. var. *simplicifolia* Cham., *V. trifolia* L. or *V. rotundifolia* L., family Verbenaceae.

Main ingredients *Man Jing Zi* contains camphene, vitricine, vitexicarpin, casticin, α- and β-pinene and α-phellandrene.

Properties Taste: acrid and bitter; nature: slightly cold.
Channels entered Bladder, Liver and Stomach.
Functions and indications Dissipates wind-heat, clears and benefits the head and eyes, dispels wind and overcomes dampness. It is indicated for the wind-heat type of common cold, headache and dizziness, red, sore and swollen eyes, pain and swelling of the gums, and Bi syndrome due to pathogenic wind-damp.
Common dosage 6-12g.
Precautions and contraindications *Man Jing Zi* should be used with caution in cases of Spleen and Stomach deficiency or headache and dizzy vision due to Blood deficiency.
Comparison of functions Both *Man Jing Zi* (Fructus Viticis) and *Gao Ben* (Rhizoma et Radix Ligustici) can dispel wind and dampness and alleviate Bi syndrome pain. They are both effective in treating headache and Bi syndrome pain due to wind-damp. *Man Jing Zi* is a key herb for treating headache and red eyes due to externally-contracted wind-heat. *Gao Ben* is better at reaching the vertex and is good at dissipating pathogenic wind-cold to treat headache in the vertex due to wind-cold in the Taiyang channel.
Toxicity *Man Jing Zi* has a very low level of toxicity. The herb has been used safely in the laboratory in amounts up to 300 times the oral dosage normally prescribed in the clinic.
Modern research

1. Decoctions of *Man Jing Zi* have a tranquillizing function and alleviate pain.[78]
2. Abates fever.[79]

Combinations and applications

Functions	Combinations	Applications
Dissipating wind-heat	*Ju Hua* (Flos Chrysanthemi Morifolii) *Bo He* (Herba Menthae Haplocalycis)	Common cold and headache due to wind-heat
Clearing and benefiting the head and eyes	*Tian Ma* (Rhizoma Gastrodiae Elatae) (see notes on legal status) *Jing Jie* (Herba Schizonepetae Tenuifoliae)	Migraine
	Chan Tui (Periostracum Cicadae) *Ju Hua* (Flos Chrysanthemi Morifolii) *Jue Ming Zi* (Semen Cassiae)	Red, sore and swollen eyes with tears
	Shi Gao (Gypsum Fibrosum) *Sheng Di Huang* (Radix Rehmanniae Glutinosae)	Pain and swelling of the gums
Dispelling wind and overcoming dampness	*Mu Gua* (Fructus Chaenomelis) *Du Huo* (Radix Angelicae Pubescentis) *Qin Jiao* (Radix Gentianae Macrophyllae)	Bi syndrome pain due to wind-damp

Sheng Ma 升麻 (Bugbane rhizome, Rhizoma Cimicifugae)

Sheng Ma is the dried rhizome of *Cimicifuga heracleifolia* Kom., *C. dahurica* (Turcz.) Maxim. or *C. foetida* L., family Ranunculaceae.
Main ingredients *Sheng Ma* contains cimicifugenol, cimigenoside, cimicifugoside, caffeic acid, ferulic acid, isoferulic acid, salicylic acid, cimicifugine, cimigenol and tannin.
Properties Taste: acrid and sweet; nature: cool.
Channels entered Lung, Spleen, Stomach and Large Intestine.

Functions and indications Releases the exterior and vents papules, clears heat and relieves toxicity, and uplifts Yang Qi. It is indicated for headache due to wind-heat, non-eruption of measles, mouth sores and toothache, sore throat, prolapse of the organs (especially the rectum and uterus) due to Qi deficiency, and enduring diarrhoea.

Common dosage 3-10g.

Precautions and contraindications As a result of its strong upward-bearing and dissipating action, *Sheng Ma* is contraindicated in cases of the wind-heat type of common cold, measles with rashes that have already erupted, effulgent Yin deficiency-fire, and ascendant hyperactivity of Liver Yang.

Remarks The raw herb is generally used for relieving toxicity and venting papules, whereas a preparation of *Sheng Ma* mix-fried with liquids is used to bear Yang Qi upwards.

Comparison of functions *Sheng Ma* (Rhizoma Cimicifugae) and *Niu Bang Zi* (Fructus Arctii Lappae) both have the function of releasing the exterior and venting papules, and clearing heat and relieving toxicity. They are also both used for non-eruption of measles.

Sheng Ma releases the exterior by bearing upwards and dissipating; however, it is not used very frequently for exterior patterns due to wind-heat. It is very effective in dispersing toxins from rashes, particularly measles, as well as in clearing heat toxins in Yangming patterns. It is also good for uplifting clear Yang Qi and can treat Qi deficiency fall, enduring dysentery and diarrhoea, and prolapse of the rectum and uterus.

Niu Bang Zi is often used for exterior patterns due to externally-contracted wind-heat and for cough due to Lung-heat with sputum that is difficult to expectorate. It also functions well in clearing heat, relieving toxicity and benefiting the throat. It is extremely effective for heat-toxin patterns accompanied by inhibited urination and defecation.

For an additional comparison, see *Ge Gen* (Radix Puerariae).

Toxicity Large dosages of *Sheng Ma* can cause headache, tetanic contraction of the limbs and tremors.

Modern research

1. Abates fever, lowers body temperature, inhibits inflammation and alleviates pain.[80]
2. Inhibited Mycobacterium tuberculosis and various dermatophytes *in vitro*.[81]

Combinations and applications

Functions	Combinations	Applications
Releasing the exterior and venting papules	*Ge Gen* (Radix Puerariae) *Niu Bang Zi* (Fructus Arctii Lappae)	Inhibited eruptions in the initial stage of measles
Clearing heat and relieving toxicity	*Shi Gao* (Gypsum Fibrosum) *Huang Lian* (Rhizoma Coptidis)	Toothache and mouth sores due to Stomach-fire
	Shi Gao (Gypsum Fibrosum) *Huang Lian* (Rhizoma Coptidis) *Bai Zhi* (Radix Angelicae Dahuricae)	Yangming headache due to wind-heat attacking upwards
	Niu Bang Zi (Fructus Arctii Lappae) *Jie Geng* (Radix Platycodi Grandiflori)	Sore throat due to wind-heat
	Da Qing Ye (Folium Isatidis seu Baphicacanthi)	Febrile diseases with papular eruptions
	Jin Yin Hua (Flos Lonicerae) *Lian Qiao* (Fructus Forsythiae Suspensae)	Swelling and toxins of abscesses and sores

Uplifting Yang Qi	*Dang Shen* (Radix Codonopsitis Pilosulae) *Huang Qi* (Radix Astragali seu Hedysari)	Shortness of breath, fatigue and prolapse of internal organs due to middle Qi fall
	Chai Hu (Radix Bupleuri)	Enduring dysentery and prolapse of the rectum due to Qi deficiency

Fu Ping 浮萍 (Common ducksmeat herb, Herba Spirodelae Polyrrhizae)

Fu Ping is the dried whole plant of *Spirodela polyrrhiza* Schleid., family Lemnaceae.

Main ingredients *Fu Ping* contains orientin, isoorientin, vitexin, isovitexin, rutin, luteolin, potassium acetate and potassium chloride.

Properties Taste: acrid; nature: cold.

Channels entered Lung and Bladder.

Functions and indications Dispels wind and releases the exterior, vents papules and alleviates itching, promotes the movement of water and disperses swelling. It is indicated for externally-contracted pathogenic wind-heat, fever without sweating, non-eruption of measles, wind-heat-type urticaria (dormant papules), itchy skin, oedema, and difficult urination.

Common dosage 10-15g, or 1-2g in pills; appropriate dosage for external application as a wash.

Precautions and contraindications *Fu Ping* is contraindicated in cases of spontaneous sweating due to exterior deficiency.

Comparison of functions Both *Fu Ping* (Herba Spirodelae Polyrrhizae) and *Ma Huang* (Herba Ephedrae) can induce sweating and release the exterior, as well as being able to promote urination and disperse swelling. *Ma Huang* is more suited to exterior full patterns due to externally-contracted wind-cold without sweating, and also has the function of stopping coughing and calming wheezing. *Fu Ping* is more effective for fever without sweating due to externally contracted wind-heat and at the initial stage of warm diseases, or for patients with externally-contracted wind-heat accompanied by oedema and inhibited urination. It also has the functions of dispelling wind, venting papules and alleviating itching and can be used for non-eruption of measles and itching due to wind-damp.

Modern research

1. Abates fever.[82]
2. Preparations of *Fu Ping* can strengthen the heart, contract the blood vessels and raise blood pressure.[83]

Combinations and applications

Functions	Combinations	Applications
Dispelling wind and releasing the exterior	*Jing Jie* (Herba Schizonepetae Tenuifoliae) *Fang Feng* (Radix Ledebouriellae Divaricatae) *Lian Qiao* (Fructus Forsythiae Suspensae)	Fever without sweating due to externally-contracted wind-heat
Venting papules and alleviating itching	*Bo He* (Herba Menthae Haplocalycis) *Chan Tui* (Periostracum Cicadae)	Non-eruption of measles

Promoting the movement of water and dispersing swelling	*Dong Gua Pi* (Epicarpium Benincasae Hispidae) *Chi Xiao Dou* (Semen Phaseoli Calcarati) *Che Qian Zi* (Semen Plantaginis)	Oedema accompanied by an exterior pattern
	Gua Lou Gen (Radix Trichosanthis)	Wasting and thirsting

Mu Zei 木贼 (Scouring rush herb, Herba Equiseti Hiemalis)

Mu Zei is the dried aerial parts of *Equisetum hiemale* L., family Equisetaceae.

Main ingredients *Mu Zei* contains succinic, fumaric, ferulic and caffeic acids, kaempferol, quercetin, vanillin and thymine.

Properties Taste: sweet and bitter; nature: neutral.

Channels entered Lung and Liver.

Functions and indications Dissipates wind-heat and removes eye screen. It is indicated for blurred vision and red eyes, profuse lacrimation induced by wind-heat, blood in the stool, haemorrhoids, and pain in the hypochondrium.

Common dosage 3-10g.

Precautions and contraindications *Mu Zei* should be used with caution in cases of eye diseases due to Qi or Blood deficiency.

Toxicity The LD_{50} for intragastric administration and intraperitoneal injection in mice of alcoholic extracts of *Mu Zei* is 249.6g/kg and 47.56g/kg respectively. The LD_{50} for intravenous injection of *Mu Zei* is 33.49g/kg.

Modern research The silicate contained in *Mu Zei* can dilate external blood vessels, lower blood pressure, inhibit inflammation, stop bleeding and have a tranquillizing function.[84]

Combinations and applications

Functions	Combinations	Applications
Dissipating wind-heat and removing eye screen	*Chan Tui* (Periostracum Cicadae) *Gu Jing Cao* (Scapus et Flos Eriocaulonis Buergeriani) *Huang Qin* (Radix Scutellariae Baicalensis)	Red eyes and profuse lacrimation due to wind-heat
	Cang Zhu (Rhizoma Atractylodis)	Blurred vision and profuse lacrimation
	Ju Hua (Flos Chrysanthemi Morifolii) *Dai Zhe Shi* (Haematitum)	Eye screen due to accumulation of wind-heat
	Huai Hua Mi (Flos Sophorae Japonicae Immaturus) *Fang Feng* (Radix Ledebouriellae Divaricatae) *Zhi Ke* (Fructus Citri Aurantii)	Intestinal haemorrhage and haemorrhoids

Modern research references

1. Fu Hangyu et al., *Zhong Yao Yao Li Yu Lin Chuang* [Pharmacology and Clinical Application of Chinese Materia Medica] 8, 1 (5) (1992): 1.
2. L.S. Goodman et al., *The Pharmacological Basis of Therapeutics*, 6th ed. (London: Macmillan, 1980), 163.
3. C. Pak et al., *Chinese J Physiol* 3, 3 (1929): 287.
4. Ding Guoming et al., *Shan Dong Zhong Yi Xue Yuan Xue Bao* [Journal of Shandong College of Traditional Chinese Medicine] 16, 1 (1992): 56.
5. Yuan Wenxue, *Yao Xue Tong Bao* [Pharmacology Bulletin] 21, 4 (1986): 235.
6. Liu Guosheng et al., *Wei Sheng Wu Xue Bao* [Microorganism Journal] 8, 2 (1960): 164.
7. Shen Yingjun, *Cheng Du Zhong Yi Xue Yuan Xue Bao* [Journal of Chengdu College of TCM] 1 (1986): 31.
8. J.C. Maruzzella, *J Pharm Pharmacol* 11 (1969): 188.
9. Yuan Axing, *Zhong Yao Tong Bao* [Bulletin of Chinese Materia Medica] 9, 3 (1984): 31.
10. Qu Shuyan et al., *Zhong Yi Za Zhi* [Journal of Traditional Chinese Medicine] 6 (1982): 72.
11. He Jialang et al., *Collection of Papers Presented to the 2nd Congress of the National Delegates of the Chinese Medicine and Pharmacology Academy*, 2 (1956): 44.
12. Pharmacology Teaching Group of Nanjing Pharmacological College, *Yao Xue Xue Bao* [Pharmacology Journal] 13, 2 (1966): 95.
13. Hu Yuejuan et al., *Zhong Guo Yao Li Xue Tong Bao* [Chinese Pharmacology Bulletin] 2, 1 (1986): 41.
14. Guan Liyun, *Bei Jing Da Xue Yi Xue Yuan Xue Bao* [Journal of Beijing University Medical College] 1 (1981): 33.
15. Cao Yi et al., *Zhong Yao Yao Li Yu Lin Chuang* [Pharmacology and Clinical Application of Chinese Materia Medica] launch issue (1985): 133.
16. Yu Zhanyang et al., *Guo Wai Yi Xue – Yao Xue Fen Ce* [Foreign Medicine – Pharmacology Fascicule] 3 (1986): 173.
17. Zhang Ziyang et al., *Zhong Guo Zhong Yao Za Zhi* [Journal of Chinese Materia Medica] 15, 2 (1990): 31.
18. Liu Yun (translator), *Zhong Yao Yao Li Yu Lin Chuang* [Pharmacology and Clinical Application of Chinese Materia Medica] 8, 3 (1992): 3.
19. Li Shurong et al., *Zhong Yao Cai* [Chinese Materia Medica] 12, 6 (1989): 37.
20. M. Matsuba et al., *CA* 115 (1991): 15578.
21. Ibid., 113 (1990): 12111.
22. Ibid., 112 (1990): 240479.
23. Ding Anwei, *Zhong Yao Tong Bao* [Bulletin of Chinese Materia Medica] 11, 3 (1986): 23.
24. Micro-organism Teaching and Research Office, *Nan Jing Yi Xue Yuan Xue Bao* [Journal of Nanjing Medical College] 5 (1960): 10.
25. Jin Dianyou, *Zhong Yi Yao Xin Xi* [Traditional Chinese Medicine and Materia Medica News] 4 (1990): 40.
26. Zhang Shuyu, *Zhong Cao Yao* [Journal of Chinese Herbs] 18, 9 (1987): 9.
27. Chen Gurong et al., *Zhong Yao Cai* [Chinese Materia Medica] 11, 1 (1985): 14.
28. Yan Yingju, *Zhong Hua Yi Xue Za Zhi* [Chinese Journal of Medicine] 57, 8 (1977): 479.
29. Wang Jianhua et al., *Zhong Guo Yao Xue Za Zhi* [Journal of Chinese Pharmacology] 26, 8 (1991): 465.
30. Lei Zaiquan and Zhang Tingmo, *Zhong Hua Lin Chuang Zhong Yao Xue* [Chinese Clinical Materia Medica] (Beijing: People's Medical Publishing House, 1998), 209.
31. He Xingdong et al., *Lin Chuang Zhong Yao Shou Ce* [Clinical Handbook of Chinese Materia Medica] (Beijing: People's Medical Publishing House, 1998), 9.
32. Feng Liangyuan et al., *An Hui Zhong Yi Xue Yuan Xue Bao* [Journal of Anhui College of Traditional Chinese Medicine] 9, 2 (1990): 56.
33. He Xingdong et al., *Lin Chuang Zhong Yao Shou Ce*, 10.
34. Deng Shixian et al., *Zhong Cao Yao* [Journal of Chinese Herbs] 19, 10 (1988): 22.
35. Li Hongyu et al., *Hua Xi Yao Xue Za Zhi* [Huaxi Pharmacology Journal] 6, 1 (1991): 16.
36. Cheng Guangjuan et al., *Zhong Yao Tong Bao* [Bulletin of Chinese Materia Medica] 12, 4 (1987): 48.
37. Shen Yaqin et al., *Zhong Xi Yi Jie He Za Zhi* [Journal of Integrated TCM and Western Medicine] 7, 12 (1987): 738.
38. He Xingdong et al., *Lin Chuang Zhong Yao Shou Ce*, 11.
39. Lei Zaiquan and Zhang Tingmo, *Zhong Hua Lin Chuang Zhong Yao Xue*, 259.
40. Jia Pinfang et al., *Nan Jing Yao Xue Yuan Xue Bao* [Journal of Nanjing Pharmacology College] 3 (1958): 1.
41. Lingling Local Health and Epidemic Prevention Station et al., *Hu Nan Yi Yao Za Zhi* [Hunan Journal of Medicine and Pharmacology] 5 (1974): 57.
42. Lei Zaiquan and Zhang Tingmo, *Zhong Hua Lin Chuang Zhong Yao Xue*, 244.
43. He Xingdong et al., *Lin Chuang Zhong Yao Shou Ce*, 6.
44. Editorial Group, *Quan Guo Zhong Cao Yao Hui Bian* [National Collection of Chinese Herbs] (Beijing: People's Medical Publishing House, 1976), 620.
45. Shen Yingjun et al., *Zhong Yao Yao Li Yu Lin Chuang* [Pharmacology and Clinical Application of Chinese Materia Medica] 8 (1992): 11.

46. Wang Zhiwei et al., *Shang Hai Yi Ke Da Xue Xue* Bao [Journal of Shanghai Medical University] 14, 5 (1987): 367.
47. Lei Zaiquan and Zhang Tingmo, *Zhong Hua Lin Chuang Zhong Yao Xue*, 253.
48. He Xingdong et al., *Lin Chuang Zhong Yao Shou Ce*, 13.
49. T.A. Sollmann, *Manual of Pharmacology*, 7th ed. (Philadelphia: W. B. Saunders & Co., 1948), 211.
50. Zhang Xiaoyun, *Zhong Hua Hu Li Za Zhi* [Chinese Journal of Nursing] 25, 10 (1990): 523.
51. He Xingdong et al., *Lin Chuang Zhong Yao Shou Ce*, 15.
52. Micro-organism Teaching and Research Group, *Shan Dong Yi Xue Yuan Xue Bao* [Journal of Shandong College of Medicine] 8 (1959): 42.
53. Jiangsu New Medical College, *Zhong Yao Da Ci Dian* [Dictionary of Chinese Materia Medica] volume 1 (Shanghai: Shanghai People's Publishing House, 1977), 429.
54. He Xingdong et al., *Lin Chuang Zhong Yao Shou Ce*, 16.
55. Lingling Local Health and Epidemic Prevention Station, *Hu Nan Yi Yao Za Zhi* [Hunan Journal of Medicine and Pharmacology] 4 (1974): 50.
56. Xuzhou Medical College, *Xin Yi Xue Zi Liao* [New Medical Documents] 1 (1971): 27.
57. T. Yoshida et al., *Biochemical Pharmacology* 20, 12 (1971): 3263.
58. Liu Yaguang, *Xin Zhong Yi* [New Journal of Traditional Chinese Medicine] 1 (1979): 50.
59. Physiology Teaching and Research Office of Zhejiang Medical University et al., *Zhe Jiang Tong Xun* [Zhejiang Newsletter] 2, 3 (1975): 70.
60. Physiology Teaching and Research Group, *Zhe Jiang Yi Ke Da Xue Xue Bao* [Journal of Zhejiang Medical University] 7, 4 (1978): 5.
61. Yuan Feng, *An Hui Yi Xue Yuan Xue Bao* [Journal of Anhui Medical College] 2 (1977): 62.
62. Pharmacology Group of the Chinese Medicine and Pharmacology Research Institute of Shandong Province, *Yao Xue Tong Bao* [Pharmacology Bulletin] 11, 12 (1965): 562.
63. Biochemical Office of Beijing Chinese Materia Medica Science and Research Institute et al., *Zhong Yao Ke Yan Jian Bao* [Chinese Materia Medica Scientific Research Briefing] 2 (1979): 1.
64. Wang Yusheng, *Zhong Yao Yao Li Yu Ying Yong* [Pharmacology and Application of Chinese Materia Medica] (Beijing; People's Medical Publishing House, 1998), 905.
65. Shanxi Medical College, *Shan Xi Yi Yao Za Zhi* [Shanxi Journal of Medicine and Pharmacology] 1 (1974): 481.
66. Zhou Chongchu et al., *Yao Xue Tong Bao* [Pharmacology Bulletin] 14, 6 (1979): 252.
67. M. Shibata, *CA* 80 (1974): 116158P.
68. Fu Hangyu, *Zhong Yao Tong Bao* [Bulletin of Chinese Materia Medica] 11, 4 (1986): 46.
69. Wu Dejiu, *Zhong Cao Yao Tong Bao* [Bulletin of Chinese Herbs] 12 (1978): 29.
70. Wang Benxiang et al., *Zhong Guo Sheng Li Ke Xue Za Zhi* [Chinese Journal of Physiological Science] 10 (1981): 964.
71. Zhang Xinghan et al., *Zhong Guo Yao Li Xue Yu Du Li Xue Za Zhi* [Chinese Journal of Pharmacology and Toxicology] 13, 1 (1989): 30.
72. Xu Hongyuan, *Zhong Yao Cai Zhi Yan Jiu* [Research on Chinese Materia Medica] (Taibei: New Medicine Publishing House, 1980), 125-126.
73. Lu Xinran et al., *Zhong Guo Yao Li Xue Bao* [Chinese Journal of Pharmacology] 7 (1986): 537.
74. Fan Lili et al., *Zhong Hua Yi Xue Za Zhi* [Chinese Journal of Medicine] 55, 10 (1975): 724.
75. Gao Guiqing et al., *Zhong Yao Tong Bao* [Bulletin of Chinese Materia Medica] 9 (1984): 432.
76. He Xingdong et al., *Lin Chuang Zhong Yao Shou Ce*, 18.
77. Wu Baojin et al., *Zhong Cao Yao* [Journal of Chinese Herbs] 17, 11 (1986): 21.
78. Ma Shiping et al., *Zhong Guo Zhong Yao Za Zhi* [Journal of Chinese Materia Medica] 14, 8 (1989): 42.
79. Chen Qi et al., *Jiang Xi Zhong Yi Yao* [Jiangxi Journal of Traditional Chinese Medicine and Materia Medica] 22, 1 (1991): 42.
80. Zhong Shitong et al., *Zhong Yao Yao Li Yu Lin Chuang* [Pharmacology and Clinical Application of Chinese Materia Medica] 12, 1 (1996): 37.
81. Chai Tianwan et al., *Yao Xue Za Zhi* [Journal of Pharmacology] 97 (1977): 911.
82. Lei Zaiquan and Zhang Tingmo, *Zhong Hua Lin Chuang Zhong Yao Xue*, 360.
83. He Xingdong et al., *Lin Chuang Zhong Yao Shou Ce*, 25.
84. Ibid., 26.

Chapter 2

Herbs for clearing heat 清热药

Herbs for clearing heat

Herbs for clearing heat are herbs which are cold or cool in nature and have the function of clearing heat, draining fire, relieving toxicity, cooling the Blood, or clearing deficiency-heat. These herbs can be used for interior heat patterns caused by heat toxins, and for heat or fire which originates from other pathogenic factors. They can also be used for warm diseases and seasonal febrile diseases due to heat toxins, dysentery, abscesses and sores, bleeding due to Blood-heat, and fever due to Yin deficiency. Additionally, they have a function in the treatment of certain diseases diagnosed according to Western medical methods such as acute infectious diseases, type-B epidemic encephalitis, epidemic cerebrospinal meningitis, septicaemia, scarlet fever and parotitis, all of which are classified as seasonal febrile diseases according to traditional Chinese medicine.

In clinical practice, particular attention should be paid to the following aspects when using herbs for clearing heat:

1. Specific differentiation must be made between Qi-level and Xue-level patterns, full-heat and deficiency-heat patterns, and disorders of the channels and Zang-Fu organs, especially between patterns of exuberant Yin repelling Yang and patterns of true cold and false heat. Appropriate herbs and prescriptions should then be used according to the circumstances of the disease.
2. It is essential to examine whether there are any other accompanying symptoms which are relevant for the therapy. During the early stages of a heat pattern combined with an exterior pattern, the external pathogenic factors may be dispelled first followed by clearance of interior heat, or alternatively the external pathogenic factors and interior heat may be cleared simultaneously so that pathogenic factors are dispelled from both the exterior and the interior. In cases of heat in both the Qi and Xue levels, herbs for clearing heat in both these levels are used in combination to dispel pathogenic factors.
3. Herbs for clearing heat are cold and therefore tend to damage the Spleen and Stomach and affect their transportation and transformation function. In cases of Spleen and Stomach deficiency, these herbs should be used together with herbs which supplement the Spleen and Stomach. Herbs for clearing heat and drying dampness are dry in nature and they also tend to damage body fluids; therefore, in cases of Yin deficiency, they should be combined with herbs for enriching Yin so that vital Qi can be supported and pathogenic factors dispelled at the same time. Attention should be paid to the dosage and course of treatment. After recovering from the disorder, a patient should no longer be treated by herbs for clearing heat, thus avoiding any damage to vital Qi.

Herbs for clearing heat can be divided into five categories according to their characteristics and clinical functions:

i. herbs for clearing heat and draining fire: these herbs are mainly used to clear heat in the Qi level; they treat full-heat patterns in this level with such manifestations as high fever, vexation and thirst;

ii. herbs for clearing heat and drying dampness: most of these herbs are cold, bitter, dry and dispersing and are used mainly for disorders of the Stomach, Intestines, Liver, Bladder and Gallbladder due to damp-heat (notably dysentery and jaundice);
iii. herbs for clearing heat and relieving toxicity: these herbs mainly enter the Qi and Xue levels and are used for abscesses, swellings, sores and other disease patterns due to exuberant heat toxins;
iv. herbs for clearing heat and cooling the Blood: these herbs are mainly used to clear heat pathogenic factors from the Ying and Xue levels; they can treat Xue-level full-heat patterns with such manifestations as vomiting of blood, nosebleeds and macular eruptions;
v. herbs for clearing deficiency-heat: these herbs clear deficiency-heat patterns and abate steaming bone disorder; they are used for fever due to Yin deficiency, steaming bone disorder and taxation heat.

HERBS FOR CLEARING HEAT AND DRAINING FIRE

Most of the herbs in this section are either sweet and cold or bitter and cold; they are very effective in clearing heat and draining fire. They can be used to clear full-heat and fire in the Qi level with such manifestations as high fever, thirst, sweating, vexation and agitation, a dry tongue with yellow fur, a full and rapid pulse, and possibly even clouded Spirit and delirious speech.

Herbs for clearing heat and draining fire are also applied when treating the following conditions: red, sore and swollen eyes due to ascendant hyperactivity of Liver-fire, coughing and wheezing due to heat attacking the Lungs, toothache due to Stomach-fire, mouth sores, insomnia and vexation due to hyperactivity of Heart-fire, scrofula and goitre due to Phlegm and fire binding together in the channels, and vexation and agitation due to lasting heat in the later stages of febrile diseases.

Herbs for clearing heat and draining fire function extremely well in removing heat. For weak patients, they are used in combination with supplementing herbs in order to support vital Qi and dispel pathogenic factors simultaneously; if the heat symptoms disappear or the condition is alleviated, these herbs should either not be taken any longer or their dosage should be reduced so as not to damage vital Qi.

In cases of full-heat in the Qi level combined with an exterior pattern, herbs for clearing heat and draining fire are used in combination with acrid, cool herbs for releasing the exterior in order to dispel both external and internal pathogenic factors. In cases of full-heat in the Qi level which has not yet attacked the Xue level, herbs that clear heat and cool the Blood should not be used too early, otherwise vital Qi will be damaged and the disease will worsen.

Tab. 2.1 Herbs for clearing heat and draining fire

Herb	Functions	Indications
Shi Gao (Gypsum Fibrosum)	Clearing heat and draining fire, eliminating vexation and allaying thirst, closing sores and generating flesh, stopping bleeding	High fever, thirst, vexation and delirious speech due to full-heat in the Qi level, toothache due to Stomach-fire, headache, mouth sores; used externally for ulcerating sores and non-closure of open sores
Zhi Mu (Rhizoma Anemarrhenae Asphodeloidis)	Clearing heat and draining fire, enriching Yin and moistening dryness	Febrile diseases due to external pathogenic factors with high fever and thirst, dry cough due to Lung-heat, steaming bone disorder, wasting and thirsting due to internal heat, Intestinal dryness with constipation
Tian Hua Fen (Radix Trichosanthis)	Clearing heat and generating body fluids, relieving toxicity and expelling pus	Vexation and thirst in febrile diseases, dry cough due to Lung-heat, wasting and thirsting due to internal heat, abscesses

Zhi Zi (Fructus Gardeniae Jasminoidis)	Draining fire and eliminating vexation, clearing heat and promoting the elimination of dampness, cooling the Blood and stopping bleeding, quickening the Blood and dispersing swelling	Vexation during various febrile diseases, jaundice, blood in the urine, vomiting of blood and bleeding due to Blood-heat, heat Lin syndrome, red, sore and swollen eyes, sores, knocks and falls
*Xia Ku Cao (*Spica Prunellae Vulgaris)	Clearing the Liver and brightening the eyes, calming the Liver and subduing Yang, dissipating lumps and dispersing swelling	Red, sore and swollen eyes caused by exuberant fire in the Liver channel, headache and dizziness due to ascendant hyperactivity of Liver Yang, scrofula due to Phlegm and Liver-fire binding together
Lu Gen (Rhizoma Phragmitis Communis)	Clearing heat and generating body fluids, stopping vomiting, venting papules, relieving toxicity	Thirst due to warm diseases, vomiting due to Stomach-heat, cough due to Lung-heat, Lung abscess and spitting of fishy-smelling sputum, pain in the chest, sore and swollen throat, difficult urination due to damp-heat, measles in children, seafood poisoning
Dan Zhu Ye (Herba Lophatheri Gracilis)	Clearing heat and eliminating vexation, generating body fluids and promoting urination	Agitation with a stifling sensation in the chest and thirst during febrile diseases, mouth sores, child fright epilepsy, painful urination
Jue Ming Zi (Semen Cassiae)	Clearing the Liver and brightening the eyes, moistening the Intestines and freeing the bowels	Red, sore and swollen eyes due to Liver-fire flaming upwards, dim vision, night blindness, dizziness due to ascendant hyperactivity of Liver Yang, recurrent constipation

Shi Gao 石膏 (Gypsum, Gypsum Fibrosum)

Shi Gao is a monoclinic mineral form of hydrated calcium sulphate.

Main ingredients Crude gypsum, *Sheng Shi Gao* (Gypsum Fibrosum Crudum), contains hydrated calcium sulphate ($CaSO_4.2H_2O$), organic acids, sulphides and a little magnesium. Calcined gypsum, *Duan Shi Gao* (Gypsum Fibrosum Calcinatum), mainly contains calcium sulphate without water.

Properties Taste: acrid and sweet; nature: extremely cold.

Channels entered Lung and Stomach.

Functions and indications Clears heat and drains fire, eliminates vexation and allays thirst, closes sores and generates flesh, and stops bleeding. It is indicated for high fever, thirst, vexation and delirious speech due to full-heat in the Qi level, toothache due to Stomach-fire, headache, and mouth sores; *Shi Gao* is used externally for ulcerating sores and non-closure of open sores (generally in its calcined form).

Common dosage 15-60g, or 200g for large dosages, decocted before other herbs; appropriate dosage of calcined *Shi Gao* for external application. *Shi Gao* should be broken up and decocted for at least 15 minutes before adding other ingredients. High dosages of *Shi Gao* are often prescribed in China; this may not be appropriate for patients in the West.

Precautions and contraindications As *Shi Gao* is extremely cold in nature, it is contraindicated in cases of Spleen and Stomach deficiency-cold, Blood deficiency or fever due to Yin deficiency.

Remarks *Sheng Shi Gao* is used to clear full-heat in the Qi level; use *Duan Shi Gao* to treat non-healing sores and to generate flesh.

Comparison of functions See *Zhi Mu* (Rhizoma Anemarrhenae Asphodeloidis) and *Hua Shi* (Talcum).

Modern research

1. Decoctions of *Shi Gao* can abate fever.[1]
2. Can inhibit convulsions and inflammation.[2]

Combinations and applications

Functions	Combinations	Applications
Clearing heat and draining fire, eliminating vexation and allaying thirst	*Zhi Mu* (Rhizoma Anemarrhenae Asphodeloidis) *Gan Cao* (Radix Glycyrrhizae) *Lu Gen* (Rhizoma Phragmitis Communis) *Tian Hua Fen* (Radix Trichosanthis)	Full-heat in the Qi level with such manifestations as high fever, thirst, vexation and a surging and large pulse (e.g. with influenza or type-B encephalitis)
	Shui Niu Jiao (Cornu Bubali) *Sheng Di Huang* (Radix Rehmanniae Glutinosae) *Xuan Shen* (Radix Scrophulariae Ningpoensis) *Mu Dan Pi* (Cortex Moutan Radicis)	Qi and Blood both ablaze, with such manifestations as high fever and thirst, faintly visible maculopapular eruptions, nosebleed
	Sheng Di Huang (Radix Rehmanniae Glutinosae) *Da Huang* (Radix et Rhizoma Rhei) *Mu Dan Pi* (Cortex Moutan Radicis) *Di Gu Pi* (Cortex Lycii Radicis)	Toothache, bad breath and constipation due to Stomach-fire

	Xing Ren (Semen Pruni Armeniacae) *Ma Huang* (Herba Ephedrae) (see notes on legal status) *Gan Cao* (Radix Glycyrrhizae)	Cough with copious sputum, wheezing and fever due to Lung-heat
	Gui Zhi (Ramulus Cinnamomi Cassiae)	Red, swollen and painful joints due to wind-damp-heat
Closing sores and generating flesh, stopping bleeding	*Huang Bai* (Cortex Phellodendri) *Qing Dai* (Indigo Naturalis) *Sheng Dan* (raw egg) (for external use)	Eczema, ulcerating sores, non-closure of open sores, burns and scalds
	Bing Pian (Borneolum Syntheticum) (for external use)	Local redness and swelling in the initial stage of sores

Zhi Mu 知母
(Anemarrhena rhizome, Rhizoma Anemarrhenae Asphodeloidis)

Zhi Mu is the rhizome of *Anemarrhena asphodeloides* Bge., family Liliaceae.

Main ingredients *Zhi Mu* contains many kinds of saponin (including timosaponins, timobiose, sarsasapogenin, markogenin, neogitogenin, asphonin and smilagenin), mangiferin, isomangiferin, choline, nicotinamide, tannic acid and nicotinic acid.

Properties Taste: bitter and sweet; nature: cold.

Channels entered Lung, Stomach and Kidney.

Functions and indications Clears heat and drains fire, enriches Yin and moistens dryness. It is indicated for febrile diseases due to external pathogenic factors with high fever and thirst, dry cough due to Lung-heat, steaming bone disorder, wasting and thirsting due to internal heat, and Intestinal dryness with constipation.

Common dosage 6-12g, or 20g for large dosages.

Precautions and contraindications Since *Zhi Mu* is bitter in taste and cold in nature and can be used to clear heat from the Intestines by purgation, it is contraindicated in cases of loose stool due to Spleen deficiency.

Remarks Raw *Zhi Mu* is commonly used for full-heat patterns, whereas brine-fried *Zhi Mu* enters the Kidney channel and is mainly used for clearing deficiency-heat and enriching Kidney Yin.

Comparison of functions Both *Zhi Mu* (Rhizoma Anemarrhenae Asphodeloidis) and *Shi Gao* (Gypsum Fibrosum) can clear heat and drain fire and are often used together to treat exuberant heat from the Lungs and Stomach at the Qi level. The difference between the two materia medica is that *Zhi Mu*, as a clearing and moistening herb, also has the function of enriching Yin and is used for wasting and thirsting disease, steaming bone disorder and night sweating due to effulgent Yin deficiency-fire, as well as for interior heat with damage to body fluids. *Sheng Shi Gao*, with its clearing and dispersing functions, is very effective for clearing full-heat in the Qi level and for strongly draining fire; it is used for dissipating pathogenic heat in the Qi level and can treat interior heat where there is no damage to body fluids.

Modern research

1. The mangiferin contained in *Zhi Mu* is very effective in inhibiting the herpes simplex virus.[3]
2. Restricts the functions of the sympathetic nervous system and the adrenal glands, lowers the heart rate and reduces the number of beta-transmitters.[4–6]
3. Preparations of *Zhi Mu* can lower the blood sugar level.[7]

Combinations and applications

Functions	Combinations	Applications
Clearing heat and draining fire	*Shi Gao* (Gypsum Fibrosum) *Tian Hua Fen* (Radix Trichosanthis) *Huang Qin* (Radix Scutellariae Baicalensis)	High fever and thirst, vexation and sweating due to full-heat in the Lungs and Stomach
	Bei Mu (Bulbus Fritillariae) *Gua Lou* (Fructus Trichosanthis) *Sang Bai Pi* (Cortex Mori Albae Radicis)	Cough and constipation with yellow sputum due to Lung-heat
Enriching Yin and moistening dryness	*Mai Men Dong* (Radix Ophiopogonis Japonici) *Sheng Di Huang* (Radix Rehmanniae Glutinosae) *Jie Geng* (Radix Platycodi Grandiflori)	Dry cough without sputum accompanied by a sore and swollen throat due to dryness in the Lungs
	Huang Bai (Cortex Phellodendri) *Sheng Di Huang* (Radix Rehmanniae Glutinosae) *Di Gu Pi* (Cortex Lycii Radicis)	Vexing heat in the five hearts, thirst and night sweating due to effulgent Yin deficiency-fire
	Tian Hua Fen (Radix Trichosanthis) *Mai Men Dong* (Radix Ophiopogonis Japonici)	Wasting and thirsting
	Suan Zao Ren (Semen Ziziphi Spinosae) *Ye Jiao Teng* (Caulis Polygoni Multiflori) *Sang Shen* (Fructus Mori Albae)	Insomnia and vexation due to insufficiency of Yin and Blood

Tian Hua Fen 天花粉 (Trichosanthes root, Radix Trichosanthis)

Tian Hua Fen is the root of *Trichosanthes kirilowii* Maxim. or *T. japonica* Regel., family Cucurbitaceae.

Legal status *Tian Hua Fen* was listed in a document entitled *A Review of Restricted Herbal Ingredients* issued by the Medicines Control Agency (MCA) in the UK in September 2001 with a view to the possible imposition of restrictions on its use at a future date. The MCA is concerned that *T. kirilowii* is used to induce abortions in China and is therefore suggesting that use of this herb may require medical supervision.

Main ingredients *Tian Hua Fen* contains trichosanthin, proteins, saponins and starch.

Properties Taste: bitter and slightly sweet; nature: cold.

Channels entered Lung and Stomach.

Functions and indications Clears heat and generates body fluids, relieves toxicity and expels pus. It is indicated for vexation and thirst in febrile diseases, dry cough due to Lung-heat, wasting and thirsting due to internal heat, and abscesses.

Common dosage 10-15g, or 30g for large dosages; appropriate dosage for external application.

Precautions and contraindications

1. *Tian Hua Fen* is contraindicated in cases of loose stool and diarrhoea due to Spleen and Stomach deficiency-cold, as well as during pregnancy.

2. *Tian Hua Fen* is incompatible with *Fu Zi* (Radix Lateralis Aconiti Carmichaeli Praeparata) and *Wu Tou* (Radix Aconiti).

Comparison of functions See *Lu Gen* (Rhizoma Phragmitis Communis).

Modern research

1. Can induce abortion in the early stages of pregnancy.[8-11]
2. Local injection of the proteins contained in *Tian Hua Fen* into cancerous tissue in mice inhibited the production of cancer cells in the breast and pelvis.[12]
3. Can inhibit HIV.[13, 14]

Combinations and applications

Functions	Combinations	Applications
Clearing heat and generating body fluids	*Bei Mu* (Bulbus Fritillariae) *Sang Bai Pi* (Cortex Mori Albae Radicis)	Fever and spitting of yellow sputum due to Lung-heat damaging body fluids
	Xuan Shen (Radix Scrophulariae Ningpoensis) *Mai Men Dong* (Radix Ophiopogonis Japonici) *Jie Geng* (Radix Platycodi Grandiflori)	Dry cough without sputum, thirst, dry throat
	Lu Gen (Rhizoma Phragmitis Communis) *Shi Gao* (Gypsum Fibrosum)	Thirst during febrile diseases
	Sheng Di Huang (Radix Rehmanniae Glutinosae) *Zhi Mu* (Rhizoma Anemarrhenae Asphodeloidis) *Yu Zhu* (Rhizoma Polygonati Odorati)	Wasting and thirsting
Relieving toxicity and expelling pus	*Gua Lou* (Fructus Trichosanthis) *Bai Zhi* (Radix Angelicae Dahuricae)	Breast abscess
	Lian Qiao (Fructus Forsythiae Suspensae) *Chi Shao* (Radix Paeoniae Rubra) *Zao Jiao Ci* (Spina Gleditsiae Sinensis)	Sores and swollen abscesses due to exuberant heat toxins
	Chi Xiao Dou (Semen Phaseoli Calcarati) (pound to powder for external use)	Non-ulcerating abscesses

Zhi Zi 栀子 (Gardenia, Fructus Gardeniae Jasminoidis)

Zhi Zi is the fruit of *Gardenia jasminoides* Ellis var. *radicans* (Thunb.) Makino, family Rubiaceae.

Main ingredients *Zhi Zi* contains gardenin, gardenoside, geniposide, gardoside, crocin, crocetin, D-mannitol and β-sitosterol. The peel of *Zhi Zi* contains ursolic acid.

Properties Taste: bitter; nature: cold.

Channels entered Heart, Liver, Lung, Stomach and San Jiao.

Functions and indications Drains fire and eliminates vexation, clears heat and promotes the elimination of dampness, cools the Blood and stops bleeding, quickens the Blood and disperses swelling. It is indicated for vexation during various febrile diseases, jaundice, blood in the urine, vomiting of blood and bleeding due to Blood-heat, heat Lin syndrome, red, sore and swollen eyes, sores, and knocks and falls.

Common dosage 3-10g; appropriate dosage for external application.

Precautions and contraindications As *Zhi Zi* is bitter and cold, it tends to damage the Spleen and Stomach; it is therefore contraindicated in cases of loose stool due to Spleen deficiency.

Remarks The peel of *Zhi Zi* dispels heat from the fleshy exterior, whereas the kernel of the fruit has the function of clearing heat from the Heart and the interior. Raw *Zhi Zi* is used to drain fire; when stir-fried, it is used to eliminate vexation, and when charred, to stop bleeding.

Modern research

1. Decoctions of *Zhi Zi* and alcoholic extracts of the herb promote the secretion of bile, reduce bilirubin levels and promote the immediate excretion of serum bilirubin.[15]
2. Can stop bleeding.[16]
3. Promotes the healing of soft tissue after contusion.[16]

Combinations and applications

Functions	Combinations	Applications
Draining fire and eliminating vexation	*Dan Dou Chi* (Semen Sojae Praeparatum) *Bo He* (Herba Menthae Haplocalycis)	Febrile diseases due to external pathogenic factors, oppression in the chest, vexation
	Shi Gao (Gypsum Fibrosum) *Zhi Mu* (Rhizoma Anemarrhenae Asphodeloidis) *Da Qing Ye* (Folium Isatidis seu Baphicacanthi)	High fever and vexation, clouded Spirit and delirious speech, and a red tongue with yellow fur in the course of seasonal febrile diseases
	Huang Lian (Rhizoma Coptidis) *Chen Pi* (Pericarpium Citri Reticulatae) *Cang Zhu* (Rhizoma Atractylodis)	Vomiting due to Stomach-fire with a sour or bitter taste in the mouth
Clearing heat and promoting the elimination of dampness	*Huang Bai* (Cortex Phellodendri) *Yin Chen Hao* (Herba Artemisiae Scopariae) *Da Huang* (Radix et Rhizoma Rhei)	Damp-heat jaundice (Yang-type jaundice)
	Huang Bai (Cortex Phellodendri) *Mu Tong* (Caulis Mutong) (see notes on legal status) *Che Qian Zi* (Semen Plantaginis)	Lin syndrome due to damp-heat, frequent urination and urinary urgency, a feeling of heat and pain when passing urine
Cooling the Blood and stopping bleeding	*Sheng Di Huang* (Radix Rehmanniae Glutinosae) *Mu Dan Pi* (Cortex Moutan Radicis) *Huang Qin Tan* (Radix Scutellariae Baicalensis Carbonisata) *Bai Mao Gen* (Rhizoma Imperatae Cylindricae) *Huai Hua* (Flos Sophorae Japonicae)	Vomiting of blood and nosebleed due to the frenetic movement of hot Blood

	Xia Ku Cao (Spica Prunellae Vulgaris) *Ju Hua* (Flos Chrysanthemi Morifolii) *Jue Ming Zi* (Semen Cassiae)	Red, sore and swollen eyes due to exuberant fire in the Liver channel
Quickening the Blood and dispersing swelling	*Huang Lian* (Rhizoma Coptidis) *Huang Bai* (Cortex Phellodendri) *Bai Zhi* (Radix Angelicae Dahuricae) *Chi Shao* (Radix Paeoniae Rubra)	Swelling and toxins of sores, fever and vexation

Note: Powdered *Zhi Zi* mixed with yellow wine, *Huang Jiu* (Vinum Aureum), is used externally for painful swelling due to knocks and falls.

Xia Ku Cao 夏枯草 (Prunella spike, Spica Prunellae Vulgaris)

Xia Ku Cao is the fruit-spike of *Prunella vulgaris* L., family Labiatae.

Main ingredients The whole plant contains triterpenes, the aglycone of which is oleanolic acid. It also contains free oleanolic acid, ursolic acid, caffeic acid, rutin, hyperoside, vitamins B_1, C and K, amaroids, alkaloids and water-soluble salts (mostly sodium chloride).

Properties Taste: acrid and bitter; nature: cold.

Channels entered Liver and Gallbladder.

Functions and indications Clears the Liver and brightens the eyes, calms the Liver and subdues Yang, dissipates lumps and disperses swelling. It is indicated for red, sore and swollen eyes caused by exuberant fire in the Liver channel, headache and dizziness due to ascendant hyperactivity of Liver Yang, and scrofula due to Phlegm and Liver-fire binding together.

Common dosage 10-15g, or 30g for large dosages; appropriate dosage for external application.

Precautions and contraindications *Xia Ku Cao* should be used with caution in cases of Stomach and Spleen deficiency.

Comparison of functions See *Jue Ming Zi* (Semen Cassiae).

Modern research

1. Preparations of *Xia Ku Cao* can lower blood pressure.[17]
2. Lowers the blood sugar level.[18]
3. A decoction of *Xia Ku Cao* inhibited the type I herpes simplex virus during *in vitro* tests.[19]

Combinations and applications

Functions	Combinations	Applications
Clearing the Liver and brightening the eyes	*Ju Hua* (Flos Chrysanthemi Morifolii) *Jue Ming Zi* (Semen Cassiae) *Qing Xiang Zi* (Semen Celosiae Argenteae)	Red, sore and swollen eyes due to exuberant fire in the Liver channel
	Shi Jue Ming (Concha Haliotidis) *Sheng Di Huang* (Radix Rehmanniae Glutinosae) *Huang Qin* (Radix Scutellariae Baicalensis)	Distending pain in the eyeball due to ascendant hyperactivity of Liver Yang caused by Yin deficiency of the Liver and Kidneys

Calming the Liver and subduing Yang	*Shi Jue Ming* (Concha Haliotidis) *Gou Teng* (Ramulus Uncariae cum Uncis) *Di Long* (Lumbricus) *Bai Shao* (Radix Paeoniae Lactiflorae)	Headache, dizziness, vexation and agitation, and a string-like pulse due to ascendant hyperactivity of Liver Yang (e.g. with hypertension)
Dissipating lumps and dispersing swelling	*Xuan Shen* (Radix Scrophulariae Ningpoensis) *Lian Qiao* (Fructus Forsythiae Suspensae)	Scrofula due to Phlegm and fire binding together
	Pu Gong Ying (Herba Taraxaci cum Radice) *Zhe Bei Mu* (Bulbus Fritillariae Thunbergii) *Mu Li* (Concha Ostreae) *Hai Zao* (Herba Sargassi) *Kun Bu* (Thallus Laminariae seu Eckloniae)	Hyperthyroidism, goitre
	Tian Men Dong (Radix Asparagi Cochinchinensis)	Breast abscess

Lu Gen 芦根
(Reed rhizome, Rhizoma Phragmitis Communis)

Lu Gen is the dried rhizome of *Phragmites communis* (L.) Trin., family Gramineae.

Main ingredients *Lu Gen* contains sugars, proteins, fats, asparagine, coixol carbohydrates, tricin and vitamins B_1, B_2 and C.

Properties Taste: sweet; nature: cold.

Channels entered Lung and Stomach.

Functions and indications Clears heat and generates body fluids, stops vomiting, vents papules, and relieves toxicity. It is indicated for thirst due to warm diseases, vomiting due to Stomach-heat, cough due to Lung-heat, Lung abscess and spitting of fishy-smelling sputum, pain in the chest, sore and swollen throat, difficult urination due to damp-heat, measles in children, and seafood poisoning.

Common dosage 15-30g; the dosage can be doubled for the fresh herb.

Precautions and contraindications *Lu Gen* is contraindicated in cases of Spleen and Stomach deficiency-cold.

Remarks The fresh herb, *Xian Lu Gen* (Rhizoma Phragmitis Communis Recens), is more effective than the dried herb in clearing heat, generating body fluids and promoting urination.

Comparison of functions Both *Lu Gen* (Rhizoma Phragmitis Communis) and *Tian Hua Fen* (Radix Trichosanthis) can clear heat in the Lungs and Stomach, and nourish Yin and generate body fluids. They are often used together for febrile diseases damaging body fluids, for vexation and thirst, and for cough due to Lung-heat. *Tian Hua Fen* has the stronger effect in generating body fluids while also relieving toxicity and dispersing swelling. *Lu Gen* is more effective for clearing heat from the Lungs and Stomach at the Qi level, although it is not as strong as *Shi Gao* (Gypsum Fibrosum) and *Zhi Mu* (Rhizoma Anemarrhenae Asphodeloidis) in this function.

For additional comparisons, see *Yu Xing Cao* (Herba Houttuyniae Cordatae) and *Bai Mao Gen* (Rhizoma Imperatae Cylindricae).

Modern research

1. The asparagine contained in *Lu Gen* is effective in stopping coughing.[20]
2. Decoctions of *Lu Gen* had a certain inhibitory effect *in vitro* on haemolytic streptococci, Streptococcus pneumoniae and Corynebacterium diphtheriae.[21]

Combinations and applications

Functions	Combinations	Applications
Clearing heat and generating body fluids, stopping vomiting	*Xuan Shen* (Radix Scrophulariae Ningpoensis) *Tian Hua Fen* (Radix Trichosanthis) *Mai Men Dong* (Radix Ophiopogonis Japonici)	Fever and thirst due to body fluids being damaged by warm diseases
	Gua Lou (Fructus Trichosanthis) *Sang Bai Pi* (Cortex Mori Albae Radicis)	Cough due to Lung-heat
	Yi Yi Ren (Semen Coicis Lachrymajobi) *Dong Gua Ren* (Semen Benincasae Hispidae) *Tao Ren* (Semen Persicae)	Lung abscess manifesting as fishy-smelling sputum, fever and pain in the chest
	Bai Mao Gen (Rhizoma Imperatae Cylindricae) *Che Qian Zi* (Semen Plantaginis)	Difficult urination due to damp-heat
	Zhu Ru (Caulis Bambusae in Taeniis) *Shi Gao* (Gypsum Fibrosum)	Vomiting due to Stomach-heat
Venting papules	*Xi He Liu* (Cacumen Tamaricis) *Chan Tui* (Periostracum Cicadae)	Measles in children accompanied by fever and thirst

Note: Frequent ingestion of the juice of fresh *Lu Gen* can relieve the toxicity of seafood poisoning.

Dan Zhu Ye 淡竹叶
(Lophatherum herb, Herba Lophatheri Gracilis)

Dan Zhu Ye is the dried aerial parts of *Lophatherum gracile* Brongn., family Gramineae.

Main ingredients *Dan Zhu Ye* contains arundoin, cylindrin, taraxerol and friedelin.

Properties Taste: sweet and bland; nature: cold.

Channels entered Heart, Stomach and Small Intestine.

Functions and indications Clears heat and eliminates vexation, generates body fluids and promotes urination. It is indicated for agitation with a stifling sensation in the chest and thirst during febrile diseases, mouth sores, child fright epilepsy, and painful urination.

Common dosage 6-15g.

Precautions and contraindications *Dan Zhu Ye* is contraindicated in cases of effulgent Yin deficiency-fire and tidal fever due to steaming bone disorder.

Remarks *Dan Zhu Ye* is good for clearing heat in the Heart and Small Intestine and can guide heat downwards.

Modern research

1. Preparations of *Dan Zhu Ye* abate fever.[22, 23]
2. Raises the blood sugar level.[23]
3. Decoctions of *Dan Zhu Ye* can inhibit Staphylococcus aureus.[24]

Combinations and applications

Functions	Combinations	Applications
Clearing heat and eliminating vexation, generating body fluids and promoting urination	*Shi Gao* (Gypsum Fibrosum) *Mai Men Dong* (Radix Ophiopogonis Japonici)	Agitation and thirst in febrile diseases

	Sheng Di Huang (Radix Rehmanniae Glutinosae) *Mu Tong* (Caulis Mutong) (see notes on legal status) *Zhi Zi* (Fructus Gardeniae Jasminoidis)	Mouth sores, scant and yellow urine due to heat in the Heart channel
	Bai Mao Gen (Rhizoma Imperatae Cylindricae) *Bian Xu* (Herba Polygoni Avicularis) *Dong Kui Zi* (Semen Malvae Verticillatae)	Heat Lin syndrome
	Gou Teng (Ramulus Uncariae cum Uncis) *Chan Tui* (Periostracum Cicadae) *Deng Xin Cao* (Medulla Junci Effusi)	Morbid night crying in infants due to Heart-heat
	Dai Zhe Shi (Haematitum) *Chan Tui* (Periostracum Cicadae)	Child fright epilepsy

Jue Ming Zi 决明子
(Cassia seed, Semen Cassiae)

Jue Ming Zi is the dried seed of *Cassia obtusifolia* L. or *C. tora* L., family Leguminosae.

Main ingredients *Jue Ming Zi* contains chrysophanol, emodin, aloe-emodin, physcion, rhein, obtusifolin, obtusin, cassiaside, torachrysone, toralactone, rubrofusarin, norrubrofusarin, fatty acids, saccharides, proteins and microelements.

Properties Taste: bitter and sweet; nature: cool.

Channels entered Liver, Kidney and Large Intestine.

Functions and indications Clears the Liver and brightens the eyes, moistens the Intestines and frees the bowels. It is indicated for red, sore and swollen eyes due to Liver-fire flaming upwards, dim vision, night blindness, dizziness due to ascendant hyperactivity of Liver Yang, and recurrent constipation.

Common dosage 10-15g.

Comparison of functions Both *Jue Ming Zi* (Semen Cassiae) and *Xia Ku Cao* (Spica Prunellae Vulgaris) can clear the Liver and brighten the eyes. *Jue Ming Zi* can treat red, sore and swollen eyes due to wind-heat and Liver-fire flaming upwards and is extremely effective when this condition is accompanied by constipation. *Xia Ku Cao* is very effective for treating red, sore and swollen eyes due to exuberant fire in the Liver channel when the condition is accompanied by dizziness.

For an additional comparison, see *Shi Jue Ming* (Concha Haliotidis).

Modern research

1. Lowers blood pressure and reduces the level of blood lipids.[25, 26]
2. Promotes bowel movement.[27]
3. Improves acuity of vision.[28]

Combinations and applications

Functions	Combinations	Applications
Clearing the Liver and brightening the eyes	*Xia Ku Cao* (Spica Prunellae Vulgaris) *Ju Hua* (Flos Chrysanthemi Morifolii)	Red, sore and swollen eyes due to Liver-fire flaming upwards

	Sang Ye (Folium Mori Albae) *Zhi Zi* (Fructus Gardeniae Jasminoidis) *Niu Bang Zi* (Fructus Arctii Lappae)	Red, sore and swollen eyes due to wind-heat
	Ju Hua (Flos Chrysanthemi Morifolii) *Mu Zei* (Herba Equiseti Hiemalis)	Acute conjunctivitis (wind-fire eye)
	Gou Teng (Ramulus Uncariae cum Uncis) *Mu Li* (Concha Ostreae) *Di Long* (Lumbricus)	Headache and dizziness due to ascendant hyperactivity of Liver Yang
	Gou Qi Zi (Fructus Lycii) *Nü Zhen Zi* (Fructus Ligustri Lucidi)	Blurred vision due to Yin deficiency of the Liver and Kidneys
Moistening the Intestines and freeing the bowels	*Huo Ma Ren* (Semen Cannabis Sativae) *Gua Lou Ren* (Semen Trichosanthis)	Intestinal dryness due to internal heat, constipation

HERBS FOR CLEARING HEAT AND DRYING DAMPNESS

Most herbs which clear heat and dry dampness are bitter and cold. Bitter herbs can perform a downward-bearing function and dry dampness, while cold herbs can clear heat. As a result, these herbs are commonly used for patterns caused by damp-heat obstruction or heat originating from dampness, mainly manifesting as vexation and a sensation of heat, a bitter taste in the mouth, diarrhoea, dysentery, jaundice, difficult and painful urination, eczema and sores.

Some of these herbs, such as *Huang Lian* (Rhizoma Coptidis), *Huang Bai* (Cortex Phellodendri), *Huang Qin* (Radix Scutellariae Baicalensis) and *Long Dan Cao* (Radix Gentianae Scabrae), can not only clear heat and dry dampness, but can also relieve toxicity by draining fire. In order to strengthen their effect in the latter function, they are often used in combination with *Shi Gao* (Gypsum Fibrosum), *Zhi Mu* (Rhizoma Anemarrhenae Asphodeloidis), *Jin Yin Hua* (Flos Lonicerae) and *Lian Qiao* (Fructus Forsythiae Suspensae).

Although herbs for clearing heat and drying dampness can treat diseases caused by damp-heat, they tend to damage Yin and the Stomach, so they are generally not used in cases of depletion of body fluids or Spleen and Stomach deficiency. Herbs for nourishing Yin and boosting the Stomach should be added according to the condition of the patient.

Tab. 2.2 Herbs for clearing heat and drying dampness

Herb	Functions	Indications
Huang Qin (Radix Scutellariae Baicalensis)	Clearing heat and drying dampness, draining fire and relieving toxicity, cooling the Blood and quieting the foetus	Diseases caused by damp-heat, such as damp-warm diseases, summerheat-warm diseases, and fullness in the chest and abdomen due to damp-heat; dysentery, diarrhoea, jaundice and heat Lin syndrome; sore and swollen throat, toothache, dry stool due to Stomach-fire, cough due to Lung-heat, bleeding, vomiting of blood, uterine bleeding, stirring foetus due to internal heat disturbing the Blood
Huang Lian (Rhizoma Coptidis)	Clearing heat and drying dampness, clearing Heart-fire and eliminating vexation, draining fire and relieving toxicity	Diarrhoea, dysentery and vomiting due to damp-heat in the Stomach and Intestines, vexation, sore and swollen throat, mouth sores, red, sore and swollen eyes in the course of warm diseases, sores
Huang Bai (Cortex Phellodendri)	Clearing heat and drying dampness, draining fire and relieving toxicity, abating deficiency-heat	Damp-heat dysentery, jaundice, red and white vaginal discharge due to damp-heat, heat Lin syndrome, wasting and thirsting, steaming bone disorder, seminal emission, leg Qi, mouth and tongue sores, itchy eczema, sores
Ku Shen (Radix Sophorae Flavescentis)	Clearing heat and drying dampness, dispelling wind and killing worms, promoting urination	Jaundice, dysentery, vaginal discharge, pudendal itch, itchy skin, scabies and tinea, eczema, haemorrhoids and blood in the stool, Lin syndrome due to damp-heat

Long Dan Cao (Radix Gentianae Scabrae)	Clearing heat and drying dampness, draining Liver-fire and settling fright	Headache and red eyes, pain in the hypochondrium due to exuberant heat in the Liver channel, jaundice due to damp-heat in the Liver and Gallbladder, vaginal discharge, Lin syndrome due to damp-heat, agitation, fright epilepsy
Qin Pi (Cortex Fraxini)	Clearing heat and relieving toxicity, clearing Liver-fire and brightening the eyes	Dysentery due to pathogenic heat toxins, red, sore and swollen eyes, blurred vision
Bai Xian Pi (Cortex Dictamni Dasycarpi Radicis)	Clearing heat and relieving toxicity, dispelling wind and drying dampness	Sores caused by pathogenic wind-heat or damp-heat toxins, scabies, wind papules, and jaundice and Bi syndrome due to pathogenic damp-heat

Huang Qin 黄芩 (Baical skullcap root, Radix Scutellariae Baicalensis)

Huang Qin is the root of *Scutellaria baicalensis* Georgi, family Labiatae.

Main ingredients *Huang Qin* contains baicalein, baicalin, wogonin, wogonoside, neobaicalein, palmitic acid, oleic acid, benzoic acid, β-sitosterol and stigmasterol.

Properties Taste: bitter; nature: cold.

Channels entered Lung, Gallbladder, Stomach and Large Intestine.

Functions and indications Clears heat and dries dampness, drains fire and relieves toxicity, cools the Blood and quiets the foetus. It is indicated for all diseases caused by damp-heat, such as damp-warm diseases, summerheat-warm diseases, and fullness in the chest and abdomen due to damp-heat, as well as for dysentery, diarrhoea, jaundice and heat Lin syndrome. It can also be used to treat sore and swollen throat, toothache, dry stool due to Stomach-fire, cough due to Lung-heat, bleeding, vomiting of blood, uterine bleeding, and stirring foetus due to internal heat disturbing the Blood.

Common dosage 3-10g, or 25g for large dosages.

Precautions and contraindications *Huang Qin* is bitter and cold and may damage vital Qi; it is therefore contraindicated in cases of Spleen and Stomach deficiency-cold without full-heat.

Remarks Raw *Huang Qin* has stronger heat-clearing properties; the stir-fried herb quiets the foetus; *Huang Qin* fried in alcohol clears heat in the Upper Jiao; and the charred herb, *Huang Qin Tan* (Radix Scutellariae Baicalensis Carbonisata) is used to stop bleeding.

Comparison of functions See *Huang Bai* (Cortex Phellodendri).

Toxicity Oral administration of 10g/kg of decoctions of *Huang Qin* and intravenous injection of 2g/kg of alcoholic extracts of the herb both had a sedative effect on rabbits, but did not cause any deaths. However, intravenous injection of 2g/kg of infusions of *Huang Qin* had a sedative and hypnotic effect on rabbits and resulted in death after 8-12 hours. The LD_{50} for intraperitoneal injection of baicalin in mice is 3.08g/kg. Tests indicate that oral preparations are much less toxic than intravenous injection of the herb.

Modern research

1. Although *Huang Qin* has proved effective in inhibiting such bacteria as Shigella shigae, Corynebacterium diphtheriae, Pseudomonas aeruginosa and Staphylococcus aureus in the clinic, the mechanism involved has yet to be explained by laboratory tests.[29]
2. Inhibits inflammation and allergy.[30-32]
3. Reduces the level of blood lipids.[33]
4. Abates fever.[34]

Combinations and applications

Functions	Combinations	Applications
Clearing heat and drying dampness	*Hua Shi* (Talcum) *Cao Dou Kou* (Semen Alpiniae Katsumadai) *Tong Cao* (Medulla Tetrapanacis Papyriferi) *Pei Lan* (Herba Eupatorii Fortunei)	Fever, oppression in the chest, a slimy sensation in the mouth, and slimy tongue fur due to damp-warm diseases
	Mu Tong (Caulis Mutong) (see notes on legal status) *Bian Xu* (Herba Polygoni Avicularis)	Heat Lin syndrome with painful urination and urinary urgency

	Zhi Zi (Fructus Gardeniae Jasminoidis) *Yin Chen Hao* (Herba Artemisiae Scopariae)	Damp-heat jaundice (Yang-type jaundice)
	Huang Lian (Rhizoma Coptidis) *Ge Gen* (Radix Puerariae) *Mu Xiang* (Radix Aucklandiae Lappae) (see notes on legal status)	Dysentery and diarrhoea due to damp-heat attacking the Lower Jiao
	Bai Zhi (Radix Angelicae Dahuricae) *Lian Qiao* (Fructus Forsythiae Suspensae) *Tian Hua Fen* (Radix Trichosanthis)	Swelling and toxins of abscesses and sores
	Chai Hu (Radix Bupleuri) *Ban Xia* (Rhizoma Pinelliae Ternatae) *Sheng Jiang* (Rhizoma Zingiberis Officinalis Recens)	Alternating chills and fever in Shaoyang diseases with a bitter taste in the mouth, dry throat, oppression in the chest and nausea
Draining fire and relieving toxicity	*Xia Ku Cao* (Spica Prunellae Vulgaris) *Gou Teng* (Ramulus Uncariae cum Uncis) *Ju Hua* (Flos Chrysanthemi Morifolii)	Dizziness and headache due to ascendant hyperactivity of Liver-fire
	Gua Lou (Fructus Trichosanthis) *Sang Bai Pi* (Cortex Mori Albae Radicis) *Yu Xing Cao* (Herba Houttuyniae Cordatae)	Cough with yellow sputum, thirst and fever due to Lung-heat
	Shan Dou Gen (Radix Sophorae Tonkinensis) *She Gan* (Rhizoma Belamcandae Chinensis) *Ban Lan Gen* (Radix Isatidis seu Baphicacanthi)	Sore and swollen throat due to Lung-heat (e.g. in tonsillitis)
	Sheng Di Huang (Radix Rehmanniae Glutinosae) *Huang Lian* (Rhizoma Coptidis) *Da Huang* (Radix et Rhizoma Rhei)	Toothache and dry stool due to Stomach-fire
Cooling the Blood and quieting the foetus	*Bai Zhu* (Rhizoma Atractylodis Macrocephalae) *Dang Gui* (Radix Angelicae Sinensis) *Zhu Ru* (Caulis Bambusae in Taeniis) *Su Geng* (Caulis Perillae Frutescentis)	Stirring foetus due to heat, nausea, vomiting, vexation and a feeling of heat in the chest, and pain and heaviness in the lower abdomen

Note: *Huang Qin* can be used on its own or in combination with *Shu Di Huang* (Radix Rehmanniae Glutinosae Conquita), *Bai Shao* (Radix Paeoniae Lactiflorae) and *Bai Zhu* (Rhizoma Atractylodis Macrocephalae) to treat vomiting of blood, nosebleed and uterine bleeding due to the frenetic movement of Blood.

Huang Lian 黄连
(Golden thread rhizome, Rhizoma Coptidis)

Huang Lian is the rhizome of *Coptis chinensis* Franch., *C. deltoidea* C. Y. Cheng et Hsiao, or *C. teetoides* C. Y. Cheng, family Ranunculaceae.

Main ingredients *Huang Lian* contains berberine, coptisine, worenine, palmatine, columbamine, jatrorrhizine, obacunone, obaculactone, magnoflorine and ferulic acid.

Properties Taste: bitter; nature: cold.

Channels entered Heart, Liver, Stomach and Large Intestine.

Functions and indications Clears heat and dries dampness, clears Heart-fire and eliminates vexation, drains fire and relieves toxicity. It is indicated for diarrhoea, dysentery and vomiting due to damp-heat in the Stomach and Intestines, vexation, sore and swollen throat, mouth sores, red, sore and swollen eyes in the course of warm diseases, and sores.

Common dosage 3-10g, or 1-1.5g in powder form for oral application; appropriate dosage for external use or external washes.

Precautions and contraindications Since *Huang Lian* is very cold and bitter, its use for a prolonged period can damage the Spleen and Stomach and the herb is therefore contraindicated in cases of Spleen and Stomach deficiency-cold and for patterns not caused by full-fire damp-heat.

Remarks Raw *Huang Lian* is used to clear Heart-fire and damp-heat in the Large Intestine; fried in alcohol, the herb is used to clear heat from the Upper Jiao and can treat red, sore and swollen eyes and mouth and tongue sores; fried with ginger juice, it can clear heat from the Middle Jiao and can fortify the Stomach and stop vomiting; when fried with brine, it can clear heat from the Lower Jiao. The charred herb is used to stop bleeding.

Comparison of functions See *Huang Bai* (Cortex Phellodendri) and *Hu Huang Lian* (Rhizoma Picrorhizae Scrophulariiflorae).

Toxicity The LD_{50} for intraperitoneal injection in mice of a 10% aqueous suspension of *Huang Lian* is 730 mg/ml. The minimum lethal dosage for intravenous injection of berberine in rats, mice, guinea pigs and rabbits is situated in the range of 27.5-250 mg/kg; intraperitoneal and subcutaneous injections did not significantly reduce toxicity. Methanol extracts of *Huang Lian* given to rats by intragastric administration for 11 weeks did not cause any changes in body weight, food intake or the weight of body organs.

Modern research

1. Different preparations of *Huang Lian* have a clearly-increased effect in inhibiting various micro-organisms such as staphylococci, streptococci, pneumococci and Bacillus anthracis.[35, 36]
2. The berberine contained in *Huang Lian* significantly inhibits the accumulation of thrombocytes,[37, 38] reduces the level of blood lipids[39, 40] and lowers the blood sugar level.[41]
3. Abates fever[42] and inhibits carcinoma.[43, 44]

Combinations and applications

Functions	Combinations	Applications
Clearing heat and drying dampness	*Bai Shao* (Radix Paeoniae Lactiflorae) *Huang Qin* (Radix Scutellariae Baicalensis) *Ma Chi Xian* (Herba Portulacae Oleraceae) *Mu Xiang* (Radix Aucklandiae Lappae) (see notes on legal status)	Damp-heat dysentery with pain in the abdomen and diarrhoea, a burning sensation in the anus, abdominal urgency and tenesmus, and yellow, slimy tongue fur
	Yu Jin (Radix Curcumae) *Yin Chen Hao* (Herba Artemisiae Scopariae) *Zi He Che* (Placenta Hominis)	Damp-heat jaundice with pain in the hypochondrium, and yellow, slimy tongue fur
Clearing Heart-fire and eliminating vexation	*Wu Zhu Yu* (Fructus Evodiae Rutaecarpae)	Vomiting due to Liver-fire or Stomach-heat
	Zhu Sha (Cinnabaris) (see notes on legal status) *Sheng Di Huang* (Radix Rehmanniae Glutinosae) *Zhi Zi* (Fructus Gardeniae Jasminoidis)	Vexation, profuse dreaming or insomnia, palpitations and fearful throbbing caused by effulgent Yin deficiency-fire

	Dan Zhu Ye (Herba Lophatheri Gracilis) *Mu Tong* (Caulis Mutong) (see notes on legal status)	Mouth sores due to flaming upwards of Heart-fire
Draining fire and relieving toxicity	*Dan Zhu Ye* (Herba Lophatheri Gracilis) *Lian Zi Xin* (Plumula Nelumbinis Nuciferae) *Lian Qiao* (Fructus Forsythiae Suspensae) *Zhi Zi* (Fructus Gardeniae Jasminoidis)	High fever, vexation and thirst in the course of warm diseases with a red tongue and yellow fur
	Bai Mao Gen (Rhizoma Imperatae Cylindricae) *Da Huang* (Radix et Rhizoma Rhei) *Huang Qin* (Radix Scutellariae Baicalensis)	Coughing of blood and nosebleed due to exuberant Heart-fire
	Da Huang (Radix et Rhizoma Rhei) *Sheng Di Huang* (Radix Rehmanniae Glutinosae) *Shi Gao* (Gypsum Fibrosum)	Painful and swollen gums, bad breath, constipation and yellow tongue fur due to exuberant Stomach-fire
	Shan Yao (Rhizoma Dioscoreae Oppositae) *Tian Hua Fen* (Radix Trichosanthis) *Ku Shen* (Radix Sophorae Flavescentis) *Sheng Di Huang* (Radix Rehmanniae Glutinosae)	Swift digestion with rapid hungering, vexation and thirst due to exuberant Stomach-fire
	Huang Qin (Radix Scutellariae Baicalensis) *Chi Shao* (Radix Paeoniae Rubra) *Mu Dan Pi* (Cortex Moutan Radicis) *Huang Bai* (Cortex Phellodendri)	Sores due to heat toxins

Note: *Huang Lian* can also clear heat in the Liver to brighten the eyes. The herbal decoction is used externally as a wash for red, sore and swollen eyes, or acute conjunctivitis (wind-fire eye).

Huang Bai 黄柏
(Amur cork tree bark, Cortex Phellodendri)

Huang Bai is the bark of *Phellodendron chinense* Schneid. or *P. amurense* Rupr., family Rutaceae.

Main ingredients *Huang Bai* contains berberine, phellodendrine, magnoflorine, palmatine, jatrorrhizine, candicine, menisperine, obacunone, obaculactone, obacunonic acid, β-sitosterol, campesterol and dictamnolide.

Properties Taste: bitter; nature: cold.

Channels entered Kidney, Bladder and Large Intestine.

Functions and indications Clears heat and dries dampness, drains fire and relieves toxicity, and abates deficiency-heat. It is indicated for damp-heat dysentery, jaundice, red and white vaginal discharge due to damp-heat, heat Lin syndrome, wasting and thirsting, steaming bone disorder, seminal emission, leg Qi, mouth and tongue sores, itchy eczema, and sores.

Common dosage 3-10g, or 20g for large dosages; appropriate dosage for external application.

Precautions and contraindications Since *Huang Bai* is bitter and cold and can easily damage Stomach Qi, it should be used with caution in cases of Spleen and Stomach deficiency-cold.

Remarks Raw *Huang Bai* is used to clear heat and dry dampness; the herb fried with brine enters the Kidney channel and can be employed to eliminate steaming bone disorder and abate deficiency-heat; and charred *Huang Bai* (*Huang Bai Tan*) is effective in clearing heat and stopping bleeding and is used to treat blood in the urine and blood in the stool.

Comparison of functions *Huang Bai* (Cortex Phellodendri), *Huang Qin* (Radix Scutellariae Baicalensis) and *Huang Lian* (Rhizoma Coptidis) can all clear heat, dry dampness, drain fire and relieve toxicity. In the clinic, two of these herbs are often used in combination to accentuate their therapeutic effects in treating disorders due to damp-heat or patterns with exuberant heat toxins. *Huang Qin* is good at draining fire in the Lungs and has the effect of quieting the foetus. *Huang Lian* can drain fire in the Heart and Stomach and stops vomiting. *Huang Bai* can drain fire at the gate of vitality and is also effective in eliminating damp-heat in the Lower Jiao. It is said that '*Huang Qin* acts on the Upper Jiao, *Huang Lian* on the Middle Jiao and *Huang Bai* on the Lower Jiao'.

For additional comparisons, see *Ku Shen* (Radix Sophorae Flavescentis), *Long Dan Cao* (Radix Gentianae Scabrae) and *Chun Pi* (Cortex Ailanthi Altissimae).

Toxicity The LD_{50} for intraperitoneal injection in mice of *Huang Bai* is 2.7g/kg, that for phellodendrine is 0.52g/kg. Overdosage manifested as cessation of activity, no response to outside stimuli and rigid limbs.

Modern research

1. A decoction of *Huang Bai* inhibited various micro-organisms *in vitro* including Staphylococcus aureus, Staphylococcus albus, Streptococcus pneumoniae and Corynebacterium diphtheriae,[45] and influenza viruses.[46]
2. Lowers blood pressure.[47, 48]
3. The function of the heart is stimulated by small dosages of *Huang Bai* and inhibited by large dosages.[49]

Combinations and applications

Functions	Combinations	Applications
Clearing heat and drying dampness	*Huang Lian* (Rhizoma Coptidis) *Mu Xiang* (Radix Aucklandiae Lappae) (see notes on legal status) *Bai Tou Weng* (Radix Pulsatillae Chinensis) *Guang Huo Xiang* (Herba Pogostemi) *Bai Zhu* (Rhizoma Atractylodis Macrocephalae)	Diarrhoea and damp-heat dysentery
	Mu Tong (Caulis Mutong) (see notes on legal status) *Dan Zhu Ye* (Herba Lophatheri Gracilis) *Bian Xu* (Herba Polygoni Avicularis)	Lin syndrome due to damp-heat
	Yin Chen Hao (Herba Artemisiae Scopariae) *Da Huang* (Radix et Rhizoma Rhei)	Damp-heat jaundice
	Ku Shen (Radix Sophorae Flavescentis) *Cang Zhu* (Rhizoma Atractylodis)	White vaginal discharge due to damp-heat
	Huai Jiao (Fructus Sophorae Japonicae) *Di Yu* (Radix Sanguisorbae Officinalis)	Blood in the stool due to haemorrhoids, bitter taste in the mouth, dry throat, desire for cold drinks

	Cang Zhu (Rhizoma Atractylodis) *Yi Yi Ren* (Semen Coicis Lachrymajobi) *Niu Xi* (Radix Achyranthis Bidentatae) *Mu Gua* (Fructus Chaenomelis)	Wei syndrome and numbness of the lower limbs, difficulty in walking due to damp-heat damaging the sinews
Draining fire and relieving toxicity	*Zhi Zi* (Fructus Gardeniae Jasminoidis) *Mu Dan Pi* (Cortex Moutan Radicis) *Huang Qin* (Radix Scutellariae Baicalensis)	Sores due to heat toxins with local redness, swelling, pain and heat
	Ku Shen (Radix Sophorae Flavescentis) *Di Fu Zi* (Fructus Kochiae Scopariae) *Cang Zhu* (Rhizoma Atractylodis)	Eczema or impetigo (yellow water sores)
Abating deficiency-heat	*Sheng Di Huang* (Radix Rehmanniae Glutinosae) *Gui Ban* (Plastrum Testudinis) (see notes on legal status) *Zhi Mu* (Rhizoma Anemarrhenae Asphodeloidis) *Xuan Shen* (Radix Scrophulariae Ningpoensis) *Nü Zhen Zi* (Fructus Ligustri Lucidi)	Steaming bone disorder with tidal fever, night sweating and seminal emission due to effulgent Yin deficiency-fire

Ku Shen 苦参 (Flavescent sophora root, Radix Sophorae Flavescentis)

Ku Shen is the root of *Sophora flavescens* Ait., family Leguminosae.

Main ingredients *Ku Shen* contains alkaloids (including matrine, oxymatrine, isomatrine, sophocarpine, isosophocarpine, sophoramine, l-methylcytisine and l-anagyrine) and flavones (including kushenols, kurarinol, kuraridinol, kurarinone and kuraridin).

Properties Taste: bitter; nature: cold.

Channels entered Heart, Liver, Stomach, Large Intestine and Bladder.

Functions and indications Clears heat and dries dampness, dispels wind and kills worms, and promotes urination. It is indicated for jaundice, dysentery, vaginal discharge, pudendal itch, itchy skin, scabies and tinea, eczema, haemorrhoids and blood in the stool, and Lin syndrome due to damp-heat.

Common dosage 3-10g, or 30g for dermatological disorders; appropriate dosage for external application.

Precautions and contraindications

1. *Ku Shen* is contraindicated in cases of Spleen and Stomach deficiency-cold because of its bitter and cold properties.
2. *Ku Shen* is incompatible with *Li Lu* (Radix et Rhizoma Veratri).

Remarks According to traditional sources, large dosages or a continuous intake of *Ku Shen* may damage the Kidneys, manifestations being pain and a feeling of heaviness in the lumbar region.

Comparison of functions Both *Ku Shen* (Radix Sophorae Flavescentis) and *Huang Bai* (Cortex Phellodendri) can clear damp-heat in the Lower Jiao and are used for dysentery, jaundice and vaginal discharge. *Ku Shen* is also good at killing worms to relieve itching and treat scabies and tinea, whereas *Huang Bai* is good at draining fire at the gate of vitality to treat fever due to Yin deficiency.

For additional comparisons, see *Bai Xian Pi* (Cortex Dictamni Dasycarpi Radicis) and *She Chuang Zi* (Fructus Cnidii Monnieri).

Toxicity The LD_{50} for extracts of *Ku Shen* given to mice via intragastric administration is 14.5g/kg; the LD_{50} for subcutaneous injection of the matrine contained in the herb is 297 ± 18 mg/kg. Dogs given intramuscular injection of 200mg/kg of matrine were observed for six days, but apart from a slight sedative effect, no significant reaction was recorded.

Modern research

1. The oxymatrine contained in *Ku Shen* inhibits arrhythmia, increases the volume of coronary blood flow, alleviates cardiac ischaemia and reduces the level of blood lipids.[50]
2. The herb itself and the oxymatrine it contains inhibit bacteria (including Shigella shigae and Staphylococcus aureus), inflammation and allergy, and calm wheezing.[51]

Combinations and applications

Functions	Combinations	Applications
Clearing heat and drying dampness	*Mu Xiang* (Radix Aucklandiae Lappae) (see notes on legal status) *Bai Shao* (Radix Paeoniae Lactiflorae)	Damp-heat dysentery
	Yin Chen Hao (Herba Artemisiae Scopariae) *Zhi Zi* (Fructus Gardeniae Jasminoidis) *Chai Hu* (Radix Bupleuri)	Damp-heat jaundice with nausea and yellow, slimy tongue fur
	Huang Bai (Cortex Phellodendri) *Tu Fu Ling* (Rhizoma Smilacis Glabrae) *She Chuang Zi* (Fructus Cnidii Monnieri)	Thick and smelly vaginal discharge due to damp-heat
Dispelling wind and killing worms	*Fang Feng* (Radix Ledebouriellae Divaricatae) *Bai Xian Pi* (Cortex Dictamni Dasycarpi Radicis) *Chan Tui* (Periostracum Cicadae)	Itchy skin and eczema due to retention of damp-heat
	Huang Bai (Cortex Phellodendri) *Ming Fan* (Alumen)	Pudendal itch
	Po Xiao (Mirabilitum Non-Purum) *Ku Lian Pi* (Cortex Meliae Radicis) *Huai Hua* (Flos Sophorae Japonicae)	Haemorrhoids or soreness in the anal region
Promoting urination	*Huang Bai* (Cortex Phellodendri) *Shi Wei* (Folium Pyrrosiae) *Bai Mao Gen* (Rhizoma Imperatae Cylindricae)	Inhibited urination and scorching heat and pain during urination due to retention of damp-heat
	Dang Gui (Radix Angelicae Sinensis) *Bei Mu* (Bulbus Fritillariae)	Difficult urination during pregnancy

Long Dan Cao 龙胆草 (Chinese gentian root, Radix Gentianae Scabrae)

Long Dan Cao is the root and rhizome of *Gentiana scabra* Bge., *G. manshurica* Kitag., *G. triflora* Pall., *G. regescens* Franch. and several other species of the same genus, family Gentianaceae.

Main ingredients *Long Dan Cao* contains gentiopicrin, swertiamarin, sweroside, gentianose, gentianine, gentianidine, gentianol and β-sitosterol.

Properties Taste: bitter; nature: cold.

Channels entered Liver, Gallbladder and Stomach.

Functions and indications Clears heat and dries dampness, drains Liver-fire and settles fright. It is indicated for headache and red eyes, pain in the hypochondrium due to exuberant heat in the Liver channel, jaundice due to damp-heat in the Liver and Gallbladder, vaginal discharge, Lin syndrome due to damp-heat, agitation, and fright epilepsy.

Common dosage 3-6g, or 15g for large dosages; appropriate dosage of the herbal decoction or powder for external application.

Precautions and contraindications *Long Dan Cao* is contraindicated in cases of loose stool due to Spleen and Stomach deficiency.

Comparison of functions Both *Long Dan Cao* (Radix Gentianae Scabrae) and *Huang Bai* (Cortex Phellodendri) can clear damp-heat in the Lower Jiao. *Long Dan Cao* is good at draining full-fire from the Liver and Gallbladder to treat dizziness and red eyes. *Huang Bai* works well in draining fire at the gate of vitality to treat tidal fever and seminal emission.

For an additional comparison, see *Qin Jiao* (Radix Gentianae Macrophyllae).

Toxicity The LD_{50} (within 96 hours) for a single intraperitoneal injection in mice of large amounts of gentiopicrin is 2770 mg/kg. Intravenous injection in dogs of 500 mg/kg of gentiopicrin caused vomiting; when the amount was raised to 1000 mg/kg, death resulted.

Modern research

1. Protects the liver.[52]
2. An injection of *Long Dan Cao* in rabbits produced a clear diuretic effect.[52]

Combinations and applications

Functions	Combinations	Applications
Clearing heat and drying dampness	*Zhi Zi* (Fructus Gardeniae Jasminoidis) *Mu Tong* (Caulis Mutong) (see notes on legal status) *Che Qian Zi* (Semen Plantaginis) *Chai Hu* (Radix Bupleuri) *Yin Chen Hao* (Herba Artemisiae Scopariae)	Fever, pain in the hypochondrium or jaundice due to damp-heat in the Liver and Gallbladder (e.g. in hepatitis or cholecystitis)
	Ku Shen (Radix Sophorae Flavescentis) *Huang Bai* (Cortex Phellodendri) *Che Qian Zi* (Semen Plantaginis)	Pudendal itch, white vaginal discharge and eczema due to damp-heat in the Lower Jiao
	Ze Xie (Rhizoma Alismatis Orientalis) *Mu Tong* (Caulis Mutong) (see notes on legal status) *Dan Zhu Ye* (Herba Lophatheri Gracilis)	Lin syndrome due to damp-heat, manifesting as frequent urination, urinary urgency and scorching heat in the urethra

	Niu Xi (Radix Achyranthis Bidentatae) *Huang Bai* (Cortex Phellodendri) *Cang Zhu* (Rhizoma Atractylodis) *Mu Gua* (Fructus Chaenomelis)	Damp-heat pouring down, manifesting as red, sore and swollen knees and feet, and oedema in leg Qi
Draining Liver-fire and settling fright	*Zhi Zi* (Fructus Gardeniae Jasminoidis) *Chai Hu* (Radix Bupleuri) *Ze Xie* (Rhizoma Alismatis Orientalis) *Mu Tong* (Caulis Mutong) (see notes on legal status) *Huang Qin* (Radix Scutellariae Baicalensis)	Headache, dizziness, pain in the hypochondrium, red eyes and deafness due to full-fire in the Liver and Gallbladder
	Gou Teng (Ramulus Uncariae cum Uncis) *Ling Yang Jiao* (Cornu Antelopis) (see notes on legal status) *Huang Lian* (Rhizoma Coptidis)	High fever and convulsions due to exuberant heat in the Liver channel
	Zi He Che (Placenta Hominis) *Niu Huang* (Calculus Bovis) *Gou Teng* (Ramulus Uncariae cum Uncis)	Fever in children, vexation and agitation
	Jue Ming Zi (Semen Cassiae) *Ju Hua* (Flos Chrysanthemi Morifolii) *Xia Ku Cao* (Spica Prunellae Vulgaris)	Red, sore and swollen eyes, aversion to light and eye discharge due to flaming upwards of Liver-fire

Qin Pi 秦皮 (Ash bark, Cortex Fraxini)

Qin Pi is the dried bark of *Fraxinus rhynchophylla* Hance., *F. chinensis* Roxb., *F. chinensis* Roxb. var. *acuminata* Lingelsh. or *F. stylosa* Lingelsh., family Oleaceae.

Main ingredients *Qin Pi* contains fraxetin, fraxin, aesculetin, aesculin and tannin.

Properties Taste: bitter; nature: cold.

Channels entered Liver, Gallbladder and Large Intestine.

Functions and indications Clears heat and relieves toxicity, clears Liver-fire and brightens the eyes. It is indicated for dysentery due to pathogenic heat toxins, red, sore and swollen eyes, and blurred vision.

Common dosage 3-12g.

Precautions and contraindications *Qin Pi* is contraindicated in cases of Spleen and Stomach deficiency-cold.

Comparison of functions Both *Qin Pi* (Cortex Fraxini) and *Ju Hua* (Flos Chrysanthemi Morifolii) can treat red, sore and swollen eyes and eye screen. *Qin Pi* is suitable for treating red, sore and swollen eyes due to depressed fire in the Liver and Gallbladder attacking upwards, whereas *Ju Hua* is good at treating this condition when it is caused by wind-heat in the Liver channel with lacrimation and aversion to light.

Toxicity The fraxetin and aesculin contained in *Qin Pi* are relatively non-toxic; the LD_{50} for intragastric administration to mice of aesculin is 11.5g/kg, that of fraxetin is 2.39g/kg. No toxic effects were observed in mice fed 1g/kg of fraxetin once a day for two weeks.

Modern research

1. Decoctions of *Qin Pi* inhibited various micro-organisms *in vitro* including Staphylococcus aureus, Bacterium coli and Shigella shigae.[53]
2. Can inhibit influenza viruses.[54]
3. The aesculetin contained in *Qin Pi* has an obvious pain-relieving action.[55]

Combinations and applications

Functions	Combinations	Applications
Clearing heat and relieving toxicity	*Bai Tou Weng* (Radix Pulsatillae Chinensis) *Huang Lian* (Rhizoma Coptidis) *Huang Bai* (Cortex Phellodendri)	Dysentery due to heat toxins, abdominal urgency and tenesmus
	Mu Dan Pi (Cortex Moutan Radicis) *Dang Gui* (Radix Angelicae Sinensis)	Red vaginal discharge due to damp-heat pouring down
Clearing Liver-fire and brightening the eyes	*Ju Hua* (Flos Chrysanthemi Morifolii) *Huang Lian* (Rhizoma Coptidis) *Dan Zhu Ye* (Herba Lophatheri Gracilis)	Red, sore and swollen eyes

Note: A decoction of *Qin Pi* on its own can be used as an external wash to treat red, sore and swollen eyes due to Liver-fire.

Bai Xian Pi 白鲜皮
(Dittany root bark, Cortex Dictamni Dasycarpi Radicis)

Bai Xian Pi is the dried root bark of *Dictamnus dasycarpus* Turcz., family Rutaceae.

Main ingredients *Bai Xian Pi* contains dictamnine, dictamnolactone (or obaculactone), obacunone, trigonelline, choline, dictamnolide, fraxinellone and sitosterols.

Properties Taste: bitter; nature: cold.

Channels entered Spleen and Stomach.

Functions and indications Clears heat and relieves toxicity, dispels wind and dries dampness. It is indicated for sores caused by pathogenic wind-heat or damp-heat toxins, scabies, wind papules, and jaundice and Bi syndrome due to pathogenic damp-heat.

Common dosage 6-10g; appropriate dosage for external application.

Precautions and contraindications As *Bai Xian Pi* is bitter and cold, it should be used with caution for patients with deficiency-cold.

Comparison of functions Both *Bai Xian Pi* (Cortex Dictamni Dasycarpi Radicis) and *Ku Shen* (Radix Sophorae Flavescentis) can dispel and eliminate damp-heat, relieve itching and abate jaundice and are used for eczema and jaundice. However, *Bai Xian Pi* can also free and benefit the joints to treat damp-heat Bi syndrome, whereas *Ku Shen* is good at treating diarrhoea, dysentery and vaginal discharge.

Modern research

1. Preparations of *Bai Xian Pi* inhibit fungi, particularly ringworm.[56]
2. The dictamnine contained in *Bai Xian Pi* can promote contraction of the uterus in rabbits and guinea pigs.[57]
3. Inhibits arrhythmia.[57]
4. The volatile oils contained in *Bai Xian Pi* inhibit carcinoma.[58, 59]

Combinations and applications

Functions	Combinations	Applications
Clearing heat and relieving toxicity, dispelling wind and drying dampness	*Ku Shen* (Radix Sophorae Flavescentis) *Huang Bai* (Cortex Phellodendri)	Itchy sores due to damp toxins

Cang Zhu (Rhizoma Atractylodis) *Huang Bai* (Cortex Phellodendri) *Niu Xi* (Radix Achyranthis Bidentatae)	Wind-damp-heat Bi syndrome, and red, swollen, hot and painful joints
Yin Chen Hao (Herba Artemisiae Scopariae) *Zhi Zi* (Fructus Gardeniae Jasminoidis)	Damp-heat jaundice

Note: A decoction of *Bai Xian Pi* and *She Chuang Zi* (Fructus Cnidii Monnieri) can be used as an external wash to treat itchy skin and scabies.

HERBS FOR CLEARING HEAT AND RELIEVING TOXICITY

Most herbs for clearing heat and relieving toxicity are cold or cool. They have the functions of clearing fire or heat pathogenic factors, relieving toxicity and dispersing swelling. They are used for disorders caused by heat toxins and fire toxins in the Zang-Fu organs and the channels and sinews; such disorders include sores, abscesses, erysipelas, sore and swollen throat, mumps, dysentery and snake bites.

Herbs for clearing heat and relieving toxicity are divided into various categories according to their characteristics. Hence, proper selection and combination are of the utmost importance:

1. in cases of heat toxins in the Xue level, these herbs should be used in combination with herbs for clearing heat and cooling the Blood;
2. in cases of full-heat and fire in the Qi level, they should be used together with herbs for clearing heat and draining fire;
3. in cases of pathogenic damp, they should be applied in combination with herbs for clearing heat and drying dampness or with aromatic herbs for transforming dampness;
4. in cases of sores due to deficiency of Qi and Blood, they should be used together with herbs for supplementing Qi and nourishing the Blood;
5. in cases of pain in the abdomen due to dysentery and tenesmus, they should be used in combination with herbs for regulating Qi, clearing heat and drying dampness;
6. in cases of abscesses and sores, or a sore, swollen throat and mouth sores, they are to be used together with substances for external application.

This kind of herb is not suitable in cases of cold-type and Yin-deficiency-type maculopapular eruptions or dysentery due to cold.

Tab. 2.3 Herbs for clearing heat and relieving toxicity

Herb	Functions	Indications
Jin Yin Hua (Flos Lonicerae)	Clearing heat and relieving toxicity, dissipating wind-heat, cooling the Blood and stopping dysentery	Sores occurring in the initial stage of warm diseases or resulting from infections caused by externally-contracted wind-heat, dysentery due to heat toxins
Lian Qiao (Fructus Forsythiae Suspensae)	Clearing Heart-fire, relieving the toxicity of sores, dissipating externally-contracted wind-heat	Headache due to wind-heat, abscesses and sores due to the retention of heat toxins, scrofula, mouth and tongue sores and a sore and swollen throat due to Heart-fire flaming upwards
Pu Gong Ying (Herba Taraxaci cum Radice)	Clearing heat and relieving toxicity, dissipating lumps and dispersing abscesses	Breast abscess, Lung abscess, Intestinal abscess, scrofula and Phlegm nodes, abscesses and sores due to heat toxins, sore and swollen throat, red, sore and swollen eyes due to an attack of heat toxins, damp-heat jaundice, heat Lin syndrome
Zi Hua Di Ding (Herba Violae Yedoensitis)	Clearing heat and relieving toxicity, dispersing swelling	Red, sore and swollen eyes, sore and swollen throat, dysentery, sores, abscesses, poisonous snake bites, scrofula

Ban Lan Gen (Radix Isatidis seu Baphicacanthi)	Clearing heat and relieving toxicity, cooling the Blood and benefiting the throat	Macular eruptions, sore and swollen throat, epidemic diseases with swollen throat, mumps, mouth sores, abscesses, erysipelas due to heat toxins
Da Qing Ye (Folium Isatidis seu Baphicacanthi)	Clearing heat and relieving toxicity, cooling the Blood and dispersing swelling	Vigorous fever, delirious speech, vexation and agitation, maculopapular eruptions caused by warm diseases invading the Xue level, vomiting of blood, abscesses, sore and swollen throat, mouth sores
Qing Dai (Indigo Naturalis)	Clearing heat and relieving toxicity, cooling the Blood and settling fright	Full-heat in the course of febrile diseases, macular eruptions, coughing of blood, child fright epilepsy, erysipelas, mouth sores
Yu Xing Cao (Herba Houttuyniae Cordatae)	Clearing heat and relieving toxicity, expelling pus and dispersing abscesses, promoting urination and freeing Lin syndrome	Lung abscess, cough due to Lung-heat, dysentery, Lin syndrome, haemorrhoids, vaginal discharge, abscesses, clove sores
She Gan (Rhizoma Belamcandae Chinensis)	Clearing heat and relieving toxicity, dispelling Phlegm and benefiting the throat, dispersing swelling and dissipating lumps	Sore and swollen throat, cough with copious sputum due to Lung-heat, scrofula, abscesses and sores
Bai Tou Weng (Radix Pulsatillae Chinensis)	Clearing heat and relieving toxicity, stopping dysentery, cooling the Blood and stopping bleeding	Dysentery due to heat toxins or damp-heat
Ye Ju Hua (Flos Chrysanthemi Indici)	Clearing heat and relieving toxicity, dispersing swelling, lowering blood pressure	Red, sore and swollen eyes, sore and swollen throat, abscesses and sores, hypertension
Chuan Xin Lian (Herba Andrographitis Paniculatae)	Clearing heat and relieving toxicity, promoting urination and dispersing swelling	Coughing and wheezing due to Lung-heat, Lung abscess, sore and swollen throat, damp-heat dysentery, Lin syndrome due to pathogenic damp-heat, eczema, sores, erysipelas, poisonous snake bites
Chong Lou (Rhizoma Paridis)	Clearing heat and relieving toxicity, dispersing swelling and alleviating pain, extinguishing wind and settling fright, transforming stasis and stopping bleeding	Swollen and toxic abscesses and sores, poisonous snake bites, fright epilepsy, convulsions, clouded Spirit, bleeding or pain due to injury caused by stasis and swelling
Ban Bian Lian (Herba Lobeliae Chinensis cum Radice)	Clearing heat and relieving toxicity, promoting urination and dispersing swelling	Poisonous snake bites, insect stings, swelling and pain in the initial stage of clove sores, ascites, puffy swelling of the face and eyes
Tu Fu Ling (Rhizoma Smilacis Glabrae)	Clearing heat and relieving toxicity, dispelling dampness and eliminating Bi syndrome	Convulsion of the limbs due to syphilis or to the mercury used to treat syphilis, abscesses and sores due to fire toxins, inhibited and painful voidings of reddish urine due to heat Lin syndrome, goitre

Guan Zhong (Rhizoma Dryopteris Crassirhizomae)	Killing worms, clearing heat and relieving toxicity, cooling the Blood and stopping bleeding	Pain in the abdomen due to worms, abscesses and sores due to heat toxins, bleeding patterns
Shan Dou Gen (Radix Sophorae Tonkinensis)	Clearing heat and relieving toxicity, benefiting the throat and alleviating pain	Sore and swollen throat, cough due to Lung-heat, sores, painful and swollen gums
Ma Bo (Sclerotium Lasiosphaerae seu Calvatiae)	Clearing heat and relieving toxicity, benefiting the throat and alleviating pain, stopping bleeding	Sore and swollen throat, loss of voice, coughing of blood, nosebleed
Ma Chi Xian (Herba Portulacae Oleraceae)	Clearing heat and relieving toxicity, stopping dysentery, cooling the Blood and stopping bleeding	Damp-heat dysentery with purulent and bloody stool, heat Lin syndrome, blood Lin syndrome, abscesses and sores
Ya Dan Zi (Fructus Bruceae Javanicae)	Clearing heat and relieving toxicity, stopping dysentery, interrupting malaria, putrefying and consuming warts	Benign tertian malaria or quartan malaria, bloody dysentery due to heat toxins, corns and warts
Bai Hua She She Cao (Herba Hedyotidis Diffusae)	Clearing heat and relieving toxicity, quickening the Blood, dispersing abscesses, promoting urination and abating jaundice	Cough due to Lung-heat, sore and swollen throat, abscesses and sores, poisonous snake bites, dysentery, jaundice, heat Lin syndrome, difficult urination
Mu Hu Die (Semen Oroxyli Indici)	Clearing the Lungs and restoring the voice, allowing constrained Liver Qi to flow freely and harmonizing the Stomach	Sore and swollen throat, hoarse voice, cough, pain in the stomach due to Liver depression and Qi stagnation
Lou Lu (Radix Rhapontici seu Echinopsis)	Clearing heat and relieving toxicity, dispersing swelling, causing milk to descend	Abscesses and sores, breast abscess and breast pain, insufficient lactation
Bai Jiang Cao (Herba Patriniae cum Radice)	Clearing heat and relieving toxicity, dispersing swelling and expelling pus, quickening the Blood and dissipating stasis	Lung abscess, Intestinal abscess, dysentery, postpartum pain in the abdomen due to Blood stasis, red, sore and swollen eyes, abscesses and sores
Hong Teng (Caulis Sargentodoxae Cuneatae)	Clearing heat and relieving toxicity, quickening the Blood and alleviating pain	Intestinal abscess with pain in the abdomen, swollen abscesses due to heat toxins, knocks and falls, painful menstruation, menstrual block, wind-damp Bi syndrome pain
Bai Lian (Radix Ampelopsis Japonicae)	Clearing heat and relieving toxicity, dispersing abscesses and dissipating lumps, generating flesh and alleviating pain	Abscesses and sores, scrofula and haemorrhoids
Lü Dou (Semen Phaseoli Radiati)	Clearing heat and relieving toxicity, clearing summerheat and promoting the movement of water	Vexation and thirst due to summerheat; abscesses and sores, oedema, diarrhoea; and relieving the toxicity caused by food poisoning and the taking of certain materia medica

Jin Yin Hua 金银花
(Honeysuckle flower, Flos Lonicerae)

Jin Yin Hua is the flower bud and flower of *Lonicera japonica* Thunb., *L. hypoglauca* Miq., *L. confusa* DC., or *L. dasystyla* Rehd., family Caprifoliaceae.

Main ingredients *Jin Yin Hua* contains inositol, flavones, saponins and tannin. The leaves contain luteolin, lonicerin and tannin. The stem contains saponins.

Properties Taste: sweet; nature: cold.

Channels entered Lung, Stomach, Heart and Large Intestine.

Functions and indications Clears heat and relieves toxicity, dissipates wind-heat, and cools the Blood and stops dysentery. It is indicated for sores occurring in the initial stage of warm diseases or resulting from infections caused by externally-contracted wind-heat, and for dysentery due to heat toxins.

Common dosage 10-30g, or 60g for large dosages (not suitable for decoction for a long period); appropriate dosage for external application.

Precautions and contraindications *Jin Yin Hua* is contraindicated in cases of diarrhoea due to Spleen and Stomach deficiency-cold, and for sores with watery pus, where these sores are not due to heat toxins.

Comparison of functions See *Lian Qiao* (Fructus Forsythiae Suspensae).

Toxicity Rabbits and dogs given aqueous preparations of *Jin Yin Hua* via intragastric administration showed no toxic reaction in terms of respiration, blood pressure or the quantity of urine produced. The LD_{50} for subcutaneous injection in mice of extracts of *Jin Yin Hua* is 53g/kg. Although the chlorogenic acid contained in *Jin Yin Hua* can produce an allergic reaction, this reaction is avoided by oral administration.

Modern research

1. Aqueous extracts of *Jin Yin Hua* can inhibit bacteria (including Staphylococcus aureus and Salmonella typhi) and influenza viruses.[60, 61]
2. Inhibits inflammation.[62]
3. Alcoholic extracts of *Jin Yin Hua* can induce abortion in the early stages of pregnancy.[63]

Combinations and applications

Functions	Combinations	Applications
Clearing heat and relieving toxicity	*Yu Xing Cao* (Herba Houttuyniae Cordatae) *Gua Lou* (Fructus Trichosanthis) *Xing Ren* (Semen Pruni Armeniacae) *Shi Gao* (Gypsum Fibrosum)	Fever, cough with yellow sputum, rapid breathing and pain in the chest
	Pu Gong Ying (Herba Taraxaci cum Radice) *Zi Hua Di Ding* (Herba Violae Yedoensitis) *Lian Qiao* (Fructus Forsythiae Suspensae) *Bai Zhi* (Radix Angelicae Dahuricae) *Gan Cao* (Radix Glycyrrhizae)	Abscesses and clove sores with local redness, swelling, pain and heat
	Huang Qi (Radix Astragali seu Hedysari)	Swollen abscesses which have not ulcerated or where discharge of pus is difficult
	Huang Qi (Radix Astragali seu Hedysari) *Dang Gui* (Radix Angelicae Sinensis) *Gan Cao* (Radix Glycyrrhizae)	Swollen and painful breast abscess

	Pu Gong Ying (Herba Taraxaci cum Radice) *Bai Jiang Cao* (Herba Patriniae cum Radice) *Mu Dan Pi* (Cortex Moutan Radicis) *Da Huang* (Radix et Rhizoma Rhei)	Intestinal abscess
	Yu Xing Cao (Herba Houttuyniae Cordatae) *Hong Teng* (Caulis Sargentodoxae Cuneatae) *Lu Gen* (Rhizoma Phragmitis Communis) *Jie Geng* (Radix Platycodi Grandiflori)	Lung abscess with coughing and spitting of pus and blood
Dissipating wind-heat	*Lian Qiao* (Fructus Forsythiae Suspensae) *Bo He* (Herba Menthae Haplocalycis) *Niu Bang Zi* (Fructus Arctii Lappae) *Jing Jie Sui* (Spica Schizonepetae Tenuifoliae)	Fever and headache, sore and swollen throat, and a floating and rapid pulse due to externally-contracted wind-heat or in the initial stage of warm diseases
	Sang Ye (Folium Mori Albae) *Niu Bang Zi* (Fructus Arctii Lappae) *Zhi Zi* (Fructus Gardeniae Jasminoidis) *Jue Ming Zi* (Semen Cassiae)	Red, sore and swollen eyes due to wind-heat attacking upwards into the eyes
	Xiang Ru (Herba Elsholtziae seu Moslae) *Hou Po* (Cortex Magnoliae Officinalis) *Lian Qiao* (Fructus Forsythiae Suspensae)	Fever, vexation and thirst, and headache without sweating due to summerheat-damp
Cooling the Blood and stopping dysentery	*Huang Qin* (Radix Scutellariae Baicalensis) *Mu Xiang* (Radix Aucklandiae Lappae) (see notes on legal status) *Bai Tou Weng* (Radix Pulsatillae Chinensis) *Huang Lian* (Rhizoma Coptidis)	Bloody dysentery due to heat toxins, fever with pain in the abdomen, blood in the stool, abdominal urgency and tenesmus
	Niu Xi (Radix Achyranthis Bidentatae) *Tu Fu Ling* (Rhizoma Smilacis Glabrae) *Gan Cao* (Radix Glycyrrhizae)	Blood Lin syndrome, stone Lin syndrome

Appendix

Ren Dong Teng 忍冬藤 (Honeysuckle stem, Caulis Lonicerae Japonicae)

Ren Dong Teng (also known as *Jin Yin Teng*) is the stem and leaves of *Lonicera japonica* Thunb. Its functions and properties are very similar to those of *Jin Yin Hua*, but its function in relieving toxicity is weaker. However, it is very effective in freeing the channels and network vessels and can eliminate wind-heat from the channels to alleviate Bi syndrome pain. It is usually used with *Sang Zhi* (Ramulus Mori Albae), *Du Huo* (Radix Angelicae Pubescentis), *Fang Ji* (Radix Stephaniae Tetrandrae) and *Yi Yi Ren* (Semen Coicis Lachrymajobi) to treat wind-damp-heat Bi syndrome with red, swollen, hot and painful joints, and inhibited bending and stretching (for *Fang Ji*, see notes on legal status). The dosage is 15-30g.

Lian Qiao 连翘
(Forsythia fruit, Fructus Forsythiae Suspensae)

Lian Qiao is the fruit of *Forsythia suspensa* (Thunb.) Vahl., family Oleaceae.

Main ingredients *Lian Qiao* contains forsythol, forsythoside, phillyrin, betulinic acid, oleanolic acid, ursolic acid, pinoresinol, matairesinoside and volatile oils.

Properties Taste: bitter; nature: slightly cold.

Channels entered Lung, Heart, Liver and Gallbladder.

Functions and indications Clears Heart-fire, relieves the toxicity of sores, and dissipates externally-contracted wind-heat. It is indicated for headache due to wind-heat, abscesses and sores due to the retention of heat toxins, scrofula, and mouth and tongue sores and a sore and swollen throat due to Heart-fire flaming upwards.

Common dosage 10-15g, or 30g for large dosages.

Precautions and contraindications *Lian Qiao* is contraindicated in cases of loose stool due to Spleen and Stomach deficiency-cold, or Yin abscesses with no pain or redness.

Comparison of functions Both *Lian Qiao* (Fructus Forsythiae Suspensae) and *Jin Yin Hua* (Flos Lonicerae) can thrust heat out towards the exterior and clear interior heat to relieve toxicity. They are often used in combination to treat externally-contracted wind-heat, the initial stage of warm diseases, and sores due to heat toxins. The difference is that *Lian Qiao*, being bitter and slightly cold, is more effective in clearing Heart-fire and relieving toxicity, as well as in dispersing abscesses and dissipating lumps and is a key herb for treating sores. On the other hand, the sweet taste and cold nature of *Jin Yin Hua* allow it to dissipate exterior heat without damage to the Stomach. Char-fried *Jin Yin Hua* can also cool the Blood and stop dysentery to treat bloody dysentery due to heat toxins.

Toxicity The LD_{50} for intraperitoneal injection of *Lian Qiao* in mice is 24.85g/kg.

Modern research

1. Decoctions of *Lian Qiao* and aqueous extracts of the herb can inhibit such bacteria as Shigella shigae and Staphylococcus aureus.[64]
2. The phillyrin contained in *Lian Qiao* can inhibit epiphytes.[65]
3. Inhibits inflammation, abates fever.[66]

Combinations and applications

Functions	Combinations	Applications
Clearing Heart-fire	*Xuan Shen* (Radix Scrophulariae Ningpoensis) *Lian Zi Xin* (Plumula Nelumbinis Nuciferae) *Shui Niu Jiao* (Cornu Bubali) *Huang Lian* (Rhizoma Coptidis)	High fever with delirious speech, clouded Spirit and vexation due to pathogenic heat invading the Heart in the course of warm-febrile diseases
	Dan Zhu Ye (Herba Lophatheri Gracilis) *Sheng Di Huang* (Radix Rehmanniae Glutinosae) *Shi Gao* (Gypsum Fibrosum) *Jin Yin Hua* (Flos Lonicerae)	Mouth sores, scant and yellow urine due to Heart-fire attacking the Small Intestine

	Mu Tong (Caulis Mutong) (see notes on legal status) *Ze Xie* (Rhizoma Alismatis Orientalis) *Bian Xu* (Herba Polygoni Avicularis) *Qing Ma Zi* (Semen Abutilonis Theophrasti)	Heat Lin syndrome (e.g. in cystitis, urethritis)
	Niu Bang Zi (Fructus Arctii Lappae) *Jie Geng* (Radix Platycodi Grandiflori) *Jin Yin Hua* (Flos Lonicerae) *Xuan Shen* (Radix Scrophulariae Ningpoensis)	Sore and swollen throat, mumps
Relieving the toxicity of sores	*Huang Lian* (Rhizoma Coptidis) *Dang Gui* (Radix Angelicae Sinensis) *Chi Shao* (Radix Paeoniae Rubra)	Hard, swollen sores due to heat toxins with no change in skin colour
	Jin Yin Hua (Flos Lonicerae) *Mu Dan Pi* (Cortex Moutan Radicis) *Pu Gong Ying* (Herba Taraxaci cum Radice) *Tian Hua Fen* (Radix Trichosanthis)	Breast abscess with local redness, pain and heat due to retention of heat toxins
	Xuan Shen (Radix Scrophulariae Ningpoensis) *Mu Li* (Concha Ostreae) *Xia Ku Cao* (Spica Prunellae Vulgaris)	Scrofula, Phlegm nodes
Dissipating externally-contracted wind-heat	*Jin Yin Hua* (Flos Lonicerae) *Jie Geng* (Radix Platycodi Grandiflori) *Lu Gen* (Rhizoma Phragmitis Communis) *Bo He* (Herba Menthae Haplocalycis)	Fever and headache, thirst and sore and swollen throat in the initial stage of febrile diseases with heat in the Upper Jiao

Pu Gong Ying 蒲公英 (Dandelion, Herba Taraxaci cum Radice)

Pu Gong Ying is the whole plant of *Taraxacum mongolicum* Hand.-Mazz. or other species of the same genus, family Compositae.

Main ingredients *Pu Gong Ying* contains taraxasterol, taraxol, taraxerol, taraxicin, inulin, choline and pectin.

Properties Taste: bitter and sweet; nature: cold.

Channels entered Liver and Stomach.

Functions and indications Clears heat and relieves toxicity, dissipates lumps and disperses abscesses. It is indicated for breast abscess, Lung abscess, Intestinal abscess, scrofula and Phlegm nodes, abscesses and sores due to heat toxins, sore and swollen throat, red, sore and swollen eyes due to an attack of heat toxins, damp-heat jaundice, and heat Lin syndrome.

Common dosage 10-30g, or 60g for large dosages; appropriate dosage for external application.

Precautions and contraindications *Pu Gong Ying* is contraindicated in cases of Yin abscesses or persistent skin sores. Overdosage may induce mild diarrhoea.

Comparison of functions See *Zi Hua Di Ding* (Herba Violae Yedoensitis) and *Bai Lian* (Radix Ampelopsis Japonicae).

Toxicity Side-effects from the use of *Pu Gong Ying* are rarely seen. However, intravenous injection in a few cases has led to shivering, a pallid complexion or symptoms of mental disorder. Intake of decoctions of *Pu Gong Ying* may cause a reaction in the gastrointestinal tract manifesting as nausea, vomiting, abdominal discomfort and diarrhoea, or urticaria (dormant papules) and generalized itching.

Modern research A decoction of *Pu Gong Ying* can inhibit such bacteria as Staphylococcus aureus and Streptococcus haemolyticus.[67]

Combinations and applications

Functions	Combinations	Applications
Clearing heat and relieving toxicity	*Long Dan Cao* (Radix Gentianae Scabrae) *Ju Hua* (Flos Chrysanthemi Morifolii) *Xia Ku Cao* (Spica Prunellae Vulgaris)	Red, sore and swollen eyes due to heat toxins
	Ban Lan Gen (Radix Isatidis seu Baphicacanthi) *Mu Dan Pi* (Cortex Moutan Radicis) *Xuan Shen* (Radix Scrophulariae Ningpoensis) *Lian Qiao* (Fructus Forsythiae Suspensae)	Sore and swollen throat due to heat toxins attacking upwards
	Jin Yin Hua (Flos Lonicerae) *Gua Lou* (Fructus Trichosanthis) *Sang Bai Pi* (Cortex Mori Albae Radicis) *Yu Xing Cao* (Herba Houttuyniae Cordatae)	Cough with yellow sputum, fever and thirst due to Lung-heat
	Jin Qian Cao (Herba Lysimachiae) *Bai Mao Gen* (Rhizoma Imperatae Cylindricae)	Heat Lin syndrome, difficult urination
Dissipating lumps and dispersing abscesses	*Ye Ju Hua* (Flos Chrysanthemi Indici) *Zi Hua Di Ding* (Herba Violae Yedoensitis) *Jin Yin Hua* (Flos Lonicerae)	Swelling and toxins of abscesses and clove sores
	Gua Lou (Fructus Trichosanthis) *Lu Lu Tong* (Fructus Liquidambaris) *Lian Qiao* (Fructus Forsythiae Suspensae) *Chuan Shan Jia* (Squama Manitis Pentadactylae) (see notes on legal status)	Breast abscess with swelling and pain
	Yu Xing Cao (Herba Houttuyniae Cordatae) *Lu Gen* (Rhizoma Phragmitis Communis) *Dong Gua Ren* (Semen Benincasae Hispidae) *Jie Geng* (Radix Platycodi Grandiflori)	Lung abscess and fever with purulent, yellow sputum
	Da Huang (Radix et Rhizoma Rhei) *Tao Ren* (Semen Persicae) *Mu Dan Pi* (Cortex Moutan Radicis) *Bai Jiang Cao* (Herba Patriniae cum Radice)	Intestinal abscess with pain in the abdomen
	Xia Ku Cao (Spica Prunellae Vulgaris) *Lian Qiao* (Fructus Forsythiae Suspensae) *Mu Li* (Concha Ostreae) *Zhe Bei Mu* (Bulbus Fritillariae Thunbergii)	Scrofula and Phlegm nodes

	Chong Lou (Rhizoma Paridis) *Ye Ju Hua* (Flos Chrysanthemi Indici) *Bai Zhi* (Radix Angelicae Dahuricae) *Lian Qiao* (Fructus Forsythiae Suspensae)	Clove sores due to heat toxins

Note: A decoction of *Pu Gong Ying* can be used as a steam-wash for the eyes to treat red, sore and swollen eyes, aversion to light and profuse lacrimation due to Liver-fire flaming upwards.

Zi Hua Di Ding 紫花地丁 (Chinese violet, Herba Violae Yedoensitis)

Zi Hua Di Ding is the dried whole plant of *Viola yedoensis* Makino, family Violaceae.

Main ingredients *Zi Hua Di Ding* contains palmitic acid, p-hydroxybenzoic acid and cerotic acid.

Properties Taste: acrid and bitter; nature: cold.

Channels entered Heart and Liver.

Functions and indications Clears heat and relieves toxicity, and disperses swelling. It is indicated for red, sore and swollen eyes, sore and swollen throat, dysentery, sores, abscesses, poisonous snake bites, and scrofula.

Common dosage 10-15g; appropriate dosage for external application.

Precautions and contraindications *Zi Hua Di Ding* is contraindicated for Yin abscesses.

Comparison of functions Both *Zi Hua Di Ding* (Herba Violae Yedoensitis) and *Pu Gong Ying* (Herba Taraxaci cum Radice) are important herbs for clearing heat and relieving toxicity to treat sores due to heat toxins and are often used together for Yang-type sores. *Pu Gong Ying* is better at dispersing swelling and dissipating lumps, and works well in the treatment of breast abscesses, whereas *Zi Hua Di Ding* is highly effective in relieving toxicity and is an important herb for dispersing abscesses and sores, being especially good at relieving the toxicity of clove sores.

For an additional comparison, see *Chong Lou* (Rhizoma Paridis).

Modern research

1. Decoctions of *Zi Hua Di Ding* can inhibit Staphylococcus aureus, Streptococcus haemolyticus, Pseudomonas aeruginosa, Salmonella typhi and Mycobacterium tuberculosis.[68]
2. Inhibits leptospirosis.[69]

Combinations and applications

Functions	Combinations	Applications
Clearing heat and relieving toxicity, dispersing swelling	*Jin Yin Hua* (Flos Lonicerae) *Ye Ju Hua* (Flos Chrysanthemi Indici)	Swollen abscesses and clove sores due to exuberant heat toxins
	Ju Hua (Flos Chrysanthemi Morifolii) *Chan Tui* (Periostracum Cicadae)	Red, sore and swollen eyes
	Pu Gong Ying (Herba Taraxaci cum Radice) *Ye Ju Hua* (Flos Chrysanthemi Indici) *Jin Yin Hua* (Flos Lonicerae)	Breast abscess
	Huang Qin (Radix Scutellariae Baicalensis) *Hong Teng* (Caulis Sargentodoxae Cuneatae)	Dysentery

Functions	Combinations	Applications
	Dan Shen (Radix Salviae Miltiorrhizae) *Che Qian Cao* (Herba Plantaginis) *Hai Jin Sha* (Spora Lygodii Japonici)	Inflammation of the prostate gland
	Hong Teng (Caulis Sargentodoxae Cuneatae) *Bai Hua She She Cao* (Herba Hedyotidis Diffusae) *Da Huang* (Radix et Rhizoma Rhei)	Intestinal abscess

Ban Lan Gen 板蓝根 (Isatis root, Radix Isatidis seu Baphicacanthi)

Ban Lan Gen is the root of *Isatis indigotica* Fort., family Cruciferae, or *Baphicacanthus cusia* (Nees) Bremek., family Acanthaceae.

Main ingredients *Ban Lan Gen* contains indoxyl-β-glucoside, isatin and β-sitosterol.

Properties Taste: bitter; nature: cold.

Channels entered Heart, Lung and Stomach.

Functions and indications Clears heat and relieves toxicity, cools the Blood and benefits the throat. It is indicated for macular eruptions, sore and swollen throat, epidemic diseases with swollen throat, mumps, mouth sores, abscesses, and erysipelas due to heat toxins.

Common dosage 15-30g, or 60-120g for large dosages.

Precautions and contraindications *Ban Lan Gen* should be used with caution for weak patients and in the absence of fire toxins.

Comparison of functions See *Qing Dai* (Indigo Naturalis) and *Guan Zhong* (Rhizoma Dryopteris Crassirhizomae).

Modern research Inhibits such bacteria as Staphylococcus aureus, Escherichia coli, Shigella shigae and Salmonella enteridis.[70, 71]

Combinations and applications

Functions	Combinations	Applications
Clearing heat and relieving toxicity	*Jin Yin Hua* (Flos Lonicerae) *Lian Qiao* (Fructus Forsythiae Suspensae) *Jing Jie* (Herba Schizonepetae Tenuifoliae)	Externally-contracted wind-heat or the initial stage of febrile diseases with such manifestations as headache, fever, and sore and swollen throat
	Shan Ci Gu (Pseudobulbus Shancigu) *Lian Qiao* (Fructus Forsythiae Suspensae) *Qing Dai* (Indigo Naturalis)	Mumps due to externally-contracted wind-heat
	Jin Yin Hua (Flos Lonicerae) *Da Huang* (Radix et Rhizoma Rhei) *Huang Bai* (Cortex Phellodendri) *Gan Cao* (Radix Glycyrrhizae)	Mouth sores, erysipelas and abscesses due to exuberant internal heat toxins

	Sheng Di Huang (Radix Rehmanniae Glutinosae) *Mu Dan Pi* (Cortex Moutan Radicis) *Chi Shao* (Radix Paeoniae Rubra) *Xuan Shen* (Radix Scrophulariae Ningpoensis) *Ma Bo* (Sclerotium Lasiosphaerae seu Calvatiae)	Macular eruptions due to warm toxins, massive febrile disorder of the head with red, sore and swollen head and face
Cooling the Blood and benefiting the throat	*Bo He* (Herba Menthae Haplocalycis) *Lian Qiao* (Fructus Forsythiae Suspensae) *Niu Bang Zi* (Fructus Arctii Lappae)	Sore and swollen throat due to the flaming upwards of heat toxins

Da Qing Ye 大青叶 (Woad leaf, Folium Isatidis seu Baphicacanthi)

Da Qing Ye is the dried leaf of *Isatis indigotica* Fort., family Cruciferae, or *Baphicacanthus cusia* (Nees) Bremek., family Acanthaceae.

Main ingredients *Da Qing Ye* contains tryptophan, isatan B, glucobrassicin, neoglucobrassicin, glucobrassicin-1-sulphonate, indigotin, adenosine, sitosterols, palmitic acid and sucrose (*Isatis indigotica*); indican, indoxyl and indirubin (*Baphicacanthus cusia*).

Properties Taste: bitter; nature: extremely cold.

Channels entered Heart, Lung and Stomach.

Functions and indications Clears heat and relieves toxicity, cools the Blood and disperses swelling. It is indicated for vigorous fever, delirious speech, vexation and agitation, maculopapular eruptions caused by warm diseases invading the Xue level, vomiting of blood, abscesses, sore and swollen throat, and mouth sores.

Common dosage 10-15g; appropriate dosage for external application.

Precautions and contraindications *Da Qing Ye* is contraindicated in cases of Spleen and Stomach deficiency-cold.

Comparison of functions See *Qing Dai* (Indigo Naturalis) and *Chuan Xin Lian* (Herba Andrographitis Paniculatae).

Toxicity Acute toxicity tests on animals indicated that the indoxyl glucoside contained in *Da Qing Ye* produced no significant toxic reaction in terms of respiration, blood pressure, cardiac function and the central nervous system.

Modern research

1. Inhibits many kinds of bacteria and viruses such as Streptococcus pneumoniae, Staphylococcus aureus and encephalitis B.[72]
2. Inhibits inflammation and abates fever.[73]

Combinations and applications

Functions	Combinations	Applications
Clearing heat and relieving toxicity, cooling the Blood and dispersing swelling	*Zhi Zi* (Fructus Gardeniae Jasminoidis) *Jin Yin Hua* (Flos Lonicerae) *Lian Qiao* (Fructus Forsythiae Suspensae)	High fever, vexation and agitation and maculopapular eruptions in warm diseases with heat invading the Xue level

Jin Yin Hua (Flos Lonicerae) *Mu Dan Pi* (Cortex Moutan Radicis)	Massive febrile disorder of the head with red, sore and swollen head and face
Shan Dou Gen (Radix Sophorae Tonkinensis) *She Gan* (Rhizoma Belamcandae Chinensis)	Sore and swollen throat
Pu Gong Ying (Herba Taraxaci cum Radice) *Chi Shao* (Radix Paeoniae Rubra)	Swelling and toxins of clove sores
Sheng Di Huang (Radix Rehmanniae Glutinosae) *Huai Hua* (Flos Sophorae Japonicae) *Zhi Zi* (Fructus Gardeniae Jasminoidis)	Coughing of blood, nosebleed and vomiting of blood due to heat disturbing the Blood in warm diseases
Dan Shen (Radix Salviae Miltiorrhizae) *Yin Chen Hao* (Herba Artemisiae Scopariae)	Jaundice, inflammation of the gallbladder

Qing Dai 青黛
(Natural indigo, Indigo Naturalis)

Qing Dai is the dried blue powder prepared from the leaf of *Baphicacanthus cusia* (Nees) Bremek., family Acanthaceae; *Indigofera tinctoria* L., family Leguminosae; *Polygonum tinctorium* Ait., family Polygonaceae; or *Isatis indigotica* Fort., family Cruciferae.

Main ingredients *Qing Dai* contains indigotin, indirubin, indigo-brown and indigo-yellow.

Properties Taste: salty and slightly bitter; nature: cold.

Channels entered Liver, Lung and Stomach.

Functions and indications Clears heat and relieves toxicity, cools the Blood and settles fright. It is indicated for full-heat in the course of febrile diseases, macular eruptions, coughing of blood, child fright epilepsy, erysipelas, and mouth sores.

Common dosage 1.5-3g of the powder taken orally with water; appropriate dosage for external application.

Precautions and contraindications *Qing Dai* should be used with caution in cases of Stomach-cold.

Comparison of functions *Qing Dai* (Indigo Naturalis), *Ban Lan Gen* (Radix Isatidis seu Baphicacanthi) and *Da Qing Ye* (Folium Isatidis seu Baphicacanthi) originate from the same plants and have similar functions. They can all clear heat and relieve toxicity, cool the Blood and disperse maculopapular eruptions. *Da Qing Ye* is an extremely cold herb and is highly effective in clearing heat, being an important herb for clearing heat toxins and cooling the Blood to disperse maculopapular eruptions. *Ban Lan Gen* has similar functions to *Da Qing Ye*, but is especially good at relieving toxicity and benefiting the throat. *Qing Dai* is good at clearing and draining fire in the Liver and Lungs and is effective for stopping bleeding.

Modern research

1. Alcoholic extracts of *Qing Dai* can inhibit such pathogenic micro-organisms as Bacillus anthracis, Staphylococcus aureus and Streptococcus pneumoniae.[74]
2. Strengthens the immune function.[75]

Combinations and applications

Functions	Combinations	Applications
Clearing heat and relieving toxicity, cooling the Blood and settling fright	*Shi Gao* (Gypsum Fibrosum) *Sheng Di Huang* (Radix Rehmanniae Glutinosae) *Sheng Ma* (Rhizoma Cimicifugae)	Macular eruptions due to heat toxins, coughing of blood, nosebleed and vomiting of blood due to the frenetic movement of hot Blood
	Niu Huang (Calculus Bovis) *Gou Teng* (Ramulus Uncariae cum Uncis)	Child fright epilepsy, fever and spasms due to heat
	Gua Lou (Fructus Trichosanthis) *Fu Hai Shi* (Os Costaziae seu Pumex) *Zhe Bei Mu* (Bulbus Fritillariae Thunbergii)	Cough due to Lung-heat with thick, yellow sputum

Note: *Qing Dai* is an important herb for external use; for example, the powdered herb can be used on its own or with *Bing Pian* (Borneolum) to treat mumps and sore and swollen throat.

Yu Xing Cao 鱼腥草 (Houttuynia, Herba Houttuyniae Cordatae)

Yu Xing Cao is the aerial parts of *Houttuynia cordata* Thunb., family Saururaceae.

Main ingredients *Yu Xing Cao* contains caryophyllene, linalool, bornyl acetate, decanoyl acetaldehyde, methyl nonylketone, lauraldehyde, capric aldehyde, potassium chloride and potassium sulphate. The leaves and spike contain quercitrin, isoquercitrin, quercetin, reynoutrin, afzerin, hyperin and rutin.

Properties Taste: acrid; nature: cool.

Channel entered Lung.

Functions and indications Clears heat and relieves toxicity, expels pus and disperses abscesses, promotes urination and frees Lin syndrome. It is indicated for Lung abscess, cough due to Lung-heat, dysentery, Lin syndrome, haemorrhoids, vaginal discharge, and abscesses and clove sores.

Common dosage 15-30g, or 60g for large dosages; not to be decocted for a long period. Use an appropriate dosage for external application of the fresh herb as a wash or paste.

Precautions and contraindications *Yu Xing Cao* is contraindicated in cases of deficiency-cold patterns and Yin abscesses.

Comparison of functions *Yu Xing Cao* (Herba Houttuyniae Cordatae) and *Lu Gen* (Rhizoma Phragmitis Communis) are commonly used to treat Lung abscesses. However, *Yu Xing Cao* tends to clear heat and relieve toxicity to disperse abscesses and expel pus, whereas *Lu Gen* tends to clear heat from the Lungs to dispel Phlegm and expel pus. The two herbs are often used in combination.

For an additional comparison, see *Bai Jiang Cao* (Herba Patriniae cum Radice).

Toxicity Intravenous injection in white mice of 75-90 mg/kg of *Yu Xing Cao* for seven days did not lead to any deaths. When mice weighing 17-20g were given an intravenous injection in the tail of 1.5 mg/kg of *Yu Xing Cao* for seven days, again no deaths occurred, but a weight increase was recorded in 90% of the mice. It has been reported that some patients complained of localized pain after intramuscular injection of the herb. There were also reports in the 1970s that injections of *Yu Xing Cao* could cause allergic shock or even death.

Modern research

1. The volatile oils contained in *Yu Xing Cao* and juice from the fresh herb have a strong action in

inhibiting bacteria (including Staphylococcus aureus, Streptococcus pneumoniae, Shigella shigae) and viruses (including type-A Asian influenza),[76, 77] but cooking the decoction for a long time can reduce its effect in inhibiting bacteria.[77]

2. Strengthens the immune function.[78]
3. Inhibits inflammation.[79]

Combinations and applications

Functions	Combinations	Applications
Clearing heat and relieving toxicity	*Jin Yin Hua* (Flos Lonicerae) *Gua Lou* (Fructus Trichosanthis) *Ting.Li Zi* (Semen Lepidii seu Descurainiae) *Xing Ren* (Semen Pruni Armeniacae)	Cough with yellow sputum, fever and thirst due to Lung-heat
	Pu Gong Ying (Herba Taraxaci cum Radice) *Qian Cao Gen* (Radix Rubiae Cordifoliae) *Bai Hua She She Cao* (Herba Hedyotidis Diffusae)	Lung abscess, coughing of blood, pain in the chest
	Bai Bu (Radix Stemonae) *E Bu Shi Cao* (Herba Centipedae) *Feng Mi* (Mel)	Paroxysmal cough due to heat toxins congesting the Lungs
	Shan Zha (Fructus Crataegi)	Dysentery due to damp-heat binding internally
Expelling pus and dispersing abscesses	*Jie Geng* (Radix Platycodi Grandiflori) *Lu Gen* (Rhizoma Phragmitis Communis) *Dong Gua Ren* (Semen Benincasae Hispidae) *Yi Yi Ren* (Semen Coicis Lachrymajobi) *Jin Yin Hua* (Flos Lonicerae)	Lung abscess with coughing of purulent and bloody sputum due to Phlegm-heat congesting the Lungs
	Lian Qiao (Fructus Forsythiae Suspensae) *Pu Gong Ying* (Herba Taraxaci cum Radice) *Chi Shao* (Radix Paeoniae Rubra)	Swelling and toxins of clove sores
	Huang Bai (Cortex Phellodendri) *Mang Xiao* (Mirabilitum) (decocted for use in a hip bath to bathe the affected area)	Haemorrhoids with painful swelling
Promoting urination and freeing Lin syndrome	*Ze Xie* (Rhizoma Alismatis Orientalis) *Che Qian Zi* (Semen Plantaginis) *Jin Qian Cao* (Herba Lysimachiae) *Sang Bai Pi* (Cortex Mori Albae Radicis)	Heat Lin syndrome, difficult urination

She Gan 射干 (Belamcanda rhizome, Rhizoma Belamcandae Chinensis)

She Gan is the rhizome of *Belamcanda chinensis* (L.) DC., family Iridaceae.

Main ingredients *She Gan* contains belamcandin, iridin, tectorigenin and tectoridin. The flower and leaves contain mangiferin.

Properties Taste: bitter; nature: cold; slightly toxic.

Channels entered Lung and Liver.

Functions and indications Clears heat and relieves toxicity, dispels Phlegm and benefits the throat, disperses swelling and dissipates lumps. It is indicated for sore and swollen throat, cough with copious sputum due to Lung-heat, scrofula, and abscesses and sores.

Common dosage 6-10g; appropriate dosage for external application.

Precautions and contraindications *She Gan* is contraindicated during pregnancy and in cases of loose stool due to Spleen deficiency.

Comparison of functions *She Gan* (Rhizoma Belamcandae Chinensis), *Shan Dou Gen* (Radix Sophorae Tonkinensis) and *Ma Bo* (Sclerotium Lasiosphaerae seu Calvatiae) can all clear heat and relieve toxicity to treat sore and swollen throat. *She Gan* is bitter and cold; in addition to its functions in clearing heat and relieving toxicity, it can also dispel Phlegm and dissipate lumps with the result that it is mainly used for treating sore and swollen throat due to Phlegm and fire binding together. *Shan Dou Gen* is extremely bitter in taste and cold in nature; it has a strong function in bearing fire downwards and relieving toxicity to benefit the throat, enabling it to be used for treating sore and swollen throat due to exuberant heat toxins. *Ma Bo* is light and dissipating; it is good at clearing and dispersing heat to benefit the throat in order to treat sore and swollen throat due to externally-contracted wind-heat.

Toxicity The LD_{50} for intragastric administration in mice of an alcoholic infusion of *She Gan* is 66.78g/kg.

Modern research

1. Inhibits inflammation.[80]
2. Abates fever.[81]
3. Promotes the secretion function of the salivary gland.[82]

Combinations and applications

Functions	Combinations	Applications
Clearing heat and relieving toxicity, dispelling Phlegm and benefiting the throat	*Ban Lan Gen* (Radix Isatidis seu Baphicacanthi) *Lian Qiao* (Fructus Forsythiae Suspensae) *Jie Geng* (Radix Platycodi Grandiflori) *Xuan Shen* (Radix Scrophulariae Ningpoensis) *Huang Qin* (Radix Scutellariae Baicalensis)	Sore and swollen throat due to congestion of Phlegm-heat
	Qian Hu (Radix Peucedani) *Gua Lou* (Fructus Trichosanthis) *Bei Mu* (Bulbus Fritillariae)	Cough with copious sputum due to Lung-heat
Dispersing swelling and dissipating lumps	*Lian Qiao* (Fructus Forsythiae Suspensae) *Xia Ku Cao* (Spica Prunellae Vulgaris)	Scrofula due to Phlegm and heat binding together

	Zhi Shi (Fructus Immaturus Citri Aurantii) *Da Huang* (Radix et Rhizoma Rhei) *E Zhu* (Rhizoma Curcumae) *Zhi Chuan Shan Jia* (Squama Manitis Pentadactylae Praeparata) (see notes on legal status) *Mu Li* (Concha Ostreae)	Abdominal masses due to Blood stasis and binding of Phlegm

Bai Tou Weng 白头翁
(Chinese pulsatilla root, Radix Pulsatillae Chinensis)

Bai Tou Weng is the root of *Pulsatilla chinensis* (Bge.) Regel, family Ranunculaceae.

Main ingredients *Bai Tou Weng* contains anemonin, rhamnose and many types of triterpenes. The whole plant without the root contains okinalein and okinalin.

Properties Taste: bitter; nature: cold.

Channels entered Large Intestine and Stomach.

Functions and indications Clears heat and relieves toxicity, stops dysentery, cools the Blood and stops bleeding. It is indicated for dysentery due to heat toxins or damp-heat.

Common dosage 10–15g, or 30g for large dosages; appropriate dosage for external application.

Precautions and contraindications *Bai Tou Weng* is contraindicated for dysentery due to deficiency-cold.

Comparison of functions See *Guan Zhong* (Rhizoma Dryopteris Crassirhizomae), *Ma Chi Xian* (Herba Portulacae Oleraceae) and *Ya Dan Zi* (Fructus Bruceae Javanicae).

Toxicity Decoctions of either *Bai Tou Weng* or of the saponins contained in the herb have a very low level of toxicity. The anemonin contained in *Bai Tou Weng* has a strong stimulatory effect on the skin and mucous membranes and can cause vomiting, pain in the abdomen, nephritis, blood in the urine and heart failure.

Modern research The fresh juice, decoction and alcoholic extract of *Bai Tou Weng* have an obvious effect in inhibiting bacteria, including Staphylococcus aureus and Shigella shigae.[83, 84]

Combinations and applications

Functions	Combinations	Applications
Clearing heat and relieving toxicity, stopping dysentery	*Huang Lian* (Rhizoma Coptidis) *Huang Bai* (Cortex Phellodendri) *Mu Xiang* (Radix Aucklandiae Lappae) (see notes on legal status) *Qing Pi* (Pericarpium Citri Reticulatae Viride) *Zhi Shi* (Fructus Immaturus Citri Aurantii)	Dysentery due to accumulation and stagnation of heat toxins in the Intestines and Stomach with such manifestations as fever, pain in the abdomen, pus and blood in the stool, and abdominal urgency and tenesmus
Cooling the Blood and stopping bleeding	*Bai Mao Gen* (Rhizoma Imperatae Cylindricae) *Zhi Zi* (Fructus Gardeniae Jasminoidis)	Bleeding due to Stomach-heat
	Di Yu (Radix Sanguisorbae Officinalis) *Huai Hua Tan* (Flos Sophorae Japonicae Carbonisatus) *Huang Qin Tan* (Radix Scutellariae Baicalensis Carbonisata)	Blood in the stool, haemorrhoidal bleeding

	Tu Fu Ling (Rhizoma Smilacis Glabrae) *Huang Bai* (Cortex Phellodendri) *Chun Pi* (Cortex Ailanthi Altissimae)	Yellow and smelly vaginal discharge due to damp-heat
	Fumigation and washing by a decoction of *Ku Shen* (Radix Sophorae Flavescentis) *Di Fu Zi* (Fructus Kochiae Scopariae) *Bing Pian* (Borneolum Syntheticum)	Trichomonas vaginalis

Ye Ju Hua 野菊花 (Wild chrysanthemum flower, Flos Chrysanthemi Indici)

Ye Ju Hua is the dried flower-head of *Chrysanthemum indicum* L., family Compositae.

Main ingredients *Ye Ju Hua* contains camphor, α-pinene, carvone, citrene, borneol, linarin, yejuhua lactone, luteolin and chrysanthemin.

Properties Taste: bitter and acrid; nature: slightly cold.

Channels entered Lung and Liver.

Functions and indications Clears heat and relieves toxicity, disperses swelling, and lowers blood pressure. It is indicated for red, sore and swollen eyes, sore and swollen throat, abscesses and sores, and hypertension.

Common dosage 10-15g; appropriate dosage for external application.

Precautions and contraindications *Ye Ju Hua* is not suitable for use in cases of loose stool due to Spleen and Stomach deficiency-cold.

Comparison of functions *Ye Ju Hua* (Flos Chrysanthemi Indici) and *Ju Hua* (Flos Chrysanthemi Morifolii) both clear heat and relieve toxicity, and can be used for red, sore and swollen eyes and for abscesses and sores. However, *Ye Ju Hua* is bitterer in taste and colder in nature than *Ju Hua*. It is extremely effective in clearing heat and relieving toxicity, whereas *Ju Hua* has stronger acrid and dissipating properties and is used for dissipating wind-heat from the head and eyes.

Toxicity Intraperitoneal injection of 52g (raw herb)/kg of aqueous solutions of extracts of *Ye Ju Hua* was given to rats revived from unconsciousness, with the result that the heart rate slowed significantly and death occurred after 4 hours. The amount causing death was nine times more than the normal effective amount. Long-term intake of *Ye Ju Hua* showed no accumulation of toxicity.

Modern research

1. Lowers blood pressure.[85, 86]
2. Inhibited certain pathogenic micro-organisms *in vitro*, including Shigella shigae and herpes and influenza viruses.[87, 88]

Combinations and applications

Functions	Combinations	Applications
Clearing heat and relieving toxicity, dispersing swelling	*Lian Qiao* (Fructus Forsythiae Suspensae) *Pu Gong Ying* (Herba Taraxaci cum Radice) *Zi Hua Di Ding* (Herba Violae Yedoensitis)	Abscesses and sores, sore and swollen throat due to heat toxins
	Chong Lou (Rhizoma Paridis)	Clove sores on the head and face

	Xia Ku Cao (Spica Prunellae Vulgaris) *Sang Ye* (Folium Mori Albae)	Red, sore and swollen eyes
	Di Yu (Radix Sanguisorbae Officinalis) *Cang Zhu* (Rhizoma Atractylodis) *Pao Jiang* (Rhizoma Zingiberis Officinalis Praeparata)	Intestinal haemorrhage
Lowering blood pressure	*Xia Ku Cao* (Spica Prunellae Vulgaris) *Huang Qin* (Radix Scutellariae Baicalensis)	Hypertension

Note: A decoction of *Ye Ju Hua* is effective for internal and external use for itchy skin.

Chuan Xin Lian 穿心莲
(Green chiretta, Herba Andrographitis Paniculatae)

Chuan Xin Lian is the dried aerial parts of *Andrographis paniculata* (Burm. f.) Nees, family Acanthaceae.

Main ingredients *Chuan Xin Lian* contains andrographolide and various andrographolide compounds, andrographan, andrographon, andrographin, daucosterol and flavone compounds.

Properties Taste: bitter; nature: cold.

Channels entered Lung, Stomach, Large Intestine and Small Intestine.

Functions and indications Clears heat and relieves toxicity, promotes urination and disperses swelling. It is indicated for coughing and wheezing due to Lung-heat, Lung abscess, sore and swollen throat, damp-heat dysentery, Lin syndrome due to pathogenic damp-heat, eczema, sores, erysipelas, and poisonous snake bites.

Common dosage 6-15g; appropriate dosage for external application.

Precautions and contraindications The bitter taste and cold nature of *Chuan Xin Lian* mean that it may damage Stomach Qi if it is used over a long period or in large dosages.

Comparison of functions Both *Chuan Xin Lian* (Herba Andrographitis Paniculatae) and *Da Qing Ye* (Folium Isatidis seu Baphicacanthi) can clear heat and relieve toxicity and have similar functions in the treatment of febrile diseases and abscesses and sores. *Chuan Xin Lian* can dispel wind-heat to clear damp-heat from the Qi and Wei levels; it also dries dampness, being employed for cough, diarrhoea, dysentery and Lin syndrome. *Da Qing Ye* can cool the Blood and disperse maculopapular eruptions, and is used to treat damp-heat in the Ying and Xue levels, seasonal epidemic toxins, maculopapular eruptions, and sore throat.

Toxicity *Chuan Xin Lian* is relatively non-toxic. Rats and rabbits fed 1g/kg of andrographolide once a day for seven days exhibited no abnormalities in terms of weight, haemogram, or kidney and liver function.

Modern research

1. A decoction of *Chuan Xin Lian* inhibited Streptococcus pneumoniae and α-haemolytic streptococci in laboratory tests.[89]
2. Strengthens the immune function.[90]
3. Induces abortion.[91]

Combinations and applications

Functions	Combinations	Applications
Clearing heat and relieving toxicity	*Di Gu Pi* (Cortex Lycii Radicis) *Sang Bai Pi* (Cortex Mori Albae Radicis)	Coughing and wheezing due to Lung-heat
	Yu Xing Cao (Herba Houttuyniae Cordatae) *Dong Gua Ren* (Semen Benincasae Hispidae) *Jie Geng* (Radix Platycodi Grandiflori)	Lung abscess, cough with purulent sputum
	Da Qing Ye (Folium Isatidis seu Baphicacanthi) *Niu Bang Zi* (Fructus Arctii Lappae)	Sore and swollen throat and fever in the initial stage of warm diseases
Promoting urination and dispersing swelling	*Ma Chi Xian* (Herba Portulacae Oleraceae) *Jin Yin Hua* (Flos Lonicerae)	Damp-heat dysentery
	Bai Mao Gen (Rhizoma Imperatae Cylindricae) *Che Qian Zi* (Semen Plantaginis)	Heat Lin syndrome, manifesting as difficult and frequent urination

Note: Powdered *Chuan Xin Lian* can be mixed with glycerin into a cream for external application in the treatment of eczema. The fresh herb can be pounded into a paste for the external treatment of snake bites.

Chong Lou 重楼
(Paris root, Rhizoma Paridis)

Chong Lou (also known as *Qi Ye Yi Zhi Hua* or *Zao Xiu*) is the dried rhizome of *Paris polyphylla* Smith var. *yunnanensis* (Franch). Hand.-Mazz. or *P. polyphylla* Smith var. *chinensis* (Franch). Hara, family Liliaceae.

Main ingredients *Chong Lou* contains pariphyllin, dioscin, diosgenin, pennogenin and other saponins, as well as alkaloids, polysaccharides, aspartic acid, asparigine, alanine, amino acids and trace elements.

Properties Taste: bitter; nature: slightly cold; slightly toxic.

Channel entered Liver.

Functions and indications Clears heat and relieves toxicity, disperses swelling and alleviates pain, extinguishes wind and settles fright, transforms stasis and stops bleeding. It is indicated for swollen and toxic abscesses and sores, poisonous snake bites, fright epilepsy, convulsions, clouded Spirit, and bleeding or pain due to injury caused by stasis and swelling.

Common dosage 5-10g, to be decocted and taken orally; 1-2g in powder or pills; appropriate dosage for external application as powder for a compress.

Precautions and contraindications *Chong Lou* is contraindicated for patients with a weak constitution, in cases of heat toxins without full-fire or where there are external abscesses in Yin patterns, and during pregnancy.

Remarks *Chong Lou* can be decocted alone and taken orally or ground to a powder and mixed with vinegar for application as a compress to treat the swelling and toxins of abscesses and sores and poisonous snake bites.

Comparison of functions Both *Chong Lou* (Rhizoma Paridis) and *Zi Hua Di Ding* (Herba Violae Yedoensitis) can treat abscesses and sores and poisonous snake bites as well as clearing heat and relieving toxicity. However, *Chong Lou* is more effective for snake bites, whereas *Zi Hua Di Ding* is an important herb for relieving toxicity to treat swollen abscesses and clove sores.

Modern research

1. Stops coughing and calms wheezing.[92]
2. Inhibits Shigella shigae, Staphylococcus aureus, paracolon bacilli and the type-A Asian influenza virus.[93]
3. Has a tranquillizing function.[94]
4. Inhibits carcinoma.[95-97]

Combinations and applications

Functions	Combinations	Applications
Clearing heat and relieving toxicity, dispersing swelling and alleviating pain	*Huang Lian* (Rhizoma Coptidis) *Chi Shao* (Radix Paeoniae Rubra) *Jin Yin Hua* (Flos Lonicerae) *Lian Qiao* (Fructus Forsythiae Suspensae)	Swelling and toxins of abscesses and clove sores
	Ban Bian Lian (Herba Lobeliae Chinensis cum Radice)	Poisonous snake bites
Extinguishing wind and settling fright	*Gou Teng* (Ramulus Uncariae cum Uncis) *Chan Tui* (Periostracum Cicadae) *Ju Hua* (Flos Chrysanthemi Morifolii)	Wind stirring internally due to Liver-heat, fright epilepsy, clouded Spirit and convulsions due to febrile diseases
Transforming stasis and stopping bleeding	*San Qi* (Radix Notoginseng) *Xue Jie* (Resina Draconis) *Zi Ran Tong* (Pyritum)	Bleeding or pain caused by stasis and swelling due to knocks and falls

Ban Bian Lian 半边莲
(Chinese lobelia, Herba Lobeliae Chinensis cum Radice)

Ban Bian Lian is the whole herb of *Lobelia chinensis* Lour., family Campanulaceae.

Main ingredients *Ban Bian Lian* contains many kinds of alkaloids, principally lobeline, lobelanine, isolobelanine and lobelanidine, as well as flavones, saponins, succinic acid, fumaric acid, p-hydroxybenzoic acid and phenols.

Properties Taste: acrid; nature: cold.

Channels entered Heart, Small Intestine and Lung.

Functions and indications Clears heat and relieves toxicity, promotes urination and disperses swelling. It is indicated for poisonous snake bites, insect stings, swelling and pain in the initial stage of clove sores (either used internally or applied externally as a compress for these indications), ascites, and puffy swelling of the face and eyes.

Common dosage 10-15g of the dried herb or 30-60g of the fresh herb as a decoction; appropriate dosage for external application mashed into a compress.

Precautions and contraindications *Ban Bian Lian* is contraindicated for oedema in deficiency patterns.

Remarks

1. Fresh *Ban Bian Lian* is usually more effective than the dried herb.
2. *Ban Bian Lian* is one of the major herbs for the treatment of poisonous snake bites and insect stings.

Toxicity The LD_{50} for intravenous injection in mice of an infusion of *Ban Bian Lian* is 6.10g/kg; for intragastric administration in rats, the LD_{50} is 75.1 ± 13.1g/kg. *Ban Bian Lian* is only slightly toxic; overdosage can lead to toxic symptoms, especially through injection of the lobeline contained in the herb.

Modern research

1. The alkaloids contained in *Ban Bian Lian* promote urination.[98]
2. Stimulates respiration.[99]
3. Induces vomiting.[100-102]
4. Has a laxative function.[99]

Combinations and applications

Functions	Combinations	Applications
Clearing heat and relieving toxicity	*Zi Hua Di Ding* (Herba Violae Yedoensitis) *Chong Lou* (Rhizoma Paridis)	Swelling and toxins of clove sores, poisonous snake bites, insect stings
	Bai Hua She She Cao (Herba Hedyotidis Diffusae) *Hu Zhang* (Radix et Rhizoma Polygoni Cuspidati) *Qian Cao Gen* (Radix Rubiae Cordifoliae)	Poisonous snake bites
Promoting urination and dispersing swelling	*Ze Xie* (Rhizoma Alismatis Orientalis) *Fu Ling* (Sclerotium Poriae Cocos) *Zhu Ling* (Sclerotium Polypori Umbellati)	Ascites, puffy swelling of the face and eyes
	Bai Mao Gen (Rhizoma Imperatae Cylindricae)	Damp-heat jaundice, inhibited urination

Note: A paste of fresh *Ban Bian Lian* can be applied externally to treat swollen and painful breast abscesses; the paste mixed with alcohol can also be used topically for the swelling and toxins of clove sores.

Tu Fu Ling 土茯苓 (Glabrous green briar rhizome, Rhizoma Smilacis Glabrae)

Tu Fu Ling is the dried root and stem tuber of *Smilax glabra* Roxb., family Liliaceae.

Main ingredients *Tu Fu Ling* contains saponins, isoengeletin, succinic acid, carotene, tannin, resin and alkaloids.

Properties Taste: sweet and bland; nature: neutral.

Channels entered Liver and Stomach.

Functions and indications Clears heat and relieves toxicity, dispels dampness and eliminates Bi syndrome. It is indicated for convulsion of the limbs due to syphilis or to the mercury used to treat syphilis, abscesses and sores due to fire toxins, inhibited and painful voidings of reddish urine due to heat Lin syndrome, and goitre.

Common dosage 15-60g.

Precautions and contraindications *Tu Fu Ling* should be used with caution in cases of Liver and Kidney Yin depletion without dampness. Some ancient texts state that taking *Tu Fu Ling* with tea may lead to hair loss.

Remarks According to *Ben Cao Gang Mu* [The Materia Medica Compendium], '*Tu Fu Ling* relieves the toxicity of mercury and silver.'

Comparison of functions Both *Tu Fu Ling* (Rhizoma Smilacis Glabrae) and *Bi Xie* (Rhizoma Dioscoreae Hypoglaucae seu Septemlobae) can treat sores. *Tu Fu Ling* is better for treating syphilitic sores, whereas *Bi Xie* is more effective for skin sores due to damp-heat. The two herbs are also used for inhibited bending and stretching, *Tu Fu Ling* being better at treating convulsion of the limbs caused by the mercury contained in medicines used in the treatment of syphilis and *Bi Xie* being more effective in treating Bi syndrome pain in the lumbar region and knees. Both herbs can also be used to treat Lin syndrome. *Tu Fu Ling* is better for heat Lin syndrome, *Bi Xie* for turbid Lin syndrome.

Modern research Inhibits carcinoma and has a detoxifying function.[103]

Combinations and applications

Functions	Combinations	Applications
Clearing heat and relieving toxicity	*Jin Yin Hua* (Flos Lonicerae) *Bai Xian Pi* (Cortex Dictamni Dasycarpi Radicis) *Wei Ling Xian* (Radix Clematidis) *Gan Cao* (Radix Glycyrrhizae)	Convulsion of the limbs due to syphilis or to the mercury used to treat syphilis, sores, swollen and painful joints
	Huang Yao Zi (Rhizoma Dioscoreae Bulbiferae)	Goitre
Dispelling dampness and eliminating Bi syndrome	*Mu Tong* (Caulis Mutong) (see notes on legal status) *Niu Xi* (Radix Achyranthis Bidentatae) *Pu Gong Ying* (Herba Taraxaci cum Radice) *Bian Xu* (Herba Polygoni Avicularis)	Inhibited and painful voidings of reddish urine due to heat Lin syndrome
	Cang Zhu (Rhizoma Atractylodis) *Huang Bai* (Cortex Phellodendri) *Ku Shen* (Radix Sophorae Flavescentis)	Vaginal discharge due to damp-heat; abscesses, swellings and scrofula
	Ze Xie (Rhizoma Alismatis Orientalis) *Bai Zhu* (Rhizoma Atractylodis Macrocephalae) *Fu Ling Pi* (Cortex Poriae Cocos)	Exuberant dampness due to Spleen deficiency, manifesting as itchy eczema

Guan Zhong 贯众
(Basket fern, Rhizoma Dryopteris Crassirhizomae)

Guan Zhong is the dried rhizome of *Dryopteris crassirhizoma* Nakai, family Dryopteridaceae.

Legal status The use of this herb is illegal in the UK as a result of its toxic nature.

Main ingredients *Guan Zhong* contains filicic acid, flavaspidic acid, albaspidin, dryocrassin, fernene, diploptene, pterosterone, tannin, volatile oils and resin.

Properties Taste: bitter; nature: cool; toxic.

Channels entered Liver and Spleen.

Functions and indications Kills worms, clears heat and relieves toxicity, cools the Blood and stops bleeding. It is indicated for pain in the abdomen due to worms, abscesses and sores due to heat toxins, and bleeding patterns.

Common dosage 10–15g.

Precautions and contraindications *Guan Zhong* is contraindicated in cases of Spleen and Stomach deficiency-cold and during pregnancy.

Remarks Charred *Guan Zhong* is used to stop bleeding, whereas the raw herb is employed to kill worms, clear heat and relieve toxicity.

Comparison of functions

1. Both *Guan Zhong* (Rhizoma Dryopteris Crassirhizomae) and *Ban Lan Gen* (Radix Isatidis seu Baphicacanthi) can clear heat and relieve toxicity. Although *Guan Zhong* can inhibit a number of viruses, it is relatively toxic, so is not used as widely as *Ban Lan Gen. Guan Zhong* is more effective in killing worms and stopping bleeding than *Ban Lan Gen*, whereas the latter is better at cooling the Blood and benefiting the throat.
2. Both *Guan Zhong* (Rhizoma Dryopteris Crassirhizomae) and *Bai Tou Weng* (Radix Pulsatillae Chinensis) can clear heat and relieve toxicity, cool the Blood and stop bleeding. *Guan Zhong* is better for treating uterine bleeding, whereas *Bai Tou Weng* is more effective for bleeding during dysentery.

Toxicity The LD_{50} for intraperitoneal injection in mice of an acetic extract of *Guan Zhong* is 1.7g/kg; for *Dong Bei Guan Zhong*, it is 640 mg/kg for intraperitoneal injection, 420 mg/kg for subcutaneous injection. The filicic acid contained in *Guan Zhong* affects the digestive and central nervous systems; when taken in large quantities, it can damage the optic nerve. Dryocrassin affects the gastrointestinal tract; when given in large quantities to animals, it led to paralysis of the limbs and death. Toxic symptoms in humans include headache, dizziness, diarrhoea, pain in the abdomen, dyspnoea and temporary loss of sight; in more serious cases, there may be delirium, coma, jaundice or kidney damage. Recovery is generally slow. The main causes of toxic side-effects are overdosage or use of the unprocessed herb. *Guan Zhong* should not be used during pregnancy, for patients with a weak constitution or with ulcers in the digestive tract, or in cases of liver and kidney malfunction.

Modern research

1. Decoctions of the species of *Guan Zhong* grown in Northeast China (*Dong Bei Guan Zhong*) can expel such parasites as tapeworm, hookworm, lumbricoids and schistosomes.[104]
2. Inhibits various bacteria and viruses, including the influenza, parainfluenza and poliomyelitis viruses[105] and HIV.[106]
3. Decoctions of *Guan Zhong* can excite the uterus and induce abortion in the early stages of pregnancy.[107]

Combinations and applications

Functions	Combinations	Applications
Killing worms	*Bing Lang* (Semen Arecae Catechu) *Shi Jun Zi* (Fructus Quisqualis Indicae)	Worms, including roundworm, hookworm and tapeworm
Clearing heat and relieving toxicity	*Jin Yin Hua* (Flos Lonicerae) *Lian Qiao* (Fructus Forsythiae Suspensae)	Abscesses, sores and mumps due to heat toxins
Cooling the Blood and stopping bleeding	*Ce Bai Ye* (Cacumen Biotae Orientalis) *Xian He Cao* (Herba Agrimoniae Pilosae) *Zong Lü Tan* (Fibra Carbonisata Trachycarpi Stipulae)	Uterine bleeding due to Blood-heat

Shan Dou Gen 山豆根 (Subprostrate sophora root, Radix Sophorae Tonkinensis)

Shan Dou Gen is the dried root and rhizome of *Sophora tonkinensis* Gagnep., also known as *Sophora subprostrata* Chun et T. Chen, family Leguminosae.

Legal status *Shan Dou Gen* was listed in a document entitled *A Review of Restricted Herbal Ingredients* issued by the Medicines Control Agency (MCA) in the UK in September 2001 with a view to the possible imposition of restrictions on its use at a future date. Use of the root of this herb is controlled in Hong Kong and the MCA is considering introducing a requirement for medical supervision in the UK.

Main ingredients *Shan Dou Gen* contains matrine, oxymatrine, methylcytisine, anagyrine, sophocarpine, sophoranone, sophoradin, sophoranochromene, sophoradochromene, genistein, pterocarpine, maackiain, trifolirhizin, sophoraflavone A, bayin and sitosterol.

Properties Taste: bitter; nature: cold.

Channel entered Lung.

Functions and indications Clears heat and relieves toxicity, benefits the throat and alleviates pain. It is indicated for sore and swollen throat, cough due to Lung-heat, sores, and painful and swollen gums.

Common dosage 6-10g; or appropriate dosage for external application.

Precautions and contraindications *Shan Dou Gen* is contraindicated in cases of loose stool due to Spleen and Stomach deficiency-cold.

Comparison of functions See *She Gan* (Rhizoma Belamcandae Chinensis).

Toxicity The LD_{50} for intraperitoneal injection in mice of aqueous extracts of *Shan Dou Gen* is 15.58g/kg; the equivalent figures for the oxymatrine and matrine contained in *Shan Dou Gen* are 572.2 mg/kg and 652.0 mg/kg respectively. Symptoms of overdose in humans start at 30-90g. The main toxic constituents are matrine and oxymatrine. The main cause of poisoning is overdosage.

Modern research

1. The matrine contained in *Shan Dou Gen* inhibits carcinoma.[108, 109]
2. Inhibits ulcers, inhibits the secretion of gastric juices.[110]
3. Calms wheezing.[111]

Combinations and applications

Functions	Combinations	Applications
Clearing heat and relieving toxicity	*Shi Gao* (Gypsum Fibrosum) *Xuan Shen* (Radix Scrophulariae Ningpoensis) *Da Huang* (Radix et Rhizoma Rhei)	Toothache and mouth sores due to Stomach-fire
	Gua Lou (Fructus Trichosanthis) *Jin Yin Hua* (Flos Lonicerae)	Cough due to Lung-heat
	Dai Zhe Shi (Haematitum) *Chuan Lian Zi* (Fructus Meliae Toosendan)	Heartburn, acid regurgitation, gastric ulcer
Benefiting the throat and alleviating pain	*She Gan* (Rhizoma Belamcandae Chinensis) *Niu Bang Zi* (Fructus Arctii Lappae) *Jie Geng* (Radix Platycodi Grandiflori)	Sore and swollen throat due to exuberant heat toxins

Note: A paste made from fresh *Shan Dou Gen* can be used externally to treat the swelling and toxins of sores.

Ma Bo 马勃 (Puff-ball, Sclerotium Lasiosphaerae seu Calvatiae)

Ma Bo is the sporophore of *Lasiosphaera fenzlii* Reich., *Calvatia gigantea* (Batsch ex Pers.) Lloyd or *C. lilacina* (Mont. et Berk.) Lloyd, family Lycoperdaceae.

Main ingredients *Ma Bo* contains calvacin, carbamide, ergosterol, leucine, tyrosine, gemmatein, lipids and sodium phosphate.

Properties Taste: acrid; nature: neutral.

Channel entered Lung.

Functions and indications Clears heat and relieves toxicity, benefits the throat and alleviates pain, and stops bleeding. It is indicated for sore and swollen throat, loss of voice, coughing of blood, and nosebleed.

Common dosage 3-6g, or 0.5-1g in powder or pills for oral use; appropriate dosage for external application.

Precautions and contraindications *Ma Bo* is contraindicated in cases of loss of voice due to wind-cold.

Comparison of functions Both *Ma Bo* (Sclerotium Lasiosphaerae seu Calvatiae) and *Xuan Shen* (Radix Scrophulariae Ningpoensis) can treat sore and swollen throat. *Ma Bo* treats sore and swollen throat due to wind-heat invading the Lungs or full-fire in the Lung channel, whereas *Xuan Shen* treats the condition when it is caused by congestion of heat toxins or deficiency-fire flaming upwards.

For an additional comparison, see *She Gan* (Rhizoma Belamcandae Chinensis).

Modern research

1. A decoction of *Ma Bo* inhibited such bacteria as Staphylococcus aureus, Pseudomonas aeruginosa and Streptococcus pneumoniae in laboratory tests.[112]
2. When peeled, stops bleeding in the nose and mouth.[112]

Combinations and applications

Functions	Combinations	Applications
Clearing heat and relieving toxicity, benefiting the throat and alleviating pain	*Xuan Shen* (Radix Scrophulariae Ningpoensis) *Ban Lan Gen* (Radix Isatidis seu Baphicacanthi) *Niu Bang Zi* (Fructus Arctii Lappae)	Sore and swollen throat and loss of voice due to wind-heat or full-fire in the Lung channel
	Huang Qin (Radix Scutellariae Baicalensis) *Jie Geng* (Radix Platycodi Grandiflori)	Cough due to Lung-heat
	Bo He (Herba Menthae Haplocalycis) *Lian Qiao* (Fructus Forsythiae Suspensae) *Xuan Shen* (Radix Scrophulariae Ningpoensis)	Mumps
Stopping bleeding	*Huang Qin Tan* (Radix Scutellariae Baicalensis Carbonisata) *Ou Jie* (Nodus Nelumbinis Nuciferae Rhizomatis) *Bai Mao Gen* (Rhizoma Imperatae Cylindricae)	Coughing of blood, nosebleed and vomiting of blood due to Lung-heat

Note: In its powdered form, *Ma Bo* can be used to treat bleeding due to external injury.

Ma Chi Xian 马齿苋
(Purslane, Herba Portulacae Oleraceae)

Ma Chi Xian is the dried aerial parts of *Portulaca oleracea* L., family Portulacaceae.

Main ingredients *Ma Chi Xian* contains noradrenaline, sylvite, dopamine and dopa; malic, citric, oxalic, linolenic, nicotinic, glutamic and aspartic acids; flavones, vitamins A, B_1 and B_2, and trace elements.

Properties Taste: sour; nature: cold.

Channels entered Large Intestine and Liver.

Functions and indications Clears heat and relieves toxicity, stops dysentery, cools the Blood and stops bleeding. It is indicated for damp-heat dysentery with purulent and bloody stool, heat Lin syndrome, blood Lin syndrome, and abscesses and sores.

Common dosage 10-15g, or 30-60g of the fresh herb; appropriate dosage for external application.

Precautions and contraindications *Ma Chi Xian* is contraindicated in cases of diarrhoea due to Spleen and Stomach deficiency-cold.

Remarks Fresh *Ma Chi Xian* has a better curative effect than the dried herb.

Comparison of functions *Ma Chi Xian* (Herba Portulacae Oleraceae) has similar functions to *Bai Tou Weng* (Radix Pulsatillae Chinensis) in clearing heat and cooling the Blood to stop dysentery. *Ma Chi Xian* is more effective in clearing heat and relieving toxicity, whereas *Bai Tou Weng* is more effective in cooling the Blood.

For an additional comparison, see *Ya Dan Zi* (Fructus Bruceae Javanicae).

Toxicity The LD_{50} for intraperitoneal injection in mice of aqueous extracts of *Ma Chi Xian* is 1040 mg/kg.

Modern research

1. Decoctions of *Ma Chi Xian* can inhibit such bacteria as Bacterium coli, Shigella shigae and Staphylococcus aureus.[113]
2. Contracts the blood vessels and promotes the healing of ulcers.[114]

Combinations and applications

Functions	Combinations	Applications
Clearing heat and relieving toxicity, stopping dysentery	*Huang Qin* (Radix Scutellariae Baicalensis) *Huang Lian* (Rhizoma Coptidis) *Mu Xiang* (Radix Aucklandiae Lappae) (see notes on legal status)	Damp-heat dysentery accompanied by pain in the abdomen, diarrhoea, and abdominal urgency and tenesmus
	Feng Mi (Mel) (add to the juice of the fresh herb)	Postpartum bloody dysentery
	Lian Qiao (Fructus Forsythiae Suspensae) *Pu Gong Ying* (Herba Taraxaci cum Radice)	Swollen and toxic clove sores due to heat toxins
	Ban Lan Gen (Radix Isatidis seu Baphicacanthi) (combine the fresh herbs for external use)	Erysipelas
Cooling the Blood and stopping bleeding	*Di Yu* (Radix Sanguisorbae Officinalis) *Huai Hua* (Flos Sophorae Japonicae)	Blood in the stool and haemorrhoidal bleeding

Additional uses:

1. *Ma Chi Xian* cooked with rice congee and taken on an empty stomach can be used for bloody dysentery due to heat toxins.
2. A paste of fresh *Ma Chi Xian* can be applied to abscesses and sores at the same time as taking a decoction of the herb.
3. A paste of fresh *Ma Chi Xian* is also used to treat snake bites and bee or wasp stings.
4. The juice of the fresh herb can be drunk to treat the frenetic movement of hot Blood and uterine bleeding.

Ya Dan Zi 鸦胆子 (Brucea fruit, Fructus Bruceae Javanicae)

Ya Dan Zi is the dried ripe fruit of *Brucea javanica* (L.) Merr., family Simarubaceae.

Main ingredients *Ya Dan Zi* contains bruceine, bruceoside, brucamarine, yatanine, brucealin, brusatol, javanicin, vanillic acid, brucenol and bruceolic acid.

Properties Taste: bitter; nature: cold; slightly toxic.

Channels entered Large Intestine and Liver.

Functions and indications Clears heat and relieves toxicity, stops dysentery, interrupts malaria, putrefies and consumes warts. It is indicated for benign tertian malaria or quartan malaria, bloody dysentery due to heat toxins, corns and warts.

Common dosage For malaria, chew 10-15 seeds, three times per day for 5-7 days; for dysentery, chew 10-30 seeds, three times a day for 10-14 days. For children, use one seed for every year of age, but do not exceed the adult dosage. The extremely bitter taste of *Ya Dan Zi* makes it unsuitable for use in a decoction. For internal use, remove the husk and place the kernel in a capsule or wrap it up in *Long Yan Rou* (Arillus Euphoriae Longanae); take after meals.

Precautions and contraindications

1. *Ya Dan Zi* irritates the gastrointestinal tract and can injure the Liver and Kidneys. Side-effects from oral intake may include vomiting, pain in the abdomen, chest distress and diarrhoea. It is therefore not suitable for taking in large dosages or over a long period of time (see *Toxicity* below).
2. *Ya Dan Zi* is contraindicated or should be administered with caution in cases of gastrointestinal bleeding or liver and kidney diseases.
3. This herb should not be used in cases of vomiting due to Spleen and Stomach deficiency, and should be used with caution during pregnancy and for infants.

Comparison of functions *Ya Dan Zi* (Fructus Bruceae Javanicae), *Bai Tou Weng* (Radix Pulsatillae Chinensis) and *Ma Chi Xian* (Herba Portulacae Oleraceae) are all important herbs for clearing heat and relieving toxicity to treat dysentery; they are especially effective for dysentery due to heat toxins. *Bai Tou Weng* and *Ma Chi Xian* can clear damp-heat and cool the Blood to stop diarrhoea and are commonly used to treat acute and chronic dysentery and amoebic dysentery. *Ya Dan Zi* is good at clearing heat and relieving toxicity and can be used on its own, subject to the contraindications above, to treat bloody dysentery due to heat toxins. However, given its strong toxic side-effects, it is now generally more commonly used as an external application for the treatment of corns and warts.

Toxicity The husk and seed of *Ya Dan Zi* are toxic. The minimum lethal dosage for *Ya Dan Zi* (after removal of its oils) given to cats via intragastric administration is 0.1g/kg, the LD_{50} for oral administration to chickens of a decoction of the seeds of *Ya Dan Zi* is 0.4g/kg. There are a number of clinical reports of toxic reaction through the misuse of this herb, for example, long-term use of small quantities resulting in chronic poisoning. The main toxic symptoms include nausea and vomiting, poor appetite, dizziness, lack of strength, pain in the abdomen, blood in the stool, hyperaemia in the gastrointestinal tract, high temperature, numbness of the limbs, and convulsions. Toxic reactions can be averted by avoidance of overdosage or long-term use and not swallowing the seeds directly.

Modern research

1. The active ingredients in *Ya Dan Zi* can kill amoeba protozoons.[115]
2. *Ya Dan Zi*, an aqueous solution of the herb and the powdered herb all inhibited malaria when injected or given orally to animals.[116-118]
3. Expels worms.[119]
4. A decoction of *Ya Dan Zi* and a chloroform extract of the herb inhibited nasopharyngeal carcinoma.[120]

Functions and applications

Functions	Applications
Clearing heat, relieving toxicity and stopping dysentery	Bloody dysentery due to heat toxins, manifesting as purulent and bloody diarrhoea and abdominal urgency and tenesmus
Interrupting malaria	Benign tertian malaria, quartan malaria
Putrefying and consuming warts	Used on its own as an external compress (the seeds should be crushed and applied as a compress on the warts, or oil from the seeds should be used directly on the affected location as an ointment)

Bai Hua She She Cao 白花蛇舌草 (Oldenlandia, Herba Hedyotidis Diffusae)

Bai Hua She She Cao is the dried whole plant of *Hedyotis diffusa* (Willd.) Roxb., family Rubiaceae.

Main ingredients *Bai Hua She She Cao* contains 3-l-alkane, stigmasterol, ursolic acid, β-sitosterol and paracoumaric acid.

Properties Taste: sweet and slightly bitter; nature: cold.

Channels entered Stomach, Large Intestine and Small Intestine.

Functions and indications Clears heat and relieves toxicity, quickens the Blood, disperses abscesses, and promotes urination and abates jaundice. It is indicated for cough due to Lung-heat, sore and swollen throat, abscesses and sores, poisonous snake bites, dysentery, jaundice, heat Lin syndrome, and difficult urination.

Common dosage 15–60g; or appropriate dosage for external application.

Precautions and contraindications *Bai Hua She She Cao* is contraindicated during pregnancy.

Remarks As it is bitter and cold, *Bai Hua She She Cao* can clear heat and relieve toxicity; as it is also sweet and cold, it can promote urination and clear damp-heat. This herb is frequently used for treating abscesses and sores.

Modern research

1. *Bai Hua She She Cao* has a non-specific inhibitory effect on carcinoma.[121]
2. A highly-concentrated decoction of *Bai Hua She She Cao* inhibited the growth *in vitro* of Pseudomonas aeruginosa, Salmonella typhi and Proteus vulgaris.[122]

Combinations and applications

Functions	Combinations	Applications
Clearing heat and relieving toxicity, quickening the Blood, dispersing abscesses	*Yu Xing Cao* (Herba Houttuyniae Cordatae) *Gua Lou* (Fructus Trichosanthis) *Xing Ren* (Semen Pruni Armeniacae)	Cough with yellow sputum and fever due to Lung-heat
	Ban Lan Gen (Radix Isatidis seu Baphicacanthi) *She Gan* (Rhizoma Belamcandae Chinensis)	Sore and swollen throat due to wind-heat or heat toxins
	Bai Jiang Cao (Herba Patriniae cum Radice) *Hong Teng* (Caulis Sargentodoxae Cuneatae)	Intestinal abscess

	Pu Gong Ying (Herba Taraxaci cum Radice) *Chi Shao* (Radix Paeoniae Rubra)	Swelling and toxins of clove sores
	Zi Hua Di Ding (Herba Violae Yedoensitis) *Ban Bian Lian* (Herba Lobeliae Chinensis cum Radice)	Poisonous snake bites
Promoting urination and abating jaundice	*Yin Chen Hao* (Herba Artemisiae Scopariae) *Zhi Zi* (Fructus Gardeniae Jasminoidis) *Chai Hu* (Radix Bupleuri)	Damp-heat jaundice
	Che Qian Zi (Semen Plantaginis) *Bai Mao Gen* (Rhizoma Imperatae Cylindricae)	Lin syndrome due to damp-heat

Note: The fresh herb can be applied externally to treat abscesses, sores and poisonous snake bites. Additionally, *Bai Hua She She Cao* can be used with *Teng Li Gen* (Radix Actinidiae Chinensis), *Ban Zhi Lian* (Herba Scutellariae Barbatae) and *San Qi* (Radix Notoginseng) to treat various tumours, including stomach cancer, cancer of the oesophagus and cancer of the rectum.

Mu Hu Die 木蝴蝶
(Oroxylum seed, Semen Oroxyli Indici)

Mu Hu Die is the dried seed of *Oroxylum indicum* (L.) Vent., family Bignoniaceae.

Main ingredients *Mu Hu Die* contains oroxin A, oroxin B, chrysin, baicalein, tetuin and scutellarein.

Properties Taste: bitter; nature: cool.

Channels entered Liver and Lung.

Functions and indications Clears the Lungs and restores the voice, allows constrained Liver Qi to flow freely and harmonizes the Stomach. It is indicated for sore and swollen throat, hoarse voice, cough, and pain in the stomach due to Liver depression and Qi stagnation.

Common dosage 3-5g.

Precautions and contraindications *Mu Hu Die* is contraindicated in cases of deficiency-cold patterns.

Comparison of functions *Mu Hu Die* (Semen Oroxyli Indici) and *Xiang Fu* (Rhizoma Cyperi Rotundi) can treat Qi pain in the Liver and Stomach. *Mu Hu Die* is better for treating pain in the Stomach due to Liver depression invading the Stomach and transforming into heat. *Xiang Fu* is better for treating pain in the Stomach due to Liver depression invading the Stomach without transforming into heat.

Combinations and applications

Functions	Combinations	Applications
Clearing the Lungs and restoring the voice	*Chan Tui* (Periostracum Cicadae) *Pang Da Hai* (Semen Sterculiae Lychnophorae)	Sore and swollen throat and hoarse voice due to wind-heat
	Sang Bai Pi (Cortex Mori Albae Radicis) *Kuan Dong Hua* (Flos Tussilaginis Farfarae) *Jie Geng* (Radix Platycodi Grandiflori)	Cough due to Lung-heat

Allowing constrained Liver Qi to flow freely and harmonizing the Stomach	*Mei Gui Hua* (Flos Rosae Rugosae)	Pain in the Liver and Stomach due to Qi stagnation

Lou Lu 漏芦 (Globethistle root, Radix Rhapontici seu Echinopsis)

Lou Lu is the dried root of *Rhaponticum uniflorum* (L.) DC. or *Echinops latifolius* Tausch., family Compositae.

Main ingredients *Lou Lu* contains arctinal, arctinol and palmitic and stearic acids (*Rhaponticum*); echinorine, echinopsine, echinine, cardopatine and β-sitosterol (*Echinops*).

Properties Taste: bitter; nature: cold.

Channels entered Stomach and Large Intestine.

Functions and indications Clears heat and relieves toxicity, disperses swelling, and causes milk to descend. It is indicated for abscesses and sores, breast abscess and breast pain, and insufficient lactation.

Common dosage 3-12g.

Precautions and contraindications *Lou Lu* is contraindicated in cases of Qi deficiency, for flat or sunken sores, and during pregnancy.

Comparison of functions Both *Lou Lu* (Radix Rhapontici seu Echinopsis) and *Yi Yi Ren* (Semen Coicis Lachrymajobi) can treat abscesses and swellings. *Lou Lu* can clear heat and relieve toxicity to treat breast abscesses due to congestion of heat toxins, whereas *Yi Yi Ren* can clear heat and expel pus to treat Lung and Intestinal abscesses due to damp-heat binding internally in the Lungs and Intestines. *Lou Lu* is good at clearing heat and *Yi Yi Ren* is extremely effective in dispelling dampness.

Toxicity The echinopsine contained in *Lou Lu* can stimulate the central nervous system in small doses and cause hypertonicity in large doses. A toxic dosage can be as little as double the normal dosage. It was reported that 30g of *Lou Lu* taken to treat breast milk stoppage led to severe poisoning.

Modern research

1. A decoction of *Lou Lu* inhibited the growth of oxidation lipids in the liver and brain of mice.[123]
2. Strengthens the immune system.[124]

Combinations and applications

Functions	Combinations	Applications
Clearing heat and relieving toxicity, dispersing swelling, causing milk to descend	*Sheng Ma* (Rhizoma Cimicifugae) *Da Qing Ye* (Folium Isatidis seu Baphicacanthi) *Da Huang* (Radix et Rhizoma Rhei)	Erysipelas, redness and swelling of the face and head
	Lian Qiao (Fructus Forsythiae Suspensae) *Pu Gong Ying* (Herba Taraxaci cum Radice)	Breast abscess without formation of pus in the interior

Wang Bu Liu Xing (Semen Vaccariae Segetalis) *Chuan Shan Jia* (Squama Manitis Pentadactylae) (see notes on legal status)	Stoppage of breast milk, painful and swollen breasts
Zhe Bei Mu (Bulbus Fritillariae Thunbergii) *Xia Ku Cao* (Spica Prunellae Vulgaris)	Scrofula
Dang Gui (Radix Angelicae Sinensis) *Fu Ping* (Herba Spirodelae Polyrrhizae) *Bai Xian Pi* (Cortex Dictamni Dasycarpi Radicis)	Scabies due to wind-heat toxins

Bai Jiang Cao 败酱草 (Patrinia, Herba Patriniae cum Radice)

Bai Jiang Cao is the dried whole plant of *Patrinia scabiosaefolia* Fisch. ex Link. or *P. villosa* (Thunb.) Juss., family Valerianaceae.

Main ingredients *Bai Jiang Cao* contains sinigrin, morroniside, loganin and villoside (*P. villosa*); patrinene, isopatrinene, patrinoside, scabioside, oleanolic acid, hederagenin and daucosterol (*P. scabiosaefolia*).

Properties Taste: acrid and bitter; nature: slightly cold.

Channels entered Stomach, Large Intestine and Liver.

Functions and indications Clears heat and relieves toxicity, disperses swelling and expels pus, quickens the Blood and dissipates stasis. It is indicated for Lung abscess, Intestinal abscess, dysentery, postpartum pain in the abdomen due to Blood stasis, red, sore and swollen eyes, and abscesses and sores.

Common dosage 6–15g; appropriate dosage for external application.

Precautions and contraindications *Bai Jiang Cao* is contraindicated in cases of Spleen and Stomach deficiency.

Comparison of functions *Bai Jiang Cao* (Herba Patriniae cum Radice), *Yu Xing Cao* (Herba Houttuyniae Cordatae) and *Hong Teng* (Caulis Sargentodoxae Cuneatae) can all clear heat, relieve toxicity, disperse swelling and expel pus. However, *Yu Xing Cao* enters the Lung channel and is an important herb for treating Lung abscess; it can also promote urination and free Lin syndrome. Both *Bai Jiang Cao* and *Hong Teng* enter the Large Intestine channel and are important for treating Intestinal abscess with pain in the abdomen. *Hong Teng* can free the channels and network vessels to quicken the Blood and alleviate pain and is used for knocks and falls, Bi syndrome pain and menstrual block. *Bai Jiang Cao* is mainly used for pain in the chest and abdomen, although it also has the function of dissipating Blood stasis to alleviate pain.

Toxicity No adverse effects were noted when 24g (raw herb)/kg of a dry extract of *Patrinia scabiosaefolia* was fed to mice via intragastric administration. Mice fed up to 1,500 times the normal human dosage of patrinoside had exhibited no abnormal reaction after seven days. There have been a few reports of patients complaining of dry mouth and discomfort in the stomach after intake of *P. scabiosaefolia*.

Modern research

1. The volatile oils contained in *Bai Jiang Cao* have a tranquillizing function.[125]
2. Preparations of *Bai Jiang Cao* had an obvious inhibitory effect in clinical experiments on the cytotoxins of acute leukaemia cells but not on those of chronic granulocyte leukaemia cells.[126]

Combinations and applications

Functions	Combinations	Applications
Clearing heat and relieving toxicity, dispersing swelling and expelling pus	*Huang Qin* (Radix Scutellariae Baicalensis) *Zhi Mu* (Rhizoma Anemarrhenae Asphodeloidis) *Xing Ren* (Semen Pruni Armeniacae)	Coughing and wheezing with yellow sputum due to Lung-heat
	Yu Xing Cao (Herba Houttuyniae Cordatae) *Jie Geng* (Radix Platycodi Grandiflori)	Lung abscess with coughing and spitting of blood and pus
	Bai Tou Weng (Radix Pulsatillae Chinensis) *Huang Lian* (Rhizoma Coptidis)	Dysentery with blood in the stool, abdominal urgency and tenesmus
	Jin Yin Hua (Flos Lonicerae) *Da Huang* (Radix et Rhizoma Rhei) *Yi Yi Ren* (Semen Coicis Lachrymajobi)	Intestinal abscess with pain in the abdomen and constipation
	Mu Dan Pi (Cortex Moutan Radicis) *Chi Shao* (Radix Paeoniae Rubra)	Swollen and toxic clove sores due to heat toxins
Quickening the Blood and dissipating stasis	*Ban Lan Gen* (Radix Isatidis seu Baphicacanthi) *Niu Bang Zi* (Fructus Arctii Lappae) *Xuan Shen* (Radix Scrophulariae Ningpoensis)	Sore and swollen throat
	Dang Gui (Radix Angelicae Sinensis) *Mu Dan Pi* (Cortex Moutan Radicis) *Chi Shao* (Radix Paeoniae Rubra) *Yi Mu Cao* (Herba Leonuri Heterophylli)	Postpartum pain in the abdomen due to Blood stasis
	Wu Ling Zhi (Excrementum Trogopteri) *Dang Gui* (Radix Angelicae Sinensis) *Xiang Fu* (Rhizoma Cyperi Rotundi)	Pain in the chest and abdomen due to internal Blood stasis

Note: Fresh *Bai Jiang Cao* used externally is effective in the treatment of abscesses and sores.

Hong Teng 红藤
(Sargentodoxa vine, Caulis Sargentodoxae Cuneatae)

Hong Teng (also known as *Da Xue Teng*) is the vine stem of *Sargentodoxa cuneata* (Oliv.) Rehd. et Wils., family Lardizabalaceae.

Main ingredients *Hong Teng* contains tannin, emodin, lignin, salidroside, carotene, β-sitosterol, protocatechuic acid and dihydroguaiaretic acid.

Properties Taste: bitter; nature: neutral.

Channels entered Large Intestine and Liver.

Functions and indications Clears heat and relieves toxicity, quickens the Blood and alleviates pain. It is indicated for Intestinal abscess with pain in the abdomen, swollen abscesses due to heat toxins, knocks and falls, painful menstruation, menstrual block, and wind-damp Bi syndrome pain.

Common dosage 15-30g, decocted or steeped in alcohol.

Precautions and contraindications *Hong Teng* should be used with caution during pregnancy.

Comparison of functions See *Bai Jiang Cao* (Herba Patriniae cum Radice).

Modern research Inhibits such bacteria as Staphylococcus aureus and Pseudomonas aeruginosa.[127]

Combinations and applications

Functions	Combinations	Applications
Clearing heat and relieving toxicity	*Jin Yin Hua* (Flos Lonicerae) *Lian Qiao* (Fructus Forsythiae Suspensae) *Mu Dan Pi* (Cortex Moutan Radicis)	Intestinal abscess with pain in the abdomen due to stagnation of heat toxins
	Jin Yin Hua (Flos Lonicerae) *Bai Zhi* (Radix Angelicae Dahuricae) *Chi Shao* (Radix Paeoniae Rubra)	Swollen abscesses and sores due to heat toxins
Quickening the Blood and alleviating pain	*Gu Sui Bu* (Rhizoma Drynariae) (crushed together into a paste)	Stasis, swelling and pain due to knocks and falls (external application on the affected area)
	Niu Xi (Radix Achyranthis Bidentatae)	Bi syndrome pain due to wind-damp, inhibited movement of the lumbar region and knees
	Yi Mu Cao (Herba Leonuri Heterophylli) *Xiang Fu* (Rhizoma Cyperi Rotundi)	Menstrual block and pain in the abdomen due to Blood deficiency

Bai Lian 白蔹
(Japanese peppervine root, Radix Ampelopsis Japonicae)

Bai Lian is the dried tuberous root of *Ampelopsis japonica* (Thunb.) Makino, family Vitaceae.

Main ingredients *Bai Lian* contains gallic, digallic, fumaric, boryonolic and tartaric acids, β-sitosterol and starch.

Properties Taste: bitter and acrid; nature: slightly cold.

Channels entered Heart, Liver, Spleen and Stomach.

Functions and indications Clears heat and relieves toxicity, disperses abscesses and dissipates lumps, generates flesh and alleviates pain. It is indicated for abscesses and sores, scrofula and haemorrhoids.

Common dosage 5-10g; appropriate dosage for external application.

Precautions and contraindications

1. *Bai Lian* is contraindicated for Spleen and Stomach deficiency-cold.
2. *Bai Lian* is incompatible with *Wu Tou* (Radix Aconiti).

Comparison of functions Both *Bai Lian* (Radix Ampelopsis Japonicae) and *Pu Gong Ying* (Herba Taraxaci cum Radice) can clear heat and relieve toxicity, and disperse abscesses and dissipate lumps to treat abscesses and sores. *Bai Lian* can disperse swelling and dissipate lumps to generate flesh and close sores; it can be used in the treatment of persistent swelling and pain in the initial stage of abscesses and sores, or for non-generation of flesh after ulceration. *Pu Gong Ying* can relieve toxicity and dissipate lumps to treat red, swollen and painful sores due to heat toxins and is especially suitable for red, swollen and painful breasts due to breast abscess.

Toxicity Decoctions of 30g/kg and 50g/kg of *Bai Lian* given to mice via intragastric administration did not result in any deaths. Accelerated respiration was recorded for the animals in the 50g/kg group.

Modern research Preparations of *Bai Lian* can inhibit bacteria and epiphytes.[128]

Combinations and applications

Functions	Combinations	Applications
Clearing heat and relieving toxicity, dispersing abscesses and dissipating lumps, generating flesh and alleviating pain	*Lian Qiao* (Fructus Forsythiae Suspensae)	The initial stage of sores
	Tian Hua Fen (Radix Trichosanthis)	Vaginal discharge and genital swelling

Note: This herb can also be used externally:
1. a powder of *Bai Lian* and *Chi Xiao Dou* (Semen Phaseoli Calcarati) can be mixed with egg white to treat the swelling and toxins of abscesses and sores;
2. a powder of *Bai Lian*, *Bai Ji* (Rhizoma Bletillae Striatae) and *Luo Shi Teng* (Caulis Trachelospermi Jasminoidis) can be used for scalds and for bleeding after injury (for *Bai Ji*, see notes on legal status);
3. a powder of *Bai Lian* with *Huang Bai* (Cortex Phellodendri) can be applied for frostbite.

Lü Dou 绿豆
(Mung bean, Semen Phaseoli Radiati)

Lü Dou is the dried seed of *Phaseolus radiatus* L., family Leguminosae.

Main ingredients *Lü Dou* contains proteins, fats, carbohydrates, iron, phosphorus, calcium, vitamins A, B and C, phosphatidylcholine, phosphatidylethanolamine, phosphatidylinositol, phosphatidylglycerol and phosphatidic acid.

Properties Taste: sweet; nature: cold.

Channels entered Heart and Stomach.

Functions and indications Clears heat and relieves toxicity, clears summerheat and promotes the movement of water. It is indicated for vexation and thirst due to summerheat, abscesses and sores, oedema and diarrhoea; and for relieving the toxicity caused by food poisoning and the taking of *Ba Dou* (Semen Crotonis Tiglii), *Fu Zi* (Radix Lateralis Aconiti Carmichaeli Praeparata) and *Pi Shuang* (Arsenicum). For *Fu Zi* and *Pi Shuang*, see notes on legal status.

Common dosage 15-30g; appropriate dosage for external application.

Precautions and contraindications *Lü Dou* is contraindicated for patients with diarrhoea due to Spleen and Stomach deficiency-cold.

Remarks *Lü Dou* can be used in summer to allay thirst due to summerheat. Boil 100g of the herb in 500 ml of water over a strong heat for 10 minutes; allow to cool before drinking.

Modern research Protects against phosphorus burns, prevents tumours, reduces the level of blood lipids.[129]

Combinations and applications

Functions	Combinations	Applications
Clearing heat and relieving toxicity, clearing summerheat and promoting the movement of water	*Huang Lian* (Rhizoma Coptidis) *Ge Gen* (Radix Puerariae) *Gan Cao* (Radix Glycyrrhizae)	Food poisoning, relieving the toxicity of *Ba Dou* (Semen Crotonis Tiglii), *Fu Zi* (Radix Lateralis Aconiti Carmichaeli Praeparata) and *Pi Shuang* (Arsenicum)
	Huang Lian (Rhizoma Coptidis) *Gan Cao* (Radix Glycyrrhizae)	Vexation and thirst due to summerheat
	Chi Xiao Dou (Semen Phaseoli Calcarati) *Chen Pi* (Pericarpium Citri Reticulatae)	Urinary stoppage, dribbling urination

Note: *Lü Dou* can be ground with *Da Huang* (Radix et Rhizoma Rhei) and applied with the juice from *Bo He* (Herba Menthae Haplocalycis) and *Feng Mi* (Mel) to treat the swelling and toxins of abscesses and sores.

Appendix

Lü Dou Yi 绿豆衣 (Mung bean skin, Testa Phaseoli Radiati)

Lü Dou Yi is the skin of *Lü Dou* (Semen Phaseoli Radiati). Sweet in taste and cold in nature, it enters the Heart and Stomach channels. Although it has the same functions as *Lü Dou*, it is more effective in clearing heat and relieving toxicity, but not as effective in dispersing summerheat. The dosage is 6-12g.

HERBS FOR CLEARING HEAT AND COOLING THE BLOOD

Herbs for clearing heat and cooling the Blood are generally bitter and cold. They clear heat from the Ying and Xue levels and are mainly used to treat Blood-heat patterns. These disorders occur when pathogenic factors invade the interior in the serious stage of warm-febrile diseases (the Ying level) and also during the critical stage of warm-febrile diseases (the Xue level), usually transmitted from the Ying level.

Clinically, herbs for clearing heat and cooling the Blood can be used to treat vexation, insomnia and delirious speech caused by pathogenic heat attacking the Ying level, accompanied by a crimson tongue with yellow fur and a fine, rapid pulse, as well as for maculopapular eruptions, vomiting of blood, coughing of blood, bleeding patterns, blood in the urine and blood in the stool caused by heat attacking the Xue level.

Heat attacks the Ying and Xue levels; it always damages Yin and consumes body fluids. Herbs for clearing heat and cooling the Blood should therefore be used in combination with herbs for nourishing Yin in order to treat fever (especially night fever), dry mouth and thirst, agitation and insomnia occurring as a consequence of heat attacking the Ying and Xue levels and consuming body fluids or as a result of latent heat in the later stages of febrile diseases. This combination is also used to treat fever, night sweating, dry throat and a crimson tongue resulting from Yin deficiency in the course of enduring illnesses. Those herbs which are also sweet and salty and nourish Yin and generate body fluids are an exception to this rule.

Herbs for clearing heat and cooling the Blood are mainly used to treat diseases caused by Blood-heat. In cases of Blood-heat combined with heat in the Qi level (the second stage of acute febrile diseases when pathogenic heat invades the interior), they are used in combination with herbs for clearing heat in the Qi level, whereas in cases of Blood patterns due to heat disturbing the Blood, they are used together with herbs for stopping bleeding and cooling the Blood. Herbs for clearing heat and cooling the Blood must not be used in the initial stage of illnesses caused by full-heat in the Qi level, otherwise Yang Qi will be damaged and heat pathogenic factors induced to invade the interior.

In addition to being cold, some of these herbs are also not easy to digest. Hence, they should be used carefully in the case of Spleen and Stomach deficiency because they may obstruct Stomach Qi.

Tab. 2.4 Herbs for clearing heat and cooling the Blood

Herb	Functions	Indications
Sheng Di Huang (Radix Rehmanniae Glutinosae)	Clearing heat and cooling the Blood, enriching Yin and nourishing the Blood to quench the upward flaming of fire	Nosebleed and vomiting of blood due to heat invading the Ying and Xue levels in warm-febrile diseases, dry mouth and vexation, high fever due to damage to Yin in febrile diseases, sore and swollen throat, wasting and thirsting with frequent urination, aching and limpness in the lumbar region and knees, night sweating, seminal emission
Xuan Shen (Radix Scrophulariae Ningpoensis)	Clearing heat and cooling the Blood, enriching Yin and bearing fire downwards, eliminating vexation, relieving toxicity and dissipating lumps	Fever and thirst, macular eruptions due to warm toxins, sore and swollen throat, abscesses and sores, scrofula, Phlegm nodes

Mu Dan Pi (Cortex Moutan Radicis)	Clearing heat and cooling the Blood, quickening the Blood and dissipating stasis	Maculopapular eruptions due to heat invading the Ying and Xue levels in warm diseases, vomiting of blood and nosebleed due to the frenetic movement of hot Blood, blood in the stool due to Blood-heat, abdominal masses, menstrual block, abscesses and sores
Chi Shao (Radix Paeoniae Rubra)	Clearing heat and cooling the Blood, dissipating Blood stasis and dispersing swelling to alleviate pain	Macular eruptions due to warm toxins, vomiting of blood and nosebleed in the course of warm diseases, abdominal masses, menstrual block due to Blood stasis, knocks and falls, abscesses and sores, pain in the abdomen and hypochondrium, fresh blood in the stool
Zi Cao (Radix Arnebiae seu Lithospermi)	Clearing heat and cooling the Blood, relieving toxicity and venting papules	High fever and vexation, measles, coughing of blood, nosebleed, sores and scabies
Shui Niu Jiao (Cornu Bubali)	Clearing heat, cooling the Blood, relieving toxicity	Coughing of blood and nosebleed due to the frenetic movement of hot Blood, dizziness due to vigorous non-abating fever, headache and sore and swollen throat due to exuberant heat and scorching fire in warm diseases, collapse due to fright, convulsions

Sheng Di Huang 生地黄 (Rehmannia root, Radix Rehmanniae Glutinosae)

Sheng Di Huang is the fresh or dried tuberous root of *Rehmannia glutinosa* (Gaertn.) Libosch., family Scrophulariaceae.

Main ingredients *Sheng Di Huang* contains catalpol, aucubin, melittoside, danmelittoside, rehmannioside, geniposide, daucosterol; caprylic, benzoic, phenylacetic, cinnamic, lauric, oleic, palmitic and linoleic acids; stachyose, raffinose, glucose, sucrose, fructose, galactose, β-sitosterol, stigmasterol, campesterol and mannitol.

Properties Taste: sweet and bitter; nature: cold.

Channels entered Heart, Liver and Kidney.

Functions and indications Clears heat and cools the Blood, and enriches Yin and nourishes the Blood to quench the upward flaming of fire. It is indicated for nosebleed and vomiting of blood due to heat invading the Ying and Xue levels in warm-febrile diseases, dry mouth and vexation, high fever due to damage to Yin in febrile diseases, sore and swollen throat, wasting and thirsting with frequent urination, aching and limpness in the lumbar region and knees, night sweating, and seminal emission.

Common dosage 10-30g; fresh *Sheng Di Huang* can be used in dosages of up to 60-100g; appropriate dosage for external application.

Precautions and contraindications *Sheng Di Huang* is contraindicated in cases of distension of the stomach and abdomen, and for loose stool due to Spleen and Stomach deficiency-cold.

Remarks Fresh *Sheng Di Huang*, also known as *Xian Di Huang* (Radix Rehmanniae Glutinosae Recens), is generally used to clear heat and cool the Blood, whereas dried *Sheng Di Huang*, or *Gan Di Huang* (Radix Rehmanniae Glutinosae Exsiccata) has the function of enriching Yin. After steaming in cooking wine, the herb is known as *Shu Di Huang* (Radix Rehmanniae Glutinosae Conquita) and is mainly used for supplementing the Essence, enriching Yin and nourishing the Blood (see also Chapter 17). The herb is most effective for stopping bleeding in its charred form, *Sheng Di Huang Tan* (Radix Rehmanniae Glutinosae Carbonisata).

Comparison of functions See *Xuan Shen* (Radix Scrophulariae Ningpoensis), *Mu Dan Pi* (Cortex Moutan Radicis) and *Shu Di Huang* (Radix Rehmanniae Glutinosae Conquita).

Modern research

1. Protects the functions of the liver.[130]
2. Regulates the blood sugar level.[131]
3. Promotes the generation of red cells and haemoglobin in animals with blood deficiency.[132]

Combinations and applications

Functions	Combinations	Applications
Clearing heat and cooling the Blood	*Ai Ye* (Folium Artemisiae Argyi) *Ce Bai Ye* (Cacumen Biotae Orientalis) *Bai Mao Gen* (Rhizoma Imperatae Cylindricae) *Huai Hua* (Flos Sophorae Japonicae) *He Ye* (Folium Nelumbinis Nuciferae)	Nosebleed, vomiting of blood and blood in the stool due to heat invading the Ying and Xue levels in the course of warm-febrile diseases
	Jing Jie Tan (Herba Schizonepetae Tenuifoliae Carbonisata) *Huang Qin* (Radix Scutellariae Baicalensis) *Da Huang Tan* (Radix et Rhizoma Rhei Carbonisatae) *Huai Hua* (Flos Sophorae Japonicae)	Dribbling urinary incontinence and uterine bleeding, vexing heat in the five hearts, and a red tongue and rapid pulse due to heat invading the Ying and Xue levels in the course of warm-febrile diseases

	Shui Niu Jiao (Cornu Bubali) *Chi Shao* (Radix Paeoniae Rubra) *Mu Dan Pi* (Cortex Moutan Radicis)	Vomiting of blood, nosebleed and dark purple maculopapular eruptions due to the frenetic movement of hot Blood
	Mu Dan Pi (Cortex Moutan Radicis) *Chan Tui* (Periostracum Cicadae) *Tu Fu Ling* (Rhizoma Smilacis Glabrae) *Jin Yin Hua* (Flos Lonicerae)	Urticaria (dormant papules) due to Blood-heat
Enriching Yin and nourishing the Blood to quench the upward flaming of fire	*Xuan Shen* (Radix Scrophulariae Ningpoensis) *Mai Men Dong* (Radix Ophiopogonis Japonici) *Shi Hu* (Herba Dendrobii) (see notes on legal status)	Fever and thirst with a crimson tongue due to damage to Yin in the course of warm diseases
	Shan Zhu Yu (Fructus Corni Officinalis) *Shu Di Huang* (Radix Rehmanniae Glutinosae Conquita)	Dizziness, tinnitus and limpness and aching in the lumbar region and knees due to insufficiency of the Liver and Kidneys
	Gui Ban (Plastrum Testudinis) (see notes on legal status) *Bai Shao* (Radix Paeoniae Lactiflorae)	Dizziness, insomnia, forgetfulness, night sweating and tidal fever caused by hyperactivity of Yang due to Yin deficiency
	Shan Yao (Rhizoma Dioscoreae Oppositae) *Wu Wei Zi* (Fructus Schisandrae)	Seminal emission, enuresis and wheezing due to Kidney deficiency
	Xuan Shen (Radix Scrophulariae Ningpoensis) *Mai Men Dong* (Radix Ophiopogonis Japonici) *Yu Zhu* (Rhizoma Polygonati Odorati) *Shan Yao* (Rhizoma Dioscoreae Oppositae)	Wasting and thirsting manifesting as vexation, thirst and profuse urination

Xuan Shen 玄参
(Figwort root, Radix Scrophulariae Ningpoensis)

Xuan Shen is the root of *Scrophularia ningpoensis* Hemsl., family Scrophulariaceae.

Main ingredients *Xuan Shen* contains harpagoside, harpagide, aucubin, ningpogoside, ningpogenin, scropoloside A, angoroside C and small amounts of volatile oils, plant sterols and alkaloids.

Properties Taste: sweet, bitter and salty; nature: cold.

Channels entered Lung, Stomach and Kidney.

Functions and indications Clears heat and cools the Blood, enriches Yin and bears fire downwards, eliminates vexation, and relieves toxicity and dissipates lumps. It is indicated for fever and thirst, macular eruptions due to warm toxins, sore and swollen throat, abscesses and sores, scrofula, and Phlegm nodes.

Common dosage 10-30g, or 60g for large dosages; appropriate dosage for external application.

Precautions and contraindications

1. *Xuan Shen* is contraindicated in cases of loose stool due to Spleen and Stomach deficiency-cold.

2. *Xuan Shen* is incompatible with *Li Lu* (Radix et Rhizoma Veratri).

Comparison of functions Both *Xuan Shen* (Radix Scrophulariae Ningpoensis) and *Sheng Di Huang* (Radix Rehmanniae Glutinosae) can clear heat and cool the Blood, enrich Yin and generate body fluids; they are often used in combination to accentuate each other's effect. However, *Xuan Shen* has a stronger effect in bearing fire downwards and relieving toxicity, while it also softens hardness and dissipates lumps so that it can be used for sore and swollen throat, scrofula and Phlegm nodes. *Sheng Di Huang* is more effective in clearing heat and cooling the Blood so that it can treat bleeding due to febrile diseases and wasting and thirsting patterns due to internal heat.

For an additional comparison, see *Ma Bo* (Sclerotium Lasiosphaerae seu Calvatiae).

Modern research

1. Preparations and alcoholic extracts of *Xuan Shen* lower blood pressure, strengthen the heart and dilate the blood vessels.[133, 134]
2. Has a tranquillizing effect, inhibits convulsions and abates fever.[133, 134]

Combinations and applications

Functions	Combinations	Applications
Clearing heat and cooling the Blood, enriching Yin and bearing fire downwards, eliminating vexation	*Sheng Di Huang* (Radix Rehmanniae Glutinosae) *Mai Men Dong* (Radix Ophiopogonis Japonici) *Lian Qiao* (Fructus Forsythiae Suspensae) *Zhi Mu* (Rhizoma Anemarrhenae Asphodeloidis) *Lian Zi Xin* (Plumula Nelumbinis Nuciferae)	Fever and thirst, vexation, maculopapular eruptions and a crimson tongue due to heat invading the Ying and Xue levels in the course of warm diseases
	Sha Shen (Radix Glehniae seu Adenophorae) *Mai Men Dong* (Radix Ophiopogonis Japonici) *Bai He* (Bulbus Lilii) *Bai Bu* (Radix Stemonae)	Dry cough without sputum, thirst, and a sore and swollen throat due to congestion of exuberant heat toxins
	Yu Zhu (Rhizoma Polygonati Odorati) *Tian Hua Fen* (Radix Trichosanthis) *Sheng Di Huang* (Radix Rehmanniae Glutinosae)	Wasting and thirsting due to effulgent Yin deficiency-fire, manifesting as dry mouth and tongue, vexation, thirst and profuse drinking
Relieving toxicity and dissipating lumps	*Bei Mu* (Bulbus Fritillariae) *Mu Li* (Concha Ostreae) *Xia Ku Cao* (Spica Prunellae Vulgaris)	Scrofula due to depression binding of Phlegm-fire
	Hai Zao (Herba Sargassi) *Kun Bu* (Thallus Laminariae seu Eckloniae) *Mu Li* (Concha Ostreae) *Dan Shen* (Radix Salviae Miltiorrhizae)	Goitre, Phlegm nodes, streaming sores
	Jin Yin Hua (Flos Lonicerae) *Lian Qiao* (Fructus Forsythiae Suspensae) *Zi Hua Di Ding* (Herba Violae Yedoensitis)	Abscesses, sores and swellings due to heat toxins
	Jin Yin Hua (Flos Lonicerae) *Dang Gui* (Radix Angelicae Sinensis) *Gan Cao* (Radix Glycyrrhizae)	Sloughing abscess due to heat toxins

Mu Dan Pi 牡丹皮 (Tree peony root bark, Cortex Moutan Radicis)

Mu Dan Pi is the peel of the root of *Paeonia suffruticosa* Andr., family Ranunculaceae.

Main ingredients *Mu Dan Pi* contains paeonol, paeonoside, paeonolide, paeoniflorin, oxypaeoniflorin, benzoylpaeoniflorin, gallic acid, volatile oils, sucrose and glucose.

Properties Taste: bitter and acrid; nature: cool.

Channels entered Heart, Liver and Kidney.

Functions and indications Clears heat and cools the Blood, quickens the Blood and dissipates stasis. It is indicated for maculopapular eruptions due to heat invading the Ying and Xue levels in warm diseases, vomiting of blood and nosebleed due to the frenetic movement of hot Blood, blood in the stool due to Blood-heat, abdominal masses, menstrual block, and abscesses and sores.

Common dosage 6-12g, or 30g for large dosages.

Precautions and contraindications *Mu Dan Pi* is contraindicated for Spleen and Stomach deficiency-cold, deficiency of Blood accompanied by coldness, as well as in cases of profuse menstruation, and during pregnancy.

Remarks Raw *Mu Dan Pi* is especially effective in clearing heat and cooling the Blood; when stir-fried with alcohol, the herb can quicken the Blood and dissipate Blood stasis; charred *Mu Dan Pi* is used for cooling the Blood to stop bleeding.

Comparison of functions Both *Mu Dan Pi* (Cortex Moutan Radicis) and *Sheng Di Huang* (Radix Rehmanniae Glutinosae) can treat fever due to Yin deficiency. *Mu Dan Pi* is aromatic and has a dispersing function so that it can not only abate fever but also dissipate stasis. *Sheng Di Huang* is sweet and cold and can enrich Yin to abate fever. The two herbs are often used together to accentuate each other's effect.

For additional comparisons, see *Chi Shao* (Radix Paeoniae Rubra) and *Di Gu Pi* (Cortex Lycii Radicis).

Modern research

1. Decoctions of *Mu Dan Pi* can inhibit such bacteria as Staphylococcus albus, Escherichia coli and Salmonella typhi.[135]
2. Inhibits the central nervous system, has a tranquillizing function, inhibits convulsions, abates fever and alleviates pain.[136]

Combinations and applications

Functions	Combinations	Applications
Clearing heat and cooling the Blood	*Shui Niu Jiao* (Cornu Bubali) *Sheng Di Huang* (Radix Rehmanniae Glutinosae) *Chi Shao* (Radix Paeoniae Rubra)	High fever and maculopapular eruptions with a crimson tongue due to heat invading the Ying and Xue levels in the course of warm diseases
	Sheng Di Huang (Radix Rehmanniae Glutinosae) *Zhi Zi* (Fructus Gardeniae Jasminoidis) *Bai Mao Gen* (Rhizoma Imperatae Cylindricae)	Vomiting of blood and nosebleed due to pathogenic heat causing the frenetic movement of hot Blood
	Qing Hao (Herba Artemisiae Chinghao) *Zhi Mu* (Rhizoma Anemarrhenae Asphodeloidis) *Bie Jia* (Carapax Amydae Sinensis) (see notes on legal status) *Bai Wei* (Radix Cynanchi Atrati)	Night fever and steaming bone disorder without sweating due to damage to Yin brought about by warm pathogenic factors

	Chai Hu (Radix Bupleuri) *Yu Jin* (Radix Curcumae) *Chuan Lian Zi* (Fructus Meliae Toosendan)	Dizziness, pain in the hypochondrium, vexing heat in the five hearts, and a string-like pulse due to depressed heat in the Lung channel
Quickening the Blood and dissipating stasis	*Dang Gui* (Radix Angelicae Sinensis) *Chuan Xiong* (Rhizoma Ligustici Chuanxiong) *Chi Shao* (Radix Paeoniae Rubra) *Tao Ren* (Semen Persicae)	Menstrual block or painful menstruation due to Blood stasis
	Da Huang (Radix et Rhizoma Rhei) *Mang Xiao* (Mirabilitum) *Bai Jiang Cao* (Herba Patriniae cum Radice)	Intestinal abscess due to Blood stasis obstructed internally
	Pu Gong Ying (Herba Taraxaci cum Radice) *Chi Shao* (Radix Paeoniae Rubra) *Zi Hua Di Ding* (Herba Violae Yedoensitis)	Clove sores and toxic abscesses with local redness, swelling, pain and heat due to internal obstruction of Qi and Blood and internally exuberant heat toxins
	Gua Lou (Fructus Trichosanthis) *Xie Bai* (Bulbus Allii Macrostemi) *Gui Zhi* (Ramulus Cinnamomi Cassiae) *Hong Hua* (Flos Carthami Tinctorii)	Pain in the chest due to Blood stasis
	Chi Shao (Radix Paeoniae Rubra) *Ru Xiang* (Gummi Olibanum) *Mo Yao* (Myrrha)	Swelling and pain due to Blood stasis caused by knocks and falls

Chi Shao 赤芍 (Red peony root, Radix Paeoniae Rubra)

Chi Shao is the root of *Paeonia lactiflora* Pall., *P. veitchii* Lynch or several other species of the same genus, family Ranunculaceae.

Main ingredients *Chi Shao* contains paeoniflorin, albiflorin, oxypaeoniflorin, benzoylpaeoniflorin, lactiflorin and benzoic acid. Recently, d-catechin and gallic acid have also been discovered as constituents.

Properties Taste: bitter; nature: slightly cold.

Channels entered Liver and Spleen.

Functions and indications Clears heat and cools the Blood, dissipates Blood stasis and disperses swelling to alleviate pain. It is indicated for macular eruptions due to warm toxins, vomiting of blood and nosebleed in the course of warm diseases, abdominal masses, menstrual block due to Blood stasis, knocks and falls, abscesses and sores, pain in the abdomen and hypochondrium, and fresh blood in the stool.

Common dosage 6-15g, or 30g for large dosages.

Precautions and contraindications

1. *Chi Shao* should be used with caution in cases of Blood deficiency and abdominal pain of the deficiency-cold type.
2. *Chi Shao* is incompatible with *Li Lu* (Radix et Rhizoma Veratri).

Comparison of functions

1. Both *Chi Shao* (Radix Paeoniae Rubra) and *Mu Dan Pi* (Cortex Moutan Radicis) can cool the

Blood and dissipate stasis and are often used in combination to treat vomiting of blood and maculopapular eruptions due to heat in the Blood. *Mu Dan Pi* is more effective in clearing heat and cooling the Blood; not only can it clear full-heat in the Xue level, but it is also effective in eliminating deficiency-heat in the Ying level to treat steaming bone disorder without sweating. *Chi Shao* is comparatively weak in clearing heat and cooling the Blood, but is more effective in quickening the Blood and dissipating stasis to alleviate pain and treat menstrual block and pain in the abdomen due to Blood stasis.

2. *Chi Shao* (Radix Paeoniae Rubra) and *Bai Shao* (Radix Paeoniae Lactiflorae) can be derived from the same plant (*Paeonia lactiflora* Pall.) and both can be used to alleviate pain. *Chi Shao* tends to clear heat, quicken the Blood and dissipate stasis to relieve pain, and is used more often for disorders due to Blood-heat and Blood stasis. On the other hand, *Bai Shao* tends to nourish the Blood, constrain Yin and calm the Liver to relieve pain, and is commonly used for disorders due to Blood and Yin deficiency. For further details, see also *Bai Shao* (Radix Paeoniae Lactiflorae).

Modern research

1. Increases the volume of coronary blood flow.[137]
2. Improves the memory.[138]
3. Protects the functions of the liver.[139, 140]

Combinations and applications

Functions	Combinations	Applications
Clearing heat and cooling the Blood	*Shui Niu Jiao* (Cornu Bubali) *Mu Dan Pi* (Cortex Moutan Radicis) *Sheng Di Huang* (Radix Rehmanniae Glutinosae)	High fever, maculopapular eruptions and a crimson tongue due to heat invading the Ying and Xue levels in the course of warm diseases
	Huang Bai (Cortex Phellodendri) *Di Yu* (Radix Sanguisorbae Officinalis) *Da Huang* (Radix et Rhizoma Rhei)	The initial stage of dysentery with significant blood and a little pus in the stool
	Xiang Fu Zi (Semen Cyperi Rotundi) *Shi Yan* (Sal, salt)	Profuse uterine bleeding or red and white vaginal discharge
	Ju Hua (Flos Chrysanthemi Morifolii) *Jue Ming Zi* (Semen Cassiae)	Red, sore and swollen eyes due to heat toxins attacking the upper body
Dissipating Blood stasis and dispersing swelling to alleviate pain	*Tao Ren* (Semen Persicae) *Dang Gui* (Radix Angelicae Sinensis) *Niu Xi* (Radix Achyranthis Bidentatae)	Menstrual block and pain in the abdomen due to Blood stasis
	Dang Gui (Radix Angelicae Sinensis) *Chuan Xiong* (Rhizoma Ligustici Chuanxiong) *Pao Jiang* (Rhizoma Zingiberis Officinalis Praeparata)	Postpartum pain in the abdomen due to Blood stasis
	Pu Gong Ying (Herba Taraxaci cum Radice) *Tian Hua Fen* (Radix Trichosanthis)	Breast abscess
	Ru Xiang (Gummi Olibanum) *Mo Yao* (Myrrha) *Xue Jie* (Resina Draconis) *Tu Bie Chong* (Eupolyphaga seu Steleophaga)	Swelling and pain due to Blood stasis after knocks and falls

	Chai Hu (Radix Bupleuri) *Xiang Fu* (Rhizoma Cyperi Rotundi) *Chen Pi* (Pericarpium Citri Reticulatae)	Pain in the hypochondrium due to Blood stasis

Zi Cao 紫草 (Arnebia or gromwell root, Radix Arnebiae seu Lithospermi)

Zi Cao is the dried root of *Arnebia euchroma* (Royle) Johnst. or *Lithospermum erythrorizon* Sieb. et Zucc., family Boraginaceae.

Main ingredients *Zi Cao* contains shikonin, teracrylshikonin, acetylshikonin and other shikonin compounds, alkannan and alkannin.

Properties Taste: sweet; nature: cold.

Channels entered Heart and Liver.

Functions and indications Clears heat and cools the Blood, relieves toxicity and vents papules. It is indicated for high fever and vexation, measles, coughing of blood, nosebleed, sores and scabies.

Common dosage 3-10g; or appropriate dosage for external application as a powder or cream.

Precautions and contraindications *Zi Cao* is contraindicated for loose stool due to Spleen deficiency because it can induce a slight purgative effect.

Modern research

1. Both the decoction of *Zi Cao* and the shikonin it contains had an obvious inhibitory effect *in vitro* on such pathogenic micro-organisms as Staphylococcus aureus, Bacterium coli and Salmonella typhi.[141]
2. The shikonin contained in *Zi Cao* can inhibit influenza and encephalitis B viruses.[142]
3. Decoctions of *Zi Cao* can abate fever.[142]

Combinations and applications

Functions	Combinations	Applications
Clearing heat and cooling the Blood, relieving toxicity and venting papules	*Huang Lian* (Rhizoma Coptidis) *Zhi Zi* (Fructus Gardeniae Jasminoidis) *Mu Dan Pi* (Cortex Moutan Radicis)	High fever, vexation and agitation, a crimson tongue and a rapid pulse due to heat invading the Ying and Xue levels in the course of warm diseases
	Sheng Di Huang (Radix Rehmanniae Glutinosae) *Mu Dan Pi* (Cortex Moutan Radicis) *Chi Shao* (Radix Paeoniae Rubra)	Coughing of blood, nosebleed and vomiting of blood due to heat
	Chan Tui (Periostracum Cicadae) *Chi Shao* (Radix Paeoniae Rubra) *Gan Cao* (Radix Glycyrrhizae)	Macular eruptions due to warm toxins, dark purple maculopapular eruptions due to exuberant toxins resulting from Blood-heat
	Bai Zhi (Radix Angelicae Dahuricae) *Xue Jie* (Resina Draconis)	Non-healing abscesses and sores
	Ku Shen (Radix Sophorae Flavescentis) *Huang Bai* (Cortex Phellodendri)	Purpura

	Gou Teng (Ramulus Uncariae cum Uncis)	Non-eruption of measles in children

Note: *Zi Cao* can also be used externally to treat abscesses, eczema, pudendal itch, and scabies and tinea. These conditions can be treated by a cream prepared from *Zi Cao* in combination with *Bai Zhi* (Radix Angelicae Dahuricae), *Dang Gui* (Radix Angelicae Sinensis) and *Xue Jie* (Resina Draconis).

Shui Niu Jiao 水牛角 (Water buffalo horn, Cornu Bubali)

Shui Niu Jiao is the horn of *Bubalus bubalis* L., family Bovidae.

Main ingredients *Shui Niu Jiao* contains cholesterol, peptides and trace elements.

Properties Taste: bitter and salty; nature: cold.

Channels entered Heart, Liver and Stomach.

Functions and indications Clears heat, cools the Blood and relieves toxicity. It is indicated for coughing of blood and nosebleed due to the frenetic movement of hot Blood, dizziness due to vigorous non-abating fever, headache and sore and swollen throat due to exuberant heat and scorching fire in warm diseases, collapse due to fright, and convulsions.

Common dosage 6-15g, prepared into powder or pills for oral use.

Precautions and contraindications *Shui Niu Jiao* is contraindicated in cases of Spleen and Stomach deficiency-cold.

Remarks *Shui Niu Jiao* is normally used these days as a substitute for *Xi Jiao* (Cornu Rhinoceri) as a result of the endangered species status of the rhinoceros.

Modern research

1. A 50% concentration of decoctions of *Shui Niu Jiao* can strengthen myocardial contractions.[143]
2. Excites the pituitary-adrenocortical system.[143]

Combinations and applications

Functions	Combinations	Applications
Clearing heat, cooling the Blood and relieving toxicity	*Sheng Di Huang* (Radix Rehmanniae Glutinosae) *Mu Dan Pi* (Cortex Moutan Radicis)	Coughing of blood, nosebleed and vomiting of blood due to the frenetic movement of hot Blood
	Lian Qiao (Fructus Forsythiae Suspensae) *Xuan Shen* (Radix Scrophulariae Ningpoensis) *Shi Gao* (Gypsum Fibrosum)	Vigorous non-abating fever, headache and sore and swollen throat due to exuberant heat and scorching fire in warm diseases
	Huang Lian (Rhizoma Coptidis) *Lian Qiao* (Fructus Forsythiae Suspensae) *Chi Shao* (Radix Paeoniae Rubra)	Sores, boils and abscesses with redness, swelling, pain and heat

HERBS FOR CLEARING DEFICIENCY-HEAT

Most of the herbs in this section are cold and can cool the Blood and clear deficiency-heat. They are mainly used for fever due to Yin deficiency, Gan disorders with fever, night fever, and absence of sweating after fever due to pathogenic heat lingering in the Ying level in the final stage of warm-febrile diseases.

Clinically, these herbs must be used in combination with other herbs depending on the nature of the disease involved:

1. in cases of pathogenic heat lingering in the Ying level in the final stage of a warm-febrile disease, they should be used together with herbs for clearing heat and cooling the Blood;
2. in cases of fever in the course of a chronic consumptive disease and steaming bone disorder due to Yin deficiency, they are to be used together with herbs for nourishing Yin, supplementing the Kidneys and moistening the Lungs;
3. in cases of Gan disorders with fever, they are used in combination with herbs which relieve indigestion and fortify the Spleen or with herbs for expelling worms.

Tab. 2.5 Herbs for clearing deficiency-heat

Herb	Functions	Indications
Qing Hao (Herba Artemisiae Chinghao)	Abating deficiency-heat and cooling the Blood, clearing and relieving summerheat, interrupting malaria	Warm diseases, fever due to summerheat or Yin deficiency, steaming bone disorder, malaria, dysentery, jaundice
Di Gu Pi (Cortex Lycii Radicis)	Cooling the Blood and eliminating steam, clearing the Lungs and draining fire	Night sweating, steaming bone disorder with sweating, cough, nosebleed, coughing of blood due to Lung-heat, vexation and thirst due to internal heat, malaria
Yin Chai Hu (Radix Stellariae Dichotomae)	Clearing deficiency-heat, eliminating Gan fever	Steaming bone disorder and other fevers due to Yin deficiency, night sweating, Gan accumulation
Hu Huang Lian (Rhizoma Picrorhizae Scrophulariiflorae)	Clearing heat and drying dampness, eliminating steam and dispersing Gan	Fever due to Yin deficiency, Gan accumulation, damp-heat dysentery
Bai Wei (Radix Cynanchi Atrati)	Clearing heat and cooling the Blood to abate fever, promoting urination and freeing Lin syndrome, relieving toxicity and treating sores	Internal heat patterns due to Yin deficiency, postpartum deficiency-heat patterns, cough due to Lung-heat, night sweating, heat Lin syndrome, blood Lin syndrome, sore and swollen throat, scrofula, poisonous snake bites

Qing Hao 青蒿
(Sweet wormwood, Herba Artemisiae Chinghao)

Qing Hao is the dried aerial parts of *Artemisia annua* L., or *A. apiacea* Hance, family Compositae.

Main ingredients *Qing Hao* contains sesquiterpenes (including arteannuin B and the anti-malarial artemisinin), flavones (including kaempferol, quercetin, luteolin, patuletin, eupatorin and rhamnetin), volatile oils (including camphene, isoartemisia ketone, β-caryophyllene, α- and β-pinene, artemisia ketone, myrcene and limonene), coumarin, stigmasterol and palmitic acid.

Properties Taste: bitter and acrid; nature: cold.

Channels entered Liver, Gallbladder and Kidney.

Functions and indications Abates deficiency-heat and cools the Blood, clears and relieves summerheat, and interrupts malaria. It is indicated for warm diseases, fever due to summerheat or Yin deficiency, steaming bone disorder, malaria, dysentery, and jaundice.

Common dosage 3-10g, or 20g for large dosages; this herb should not be decocted for a long period.

Precautions and contraindications *Qing Hao* is contraindicated in cases of loose stool due to Spleen and Stomach deficiency-cold, or postpartum wheezing due to Qi deficiency.

Comparison of functions Both *Qing Hao* (Herba Artemisiae Chinghao) and *Chai Hu* (Radix Bupleuri) enter the Liver and Gallbladder channels and can treat malaria and alternating chills and fever. The difference is that *Chai Hu* has an upward-bearing and dispersing nature and is good at allowing constrained Liver Qi to flow freely, relieving depression and uplifting clear Yang. Overdosage of this herb can damage Yin. *Qing Hao*, with its aromatic clearing and cooling functions, is good at clearing and expelling deep-lying heat, cooling the Blood, eliminating steaming bone disorder and relieving summerheat; in performing these functions, it does not damage Yin.

For an additional comparison, see *Yin Chen Hao* (Herba Artemisiae Scopariae).

Modern research

1. The artemisinin contained in *Qing Hao* has a direct effect in the treatment of malaria.[144, 145]
2. Slows the heart rate, and reduces the volume of the coronary arteries.[146]

Combinations and applications

Functions	Combinations	Applications
Abating deficiency-heat and cooling the Blood	*Zhi Mu* (Rhizoma Anemarrhenae Asphodeloidis) *Bie Jia* (Carapax Amydae Sinensis) (see notes on legal status) *Sheng Di Huang* (Radix Rehmanniae Glutinosae) *Mu Dan Pi* (Cortex Moutan Radicis)	The final stage of warm diseases with residual heat and damage to Yin, night fever abating at dawn, abatement of fever without sweating or unremitting low-level fever in the aftermath of febrile diseases
	Bie Jia (Carapax Amydae Sinensis) (see notes on legal status) *Qin Jiao* (Radix Gentianae Macrophyllae) *Di Gu Pi* (Cortex Lycii Radicis)	Steaming bone disorder with taxation fever, night sweating and cough due to effulgent Yin deficiency-fire

Clearing and relieving summerheat	*Shi Gao* (Gypsum Fibrosum) *Zhi Mu* (Rhizoma Anemarrhenae Asphodeloidis) *Xi Gua Cui Yi* (Epicarpium Citrulli Vulgaris)	Fever and thirst, vexation and scant urine due to an invasion of summerheat
	Guang Huo Xiang (Herba Pogostemi) *Pei Lan* (Herba Eupatorii Fortunei) *Bai Bian Dou* (Semen Dolichoris Lablab) *Hua Shi* (Talcum)	Fever and thirst, and focal distension and fullness in the chest and stomach due to summerheat-damp
Interrupting malaria	*Huang Qin* (Radix Scutellariae Baicalensis) *Chang Shan* (Radix Dichroae Febrifugae) *Ban Xia* (Rhizoma Pinelliae Ternatae) *Zhu Ru* (Caulis Bambusae in Taeniis)	Alternating chills and fever, or high fever with a slight chill due to latent pathogenic factors in the Shaoyang channel during warm-febrile diseases

Di Gu Pi 地骨皮 (Wolfberry root bark, Cortex Lycii Radicis)

Di Gu Pi is the bark of the root of *Lycium chinense* Mill. and *L. barbarum* L., family Solanaceae.

Main ingredients *Di Gu Pi* contains cinnamic acid and many types of phenol, betaine, kukoamine A, β-sitosterol, linoleic acid and linolenic acid.

Properties Taste: sweet and bland; nature: cold.

Channels entered Lung, Liver and Kidney.

Functions and indications Cools the Blood and eliminates steam, clears the Lungs and drains fire. It is indicated for night sweating, steaming bone disorder with sweating, cough, nosebleed, coughing of blood due to Lung-heat, vexation and thirst due to internal heat, and malaria.

Common dosage 10-15g, or 30g for large dosages.

Precautions and contraindications *Di Gu Pi* is contraindicated in cases of loose stool due to Spleen and Stomach deficiency-cold, and in cases of fever due to externally-contracted wind-cold.

Comparison of functions Both *Di Gu Pi* (Cortex Lycii Radicis) and *Mu Dan Pi* (Cortex Moutan Radicis) can cool the Blood and abate deficiency-heat. *Di Gu Pi* is good at treating steaming bone disorder with sweating, and coughing and wheezing due to Lung-heat, whereas *Mu Dan Pi* is better for treating steaming bone disorder without sweating.

Modern research

1. Abates fever.[147]
2. Lowers blood pressure and slows the heart rate.[148]
3. In laboratory tests, a decoction of *Di Gu Pi* inhibited Salmonella typhi, Salmonella paratyphi A and Shigella flexneri, but not Staphylococcus aureus.[149]

Combinations and applications

Functions	Combinations	Applications
Cooling the Blood and eliminating steam	*Tian Men Dong* (Radix Asparagi Cochinchinensis) *Mai Men Dong* (Radix Ophiopogonis Japonici) *Yin Chai Hu* (Radix Stellariae Dichotomae) *Bie Jia* (Carapax Amydae Sinensis) (see notes on legal status) *Sheng Di Huang* (Radix Rehmanniae Glutinosae) *Zhi Mu* (Rhizoma Anemarrhenae Asphodeloidis)	Tidal fever, night sweating and steaming bone disorder due to effulgent Yin deficiency-fire
	Tian Hua Fen (Radix Trichosanthis) *Mai Men Dong* (Radix Ophiopogonis Japonici) *Yu Zhu* (Rhizoma Polygonati Odorati) *Ze Xie* (Rhizoma Alismatis Orientalis)	Wasting and thirsting due to internal heat, agitation
	Bai Mao Gen (Rhizoma Imperatae Cylindricae) *Mu Dan Pi* (Cortex Moutan Radicis) *Ce Bai Ye* (Cacumen Biotae Orientalis)	Nosebleed and coughing and vomiting of blood due to the frenetic movement of hot Blood
Clearing the Lungs and draining fire	*Sang Bai Pi* (Cortex Mori Albae Radicis) *Huang Qin* (Radix Scutellariae Baicalensis) *Bei Mu* (Bulbus Fritillariae) *Zhi Mu* (Rhizoma Anemarrhenae Asphodeloidis) *Shi Gao* (Gypsum Fibrosum)	Cough, shortness of breath, copious sputum and thirst due to Lung-heat

Yin Chai Hu 银柴胡 (Stellaria root, Radix Stellariae Dichotomae)

Yin Chai Hu is the dried root of *Stellaria dichotoma* L. var. *lanceolata* Bge., family Caryophyllaceae.

Legal status *Yin Chai Hu* was listed in a document entitled *A Review of Restricted Herbal Ingredients* issued by the Medicines Control Agency (MCA) in the UK in September 2001 with a view to the possible imposition of restrictions on its use at a future date. Use of this herb is controlled in Hong Kong and the MCA is considering introducing a requirement for medical supervision in the UK.

Main ingredients *Yin Chai Hu* contains α-spinasterol, β-sitosterol, stigmasterol, wogonin, valeric acid, caproic acid, heptylic acid, octaroic acid and stellaria cyclopeptide.

Properties Taste: sweet; nature: slightly cold.

Channels entered Liver and Stomach.

Functions and indications Clears deficiency-heat and eliminates Gan fever. It is indicated for steaming bone disorder and other fevers due to Yin deficiency, night sweating, and Gan accumulation.

Common dosage 3-10g.

Precautions and contraindications *Yin Chai Hu* is contraindicated in cases of externally-contracted wind-cold or Blood deficiency without fever.

Comparison of functions Despite the similarity of name, *Yin Chai Hu* (Radix Stellariae Dichotomae) and *Chai Hu* (Radix Bupleuri) are not from the same family. Although both have the function of abating fever, *Yin Chai Hu* is used for clearing and abating deficiency-heat and is employed specifically to treat fever due to Yin deficiency as well as Gan accumulation. It does not have an upward-bearing and dispersing nature. *Chai Hu* can abate fever through harmonization and is effective in treating alternating chills and fever due to Shaoyang diseases. It does have an upward-bearing and dispersing nature, but does not have the function of eliminating steaming bone disorder and dispersing Gan accumulation.

For an additional comparison, see *Qin Jiao* (Radix Gentianae Macrophyllae).

Modern research Can reduce serum cholesterol and the lipoid content in the aorta.[150]

Combinations and applications

Functions	Combinations	Applications
Clearing deficiency-heat, eliminating Gan fever	*Qing Hao* (Herba Artemisiae Chinghao) *Di Gu Pi* (Cortex Lycii Radicis)	Steaming bone disorder, tidal fever and night sweating resulting from internal heat due to Yin deficiency
	Bie Jia (Carapax Amydae Sinensis) (see notes on legal status)	Warm pathogenic factors damaging Yin, manifesting as dry skin and thin body, and tidal fever due to Yin deficiency
	Dan Shen (Radix Salviae Miltiorrhizae) *Huang Qin* (Radix Scutellariae Baicalensis) *Zhi Zi* (Fructus Gardeniae Jasminoidis)	Fever due to Gan accumulation

Hu Huang Lian 胡黄连 (Picrorhiza rhizome, Rhizoma Picrorhizae Scrophulariiflorae)

Hu Huang Lian is the dried rhizome of *Picrhoriza scrophulariiflora* Pennell, family Scrophulariaceae.

Main ingredients *Hu Huang Lian* contains catalpol, kutkoside, kutkin, picrosides I, II and III, d-mannitol, vanillic acid, cinnamic acid, ferulic acid, kutkinol and kutkisterol.

Properties Taste: bitter; nature: cold.

Channels entered Liver, Stomach and Large Intestine.

Functions and indications Clears heat and dries dampness, eliminates steam and disperses Gan. It is indicated for fever due to Yin deficiency, Gan accumulation, and damp-heat dysentery.

Common dosage 3-10g.

Precautions and contraindications *Hu Huang Lian* is contraindicated in cases of Spleen and Stomach deficiency-cold.

Comparison of functions Both *Hu Huang Lian* (Rhizoma Picrorhizae Scrophulariiflorae) and *Huang Lian* (Rhizoma Coptidis) are bitter and cold, and can clear heat and dry dampness to treat damp-heat dysentery. Since their functions are similar, *Hu Huang Lian* is often used as a cheaper substitute for *Huang Lian*. *Hu Huang Lian* is good at abating deficiency fever and eliminating Gan fever, whereas *Huang Lian* is effective for clearing Heart-fire and draining Stomach-fire and is an important herb for relieving toxicity.

Modern research Soothes the gallbladder and inhibits epiphytes.[151]

Combinations and applications

Functions	Combinations	Applications
Clearing heat and drying dampness, eliminating steam and dispersing Gan	*Huang Qin* (Radix Scutellariae Baicalensis) *Mu Xiang* (Radix Aucklandiae Lappae) (see notes on legal status)	Damp-heat dysentery
	Wu Mei (Fructus Pruni Mume) *He Zi* (Fructus Terminaliae Chebulae)	Chronic diarrhoea
	Di Yu (Radix Sanguisorbae Officinalis) *Huang Bai* (Cortex Phellodendri) *Huai Hua* (Flos Sophorae Japonicae)	Bleeding and painful swelling in the anus due to haemorrhoids
	Xuan Shen (Radix Scrophulariae Ningpoensis) *Yin Chai Hu* (Radix Stellariae Dichotomae) *Shi Da Gong Lao Ye* (Folium Mahoniae)	Fever, dry mouth and night sweating due to Yin deficiency
	Di Gu Pi (Cortex Lycii Radicis) *Qin Jiao* (Radix Gentianae Macrophyllae) *Bie Jia* (Carapax Amydae Sinensis) (see notes on legal status)	Steaming bone disorder, tidal fever and night sweating, fever due to Yin deficiency
	Dang Shen (Radix Codonopsitis Pilosulae) *Shi Jun Zi* (Fructus Quisqualis Indicae) *Shan Zha* (Fructus Crataegi)	Fever due to Gan accumulation, indigestion

Bai Wei 白薇
(Black-end swallowwort root, Radix Cynanchi Atrati)

Bai Wei is the dried root and rhizome of *Cynanchum atratum* Bge. or *C. versicolor* Bge., family Asclepiadaceae.

Main ingredients *Bai Wei* contains cynanchol, cynatratoside A to F, cynanversicoside, neocynanversicoside, cardiac glycosides and volatile oils.

Properties Taste: bitter and salty; nature: cold.

Channels entered Lung, Stomach and Kidney.

Functions and indications Clears heat and cools the Blood to abate fever, promotes urination and frees Lin syndrome, relieves toxicity and treats sores. It is indicated for internal heat patterns due to Yin deficiency, postpartum deficiency-heat patterns, cough due to Lung-heat, night sweating, heat Lin syndrome, blood Lin syndrome, sore and swollen throat, scrofula, and poisonous snake bites.

Common dosage 3-12g; appropriate dosage for external application.

Precautions and contraindications *Bai Wei* is contraindicated in cases of loose stool due to Spleen and Stomach deficiency-cold.

Remarks As *Bai Wei* can enter the Xue level, it is an excellent herb for clearing heat and draining fire.

Modern research

1. Strengthens contraction of the cardiac muscle, slows the heart rate and is effective against haematose heart failure.[152]
2. Inhibits inflammation and abates fever.[153, 154]
3. Expels sputum and calms wheezing.[154]

Combinations and applications

Functions	Combinations	Applications
Clearing heat and cooling the Blood to abate fever	*Sheng Di Huang* (Radix Rehmanniae Glutinosae) *Xuan Shen* (Radix Scrophulariae Ningpoensis) *Dan Zhu Ye* (Herba Lophatheri Gracilis)	Enduring fever with vexation and thirst due to heat invading the Ying and Xue levels in the course of warm diseases
	Di Gu Pi (Cortex Lycii Radicis) *Mai Men Dong* (Radix Ophiopogonis Japonici)	The final stage of febrile diseases with a reduced level of fever and sweating
	Zhe Bei Mu (Bulbus Fritillariae Thunbergii) *Hai Ge Ke* (Concha Meretricis seu Cyclinae)	Cough due to Lung-heat
	Zhu Ru (Caulis Bambusae in Taeniis) *Shi Gao* (Gypsum Fibrosum)	Vexation and vomiting due to postpartum deficiency-heat
Promoting urination and freeing Lin syndrome	*Mu Tong* (Caulis Mutong) (see notes on legal status) *Hua Shi* (Talcum) *Sheng Di Huang* (Radix Rehmanniae Glutinosae)	Heat Lin syndrome, blood Lin syndrome
Relieving toxicity and treating sores	*Tian Men Dong* (Radix Asparagi Cochinchinensis)	Scrofula

Note: A powder of *Bai Wei* can be applied externally to treat bleeding due to external injury.

Modern research references

1. Wang Aifang et al., *Yao Xue Tong Bao* [Pharmacology Bulletin] 3 (1981): 61.
2. He Xingdong et al., *Lin Chuang Zhong Yao Shou Ce* [Clinical Handbook of Chinese Materia Medica] (Beijing: People's Medical Publishing House, 1998), 28.
3. Zhen Shimin et al., *Zhong Guo Yao Li Xue Bao* [Chinese Journal of Pharmacology] 10, 1 (1989): 85.
4. Liang Yuehua et al., *Zhong Yi Za Zhi* [Journal of Traditional Chinese Medicine] 23, 11 (1982): 68.
5. Liang Yuehua et al., *Bei Jing Yi Ke Da Xue Xue Bao* [Journal of Beijing Medical University] 19, 1 (1987): 54.
6. Liang Yuehua et al., *Zhong Yao Tong Bao* [Bulletin of Chinese Materia Medica] 13, 11 (1988): 48.
7. Zhou Qun et al., *Zhong Cao Yao* [Journal of Chinese Herbs] 19, 3 (1988): 35.
8. Birth Control Research Office of Wuhan Medical College, *Ji Hua Sheng Yu Ke Yan Zi Liao* [Scientific Research Document on Birth Control] (1978): 26.
9. Zeng Mibai et al., *Shi Yan Sheng Wu Xue Bao* [Journal of Experimental Biology] 12, 3 (1979): 267.
10. Shu Huaibai et al., *Sheng Li Xue Bao* [Physiology Journal] 31, 1 (1979): 21.
11. Liu Guowu et al., *Sheng Zhi Yu Bi Yun* [Reproduction and Contraception] 1, 3 (1981): 20.
12. Geng Baoqin et al., *Zhe Jiang Zhong Liu Tong Xun* [Zhejiang Tumour Newsletter] 4 (1980): 166.

13. Michael S. McGrath et al., *Proc Natl Acad Sci USA* 86, 8 (1989): 2844.
14. Hu Yunsheng (translator), *Guo Wai Yao Xun* [Foreign Pharmacology Newsletter] 6 (1993): 31.
15. Lei Zaiquan and Zhang Tingmo, *Zhong Hua Lin Chuang Zhong Yao Xue* [Chinese Clinical Materia Medica] (Beijing: People's Medical Publishing House, 1998), 452.
16. He Xingdong et al., *Lin Chuang Zhong Yao Shou Ce*, 33.
17. Wang Haibo et al., *Zhong Cao Yao* [Journal of Chinese Herbs] 25, 6 (1994): 302.
18. Liu Baolin et al., *Zhong Guo Yao Ke Da Xue Xue Bao* [Journal of Chinese Pharmacology University] 26, 1 (1995): 44.
19. Zheng Nishi et al., *Jiang Xi Yi Xue Yuan Xue Bao* [Journal of Jiangxi Medical College] 31, 2 (1991): 15.
20. Lei Zaiquan and Zhang Tingmo, *Zhong Hua Lin Chuang Zhong Yao Xue*, 381.
21. He Xingdong et al., *Lin Chuang Zhong Yao Shou Ce*, 30.
22. L.G. Hutchins et al., *Chim J Physiol* 11 (1937): 35.
23. Zhu Hengbi et al., *Abstract of Papers Presented to the First Congress of the Chinese Physiological Science Association*, 1958, medical papers: 65, 67.
24. Experimental Group of Guangdong College of TCM, *Xin Zhong Yi* [New Journal of Traditional Chinese Medicine] 920 (1971): 30.
25. Xu Shibo et al., *Zhong Yao Yao Li Yu Lin Chuang* [Pharmacology and Clinical Application of Chinese Materia Medica], supplement to issue no. 3 (1987): 90.
26. Shen Qigui et al., *Zhe Jiang Yi Ke Da Xue Xue Bao* [Journal of Zhejiang Medical University] 22, 6 (1993): 246.
27. Zhang Qiwei et al., *Guo Wai Yi Xue – Zhong Yi Zhong Yao Fen Ce* [Foreign Medicine – TCM Fascicule] 17, 1 (1995): 5.
28. Han Changzhi, *Tong Ji Yi Ke Da Xue Xue Bao* [Journal of Tongji Medical University] 23, 6 (1994): 470.
29. Wu Guorong, *Hu Nan Zhong Yi Za Zhi* [Hunan Journal of Traditional Chinese Medicine] 2, 6 (1986): 7.
30. Huang Li et al., *Zhong Guo Zhong Yao Za Zhi* [Journal of Chinese Materia Medica] 15, 2 (1990): 115.
31. Jia Xiurong et al., *Wei Liang Yuan Su* [Trace Elements] supplement (1991): 42.
32. Huang Li et al., *Zhong Guo Zhong Yao Za Zhi* [Journal of Chinese Materia Medica] 16, 3 (1991): 177.
33. Y. Kimura et al., *Chem Phar Bull* 30, 1 (1982): 219.
34. Zhou Xiansu et al., *Tai Wan Yi Xue Hui Za Zhi* [Journal of Taiwan Medical Association] 76, 4 (1977): 46.
35. Xu Zhonglu, *Zhong Hua Yi Xue Za Zhi* [Chinese Journal of Medicine] 33, 3-4 (1947): 71.
36. Chen Xingke et al., *Zhong Cheng Yao Yan Jiu* [Chinese Medicinal Preparation Research] 5 (1987): 18.
37. Chu Zhonglu et al., *Di Er Jun Yi Da Xue Xue Bao* [Journal of Second Military Medical University] 10, 2 (1989): 193.
38. Huang Weimin et al., *Zhong Hua Xue Ye Xue Za Zhi* [Chinese Journal of Haematology] 10, 5 (1989): 228.
39. Shan Ailian et al., *Yao Xue Tong Bao* [Pharmacology Bulletin] 21, 3 (1986): 141.
40. Chen Qiming et al., *Yao Xue Xue Bao* [Pharmacology Journal] 21, 6 (1986): 401.
41. Ibid., 22, 3 (1987): 161.
42. Tan Yuzhi et al., *Zhong Guo Zhong Yao Za Zhi* [Journal of Chinese Materia Medica] 14, 5 (1989): 50.
43. Huang Qirong et al., *Guo Wai Yi Xue – Zhong Yi Zhong Yao Fen Ce* [Foreign Medicine – TCM Fascicule] 10, 10 (1988): 43.
44. Wang Guangde (translator), *Guo Wai Yi Xue – Zhong Yi Zhong Yao Fen Ce* 10, 5 (1988): 36.
45. Xu Zhonglu, *Zhong Hua Yi Xue Za Zhi* [Chinese Journal of Medicine] 33, 3-4 (1974): 71.
46. Jing Qing et al., *Tian Jin Yi Yao* [Tianjin Journal of Medicine and Pharmacology] 6 (1976): 283.
47. Feng Gaohong et al., *Jiang Xi Yi Yao* [Jiangxi Journal of Medicine and Pharmacology] 7 (1961): 29.
48. Zhu Qiaozhen et al., *Yao Xue Xue Bao* [Pharmacology Journal] 9, 5 (1962): 281.
49. He Xingdong et al., *Lin Chuang Zhong Yao Shou Ce*, 42.
50. Lei Zaiquan and Zhang Tingmo, *Zhong Hua Lin Chuang Zhong Yao Xue*, 458.
51. He Xingdong et al., *Lin Chuang Zhong Yao Shou Ce*, 44.
52. Central Laboratory of the Hospital Affiliated to Hubei TCM College, *Collection of Documents Relating to Integrated Western and Traditional Chinese Medicine* (1979): 96.
53. Mei Binfu, *Hua Xue Xue Bao* [Chemistry Journal] 28, 1 (1962): 25.
54. Wang Yuliang et al., *Zhong Guo Yi Yao Xue Bao* [Chinese Journal of Medicine and Pharmacology] 6, 3 (1991): 32.
55. Hu Yinheng et al., *Xin Yi Yao Xue Za Zhi* [New Medicine and Pharmacology Journal] 8 (1975): 41.
56. Huang Qinghua et al., *Zhong Yi Yan Jiu* [Traditional Chinese Medicine Research] 6, 2 (1993): 27.
57. Wang Yusheng et al., *Zhong Yao Yao Li Yu Ying Yong* [Pharmacology and Application of Chinese Materia Medica] (Beijing: People's Medical Publishing House, 1988), 382.
58. Kang Shengli et al., *Shen Yang Yao Xue Yuan Xue Bao* [Journal of Shenyang Pharmacology College] 18 (1983): 11.
59. Liu Jinfang et al., *Zhong Xi Yi Jie He Za Zhi* [Journal of Integrated TCM and Western Medicine] 10, 7 (1990): 429.
60. Liu Jiaquan, *Xin Yi Xue Bao* [New Medical Journal] 6, 3 (1957): 155.

61. Fu Hangyu et al., *Quan Guo Qing Re Jie Du Yao Hui Yi Lun Wen Ji* [Collection of Papers from the National Conference on Materia Medica for Clearing Heat and Relieving Toxicity] (1986): 74.
62. Liu Jie et al., *Zhong Guo Yao Li Xue Bao* [Chinese Journal of Pharmacology] 9, 5 (1988) 395.
63. Cao Caiping et al., *Yi Yao Gong Ye* [Medical and Pharmaceutical Industry Journal] 17, 3 (1986): 115.
64. Kuang Xuehai et al., *Zhong Yi Yao Xin Xi* [Traditional Chinese Medicine and Materia Medica News] 3 (1985): 25.
65. Ma Zhenya, *Shan Xi Xin Yi Yao* [Shaanxi New Medical Journal] 4 (1982): 58.
66. Ma Shoujiang et al., *Zhong Yao Yao Li Yu Lin Chuang* [Pharmacology and Clinical Application of Chinese Materia Medica], supplement to issue no. 8 (1992): 170.
67. Liu Guangxi et al., *Zhong Xi Yi Jie He Za Zhi* [Journal of Integrated TCM and Western Medicine] 6, 12 (1986): 737.
68. Lei Zaiquan and Zhang Tingmo, *Zhong Hua Lin Chuang Zhong Yao Xue*, 550.
69. He Xingdong et al., *Lin Chuang Zhong Yao Shou Ce*, 55.
70. Li Qinghua, *Zhong Cao Yao* [Journal of Chinese Herbs] 11, 10 (1983): 8.
71. Xu Zhencan et al., *Zhong Cheng Yao Yan Jiu* [Chinese Medicinal Preparation Research] 12 (1987): 9.
72. Lingling Local Health and Epidemic Prevention Station et al., *Hu Nan Yi Yao Za Zhi* [Hunan Journal of Medicine and Pharmacology] 2, 1 (1975): 46.
73. Pharmacology Teaching and Research Office of Shandong College of Medicine, *Shan Dong Yi Xue Yuan Xue Bao* [Journal of Shandong College of Medicine] 11 (1960): 52.
74. Lei Zaiquan and Zhang Tingmo, *Zhong Hua Lin Chuang Zhong Yao Xue*, 503.
75. He Xingdong et al., *Lin Chuang Zhong Yao Shou Ce*, 57.
76. Li Guoli et al., *Wei Sheng Wu Xue Tong Bao* [Microorganism Bulletin] 16, 3 (1989): 153.
77. Yan Guihua et al., *Yao Xue Tong Bao* [Pharmacology Bulletin] 8, 2 (1960): 57.
78. Song Zhijun et al., *Zhong Cao Yao* [Journal of Chinese Herbs] 24, 12 (1993): 643.
79. Wang Yusheng et al., *Zhong Yao Yao Li Yu Ying Yong*, 740.
80. Wu Zefang et al., *Yao Wu Fen Xi Za Zhi* [Chinese Journal of Pharmacological Analysis] 5, 3 (1985): 167.
81. Wu Zefang et al., *Zhong Yao Yao Li Yu Lin Chuang* [Pharmacology and Clinical Application of Chinese Materia Medica] 6, 6 (1990): 28.
82. He Xingdong et al., *Lin Chuang Zhong Yao Shou Ce*, 64.
83. Yan Guihua et al., *Yao Xue Tong Bao* [Pharmacology Bulletin] 8, 2 (1960): 57.
84. Wang Weisi, *Yao Xue Tong Bao* 7, 10 (1959): 522.
85. Sun Qixun et al., *Sheng Li Xue Bao* [Physiology Journal] 23, 3 (1959): 254.
86. Liu Jufang et al., *Yao Xue Xue Bao* [Pharmacology Journal] 9, 3 (1962): 151.
87. Dai Guiwei et al., *Zhong Yi Za Zhi* [Journal of Traditional Chinese Medicine] 23, 5 (1982): 65.
88. Beijing Sixth Pharmaceutical Factory, *Zhong Yao Tong Bao* [Bulletin of Chinese Materia Medica] 10, 7 (1985): 45.
89. Meng Zhenmu, *Yao Xue Xue Bao* [Pharmacology Journal] 8 (1981): 571.
90. Huang Tianyou et al., *Di Yi Jun Yi Da Xue Xue Bao* [Journal of First Military Medical University] 8, 1 (1986): 37.
91. Zhou Shiqing et al., *Dong Wu Xue Za Zhi* [Zoology Journal] 21, 6 (1986): 22.
92. Editorial Committee, *Quan Guo Zhong Cao Yao Hui Bian* [National Collection of Chinese Herbs] volume 1 (Beijing: People's Medical Publishing House, 1996), 5.
93. Wang Qiang et al., *Zhong Guo Yao Ke Da Xue Xue Bao* [Journal of Chinese Pharmacology University] 20, 4 (1989): 251.
94. Wang Qiang et al., *Zhong Guo Zhong Yao Za Zhi* [Journal of Chinese Materia Medica] 2 (1990): 45.
95. Wang Qiang et al., *Zhong Cao Yao* [Journal of Chinese Herbs] 18, 11 (1987): 48.
96. Fan Yihua et al., *Guang Zhou Yi Yao* [Guangzhou Journal of Medicine and Pharmacology] 3 (1987): 53.
97. Su Chengye et al., *Da Lian Yi Xue Yuan Xue Bao* [Journal of Dalian College of Medicine], 5, 2 (1983): 1.
98. Xing Wenrong et al., *Zhong Hua Yi Xue Za Zhi* [Chinese Journal of Medicine] 44, 12 (1985): 137.
99. H. Wiland et al., *Arch Exptl Path Pharm* 92 (1922): 195.
100. J.R. Dipalma (ed.), *Drill's Pharmacology in Medicine*, 4th ed. (New York: McGraw-Hill, 1971), 713.
101. R. Laffan et al., *J Pharm Exptl Therapy* 121, 4 (1957): 418.
102. R. Richter, *Arch Exptl Path Pharm*, 193 (1939): 117.
103. Yan Ruiqi et al., *Ai Zheng* [Journal of Cancer] 5, 2 (1986): 14.
104. Sheng Jingfen et al., *Yao Xue Tong Bao* [Pharmacology Bulletin] 16, 2 (1981): 15.
105. Fu Hangyu et al., *Quan Guo Qing Re Jie Du Yao Hui Yi Lun Wen Ji* [Collection of Papers from the National Conference on Materia Medica for Clearing Heat and Relieving Toxicity] (1986): 75.
106. Liu Jingyu et al., *Zhong Guo Yi Yao Xue Bao* [Chinese Journal of Medicine and Pharmacology] 6, 2 (1991): 116.
107. Chen Yi et al., *Tian Jin Yi Yao* [Tianjin Journal of Medicine and Pharmacology] 8 (1980): 488.

108. Yang Yican et al., *Shan Xi Xin Yi Yao* [Shaanxi New Medical Journal] 10 (1983): 49.
109. Yuan Cai et al., *Yao Xue Xue Bao* [Pharmacology Journal] 22, 4 (1987): 245.
110. Sejima Dotyu et al., *Ri Ben Yao Li Xue Za Zhi* [Japanese Journal of Pharmacology] 74, 8 (1978): 897.
111. Shen Yaqin et al., *Xi Bei Yao Xue Za Zhi* [Northwest Journal of Pharmacology] 4, 4 (1989): 12.
112. He Xingdong et al., *Lin Chuang Zhong Yao Shou Ce*, 66.
113. Lei Zaiquan and Zhang Tingmo, *Zhong Hua Lin Chuang Zhong Yao Xue*, 533.
114. He Xingdong et al., *Lin Chuang Zhong Yao Shou Ce*, 67.
115. Quan Ciguang, *Zhong Hua Yi Xue Za Zhi* [Chinese Journal of Medicine (published in Shanghai)] 63, 2 (1944): 89.
116. M.J. O'Neill et al., *J Pharm Pharmacol* 37 (Suppl.) (1985): 49.
117. M.J. O'Neill et al., *J Nat Prod* 50, 1 (1987): 41.
118. Lee Kuohsing et al., *J Nat Prod* 50, 5 (1987): 847.
119. Zhang Yuede, *Zhong Hua Yi Xue Za Zhi* [Chinese Journal of Medicine] 37, 6 (1951): 480.
120. Wang Benxian, *Xin Bian Zhong Yao Xue Ci Dian* [New Dictionary of Chinese Materia Medica] (Tianjin: Tianjin Science and Technology Publishing House, 1996), 889.
121. Tumour Research Group of Chinese Materia Medica Institute, Chinese Academy of Traditional Chinese Medicine, *Ke Ji Zi Liao Hui Bian* [Collection of Scientific Papers] (1972): 140.
122. Lin Peixia et al., *Zhong Xi Yi Jie He Zi Liao Hui Bian* [Collection of Scientific Papers on Integrated TCM and Western Medicine] 2 (1978): 205.
123. Lei Zaiquan and Zhang Tingmo, *Zhong Hua Lin Chuang Zhong Yao Xue*, 565.
124. He Xingdong et al., *Lin Chuang Zhong Yao Shou Ce*, 76.
125. Ma Yuemei et al., *Zhong Yao Tong Bao* [Bulletin of Chinese Materia Medica] 12, 6 (1987): 38.
126. Sun Wanli et al., *Gan Su Zhong Yi Xue Yuan Xue Bao* [Journal of Gansu College of TCM] 3 (1990): 34.
127. Wang Benxian, *Xin Bian Zhong Yao Xue Ci Dian*, 65.
128. Gao Xiaoshan, *Zhong Yi Za Zhi* [Journal of Traditional Chinese Medicine] 32, 1 (1991): 36.
129. Lei Zaiquan and Zhang Tingmo, *Zhong Hua Lin Chuang Zhong Yao Xue*, 434.
130. Yan Yinwu et al., *Collection of Abstracts of Papers Presented to the 1962 Academic Congress of the Chinese Pharmaceutical Association,* 1963: 332.
131. Huang Liangyue et al., *Zhong Cao Yao Yan Jiu Zi Liao* [Chinese Medicinal Herbs Research Documentation] 15 (1979): 25.
132. Yuan Yuan et al., *Zhong Guo Zhong Yao Za Zhi* [Journal of Chinese Materia Medica] 17, 6 (1992): 366.
133. Li Guangcui et al., *Abstract of Papers Reporting to the Congress of the Chinese Medical Science Academy* II (1956): 70.
134. Zang Baoheng, *Bei Jing Yi Xue Yuan Xue Bao* [Journal of Beijing Medical College] 1 (1959): 52.
135. Lei Zaiquan and Zhang Tingmo, *Zhong Hua Lin Chuang Zhong Yao Xue*, 481.
136. He Xingdong et al., *Lin Chuang Zhong Yao Shou Ce*, 48.
137. Wang Yuying et al., *Zhong Cheng Yao Yan Jiu* [Chinese Medicinal Preparation Research] 1 (1980): 31.
138. Chu Zhengxu et al., *Di Er Jun Yi Da Xue Xue Bao* [Journal of Second Military Medical University] 12, 5 (1991): 465.
139. Qi Xinguan et al., *Zhong Guo Yi Ke Da Xue Xue Bao* [Journal of Chinese Medical University] 19, 3 (1990): 165.
140. Qi Xinguan et al., *Zhong Xi Yi Jie He Za Zhi* [Journal of Integrated TCM and Western Medicine] 11, 2 (1991): 102.
141. Lei Zaiquan and Zhang Tingmo, *Zhong Hua Lin Chuang Zhong Yao Xue*, 489.
142. He Xingdong et al., *Lin Chuang Zhong Yao Shou Ce*, 51.
143. Lei Zaiquan and Zhang Tingmo, *Zhong Hua Lin Chuang Zhong Yao Xue*, 471.
144. Chinese Research Group on Arteannuin, *Zhong Yi Za Zhi* [Journal of Traditional Chinese Medicine] 2, 1 (1982): 17.
145. Lian Fubao et al., *Zhong Guo Yi Xue Ke Xue Yuan Xue Bao* [Journal of the Chinese Academy of Medical Science] 11, 3 (1989): 180.
146. Huang Jiazhang et al., *Zhong Guo Yao Li Xue Yu Du Li Xue Za Zhi* [Chinese Journal of Pharmacology and Toxicology] 1, 4 (1987): 283.
147. Ye Kouwei et al., *Yi Xue Zhong Yang Za Zhi* [Medical Centre Journal] 233 (1967): 664.
148. Shanxi Public Health Bureau, *Shan Xi Yi Yao* [Shanxi Medical Journal] 9 (1973): 48.
149. Chen Bingtong, *Zhong Hua Yi Xue Za Zhi* [Chinese Journal of Medicine] 50, 8 (1964): 524.
150. He Xingdong et al., *Lin Chuang Zhong Yao Shou Ce*, 83.
151. Lei Zaiquan and Zhang Tingmo, *Zhong Hua Lin Chuang Zhong Yao Xue*, 643.
152. He Xingdong et al., *Lin Chuang Zhong Yao Shou Ce*, 81.
153. Liang Aihua et al., *Zhong Guo Zhong Yao Za Zhi* [Journal of Chinese Materia Medica] 21, 10 (1996): 622.
154. Xue Baoyun et al., *Zhong Guo Zhong Yao Za Zhi* 20, 12 (1995): 751.

Chapter 3

Downward-draining herbs

泻下药

Downward-draining herbs

Most downward-draining herbs with a moist, offensive or drastic function are cold or cool in nature. Their function is to free the bowels or moisten the Large Intestine. They have the effects of facilitating the expulsion of stool, clearing heat, draining fire and percolating accumulated water, and are mainly used for interior full patterns.

Downward-draining herbs are generally divided into three categories depending on their effect: moist downward-draining herbs (or moist laxatives), offensive downward-draining herbs (or purgatives) and drastic downward-draining and water-expelling herbs (or cathartics).

Clinically, attention should be paid to the following aspects:

1. Although offensive downward-draining herbs can clear and drain pathogenic factors rapidly, it is easy for them to damage vital Qi; they are therefore most appropriate for full patterns. This type of herb is not suitable for elderly or weak patients, or during pregnancy or menstruation. In cases with full pathogenic factors and vital Qi deficiency, herbs to supplement Qi must be applied in combination with downward-draining herbs. In this way, they can not only dispel the pathogenic factors but simultaneously support vital Qi in order to avoid it being damaged. In cases with an interior full pattern combined with an exterior pattern, either release the exterior first and then relieve the interior full pattern, or treat the interior and exterior pathogenic factors at the same time in order to avoid inward fall of the exterior pathogenic factor, which will make the disease worse.
2. Select the downward-draining herb according to the nature of the disease and increase or reduce the dosage appropriately. If the disease is very serious, select a large dosage of offensive downward-draining herbs for intake as a decoction; if the disease is chronic and steady, select a small dosage of mild downward-draining herbs for oral intake in pill form.
3. The effect of different downward-draining herbs is closely related to the dosage. A large dosage of mild downward-draining herbs has the same effect as a normal dosage of strong ones; conversely, a small dosage of strong downward-draining herbs has the same effect as a normal dosage of mild ones.

MOIST DOWNWARD-DRAINING HERBS (MOIST LAXATIVES)

Moist downward-draining herbs are derived from the seed or nut of plants with a high lipid content. They are sweet in taste and neutral in nature, and have the functions of moistening dryness and freeing the bowels. They can be used for Intestinal dryness with constipation caused by damage to Yin after a febrile disease, desiccation of body fluids in elderly patients, or postpartum Yin and Blood deficiency.

Since the cause and accompanying symptoms of constipation differ from case to case, care must be taken to use the appropriate combination. For constipation due to damage to body fluids in febrile diseases, use these herbs together with herbs for clearing heat and enriching Yin; for Blood deficiency, use them in combination with herbs for nourishing the Blood; and for Qi stagnation and distension, use them together with herbs for moving Qi and alleviating pain.

Tab. 3.1 Moist downward-draining herbs (moist laxatives)

Herb	Functions	Indications
Huo Ma Ren (Semen Cannabis Sativae)	Moistening dryness and lubricating the Intestines, nourishing Yin and supplementing deficiency	Intestinal dryness with constipation in the elderly and infirm, and in other patients in the aftermath of a febrile disease or postpartum
Yu Li Ren (Semen Pruni)	Moistening the Intestines and freeing the bowels, promoting urination and dispersing swelling	Intestinal dryness with constipation associated with Qi stagnation in the Large Intestine, oedema and leg Qi

Huo Ma Ren 火麻仁 (Hemp seed, Semen Cannabis Sativae)

Huo Ma Ren is the dried fruit of *Cannabis sativa* L., family Moraceae.

Main ingredients *Huo Ma Ren* contains 30% of lipids (10% of which are saturated fatty acids, 12% oleic acid, 53% linoleic acid and 25% linolenic acid), trigonelline, cannabinol, phytin, muscarin and edestinase.

Properties Taste: sweet; nature: neutral.

Channels entered Spleen, Stomach and Large Intestine.

Functions and indications Moistens dryness and lubricates the Intestines, nourishes Yin and supplements deficiency. It is indicated for Intestinal dryness with constipation in the elderly and infirm, and in other patients in the aftermath of a febrile disease or postpartum.

Common dosage 10–30g; crush before decocting.

Precautions and contraindications *Huo Ma Ren* should not be used for patients with loose stool or diarrhoea.

Comparison of functions See *Yu Li Ren* (Semen Pruni).

Toxicity *Huo Ma Ren* contains a significant proportion of lipids; misuse can result in a toxic reaction, which normally occurs within one to two hours of intake. Clinical reports on 332 and 122 cases respectively of poisoning due to overdosage of the oils in *Huo Ma Ren* stated that no deaths occurred. The main toxic constituent of *Huo Ma Ren* is cannabinol. Intake of 60–100g can produce a toxic reaction, manifesting as nausea, vomiting, diarrhoea, dizziness and headache, or in more serious cases, numbness of the limbs, vexation and agitation, delirium, palpitations, higher blood pressure, convulsions or even death.

Modern research Stimulates the mesentery, promotes peristalsis, reduces intestinal absorption of water to perform a purgative function.[1]

Combinations and applications

Functions	Combinations	Applications
Moistening dryness and lubricating the Intestines, nourishing Yin and supplementing deficiency	*Dang Gui* (Radix Angelicae Sinensis) *Xing Ren* (Semen Pruni Armeniacae) *Shu Di Huang* (Radix Rehmanniae Glutinosae Conquita)	Intestinal dryness with constipation during the prenatal and postpartum periods and in the elderly and infirm due to depletion of the Blood and body fluids
	Huang Qi (Radix Astragali seu Hedysari) *Sheng Di Huang* (Radix Rehmanniae Glutinosae) *Mai Men Dong* (Radix Ophiopogonis Japonici)	Constipation due to Qi and Yin deficiency
	Da Huang (Radix et Rhizoma Rhei) *Hou Po* (Cortex Magnoliae Officinalis)	Constipation due to heat damaging Yin

Yu Li Ren 郁李仁
(Bush cherry stone, Semen Pruni)

Yu Li Ren is the dried seed of *Prunus humilis* Bge., *P. japonica* Thunb. or *P. pedunculata* Maxim., family Rosaceae.

Main ingredients *Yu Li Ren* contains 58-74% of lipids, and volatile oils, proteins, starch, saponins, phytosterol and vitamin B_1.

Properties Taste: acrid, bitter and sweet; nature: neutral.

Channels entered Spleen, Large Intestine and Small Intestine.

Functions and indications Moistens the Intestines and frees the bowels, promotes urination and disperses swelling. It is indicated for Intestinal dryness with constipation associated with Qi stagnation in the Large Intestine, and for oedema and leg Qi.

Common dosage 5-10g.

Precautions and contraindications *Yu Li Ren* should be used with caution during pregnancy.

Comparison of functions Both *Yu Li Ren* (Semen Pruni) and *Huo Ma Ren* (Semen Cannabis Sativae) can moisten the Intestines and free the bowels to treat Intestinal dryness with constipation. As *Huo Ma Ren* is sweet, neutral, oily and lubricating, it has enriching and nourishing functions and can supplement deficiency; it is therefore an excellent herb for treating Intestinal dryness with constipation due to depletion of body fluids and Blood deficiency in elderly patients, those with deficiency patterns, and postpartum. *Yu Li Ren* is lubricating, bitter and downward-bearing and can move Qi stagnation in the Large Intestine, promote urination and disperse swelling. It does not supplement deficiency and is therefore generally used for constipation due to Qi stagnation in full patterns; it can also treat oedema, leg Qi and puffy swelling.

Modern research Lowered blood pressure in tests on animals.[2]

Combinations and applications

Functions	Combinations	Applications
Moistening the Intestines and freeing the bowels	*Tao Ren* (Semen Persicae) *Xing Ren* (Semen Pruni Armeniacae) *Bai Zi Ren* (Semen Biotae Orientalis) *Song Zi Ren* (Semen Pini)	Constipation due to Blood depletion postpartum or in the elderly and those with a weak constitution
	Jiao Bing Lang (Semen Arecae Catechu, scorch-fried) *Qing Pi* (Pericarpium Citri Reticulatae Viride)	Constipation due to Qi stagnation
Promoting urination and dispersing swelling	*Sang Bai Pi* (Cortex Mori Albae Radicis) *Chi Xiao Dou* (Semen Phaseoli Calcarati) *Bai Mao Gen* (Rhizoma Imperatae Cylindricae)	Oedema, fullness and distension in the abdomen
	Bai Zhu (Rhizoma Atractylodis Macrocephalae) *Fu Ling* (Sclerotium Poriae Cocos)	Oedema, inhibited urination

OFFENSIVE DOWNWARD-DRAINING HERBS (PURGATIVES)

Most of the herbs in this section are bitter and cold, and have a strong purgative effect. They can clear heat and drain fire, expel toxins from the Stomach and Intestines, and treat constipation. In addition, they can be used for food accumulation, the presence of hard and dry stool, distension in the abdomen, or even high fever with delirious speech. These conditions are accompanied by a dry tongue with yellow fur and a slippery, rapid pulse due to the stagnation of full-heat.

Clinically, offensive downward-draining herbs are used in the following combinations:

1. for full-cold-type constipation, use them with herbs for warming the interior;
2. for constipation and abdominal distension due to Qi stagnation, use them in combination with herbs for moving Qi;
3. for patients not able to tolerate purgation as a result of vital Qi deficiency, use these offensive downward-draining herbs together with supplementing herbs;
4. for interior full patterns in conjunction with an exterior pattern, release the exterior first, then treat the interior heat; combine offensive downward-draining herbs with herbs for releasing the exterior so that both exterior and interior pathogenic factors are dispelled.

Offensive downward-draining herbs of a cold nature can also be used for febrile diseases, persistent high fever and delirious speech; for dizziness, headache and vomiting of blood due to the flaming upwards of heat and fire; for bleeding caused by Blood-heat; and for dysentery and Intestinal abscess due to the accumulation and stagnation of damp-heat in the Large Intestine.

Tab. 3.2 Offensive downward-draining herbs (purgatives)

Herb	Functions	Indications
Da Huang (Radix et Rhizoma Rhei)	Draining downwards and attacking accumulation, draining fire and cooling the Blood, quickening the Blood and freeing menstruation, dispersing swelling and alleviating pain, clearing heat and drying dampness	Food accumulation, constipation due to binding of heat, distension and pain in the abdomen, high fever with delirious speech, abdominal urgency and tenesmus, bleeding and vomiting of blood, pain in the abdomen due to postpartum Blood stasis, menstrual block due to Blood stasis, abdominal masses, knocks and falls, abscesses and sores, damp-heat jaundice, acute conjunctivitis (wind-fire eye), painful and swollen gums
Mang Xiao (Mirabilitum)	Clearing heat, freeing the bowels and guiding out stagnation, moistening dryness, softening hardness and breaking up Blood stasis	Constipation and mania due to full-heat accumulation in the Intestines and Stomach, red, sore and swollen eyes, sore throat and mouth sores due to full-heat toxins, and abscesses and sores
Fan Xie Ye (Folium Sennae)	Guiding out stagnation and freeing the bowels	Constipation due to binding of heat, oppression in the chest, distension in the abdomen

Lu Hui (Herba Aloes)	Clearing heat and freeing the bowels, dispersing accumulation and killing worms	Constipation due to heat in the Intestines, menstrual block, child Gan accumulation, roundworm, headache due to Liver-fire, red eyes, toothache, haemorrhoids, scrofula

Da Huang 大黄 (Rhubarb root and rhizome, Radix et Rhizoma Rhei)

Da Huang is the root and rhizome of *Rheum palmatum* L., *R. tanguticum* Maxim. ex Balf. or *R. officinale* Baill., family Polygonaceae.

Main ingredients The active ingredients in *Da Huang* include anthraquinone glycosol derivatives (including chrysophanol, aloe-emodin, rhein, emodin and physcion) and tannins (mainly contained in glucose pyrogallol tannins, catechu tannin and free gallic acid).

Properties Taste: bitter; nature: cold.

Channels entered Spleen, Stomach, Large Intestine, Liver and Heart.

Functions and indications Drains downwards and attacks accumulation, drains fire and cools the Blood, quickens the Blood and frees menstruation, disperses swelling and alleviates pain, clears heat and dries dampness. It is indicated for food accumulation, constipation due to binding of heat, distension and pain in the abdomen, high fever with delirious speech, abdominal urgency and tenesmus, bleeding and vomiting of blood, pain in the abdomen due to postpartum Blood stasis, menstrual block due to Blood stasis, abdominal masses, knocks and falls, abscesses and sores, damp-heat jaundice, acute conjunctivitis (wind-fire eye), and painful and swollen gums.

Common dosage 3-15g, added towards the end of the decoction process; appropriate dosage for external application.

Precautions and contraindications *Da Huang* is contraindicated in cases of Stomach Qi deficiency, cases without full-heat in the Xue level, or cases without accumulation and stagnation in the Stomach and Intestines; and also during pregnancy or menstruation, or for nursing mothers.

Remarks Raw *Da Huang* is a cathartic; it should be decocted later than other ingredients or dipped in boiling water to strengthen its effect (its purgative power will be reduced by prolonged decoction). *Da Huang* processed with alcohol (*Jiu Zhi Da Huang*) is a mild purgative and quickens the Blood; it should be used in cases with Blood stasis and for patients for whom drastic purging is not suitable. Charred *Da Huang*, or *Da Huang Tan* (Radix et Rhizoma Rhei Carbonisatae), is commonly used to stop bleeding. External application of the herb can disperse abscesses and relieve toxicity.

Comparison of functions See *Mang Xiao* (Mirabilitum).

Toxicity The LD_{50} for subcutaneous injection in mice of preparations of *Da Huang* is 4.05g/kg. The LD_{50} for intragastric administration to mice of the emodin and physcion contained in *Da Huang* is 0.56g/kg and 1.15g/kg respectively. Intraperitoneal injection in mice of 40g (raw herb)/kg of acetic extracts of *Da Huang* had caused no deaths or abnormality of function after 72 hours. Fresh *Da Huang* is generally more toxic than the raw herb. Overdosage can cause such toxic symptoms as nausea, vomiting, dizziness, distension in the abdomen and jaundice.

Modern research

1. The purgative effect of *Da Huang* is the result of stimulation of the middle part of the colon without this influencing absorption by the small intestine.[3, 4]
2. Increases the secretion of bile and the volume of flow.[5, 6]
3. Abates fever, inhibits inflammation.[7-9]
4. Strengthens the immune function.[10, 11]

Combinations and applications

Functions	Combinations	Applications
Draining downwards and attacking accumulation	*Mang Xiao* (Mirabilitum) *Hou Po* (Cortex Magnoliae Officinalis) *Zhi Shi* (Fructus Immaturus Citri Aurantii)	Fever and vexation, pain in the abdomen and constipation, and thick, yellow tongue fur due to full-heat accumulation in the Intestines and Stomach
	Mu Xiang (Radix Aucklandiae Lappae) (see notes on legal status) *Bing Lang* (Semen Arecae Catechu) *Hou Po* (Cortex Magnoliae Officinalis) *Lai Fu Zi* (Semen Raphani Sativi)	Food accumulation, distension in the abdomen and constipation, acid vomiting, vomiting
	Bai Shao (Radix Paeoniae Lactiflorae) *Fang Feng* (Radix Ledebouriellae Divaricatae)	Constipation, cold in the abdomen, rumbling intestines, cold limbs, white tongue fur and a slippery pulse due to full-cold accumulation and stagnation
Draining fire and cooling the Blood (with *Da Huang Tan*)	*Huang Lian* (Rhizoma Coptidis) *Huang Qin* (Radix Scutellariae Baicalensis)	Bleeding patterns due to the frenetic movement of hot Blood
	Bai Mao Gen (Rhizoma Imperatae Cylindricae)	Nosebleed due to Blood-heat
	Ce Bai Ye (Cacumen Biotae Orientalis) *Qian Cao Gen* (Radix Rubiae Cordifoliae)	Coughing of blood due to Blood-heat
	Bai Ji (Rhizoma Bletillae Striatae) (see notes on legal status)	Vomiting of blood due to Blood-heat
	Di Yu (Radix Sanguisorbae Officinalis)	Blood in the stool due to Blood-heat
	Han Lian Cao (Herba Ecliptae Prostratae) *Da Ji* (Herba seu Radix Cirsii Japonici) *Xiao Ji* (Herba Cephalanoploris seu Cirsii)	Blood in the urine due to Blood-heat
Quickening the Blood and freeing menstruation	*Tao Ren* (Semen Persicae) *Hong Hua* (Flos Carthami Tinctorii) *Niu Xi* (Radix Achyranthis Bidentatae)	Postpartum pain in the abdomen and retention of lochia due to Blood stasis
	Chuan Xiong (Rhizoma Ligustici Chuanxiong) *Mo Yao* (Myrrha) *Hong Hua* (Flos Carthami Tinctorii)	Painful menstruation due to Blood stasis, or menstruation with clotted dark discharge, accompanied by a purple tongue
	Huang Qin (Radix Scutellariae Baicalensis) *Tao Ren* (Semen Persicae) *Shui Zhi* (Hirudo seu Whitmania) *Tu Bie Chong* (Eupolyphaga seu Steleophaga)	Menstrual block due to Blood stasis

Dispersing swelling and alleviating pain	*Ru Xiang* (Gummi Olibanum) *Mo Yao* (Myrrha) *Su Mu* (Lignum Sappan)	Local swelling and pain due to knocks and falls
	Jin Yin Hua (Flos Lonicerae) *Lian Qiao* (Fructus Forsythiae Suspensae) *Pu Gong Ying* (Herba Taraxaci cum Radice)	Swollen abscesses and clove sores due to heat toxins
	Mu Dan Pi (Cortex Moutan Radicis) *Mang Xiao* (Mirabilitum) *Tao Ren* (Semen Persicae) *Chi Shao* (Radix Paeoniae Rubra)	Intestinal abscess due to Qi and Blood stagnation and accumulation of heat toxins
Clearing heat and drying dampness	*Yin Chen Hao* (Herba Artemisiae Scopariae) *Zhi Zi* (Fructus Gardeniae Jasminoidis) *Che Qian Zi* (Semen Plantaginis)	Damp-heat jaundice (Yang-type jaundice), oppression in the chest, a bitter taste in the mouth, yellow urine
	Huang Bai (Cortex Phellodendri) *Bian Xu* (Herba Polygoni Avicularis) *Dong Kui Zi* (Semen Malvae Verticillatae)	Lin syndrome due to damp-heat
	Huang Bai (Cortex Phellodendri) *Tu Fu Ling* (Rhizoma Smilacis Glabrae) *Bai Guo* (Semen Ginkgo Bilobae)	Yellow and smelly vaginal discharge due to damp-heat
	Huang Lian (Rhizoma Coptidis) *Zhi Shi* (Fructus Immaturus Citri Aurantii) *Mu Xiang* (Radix Aucklandiae Lappae) (see notes on legal status)	Dysentery and abdominal urgency and tenesmus due to damp-heat

Mang Xiao 芒硝 (Mirabilite, Mirabilitum)

Mang Xiao is a mineral form of sodium sulphate.

Main ingredients *Mang Xiao* contains around 98% of sodium sulphate ($Na_2SO_4.10H_2O$) along with such impurities as calcium sulphate, sodium chloride and magnesium sulphate.

Properties Taste: salty and bitter; nature: cold.

Channels entered Stomach and Large Intestine.

Functions and indications Clears heat, frees the bowels and guides out stagnation, and moistens dryness, softens hardness and breaks up Blood stasis. It is indicated for constipation and mania due to full-heat accumulation in the Intestines and Stomach, red, sore and swollen eyes, sore throat and mouth sores due to full-heat toxins, and abscesses and sores.

Common dosage 3-15g, or 30g for large dosages; used as pills or powder, or dissolved in decoctions. Appropriate dosage for external application.

Precautions and contraindications *Mang Xiao* is contraindicated during pregnancy and in cases of Spleen and Stomach deficiency-cold without accumulation and stagnation of pathogenic heat.

Remarks Depending on the processing of the mineral, there are three different products: *Po Xiao* (Mirabilitum Non-Purum), *Mang Xiao* and *Xuan*

Ming Fen (Mirabilitum Depuratum). Although these three types of sodium sulphate have the same function, their purgative effect differs: *Po Xiao* is not as pure as the other two and therefore has the strongest purgative function, being normally reserved for external use; *Mang Xiao* is a mild purgative; *Xuan Ming Fen* is purer in quality, and is even milder as a purgative, so it is normally used as a medicinal in stomatology and ophthalmology.

Comparison of functions Both *Mang Xiao* (Mirabilitum) and *Da Huang* (Radix et Rhizoma Rhei) have a strong downward-draining effect in freeing the bowels and can treat full-heat accumulation and constipation. They also have an external use for clearing heat and dispersing swelling to treat the swelling and toxins of abscesses and sores. *Da Huang* is bitter and cold and can be combined with other herbs to treat constipation due to accumulation and stagnation. It can also be used to clear heat and drain fire, relieve toxicity, stop bleeding, quicken the Blood and dispel stasis, as well as for clearing and draining damp-heat; it can be employed for high fever in warm-febrile diseases, constipation due to binding of heat, bleeding patterns due to Blood-heat, Blood stasis patterns, and damp-heat jaundice and Lin syndrome. *Mang Xiao* is effective in moistening dryness and softening hardness while draining heat and freeing the bowels. It is used for constipation with dry stool due to full-heat accumulation and can be applied externally to treat sore and swollen throat, mouth ulcers and red eyes.

Modern research

1. Has a purgative function.[12]
2. Dissolves gallbladder stones.[13]
3. Inhibits inflammation.[13, 14]

Combinations and applications

Functions	Combinations	Applications
Clearing heat, freeing the bowels and guiding out stagnation	*Da Huang* (Radix et Rhizoma Rhei) *Hou Po* (Cortex Magnoliae Officinalis) *Zhi Shi* (Fructus Immaturus Citri Aurantii)	Fever, constipation, delirious speech, mania and yellow tongue fur due to full-heat accumulation in the Stomach and Intestines
	Xi Gua Shuang (Pulvis Fructus Citrulli Vulgaris) *Bing Pian* (Borneolum Syntheticum) *Peng Sha* (Borax) (grind to a powder for external use)	Mouth sores due to full-heat toxins
	Da Huang (Radix et Rhizoma Rhei) *Shan Dou Gen* (Radix Sophorae Tonkinensis) *Xuan Shen* (Radix Scrophulariae Ningpoensis) *Gan Cao* (Radix Glycyrrhizae)	Sore throat, high fever and constipation due to full-heat toxins
Moistening dryness, softening hardness and breaking up Blood stasis	*Dang Gui* (Radix Angelicae Sinensis) *Tao Ren* (Semen Persicae) *Hong Hua* (Flos Carthami Tinctorii)	Menstrual block due to Blood stasis
	San Leng (Rhizoma Sparganii Stoloniferi) *E Zhu* (Rhizoma Curcumae) *Cang Zhu* (Rhizoma Atractylodis) *Yu Jin* (Radix Curcumae)	Abdominal masses due to Qi stagnation and Blood stasis

Note: *Mang Xiao* can also be dissolved in water for external use to treat breast abscess and swollen abscesses.

Fan Xie Ye 番泻叶
(Senna leaf, Folium Sennae)

Fan Xie Ye is the dried small leaf of *Cassia angustifolia* Vahl or *C. acutifolia* Del., family Leguminosae.

Main ingredients *Fan Xie Ye* contains sennoside A, B, C and D, chrysophanol, aloe-emodin, barbaloin and rhein.

Properties Taste: sweet and bitter; nature: cold.

Channel entered Large Intestine.

Functions and indications Guides out stagnation and frees the bowels. It is indicated for constipation due to binding of heat, oppression in the chest, and distension in the abdomen.

Common dosage 1.5-9g, added towards the end of the decoction process; 1.5-3g when steeped in warm water.

Precautions and contraindications

1. *Fan Xie Ye* is contraindicated during menstruation and pregnancy and for nursing mothers.
2. A large dosage of the herb may induce nausea, vomiting and pain in the abdomen.

Modern research

1. Has a purgative function.[15]
2. A 10% concentration of the steep of *Fan Xie Ye* can inhibit Bacterium coli, Proteus vulgaris and Corynebacterium dysenteriae.[16]

Combinations and applications

Functions	Combinations	Applications
Guiding out stagnation and freeing the bowels	*Zhi Shi* (Fructus Immaturus Citri Aurantii) *Hou Po* (Cortex Magnoliae Officinalis)	Constipation and pain in the abdomen due to binding of heat
	Chen Pi (Pericarpium Citri Reticulatae) *Ding Xiang* (Flos Caryophylli)	Distension in the abdomen, oppression in the chest, constipation

Note: *Fan Xie Ye* can also be used as a warm-water infusion to treat constipation.

Lu Hui 芦荟
(Aloe, Herba Aloes)

Lu Hui is the solid residue obtained by evaporating the liquid drained from the leaves of various species of aloe such as *Aloe vera* L. or *A. ferox* Mill., family Liliaceae.

Legal status *Lu Hui* is a restricted substance listed in Appendix II of the Convention on International Trade in Endangered Species of Wild Fauna and Flora (CITES). Appropriate import and export permits are required for trade in this materia medica.

Main ingredients *Lu Hui* contains aloin, isobarbaloin, aloe-emodin, β-barbaloin, aloeresitannol, cinnamic acid, malic acid, succinic acid, lactic acid and p-coumaric acid.

Properties Taste: bitter; nature: cold.

Channels entered Stomach, Large Intestine and Liver.

Functions and indications Clears heat and frees the bowels, disperses accumulation and kills worms. It is indicated for constipation due to heat in the Intestines, menstrual block, child Gan accumulation, roundworm, headache due to Liver-fire, red eyes, toothache, haemorrhoids, and scrofula.

Common dosage 1-2 g, prepared in pills (not for decoction); appropriate dosage for external application.

Precautions and contraindications *Lu Hui* is contraindicated in cases of Spleen and Stomach deficiency-cold with reduced appetite and loose stool, as well as during pregnancy.

Modern research Preparations of *Lu Hui* can inhibit various dermatophytes and Mycobacterium tuberculosis var. hominis.[17]

Combinations and applications

Functions	Combinations	Applications
Clearing heat and freeing the bowels	*Zhu Sha* (Cinnabaris) (see notes on legal status)	Constipation, vexation, red eyes and insomnia due to heat accumulation in the Stomach and Intestines
	Long Dan Cao (Radix Gentianae Scabrae) *Zhi Zi* (Fructus Gardeniae Jasminoidis) *Qing Dai* (Indigo Naturalis)	Constipation accompanied by headache, dizziness, vexation, agitation and irascibility, and fright wind and epilepsy due to exuberant fire in the Liver channel
Dispersing accumulation and killing worms	*Chen Pi* (Pericarpium Citri Reticulatae) *Bai Zhu* (Rhizoma Atractylodis Macrocephalae) *Yin Chai Hu* (Radix Stellariae Dichotomae)	Child Gan accumulation
	Shi Jun Zi (Fructus Quisqualis Indicae) *Lei Wan* (Sclerotium Omphalia Lapidescens)	Roundworm

Note: *Lu Hui* can also be used externally for scabies.

DRASTIC DOWNWARD-DRAINING AND WATER-EXPELLING HERBS (CATHARTICS)

Drastic downward-draining and water-expelling herbs are the strongest purgatives. Internal use will result in drastic diarrhoea that drains out water from the body. Some of these herbs can promote urination, thus dispersing swelling. Clinically, they are mainly used for constipation due to abnormal accumulation of fluids in the peritoneal or thoracic cavities and for wheezing due to Phlegm accumulation in the chest and abdomen. In recent years, they have also been used for schistosomal ascites and ascites due to cirrhosis of the liver, producing good effects in relieving the symptoms.

Not only do most of these herbs have a drastic effect, they are also toxic, so they cannot be taken for a long time in large dosages. For chronic diseases and cases of full pathogenic factors with vital Qi deficiency, one of the following methods can be applied:

- eliminate the pathogenic factors first and then supplement vital Qi;
- alternatively, supplement vital Qi first and then eliminate the pathogenic factors; or
- eliminate the pathogenic factors and supplement vital Qi at the same time.

The processing, combination, dosage, pharmaceutical forms and administration of these herbs must be strictly controlled in order to ensure their safe use. They are contraindicated during pregnancy.

Tab. 3.3 Drastic downward-draining and water-expelling herbs (cathartics)

Herb	Functions	Indications
Gan Sui (Radix Euphorbiae Kansui)	Draining water and expelling fluids, clearing heat and dispersing swelling, freeing the bowels and promoting urination	Distension and fullness due to oedema, water accumulation in the chest and abdomen, difficult urination and defecation, Phlegm-fluid patterns, mumps and abscesses
Jing Da Ji (Radix Euphorbiae Pekinensis)	Draining water and expelling fluids, dispersing swelling and dissipating lumps	Oedema, ascites, Phlegm-fluid patterns, scrofula, abscesses and sores
Qian Niu Zi (Semen Pharbitidis)	Draining downwards and expelling water, killing worms and dispersing accumulation	Oedema, ascites, difficult urination and defecation, constipation, coughing and wheezing due to Phlegm-fluids, pain in the abdomen due to worm accumulation
Yuan Hua (Flos Daphnes Genkwa)	Draining water and eliminating dampness, freeing Phlegm and dispersing fluids, killing worms and treating sores	Oedema, Phlegm-fluid patterns, masses in the stomach and abdomen, cough due to counterflow Qi, pain in the hypochondrium, malaria, sores
Ba Dou (Semen Crotonis Tiglii)	Draining cold accumulation downwards, expelling water and reducing swelling, dispelling Phlegm and benefiting the throat	Cold accumulation in the gastrointestinal tract, drum distension and ascites, Phlegm-fluid patterns, full-cold binding in the chest, diarrhoea, pain in the abdomen and abdominal urgency, diphtheria, throat Bi syndrome, sores, scabies and tinea

Gan Sui 甘遂
(Kansui root, Radix Euphorbiae Kansui)

Gan Sui is the dried tuberous root of *Euphorbia kansui* T. N. Liou ex T. P. Wang, family Euphorbiaceae.

Legal status *Gan Sui* was listed in a document entitled *A Review of Restricted Herbal Ingredients* issued by the Medicines Control Agency (MCA) in the UK in September 2001 with a view to the possible imposition of restrictions on its use at a future date. This herb is controlled in Hong Kong and the MCA is concerned by the fact that it contains toxic diterpenes.

Main ingredients *Gan Sui* contains euphorbon, kansuiol, α-euphorbol, β-euphorbol, euphadienol, 2-O-deoxyingenol, ingenol, kansuinine A, kansuinine B, vitamin B_1, citric acid, palmitic acid, tannin, D-glucose and oxalic acid.

Properties Taste: bitter; nature: cold; toxic.

Channels entered Lung, Kidney and Large Intestine.

Functions and indications Drains water and expels fluids, clears heat and disperses swelling, frees the bowels and promotes urination. It is indicated for distension and fullness due to oedema, water accumulation in the chest and abdomen, difficult urination and defecation, Phlegm-fluid patterns, mumps and abscesses.

Remarks Water accumulation in the chest and abdomen is a pattern arising from the accumulation of pathogenic heat with stagnation of fluids in the chest, pain below the heart, fullness and stiffness as major manifestations; it results from the early administration of a purgative for a Taiyang disease leading to exterior heat pathogenic factors attacking the interior and binding with the fluids pre-existing in the thorax, or from vigorous and forceful heat in the Yangming channel coming from the Taiyang channel and binding with the fluids originally existing in the abdomen.

Common dosage 0.5-1g for internal use; appropriate dosage for external application. Clinically, *Gan Sui* should be used in pill form, since the active ingredients are not easily dissolved in water. Preparation with vinegar can reduce toxicity.

Precautions and contraindications

1. *Gan Sui* is contraindicated for weak patients and during pregnancy.
2. *Gan Sui* is incompatible with *Gan Cao* (Radix Glycyrrhizae).

Comparison of functions See *Yuan Hua* (Flos Daphnes Genkwa).

Toxicity The LD_{50} for intraperitoneal injection of *Gan Sui* in mice is 346.1 ± 28.6mg/kg. *Gan Sui* strongly irritates the mucous membrane of the digestive tract. Symptoms of overdose include severe diarrhoea, nausea, vomiting, pain in the abdomen, palpitations, dizziness, lower blood pressure, vexation and agitation, and in severe cases, shock, convulsions, coma or even death. Overdose is generally due to direct swallowing of excessive quantities of the powdered herb on its own or use of the unprocessed herb.

Modern research

1. Strongly stimulates the intestines, thus causing diarrhoea.[18]
2. Induces abortion.[19]
3. Promotes urination.[20]

Combinations and applications

Functions	Combinations	Applications
Draining water and expelling fluids	*Da Huang* (Radix et Rhizoma Rhei) *Mang Xiao* (Mirabilitum)	Water accumulation in the chest due to binding of pathogenic heat
	Jing Da Ji (Radix Euphorbiae Pekinensis) *Bai Jie Zi* (Semen Sinapis Albae)	Suspended fluids, cough, and pain in the hypochondrium

Clearing heat and dispersing swelling	*Da Huang* (Radix et Rhizoma Rhei) *Pu Gong Ying* (Herba Taraxaci cum Radice)	The initial stage of mumps and abscesses due to damp-heat

Note: A paste prepared from powdered *Gan Sui* and wheat flour can be applied to the navel for inhibited urination and defecation.

Jing Da Ji 京大戟 (Peking spurge root, Radix Euphorbiae Pekinensis)

Jing Da Ji is the dried root of *Euphorbia pekinensis* Rupr., family Euphorbiaceae.

Legal status *Jing Da Ji* was listed in a document entitled *A Review of Restricted Herbal Ingredients* issued by the Medicines Control Agency (MCA) in the UK in September 2001 with a view to the possible imposition of restrictions on its use at a future date. This herb is controlled in Hong Kong and the MCA is concerned by the fact that it contains toxic diterpenes.

Main ingredients *Jing Da Ji* contains euphorbon (consisting of euphorbetin, d-glucose and l-arabinose), euphorbia A, B, C, alkaloids and anthraquinone derivatives.

Properties Taste: bitter and acrid; nature: cold; toxic.

Channels entered Lung, Kidney and Large Intestine.

Functions and indications Drains water and expels fluids, disperses swelling and dissipates lumps. It is indicated for oedema, ascites, Phlegm-fluid patterns, scrofula, abscesses and sores.

Common dosage 1.5-3g; or 1g of powder for oral use. Preparation with vinegar can reduce toxicity.

Precautions and contraindications

1. *Jing Da Ji* is contraindicated during pregnancy and for persons of a weak constitution.
2. *Jing Da Ji* is incompatible with *Gan Cao* (Radix Glycyrrhizae).

Comparison of functions See *Yuan Hua* (Flos Daphnes Genkwa).

Toxicity The main toxic ingredients of *Jing Da Ji* include euphorbon and anthraquinone derivatives. This herb has a strong stimulatory effect and can cause inflammation on contact. Internal administration can lead to swelling, distension and hyperaemia of the mucous membrane of the mouth, throat, stomach and intestines. Toxic symptoms can arise through internal administration of as little as 9-15g.

Modern research Strongly stimulates the intestines to induce purgation.[21]

Combinations and applications

Functions	Combinations	Applications
Draining water and expelling fluids, dispersing swelling and dissipating lumps	*Da Zao* (Fructus Ziziphi Jujubae) *Qian Niu Zi* (Semen Pharbitidis) *Mu Xiang* (Radix Aucklandiae Lappae) (see notes on legal status)	Full-pattern oedema, ascites
	Yuan Hua (Flos Daphnes Genkwa) *Gan Sui* (Radix Euphorbiae Kansui)	Suspended fluids
	Shan Ci Gu (Pseudobulbus Shancigu) *Xiong Huang* (Realgar) (see notes on legal status)	Swollen and toxic abscesses and sores due to congestion and stagnation of heat toxins, scrofula and Phlegm nodes due to Phlegm-fire congealing

Qian Niu Zi 牵牛子 (Morning glory seed, Semen Pharbitidis)

Qian Niu Zi is the dried seed of *Pharbitis nil* (L.) Choisy or *P. purpurea* (L.) Voigt, family Convolvulaceae.

Main ingredients *Qian Niu Zi* contains pharbitin (whose constituents include pharbitic acid and ipurolic acid), nilic acid, lysergol, elymoclavine, agroclarine, ergonorine, ergosine and ergosinine.

Properties Taste: bitter; nature: cold; toxic.

Channels entered Lung, Kidney and Large Intestine.

Functions and indications Drains downwards and expels water, kills worms and disperses accumulation. It is indicated for oedema, ascites, difficult urination and defecation, constipation, coughing and wheezing due to Phlegm-fluids, and pain in the abdomen due to worm accumulation.

Common dosage 3-10g in decoction; or 1.5-3g of powder for oral use.

Precautions and contraindications

1. *Qian Niu Zi* is contraindicated during pregnancy and in cases of oedema due to Spleen deficiency.
2. *Qian Niu Zi* antagonizes *Ba Dou* (Semen Crotonis Tiglii).

Remarks

1. Stir-frying *Qian Niu Zi* moderates its effect.
2. *Qian Niu Zi* should be broken into pieces before decoction.

Comparison of functions *Qian Niu Zi* (Semen Pharbitidis) is less drastic in nature than *Gan Sui* (Radix Euphorbiae Kansui), *Jing Da Ji* (Radix Euphorbiae Pekinensis) and *Yuan Hua* (Flos Daphnes Genkwa) and can also be used to kill worms and disperse food accumulation.

Toxicity The LD_{50} for subcutaneous injection in mice of the resins contained in *Qian Niu Zi* is 37.5mg/kg. Overdosage of the herb strongly irritates the gastrointestinal tract and stimulates the kidneys to cause bleeding; in severe cases, it damages the central nervous system to cause aphasia. The main toxic symptoms include dizziness, headache, profuse vomiting, pain in the abdomen, diarrhoea and blood in the stool, and in severe cases, dehydration, blood in the urine, aphasia and shock.

Modern research

1. Both the pharbitin contained in *Qian Niu Zi* and the decoction of the herb have a strong purgative effect.[22]
2. Inhibited parasites *in vitro*, notably roundworm and tapeworm.[23]

Combinations and applications

Functions	Combinations	Applications
Draining downwards and expelling water	*Gan Sui* (Radix Euphorbiae Kansui) *Yuan Hua* (Flos Daphnes Genkwa) *Jing Da Ji* (Radix Euphorbiae Pekinensis)	Ascites, distension in the abdomen, scant urine
	Chen Xiang (Lignum Aquilariae Resinatum) *Guan Gui* (Cortex Tubiformis Cinnamomi Cassiae)	Oedema and distension in the abdomen due to Yang deficiency of the Spleen and Stomach
	Ting Li Zi (Semen Lepidii seu Descurainiae) *Xing Ren* (Semen Pruni Armeniacae) *Chen Pi* (Pericarpium Citri Reticulatae)	Congestion of Lung Qi, manifesting as coughing and wheezing due to Phlegm-fluids and puffy swelling of the face and eyes

Killing worms and dispersing accumulation	*Shi Jun Zi* (Fructus Quisqualis Indicae) *Bing Lang* (Semen Arecae Catechu)	Worms (including roundworm, threadworm and tapeworm)
	Zhi Shi (Fructus Immaturus Citri Aurantii) *Lai Fu Zi* (Semen Raphani Sativi)	Food accumulation in infants

Note: *Qian Niu Zi* can be ground and added to *Sheng Jiang Zhi* (Succus Rhizomatis Zingiberis Officinalis Recens) to treat constipation due to full-heat accumulation and stagnation.

Yuan Hua 芫花
(Genkwa flower, Flos Daphnes Genkwa)

Yuan Hua is the dried flower-bud of *Daphne genkwa* Sieb. et Zucc., family Thymelaeaceae.

Main ingredients *Yuan Hua* contains genkwanin, hydroxygenkwanin, yuanhuacine, yuanhuapine, yuanhuafine, yuanhuatine, apigenin, luteolin, benzoic acid, sterols and coumarin.

Properties Taste: acrid and bitter; nature: warm; toxic.

Channels entered Lung, Kidney and Large Intestine.

Functions and indications Drains water and eliminates dampness, frees Phlegm and disperses fluids, kills worms and treats sores. It is indicated for oedema, Phlegm-fluid patterns, masses in the stomach and abdomen, cough due to counterflow Qi, pain in the hypochondrium, malaria, and sores.

Common dosage 1.5-3g; or 0.5g of powder for oral use; appropriate dosage for external application. For internal use, process with vinegar to reduce the toxicity of the herb.

Precautions and contraindications

1. *Yuan Hua* is contraindicated during pregnancy and for patients with a weak constitution.
2. *Yuan Hua* is incompatible with *Gan Cao* (Radix Glycyrrhizae).

Comparison of functions *Yuan Hua* (Flos Daphnes Genkwa), *Gan Sui* (Radix Euphorbiae Kansui) and *Jing Da Ji* (Radix Euphorbiae Pekinensis) are all toxic herbs that can drain downwards drastically and expel water. They are used for severe oedema, water accumulation and Phlegm-fluid accumulation. Their effect is strengthened when they are used together. *Jing Da Ji* has a stronger effect than *Yuan Hua* and *Gan Sui* in draining water, dispersing swelling and dissipating abscesses, and mainly drains water from the Zang-Fu organs; *Gan Sui* is effective in draining water by freeing the channels; *Yuan Hua* is better for draining Phlegm-fluids in the chest and Lungs. *Yuan Hua* is more toxic than the other two herbs.

Toxicity The LD_{50} for intraperitoneal injection in rats of a *Yuan Hua* decoction is 9.25g/kg. The main toxic ingredients are genkwanin, apigenin and benzoic acid. Overdosage can stimulate the mucous membrane of the gastrointestinal tract, leading to irritation of the digestive tract, and can also stimulate the central nervous system to cause convulsions and respiratory failure. Toxic symptoms include dry mouth, slight nausea, severe vomiting and pain in the abdomen, and watery diarrhoea, and in more severe cases, bloody dysentery, dehydration and low blood pressure. The main causes of toxicity are overdosage or internal administration of the unprocessed herb. Toxicity is significantly reduced after processing with vinegar.

Modern research

1. Stops coughing and expels sputum.[24]
2. Induces urination.[24]
3. Preparations of *Yuan Hua* inhibited Streptococcus pneumoniae and Haemophilus influenzae *in vitro*.[24]
4. Preparations from the root of *Yuan Hua* can induce abortion.[25]

Combinations and applications

Functions	Combinations	Applications
Draining water and eliminating dampness, freeing Phlegm and dispersing fluids	*Gan Sui* (Radix Euphorbiae Kansui) *Jing Da Ji* (Radix Euphorbiae Pekinensis)	Ascites, scant urine
	Da Zao (Fructus Ziziphi Jujubae)	Cough due to damp-cold
	Gan Sui (Radix Euphorbiae Kansui) *Bai Jie Zi* (Semen Sinapis Albae)	Water collecting in the chest and hypochondrium

Notes:

1. External use of *Yuan Hua* has the function of killing worms and treating sores to treat porrigo and stubborn tinea.
2. *Yuan Hua* can be used as an external wash to treat frostbite.

Ba Dou 巴豆 (Croton seed, Semen Crotonis Tiglii)

Ba Dou is the ripe seed of *Croton tiglium* L., family Euphorbiaceae.

Legal status Under the Prescription Only Medicines (Products Other Than Veterinary Drugs) Order 1997, prescription of the use of this herb in the UK is restricted to medical practitioners.

Main ingredients *Ba Dou* contains 34-57% of croton oils (consisting of crotonic acid, tiglic acid and glycerides), phorbol, crotonoside, crotin, arginine, lysine and anthocyanidin.

Properties Taste: acrid; nature: hot; extremely toxic.

Channels entered Stomach, Lung and Large Intestine.

Functions and indications Drains cold accumulation downwards, expels water and reduces swelling, dispels Phlegm and benefits the throat. It is indicated for cold accumulation in the gastrointestinal tract, drum distension and ascites, Phlegm-fluid patterns, full-cold binding in the chest, diarrhoea, pain in the abdomen and abdominal urgency, diphtheria, throat Bi syndrome, sores, scabies and tinea.

Common dosage 0.1-0.3g in pills orally; appropriate dosage for external application. *Ba Dou* is usually made into a defatted powder known as croton frost (*Ba Dou Shuang*, Pulvis Crotonis Semenis) in order to attenuate its toxicity.

Precautions and contraindications

1. *Ba Dou* is contraindicated for patients with a weak constitution and during pregnancy.
2. *Ba Dou* antagonizes *Qian Niu Zi* (Semen Pharbitidis).
3. The oil contained in *Ba Dou* is very irritating to the skin and the mucosa of the mouth and stomach and ingestion of 20 drops of oil may cause death (see *Toxicity* below).

Remarks *Ba Dou* has the characteristic that its draining (diarrhoea-inducing) function will be enhanced when it meets warmth and checked when it meets cold. Therefore, if the draining function of *Ba Dou* is not powerful enough, hot congee or water can be drunk to promote the efficacy of the herb. Cold congee or water, or a cold decoction of *Huang Lian* (Rhizoma Coptidis) or *Lü Dou* (Semen Phaseoli Radiati) can be taken to relieve persistent diarrhoea caused by administration of the herb.

Toxicity Administration of 20 drops of croton oil can cause death in humans. The LD_{50} for oral administration to mice of a paste of raw *Ba Dou* is 1.6g/kg; that for oral administration of crotonic acid to rats is 1g/kg. The LD_{50} for subcutaneous injection of crotin in rabbits is 50-80mg/kg. The most toxic constituent of *Ba Dou* is croton oil, which strongly stimulates the mucous membrane in the stomach and intestines. It also stimulates the kidneys and causes acute dermatitis on contact with the skin. External application of *Ba Dou Shuang* can lead to contact dermatitis, pustules and blisters.

Modern research

1. Stimulates the intestinal mucous membrane.[26]
2. Inhibits Staphylococcus aureus, Pseudomonas aeruginosa and Corynebacterium diphtheriae.[27]
3. Alleviates pain.[28]
4. Inhibits the immune function.[29]

Combinations and applications

Functions	Combinations	Applications
Draining cold accumulation downwards	*Gan Jiang* (Rhizoma Zingiberis Officinalis) *Da Huang* (Radix et Rhizoma Rhei)	Constipation with sudden fullness, distension and pain in the abdomen due to cold accumulation in the gastrointestinal tract
	Jie Geng (Radix Platycodi Grandiflori) *Zhe Bei Mu* (Bulbus Fritillariae Thunbergii)	Full-cold binding in the chest, focal distension and pain in the chest and hypochondrium, constipation
	Dan Nan Xing (Pulvis Arisaematis cum Felle Bovis) *Shen Qu* (Massa Fermentata) *Shan Zha* (Fructus Crataegi)	Infantile Phlegm and food accumulation, manifesting as pain in the abdomen and constipation, fright palpitation with disquiet
Expelling water and reducing swelling	*Xing Ren* (Semen Pruni Armeniacae)	Drum distension and ascites, water-damp full patterns due to inhibited urination and defecation

External uses:

1. Scorch-fried *Ba Dou* mixed with *Ru Xiang* (Gummi Olibanum) can be pounded into a cream and applied to sores and clove sores.
2. Insufflating *Ba Dou Shuang* into the throat to treat diphtheria and throat obstruction due to diphtheria will induce vomiting to remove the sputum or cause diarrhoea to relieve the obstruction.

Modern research references

1. He Xingdong et al., *Lin Chuang Zhong Yao Shou Ce* [Clinical Handbook of Chinese Materia Medica] (Beijing, People's Medical Publishing House, 1998), 91.
2. Lei Zaiquan and Zhang Tingmo, *Zhong Hua Lin Chuang Zhong Yao Xue* [Chinese Clinical Materia Medica] (Beijing: People's Medical Publishing House, 1998), 652.
3. Yang Wenxiu et al., *Zhong Xi Yi Jie He Za Zhi* [Journal of Integrated TCM and Western Medicine] 13, 1 (1993): 33.
4. Cui Zhiqing et al., *Zhong Cao Yao* [Journal of Chinese Herbs] 24, 12 (1993): 635.
5. Pei Dekai et al., *Zhong Yi Za Zhi* [Journal of Traditional Chinese Medicine] 23, 7 (1982): 552.
6. Wang Lidong et al., *Sheng Li Ke Xue* [Physiological Science] 9, 3 (1989): 158.
7. Guo Changyan et al., *Zhong Xi Yi Jie He Za Zhi* [Journal of Integrated TCM and Western Medicine] 6, 2 (1986): 106; 9, 3 (1989): 161.
8. Zhao Shuying et al., *Zhong Xi Yi Jie He Za Zhi* 2, 2 (1982): 90.
9. Weng Fuhai et al., *Tian Jin Yi Ke Da Xue Xue Bao* [Journal of Tianjin Medical University] 21, 1 (1996): 1-3.
10. Xu Ping et al., *Jiang Su Zhong Yi Za Zhi* [Jiangsu Journal of Traditional Chinese Medicine] 11, 12 (1990): 38.
11. Lin Xiuzhen et al., *Zhong Yao Yao Li Yu Lin Chuang* [Pharmacology and Clinical Application of Chinese Materia Medica] 11, 2 (1995): 27.
12. Li Letian et al., *Zhong Yi Za Zhi* [Journal of Traditional Chinese Medicine] 21, 6 (1980): 471.
13. Zhang Xiangde et al., *Zhong Yi Za Zhi* 29, 3 (1988): 32.
14. Deng Wenlong, *Zhong Yi Fang Ji Yao Li Yu Ying Yong* [Pharmacology and Application of TCM Prescriptions] (Chongqing: Chongqing Publishing House, 1990), 180-207.

15. Cui Zhiqing et al., *Zhong Guo Yao Li Xue Tong Bao* [Chinese Pharmacology Bulletin] 8, 4 (1992): 269.
16. Jin Yacheng, *Zhong Yi Za Zhi* [Journal of Traditional Chinese Medicine] 21, 6 (1980): 24.
17. Lei Zaiquan and Zhang Tingmo, *Zhong Hua Lin Chuang Zhong Yao Xue*, 664.
18. Kuang Qiyin, *Yao Xue Tong Bao* [Pharmacology Bulletin] 2 (1960): 57.
19. Shi Dawei, *Ha Er Bin Yi Ke Da Xue Xue Bao* [Journal of Harbin Medical University] 24, 3 (1990): 166.
20. Zhang Shouquan, *Si Chuan Yi Xue* [Sichuan Journal of Medicine] 3, 9 (1985): 21.
21. He Xingdong et al., *Lin Chuang Zhong Yao Shou Ce*, 93.
22. Zhu Yan, *Zhong Yao Yao Li Yu Ying Yong* [Pharmacology and Application of Chinese Materia Medica] (Beijing: People's Medical Publishing House, 1958), 201.
23. Jiangsu New Medical College, *Zhong Yao Da Ci Dian* [Dictionary of Chinese Materia Medica], volume 2 (Shanghai: Shanghai People's Publishing House, 1989), 1626.
24. Chi Qun, *Shan Xi Xin Yi Yao* [Shaanxi New Medical Journal] 7 (1979): 56.
25. Cao Renlie, *Zhong Hua Pi Fu Ke Za Zhi* [Chinese Dermatology Journal] 4 (1957): 286.
26. T.A. Sollmann, *Manual of Pharmacology*, 8th ed. (Philadelphia: W. B. Saunders & Co., 1957), 214.
27. R.K. Boutweli et al., *Cancer Res* 17, 1 (1957): 71.
28. J.H. Hitchens et al., *Arch Int Pharmacodyn*, 169, 2 (1967): 384.
29. L.F. Fuh et al., *CA* 97 (1982): 179970.

Chapter 4

Herbs for dispelling wind-damp

祛风湿药

Herbs for dispelling wind-damp

Many of the herbs in this chapter are acrid in taste and warm in nature. They can dispel wind and eliminate dampness, treat Bi (painful obstruction) syndrome, and soothe the sinews and free the channels to promote the movement of Qi. Some of them can also supplement or boost the Kidneys and strengthen the bones.

Herbs for dispelling wind-damp are indicated for Bi syndromes caused by wind, cold and damp pathogenic factors blocking the channels, or by the obstruction of Qi and Blood, where these syndromes mainly manifest as pain in the limbs and joints, soreness, numbness and spasm of the sinews, and inhibited bending and stretching. These herbs can also be used to treat pain in the lumbar region and painful knee joints caused by Liver and Kidney deficiency.

Clinically, the appropriate combinations of herbs are selected according to the type of Bi syndrome involved:

1. in cases of invasion by wind pathogenic factors, select those herbs for dispelling wind-damp whose principal function is to extinguish wind and combine them with herbs for nourishing the Blood and herbs for quickening the Blood;
2. in cases of invasion by cold pathogenic factors, select those herbs for dispelling wind-damp which have a pronounced warm nature and combine them with herbs for warming the channels and freeing Yang; in this way, the pain is stopped by dispelling cold;
3. in cases of invasion by dampness, select those herbs for dispelling wind-damp which have a warm, dry nature and combine them with herbs for fortifying the Spleen, thus eliminating the dampness;
4. for heat-type Bi syndrome caused by internal heat due to Yin deficiency or heat due to stagnated wind, cold or damp pathogenic factors, select those herbs for dispelling wind-damp which have a cold nature and combine them with herbs for clearing heat and relieving toxicity;
5. for cases in the early stages of a Bi syndrome, use herbs for dispelling wind-damp in combination with herbs for releasing the exterior in order to eliminate dampness and dispel wind by sweating;
6. for cases due to the obstruction of pathogenic factors in the channels and sinews, use herbs for dispelling wind-damp in combination with herbs for quickening the Blood in order to clear the pathogenic factors from the channels;
7. for weak patients with a chronic disease, use herbs for dispelling wind-damp together with herbs for supplementing Qi and nourishing the Blood;
8. for chronic rheumatic diseases involving the Liver and Kidneys and manifesting as pain in the lumbar region, sore knees and difficulty in walking, use herbs for dispelling wind-damp together with herbs for supplementing the Liver and Kidneys and strengthening the sinews and bones. This combination will support vital Qi in eliminating pathogenic factors.

Since most of the herbs for dispelling wind-damp are acrid in taste and warm and dry in nature, they can easily damage Yin and consume the Blood. They should therefore be used with caution for patients with Yin or Blood deficiency.

Tab. 4.1 Herbs for dispelling wind, eliminating dampness and dissipating cold

Herb	Functions	Indications
Du Huo (Radix Angelicae Pubescentis)	Dispelling wind and overcoming dampness, freeing Bi syndrome and alleviating pain	Wind-cold-damp Bi syndrome, pain in the lumbar region and knees, pain in the hands and feet, numbness and paralysis
Mu Gua (Fructus Chaenomelis)	Soothing the sinews and quickening the network vessels, harmonizing the Stomach and transforming dampness	Wind-damp Bi syndrome pain, cramp due to vomiting and diarrhoea, oedema in leg Qi, dysentery, indigestion
Qi She (Agkistrodon)	Dispelling wind and freeing the network vessels to promote the movement of Qi, settling fright and alleviating tetany, dispelling wind and relieving toxicity	Paralysis and wind-stroke, facial paralysis, stubborn wind-damp Bi syndrome, numbness of the limbs, opisthotonos, child fright epilepsy, itchy skin, toxic sores due to syphilis, scrofula, headache due to pathogenic wind
Wei Ling Xian (Radix Clematidis)	Dispelling wind-damp and alleviating Bi syndrome pain	Wind-damp Bi syndrome, numbness, convulsions, inhibited bending and stretching
Shen Jin Cao (Herba Lycopodii Japonici)	Soothing the sinews and quickening the network vessels, dispelling wind and dissipating cold, eliminating dampness and dispersing swelling	Wind-cold-damp Bi syndrome, painful joints, numbness of the skin, swelling and pain due to sprain
Hai Feng Teng (Caulis Piperis Kadsurae)	Dispelling wind and eliminating dampness, freeing the channels and quickening the network vessels	Wind-damp Bi syndrome, inhibited bending and stretching, convulsions, pain in the lumbar region and knees, sprains, knocks and falls
Lu Lu Tong (Fructus Liquidambaris)	Dispelling wind, freeing the channels and quickening the network vessels, promoting urination and eliminating dampness	Wind-damp Bi syndrome, numbness of the limbs, hypertonicity of the hands and feet, knocks and falls, menstrual block, stoppage of breast milk, oedema, difficult urination, scabies, itching due to wind papules

Tab. 4.2 Herbs for dispelling wind, eliminating dampness and clearing heat

Herb	Functions	Indications
Qin Jiao (Radix Gentianae Macrophyllae)	Dispelling wind-damp and alleviating pain, abating jaundice, clearing deficiency-heat	Wind-damp Bi syndrome pain, hypertonicity of the sinews and vessels, tidal fever due to Yin deficiency, damp-heat jaundice, facial paralysis due to wind-stroke

Fang Ji (Radix Stephaniae Tetrandrae)	Dispelling wind and eliminating dampness to alleviate pain, promoting urination and dispersing swelling	Oedema and swelling of the abdomen, painful urination, wind-damp Bi syndrome pain, oedema in leg Qi
Sang Zhi (Ramulus Mori Albae)	Dispelling wind, freeing the channels and benefiting the joints	Wind-damp Bi syndrome, pain in the limbs, vitiligo (white patch wind)
Xi Xian Cao (Herba Siegesbeckiae)	Dispelling wind-damp and freeing the network vessels, clearing heat and relieving toxicity	Wind-damp Bi syndrome, limb joint pain, paralysis of the limbs due to wind-stroke, sores, eczema
Hai Tong Pi (Cortex Erythrinae)	Dispelling wind and overcoming dampness, freeing the channels and quickening the network vessels, alleviating itching	Wind-damp Bi syndrome, numbness of the limbs, pain in the lumbar region and knees, scabies and tinea, eczema
Luo Shi Teng (Caulis Trachelospermi Jasminoidis)	Dispelling wind and freeing the network vessels, cooling the Blood and dispersing abscesses	Wind-damp Bi syndrome, hypertonicity of the sinews and vessels, sore throat, abscesses and sores
Xu Chang Qing (Radix Cynanchi Paniculati)	Dispelling wind, eliminating dampness and alleviating pain, dispelling wind and alleviating itching	Wind-damp Bi syndrome pain, pain in the lumbar region, knocks and falls, pain in the stomach and abdomen, toothache, and skin diseases such as eczema, urticaria (dormant papules) and stubborn tinea

Tab. 4.3 Herbs for dispelling wind-damp and strengthening the sinews and bones

Herb	Functions	Indications
Sang Ji Sheng (Ramulus Loranthi)	Dispelling wind and overcoming dampness, supplementing the Liver and boosting the Kidneys, strengthening the sinews and bones, nourishing the Blood and quieting the foetus	Wind-damp Bi syndrome pain, limpness and aching in the lumbar region and knees, lack of strength in the sinews and bones, bleeding during pregnancy, stirring foetus, numbness of the limbs, hemiplegia
Wu Jia Pi (Cortex Acanthopanacis Gracilistyli Radicis)	Dispelling wind and eliminating dampness, strengthening the sinews and bones, promoting urination and dispersing swelling	Wind-cold-damp Bi syndrome, Wei syndrome of the sinews and bones, oedema, leg Qi, pain in the lumbar region
Gou Ji (Rhizoma Cibotii Barometz)	Supplementing and boosting the Liver and Kidneys, strengthening the sinews and bones, dispelling wind and eliminating dampness, warming and supplementing the Kidneys to secure the Essence and stop vaginal discharge	Limpness and aching in the lumbar region and knees, pain in the knees and feet, frequent urination, enuresis, vaginal discharge, wind-cold-damp Bi syndrome

HERBS FOR DISPELLING WIND, ELIMINATING DAMPNESS AND DISSIPATING COLD

Du Huo 独活 (Pubescent angelica root, Radix Angelicae Pubescentis)

Du Huo is the root of *Angelica pubescens* Maxim. f. *biserrata* Shan et Yuan, family Umbelliferae.

Main ingredients *Du Huo* contains furanocoumarins (including angelicol, angelicone and bergapten), as well as angelic, palmitic, stearic, oleic, tiglic and linolenic acids, phytosterols, glucose and essential oils.

Properties Taste: acrid and bitter; nature: warm.

Channels entered Kidney and Bladder.

Functions and indications Dispels wind and overcomes dampness, frees Bi syndrome and alleviates pain. It is indicated for wind-cold-damp Bi syndrome, pain in the lumbar region and knees, pain in the hands and feet, and numbness and paralysis.

Common dosage 3-10g, or appropriate dosage for external washes.

Precautions and contraindications *Du Huo* is contraindicated in cases of internal heat due to Yin deficiency, or conditions not caused by wind-cold-damp pathogenic factors.

Comparison of functions See *Qiang Huo* (Rhizoma et Radix Notopterygii), *Wei Ling Xian* (Radix Clematidis) and *Qin Jiao* (Radix Gentianae Macrophyllae).

Toxicity The LD_{50} for intramuscular injection in rats of the bergapten contained in *Du Huo* is 945mg/kg. It has been reported that a *Du Huo* decoction used to treat a patient with tracheitis caused numbness of the tongue, nausea, vomiting and gastric discomfort.

Modern research

1. The steep and decoction of *Du Huo* inhibit inflammation and alleviate pain.[1]
2. Inhibited Mycobacterium tuberculosis, Staphylococcus aureus and Escherichia coli during *in vitro* tests.[2]

Combinations and applications

Functions	Combinations	Applications
Dispelling wind and overcoming dampness, freeing Bi syndrome and alleviating pain	*Fang Feng* (Radix Ledebouriellae Divaricatae) *Mu Gua* (Fructus Chaenomelis) *Niu Xi* (Radix Achyranthis Bidentatae) *Du Zhong* (Cortex Eucommiae Ulmoidis) *Xu Duan* (Radix Dipsaci)	Numbness of the lower limbs and pain in the lumbar region and knees due to obstruction of wind-cold-damp pathogenic factors in the channels
	Qiang Huo (Rhizoma et Radix Notopterygii) *Gao Ben* (Rhizoma et Radix Ligustici) *Man Jing Zi* (Fructus Viticis)	Headache due to externally-contracted wind-cold-damp with slimy, white tongue fur and a soggy and moderate pulse

Combinations	Applications
Xi Xin (Herba cum Radice Asari) *Fang Feng* (Radix Ledebouriellae Divaricatae) *Bai Fu Zi* (Rhizoma Typhonii Gigantei) *Chuan Xiong* (Rhizoma Ligustici Chuanxiong)	Headache and toothache due to an invasion of wind
Sang Ji Sheng (Ramulus Loranthi) *Dang Gui* (Radix Angelicae Sinensis) *Ren Shen* (Radix Ginseng) *Du Zhong* (Cortex Eucommiae Ulmoidis) *Xi Xin* (Herba cum Radice Asari)	Prolonged Bi syndrome with insufficiency of Qi and Blood and depletion of the Liver and Kidneys

Mu Gua 木瓜 (Chinese quince fruit, Fructus Chaenomelis)

Mu Gua is the fruit of *Chaenomeles speciosa* (Sweet) Nakai, *C. lagenaria* (Loisel.) Koidz. or *C. sinensis* (Thouin) Koehne, family Rosaceae.

Main ingredients *Mu Gua* contains saponins, malic, tartaric, citric, ascorbic, fumaric and oleanolic acids, flavones and tannin.

Properties Taste: sour; nature: warm.

Channels entered Liver and Spleen.

Functions and indications Soothes the sinews and quickens the network vessels, harmonizes the Stomach and transforms dampness. It is indicated for wind-damp Bi syndrome pain, cramp due to vomiting and diarrhoea, oedema in leg Qi, dysentery, and indigestion.

Common dosage 6-12g for internal use in decoctions, pills or powders; or for external washes.

Precautions and contraindications *Mu Gua* should be used with caution in cases of food damaging the Spleen and Stomach.

Remarks *Mu Gua* can transform dampness and soothe the sinews and is an important herb for Bi syndrome due to damp and for hypertonicity of the sinews and vessels.

Modern research

1. Protects the functions of the liver.[3]
2. Can be used to treat bacillary dysentery.[4, 5]
3. Decoctions of *Mu Gua* can inhibit carcinoma.[6, 7]

Combinations and applications

Functions	Combinations	Applications
Soothing the sinews and quickening the network vessels	*Niu Xi* (Radix Achyranthis Bidentatae) *Du Huo* (Radix Angelicae Pubescentis) *He Shou Wu* (Radix Polygoni Multiflori) *Dang Gui* (Radix Angelicae Sinensis) *Wei Ling Xian* (Radix Clematidis)	Hypertonicity of the sinews and vessels due to damp obstruction in the channels and network vessels
	Ru Xiang (Gummi Olibanum) *Mo Yao* (Myrrha)	Damp Bi syndrome, stiffness in the neck
	Niu Xi (Radix Achyranthis Bidentatae) *Ba Ji Tian* (Radix Morindae Officinalis) *Xu Duan* (Radix Dipsaci)	Pain in the lumbar region due to wind-damp

	Wu Zhu Yu (Fructus Evodiae Rutaecarpae) *Zi Su Ye* (Folium Perillae Frutescentis) *Bing Lang* (Semen Arecae Catechu)	Leg Qi, swelling of the sinews and pain in the feet due to cold-damp
	Huang Bai (Cortex Phellodendri) *Yi Yi Ren* (Semen Coicis Lachrymajobi) *Niu Xi* (Radix Achyranthis Bidentatae)	Leg Qi, swelling of the sinews and pain in the feet due to damp-heat
Harmonizing the Stomach and transforming dampness	*Xiao Hui Xiang* (Fructus Foeniculi Vulgaris) *Gan Cao* (Radix Glycyrrhizae) *Sheng Jiang* (Rhizoma Zingiberis Officinalis Recens) *Zi Su Ye* (Folium Perillae Frutescentis) *Wu Zhu Yu* (Fructus Evodiae Rutaecarpae)	Diarrhoea, vomiting and pain in the abdomen, hypertonicity of the sinews due to abnormal upward and downward bearing of Qi in the Zang organs caused by dampness obstructing the Spleen and Stomach
	Sang Ye (Folium Mori Albae) *Da Zao* (Fructus Ziziphi Jujubae)	Pain in the lower abdomen
	Che Qian Zi (Semen Plantaginis) *Ying Su Ke* (Pericarpium Papaveris Somniferi) (see notes on legal status)	Dysentery with purulent and bloody stool due to damp-heat binding internally

Qi She 蕲蛇 (Long-noded pit viper, Agkistrodon)

Qi She (also known as *Bai Hua She*) is the whole body, with viscera discarded, of *Agkistrodon acutus* (Guenther), family Viperidae.

Main ingredients *Qi She* contains glycoprotein thrombin, bungarotoxin, coagulase and lipase.

Properties Taste: sweet and salty; nature: warm; toxic.

Channel entered Liver.

Functions and indications Dispels wind and frees the network vessels to promote the movement of Qi, settles fright and alleviates tetany, dispels wind and relieves toxicity. It is indicated for paralysis and wind-stroke, facial paralysis, stubborn wind-damp Bi syndrome, numbness of the limbs, opisthotonos, child fright epilepsy, itchy skin, toxic sores due to syphilis, scrofula, and headache due to pathogenic wind.

Common dosage 3-10g; or 1-1.5g of powder for oral usage; or 30g for preparing 500-1000ml of a herbal medicinal wine.

Precautions and contraindications *Qi She* is contraindicated for internal heat due to Yin deficiency, or for internal wind patterns due to Blood deficiency.

Remarks *Qi She* can act internally on the channels and network vessels and externally to dispel wind. It is highly effective in dispelling wind and freeing the channels and is therefore used for severe wind patterns.

Toxicity The LD_{50} for subcutaneous injection in mice of *Qi She* venom is less than 8.9mg/kg. After processing and removal of the head, the substance is no longer toxic. There have been no reports of toxic symptoms following oral intake of *Qi She* preparations.

Modern research After processing to eliminate its toxins, *Qi She* can be an effective medicinal in the treatment of neuralgia and pain in cancer.[8]

Combinations and applications

Functions	Combinations	Applications
Dispelling wind and freeing the network vessels to promote the movement of Qi	*Quan Xie* (Buthus Martensi) *Sang Zhi* (Ramulus Mori Albae) *Di Long* (Lumbricus) *Tao Ren* (Semen Persicae) *Dang Gui* (Radix Angelicae Sinensis)	Paralysis, hemiplegia or facial paralysis due to wind-stroke
	Wu Gong (Scolopendra Subspinipes) *Huang Qi* (Radix Astragali seu Hedysari) *Gui Zhi* (Ramulus Cinnamomi Cassiae) *Dang Gui* (Radix Angelicae Sinensis)	Wind-damp Bi syndrome, hypertonicity of the sinews
Settling fright and alleviating tetany	*Zhu Sha* (Cinnabaris) (see notes on legal status) *Shi Chang Pu* (Rhizoma Acori Graminei) *Dan Nan Xing* (Pulvis Arisaematis cum Felle Bovis) *Chan Tui* (Periostracum Cicadae)	Child fright wind, convulsions, fright epilepsy
	Wu Shao She (Zaocys Dhumnades) *Wu Gong* (Scolopendra Subspinipes) (taken in powder form)	Tetanus
Dispelling wind and relieving toxicity	*Tian Ma* (Rhizoma Gastrodiae Elatae) (see notes on legal status) *Bo He* (Herba Menthae Haplocalycis) *Jing Jie* (Herba Schizonepetae Tenuifoliae) *Ku Shen* (Radix Sophorae Flavescentis) *Bai Xian Pi* (Cortex Dictamni Dasycarpi Radicis)	Tinea, abscesses and sores, itchy papules, wind papules
	Di Gu Pi (Cortex Lycii Radicis) *Jing Jie Sui* (Spica Schizonepetae Tenuifoliae) *Shi Gao* (Gypsum Fibrosum) *Tian Nan Xing* (Rhizoma Arisaematis)	Headache due to pathogenic wind
	Ban Xia (Rhizoma Pinelliae Ternatae) *Jiang Can* (Bombyx Batryticatus) *Hai Zao* (Herba Sargassi) *Kun Bu* (Thallus Laminariae seu Eckloniae)	Scrofula and Phlegm nodes

Wei Ling Xian 威灵仙 (Chinese clematis root, Radix Clematidis)

Wei Ling Xian is the dried root and rhizome of *Clematis chinensis* Osbeck, *C. hexapetala Pall.* or *C. manshurica* Rupr., family Ranunculaceae.

Main ingredients *Wei Ling Xian* contains anemonin, anemonol, sterols, phenols, saponins and oleanolic acid.

Properties Taste: acrid and salty; nature: warm; slightly toxic.
Channel entered Bladder.
Functions and indications Dispels wind-damp and alleviates Bi syndrome pain. It is indicated for wind-damp Bi syndrome, numbness, convulsions, and inhibited bending and stretching.
Common dosage 5-10g; or up to 30g for dislodging fish bones stuck in the throat.
Precautions and contraindications *Wei Ling Xian* should be used with caution for weak patients, since it will damage vital Qi if used over a long period. It is contraindicated in cases of Qi and Blood deficiency and for treating patients in the absence of wind, cold or damp pathogenic factors.
Remarks *Wei Ling Xian* is effective in treating Bi syndrome pain; to strengthen the effect, it should be combined with other herbs depending on the location of the affected part. For pain in the upper part of the body, it is used with *Qiang Huo* (Rhizoma et Radix Notopterygii); for pain in the lower part of the body, use with *Du Huo* (Radix Angelicae Pubescentis) and *Niu Xi* (Radix Achyranthis Bidentatae); and for limb joint pain, use with *Gui Zhi* (Ramulus Cinnamomi Cassiae).
Comparison of functions Both *Wei Ling Xian* (Radix Clematidis) and *Du Huo* (Radix Angelicae Pubescentis) are used for Bi syndrome. *Du Huo* is better at acting downwards and is suitable for patterns in the lower part of the body, especially prolonged Bi syndrome pain; it can also be used for releasing the exterior. *Wei Ling Xian* is a mobile herb and is used more often for migratory joint pain due to wind-damp.

For an additional comparison, see *Qin Jiao* (Radix Gentianae Macrophyllae).
Modern research Alcoholic extracts of *Wei Ling Xian* can protect the cardiac muscle, and alcoholic and aqueous extracts of the herb can promote the secretion of bile.[9]

Combinations and applications

Functions	Combinations	Applications
Dispelling wind-damp and alleviating Bi syndrome pain	*Rou Gui* (Cortex Cinnamomi Cassiae) *Dang Gui* (Radix Angelicae Sinensis)	Pain in the lumbar region due to wind-damp
	Du Huo (Radix Angelicae Pubescentis) *Fang Feng* (Radix Ledebouriellae Divaricatae) *Dang Gui* (Radix Angelicae Sinensis)	Wind-damp Bi syndrome pain

Note: Slowly swallowing a decoction of *Wei Ling Xian* prepared on its own or with vinegar and brown sugar can dislodge fish bones stuck in the throat.

Shen Jin Cao 伸筋草
(Club moss, Herba Lycopodii Japonici)

Shen Jin Cao is the dried whole plant of *Lycopodium japonicum* Thunb., family Lycopodiaceae.
Main ingredients *Shen Jin Cao* contains lycopodine, clavatine, vanillic acid, ferulic acid, α-onocerin and clavatol.
Properties Taste: acrid and bitter; nature: warm.
Channels entered Liver, Spleen and Kidney.
Functions and indications Soothes the sinews and quickens the network vessels, dispels wind and dissipates cold, eliminates dampness and disperses swelling. It is indicated for wind-cold-damp Bi syndrome, painful joints, numbness of the skin, and swelling and pain due to sprain.
Common dosage 9-15g.
Precautions and contraindications *Shen Jin Cao* is contraindicated during pregnancy.
Modern research Aqueous extracts of *Shen Jin Cao* can lower body temperature, and induce stiff and clonic spasm, palsy and asphyxia in animals.[10]

Combinations and applications

Functions	Combinations	Applications
Soothing the sinews and quickening the network vessels, dispelling wind and dissipating cold, eliminating dampness and dispersing swelling	*Hu Zhang* (Radix et Rhizoma Polygoni Cuspidati) *Ji Xue Teng* (Caulis Spatholobi)	Wind-cold-damp Bi syndrome pain
	Sang Ji Sheng (Ramulus Loranthi) *Luo Shi Teng* (Caulis Trachelospermi Jasminoidis) *Fang Feng* (Radix Ledebouriellae Divaricatae)	Generalized pain due to wind
	Shu Di Huang (Radix Rehmanniae Glutinosae Conquita) *Shan Zhu Yu* (Fructus Corni Officinalis) *Qian Nian Jian* (Rhizoma Homalomenae Occultae) *Dang Gui* (Radix Angelicae Sinensis)	Inhibited bending and stretching due to insufficiency of the Liver and Kidneys and improper nourishment of the sinews and vessels
	Chen Hu Lu (Fructus Lagenariae Depressae) *Bing Lang* (Semen Arecae Catechu)	Oedema

Hai Feng Teng 海风藤
(Kadsura pepper stem, Caulis Piperis Kadsurae)

Hai Feng Teng is the dried stem of *Piper kadsura* (Choisy) Ohwi, also known as *Piper futokadsura* Sieb. et Zucc., family Piperaceae.

Main ingredients *Hai Feng Teng* contains futoamide, futoquinol, futoenone, futoxide, piperenone, kadsurenone, kadsurenin, β-sitosterol, stigmasterol and volatile oils (including α-pinene, β-pinene, isoasarone, limonene, sabinene and camphene).

Properties Taste: acrid and bitter; nature: slightly warm.

Channel entered Liver.

Functions and indications Dispels wind and eliminates dampness, frees the channels and quickens the network vessels. It is indicated for wind-damp Bi syndrome, inhibited bending and stretching, convulsions, pain in the lumbar region and knees, sprains, knocks and falls.

Common dosage 5-15g.

Comparison of functions See *Luo Shi Teng* (Caulis Trachelospermi Jasminoidis).

Modern research Reduces swelling and alleviates pain, calms wheezing, and increases the supply of blood to the heart.[11]

Combinations and applications

Functions	Combinations	Applications
Dispelling wind and eliminating dampness, freeing the channels and quickening the network vessels	*Wei Ling Xian* (Radix Clematidis) *Qin Jiao* (Radix Gentianae Macrophyllae) *Gui Zhi* (Ramulus Cinnamomi Cassiae)	Wind-damp Bi syndrome pain
	Ji Xue Teng (Caulis Spatholobi) *Niu Xi* (Radix Achyranthis Bidentatae)	Knocks and falls

Lu Lu Tong 路路通 (Sweetgum fruit, Fructus Liquidambaris)

Lu Lu Tong is the dried fruit of *Liquidambar formosana* Hance, family Hamamelidaceae.

Main ingredients *Lu Lu Tong* contains terpenes, borneol, cinnamic acid, liquidambaric acid, resin, balsam and benzine.

Properties Taste: acrid and bitter; nature: neutral.

Channels entered Liver, Stomach and Bladder.

Functions and indications Dispels wind, frees the channels and quickens the network vessels, promotes urination and eliminates dampness. It is indicated for wind-damp Bi syndrome, numbness of the limbs, hypertonicity of the hands and feet, knocks and falls, menstrual block, stoppage of breast milk, oedema, difficult urination, scabies, and itching due to wind papules.

Common dosage 3-9g.

Precautions and contraindications *Lu Lu Tong* is contraindicated during pregnancy.

Modern research The balsam contained in *Lu Lu Tong*, mixed with 60% of alcohol and used externally, can prevent hookworm larvae from penetrating the skin of mice.[10]

Combinations and applications

Functions	Combinations	Applications
Dispelling wind	*Luo Shi Teng* (Caulis Trachelospermi Jasminoidis) *Qin Jiao* (Radix Gentianae Macrophyllae) *Shen Jin Cao* (Herba Lycopodii Japonici)	Wind-damp Bi syndrome pain, spasms of the limbs
	Di Fu Zi (Fructus Kochiae Scopariae) *Chi Shao* (Radix Paeoniae Rubra)	Wind papules
Freeing the channels and quickening the network vessels	*Qing Pi* (Pericarpium Citri Reticulatae Viride) *Chuan Shan Jia* (Squama Manitis Pentadactylae) (see notes on legal status)	Stoppage of breast milk
	Dang Gui (Radix Angelicae Sinensis) *Chuan Xiong* (Rhizoma Ligustici Chuanxiong) *Chong Wei Zi* (Semen Leonuri Heterophylli)	Menstrual block or scant menstruation due to Qi stagnation and Blood stasis with distension and pain in the abdomen
	Su Mu (Lignum Sappan) *Chi Shao* (Radix Paeoniae Rubra) *Hong Hua* (Flos Carthami Tinctorii)	Swelling and pain due to Blood stasis resulting from knocks and falls
Promoting urination and eliminating dampness	*Fu Ling Pi* (Cortex Poriae Cocos) *Sang Bai Pi* (Cortex Mori Albae Radicis) *Di Gu Pi* (Cortex Lycii Radicis) *Ze Xie* (Rhizoma Alismatis Orientalis)	Oedema, inhibited urination

HERBS FOR DISPELLING WIND, ELIMINATING DAMPNESS AND CLEARING HEAT

Qin Jiao 秦艽 (Large-leaf gentian root, Radix Gentianae Macrophyllae)

Qin Jiao is the root of *Gentiana macrophylla* Pall., *G. straminea* Maxim., *G. crassicaulis* Duthie ex Burk., or *G. dahurica* Fisch., family Gentianaceae.

Main ingredients *Qin Jiao* contains gentianine, gentianidine, gentianol, gentiopicroside, alkaloids, volatile oils and carbohydrates.

Properties Taste: acrid and bitter; nature: slightly cold.

Channels entered Stomach, Liver and Gallbladder.

Functions and indications Dispels wind-damp and alleviates pain, abates jaundice, and clears deficiency-heat. It is indicated for wind-damp Bi syndrome pain, hypertonicity of the sinews and vessels, tidal fever due to Yin deficiency, damp-heat jaundice, and facial paralysis due to wind-stroke.

Common dosage 6-15g, or 30g for large dosages; appropriate dosage for external application.

Precautions and contraindications *Qin Jiao* is contraindicated in cases of weakness, frequent urination, or loose stool due to Spleen deficiency.

Comparison of functions

1. *Qin Jiao* (Radix Gentianae Macrophyllae) and *Long Dan Cao* (Radix Gentianae Scabrae) can dispel damp and abate fever to treat damp-heat jaundice. Despite being slightly cold, *Qin Jiao* is not a dry herb and, although it can dispel wind and eliminate dampness, it does not damage Yin liquids. It is often used therefore for wind-damp Bi syndrome pain as well as for steaming bone disorder and tidal fever. *Long Dan Cao*, being extremely bitter and cold, can drain full-fire in the Liver channel and damp-heat in the Lower Jiao. It is used to treat red eyes due to Liver-fire, dizziness and deafness, and pudendal itch and vaginal discharge.
2. Both *Qin Jiao* and *Wei Ling Xian* (Radix Clematidis) can treat wind-damp Bi syndrome pain, but *Qin Jiao* trends to treat this pain in the Yangming channel, whereas *Wei Ling Xian* tends to treat it in the Taiyang channel.
3. Both *Qin Jiao* and *Yin Chai Hu* (Radix Stellariae Dichotomae) can treat steaming bone disorder due to deficiency taxation, but *Qin Jiao* is more effective in treating the disorder with tidal fever, whereas *Yin Chai Hu* functions better when it is due to internal heat and manifests with intermittent fever and chills.
4. *Qin Jiao* and *Du Huo* (Radix Angelicae Pubescentis) can treat wind-damp pain in the lower part of the body, but *Qin Jiao* is more effective in treating heat pain due to wind-damp, whereas *Du Huo* is better for cold pain due to wind-damp.

Toxicity The LD_{50} for intragastric administration and intraperitoneal injection of gentianine in mice is 486mg/kg and 300mg/kg respectively. There was a report of nausea and vomiting in four patients with rheumatic arthritis who took 100mg of gentianine orally three times a day; one of the patients suffered from palpitations and a reduced heart rate, which quickly returned to normal.

Modern research

1. Stimulates the pituitary-adrenocortical function through the nervous system to inhibit inflammation.[12]
2. Inhibits allergy.[13]
3. Lowers blood pressure,[12] and raises the blood sugar level.[13]

Combinations and applications

Functions	Combinations	Applications
Dispelling wind-damp and alleviating pain	*Wei Ling Xian* (Radix Clematidis) *Chuan Wu* (Radix Aconiti Carmichaeli) (see notes on legal status) *Ma Huang* (Herba Ephedrae) (see notes on legal status) *Xi Xin* (Herba cum Radice Asari)	Limb joint pain and hypertonicity of the sinews and vessels due to wind-cold-damp Bi syndrome
	Ren Dong Teng (Caulis Lonicerae Japonicae) *Yi Yi Ren* (Semen Coicis Lachrymajobi) *Sang Zhi* (Ramulus Mori Albae) *Fang Ji* (Radix Stephaniae Tetrandrae) (see notes on legal status)	Wind-damp-heat Bi syndrome, limb joint pain
	Fang Feng (Radix Ledebouriellae Divaricatae) *Sheng Di Huang* (Radix Rehmanniae Glutinosae) *Huang Qin* (Radix Scutellariae Baicalensis)	Hemiplegia due to wind pathogenic factors invading the channels and network vessels
	Dang Gui (Radix Angelicae Sinensis) *Shu Di Huang* (Radix Rehmanniae Glutinosae Conquita) *Bai Shao* (Radix Paeoniae Lactiflorae) *Chuan Xiong* (Rhizoma Ligustici Chuanxiong)	Wind-stroke due to Blood deficiency
Abating jaundice	*Yin Chen Hao* (Herba Artemisiae Scopariae) *Zhi Zi* (Fructus Gardeniae Jasminoidis) *Mu Tong* (Caulis Mutong) (see notes on legal status) *Bai Mao Gen* (Rhizoma Imperatae Cylindricae)	Damp-heat jaundice
Clearing deficiency-heat	*Zhi Mu* (Rhizoma Anemarrhenae Asphodeloidis) *Di Gu Pi* (Cortex Lycii Radicis) *Qing Hao* (Herba Artemisiae Chinghao) *Bie Jia* (Carapax Amydae Sinensis) (see notes on legal status)	Steaming bone disorder and tidal fever due to Yin deficiency, night sweating
	Gan Cao (Radix Glycyrrhizae)	Wasting and thirsting, vexation
	Zhi Mu (Rhizoma Anemarrhenae Asphodeloidis) *Chai Hu* (Radix Bupleuri) *Zhi Gan Cao* (Radix Glycyrrhizae Praeparata)	Cough due to deficiency taxation

Fang Ji 防己
(Stephania root, Radix Stephaniae Tetrandrae)

Han Fang Ji is the root of *Stephania tetrandra* S. Moore, family Menispermaceae; *Guang Fang Ji* (aristolochia root, Radix Aristolochiae Fangchi) is the root of *Aristolochia fangchi* Y. C. Wu ex L. D. Chou et S. M. Hwang, family Aristolochiaceae.

Legal status At the time of publication, the Medicines (*Aristolochia* and Mu Tong etc.) (Prohibition) Order 2001 renders illegal in the UK the sale, supply and importation of unlicensed medicines for human use containing or presented as containing this herb. The restricted status of *Han Fang Ji* may only be of temporary duration, as the motivation for the import ban can be attributed to contamination of supplies by the toxic herb, *Guang Fang Ji*.

Main ingredients *Han Fang Ji* contains 1.2% of alkaloids (including tetrandrine, dimethyltetrandrine, fangchinoline and cyclanoline), flavones, phenols and volatile oils. *Guang Fang Ji* contains many types of alkaloids such as trilobine and magnoflorine.

Properties Taste: acrid and bitter; nature: cold.

Channels entered Bladder, Kidney and Spleen.

Functions and indications Dispels wind and eliminates dampness to alleviate pain, promotes urination and disperses swelling. It is indicated for oedema and swelling of the abdomen, painful urination, wind-damp Bi syndrome pain, and oedema in leg Qi.

Common dosage 6-15g.

Precautions and contraindications *Fang Ji* is contraindicated in cases of Yin deficiency and patterns without full damp-heat.

Remarks *Fang Ji* can be divided into *Han Fang Ji* and *Guang Fang Ji* (or *Mu Fang Ji*), both of which can dispel wind and eliminate dampness, and disperse swelling by promoting urination. *Guang Fang Ji* is used to alleviate pain and treat Bi syndromes in the upper part of the body when combined with wind pathogenic factors. *Han Fang Ji* is used to disperse swelling by promoting urination and to treat Bi syndromes in the lower part of the body when combined with dampness. In a prescription, *Fang Ji* generally refers to *Han Fang Ji*.

Toxicity The LD_{50} for abdominal injection of the alkaloids contained in *Han Fang Ji* is 113.1mg/kg. Most rabbits died after intravenous injection of 20mg/kg, but there were no significant side-effects after intravenous injection of 23-25mg/kg in dogs. The LD_{50} for intravenous injection of tetrandrine in rats is 38.0mg/kg; for mice, it is 82.5mg/kg; for oral administration, it is 2230mg/kg for rats and 3700mg/kg for mice. When rats were given 20mg/kg per day of the herb via oral administration for 21 days, most of them suffered degeneration of the parenchymal cells in the liver, kidneys and adrenal gland. When the dosage was increased to 40mg/kg and 80mg/kg, toxic damage to the liver, kidneys and adrenal gland became severe. After the dosage was increased to 400mg/kg, all rats died within seven days.

Modern research

1. Inhibits inflammation.[14, 15]
2. Lowers blood pressure,[16] inhibits arrhythmia[17] and increases the volume of blood flow to the coronary arteries.[18]

Combinations and applications

Functions	Combinations	Applications
Dispelling wind and eliminating dampness to alleviate pain	*Qin Jiao* (Radix Gentianae Macrophyllae) *Sang Zhi* (Ramulus Mori Albae) *Ren Dong Teng* (Caulis Lonicerae Japonicae)	Damp-heat Bi syndrome

	Qiang Huo (Rhizoma et Radix Notopterygii) *Du Huo* (Radix Angelicae Pubescentis) *Wei Ling Xian* (Radix Clematidis)	Wind-cold-damp Bi syndrome
	Ku Shen (Radix Sophorae Flavescentis) *Bai Xian Pi* (Cortex Dictamni Dasycarpi Radicis) *Tu Fu Ling* (Rhizoma Smilacis Glabrae)	Eczema, boils
Promoting urination and dispersing swelling	*Huang Qi* (Radix Astragali seu Hedysari) *Gui Zhi* (Ramulus Cinnamomi Cassiae) *Fu Ling* (Sclerotium Poriae Cocos)	Oedema of the limbs
	Mu Tong (Caulis Mutong) (see notes on legal status) *Ze Xie* (Rhizoma Alismatis Orientalis) *Zhu Ling* (Sclerotium Polypori Umbellati)	Inhibited urination due to damp-heat in the Bladder
	Dong Kui Zi (Semen Malvae Verticillatae) *Fang Feng* (Radix Ledebouriellae Divaricatae)	Enuresis
	Mu Gua (Fructus Chaenomelis) *Niu Xi* (Radix Achyranthis Bidentatae) *Mu Tong* (Caulis Mutong) (see notes on legal status) *Bing Lang* (Semen Arecae Catechu)	Swollen and painful lower limbs due to damp-heat obstruction
	Wu Zhu Yu (Fructus Evodiae Rutaecarpae) *Bing Lang* (Semen Arecae Catechu) *Mu Gua* (Fructus Chaenomelis)	Leg Qi with swelling and pain in the feet and shins, accompanied by numbness in severe cases

Sang Zhi 桑枝 (Mulberry twig, Ramulus Mori Albae)

Sang Zhi is the dried young twig of *Morus alba* L., family Moraceae.

Main ingredients *Sang Zhi* contains mulberrin, mulberrochromene, cyclomulberrin, morin, maclurin, 2,4,6,4′-tetrahydroxybenzophenone, pectin, succinic acid, glucose and adenine.

Properties Taste: bitter; nature: neutral.

Channel entered Liver.

Functions and indications Dispels wind, frees the channels and benefits the joints. It is indicated for wind-damp Bi syndrome, pain in the limbs, and vitiligo (white patch wind).

Common dosage 10-30g.

Comparison of functions Both *Sang Zhi* (Ramulus Mori Albae) and *Gui Zhi* (Ramulus Cinnamomi Cassiae) can free the channels and network vessels. *Sang Zhi* frees the channels by dispelling wind and eliminating dampness, whereas *Gui Zhi* performs this function by warming Yang. The two herbs are often combined for wind-damp Bi syndrome pain in the upper limbs. *Sang Zhi* is good for heat patterns due to wind-damp, while *Gui Zhi* tends to be used to treat Bi syndrome due to cold.

For an additional comparison, see *Sang Bai Pi* (Cortex Mori Albae Radicis).

Modern research

1. Effective in the treatment of patients with a low lymphocyte transformation rate.[19]
2. Inhibited Staphylococcus aureus in clinical tests.[20]

Combinations and applications

Functions	Combinations	Applications
Dispelling wind, freeing the channels and benefiting the joints	*Wei Ling Xian* (Radix Clematidis) *Fang Ji* (Radix Stephaniae Tetrandrae) (see notes on legal status) *Dang Gui* (Radix Angelicae Sinensis)	Numbness due to wind-damp
	Luo Shi Teng (Caulis Trachelospermi Jasminoidis) *Ren Dong Teng* (Caulis Lonicerae Japonicae) *Di Long* (Lumbricus)	Wind-damp-heat Bi syndrome with red and swollen joints
	Yi Mu Cao (Herba Leonuri Heterophylli)	Vitiligo (white patch wind)
	Gui Zhi (Ramulus Cinnamomi Cassiae) *Wei Ling Xian* (Radix Clematidis)	Wind-damp Bi syndrome pain in the upper limbs

Xi Xian Cao 豨莶草 (Siegesbeckia herb, Herba Siegesbeckiae)

Xi Xian Cao is the dried aerial parts of *Siegesbeckia orientalis* L., *S. pubescens* Mak. or *S. glabrescens* Mak., family Compositae.

Main ingredients *Siegesbeckia orientalis* contains darutoside, darutigenol, orientin, orientalide, stigmasterol and β-sitosterol; *S. pubescens* contains darutoside, darutigenol, alkaloids, amaroids and volatile oils; *S. glabrescens* contains darutoside, darutigenol, neodarutoside, 16-acetylkirenol and isopropylidenekirenol.

Properties Taste: bitter; nature: cold.

Channels entered Liver and Kidney.

Functions and indications Dispels wind-damp and frees the network vessels, clears heat and relieves toxicity. It is indicated for wind-damp Bi syndrome, limb joint pain, paralysis of the limbs due to wind-stroke, sores, and eczema.

Common dosage 10-15g.

Precautions and contraindications *Xi Xian Cao* is contraindicated in cases of Yin or Blood insufficiency.

Remarks

1. *Xi Xian Cao* is also effective in reducing hypertension.
2. Fresh *Xi Xian Cao* is good for abscesses, sores and eczema; after processing with wine, the prepared herb is used for treating Bi syndrome.

Toxicity The LD_{50} for intravenous injection in mice of *Xi Xian Cao* is 45.5g/kg. The maximum safe dosage for intraperitoneal injection in rats was 400 times that of the normal dosage for humans.

Modern research

1. Inhibits inflammation.[21]
2. In laboratory tests, *Xi Xian Cao* was very effective in inhibiting Staphylococcus aureus and fairly effective in inhibiting Shigella shigae, Pseudomonas aeruginosa and Salmonella typhi.[22]
3. Lowers blood pressure.[23]
4. Improves microcirculation.[24, 25]

Combinations and applications

Functions	Combinations	Applications
Dispelling wind-damp and freeing the network vessels	*Sang Zhi* (Ramulus Mori Albae) *Ren Dong Teng* (Caulis Lonicerae Japonicae) *Fang Ji* (Radix Stephaniae Tetrandrae) (see notes on legal status)	Damp-heat Bi syndrome with red, sore and swollen joints
	Sang Ji Sheng (Ramulus Loranthi) *Mu Gua* (Fructus Chaenomelis) *Shu Di Huang* (Radix Rehmanniae Glutinosae Conquita)	Wind-damp Bi syndrome pain involving the Liver and Kidneys
	Huang Qi (Radix Astragali seu Hedysari) *Qi She* (Agkistrodon) *Gou Qi Zi* (Fructus Lycii)	Facial paralysis, hemiplegia, inhibited speech
Clearing heat and relieving toxicity	*Ku Shen* (Radix Sophorae Flavescentis) *Bai Xian Pi* (Cortex Dictamni Dasycarpi Radicis)	Sore toxins due to damp-heat, eczema

Notes:
1. A decoction of *Xi Xian Cao* is effective in the treatment of malaria.
2. The fresh herb can be used externally for snake bites.

Hai Tong Pi 海桐皮
(Erythrina bark, Cortex Erythrinae)

Hai Tong Pi is the dried bark of *Erythrina variegata* L. var. *orientalis* (L.) Merr. or *E. arborescens* Roxb., family Leguminosae.

Main ingredients *Hai Tong Pi* contains erythraline, hypaphorine, amino acids, organic acids, erythrinin, erybidin and saponins.

Properties Taste: bitter and acrid; nature: neutral.

Channel entered Liver, Kidney and Spleen.

Functions and indications Dispels wind and overcomes dampness, frees the channels and quickens the network vessels, and alleviates itching. It is indicated for wind-damp Bi syndrome, numbness of the limbs, pain in the lumbar region and knees, scabies and tinea, and eczema.

Common dosage 6-12g as a decoction or steeped in wine; external application as a gargle or powder.

Modern research
1. Relieves spasm of the smooth muscle.[26]
2. Alleviates pain.[27]

Combinations and applications

Functions	Combinations	Applications
Dispelling wind and overcoming dampness, freeing the channels and quickening the network vessels	*Huang Bai* (Cortex Phellodendri) *Fang Ji* (Radix Stephaniae Tetrandrae) (see notes on legal status) *Bi Xie* (Rhizoma Dioscoreae)	Swelling and pain in the knees due to damp-heat pouring down

Yi Yi Ren (Semen Coicis Lachrymajobi) *Fang Feng* (Radix Ledebouriellae Divaricatae) *Qiang Huo* (Rhizoma et Radix Notopterygii) *Rou Gui* (Cortex Cinnamomi Cassiae) *Shu Di Huang* (Radix Rehmanniae Glutinosae Conquita) *Bing Lang* (Semen Arecae Catechu)	Wind-damp Bi syndrome with pain in the joints of the lower limbs
Dang Gui (Radix Angelicae Sinensis) *Chi Shao* (Radix Paeoniae Rubra) *Bai Zhu* (Rhizoma Atractylodis Macrocephalae)	Pain in the upper limbs due to obstruction of Qi and Blood in the channels and network vessels

Note: A decoction of *Hai Tong Pi* on its own or in combination with *She Chuang Zi* (Fructus Cnidii Monnieri), *Ku Shen* (Radix Sophorae Flavescentis), *Tu Fu Ling* (Rhizoma Smilacis Glabrae) and *Huang Bai* (Cortex Phellodendri) can be used externally to treat eczema, itchy skin, and scabies and tinea.

Luo Shi Teng 络石藤
(Chinese star jasmine stem, Caulis Trachelospermi Jasminoidis)

Luo Shi Teng is the dried leafy stem of *Trachelospermum jasminoides* (Lindl.) Lem., family Apocynaceae.

Main ingredients *Luo Shi Teng* contains tracheloside, arctiin, matairesinoside and quercetin.

Properties Taste: bitter; nature: slightly cold.

Channels entered Heart and Liver.

Functions and indications Dispels wind and frees the network vessels, cools the Blood and disperses abscesses. It is indicated for wind-damp Bi syndrome, hypertonicity of the sinews and vessels, sore throat, and abscesses and sores.

Common dosage 6–15g.

Comparison of functions Both *Luo Shi Teng* (Caulis Trachelospermi Jasminoidis) and *Hai Feng Teng* (Caulis Piperis Kadsurae) are good at dispelling wind and freeing the network vessels and are commonly used for inhibited bending and stretching of the joints due to wind-damp as well as for hypertonicity of the sinews and vessels. However, *Hai Feng Teng* tends to be slightly warm and is suitable for severe wind, cold and damp patterns without heat, whereas *Luo Shi Teng*, being slightly cold, can treat Bi syndrome pain due to wind-damp accompanied by heat.

Modern research

1. The arctiin contain in *Luo Shi Teng* can dilate the blood vessels and lower blood pressure.[28]
2. A large dosage of decoctions of *Luo Shi Teng* can induce respiratory failure.[28]

Combinations and applications

Functions	Combinations	Applications
Dispelling wind and freeing the network vessels	*Qian Nian Jian* (Rhizoma Homalomenae Occultae) *Du Huo* (Radix Angelicae Pubescentis) *Wei Ling Xian* (Radix Clematidis) *Fang Feng* (Radix Ledebouriellae Divaricatae) *Qin Jiao* (Radix Gentianae Macrophyllae) *Fang Ji* (Radix Stephaniae Tetrandrae) (see notes on legal status)	Hypertonicity of the sinews and vessels due to wind-damp
	Ren Dong Teng (Caulis Lonicerae Japonicae) *Bai Wei* (Radix Cynanchi Atrati) *Dan Shen* (Radix Salviae Miltiorrhizae) *Hai Tong Pi* (Cortex Erythrinae) *Cang Zhu* (Rhizoma Atractylodis) *Huang Bai* (Cortex Phellodendri) *Niu Xi* (Radix Achyranthis Bidentatae)	Wind-damp-heat Bi syndrome with red, sore and swollen joints
Cooling the Blood and dispersing abscesses	*Jin Yin Hua* (Flos Lonicerae) *Pu Gong Ying* (Herba Taraxaci cum Radice) *Zi Hua Di Ding* (Herba Violae Yedoensitis)	Swelling and toxins of sores
	Zao Jiao Ci (Spina Gleditsiae Sinensis) *Ru Xiang* (Gummi Olibanum)	Abscesses, swelling and toxins of clove sores
	Jie Geng (Radix Platycodi Grandiflori) *She Gan* (Rhizoma Belamcandae Chinensis) *Mu Tong* (Caulis Mutong) (see notes on legal status)	Sore throat

Xu Chang Qing 徐长卿
(Paniculate swallowwort root, Radix Cynanchi Paniculati)

Xu Chang Qing is the root and rhizome of *Cynanchum paniculatum* (Bge.) Kitag., family Asclepiadaceae.

Main ingredients *Xu Chang Qing* contains paeonol, flavones and a small amount of alkaloids.

Properties Taste: acrid; nature: warm.

Channels entered Liver and Stomach.

Functions and indications Dispels wind, eliminates dampness and alleviates pain, and dispels wind and alleviates itching. It is indicated for wind-damp Bi syndrome pain, pain in the lumbar region, knocks and falls, pain in the stomach and abdomen, toothache, and skin diseases such as eczema, urticaria (dormant papules) and stubborn tinea.

Common dosage 3-10g in an oral decoction; 1.5-3g in a powder preparation.

Remarks *Xu Chang Qing* should not be decocted for a long time because of its strong aroma.

Modern research

1. Has a tranquillizing function and alleviates pain.[29]
2. Reduces the level of blood fats.[29]
3. Lowers blood pressure.[30]
4. Inhibited such bacteria as Staphylococcus aureus, Escherichia coli, Pseudomonas aeruginosa and Salmonella typhi *in vitro*.[31]

Combinations and applications

Functions	Combinations	Applications
Dispelling wind, eliminating dampness and alleviating pain	*Wei Ling Xian* (Radix Clematidis) *Wu Jia Pi* (Cortex Acanthopanacis Gracilistyli Radicis)	Wind-damp Bi syndrome
	Xu Duan (Radix Dipsaci) *Du Zhong* (Cortex Eucommiae Ulmoidis)	Pain in the lumbar region
	Du Huo (Radix Angelicae Pubescentis) *Niu Xi* (Radix Achyranthis Bidentatae)	Wind-damp Bi syndrome and pain in the lumbar region
	Yan Hu Suo (Rhizoma Corydalis Yanhusuo)	Pain in the stomach and abdomen
	Chuan Xiong (Rhizoma Ligustici Chuanxiong)	Pain in the abdomen during menstruation
	Tao Ren (Semen Persicae) *Wu Ling Zhi* (Excrementum Trogopteri)	Knocks and falls
Dispelling wind and alleviating itching	*Ku Shen* (Radix Sophorae Flavescentis) *Di Fu Zi* (Fructus Kochiae Scopariae) *Bai Xian Pi* (Cortex Dictamni Dasycarpi Radicis)	Eczema, urticaria (dormant papules) and stubborn tinea

Notes:

1. A decoction of *Xu Chang Qing* can be used as a gargle for toothache.
2. *Xu Chang Qing* can also relieve the toxicity of poisonous snake bites. It is usually taken orally or used externally in combination with *Ban Bian Lian* (Herba Lobeliae Chinensis cum Radice).

HERBS FOR DISPELLING WIND-DAMP AND STRENGTHENING THE SINEWS AND BONES

Sang Ji Sheng 桑寄生
(Mulberry mistletoe, Ramulus Loranthi)

Sang Ji Sheng is the leafy stem and branch of *Loranthus parasiticus* (L.) Merr., *Taxillus chinensis* (DC.) Danser (also known as Herba Taxilli) or *Viscum coloratum* (Kom.) Nakai, family Loranthaceae.

Legal status *Sang Ji Sheng* was listed in a document entitled *A Review of Restricted Herbal Ingredients* issued by the Medicines Control Agency (MCA) in the UK in September 2001 with a view to the possible imposition of restrictions on its use at a future date. The MCA is concerned that some other countries restrict the use for therapeutic purposes of another possible source for this herb, *Viscum album*, and is therefore considering imposing a requirement for medical supervision in use.

Main ingredients *Sang Ji Sheng* contains quercetin, avicularin, viscotoxins, acetylcholine, histamine, triterpenes and phospholipids (Taxillus); oleanolic acid, β-amyrin and flavone compounds (*Viscum*).

Properties Taste: bitter; nature: neutral.

Channels entered Liver and Kidney.

Functions and indications Dispels wind and overcomes dampness, supplements the Liver and boosts the Kidneys, strengthens the sinews and bones, nourishes the Blood and quiets the foetus. It is indicated for wind-damp Bi syndrome pain, limpness and aching in the lumbar region and knees, lack of strength in the sinews and bones, bleeding during pregnancy, stirring foetus, numbness of the limbs, and hemiplegia.

Common dosage 10-20g, or 30-60g for large dosages.

Comparison of functions See *Wu Jia Pi* (Cortex Acanthopanacis Gracilistyli Radicis).

Modern research Both the avicularin contained in *Sang Ji Sheng* and decoctions of the herb can lower blood pressure, enlarge the coronary arteries and increase the volume of blood supply to the heart.[32]

Combinations and applications

Functions	Combinations	Applications
Dispelling wind and overcoming dampness	*Du Huo* (Radix Angelicae Pubescentis) *Niu Xi* (Radix Achyranthis Bidentatae) *Xu Duan* (Radix Dipsaci) *Fang Ji* (Radix Stephaniae Tetrandrae) (see notes on legal status) *Wu Jia Pi* (Cortex Acanthopanacis Gracilistyli Radicis)	Wind-cold-damp Bi syndrome, manifesting as limb joint pain due to wind, especially used for pain and stiffness in the lumbar region and knees and inhibited bending and stretching
Supplementing the Liver and boosting the Kidneys, strengthening the sinews and bones	*Xu Duan* (Radix Dipsaci) *He Shou Wu* (Radix Polygoni Multiflori) *Tu Si Zi* (Semen Cuscutae)	Aching in the lumbar region due to insufficiency of the Liver and Kidneys, Wei syndrome of the sinews and bones
Nourishing the Blood and quieting the foetus	*Ai Ye* (Folium Artemisiae Argyi) *E Jiao* (Gelatinum Corii Asini) *Du Zhong* (Cortex Eucommiae Ulmoidis) *Xu Duan* (Radix Dipsaci)	Vaginal bleeding during pregnancy, stirring foetus due to Liver and Kidney deficiency resulting in insecurity of the Ren and Du vessels

Wu Jia Pi 五加皮 (Acanthopanax root bark, Cortex Acanthopanacis Gracilistyli Radicis)

Wu Jia Pi is the dried root-bark of *Acanthopanax gracilistylus* W. W. Smith, family Araliaceae.

Main ingredients *Wu Jia Pi* contains volatile oils (including 4-methyl-salicylaldehyde), vitamins A and B, tannin, fatty acids and palmitic acid.

Properties Taste: acrid and bitter; nature: warm.

Channels entered Liver and Kidney.

Functions and indications Dispels wind and eliminates dampness, strengthens the sinews and bones, promotes urination and disperses swelling. It is indicated for wind-cold-damp Bi syndrome, Wei syndrome of the sinews and bones, oedema, leg Qi, and pain in the lumbar region.

Common dosage 5-10g as a decoction or steeped in alcohol.

Precautions and contraindications *Wu Jia Pi* is contraindicated in cases of effulgent Yin deficiency-fire.

Remarks In classical TCM texts, *Wu Jia Pi* is subdivided into two species:

1. *Nan Wu Jia* (*Acanthopanax giraldii* Harms), which is good for supplementing the Liver and Kidneys and for strengthening the sinews and bones.
2. *Bei Wu Jia* (*Periploca sepium* Bge.), which is good for strengthening the functions of the Heart and for promoting urination. As this herb is toxic, it is not advisable to use it in large dosages.

Comparison of functions Both *Wu Jia Pi* (Cortex Acanthopanacis Gracilistyli Radicis) and *Sang Ji Sheng* (Ramulus Loranthi) can dispel wind and eliminate dampness, supplement the Liver and Kidneys, and strengthen the sinews and bones. They are used for wind-damp Bi syndrome pain, limpness and aching in the lumbar region and knees, and lack of strength in the sinews and bones. However, *Sang Ji Sheng* can also nourish the Blood and quiet the foetus and is used for stirring foetus due to Liver and Kidney deficiency. *Wu Jia Pi* can promote urination and is used for oedema and difficult urination. *Wu Jia Pi* is more effective in freeing the channels to alleviate pain.

Modern research

1. Inhibits inflammation.[33]
2. An injection of the herb can inhibit the immune function.[34, 35]

Combinations and applications

Functions	Combinations	Applications
Dispelling wind and overcoming dampness, strengthening the sinews and bones	*Mu Gua* (Fructus Chaenomelis) *Niu Xi* (Radix Achyranthis Bidentatae)	Limpness and aching in the lumbar region and knees due to Liver and Kidney deficiency
	Du Zhong (Cortex Eucommiae Ulmoidis) *Sang Ji Sheng* (Ramulus Loranthi)	Pain in the lumbar region and heaviness of the legs
	Fang Feng (Radix Ledebouriellae Divaricatae) *Wei Ling Xian* (Radix Clematidis)	Wind-cold-damp Bi syndrome pain
	Zi Su Ye (Folium Perillae Frutescentis) *Wu Zhu Yu* (Fructus Evodiae Rutaecarpae) *Bing Lang* (Semen Arecae Catechu) *Sheng Jiang* (Rhizoma Zingiberis Officinalis Recens)	Swelling and pain in leg Qi

Promoting urination and dispersing swelling	*Fu Ling Pi* (Cortex Poriae Cocos) *Da Fu Pi* (Pericarpium Arecae Catechu) *Sheng Jiang Pi* (Cortex Zingiberis Officinalis Recens)	Oedema and inhibited urination

Gou Ji 狗脊 (Cibot rhizome, Rhizoma Cibotii Barometz)

Gou Ji is the dried rhizome of *Cibotium barometz* (L.) J. Sm., family Dicksoniaceae.

Legal status *Gou Ji* is a restricted substance listed in Appendix II of the Convention on International Trade in Endangered Species of Wild Fauna and Flora (CITES). Appropriate import and export permits are required for trade in this materia medica.

Main ingredients *Gou Ji* contains aspidinol and starch.

Properties Taste: bitter and sweet; nature: warm.

Channels entered Liver and Kidney.

Functions and indications Supplements and boosts the Liver and Kidneys, strengthens the sinews and bones, dispels wind and eliminates dampness, and warms and supplements the Kidneys to secure the Essence and stop vaginal discharge. It is indicated for limpness and aching in the lumbar region and knees, pain in the knees and feet, frequent urination, enuresis, vaginal discharge, and wind-cold-damp Bi syndrome.

Common dosage 10-15g.

Precautions and contraindications Since *Gou Ji* has the action of warming and supplementing the Kidneys, it is contraindicated in cases of scant, irregular and yellow urine, painful urination, dry mouth with a bitter taste, and Yin deficiency with heat signs.

Comparison of functions See *Xu Duan* (Radix Dipsaci).

Modern research

1. Inhibits carcinoma.[36]
2. Stops bleeding.[37]

Combinations and applications

Functions	Combinations	Applications
Supplementing and boosting the Liver and Kidneys, strengthening the sinews and bones, dispelling wind and eliminating dampness	*Du Zhong* (Cortex Eucommiae Ulmoidis) *Xu Duan* (Radix Dipsaci) *Niu Xi* (Radix Achyranthis Bidentatae)	Pain in the lumbar region, stiffness in the spine and limpness of the feet and knees due to insufficiency of the Liver and Kidneys
	Du Huo (Radix Angelicae Pubescentis) *Sang Ji Sheng* (Ramulus Loranthi) *Wei Ling Xian* (Radix Clematidis)	Pain in the legs and knees and numbness of the hands and feet due to externally-contracted wind-cold-damp and insufficiency of the Liver and Kidneys
	Xian Mao (Rhizoma Curculiginis Orchioidis) *Dang Gui* (Radix Angelicae Sinensis) *Chuan Xiong* (Rhizoma Ligustici Chuanxiong) *Mu Gua* (Fructus Chaenomelis)	Limb joint pain due to wind-cold-damp

Warming and supplementing the Kidneys to secure the Essence and stop vaginal discharge	*Mu Gua* (Fructus Chaenomelis) *Wu Jia Pi* (Cortex Acanthopanacis Gracilistyli Radicis)	Pain in the lumbar region with frequent urination
	Tu Si Zi (Semen Cuscutae) *Fu Pen Zi* (Fructus Rubi Chingii)	White vaginal discharge and enuresis due to insecurity of the Chong and Ren vessels caused by deficiency-cold in the Lower Jiao

Modern research references

1. Zhu Shou et al., *Zhong Yao Yao Li Yu Lin Chuang* [Pharmacology and Clinical Application of Chinese Materia Medica] launch issue (1985): 93.
2. Lei Zaiquan and Zhang Tingmo, *Zhong Hua Lin Chuang Zhong Yao Xue* [Chinese Clinical Materia Medica] (Beijing: People's Medical Publishing House, 1998), 687.
3. Tian Qiwei, *Zhong Cao Yao* [Journal of Chinese Herbs] 20, 2 (1989): 4.
4. Guo Chengli, *Zhong Hua Yi Xue Za Zhi* [Chinese Journal of Medicine] 64, 11 (1984): 689.
5. Tian Qiwei, *Hu Nan Yi Xue Qing Bao* [Hunan Medical Information] 3 (1984): 70.
6. Yu Zhongren, *Zhong Cao Yao Tong Xun* [Chinese Herbs Newsletter] 3 (1975): 70.
7. The Third Military Medical University, *Zhong Cao Yao Tong Xun* 6 (1976): 15.
8. Lei Zaiquan and Zhang Tingmo, *Zhong Hua Lin Chuang Zhong Yao Xue*, 753.
9. He Xingdong et al., *Lin Chuang Zhong Yao Shou Ce* [Clinical Handbook of Chinese Materia Medica] (Beijing: People's Medical Publishing House, 1998), 101.
10. Lei Zaiquan and Zhang Tingmo, *Zhong Hua Lin Chuang Zhong Yao Xue*, 765.
11. He Xingdong et al., *Lin Chuang Zhong Yao Shou Ce*, 112.
12. Song Zhenyu et al., *Sheng Li Xue Bao* [Physiology Journal] 22, 3 (1958): 201.
13. Liu Gengtao et al., *Sheng Li Xue Bao* 23, 3 (1959): 203.
14. Xu Lina et al., *Yao Xue Xue Bao* [Pharmacology Journal] 12, 6 (1965): 357.
15. He Fengci et al., *Zhong Guo Yao Li Xue Bao* [Chinese Journal of Pharmacology] 10, 3 (1989): 249.
16. Zhang Min et al., *Di San Jun Yi Da Xue Xue Bao* [Journal of Third Military Medical University] 14, 4 (1992): 327.
17. Ying Shida et al., *Shan Dong Yi Ke Da Xue Xue Bao* [Journal of Shandong Medical University] 29, 3 (1991): 22.
18. Tang Jinzhong et al., *Di Er Jun Yi Da Xue Xue Bao* [Journal of Second Military Medical University] 13, 3 (1992): 251.
19. Qu Benling et al., *He Nan Yi Xue Yuan Xue Bao* [Journal of Henan Medical College] 16, 1 (1981): 287.
20. Micro-organism Group of the General Military Hospital Clinical Medical Laboratory, *Jiang Su Yi Yao* [Jiangsu Journal of Medicine and Pharmacology] 10 (1978): 45.
21. Sun Jiemin, *Zhong Yi Yao Yan Jiu* [Traditional Chinese Medicine and Materia Medica Research] 3 (1991): 50.
22. Liu Gengtao et al., *Yao Xue Xue Bao* [Pharmacology Journal] 11, 10 (1964): 708.
23. Wang Yusheng et al., *Zhong Yao Yao Li Yu Ying Yong* [Pharmacology and Application of Chinese Materia Medica] (Beijing: People's Medical Publishing House, 1998), 1219.
24. Xu Wen, *Zhong Hua Nei Ke Za Zhi* [Chinese Journal of Internal Medicine] 2 (1960): 115.
25. Jiang Lin et al., *Guang Xi Zhong Yi Yao* [Guangxi Journal of Traditional Chinese Medicine and Materia Medica] 13, 4 (1990): 188.
26. Jiang Lin, *Zhong Cheng Yao* [Journal of Chinese Medicinal Preparations] 9 (1988): 45.
27. Huang Liangyue et al., *Zhong Yao Cai* [Chinese Materia Medica] 15, 6 (1992): 29.
28. Lei Zaiquan and Zhang Tingmo, *Zhong Hua Lin Chuang Zhong Yao Xue*, 762.
29. Hebei New Medical University, *Xin Yi Yao Yan Jiu* [New Medicine and Materia Medica Research Journal] 1 (1975): 36.
30. Hebei New Medical University, *Xin Yi Yao Xue Za Zhi* [New Medicine and Pharmacology Journal] 10 (1973): 30.
31. Hubei Science and Technology Documents (Medical Volume), 2 (1971): 211.
32. He Xingdong et al., *Lin Chuang Zhong Yao Shou Ce*, 108.
33. Shen Yingjun et al., *Cheng Du Zhong Yi Xue Yuan Xue Bao* [Journal of Chengdu College of TCM] 4 (1983): 43.
34. Chen Ping et al., *Zhong Guo Yao Xue Za Zhi* [Journal of Chinese Pharmacology] 6 (1993): 351.
35. Chen Ping et al., *Zhong Yao Yao Li Yu Lin Chuang* [Pharmacology and Clinical Application of Chinese Materia Medica] 3 (1994): 17.
36. Editorial Group of Nanjing College of Pharmacy, *Chinese Materia Medica* (Nanjing: Jiangsu People's Publishing House, 1978), 40.
37. Surgical Teaching and Research Group, Second Hospital Affiliated to No. 2 Military Medical University et al., *Zhong Hua Wai Ke Za Zhi* [Chinese Journal of Surgery] 8 (1962): 504.

Chapter 5

Aromatic herbs for transforming dampness

芳香化湿药

Aromatic herbs for transforming dampness

All the herbs for transforming dampness listed in this chapter have a fragrant smell, and are mostly warm and dry in nature. They can eliminate dampness and arouse the Spleen. They are indicated for fullness in the chest and abdomen, heaviness of the head and body, reduced appetite, a greasy and sweet taste in mouth, excessive saliva, nausea and vomiting, loose stool and urinary turbidity, white vaginal discharge caused by obstruction of dampness, and disorders of the transportation and transformation functions of the Spleen, as well as for warm-febrile diseases and summerheat-damp.

Clinically, the patterns and symptoms involved determine the appropriate combination of herbs that should be selected:

1. in cases of distension in the abdomen and diarrhoea due to Qi stagnation and damp obstruction, combine with herbs for moving Qi;
2. in cases of exterior patterns, combine with herbs for releasing the exterior;
3. for cold and pain in the stomach and abdomen due to cold-damp obstruction, combine with herbs for dispelling cold and warming the Middle Jiao;
4. for poor appetite and distension in the stomach after eating, combine with herbs for moving Qi and herbs for dispersing food accumulation and guiding out stagnation;
5. for vomiting, combine with herbs for regulating Stomach Qi and stopping vomiting;
6. for Spleen and Stomach deficiency and damp obstruction, combine with herbs for fortifying the Spleen and Stomach.

Aromatic herbs for transforming dampness are particularly warm and dry, and tend to damage body fluids and consume vital Qi. Hence, they should be used cautiously in cases of Yin deficiency and depletion of body fluids, and in cases of Qi deficiency. As most of these herbs contain volatile oils, they must not be decocted for a long time, otherwise their effect will be reduced.

Tab. 5 Aromatic herbs for transforming dampness

Herb	Functions	Indications
Huo Xiang (Herba Agastaches seu Pogostemi)	Transforming dampness, harmonizing the Stomach and stopping vomiting, relieving summerheat and releasing the exterior	Common colds due to externally-contracted summerheat-damp, headache due to cold or heat, food accumulation, focal distension and fullness in the chest and stomach, vomiting, and cholera, dysentery and malaria
Hou Po (Cortex Magnoliae Officinalis)	Moving Qi and dispersing stagnation, drying dampness and dispersing accumulation, bearing counterflow Lung Qi downwards and calming wheezing	Distension and fullness in the chest and stomach, food accumulation due to Qi stagnation, distension in the abdomen and constipation, nausea and vomiting, coughing and wheezing due to Phlegm-fluids, diarrhoea and dysentery due to cold-damp
Cang Zhu (Rhizoma Atractylodis)	Drying dampness and fortifying the Spleen, dispelling wind and overcoming dampness	Distension and fullness in the stomach and abdomen due to damp obstruction in the Middle Jiao, reduced appetite, nausea and vomiting, wind-cold-damp Bi syndrome, limpness of the legs caused by damp-heat pouring down, blood in the stool, vaginal discharge, night blindness
Pei Lan (Herba Eupatorii Fortunei)	Fortifying the Spleen and transforming dampness, clearing summerheat and repelling turbidity	Damp turbidity obstruction in the Middle Jiao, a sweet and greasy taste in the mouth, distension of the stomach, patterns caused by externally-contracted summerheat-damp, and the initial stage of damp warm-febrile diseases
Sha Ren (Fructus Amomi)	Transforming dampness and arousing the Spleen, moving Qi to diffuse damp obstruction in the Middle Jiao, quieting the foetus	Fullness and distension in the stomach and abdomen due to damp turbidity obstruction in the Middle Jiao or Qi and food stagnation, diarrhoea due to deficiency-cold, morning sickness, stirring foetus
Bai Dou Kou (Fructus Amomi Kravanh)	Moving Qi, fortifying the Spleen and transforming dampness, warming the Middle Jiao and stopping vomiting	Pain in the stomach, distension and fullness in the chest and abdomen, vomiting, acid vomiting
Cao Dou Kou (Semen Alpiniae Katsumadai)	Fortifying the Spleen and drying dampness, warming the Middle Jiao and stopping vomiting, moving Qi	Cold and pain in the stomach and abdomen, vomiting and diarrhoea due to cold-damp, Phlegm-fluid accumulation
Cao Guo (Fructus Amomi Tsaoko)	Drying dampness and warming the Middle Jiao, dissipating cold and interrupting malaria	Distension, fullness and pain in the stomach and abdomen, vomiting and diarrhoea due to cold-damp obstructing the Spleen and Stomach, malaria due to cold-damp

Huo Xiang 藿香 (Agastache or patchouli, Herba Agastaches seu Pogostemi)

Huo Xiang (Herba Agastaches) is the branch and leaf of *Agastache rugosa* (Fisch. et Mey.) O. Ktze., family Labiatae. Alternatively, *Guang Huo Xiang* (Herba Pogostemi) may be used as this herb. *Guang Huo Xiang* is the aerial parts of *Pogostemon cablin* (Blanco) Benth., family Labiatae.

Main ingredients Both *Huo Xiang* and *Guang Huo Xiang* contain volatile oils. *Huo Xiang* contains 0.28% of volatile oils (principally methyl chavicol) as well as anethole, anisaldeyde, p-methoxycinnamaldehyde and various flavone compounds, including acacetin, tilianine, linarin, agastachoside and agastachin; *Guang Huo Xiang* contains 1.5% of volatile oils (including pogostone and patchouli alcohol), as well as benzaldehyde, eugenol, cinnamic aldehyde and various flavone compounds (principally apigenin, rhamnetin and ombuine).

Properties Taste: acrid; nature: slightly warm.

Channels entered Spleen, Stomach and Lung.

Functions and indications Transforms dampness, harmonizes the Stomach and stops vomiting, relieves summerheat and releases the exterior. It is indicated for common colds due to externally-contracted summerheat-damp, headache due to cold or heat, food accumulation, focal distension and fullness in the chest and stomach, vomiting, and cholera, dysentery and malaria.

Common dosage 6–10g; double the dosage for fresh *Huo Xiang*; do not decoct for a long period; appropriate dosage for external application.

Precautions and contraindications As this herb is aromatic and dry, it tends to consume Qi and damage body fluids. It must therefore not be used in cases of effulgent Yin deficiency-fire with a crimson tongue and no fur.

Remarks The leaves of this herb are light in nature and good at dispelling external pathogenic factors, whereas the stem can regulate the movement of vital Qi and bear Stomach Qi downwards to stop vomiting. Fresh *Huo Xiang* is mainly used for relieving summerheat and transforming dampness.

Comparison of functions Both *Huo Xiang* (Herba Agastaches seu Pogostemi) and *Zi Su Ye* (Folium Perillae Frutescentis) have the functions of releasing the exterior, harmonizing the Stomach and moving Qi. Since *Huo Xiang* is aromatic and dry, it is better at transforming dampness, arousing the Spleen and stopping vomiting. *Zi Su Ye* is acrid and dissipating and is more effective for inducing sweating, dissipating cold and releasing the exterior.

For an additional comparison, see *Pei Lan* (Herba Eupatorii Fortunei).

Modern research

1. Relieves gastrointestinal spasm and stops diarrhoea.[1-3]
2. Inhibits pathogenic fungi and kills Leptospira.[2-4]

Combinations and applications

Functions	Combinations	Applications
Transforming dampness, harmonizing the Stomach and stopping vomiting	*Chen Pi* (Pericarpium Citri Reticulatae) *Ban Xia* (Rhizoma Pinelliae Ternatae) *Cang Zhu* (Rhizoma Atractylodis) *Hou Po* (Cortex Magnoliae Officinalis)	Reduced appetite, fullness in the chest, nausea and vomiting, and white, slimy tongue fur due to damp obstruction in the Spleen and Stomach
	Gan Jiang (Rhizoma Zingiberis Officinalis) *Sha Ren* (Fructus Amomi) *Cang Zhu* (Rhizoma Atractylodis)	Reduced appetite, focal distension and fullness in the chest or upper abdomen, and nausea and vomiting due to Spleen and Stomach deficiency-cold

	Hua Shi (Talcum) *Ding Xiang* (Flos Caryophylli)	Vomiting and diarrhoea in summertime
	Sha Ren (Fructus Amomi) *Ban Xia* (Rhizoma Pinelliae Ternatae)	Morning sickness
	Huang Lian (Rhizoma Coptidis) *Zhu Ru* (Caulis Bambusae in Taeniis)	Vomiting due to damp-heat obstruction in the Middle Jiao
Relieving summerheat and releasing the exterior	*Chen Pi* (Pericarpium Citri Reticulatae) *Ban Xia* (Rhizoma Pinelliae Ternatae) *He Ye* (Folium Nelumbinis Nuciferae) *Pei Lan* (Herba Eupatorii Fortunei) *Xiang Ru* (Herba Elsholtziae seu Moslae)	Summerheat-damp with oppression in the chest, fatigue, fever and chills, nausea and diarrhoea
	Zi Su Ye (Folium Perillae Frutescentis) *Jing Jie* (Herba Schizonepetae Tenuifoliae) *Hou Po* (Cortex Magnoliae Officinalis) *Pei Lan* (Herba Eupatorii Fortunei)	Common cold combined with an invasion of damp, fever, a thick feeling in the head, headache, heaviness of the body, and slimy tongue fur
	Ban Xia (Rhizoma Pinelliae Ternatae) *Xing Ren* (Semen Pruni Armeniacae) *Fu Ling* (Sclerotium Poriae Cocos) *Hou Po* (Cortex Magnoliae Officinalis)	The initial stage of damp-warm diseases manifesting as generalized fever without thirst, fatigued limbs, oppression in the chest, a slimy sensation in the mouth, and a soggy and moderate pulse

Hou Po 厚朴 (Magnolia bark, Cortex Magnoliae Officinalis)

Hou Po is the dried bark of *Magnolia officinalis* Rehd. et Wils. or *M. officinalis* Rehd. et Wils. var. *biloba* Rehd. et Wils., family Magnoliaceae.

Main ingredients *Hou Po* contains magnolol, tetrahydromagnolol, isomagnolol, honokiol, syringaresinol, magnaldehyde, magnatriol, eudesmol and magnocurarine.

Properties Taste: acrid and bitter; nature: warm.

Channels entered Spleen, Stomach, Lung and Large Intestine.

Functions and indications Moves Qi and disperses stagnation, dries dampness and disperses accumulation, bears counterflow Lung Qi downwards and calms wheezing. It is indicated for distension and fullness in the chest and stomach, food accumulation due to Qi stagnation, distension in the abdomen and constipation, nausea and vomiting, coughing and wheezing due to Phlegm-fluids, and diarrhoea and dysentery due to cold-damp.

Common dosage 3-10g.

Precautions and contraindications As *Hou Po* is bitter in taste and dry in nature and can bear counterflow Qi downwards, it should be used with caution in cases of Qi deficiency of the Spleen and Stomach and insufficiency of body fluids, as well as during pregnancy.

Comparison of functions See *Cang Zhu* (Rhizoma Atractylodis).

Toxicity Oral administration of *Hou Po* is relatively non-toxic. The main toxic ingredient in the herb is magnocurarine, which is absorbed very slowly in the gastrointestinal tract and is then excreted by the kidneys leaving a comparatively low concentration in the blood. A 60g/kg decoction of *Hou Po* given to mice via intragastric administration had not resulted in any deaths after three days.

Modern research

1. In small dosages, *Hou Po* increases duodenal tension; in large dosages, it inhibits intestinal contraction.[5]
2. Decoctions of *Hou Po* inhibited staphylococci, haemolytic streptococci, pneumococci and Bordetella pertussis *in vitro*.[6]
3. Inhibits carcinoma.[7]
4. Inhibits allergies.[8]
5. Lowers blood pressure and inhibits haematoblastic concentration.[9, 10]

Combinations and applications

Functions	Combinations	Applications
Moving Qi and dispersing stagnation, drying dampness and dispersing accumulation	*Cang Zhu* (Rhizoma Atractylodis) *Chen Pi* (Pericarpium Citri Reticulatae) *Mu Xiang* (Radix Aucklandiae Lappae) (see notes on legal status) *Huo Xiang* (Herba Agastaches seu Pogostemi)	Damp obstruction in the Spleen and Stomach, distension in the abdomen, poor appetite, and thick and slimy tongue fur
	Zhi Shi (Fructus Immaturus Citri Aurantii) *Da Huang* (Radix et Rhizoma Rhei) *Lai Fu Zi* (Semen Raphani Sativi)	Food accumulation, distension and pain in the abdomen, constipation, acid vomiting
	Ren Shen (Radix Ginseng) *Sheng Jiang* (Rhizoma Zingiberis Officinalis Recens)	Distension in the abdomen due to deficiency-cold
Bearing counterflow Lung Qi downwards and calming wheezing	*Su Zi* (Fructus Perillae Frutescentis) *Xing Ren* (Semen Pruni Armeniacae) *Ban Xia* (Rhizoma Pinelliae Ternatae) *Xuan Fu Hua* (Flos Inulae)	Cough due to Phlegm-fluids with copious white sputum, fullness in the chest
	Ban Xia (Rhizoma Pinelliae Ternatae) *Fu Ling* (Sclerotium Poriae Cocos) *Sheng Jiang* (Rhizoma Zingiberis Officinalis Recens) *Zi Su Ye* (Folium Perillae Frutescentis)	A sensation of suffocation in the throat, plum pit Qi (globus hystericus), difficulty in swallowing or expectorating

Cang Zhu 苍术 (Atractylodes rhizome, Rhizoma Atractylodis)

Cang Zhu is the rhizome of *Atractylodes lancea* (Thunb.) DC. or *A. chinensis* (DC.) Koidz., family Compositae.

Main ingredients *Cang Zhu* (*A. lancea*) contains 5-9% of volatile oils (mainly atractylol, hinesol, β-eudesmol and β-selinene), atractylodine and furaldehyde; *A. chinensis* contains 1.5% of volatile oils (mainly atractylol, atractylone, cineol and α-bisabolol), atractylodinol and acetyl atractylodinol.

Properties Taste: acrid and bitter; nature: warm.

Channels entered Spleen and Stomach.

Functions and indications Dries dampness and fortifies the Spleen, dispels wind and overcomes dampness. It is indicated for distension and fullness in the stomach and abdomen due to damp obstruction in the Middle Jiao, reduced appetite, nausea and vomiting, wind-cold-damp Bi syndrome, limpness of the legs caused by damp-heat pouring down, blood in the stool, vaginal discharge, and night blindness.

Common dosage 6-10g, or 20g for large dosages.

Precautions and contraindications *Cang Zhu* is contraindicated for heat patterns due to Yin deficiency and in cases of profuse sweating due to Qi deficiency.

Remarks Raw *Cang Zhu* has a strong dissipating function due to its acrid taste, and it is normally used for exterior damp patterns; stir-fried *Cang Zhu* is effective in drying dampness and is suitable for interior damp patterns.

Comparison of functions Both *Cang Zhu* (Rhizoma Atractylodis) and *Hou Po* (Cortex Magnoliae Officinalis) are acrid and bitter and enter the Spleen and Stomach channels to treat distension and fullness in the stomach due to damp obstruction in the Spleen and Stomach, nausea and vomiting, and reduced appetite and fatigue. They are often used in combination. *Cang Zhu* can transform internal damp turbidity to dry dampness and fortify the Spleen; it is effective for exterior patterns due to wind-cold with damp, for wind-cold-damp Bi syndrome, and for vaginal discharge due to damp turbidity. It can be used for all disorders due to damp turbidity or exterior and interior cold-damp. In addition to its ability to transform dampness, *Hou Po* is good at moving Qi and dispersing stagnation as well as for dispersing accumulation and calming wheezing. It is an important herb for eliminating distension and fullness in the abdomen (mainly of the full type) with palpable or impalpable masses.

For an additional comparison, see *Bai Zhu* (Rhizoma Atractylodis Macrocephalae).

Toxicity This herb is very safe in normal use. More than 4,000 healthy people exposed to incense smoke from *Cang Zhu* and *Ai Ye* (Folium Artemisiae Argyi) for 30 consecutive evenings indoors did not suffer any adverse effects.

Modern research

1. The volatile oils contained in *Cang Zhu* support the stomach and dispel wind, thus benefiting the appetite.[11]
2. Inhibited gastric ulcers under laboratory conditions.[11]

Combinations and applications

Functions	Combinations	Applications
Drying dampness and fortifying the Spleen	*Hou Po* (Cortex Magnoliae Officinalis) *Chen Pi* (Pericarpium Citri Reticulatae) *Ban Xia* (Rhizoma Pinelliae Ternatae) *Su Geng* (Caulis Perillae Frutescentis)	Distension and fullness in the stomach and abdomen, nausea and vomiting due to damp obstruction in the Middle Jiao
	Huo Xiang (Herba Agastaches seu Pogostemi) *Zi Su Ye* (Folium Perillae Frutescentis) *Xiang Ru* (Herba Elsholtziae seu Moslae)	Common cold with dampness
	Bai Zhu (Rhizoma Atractylodis Macrocephalae) *Sheng Ma* (Rhizoma Cimicifugae) *Zhi Gan Cao* (Radix Glycyrrhizae Praeparata)	Enduring diarrhoea due to damp obstruction caused by Qi deficiency of the Spleen and Stomach

	Bai Zhu (Rhizoma Atractylodis Macrocephalae) *Ban Xia* (Rhizoma Pinelliae Ternatae) *Fu Ling* (Sclerotium Poriae Cocos)	Vaginal discharge and pudendal itch due to Spleen deficiency with exuberant dampness
	Di Yu (Radix Sanguisorbae Officinalis)	Blood in the stool
Dispelling wind and overcoming dampness	*Huang Bai* (Cortex Phellodendri) *Qin Jiao* (Radix Gentianae Macrophyllae) *Fang Ji* (Radix Stephaniae Tetrandrae) (see notes on legal status) *Du Huo* (Radix Angelicae Pubescentis)	Swollen and painful foot and knee joints, limpness of the lower limbs due to damp-heat pouring down
	Du Huo (Radix Angelicae Pubescentis) *Yi Yi Ren* (Semen Coicis Lachrymajobi) *Chuan Wu* (Radix Aconiti Carmichaeli) (see notes on legal status)	Wind-cold-damp Bi syndrome, painful muscles and joints
	Qiang Huo (Rhizoma et Radix Notopterygii) *Fang Feng* (Radix Ledebouriellae Divaricatae)	Headache and pain in the limbs due to externally contracted wind-cold-damp

Note: When combined with calves' or pig's liver or *Hei Zhi Ma* (Semen Sesami Indici), *Cang Zhu* can also brighten the eyes and is used for treating night blindness and softening of the cornea.

Pei Lan 佩兰
(Eupatorium, Herba Eupatorii Fortunei)

Pei Lan is the dried aerial parts of *Eupatorium fortunei* Turcz., family Compositae.

Main ingredients *Pei Lan* contains 0.5-2.0% of volatile oils (including p-cymene, neryl acetate and mannitol), coumarin, coumaric acid, thymohydroquinone, taraxasterol, stigmasterol and palmitic acid.

Properties Taste: acrid; nature: neutral.

Channels entered Spleen and Stomach.

Functions and indications Fortifies the Spleen and transforms dampness, clears summerheat and repels turbidity. It is indicated for damp turbidity obstruction in the Middle Jiao, a sweet and greasy taste in the mouth, distension of the stomach, patterns caused by externally-contracted summerheat-damp, and the initial stage of damp warm-febrile diseases.

Common dosage 5-10g; double the dosage for the fresh herb.

Precautions and contraindications As *Pei Lan* is acrid and strongly dissipating, it can damage Yin and consume Qi; it is therefore contraindicated in cases of Yin and Qi deficiency.

Comparison of functions *Pei Lan* (Herba Eupatorii Fortunei), *Huo Xiang* (Herba Agastaches seu Pogostemi) and *Xiang Ru* (Herba Elsholtziae seu Moslae) are aromatic and can transform dampness, clear summerheat and release the exterior; they are often used in combination to accentuate each other's effect. *Huo Xiang* can harmonize the Middle Jiao and stop vomiting and is a key herb for treating nausea and vomiting due to damp depression and Qi stagnation. It is especially suitable for externally-contracted summerheat-damp or vomiting due to dampness. *Pei Lan* is effective in eliminating putridity and repelling foulness and turbidity and is an important herb in the treatment of conditions with a sweet and greasy taste in the mouth due to dampness in the Spleen. *Xiang Ru* can harmonize the Middle Jiao, transform dampness and promote the movement of water. In terms of inducing sweating and releasing the exterior, *Xiang Ru* is the most effective and *Pei Lan* the least effective.

Modern research

1. A non-diluted solution of a decoction of *Pei Lan* inhibited Staphylococcus aureus, Salmonella typhi, Proteus vulgaris and Shigella shigae in laboratory tests.[12]
2. The volatile oils contained in *Pei Lan* can inhibit influenza viruses.[12]
3. Inhibits the egg discharge of animals so as to interrupt oestrus.[13]

Combinations and applications

Functions	Combinations	Applications
Fortifying the Spleen and transforming dampness, clearing summerheat and repelling turbidity	*Huo Xiang* (Herba Agastaches seu Pogostemi) *Cang Zhu* (Rhizoma Atractylodis) *He Ye* (Folium Nelumbinis Nuciferae)	Fullness and distension in the chest and stomach, and reduced appetite due to damp obstruction in the Spleen and Stomach
	Huang Lian (Rhizoma Coptidis) *Bai Dou Kou* (Fructus Amomi Kravanh)	A sweet and greasy taste in the mouth due to damp-heat in the Spleen and Stomach
	Hua Shi (Talcum) *Yi Yi Ren* (Semen Coicis Lachrymajobi)	The initial stage of damp warm-febrile diseases
	He Ye (Folium Nelumbinis Nuciferae) *Chen Pi* (Pericarpium Citri Reticulatae) *Ban Xia* (Rhizoma Pinelliae Ternatae) *Zi Su Ye* (Folium Perillae Frutescentis)	Fever and chills, fullness in the abdomen, and reduced appetite due to an invasion of summerheat-damp

Sha Ren 砂仁 (Amomum fruit, Fructus Amomi)

Sha Ren is the dried fruit of *Amomum villosum* Lour. or *A. longiligulare* T. L. Wu, family Zingiberaceae.

Main ingredients *Sha Ren* contains 3% of volatile oils (including camphor, borneol, bornyl acetate, linalool and nerolidol), saponins, potassium, calcium, magnesium, zinc and manganese.

Properties Taste: acrid; nature: warm.

Channels entered Spleen and Stomach.

Functions and indications Transforms dampness and arouses the Spleen, moves Qi to diffuse damp obstruction in the Middle Jiao, and quiets the foetus. It is indicated for fullness and distension in the stomach and abdomen due to damp turbidity obstruction in the Middle Jiao or Qi and food stagnation, diarrhoea due to deficiency-cold, morning sickness, and stirring foetus.

Common dosage 3-6g, added towards the end of the decocting process.

Precautions and contraindications *Sha Ren* is contraindicated in cases of Yin deficiency with heat.

Comparison of functions See *Bai Dou Kou* (Fructus Amomi Kravanh).

Toxicity Clinical tests, animal experiments and pathological examinations indicated that dosages of *Sha Ren* based on normal clinical usage are very safe and produced no significant toxic reaction.

Modern research

1. Promotes movement in the intestinal tract.[14]
2. Inhibits haematoblastic concentration.[15]
3. Has a clear effect in preventing the death of animals induced by cortin and collagen.[15]
4. Inhibits the growth of Proteus vulgaris, Shigella shigae and Bacterium coli.[16]

Combinations and applications

Functions	Combinations	Applications
Transforming dampness and arousing the Spleen, moving Qi to diffuse damp obstruction in the Middle Jiao	*Hou Po* (Cortex Magnoliae Officinalis) *Cang Zhu* (Rhizoma Atractylodis) *Bai Dou Kou* (Fructus Amomi Kravanh)	Distension in the abdomen and reduced appetite due to Qi stagnation and damp obstruction in the Middle Jiao
	Mu Xiang (Radix Aucklandiae Lappae) (see notes on legal status) *Bai Zhu* (Rhizoma Atractylodis Macrocephalae)	Food accumulation due to Qi stagnation
	Cao Guo (Fructus Amomi Tsaoko) *Gan Jiang* (Rhizoma Zingiberis Officinalis)	Distension in the abdomen, nausea and vomiting due to cold-damp obstruction
Quieting the foetus	*Su Geng* (Caulis Perillae Frutescentis) *Ban Xia* (Rhizoma Pinelliae Ternatae)	Morning sickness, stirring foetus
	Du Zhong (Cortex Eucommiae Ulmoidis) *Xu Duan* (Radix Dipsaci) *Sang Ji Sheng* (Ramulus Loranthi)	Stirring foetus accompanied by aching in the lumbar region due to Kidney deficiency and Qi stagnation

Note: *Sha Ren* is also used in herbal prescriptions with supplementing herbs, notably *Shu Di Huang* (Radix Rehmanniae Glutinosae Conquita), to safeguard Stomach Qi and prevent stagnation.

Bai Dou Kou 白豆蔻 (Round cardamom fruit, Fructus Amomi Kravanh)

Bai Dou Kou is the dried seed of *Amomum kravanh* Pierre ex Gagnep. or *A. cardamomum* L. (also known as *Elettaria cardamomum* Maton.), family Zingiberaceae.

Main ingredients *Bai Dou Kou* contains d-camphor, d-borneol, eucalyptole, terpinene, caryophyllene, myrcene and myrtenal.

Properties Taste: acrid; nature: warm.

Channels entered Lung, Spleen and Stomach.

Functions and indications Moves Qi, fortifies the Spleen and transforms dampness, warms the Middle Jiao and stops vomiting. It is indicated for pain in the stomach, distension and fullness in the chest and abdomen, vomiting and acid vomiting.

Common dosage 3-6g, added towards the end of the decocting process.

Precautions and contraindications *Bai Dou Kou* is contraindicated in cases of Blood dryness due to Yin deficiency, for patients with exuberant fire in the Lungs and Stomach, and in the absence of cold-damp.

Comparison of functions Both *Bai Dou Kou* (Fructus Amomi Kravanh) and *Sha Ren* (Fructus Amomi) are acrid and warm and can transform dampness, move Qi and warm the Middle Jiao. They are key herbs for arousing the Spleen and harmonizing the Stomach and are used for cold-damp and Qi stagnation in the Spleen and Stomach, for distension, fullness and pain in the stomach, and for nausea, vomiting and diarrhoea. The two herbs are often used in combination for these applications. *Bai Dou Kou* tends to work in the Upper and Middle Jiao and is very effective in transforming dampness in that area; it also regulates Qi in the Spleen and Lungs, stops vomiting and treats mild symptoms such as oppression in the chest and internal encumbering of cold-damp. *Sha Ren* is more effective in moving Qi and is therefore suitable for treating Qi stagnation in the Spleen and Stomach, being commonly used for severe patterns such as cold-damp stagnation and obstruction of cold in the Middle Jiao.

For an additional comparison, see *Cao Dou Kou* (Semen Alpiniae Katsumadai).

Modern research

1. The seeds of *Bai Dou Kou* can benefit the stomach.[17]
2. A small dosage of the volatile oils contained in *Bai Dou Kou* can enhance the anti-tuberculosis function of streptomycin.[17]

Combinations and applications

Functions	Combinations	Applications
Moving Qi, fortifying the Spleen and transforming dampness	*Hou Po* (Cortex Magnoliae Officinalis) *Mu Xiang* (Radix Aucklandiae Lappae) (see notes on legal status)	Distension and pain in the chest and abdomen due to Qi stagnation
	Chen Pi (Pericarpium Citri Reticulatae) *Huo Xiang* (Herba Agastaches seu Pogostemi) *Hou Po Hua* (Flos Magnoliae Officinalis)	Distension and fullness in the stomach and abdomen with a sticky sensation in the mouth and slimy tongue fur due to dampness obstructing the Middle Jiao
	Yi Yi Ren (Semen Coicis Lachrymajobi) *Hua Shi* (Talcum) *Dan Zhu Ye* (Herba Lophatheri Gracilis)	Fever obscured by pathogenic dampness and accompanied by nausea and a desire to vomit in the initial stage of damp warm-febrile diseases
	Huang Lian (Rhizoma Coptidis) *Huang Qin* (Radix Scutellariae Baicalensis)	Exuberant heat, vexation and thirst in damp warm-febrile diseases
	Chen Pi (Pericarpium Citri Reticulatae) *He Zi* (Fructus Terminaliae Chebulae)	Dysentery with pain in the abdomen
Warming the Middle Jiao and stopping vomiting	*Chen Pi* (Pericarpium Citri Reticulatae) *Ban Xia* (Rhizoma Pinelliae Ternatae)	Vomiting due to Stomach-cold
	Sha Ren (Fructus Amomi) *Gan Cao* (Radix Glycyrrhizae)	Infantile vomiting of milk due to Stomach-cold
	Zhu Ru (Caulis Bambusae in Taeniis) *Da Zao* (Fructus Ziziphi Jujubae) *Sheng Jiang* (Rhizoma Zingiberis Officinalis Recens)	Vomiting in pregnancy

Cao Dou Kou 草豆蔻 (Katsumada galangal seed, Semen Alpiniae Katsumadai)

Cao Dou Kou is the dried seed of *Alpinia katsumadai* Hayata, family Zingiberaceae.

Main ingredients *Cao Dou Kou* contains borneol, camphor, alpinetin, cardamomin, terpinol and nerolidol.

Properties Taste: acrid; nature: warm.

Channels entered Spleen and Stomach.

Functions and indications Fortifies the Spleen and dries dampness, warms the Middle Jiao and stops vomiting, and moves Qi. It is indicated for cold and pain in the stomach and abdomen, vomiting and diarrhoea due to cold-damp, and Phlegm-fluid accumulation.

Common dosage 3-6g, added towards the end of the decocting process.

Precautions and contraindications Since *Cao Dou Kou* is warm and dry and can damage and consume body fluids, it is contraindicated in cases of Yin deficiency, insufficiency of body fluids, and deficiency-cold.

Comparison of functions *Cao Dou Kou* (Semen Alpiniae Katsumadai) basically has the same functions as *Bai Dou Kou* (Fructus Amomi Kravanh). *Cao Dou Kou* can be used in the clinic as a substitute for *Bai Dou Kou* when the latter is in short supply. Although *Cao Dou Kou* is not as effective in moving Qi as *Bai Dou Kou*, its warming and drying properties are slightly stronger. As a result, *Cao Dou Kou* is mainly used to treat Qi stagnation due to cold-damp in the Spleen and Stomach, whereas *Bai Dou Kou* is better for treating Qi stagnation of the Spleen and Lungs and obstruction of cold-damp in the Middle Jiao.

For an additional comparison, see *Cao Guo* (Fructus Amomi Tsaoko).

Toxicity This herb is very safe for normal use in the clinic. There have been no reports of toxic side-effects.

Modern research

1. Increases the activity of pepsins to promote digestion.[18]
2. A low-concentration decoction (0.25-0.75%) of *Cao Dou Kou* excited the intestinal tract of guinea pigs; higher concentrations (1.00-1.25%) had an inhibiting effect.[19]
3. The volatile oils contained in *Cao Dou Kou* inhibit the intestinal tract.[19]

Combinations and applications

Functions	Combinations	Applications
Fortifying the Spleen and drying dampness, warming the Middle Jiao and stopping vomiting, moving Qi	*Chen Pi* (Pericarpium Citri Reticulatae) *Hou Po* (Cortex Magnoliae Officinalis) *Huo Xiang* (Herba Agastaches seu Pogostemi)	Oppression in the stomach and reduced appetite due to cold-damp in the Spleen
	Rou Gui (Cortex Cinnamomi Cassiae) *Gan Jiang* (Rhizoma Zingiberis Officinalis) *Gan Cao* (Radix Glycyrrhizae) *Chen Pi* (Pericarpium Citri Reticulatae)	Incessant thin, watery diarrhoea and reduced food intake due to Stomach-cold
	Cang Zhu (Rhizoma Atractylodis) *Gao Liang Jiang* (Rhizoma Alpiniae Officinari) *Hou Po* (Cortex Magnoliae Officinalis)	Diarrhoea and distension and pain in the stomach and abdomen due to Stomach-cold
	Wu Zhu Yu (Fructus Evodiae Rutaecarpae) *Gan Jiang* (Rhizoma Zingiberis Officinalis) *Ban Xia* (Rhizoma Pinelliae Ternatae)	Vomiting and pain in the stomach due to cold-damp stagnation resulting in impaired harmonious downward-bearing of Stomach Qi

Cao Guo 草果
(Tsaoko fruit, Fructus Amomi Tsaoko)

Cao Guo is the dried ripe fruit of *Amomum tsao-ko* Crevost et Lemaire, family Zingiberaceae.

Main ingredients *Cao Guo* contains α- and β-pinene, 1,8 cineol, n-nonyl aldehyde, capraldehyde, camphor, geraniol and nerolidol.

Properties Taste: acrid; nature: warm.

Channels entered Spleen and Stomach.

Functions and indications Dries dampness and warms the Middle Jiao, dissipates cold and interrupts malaria. It is indicated for distension, fullness and pain in the stomach and abdomen, vomiting and diarrhoea due to cold-damp obstructing the Spleen and Stomach, and malaria due to cold-damp.

Common dosage 3-6g.

Precautions and contraindications *Cao Guo* is contraindicated for patients with insufficiency of Yin and Blood, and should be used with caution for elderly, weak or fearful patients.

Comparison of functions Both *Cao Guo* (Fructus Amomi Tsaoko) and *Cao Dou Kou* (Semen Alpiniae Katsumadai) can dry dampness, dissipate cold and warm the Middle Jiao, and are used to treat patterns due to cold and damp pathogenic factors obstructing the Spleen and Stomach. They are often combined with herbs for clearing heat and drying dampness or with other aromatic herbs for transforming dampness in order to treat damp-warm diseases.

Cao Guo is acrid, warm and dry. It is good for transforming dampness and turbidity in the Spleen and Stomach, eliminating Phlegm and interrupting malaria. It is often used for malaria due to cold-damp stagnating in the Spleen and Stomach, as well as for epidemic febrile diseases caused by stagnation of dampness and turbidity manifesting as chills and fever, focal distension in the chest, nausea and vomiting, and thick and slimy tongue fur. *Cao Guo* is more effective in treating malaria when used in combination with *Zhi Mu* (Rhizoma Anemarrhenae Asphodeloidis). *Cao Dou Kou* is acrid and aromatic, but its drying properties are not as strong as those of *Cao Guo*. It has the functions of fortifying the Spleen, drying dampness and moving Qi, and is effective in treating pain in the stomach and vomiting due to cold-damp. Both of these herbs are dry in nature and can easily damage Yin. They are suitable for full patterns due to cold and damp, but are not applicable in cases of Yin deficiency or weakness of the Spleen and Stomach in the absence of cold-damp.

Toxicity This herb is very safe for normal use in the clinic. There have been no reports of toxic side-effects.

Combinations and applications

Functions	Combinations	Applications
Drying dampness and warming the Middle Jiao	*Gao Liang Jiang* (Rhizoma Alpiniae Officinari) *Hou Po* (Cortex Magnoliae Officinalis) *Ding Xiang* (Flos Caryophylli)	Distension and fullness in the stomach and abdomen due to cold-damp obstruction
	Cang Zhu (Rhizoma Atractylodis) *Hou Po* (Cortex Magnoliae Officinalis)	Distension and fullness in the stomach and abdomen, vomiting
	Ban Xia (Rhizoma Pinelliae Ternatae) *Chen Pi* (Pericarpium Citri Reticulatae) *Dan Nan Xing* (Pulvis Arisaematis cum Felle Bovis)	Phlegm-fluid patterns due to damp stagnation, headache and backache, and a desire to vomit after eating

Dissipating cold and interrupting malaria	*Chang Shan* (Radix Dichroae Febrifugae) *Chai Hu* (Radix Bupleuri) *Zhi Mu* (Rhizoma Anemarrhenae Asphodeloidis)	Malaria due to cold-damp

Modern research references

1. Sun Zheng et al., *Zhong Cheng Yao* [Journal of Chinese Medicinal Preparations] 12, 1 (1990): 2.
2. Liu Zhongyu et al., *Zhong Cao Yao* [Journal of Chinese Herbs] 15, 12 (1984): 15.
3. Tian Wenyi et al., *Zhong Cheng Yao* [Journal of Chinese Medicinal Preparations] 12, 4 (1990): 31.
4. Kong Gengxing, *Zhong Cao Yao* [Journal of Chinese Herbs] 15, 3 (1984): 16.
5. Basic Medicine Teaching and Research Office of Shanghai No. 1 Medical College, *Xin Yi Yao Xue Za Zhi* [New Medicine and Pharmacology Journal] 4 (1974): 31.
6. Chen Linfang, *Yao Jian Gong Ye Tong Xun* [Medicine Inspection Industry Newsletter] 4 (1980): 209.
7. T. Konoshima, *Planta Medica* 56, 6 (1990): 653.
8. Du Deji, *Zhong Yao Yao Li Yu Lin Chuang* [Pharmacology and Clinical Application of Chinese Materia Medica] 6, 6 (1990): 42.
9. Pharmacological Teaching and Research Office of Shanghai College of TCM, *Xin Yi Yao Xue Za Zhi* [New Medicine and Pharmacology Journal] 5 (1974): 41.
10. Teng Che Ming et al., *Throm Res* 50, 6 (1988): 757.
11. He Xingdong et al., *Lin Chuang Zhong Yao Shou Ce* [Clinical Handbook of Chinese Materia Medica] (Beijing: People's Medical Publishing House, 1998), 115.
12. Lei Zaiquan and Zhang Tingmo, *Zhong Hua Lin Chuang Zhong Yao Xue* [Chinese Clinical Materia Medica] (Beijing: People's Medical Publishing House, 1998), 805.
13. He Xingdong et al., *Lin Chuang Zhong Yao Shou Ce*, 118.
14. Huang Yiming et al., *Zhong Yao Cai* [Chinese Materia Medica] 3 (1985): 40.
15. Wu Shizhu, *Zhong Yao Yao Li Yu Lin Chuang* [Pharmacology and Clinical Application of Chinese Materia Medica] 6, 5 (1990): 32.
16. Chen Yongpei et al., *Fu Jian Zhong Yi Yao* [Fujian Journal of Traditional Chinese Medicine and Materia Medica] 21, 5 (1990): 25.
17. He Xingdong et al., *Lin Chuang Zhong Yao Shou Ce*, 119.
18. Lei Zaiquan and Zhang Tingmo, *Zhong Hua Lin Chuang Zhong Yao Xue*, 818.
19. He Xingdong et al., *Lin Chuang Zhong Yao Shou Ce*, 120.

Chapter 6

Herbs for promoting the movement of water and percolating dampness

利水渗湿药

Herbs for promoting the movement of water and percolating dampness

Most herbs for promoting the movement of water and percolating dampness are sweet and bland in taste, and cool or cold in nature. These herbs can percolate dampness and disperse swelling by promoting urination; they can also stop diarrhoea, benefit the Gallbladder, free Lin syndrome and expel stones from the gallbladder. They are mainly used for disorders caused by dysfunction of the Bladder or Yang deficiency of the Spleen and Kidneys resulting in failure to regulate the flow of Qi and water, as well as for water accumulation in the body or for various disorders caused by the combination of dampness with heat or cold pathogenic factors.

Herbs for promoting the movement of water and percolating dampness can be divided into three categories according to their functional characteristics:

1. herbs for promoting the movement of water and dispersing swelling: mainly used for dampness obstruction, inhibited urination, and oedema;
2. herbs for promoting urination and freeing Lin syndrome: mainly used for various types of Lin syndrome and for inhibited urination;
3. herbs for promoting the elimination of dampness and abating jaundice: mainly used for damp-heat jaundice and gallbladder stones.

Some of these herbs can also be used to treat Phlegm patterns, sores and eczema, limb joint pain, and diarrhoea.

The main combinations of herbs for promoting the movement of water and percolating dampness are listed below:

i. for oedema and Lin syndrome combined with an exterior pattern, they should be used with herbs for releasing the exterior;
ii. for Lin syndrome due to the combination of dampness and heat, they should be used with herbs for clearing heat and drying dampness;
iii. for disorders due to Kidney Yang deficiency, breakdown of Qi transformation and dampness obstruction, they should be used with herbs for supplementing the Kidneys;
iv. for oedema due to deficiency of the Spleen, which is thus impaired in its function of transforming and transporting water and dampness, they should be used with herbs for supplementing Qi and fortifying the Spleen;
v. for full-heat patterns, they should be used with herbs for clearing heat;
vi. for diarrhoea due to Yang deficiency, they should be used with herbs for supplementing Qi and fortifying the Spleen, and with herbs for warming the Middle Jiao and dispelling cold;
vii. for Phlegm-fluids in the Lungs, they should be used with herbs for warming the Lungs to dispel Phlegm-cold;
viii. for body fluid accumulation in the chest and swelling of the abdomen, they should be used with drastic downward-draining and water-expelling herbs (cathartics).

Improper use of these herbs can damage body fluids, so they should be used with caution in cases of Yin deficiency and consumption of body fluids.

Tab. 6.1 Herbs for promoting the movement of water and dispersing swelling

Herb	Functions	Indications
Fu Ling (Sclerotium Poriae Cocos)	Promoting the movement of water and percolating dampness, fortifying the Spleen and harmonizing the Stomach, quieting the Heart and Spirit	Oedema due to Spleen deficiency with prevalence of dampness, inhibited urination, diarrhoea, Phlegm-fluid patterns, palpitations, forgetfulness, insomnia
Yi Yi Ren (Semen Coicis Lachrymajobi)	Promoting the movement of water and percolating dampness, fortifying the Spleen and stopping diarrhoea, eliminating Bi syndrome and alleviating pain, clearing heat and expelling pus	Diarrhoea due to Spleen deficiency, numbness of the muscles, hypertonicity of the sinews and vessels, inhibited bending and stretching, inhibited urination, oedema in leg Qi, wind-damp Bi syndrome, Lung abscess, Intestinal abscess
Ze Xie (Rhizoma Alismatis Orientalis)	Promoting the movement of water and percolating dampness, clearing heat and draining fire	Inhibited urination, oedema, distension in the abdomen, diarrhoea, blood Lin syndrome, vaginal discharge due to damp-heat, dizziness due to Phlegm-fluids
Zhu Ling (Sclerotium Polypori Umbellati)	Promoting the movement of water and percolating dampness	Dribbling and painful urination, oedema, vaginal discharge, turbid Lin syndrome, diarrhoea
Dong Gua Pi (Epicarpium Benincasae Hispidae)	Promoting the movement of water and dispersing swelling	Oedema
Chi Xiao Dou (Semen Phaseoli Calcarati)	Promoting the movement of water and dispersing swelling, promoting the elimination of dampness and abating jaundice, relieving toxicity and expelling pus	Oedema and abdominal fullness, puffy swelling in leg Qi, abscesses and sores due to heat toxins, damp-heat jaundice

Tab. 6.2 Herbs for promoting urination and freeing Lin syndrome

Herb	Functions	Indications
Che Qian Zi (Semen Plantaginis)	Promoting urination and freeing Lin syndrome, percolating dampness and stopping diarrhoea, clearing the Liver and brightening the eyes, dispelling Phlegm and stopping coughing	Inhibited urination, heat Lin syndrome, blood Lin syndrome, stone Lin syndrome, oedema, diarrhoea, cough with copious sputum, vaginal discharge, red eyes, blurred vision
Hua Shi (Talcum)	Promoting urination and freeing Lin syndrome, clearing heat and relieving summerheat, dispelling dampness and closing sores	Inhibited urination, dribbling and painful urination, vexation and thirst due to summerheat, eczema, prickly heat

Mu Tong (Caulis Mutong)	Promoting urination and freeing Lin syndrome, clearing the Heart and draining fire, freeing the Blood vessels, freeing menstruation and causing milk to descend	Short voidings of reddish urine, difficult and painful urination, vexation in the Heart, mouth sores, sore throat, damp-heat Bi syndrome, stoppage of breast milk
Hai Jin Sha (Spora Lygodii Japonici)	Promoting urination and freeing Lin syndrome, expelling stones from the urinary tract	All types of Lin syndrome, oedema, drum-like abdominal distension
Tong Cao (Medulla Tetrapanacis Papyriferi)	Clearing heat and promoting urination, freeing Qi and causing milk to descend	Inhibited urination, Lin syndrome, stoppage of breast milk
Qu Mai (Herba Dianthi)	Promoting urination and freeing Lin syndrome, breaking up Blood stasis and freeing menstruation	Inhibited urination, the five types of Lin syndrome (stone, blood, heat, Qi and turbid Lin), menstrual block due to Blood stasis, and red, sore and swollen eyes
Bian Xu (Herba Polygoni Avicularis)	Promoting urination and freeing Lin syndrome, killing worms and alleviating itching	Scant and dark urine, Lin syndrome, inhibited urination, oedema, eczema, pudendal itch
Di Fu Zi (Fructus Kochiae Scopariae)	Clearing damp-heat and promoting urination, alleviating itching	Inhibited urination, Lin syndrome, itchy skin due to pathogenic damp-heat pouring down into the Lower Jiao
Shi Wei (Folium Pyrrosiae)	Promoting urination and freeing Lin syndrome, cooling the Blood and stopping bleeding, clearing the Lungs and stopping coughing	Heat and blood Lin syndromes, inhibited urination, vomiting of blood and uterine bleeding due to the frenetic movement of hot Blood, and cough due to Lung-heat
Bi Xie (Rhizoma Dioscoreae Hypoglaucae seu Septemlobae)	Separating the clear and the turbid, eliminating Bi syndrome pain, clearing damp-heat from the skin	Turbid Lin syndrome, urinary turbidity, vaginal discharge, wind-damp Bi syndrome, inhibited bending and stretching, aching in the lumbar region and knees, shank sores due to damp-heat
Deng Xin Cao (Medulla Junci Effusi)	Clearing the Heart and draining fire, promoting urination and freeing Lin syndrome	The five types of Lin syndrome (stone, blood, heat, Qi and turbid Lin), inhibited urination, vexation and insomnia, night crying in infants, mouth and tongue sores
Yu Mi Xu (Stylus Zeae Mays)	Promoting urination and freeing Lin syndrome, calming the Liver, benefiting the Gallbladder and abating jaundice	Inhibited urination, oedema due to water collecting internally, jaundice, dizziness due to hyperactivity of Liver Yang or heat in the Liver channel

Tab. 6.3 Herbs for promoting the elimination of dampness and abating jaundice

Herb	Functions	Indications
Yin Chen Hao (Herba Artemisiae Scopariae)	Clearing damp-heat, benefiting the Gallbladder and abating jaundice	Damp-heat or damp-cold jaundice, inhibited urination, eczema, itchy skin
Jin Qian Cao (Herba Lysimachiae)	Promoting urination and freeing Lin syndrome, benefiting the Gallbladder and expelling stones, relieving toxicity and dispersing swelling	Stone Lin syndrome, heat Lin syndrome, damp-heat jaundice, obstinate sores, urinary urgency and painful urination, yellow vaginal discharge, snake bites
Hu Zhang (Radix et Rhizoma Polygoni Cuspidati)	Dispelling wind and promoting the elimination of dampness, clearing heat and freeing Lin syndrome, quickening the Blood and freeing menstruation, transforming Phlegm and stopping coughing	Damp-heat jaundice, turbid Lin syndrome, vaginal discharge, pain in the sinews and bones due to wind-damp, menstrual block, retention of lochia, knocks and falls

HERBS FOR PROMOTING THE MOVEMENT OF WATER AND DISPERSING SWELLING

Fu Ling 茯苓 (Poria, Sclerotium Poriae Cocos)

Fu Ling is the sclerotium of the fungus *Poria cocos* (Schw.) Wolf, family Polyporaceae.

Main ingredients *Fu Ling* contains pachymic, eburicoic, tumulosic and pinicolic acids, β-pachyman, proteins, fats, lecithin, choline, ergosterol and sylvite.

Properties Taste: sweet and bland; nature: neutral.

Channels entered Heart, Lung, Spleen and Kidney.

Functions and indications Promotes the movement of water and percolates dampness, fortifies the Spleen and harmonizes the Stomach, and quiets the Heart and Spirit. It is indicated for oedema due to Spleen deficiency with prevalence of dampness, inhibited urination, diarrhoea, Phlegm-fluid patterns, palpitations, forgetfulness, and insomnia.

Common dosage 10-15g, or 30g for large dosages.

Precautions and contraindications *Fu Ling* is contraindicated in cases of seminal emission due to deficiency-cold, or for patients with Qi deficiency fall.

Comparison of functions See *Yi Yi Ren* (Semen Coicis Lachrymajobi), *Zhu Ling* (Sclerotium Polypori Umbellati) and *Lei Wan* (Sclerotium Omphaliae Lapidescens).

Toxicity The LD_{50} for intragastric administration and intraperitoneal injection in mice of a warm aqueous extract of *Fu Ling* is at least 10g/kg and 2g/kg respectively.

Modern research

1. Promotes urination; increases the amount of urine and sodium and potassium discharge.[1]
2. Strengthens the immune function and inhibits carcinoma.[2-6]
3. Has a tranquillizing function.[7]

Combinations and applications

Functions	Combinations	Applications
Promoting the movement of water and percolating dampness	*Gui Zhi* (Ramulus Cinnamomi Cassiae) *Bai Zhu* (Rhizoma Atractylodis Macrocephalae) *Ze Xie* (Rhizoma Alismatis Orientalis)	Oedema with distension and fullness, and inhibited urination due to poor Qi transformation in the Bladder and stagnation of water and dampness
	Bai Zhu (Rhizoma Atractylodis Macrocephalae) *Dang Shen* (Radix Codonopsitis Pilosulae) *Chen Pi* (Pericarpium Citri Reticulatae) *Ze Xie* (Rhizoma Alismatis Orientalis)	Generalized oedema due to Spleen deficiency with collection of dampness
	Huang Bai (Cortex Phellodendri) *Mu Tong* (Caulis Mutong) (see notes on legal status) *Che Qian Zi* (Semen Plantaginis)	Oedema, inhibited urination and a burning pain in the urethra due to damp-heat

Fortifying the Spleen and harmonizing the Stomach	*Bai Zhu* (Rhizoma Atractylodis Macrocephalae) *Shan Yao* (Rhizoma Dioscoreae Oppositae) *Chen Pi* (Pericarpium Citri Reticulatae) *Jiao San Xian* (scorch-fried combination of Fructus Crataegi, Massa Fermentata and Fructus Hordei Vulgaris Germinatus)	Loose stool, poor appetite and indigestion due to Spleen and Stomach deficiency
	Chao Bai Zhu (Rhizoma Atractylodis Macrocephalae, stir-fried) *Rou Dou Kou* (Semen Myristicae Fragrantis) *Che Qian Zi* (Semen Plantaginis)	Watery diarrhoea
	Gui Zhi (Ramulus Cinnamomi Cassiae) *Bai Zhu* (Rhizoma Atractylodis Macrocephalae) *Gan Cao* (Radix Glycyrrhizae) *Gan Jiang* (Rhizoma Zingiberis Officinalis) *Ban Xia* (Rhizoma Pinelliae Ternatae)	Reduced food intake and distension in the stomach due to Spleen deficiency with Phlegm-fluids and water-fluids collecting in the Stomach
	Su Zi (Fructus Perillae Frutescentis) *Bai Jie Zi* (Semen Sinapis Albae) *Gan Jiang* (Rhizoma Zingiberis Officinalis) *Xi Xin* (Herba cum Radice Asari)	Phlegm-fluids gathering in the Lungs, cough with thin sputum
	Fu Zi (Radix Lateralis Aconiti Carmichaeli Praeparata) (see notes on legal status) *Wu Jia Pi* (Cortex Acanthopanacis Gracilistyli Radicis) *Huang Qi* (Radix Astragali seu Hedysari) *Gan Jiang* (Rhizoma Zingiberis Officinalis)	Water Qi assaulting the Heart, manifesting as palpitations and disquiet, oedema
	Ban Xia (Rhizoma Pinelliae Ternatae) *Sheng Jiang* (Rhizoma Zingiberis Officinalis Recens)	Incessant vomiting due to water collecting in the Middle Jiao
Quieting the Heart and Spirit	*Dang Gui* (Radix Angelicae Sinensis) *Bai Zi Ren* (Semen Biotae Orientalis) *Bai Zhu* (Rhizoma Atractylodis Macrocephalae) *Suan Zao Ren* (Semen Ziziphi Spinosae) *Zhu Sha* (Cinnabaris) (see notes on legal status)	Disquieted Heart and Spirit, insomnia and forgetfulness due to Heart and Spleen deficiency
	Ren Shen (Radix Ginseng) *Long Gu* (Os Draconis) *Shi Chang Pu* (Rhizoma Acori Graminei) *Yuan Zhi* (Radix Polygalae)	Palpitations and insomnia due to non-interaction of the Heart and Kidneys

Note: *Fu Ling* can be used with *Huang Bai* (Cortex Phellodendri), *Che Qian Zi* (Semen Plantaginis) and *Ze Xie* (Rhizoma Alismatis Orientalis) to treat vaginal discharge due to damp toxins or damp-heat.

Appendix

Fu Ling Pi 茯苓皮 (Poria skin, Cortex Poriae Cocos)

Fu Ling Pi is the black outer layer of *Fu Ling*; it has the same nature and properties as *Fu Ling*. Its function is to disperse swelling by promoting the movement of water and it is normally used for oedema in combination with *Sheng Jiang Pi* (Cortex Zingiberis Officinalis Recens), *Sang Bai Pi* (Cortex Mori Albae Radicis), *Da Fu Pi* (Pericarpium Arecae Catechu) and *Chen Pi* (Pericarpium Citri Reticulatae). The dosage is 10-15g.

Chi Fu Ling 赤茯苓 (Red poria, Sclerotium Poriae Cocos Rubrae)

Chi Fu Ling is the red variety of *Fu Ling*. It is used for damp-heat patterns such as short voidings of reddish urine with dribbling, often in combination with *Che Qian Zi* (Semen Plantaginis) and *Zhi Zi* (Fructus Gardeniae Jasminoidis). The dosage is 10-15g.

Fu Shen 茯神 (Poria with hostwood, Sclerotium Poriae Cocos cum Ligno Hospite)

Fu Shen is the white part of the core of *Fu Ling*. It is sweet and bland in taste and neutral in nature, and enters the Heart and Spleen channels. Its function in quieting the Heart and Spirit makes it particularly suitable for treating vexation and insomnia, often in combination with *Yuan Zhi* (Radix Polygalae) and *Long Chi* (Dens Draconis). The dosage is 6-10g.

Yi Yi Ren 薏苡仁
(Coix seed, Semen Coicis Lachrymajobi)

Yi Yi Ren is the dried mature seed of *Coix lachrymajobi* L. var. *ma-yuen* (Roman.) Stapf, family Gramineae.

Main ingredients *Yi Yi Ren* contains coixol, coixenolide, vitamin B_1, carbohydrates, proteins and fats.

Properties Taste: sweet and bland; nature: slightly cold.

Channels entered Spleen, Stomach and Lung.

Functions and indications Promotes the movement of water and percolates dampness, fortifies the Spleen and stops diarrhoea, eliminates Bi syndrome and alleviates pain, clears heat and expels pus. It is indicated for diarrhoea due to Spleen deficiency, numbness of the muscles, hypertonicity of the sinews and vessels, inhibited bending and stretching, inhibited urination, oedema in leg Qi, wind-damp Bi syndrome, Lung abscess, and Intestinal abscess.

Common dosage 10-30g, or 60g for large dosages. As *Yi Yi Ren* is a mild herb, it can be used in large dosages over a long period of time.

Precautions and contraindications *Yi Yi Ren* is contraindicated in cases of seminal emission and profuse urination, and during pregnancy.

Remarks Raw *Yi Yi Ren* is normally used to eliminate dampness, whereas the stir-fried herb is usually employed to fortify the Spleen and stop diarrhoea.

Comparison of functions *Yi Yi Ren* (Semen Coicis Lachrymajobi) and *Fu Ling* (Sclerotium Poriae Cocos) have similar functions in promoting the movement of water and fortifying the Spleen and are used for inhibited urination and for oedema due to Spleen deficiency and exuberant dampness. However, *Yi Yi Ren* is more effective in percolating dampness; being slightly cold, it can also clear heat to treat Lung and Intestinal abscesses and can dispel pathogenic dampness in the sinews and bones. *Fu Ling* has a stronger function in fortifying the Spleen and can also harmonize the Stomach and quiet the Heart and Spirit, being neutral in nature.

For an additional comparison, see *Lou Lu* (Radix Rhapontici seu Echinopsis).

Modern research

1. Abates fever, alleviates pain and has a tranquillizing function.[8]
2. Excites the intestinal tract and uterus.[8]
3. Induces ovulation.[8]
4. The amyloses contained in *Yi Yi Ren* strengthen the immune function.[9]

Combinations and applications

Functions	Combinations	Applications
Promoting the movement of water and percolating dampness	*Fu Ling* (Sclerotium Poriae Cocos) *Zhu Ling* (Sclerotium Polypori Umbellati) *Che Qian Zi* (Semen Plantaginis) *Ze Xie* (Rhizoma Alismatis Orientalis)	Oedema and inhibited urination due to Spleen deficiency with exuberant dampness
	Mu Gua (Fructus Chaenomelis) *Niu Xi* (Radix Achyranthis Bidentatae) *Fang Ji* (Radix Stephaniae Tetrandrae) (see notes on legal status)	Swollen and painful feet and knees, damp leg Qi
	Xing Ren (Semen Pruni Armeniacae) *Cao Dou Kou* (Semen Alpiniae Katsumadai) *Hou Po* (Cortex Magnoliae Officinalis)	Headache, heavy body and oppression in the chest resulting from damp-warmth due to pathogenic factors invading the Qi level
	Huang Bai (Cortex Phellodendri) *Lian Zi Xin* (Plumula Nelumbinis Nuciferae)	Yellow vaginal discharge due to damp-heat pouring down
Fortifying the Spleen and stopping diarrhoea	*Dang Shen* (Radix Codonopsitis Pilosulae) *Guang Huo Xiang* (Herba Pogostemi) *Bai Zhu* (Rhizoma Atractylodis Macrocephalae) *Fu Ling* (Sclerotium Poriae Cocos) *Mu Xiang* (Radix Aucklandiae Lappae) (see notes on legal status)	Diarrhoea, reduced food intake, distension in the abdomen and white, slimy tongue fur due to Spleen deficiency
Eliminating Bi syndrome and alleviating pain	*Gu Sui Bu* (Rhizoma Drynariae) *Mu Gua* (Fructus Chaenomelis) *Shen Jin Cao* (Herba Lycopodii Japonici) *Xu Duan* (Radix Dipsaci) *Zhi Chuan Shan Jia* (Squama Manitis Pentadactylae Praeparata)	Hypertonicity of the sinews and vessels and inhibited bending and stretching due to wind-damp
	Ma Huang (Herba Ephedrae) (see notes on legal status) *Xing Ren* (Semen Pruni Armeniacae) *Gan Cao* (Radix Glycyrrhizae)	Generalized pain due to wind-damp, fever intensifying in the late afternoon

Clearing heat and expelling pus	*Dong Gua Ren* (Semen Benincasae Hispidae) *Lu Gen* (Rhizoma Phragmitis Communis) *Tao Ren* (Semen Persicae) *Yu Xing Cao* (Herba Houttuyniae Cordatae)	Lung abscess due to damp-heat binding internally with coughing and spitting of purulent sputum
	Da Huang (Radix et Rhizoma Rhei) *Mu Dan Pi* (Cortex Moutan Radicis) *Bai Jiang Cao* (Herba Patriniae cum Radice)	Intestinal abscess due to damp-heat binding internally

Ze Xie 泽泻
(Water plantain rhizome, Rhizoma Alismatis Orientalis)

Ze Xie is the rhizome of *Alisma orientalis* (Sam.) Juzep., family Alismataceae.

Main ingredients *Ze Xie* contains alisol A, alisol B, choline, lecithin, methionine, thyronine, volatile oils, alkaloids and vitamin B_{12}.

Properties Taste: sweet and bland; nature: cold.

Channels entered Kidney and Bladder.

Functions and indications Promotes the movement of water and percolates dampness, clears heat and drains fire. It is indicated for inhibited urination, oedema, distension in the abdomen, diarrhoea, blood Lin syndrome, vaginal discharge due to damp-heat, and dizziness due to Phlegm-fluids.

Common dosage 6-10g, or 30g for large dosages.

Precautions and contraindications Taking *Ze Xie* over a long period may damage Yin, so it must not be used in cases of Yin deficiency without damp-heat or in cases of seminal emission due to Kidney deficiency.

Comparison of functions *Ze Xie* (Rhizoma Alismatis Orientalis) has a similar function to *Zhu Ling* (Sclerotium Polypori Umbellati) in promoting the movement of water and percolating dampness. However, *Ze Xie* can also drain fire from the Kidneys and eliminate dampness from the Bladder; it is particularly effective for treating damp-heat in the Lower Jiao. It is also used for dizziness due to Phlegm-fluids. *Zhu Ling* is used for patterns of accumulation of water within the body, especially when accompanied by heat signs.

For an additional comparison, see *Mu Tong* (Caulis Mutong).

Modern research

1. Promotes urination.[10]
2. Inhibits inflammation.[10]
3. Lowers cell immunity.[10]

Combinations and applications

Functions	Combinations	Applications
Promoting the movement of water and percolating dampness	*Fu Ling* (Sclerotium Poriae Cocos) *Zhu Ling* (Sclerotium Polypori Umbellati)	Oedema and inhibited urination due to collection of water and dampness

	Sheng Di Huang (Radix Rehmanniae Glutinosae) *Mu Tong* (Caulis Mutong) (see notes on legal status) *Huang Bai* (Cortex Phellodendri) *Shi Wei* (Folium Pyrrosiae)	Burning heat in the urethra, and dribbling and painful urination due to damp-heat in the Lower Jiao
	Fen Bi Xie (Rhizoma Dioscoreae Hypoglaucae) *Hua Shi* (Talcum) *Hai Jin Sha* (Spora Lygodii Japonici)	Urinary turbidity
	Sang Bai Pi (Cortex Mori Albae Radicis) *Da Fu Pi* (Pericarpium Arecae Catechu) *Fu Ling* (Sclerotium Poriae Cocos) *Sang Ji Sheng* (Ramulus Loranthi)	Oedema during pregnancy with wheezing and rough breathing, and difficult urination and defecation
	Bai Zhu (Rhizoma Atractylodis Macrocephalae) *Fu Ling* (Sclerotium Poriae Cocos)	Diarrhoea due to water and dampness
	Ban Xia (Rhizoma Pinelliae Ternatae) *Bai Zhu* (Rhizoma Atractylodis Macrocephalae)	Dizziness due to Phlegm-fluids
Clearing heat and draining fire	*Long Dan Cao* (Radix Gentianae Scabrae) *Yin Chen Hao* (Herba Artemisiae Scopariae) *Qing Dai* (Indigo Naturalis) *Chai Hu* (Radix Bupleuri) *Che Qian Zi* (Semen Plantaginis)	Red eyes, pain in the hypochondrium, jaundice and yellow urine
	Huang Bai (Cortex Phellodendri) *Zhi Mu* (Rhizoma Anemarrhenae Asphodeloidis) *Sheng Di Huang* (Radix Rehmanniae Glutinosae) *Mu Dan Pi* (Cortex Moutan Radicis)	Dizziness and steaming bone disorder caused by deficiency-fire flaming upwards
	Shu Di Huang (Radix Rehmanniae Glutinosae Conquita) *Shan Zhu Yu* (Fructus Corni Officinalis)	Seminal emission, night sweating, tinnitus and aching in the lumbar region due to hyperactivity of the ministerial fire and insufficiency of Kidney Yin

Zhu Ling 猪苓
(Umbellate pore, Sclerotium Polypori Umbellati)

Zhu Ling is the sclerotium of *Polyporus umbellatus* (Pers.) Fries., family Polyporaceae.

Main ingredients *Zhu Ling* contains ergosterol, α-hydroxytetracosanoic acid and biotin.

Properties Taste: sweet and bland; nature: neutral.

Channels entered Kidney and Bladder.

Functions and indications Promotes the movement of water and percolates dampness. It is indicated for dribbling and painful urination, oedema, vaginal discharge, turbid Lin syndrome, and diarrhoea.

Common dosage 5-10g.

Precautions and contraindications *Zhu Ling* should be used with caution in cases without dampness.

Comparison of functions Both *Zhu Ling* (Sclerotium Polypori Umbellati) and *Fu Ling* (Sclerotium Poriae Cocos) have the function of promoting the movement of water and percolating dampness and can treat inhibited urination, Lin syndrome pain and oedema. They are often used together to strengthen the function of promoting the movement of water. *Zhu Ling* has a stronger effect than *Fu Ling* in promoting the movement of water and percolating dampness. It can be used for patterns of accumulation of water within the body, especially when accompanied by heat signs. Although *Fu Ling* is weaker in percolating dampness and promoting the movement of water, it has the concurrent properties of fortifying the Spleen, harmonizing the Stomach and quieting the Heart and Spirit. It can be used for Spleen deficiency patterns accompanied by dampness.

For additional comparisons, see *Ze Xie* (Rhizoma Alismatis Orientalis) and *Lei Wan* (Sclerotium Omphaliae Lapidescens).

Modern research

1. Strongly promotes urination; promotes the discharge of sodium, potassium, calcium, manganese, zinc and copper.[11]
2. Protects the functions of the liver.[12]
3. Inhibits carcinoma.[13]

Combinations and applications

Functions	Combinations	Applications
Promoting the movement of water and percolating dampness	*Fu Ling* (Sclerotium Poriae Cocos) *Bai Zhu* (Rhizoma Atractylodis Macrocephalae) *Ze Xie* (Rhizoma Alismatis Orientalis)	Oedema and diarrhoea due to Spleen deficiency with exuberant dampness
	Hua Shi (Talcum) *Mu Tong* (Caulis Mutong) (see notes on legal status) *Dong Kui Zi* (Semen Malvae Verticillatae)	Dribbling and painful urination, heat Lin syndrome
	Huang Bai (Cortex Phellodendri) *Rou Dou Kou* (Semen Myristicae Fragrantis)	Diarrhoea, somnolence and no desire for food and drink
	Che Qian Zi (Semen Plantaginis) *Huang Bai* (Cortex Phellodendri)	Red and white vaginal discharge
	Cang Zhu (Rhizoma Atractylodis) *Gan Jiang* (Rhizoma Zingiberis Officinalis)	Continuous diarrhoea due to cold-damp in the Intestines and Stomach

Dong Gua Pi 冬瓜皮 (Wax gourd peel, Epicarpium Benincasae Hispidae)

Dong Gua Pi is the dried epicarp of *Benincasa hispida* (Thunb.) Cogn., family Cucurbitaceae.

Main ingredients *Dong Gua Pi* contains wax and resin.

Properties Taste: sweet; nature: slightly cold.
Channels entered Lung and Small Intestine.
Functions and indications Promotes the movement of water and disperses swelling. It is indicated for oedema.
Common dosage 15-30g.
Modern research Increases the amount of urine in the recovery stage of non-renal oedema; the amount of urine increases two hours after intake and then decreases.[14]

Combinations and applications

Functions	Combinations	Applications
Promoting the movement of water and dispersing swelling	*Fu Ling* (Sclerotium Poriae Cocos) *Ze Xie* (Rhizoma Alismatis Orientalis) *Bai Zhu* (Rhizoma Atractylodis Macrocephalae)	Oedema
	Chi Xiao Dou (Semen Phaseoli Calcarati)	Wheezing, fullness in the chest, oedema
	Yi Yi Ren (Semen Coicis Lachrymajobi) *Hua Shi* (Talcum) *Bai Bian Dou* (Semen Dolichoris Lablab)	Summerheat-damp

Appendix

Dong Gua Ren 冬瓜仁 (Wax gourd seed, Semen Benincasae Hispidae)

Dong Gua Ren is the seed of *Benincasa hispida* (Thunb.) Cogn., family Cucurbitaceae. It is sweet in taste and cold in nature and enters the Lung, Stomach, Large Intestine and Small Intestine channels. It has the functions of clearing heat and transforming Phlegm, and expelling pus and dispersing abscesses; it is indicated for cough due to Lung-heat, Lung abscess, Intestinal abscess, white vaginal discharge, and inhibited urination. The dosage is 9-15g. *Dong Gua Ren* can be used in combination with *Lu Gen* (Rhizoma Phragmitis Communis), *Tao Ren* (Semen Persicae) and *Yi Yi Ren* (Semen Coicis Lachrymajobi) for Lung abscess; with *Da Huang* (Radix et Rhizoma Rhei) and *Mu Dan Pi* (Cortex Moutan Radicis) for Intestinal abscess; and with *Huang Bai* (Cortex Phellodendri) and *Bi Xie* (Rhizoma Dioscoreae) for white, turbid vaginal discharge due to damp-heat in the Lower Jiao and for inhibited urination.

Chi Xiao Dou 赤小豆 (Aduki bean, Semen Phaseoli Calcarati)

Chi Xiao Dou is the dried ripe seed of *Phaseolus calcaratus* Roxb. or *P. angularis* Wight, family Leguminosae.
Main ingredients *Chi Xiao Dou* contains proteins, nicotinic acid, vitamins A, B_1 and B_2, phytosterol and triterpene saponins.
Properties Taste: sweet and sour; nature: neutral.
Channels entered Heart and Small Intestine.
Functions and indications Promotes the movement of water and disperses swelling, promotes the elimination of dampness and abates jaundice, relieves toxicity and expels pus. It is indicated for oedema and abdominal fullness, puffy swelling in leg Qi, abscesses and sores due to heat toxins, and damp-heat jaundice.
Common dosage 10-30g; appropriate dosage for external application.

Combinations and applications

Functions	Combinations	Applications
Promoting the movement of water and dispersing swelling	*Bai Mao Gen* (Rhizoma Imperatae Cylindricae) *Sang Bai Pi* (Cortex Mori Albae Radicis)	Oedema due to nephritis, cirrhosis or malnutrition, inhibited urination
	Chen Hu Lu (Fructus Lagenariae Depressae) *Sheng Jiang* (Rhizoma Zingiberis Officinalis Recens) *Shang Lu* (Radix Phytolaccae)	Leg Qi
Promoting the elimination of dampness and abating jaundice	*Ma Huang* (Herba Ephedrae) (see notes on legal status) *Lian Qiao* (Fructus Forsythiae Suspensae) *Sang Bai Pi* (Cortex Mori Albae Radicis)	Mild cases of damp-heat jaundice, manifesting as yellow skin, fever and absence of sweating

Note: *Chi Xiao Dou* can be ground with egg white, honey or vinegar for external application on abscesses to relieve toxicity and expel pus.

HERBS FOR PROMOTING URINATION AND FREEING LIN SYNDROME

Che Qian Zi 车前子
(Plantain seed, Semen Plantaginis)

Che Qian Zi is the seed of *Plantago asiatica* L., *P. depressa* Willd. or *P. major* L., family Plantaginaceae.

Main ingredients *Che Qian Zi* contains plantasan, mucilage, plantenolic acid, succinic acid, adenine, choline, vitamin A and vitamin B. The whole plant contains aucubin, plantagin and ursolic acid.

Properties Taste: sweet; nature: cold.

Channels entered Kidney, Liver, Lung and Small Intestine.

Functions and indications Promotes urination and frees Lin syndrome, percolates dampness and stops diarrhoea, clears the Liver and brightens the eyes, dispels Phlegm and stops coughing. It is indicated for inhibited urination, heat Lin syndrome, blood Lin syndrome, stone Lin syndrome, oedema, diarrhoea, cough with copious sputum, vaginal discharge, red eyes, and blurred vision.

Common dosage 6-10g, or 30g for large dosages; decoct in a cloth wrapping.

Precautions and contraindications *Che Qian Zi* is contraindicated in cases of seminal emission due to Kidney deficiency and in cases without damp-heat, as well as during pregnancy.

Comparison of functions Both *Che Qian Zi* (Semen Plantaginis) and *Hua Shi* (Talcum) can clear heat and promote urination to free Lin syndrome. *Che Qian Zi* is cold in nature and has downward-bearing and sinking actions; it is especially suitable for heat Lin syndrome. It also clears Lung-heat to transform Phlegm and stop coughing, clears Liver-heat to brighten the eyes, and percolates dampness to stop diarrhoea. *Hua Shi* is a lubricating herb and promotes urination; it is especially suitable for stone Lin syndrome. It can also dispel dampness and close sores when used externally.

For an additional comparison, see *Yin Chen Hao* (Herba Artemisiae Scopariae).

Modern research

1. Small dosages of *Che Qian Zi* can raise blood pressure, whereas large dosages of the herb can lower blood pressure and induce cardiac paralysis.[15]
2. Promotes urination.[16]
3. Aqueous extracts of *Che Qian Zi* had an inhibitory effect on Staphylococcus aureus and Shigella sonnei in laboratory experiments.[17]

Combinations and applications

Functions	Combinations	Applications
Promoting urination and freeing Lin syndrome	*Bian Xu* (Herba Polygoni Avicularis) *Mu Tong* (Caulis Mutong) (see notes on legal status) *Hua Shi* (Talcum) *Zhi Zi* (Fructus Gardeniae Jasminoidis)	Dribbling, difficult and painful urination due to heat binding the Bladder in heat Lin syndrome patterns
	Hai Jin Sha (Spora Lygodii Japonici) *Jin Qian Cao* (Herba Lysimachiae)	Stone Lin syndrome
	Yin Chen Hao (Herba Artemisiae Scopariae) *Da Huang* (Radix et Rhizoma Rhei)	Damp-heat jaundice

	Ze Xie (Rhizoma Alismatis Orientalis) *Fu Ling Pi* (Cortex Poriae Cocos) *Dong Gua Pi* (Epicarpium Benincasae Hispidae)	All types of oedema
Percolating dampness and stopping diarrhoea	*Hua Shi* (Talcum) *Ze Xie* (Rhizoma Alismatis Orientalis) *He Ye* (Folium Nelumbinis Nuciferae)	Diarrhoea due to summerheat-damp, watery stool, vexation and thirst, blood in the urine
	Fu Ling (Sclerotium Poriae Cocos) *Yi Yi Ren* (Semen Coicis Lachrymajobi) *Sha Ren* (Fructus Amomi)	Diarrhoea due to Spleen deficiency, indigestion
Clearing the Liver and brightening the eyes	*Long Dan Cao* (Radix Gentianae Scabrae) *Ju Hua* (Flos Chrysanthemi Morifolii) *Jue Ming Zi* (Semen Cassiae)	Red, sore and swollen eyes and eye screen due to exuberant heat in the Liver channel
	Gou Qi Zi (Fructus Lycii) *Sang Shen* (Fructus Mori Albae) *He Shou Wu* (Radix Polygoni Multiflori)	Blurred vision due to insufficiency of the Liver and Kidneys
Dispelling Phlegm and stopping coughing	*Xing Ren* (Semen Pruni Armeniacae) *Sang Bai Pi* (Cortex Mori Albae Radicis) *Huang Qin* (Radix Scutellariae Baicalensis)	Cough with yellow sputum due to Lung-heat
	Bi Ba (Fructus Piperis Longi) *Chan Tui* (Periostracum Cicadae)	Whooping cough

Appendix

Che Qian Cao 车前草 (Plantain herb, Herba Plantaginis)

Che Qian Cao is the whole plant of *Plantago asiatica* L., *P. depressa* Willd. or *P. major* L. Its nature and properties are similar to those of *Che Qian Zi*. It is good for clearing heat and dispelling dampness, cooling the Blood and relieving toxicity. It is indicated for blood in the urine, bleeding due to Blood-heat, diarrhoea due to damp-heat, and sores and swellings due to heat toxins. The common dosage is 10-15g, or double the dosage when the fresh herb is used; appropriate dosage for external application.

Hua Shi 滑石 (Talc, Talcum)

Hua Shi is the mineral form of magnesium silicate, crystallizing in the triclinic system; it is usually prepared as a powder.

Main ingredients *Hua Shi* contains magnesium silicate [$Mg_3(Si_4O_{10})(OH)_2$], a little aluminium oxide and nickel oxide.

Properties Taste: sweet and bland; nature: cold.

Channels entered Stomach and Bladder.

Functions and indications Promotes urination and frees Lin syndrome, clears heat and relieves summerheat, dispels dampness and closes sores. It is indicated for inhibited urination, dribbling and painful urination, vexation and thirst due to summerheat, eczema, and prickly heat.

Common dosage 10-15g, or 30g for large dosages (wrap in a cloth before decoction); appropriate dosage for external application.

Precautions and contraindications *Hua Shi* is contraindicated in cases of Spleen and Stomach deficiency-cold, seminal emission, damage to body fluids due to febrile diseases, profuse urination, and during pregnancy.

Comparison of functions Both *Hua Shi* (Talcum) and *Shi Gao* (Gypsum Fibrosum) can clear heat and allay thirst. *Hua Shi* allays thirst through benefiting the orifices and dispelling dampness to harmonize the Spleen and Stomach. It is suitable for summerheat with dampness accompanied by short, inhibited voidings of reddish urine, vexation and thirst. *Shi Gao* allays thirst by clearing fever from the Yangming channel to dispel heat and secure body fluids. It is therefore suitable for vexation and thirst due to exuberant heat in the Yangming channel. For external use, both herbs can dispel dampness and promote contraction. Powdered *Hua Shi* treats eczema and prickly heat with itching, whereas calcined *Shi Gao* is often used for non-closure of open sores.

For an additional combination, see *Che Qian Zi* (Semen Plantaginis).

Modern research

1. Magnesium silicate can protect against inflammation of the internal surface of the gastrointestinal mucous membrane.[18]
2. Stops vomiting and diarrhoea, and inhibits the absorption of toxins in the gastrointestinal tract.[19]

Combinations and applications

Functions	Combinations	Applications
Promoting urination and freeing Lin syndrome	*Mu Tong* (Caulis Mutong) (see notes on legal status) *Che Qian Zi* (Semen Plantaginis) *Ze Xie* (Rhizoma Alismatis Orientalis) *Hai Jin Sha* (Spora Lygodii Japonici)	Pain in the urethra, inhibited urination, dribbling and painful urination due to Lin syndrome
	Yi Yi Ren (Semen Coicis Lachrymajobi) *Zhu Ling* (Sclerotium Polypori Umbellati) *Che Qian Zi* (Semen Plantaginis)	Watery diarrhoea due to damp-heat, accompanied by short voidings of reddish urine
	Mu Tong (Caulis Mutong) (see notes on legal status) *Qu Mai* (Herba Dianthi) *Zhi Zi* (Fructus Gardeniae Jasminoidis)	Heat Lin syndrome
	Hai Jin Sha (Spora Lygodii Japonici) *Jin Qian Cao* (Herba Lysimachiae)	Stone Lin syndrome
	Pu Huang (Pollen Typhae) *Dong Kui Zi* (Semen Malvae Verticillatae)	Inhibited urination, pain in the penis or lower abdomen due to damp-heat smouldering internally
Clearing heat and relieving summerheat	*Shi Gao* (Gypsum Fibrosum) *Gan Cao* (Radix Glycyrrhizae) *Dan Zhu Ye* (Herba Lophatheri Gracilis)	Vexation, thirst and scant and reddish urine due to summerheat-heat
	Guang Huo Xiang (Herba Pogostemi) *Pei Lan* (Herba Eupatorii Fortunei) *Ban Xia* (Rhizoma Pinelliae Ternatae) *Fu Ling* (Sclerotium Poriae Cocos)	Vomiting and diarrhoea due to summerheat-stroke
	Yi Yi Ren (Semen Coicis Lachrymajobi) *Bai Dou Kou* (Fructus Amomi Kravanh)	The initial stage of damp-warm diseases or summerheat-damp pathogenic factors in the Qi level

Dispelling dampness and closing sores (external use)	*Shi Gao* (Gypsum Fibrosum) *Ku Fan* (Alumen Praeparatum) *Huang Bai* (Cortex Phellodendri)	Eczema, damp and itchy toes, prickly heat

Mu Tong 木通 (Mutong stem, Caulis Mutong)

Mu Tong is the vine of *Aristolochia manshuriensis* Kom., family Aristolochiaceae (*Guan Mu Tong*), or *Clematis armandi* Franch. and *C. montana* Buch.-Ham., family Ranunculaceae (*Chuan Mu Tong*).

Legal status At the time of publication, the Medicines *(Aristolochia* and Mu Tong etc.) (Prohibition) Order 2001 prohibits in the UK the sale, supply and importation of unlicensed medicines for human use containing or presented as containing this herb.

Main ingredients *Guan Mu Tong* contains aristolochic acid, aristoloside, magnoflorine, oleanolic acid, hederagenin, tannic acid and calcium.

Properties Taste: bitter; nature: cold.

Channels entered Heart, Small Intestine and Bladder.

Functions and indications Promotes urination and frees Lin syndrome, clears the Heart and drains fire, frees the Blood vessels, frees menstruation and causes milk to descend. It is indicated for short voidings of reddish urine, difficult and painful urination, vexation in the Heart, mouth sores, sore throat, damp-heat Bi syndrome, and stoppage of breast milk.

Common dosage 3-10g.

Precautions and contraindications *Mu Tong* is contraindicated in cases of seminal emission, damage to body fluids and diseases without damp-heat, as well as during pregnancy.

Remarks In the past, *Akebia guinata* (Thunb.) Decne. was used for this herb, but this plant is employed very rarely nowadays.

Comparison of functions Both *Mu Tong* (Caulis Mutong) and *Ze Xie* (Rhizoma Alismatis Orientalis) have the function of promoting the movement of water and clearing heat, but *Mu Tong* tends to clear fire in the Heart channel and drain heat in the Small Intestine channel, whereas *Ze Xie* tends to drain damp-heat in the Kidney and Bladder channels.

For an additional comparison, see *Tong Cao* (Medulla Tetrapanacis Papyriferi).

Toxicity Intravenous injection of 60mg/kg of aristolochic acid in mice resulted in death. Rabbits given a daily intravenous injection of 1.5mg/kg died between the third and ninth days. Examination revealed pathological changes in the blood capillaries of the internal organs as well as haemorrhaging and oedema, with extensive damage to the kidneys. Symptoms of toxic overdose in humans appear after 3-6 hours, manifesting initially as discomfort in the upper abdomen, vomiting, pain in the abdomen and diarrhoea, subsequently developing into urinary frequency and urinary urgency, facial oedema, higher blood pressure and, in severe cases, resulting in acute renal failure, uraemia and death.

Modern research

1. The potassium and other active ingredients contained in *Mu Tong* can promote urination.[20]
2. Large dosages (over 60g) may cause acute renal failure (see *Toxicity*).[21-25]

Combinations and applications

Functions	Combinations	Applications
Promoting urination and freeing Lin syndrome	*Bian Xu* (Herba Polygoni Avicularis) *Che Qian Zi* (Semen Plantaginis) *Qu Mai* (Herba Dianthi) *Zhi Zi* (Fructus Gardeniae Jasminoidis)	Short voidings of reddish urine, dribbling and painful urination due to heat Lin syndrome
	Zhu Ling (Sclerotium Polypori Umbellati) *Zi Su Ye* (Folium Perillae Frutescentis) *Bing Lang* (Semen Arecae Catechu) *Sang Bai Pi* (Cortex Mori Albae Radicis)	Leg Qi due to dampness, generalized oedema, inhibited urination, wheezing
Clearing the Heart and draining fire	*Dan Zhu Ye* (Herba Lophatheri Gracilis) *Sheng Di Huang* (Radix Rehmanniae Glutinosae) *Gan Cao* (Radix Glycyrrhizae)	Mouth sores, vexation and insomnia due to Heart-fire flaming upwards
Freeing the Blood vessels	*Fang Ji* (Radix Stephaniae Tetrandrae) (see notes on legal status) *Sang Zhi* (Ramulus Mori Albae) *Wei Ling Xian* (Radix Clematidis)	Swollen and painful limb joints with inhibited bending and stretching due to damp-heat
Freeing menstruation and causing milk to descend	*Lu Lu Tong* (Fructus Liquidambaris) *Wang Bu Liu Xing* (Semen Vaccariae Segetalis) *Chuan Shan Jia* (Squama Manitis Pentadactylae) (see notes on legal status)	Stoppage of breast milk
	Hong Hua (Flos Carthami Tinctorii) *Niu Xi* (Radix Achyranthis Bidentatae) *Yan Hu Suo* (Rhizoma Corydalis Yanhusuo) *Sheng Di Huang* (Radix Rehmanniae Glutinosae)	Menstrual block due to Qi stagnation and Blood stasis

Hai Jin Sha 海金沙 (Climbing fern spore, Spora Lygodii Japonici)

Hai Jin Sha is the spore of *Lygodium japonicum* (Thunb.) Sw., family Lygodiaceae.

Main ingredients The spores of *Hai Jin Sha* contain fatty oils; the leaves of the vine contain trans p-coumaric acid, caffeic acid and flavones.

Properties Taste: sweet; nature: cold.

Channels entered Bladder and Small Intestine.

Functions and indications Promotes urination and frees Lin syndrome, and expels stones from the urinary tract. It is indicated for all types of Lin syndrome, as well as for oedema and drum-like abdominal distension.

Common dosage 6-12g, decocted in a cloth wrapping.

Precautions and contraindications *Hai Jin Sha* is contraindicated in cases of Yin deficiency in the absence of damp-heat.

Comparison of functions Both *Hai Jin Sha* (Spora Lygodii Japonici) and *Shi Wei* (Folium Pyrrosiae) can clear heat and free Lin syndrome and are often used to treat heat, stone and blood Lin syndromes. *Hai Jin Sha* is used more frequently for stone Lin syndrome, *Shi Wei* for blood and heat Lin syndromes. *Shi Wei* can also clear the Lungs and stop coughing in the upper body, and cool the Blood and stop uterine bleeding in the lower body.

For an additional comparison, see *Jin Qian Cao* (Herba Lysimachiae).

Modern research

1. The caffeic acid contained in *Hai Jin Sha* protects the liver and gallbladder.[26]
2. Increases the water content in bile without increasing the secretion of cholesterol.[26]

Combinations and applications

Functions	Combinations	Applications
Promoting urination and freeing Lin syndrome, expelling stones from the urinary tract	*Dong Kui Zi* (Semen Malvae Verticillatae) *Shi Wei* (Folium Pyrrosiae) *Jin Qian Cao* (Herba Lysimachiae) *Ji Nei Jin* (Endothelium Corneum Gigeriae Galli)	Stone Lin syndrome
	Che Qian Zi (Semen Plantaginis) *Qu Mai* (Herba Dianthi) *Zhi Zi* (Fructus Gardeniae Jasminoidis)	Heat Lin syndrome
	Bai Mao Gen (Rhizoma Imperatae Cylindricae) *Ze Xie* (Rhizoma Alismatis Orientalis) *Huang Bai Tan* (Cortex Phellodendri Carbonisatus)	Blood Lin syndrome
	Bai Zhu (Rhizoma Atractylodis Macrocephalae) *Gan Cao* (Radix Glycyrrhizae)	Drum-like abdominal distension due to Spleen-damp
	Qian Niu Zi (Semen Pharbitidis) *Gan Sui* (Radix Euphorbiae Kansui)	Generalized oedema due to Spleen deficiency

Appendix

Hai Jin Sha Teng 海金沙藤 (Climbing fern, Herba Lygodii Japonici)

Hai Jin Sha Teng is the whole plant of *Lygodium japonicum* (Thunb.) Sw., family Lygodiaceae. It is similar in taste, properties and functions to *Hai Jin Sha*, but it can also clear heat and relieve toxicity. It is indicated for Lin syndrome, damp-heat jaundice, dysentery, white vaginal discharge, and abscesses and swellings. The dosage is 15-30g in a decoction, or an appropriate amount for external application topically as a wash or compress.

Tong Cao 通草 (Rice paper pith, Medulla Tetrapanacis Papyriferi)

Tong Cao is the pith of *Tetrapanax papyriferus* (Hook.) K. Koch, family Araliaceae.

Main ingredients *Tong Cao* contains uronic acid, proteins and polysaccharides.

Properties Taste: sweet and bland; nature: slightly cold.

Channels entered Lung and Stomach.

Functions and indications Clears heat and promotes urination, frees Qi and causes milk to descend. It is indicated for inhibited urination, Lin syndrome, and stoppage of breast milk.

Common dosage 2-5g.

Precautions and contraindications *Tong Cao* should be used with caution in cases of Qi and Yin deficiency, and during pregnancy.

Comparison of functions Both *Tong Cao* (Medulla Tetrapanacis Papyriferi) and *Mu Tong* (Caulis Mutong) can clear heat, promote urination and cause milk to descend. *Tong Cao* is sweet and bland in taste and slightly cold in nature, whereas *Mu Tong* is bitter and cold and has a stronger effect than *Tong Cao* in clearing heat and promoting urination. *Tong Cao* is light in quality and cannot be used in large dosages; since *Mu Tong* can drain original Qi, it must not be used in large dosages either.

For an additional comparison, see *Deng Xin Cao* (Medulla Junci Effusi).

Modern research

1. The potassium contained in *Tong Cao* promotes urination.[27]
2. Preliminary results indicate that *Tong Cao* promotes lactation, but this requires further research.[28]

Combinations and applications

Functions	Combinations	Applications
Clearing heat and promoting urination	*Yi Yi Ren* (Semen Coicis Lachrymajobi) *Dan Zhu Ye* (Herba Lophatheri Gracilis) *Hua Shi* (Talcum)	Inhibited urination and dribbling and painful urination due to damp-heat Lin syndrome
	Zhu Ling (Sclerotium Polypori Umbellati) *Ze Xie* (Rhizoma Alismatis Orientalis) *Mu Tong* (Caulis Mutong) (see notes on legal status)	Oedema due to collection of water and dampness, inhibited urination
	Xing Ren (Semen Pruni Armeniacae) *Hua Shi* (Talcum) *Chen Pi* (Pericarpium Citri Reticulatae)	Oppression in the chest, nausea and reddish urine in the initial stage of warm diseases
Freeing Qi and causing milk to descend	*Chuan Shan Jia* (Squama Manitis Pentadactylae) (see notes on legal status) *Wang Bu Liu Xing* (Semen Vaccariae Segetalis)	Stoppage of breast milk

Qu Mai 瞿麦 (Chinese pink herb, Herba Dianthi)

Qu Mai is the dried aerial parts of *Dianthus superbus* L. or *D. chinensis* L., family Caryophyllaceae.

Main ingredients *Qu Mai* contains dianthus saponins, sylvite, volatile oils (including eugenol, phenylethylalcohol, methyl salicylate and benzyl benzoate), phosphoric acid, vitamin A, alkaloids and flavones.

Properties Taste: bitter; nature: cold.

Channels entered Heart, Kidney, Small Intestine and Bladder.

Functions and indications Promotes urination and frees Lin syndrome, breaks up Blood stasis and frees menstruation. It is indicated for inhibited urination, the five types of Lin syndrome (stone, blood, heat, Qi and turbid Lin), menstrual block due to Blood stasis, and red, sore and swollen eyes.

Common dosage 10-15g.

Precautions and contraindications *Qu Mai* is contraindicated in cases of Spleen Qi deficiency and during pregnancy.

Comparison of functions See *Bian Xu* (Herba Polygoni Avicularis).

Modern research

1. Decoctions of *Qu Mai* clearly promoted urination and the discharge of sodium and potassium in laboratory tests.[29]
2. Inhibits Staphylococcus aureus and Bacterium coli.[30]

Combinations and applications

Functions	Combinations	Applications
Promoting urination and freeing Lin syndrome	*Mu Tong* (Caulis Mutong) (see notes on legal status) *Hua Shi* (Talcum) *Che Qian Zi* (Semen Plantaginis)	Heat Lin syndrome and short voidings of reddish urine
	Shi Wei (Folium Pyrrosiae) *Hua Shi* (Talcum) *Dong Kui Zi* (Semen Malvae Verticillatae) *Che Qian Zi* (Semen Plantaginis)	Stone Lin syndrome
	Pu Huang (Pollen Typhae)	Postpartum Lin syndrome
Breaking up Blood stasis and freeing menstruation	*Ze Xie* (Rhizoma Alismatis Orientalis)	Red, sore and swollen eyes
	Yi Mu Cao (Herba Leonuri Heterophylli) *Dan Shen* (Radix Salviae Miltiorrhizae) *Hong Hua* (Flos Carthami Tinctorii)	Menstrual block or menstrual irregularities due to Blood stasis

Bian Xu 扁蓄
(Prostrate knotweed, Herba Polygoni Avicularis)

Bian Xu is the dried aerial parts of *Polygonum aviculare* L., family Polygonaceae.

Main ingredients *Bian Xu* contains avicularin, quercitrin, d-catechol; gallic, caffeic, oxalic, silicic, chlorogenic and p-coumaric acids; glucose, fructose and sucrose.

Properties Taste: bitter; nature: slightly cold.

Channel entered Bladder.

Functions and indications Promotes urination and frees Lin syndrome, kills worms and alleviates itching. It is indicated for scant and dark urine, Lin syndrome, inhibited urination, oedema, eczema, and pudendal itch.

Common dosage 10-15g; or appropriate dosage for external application.

Precautions and contraindications *Bian Xu* should be used with caution in cases of Spleen deficiency and in the absence of damp-heat.

Comparison of functions *Bian Xu* (Herba Polygoni Avicularis) and *Qu Mai* (Herba Dianthi) have similar functions in promoting urination and freeing Lin syndrome and can be used together to strengthen their effect. *Bian Xu* tends to be more effective in treating Lin syndrome with equal severity of damp and heat, while concurrently drying dampness and killing worms. *Qu Mai*, bitter in taste and cold in nature, is better for Lin syndrome where heat is more severe than damp. It can also break up Blood stasis to free menstruation and treat menstrual block.

Modern research

1. Promotes urination and the discharge of sodium and potassium, soothes the gallbladder.[31]
2. Strengthens contraction of the uterus.[31]
3. An intravenous injection of *Bian Xu* lowered blood pressure in cats, rabbits and dogs.[31]
4. A steep of *Bian Xu* inhibited pathogenic fungi *in vitro*.[31]

Combinations and applications

Functions	Combinations	Applications
Promoting urination and freeing Lin syndrome	*Qu Mai* (Herba Dianthi) *Che Qian Zi* (Semen Plantaginis) *Hua Shi* (Talcum) *Zhi Zi* (Fructus Gardeniae Jasminoidis)	Heat Lin syndrome with pain in the lower abdomen and reddish urine with burning heat
	Dong Gua Pi (Epicarpium Benincasae Hispidae) *Fu Ling Pi* (Cortex Poriae Cocos) *Ze Xie* (Rhizoma Alismatis Orientalis)	Oedema, inhibited urination
Killing worms and alleviating itching	*Di Fu Zi* (Fructus Kochiae Scopariae) *Ku Shen* (Radix Sophorae Flavescentis)	Pudendal itch, eczema
	Fei Zi (Semen Torreyae Grandis)	Hookworm
	Mi Cu (Acetum Oryzae, rice vinegar)	Roundworm

Note: A decoction of *Bian Xu* can also be used as an external wash to treat eczema and pudendal itch.

Di Fu Zi 地肤子 (Broom cypress fruit, Fructus Kochiae Scopariae)

Di Fu Zi is the dried fruit of *Kochia scoparia* (L.) Schrad., family Chenopodiaceae.

Main ingredients *Di Fu Zi* contains triterpene saponins, fatty oils, alkaloids and vitamin A.

Properties Taste: sweet and bitter; nature: cold.

Channel entered Bladder.

Functions and indications Clears damp-heat and promotes urination, and alleviates itching. It is indicated for inhibited urination, Lin syndrome, and itchy skin due to pathogenic damp-heat pouring down into the Lower Jiao.

Common dosage 10–15g; or appropriate dosage for external application.

Modern research Inhibits dermatophytes.[32]

Combinations and applications

Functions	Combinations	Applications
Clearing damp-heat and promoting urination	*Zhi Mu* (Rhizoma Anemarrhenae Asphodeloidis) *Huang Lian* (Rhizoma Coptidis) *Qu Mai* (Herba Dianthi) *Tong Cao* (Medulla Tetrapanacis Papyriferi)	Lin syndrome and inhibited urination due to damp-heat in the Bladder
Alleviating itching	*Huang Bai* (Cortex Phellodendri) *Bai Xian Pi* (Cortex Dictamni Dasycarpi Radicis)	Eczema and itchy skin
	Ku Shen (Radix Sophorae Flavescentis) *She Chuang Zi* (Fructus Cnidii Monnieri) *Ming Fan* (Alumen)	Itching in the female genitalia due to damp

Shi Wei 石韦 (Pyrrosia leaf, Folium Pyrrosiae)

Shi Wei is the dried leaf of *Pyrrosia sheareri* (Bak.) Ching, *P. lingua* (Thunb.) Farw. or *P. petiolosa* (Christ) Ching, family Polypodiaceae.

Main ingredients *Shi Wei* contains isomangiferin, fumaric acid and caffeic acid (*P. sheareri*); diploptene, β-sitosterol, saponins, anthraquinones and tannin (*P. lingua*).

Properties Taste: sweet and bitter; nature: slightly cold.

Channels entered Lung and Bladder.

Functions and indications Promotes urination and frees Lin syndrome, cools the Blood and stops bleeding, clears the Lungs and stops coughing. It is indicated for heat and blood Lin syndromes, inhibited urination, vomiting of blood and uterine bleeding due to the frenetic movement of hot Blood, and cough due to Lung-heat.

Common dosage 5-10g; in large dosages, up to 30g.

Precautions and contraindications *Shi Wei* should be used with caution in cases of Spleen and Stomach deficiency-cold or in the absence of damp-heat.

Comparison of functions See *Hai Jin Sha* (Spora Lygodii Japonici) and *Jin Qian Cao* (Herba Lysimachiae).

Modern research

1. Stops coughing, calms wheezing and expels sputum.[33]
2. Has a certain inhibitory effect on influenza viruses.[34]

Combinations and applications

Functions	Combinations	Applications
Promoting urination and freeing Lin syndrome	*Mu Tong* (Caulis Mutong) (see notes on legal status) *Hua Shi* (Talcum) *Qu Mai* (Herba Dianthi)	Heat Lin syndrome, blood Lin syndrome, reddish urine with painful urination
	Zhi Zi (Fructus Gardeniae Jasminoidis) *Che Qian Cao* (Herba Plantaginis) *Gan Cao* (Radix Glycyrrhizae)	Stone Lin syndrome

	Dang Gui (Radix Angelicae Sinensis) *Chi Shao* (Radix Paeoniae Rubra) *Pu Huang* (Pollen Typhae)	Blood Lin syndrome
Cooling the Blood and stopping bleeding	*Di Yu* (Radix Sanguisorbae Officinalis) *Zong Lü Tan* (Fibra Carbonisata Trachycarpi Stipulae)	Vomiting of blood and uterine bleeding due to Lung-heat
Clearing the Lungs and stopping coughing	*Gan Cao* (Radix Glycyrrhizae) *Che Qian Zi* (Semen Plantaginis)	Cough with yellow sputum due to Lung-heat
	Bai Ji (Rhizoma Bletillae Striatae) *Di Yu* (Radix Sanguisorbae Officinalis) *Ce Bai Ye* (Cacumen Biotae Orientalis)	Cough with expectoration of blood

Bi Xie 萆薢 (Collett yam rhizome or seven-lobed yam rhizome, Rhizoma Dioscoreae Hypoglaucae seu Septemlobae)

Bi Xie is the dried rhizome of *Dioscorea hypoglauca* Palib. (Rhizoma Dioscoreae Hypoglaucae) or *D. septemloba* Thunb. (Rhizoma Dioscoreae Septemlobae), family Dioscoreaceae. *D. hypoglauca* is also known as *Fen Bi Xie*, *D. septemloba* as *Mian Bi Xie*.

Main ingredients *Bi Xie* contains steroid saponins, dioscorea saponins (including dioscin and diosgenin), tannins and starch.

Properties Taste: bitter; nature: neutral.

Channels entered Liver, Stomach and Bladder.

Functions and indications Separates the clear and the turbid, eliminates Bi syndrome pain, and clears damp-heat from the skin. It is indicated for turbid Lin syndrome, urinary turbidity, vaginal discharge, wind-damp Bi syndrome, inhibited bending and stretching, aching in the lumbar region and knees, and shank sores due to damp-heat.

Common dosage 10-15g.

Precautions and contraindications *Bi Xie* is contraindicated in cases of seminal emission due to Kidney deficiency.

Comparison of functions See *Jin Qian Cao* (Herba Lysimachiae) and *Tu Fu Ling* (Rhizoma Smilacis Glabrae).

Modern research Inhibits dermatophytes, has a tranquillizing function and promotes urination.[35]

Combinations and applications

Functions	Combinations	Applications
Separating the clear and the turbid	*Shi Chang Pu* (Rhizoma Acori Graminei) *Huang Bai* (Cortex Phellodendri)	Turbid Lin syndrome
	Yi Zhi Ren (Fructus Alpiniae Oxyphyllae) *Wu Yao* (Radix Linderae Strychnifoliae)	Frequent urination and limpness and aching in the lumbar region and knees
Eliminating Bi syndrome pain	*Gui Zhi* (Ramulus Cinnamomi Cassiae) *Fu Zi* (Radix Lateralis Aconiti Carmichaeli Praeparata) (see notes on legal status)	Damp-cold Bi syndrome

	Sang Zhi (Ramulus Mori Albae) *Qin Jiao* (Radix Gentianae Macrophyllae) *Yi Yi Ren* (Semen Coicis Lachrymajobi)	Damp-heat Bi syndrome
	Du Zhong (Cortex Eucommiae Ulmoidis) *Niu Xi* (Radix Achyranthis Bidentatae) *Bai Mao Gen* (Rhizoma Imperatae Cylindricae)	Inhibited bending and stretching, aching in the lumbar region and knees
Clearing damp-heat from the skin	*Huang Bai* (Cortex Phellodendri) *Yi Yi Ren* (Semen Coicis Lachrymajobi)	Shank sores and ulcerating sores due to damp-heat pouring down

Note: *Bi Xie* can also be used to treat vaginal discharge due to damp turbidity in the Lower Jiao.

Deng Xin Cao 灯心草 (Rush pith, Medulla Junci Effusi)

Deng Xin Cao is the dried stem pulp of *Juncus effusus* L., family Juncaceae.

Main ingredients *Deng Xin Cao* contains fibres, fatty oils, proteins and polysaccharides.

Properties Taste: sweet and bland; nature: slightly cold.

Channels entered Heart, Lung and Small Intestine.

Functions and indications Clears the Heart and drains fire, promotes urination and frees Lin syndrome. It is indicated for the five types of Lin syndrome (stone, blood, heat, Qi and turbid Lin), inhibited urination, vexation and insomnia, night crying in infants, and mouth and tongue sores.

Precautions and contraindications *Deng Xin Cao* is contraindicated in cases of deficiency-cold.

Common dosage 1.5-2.5g, used in decoction or pills.

Comparison of functions Both *Deng Xin Cao* (Medulla Junci Effusi) and *Tong Cao* (Medulla Tetrapanacis Papyriferi) can clear heat in the Heart and promote urination to treat painful and difficult urination. *Deng Xin Cao* is mainly used for Heart vexation and insomnia, and night crying in infants, whereas *Tong Cao* can also cause milk to descend.

Modern research Promotes urination and stops bleeding.[36]

Combinations and applications

Functions	Combinations	Applications
Clearing the Heart and draining fire, promoting urination and freeing Lin syndrome	*Hua Shi* (Talcum) *Zhi Zi* (Fructus Gardeniae Jasminoidis) *Che Qian Zi* (Semen Plantaginis)	Heat Lin syndrome
	Dan Zhu Ye (Herba Lophatheri Gracilis)	Child fright heat, night crying in infants
	Mu Tong (Caulis Mutong) (see notes on legal status) *Sheng Di Huang* (Radix Rehmanniae Glutinosae) *Gan Cao* (Radix Glycyrrhizae)	Short voidings of reddish urine, mouth and tongue sores

Yu Mi Xu 玉米须
(Corn silk, Stylus Zeae Mays)

Yu Mi Xu is dried style of *Zea mays* L., family Gramineae.

Main ingredients *Yu Mi Xu* contains vitamin K, α-tocophenolquinone, β-sitosterol, stigmasterol, malic acid, citric acid, tartaric acid, oxalic acid, cryptoxanthin, fatty oils and potassium nitrate.

Properties Taste: sweet; nature: neutral.

Channels entered Liver, Bladder and Gallbladder.

Functions and indications Promotes urination and frees Lin syndrome, calms the Liver, benefits the Gallbladder and abates jaundice. It is indicated for inhibited urination, oedema due to water collecting internally, jaundice, and dizziness due to hyperactivity of Liver Yang or heat in the Liver channel.

Common dosage 30-60g.

Remarks Boiled on its own and drunk as a decoction, *Yu Mi Xu* can promote urination, disperse oedema and reduce high blood pressure.

Modern research

1. Aqueous solutions, alcoholic solutions and decoctions of *Yu Mi Xu* can reduce high blood pressure.[37]
2. A decoction of 8-10g of *Yu Mi Xu* had a slight effect in promoting urination in healthy people, whereas drinking the juice on its own had a significant effect.[38]
3. Can significantly increase the secretion of bile and promote its excretion.[39]
4. Since vitamin K is a major ingredient of *Yu Mi Xu*, the herb can be used in the treatment of blood coagulation dysfunction caused by vitamin K deficiency.[39]

Combinations and applications

Functions	Combinations	Applications
Promoting urination and freeing Lin syndrome	*Che Qian Cao* (Herba Plantaginis) *Hai Jin Sha* (Spora Lygodii Japonici) *Jin Qian Cao* (Herba Lysimachiae)	Short voidings of reddish urine and difficult and painful urination due to damp-heat in the Bladder
	Dong Gua Pi (Epicarpium Benincasae Hispidae) *Chi Xiao Dou* (Semen Phaseoli Calcarati) *Yi Yi Ren* (Semen Coicis Lachrymajobi)	Oedema due to water and dampness collecting internally, inhibited urination
	Shi Wei (Folium Pyrrosiae) *Pu Gong Ying* (Herba Taraxaci cum Radice) *Ma Chi Xian* (Herba Portulacae Oleraceae)	Infection of the urinary tract
Calming the Liver, benefiting the Gallbladder and abating jaundice	*Jin Qian Cao* (Herba Lysimachiae) *Yu Jin* (Radix Curcumae) *Yin Chen Hao* (Herba Artemisiae Scopariae)	Various types of jaundice
	Gou Teng (Ramulus Uncariae cum Uncis) *Shi Jue Ming* (Concha Haliotidis) *Ju Hua* (Flos Chrysanthemi Morifolii)	Dizziness due to hyperactivity of Liver Yang or heat in the Liver channel

HERBS FOR PROMOTING THE ELIMINATION OF DAMPNESS AND ABATING JAUNDICE

Yin Chen Hao 茵陈蒿 (Oriental wormwood, Herba Artemisiae Scopariae)

Yin Chen Hao is the shoots and leaves of *Artemisia scoparia* Waldst. et Kit., or *A. capillaris* Thunb., family Compositae.

Main ingredients *Yin Chen Hao* contains scoparone, volatile oils (including β-pinene, capillin, capillon, capillone, capillene and capillarin), chlorogenic acid, caffeic acid, capillarisin and methyl capillarisin.

Properties Taste: bitter; nature: slightly cold.

Channels entered Spleen, Stomach, Liver and Gallbladder.

Functions and indications Clears damp-heat, benefits the Gallbladder and abates jaundice. It is indicated for damp-heat or damp-cold jaundice, inhibited urination, eczema and itchy skin.

Common dosage 10-30g, or 60-90g for large dosages; appropriate dosage for external washes.

Precautions and contraindications *Yin Chen Hao* is contraindicated for patients with a generalized yellowish skin colour due to Blood deficiency.

Comparison of functions

1. Both *Yin Chen Hao* (Herba Artemisiae Scopariae) and *Che Qian Zi* (Semen Plantaginis) have the functions of clearing heat and dispelling dampness. However, *Yin Chen Hao* tends to clear damp-heat in the Liver and Gallbladder and is more effective in abating jaundice, whereas *Che Qian Zi* is more effective in clearing Heat in the Liver and Lungs and can concurrently stop coughing and dispel Phlegm.
2. Both *Yin Chen Hao* (Herba Artemisiae Scopariae) and *Qing Hao* (Herba Artemisiae Chinghao) can clear damp-heat and are used for damp-warmth and summerheat-warmth patterns. *Yin Chen Hao* is a key herb for abating jaundice. *Qing Hao* treats taxation fever due to steaming bone disorder and drains summerheat-heat; it is commonly used for the treatment of tidal fever due to steaming bone disorder, fever and chills due to malaria, and vigorous fever due to an invasion of summerheat-warmth.

Modern research

1. Decoctions of *Yin Chen Hao* can protect the liver and soothe the gallbladder.[40, 41]
2. Decoctions of *Yin Chen Hao* inhibited Staphylococcus aureus, Corynebacterium diphtheriae, Pseudomonas aeruginosa and Escherichia coli *in vitro*.[42]
3. Lowers blood pressure, reduces the level of blood lipids.[43]
4. Abates fever and inhibits inflammation, strengthens the immune function.[44, 45]

Combinations and applications

Functions	Combinations	Applications
Clearing damp-heat, benefiting the Gallbladder and abating jaundice	*Zhi Zi* (Fructus Gardeniae Jasminoidis) *Huang Bai* (Cortex Phellodendri) *Da Huang* (Radix et Rhizoma Rhei) *Che Qian Zi* (Semen Plantaginis)	Damp-heat jaundice (Yang-type jaundice) with fullness in the abdomen and constipation

Fu Zi (Radix Lateralis Aconiti Carmichaeli Praeparata) (see notes on legal status) *Gan Jiang* (Rhizoma Zingiberis Officinalis) *Bai Zhu* (Rhizoma Atractylodis Macrocephalae) *Ze Xie* (Rhizoma Alismatis Orientalis)	Damp-cold jaundice (Yin-type jaundice) with a dull skin
Guang Huo Xiang (Herba Pogostemi) *Bai Dou Kou* (Fructus Amomi Kravanh) *Tong Cao* (Medulla Tetrapanacis Papyriferi) *Hou Po* (Cortex Magnoliae Officinalis)	The initial stage of damp-warm diseases, slight fever, nausea and oppression in the chest
Huang Bai (Cortex Phellodendri) *Di Fu Zi* (Fructus Kochiae Scopariae) *Tu Fu Ling* (Rhizoma Smilacis Glabrae)	Itchy skin, eczema, damp sores

Note: A decoction of *Yin Chen Hao* can be used on its own as an external wash to treat damp sores and itchy skin.

Jin Qian Cao 金钱草 (Lysimachia, Herba Lysimachiae)

Jin Qian Cao is the whole plant of *Lysimachia christinae* Hance, family Primulaceae.

Main ingredients *Jin Qian Cao* contains flavones, glucosides, tannins, volatile oils, amino acids, choline, potassium chloride and lactone.

Properties Taste: sweet and bland; nature: neutral.

Channels entered Liver, Gallbladder, Kidney and Bladder.

Functions and indications Promotes urination and frees Lin syndrome, benefits the Gallbladder and expels stones, relieves toxicity and disperses swelling. It is indicated for stone Lin syndrome, heat Lin syndrome, damp-heat jaundice, obstinate sores, urinary urgency and painful urination, yellow vaginal discharge, and snake bites.

Common dosage 30-60g, or double the dosage of the fresh herb; for external application, pound the fresh herb into a paste.

Comparison of functions *Jin Qian Cao* (Herba Lysimachiae), *Hai Jin Sha* (Spora Lygodii Japonici), *Shi Wei* (Folium Pyrrosiae) and *Bi Xie* (Rhizoma Dioscoreae Hypoglaucae seu Septemlobae) can all promote urination and free Lin syndrome to treat various types of Lin syndrome. *Hai Jin Sha* clears damp-heat in the Small Intestine and Bladder and is especially suitable for stone Lin syndrome. Since *Shi Wei* can cool the Blood and stop bleeding, it is often used for blood and heat Lin syndromes; it also clears the Lungs to stop coughing. *Bi Xie* is used more for turbid Lin syndrome, as it can separate the clear and the turbid; it can also treat wind-damp Bi syndrome. *Jin Qian Cao* is also highly suitable for stone Lin syndrome; in addition, it can relieve toxicity and disperse swelling.

Modern research

1. Soothes the gallbladder and protects the liver.[46]
2. Inhibits inflammation.[47]
3. Reduces the level of blood lipids.[48]
4. Stops bleeding.[49]

Combinations and applications

Functions	Combinations	Applications
Promoting urination and freeing Lin syndrome	*Che Qian Zi* (Semen Plantaginis) *Mu Tong* (Caulis Mutong) (see notes on legal status) *Dong Kui Zi* (Semen Malvae Verticillatae)	Heat Lin syndrome, urinary urgency and painful urination
	Hua Shi (Talcum) *Hai Jin Sha* (Spora Lygodii Japonici) *Che Qian Zi* (Semen Plantaginis)	Stone Lin syndrome
Benefiting the Gallbladder and expelling stones	*Yin Chen Hao* (Herba Artemisiae Scopariae) *Zhi Zi* (Fructus Gardeniae Jasminoidis)	Damp-heat jaundice
	Pu Gong Ying (Herba Taraxaci cum Radice) *Hu Zhang* (Radix et Rhizoma Polygoni Cuspidati)	Stones in the urinary system
	Shi Wei (Folium Pyrrosiae) *Fu Ling* (Sclerotium Poriae Cocos) *Niu Xi* (Radix Achyranthis Bidentatae)	Stones in the biliary tract and the urethra
	Huang Bai (Cortex Phellodendri) *Mu Tong* (Caulis Mutong) (see notes on legal status)	Yellow vaginal discharge due to damp-heat pouring down
Relieving toxicity and dispersing swelling	*Bai Hua She She Cao* (Herba Hedyotidis Diffusae)	Snake bites, obstinate swollen and toxic sores, swollen boils

Hu Zhang 虎杖
(Giant knotweed root and rhizome, Radix et Rhizoma Polygoni Cuspidati)

Hu Zhang is the root and rhizome of *Polygonum cuspidatum* Sieb. et Zucc., family Polygonaceae.

Main ingredients *Hu Zhang* contains emodin, chrysophanol, rheic acid, physcion and polydatin.

Properties Taste: bitter; nature: cold.

Channels entered Liver, Gallbladder and Lung.

Functions and indications Dispels wind and promotes the elimination of dampness, clears heat and frees Lin syndrome, quickens the Blood and frees menstruation, transforms Phlegm and stops coughing. It is indicated for damp-heat jaundice, turbid Lin syndrome, vaginal discharge, pain in the sinews and bones due to wind-damp, menstrual block, retention of lochia, and knocks and falls.

Common dosage 10-30g; appropriate dosage for external application.

Precautions and contraindications *Hu Zhang* is contraindicated during pregnancy.

Toxicity *Hu Zhang* and its preparations can give rise to very slight side-effects. Oral administration can cause a reaction in the digestive tract with such symptoms as dry mouth, a bitter taste in the mouth, nausea, vomiting, pain in the abdomen and diarrhoea. External application does not have a stimulatory effect, but occasionally induces aversion to cold.

Modern research

1. Protects the functions of the liver.[50]
2. Has an anti-viral effect, inhibits hepatitis B-type virus.[51, 52]
3. Inhibits carcinoma.[53]
4. Decoctions of *Hu Zhang* inhibited various bacteria *in vitro*, including Staphylococcus aureus, Escherichia coli, Pseudomonas aeruginosa and Proteus vulgaris.[54]

Combinations and applications

Functions	Combinations	Applications
Dispelling wind and promoting the elimination of dampness	*Niu Xi* (Radix Achyranthis Bidentatae) *Fang Feng* (Radix Ledebouriellae Divaricatae) *Mu Gua* (Fructus Chaenomelis) *Gui Zhi* (Ramulus Cinnamomi Cassiae)	Pain in the sinews and bones due to wind-damp, numbness of the limbs
	Yin Chen Hao (Herba Artemisiae Scopariae) *Zhi Zi* (Fructus Gardeniae Jasminoidis)	Damp-heat jaundice
Clearing heat and freeing Lin syndrome	*Jin Qian Cao* (Herba Lysimachiae) *Chai Hu* (Radix Bupleuri)	Stones in the urinary or biliary systems
	Huang Bai (Cortex Phellodendri) *Yi Yi Ren* (Semen Coicis Lachrymajobi) *Bi Xie* (Rhizoma Dioscoreae Hypoglaucae seu Septemlobae)	Turbid Lin syndrome and vaginal discharge due to damp-heat in the Lower Jiao
Quickening the Blood and freeing menstruation	*Tao Ren* (Semen Persicae) *Hong Hua* (Flos Carthami Tinctorii) *Niu Xi* (Radix Achyranthis Bidentatae) *Tu Gua Ren* (Semen Trichosanthis Cucumeroidis)	Menstrual block and painful menstruation due to Blood stasis
	Ru Xiang (Gummi Olibanum) *Mo Yao* (Myrrha)	Knocks and falls, pain due to Blood stasis and stagnation
Transforming Phlegm and stopping coughing	*Huang Qin* (Radix Scutellariae Baicalensis) *Xing Ren* (Semen Pruni Armeniacae) *Pi Pa Ye* (Folium Eriobotryae Japonicae) (or used alone)	Cough due to Lung-heat

Note: *Hu Zhang* can also be used on its own internally as a decoction or ground for external application to treat swollen abscesses and the toxins of snake bites.

Modern research references

1. Lu Ding et al., *Zhong Guo Yi Xue Ke Xue Yuan Xue Bao* [Journal of the Chinese Academy of Medical Science] 10, 8 (1988): 194.
2. Chen Chunxia, *Zhong Cao Yao* [Journal of Chinese Herbs] 15, 4 (1985): 40.
3. Song Fangji et al., *Xin Yi Yao Xue Za Zhi* [New Medicine and Pharmacology Journal] 6 (1979): 61.
4. Xu Jin et al., *Zhong Guo Yi Xue Ke Xue Yuan Xue Bao* [Journal of the Chinese Academy of Medical Science] 10, 1 (1988): 45.
5. Lu Ding et al., *Zhong Guo Yi Xue Ke Xue Yuan Xue Bao* 9, 6 (1987): 433.
6. Cao Qiaoli et al., *Di Yi Jun Yi Da Xue Xue Bao* [Journal of First Military Medical University] 11, 3 (1991): 263.

7. Long Zhenzhou, *Zhong Hua Wei Sheng Wu He Mian Yi Za Zhi* [Chinese Micro-organism and Immunization Journal] 5, 5 (1985): 280.
8. He Xingdong et al., *Lin Chuang Zhong Yao Shou Ce* [Clinical Handbook of Chinese Materia Medica] (Beijing: People's Medical Publishing House, 1998), 126.
9. Lei Zaiquan and Zhang Tingmo, *Zhong Hua Lin Chuang Zhong Yao Xue* [Chinese Clinical Materia Medica] (Beijing: People's Medical Publishing House, 1998), 839.
10. He Xingdong et al., *Lin Chuang Zhong Yao Shou Ce*, 125.
11. Wang Liwen et al., *Yao Xue Xue Bao* [Pharmacology Journal] 11, 12 (1964): 815.
12. Yan Shuchang et al., *Zhong Xi Yi Jie He Za Zhi* [Journal of Integrated TCM and Western Medicine], special issue on basic theory research (1988): 30, 126.
13. Sha Jingmei et al., *Yao Xue Tong Bao* [Pharmacology Bulletin] 20, 2 (1985): 74.
14. He Xingdong et al., *Lin Chuang Zhong Yao Shou Ce*, 136.
15. Jiangsu New Medical College, *Zhong Yao Da Ci Dian* [Dictionary of Chinese Materia Medica], volume 1 (Shanghai: Shanghai People's Publishing House, 1977), 401.
16. Lu Xianghua, *Yao Xue Xue Bao* [Pharmacology Journal] 13, 6 (1966): 454.
17. Xuzhou Medical College, *Xin Yi Xue Zi Liao* [New Medical Documents] 1 (1971): 27.
18. Lei Zaiquan and Zhang Tingmo, *Zhong Hua Lin Chuang Zhong Yao Xue*, 866.
19. He Xingdong et al., *Lin Chuang Zhong Yao Shou Ce*, 128.
20. Y. Johji et al., *Chem Pharm Bull* 27, 6 (1979): 1464.
21. Wu Songhan, *Jiang Su Zhong Yi Za Zhi* [Jiangsu Journal of Traditional Chinese Medicine] 10 (1964): 12.
22. Zhu Tianzhong et al., *Zhong Yao Tong Bao* [Bulletin of Chinese Materia Medica] 12, 10 (1987): 55.
23. Wei Taqing, *Guang Xi Zhong Yi Yao* [Guangxi Journal of Traditional Chinese Medicine and Materia Medica] 1 (1981): 33.
24. Li Qing, *Zhong Yi Za Zhi* [Journal of Traditional Chinese Medicine] 38, 7 (1997): 420.
25. Hong Yongsen et al., *Zhe Jiang Zhong Yi Za Zhi* [Zhejiang Journal of Traditional Chinese Medicine] 8, 2 (1965): 32.
26. He Xingdong et al., *Lin Chuang Zhong Yao Shou Ce*, 132.
27. Lei Zaiquan and Zhang Tingmo, *Zhong Hua Lin Chuang Zhong Yao Xue*, 871.
28. He Xingdong et al., *Lin Chuang Zhong Yao Shou Ce*, 130.
29. Wang Liwen et al., *Zhong Cao Yao* [Journal of Chinese Herbs] 5 (1980): 272.
30. Wu Baojie, *Pharmacology of Chinese Herbal Medicine* (Beijing: People's Medical Publishing House, 1983), 185.
31. He Xingdong et al., *Lin Chuang Zhong Yao Shou Ce*, 138.
32. Lei Zaiquan and Zhang Tingmo, *Zhong Hua Lin Chuang Zhong Yao Xue*, 882.
33. Tracheitis Group of Shanghai No. 1 Medical College, *Yi Yao Gong Ye* [Medical and Pharmaceutical Industry Journal] 6 (1973): 1.
34. Zhao Yunhua, *Zhong Xi Yi Jie He Za Zhi* [Journal of Integrated TCM and Western Medicine] 5, 9 (1985): 503.
35. He Xingdong et al., *Lin Chuang Zhong Yao Shou Ce*, 134.
36. Lei Zaiquan and Zhang Tingmo, *Zhong Hua Lin Chuang Zhong Yao Xue*, 873.
37. Li Guancui et al., *Zhong Guo Yi Xue Ke Xue Yuan Lun Wen Zhai Yao* [Digest of Chinese Academy of Medical Science Discussion Papers] (1956): 70.
38. Rao Manren et al., *Shanghai Di Yi Yi Xue Yuan Xue Bao* [Journal of Shanghai No. 1 Medical College] 1 (1958): 59.
39. Wang Benxian, *Xin Bian Zhong Yao Xue Ci Dian* [New Dictionary of Chinese Materia Medica] (Tianjin: Tianjin Science and Technology Publishing House, 1996), 273.
40. Han Dewu et al., *Zhong Cao Yao Tong Xun* [Chinese Herbs Newsletter] 8 (1976): 23.
41. Zhao Junhong et al., *Nan Jing Yi Xue Yuan Xue Bao* [Journal of Nanjing Medical College] 8, 4 (1992): 221.
42. Cheng Hai et al., *Xin Yi Xue* [New Journal of Medicine] 8 (1970): 35.
43. Yuan Feng, *An Hui Yi Xue Yuan Xue Bao* [Journal of Anhui Medical College] 2 (1976): 68.
44. Wan Raode et al., *Yao Xue Tong Bao* [Pharmacology Bulletin] 22, 10 (1987): 590.
45. Xu Qiang, *Guo Wai Yi Xue – Zhong Yi Zhong Yao Fen Ce* [Foreign Medicine – TCM Fascicule] 11, 2 (1989): 59.
46. Shi Jingzhen et al., *Zhong Yao Yao Li Yu Lin Chuang* [Pharmacology and Clinical Application of Chinese Materia Medica] 6, 1 (1990): 33.
47. Liu Jie et al., *Zhong Guo Yao Li Xue Bao* [Chinese Journal of Pharmacology] 9, 5 (1988): 395.
48. Lu Zhenchu et al., *Jiang Su Sheng Zhong Yao Yan Jiu Suo Suo Kan* [Internal Journal of Jiangsu Chinese Materia Medica Research Institute] (1985): 215.
49. Nan Yunsheng et al., *Zhong Cheng Yao* [Journal of Chinese Medicinal Preparations] 11, 8 (1989): 17.
50. Yan Shunqin, *Guo Wai Yi Xue – Zhong Yi Zhong Yao Fen Ce* [Foreign Medicine – TCM Fascicule] 4 (1984): 52.
51. Zhou Jinhuang et al., *Pharmacology of Chinese Materia Medica* (Shanghai: Shanghai Science and Technology Publishing House, 1986), 196.
52. Infectious Diseases Group of Internal Medicine Dept., No. 2 Hospital of Chongqing Medical College, *Zhong Hua Nei Ke Za Zhi* [Chinese Journal of Internal Medicine] 3 (1976): 192.

53. Fu Naiwu et al., *Zhong Yao Yao Li Yu Lin Chuang* [Pharmacology and Clinical Application of Chinese Materia Medica] 10, 2 (1994): 13.

54. Zhang Yuhua (translator), *Guo Wai Yi Xue – Zhi Wu Yao Fen Ce* [Foreign Medicine – Herbs Fascicule] 3, 2 (1982): 24.

Chapter 7

Herbs for warming the interior

温里药

Herbs for warming the interior

Most of the herbs for warming the interior are acrid in taste and warm or hot in nature. They have the functions of warming the interior and dissipating cold, returning Yang and stemming counterflow (especially useful for weak patients with Yang collapse), and warming the channels and alleviating pain by promoting the movement of Qi.

These herbs are used to treat interior cold patterns manifesting as vomiting, diarrhoea, cold and pain in the abdomen, a pale complexion, cold limbs, reduced appetite, white tongue fur, and a sunken, slow pulse due to external cold pathogenic factors attacking the body over a long period; they also treat primary Yang depletion patterns manifesting as sweating, chills and fatigue, cold mouth and nose, watery diarrhoea with non-transformation of food, cold limbs, and a weak pulse due to exhaustion of the functions of the Zang-Fu organs.

Herbs for warming the interior produce different effects depending on the main channel or channels which they enter:

1. Herbs which mainly enter the Spleen and Stomach channels can warm the Middle Jiao, dissipate cold and alleviate pain; they are used to treat Spleen and Stomach deficiency-cold and cold affecting the Spleen and Stomach, where these patterns manifest as cold and pain in the stomach and abdomen, vomiting and diarrhoea, and a pale tongue with white fur.
2. Herbs which mainly enter the Lung channel can warm the Lungs and transform fluids to treat Lung-cold Phlegm-fluid patterns manifesting as Phlegm rale, coughing and wheezing, thin, clear and white sputum, and a pale tongue with white fur.
3. Herbs which mainly enter the Liver channel can warm the Liver, dissipate cold and alleviate pain and are used to treat patterns of cold affecting the Liver channel, manifesting as pain in the lower abdomen, pain due to cold Shan disorders and reverting Yin headache.
4. Herbs which mainly enter the Kidney channel can warm the Kidneys and reinforce Yang to treat patterns with insufficiency of Kidney Yang manifesting as impotence, cold uterus, cold and pain in the lower back and knees, frequent urination at night, seminal emission and enuresis.
5. Herbs which mainly enter the Heart and Kidney channels can warm Yang and free the network vessels to treat patterns of Yang deficiency of the Heart and Kidneys manifesting as palpitations, fearful throbbing, fear of cold, cold limbs, inhibited urination and puffy swelling of the limbs; these herbs can also return Yang and stem counterflow to treat Yang collapse with such symptoms as fear of cold with a curled-up lying posture, sweating, fatigued Spirit, cold limbs and a faint pulse verging on expiry.

Some of these herbs also have the functions of expelling wind-damp, quickening the Blood, bearing counterflow Qi downwards and killing worms and can therefore be used to treat wind-damp Bi syndrome, menstrual block and painful menstruation, vomiting and hiccups, and pain in the abdomen due to worm accumulation.

The different combinations of herbs for warming the interior are categorized below:

i. for Yang deficiency patterns of the Spleen and Kidneys, use them with herbs for warming and supplementing the Spleen and Kidneys;
ii. for vomiting and diarrhoea due to Yang deficiency of the Spleen and Stomach, use them with herbs for supplementing Qi, fortifying the Spleen and harmonizing the Stomach;
iii. for Shaoyin patterns combined with Qi deficiency, use them with herbs for supplementing Qi;
iv. for cold congealing and Qi stagnation in the Middle Jiao, use them with herbs for regulating Qi;
v. for interior cold patterns combined with an exterior pattern, use them with acrid, warm herbs for releasing the exterior;
vi. for limb joint pain due to damp-cold congealing in the channels, use them with herbs for eliminating dampness and alleviating pain.

Herbs for warming the interior are warm and dry in nature. They tend to damage Yin and reinforce fire, so they are contraindicated or should be used with caution in cases of full-heat patterns, effulgent Yin deficiency-fire, depletion of Blood and body fluids, and during pregnancy. The dosage of these herbs should be adjusted according to the climate.

Tab. 7 Herbs for warming the interior

Herb	Functions	Indications
Fu Zi (Radix Lateralis Aconiti Carmichaeli Praeparata)	Returning Yang and stemming counterflow, warming the Spleen and Kidneys to reinforce Yang, dissipating cold and alleviating pain	Yang collapse and deficiency desertion, cold limbs with a faint pulse, vomiting and diarrhoea, cold and pain in the Heart and abdomen, oedema due to Yang deficiency, wind-cold-damp Bi syndrome, impotence and frequent urination, and other obstinate cold patterns
Gan Jiang (Rhizoma Zingiberis Officinalis)	Warming the Middle Jiao and dissipating cold, warming the Lungs and transforming fluids, returning Yang and freeing the vessels	Spleen and Stomach deficiency-cold, pain in the stomach and abdomen, diarrhoea, nausea and vomiting, cold-damp Phlegm-fluids, coughing and wheezing, scant urine and oedema due to insufficiency of Kidney Yang, cold limbs
Rou Gui (Cortex Cinnamomi Cassiae)	Supplementing fire and reinforcing Yang, dissipating cold and alleviating pain, warming and freeing the channels and vessels	Insufficiency of Kidney Yang, oedema and inhibited urination due to Kidney Yang deficiency, cold limbs, cold and pain in the stomach and abdomen, infertility, menstrual block due to Yang deficiency, non-healing abscesses and sores
Wu Zhu Yu (Fructus Evodiae Rutaecarpae)	Allowing constrained Liver Qi to flow freely, bearing counterflow Qi downwards and stopping vomiting, warming the Middle Jiao, dissipating cold and alleviating pain, drying dampness	Reverting Yin headache, cold and pain in the stomach and abdomen, painful menstruation due to Yang deficiency, vomiting and acid vomiting, acid regurgitation and heartburn, early-morning diarrhoea, eczema

Hua Jiao (Pericarpium Zanthoxyli)	Warming the Middle Jiao, dissipating cold and drying dampness, killing worms and alleviating pain	Spleen and Stomach deficiency-cold, cold and pain in the stomach and abdomen with vomiting and diarrhoea, pain in the abdomen and vomiting due to roundworm
Xiao Hui Xiang (Fructus Foeniculi Vulgaris)	Dissipating cold and alleviating pain, regulating Qi and harmonizing the Stomach	Cold and pain in the lower abdomen, cold Shan disorders, unilateral sagging of the testicles with distension and pain, pain in the lumbar region due to Kidney deficiency, painful menstruation due to cold
Ding Xiang (Flos Caryophylli)	Warming the Middle Jiao and bearing counterflow Qi downwards, warming the Kidneys and reinforcing Yang, alleviating pain	Vomiting due to Stomach-cold, hiccups due to deficiency-cold, reduced appetite, diarrhoea, pain in the lower abdomen, impotence and a feeling of cold in the genitalia due to Kidney deficiency
Gao Liang Jiang (Rhizoma Alpiniae Officinari)	Warming the Middle Jiao and dissipating cold, moving Qi and alleviating pain	Cold and pain in the stomach and abdomen, vomiting, cold Shan disorders

Fu Zi 附子
(Prepared Sichuan aconite daughter root, Radix Lateralis Aconiti Carmichaeli Praeparata)

Fu Zi is the daughter root of *Aconitum carmichaeli* Debx., family Ranunculaceae.

Legal status For external application only; under the Prescription Only Medicines (Human Use) Order 1997, the internal use of this herb is illegal in the UK unless made available by a prescription from a registered doctor or dentist. Where the functions, indications, combinations and applications described below refer to internal use, they should be considered as being included for information only. In addition, when used externally, the herb cannot make up any more than 1.3% of the preparation applied.

Main ingredients *Fu Zi* contains hypaconitine, aconitine, mesaconitine, talatisamine, chuan-wubase A and B, carmichaeline, artisines, aminophenols and higenamine.

Properties Taste: acrid and sweet; nature: extremely hot; toxic.

Channels entered Heart, Kidney and Spleen.

Functions and indications Returns Yang and stems counterflow, warms the Spleen and Kidneys to reinforce Yang, dissipates cold and alleviates pain. It is indicated for Yang collapse and deficiency desertion, cold limbs with a faint pulse, vomiting and diarrhoea, cold and pain in the Heart and abdomen, oedema due to Yang deficiency, wind-cold-damp Bi syndrome, impotence and frequent urination, and other obstinate cold patterns.

Common dosage Normally 3-10g, never more than 15g. *Fu Zi* should be decocted for 30-60 minutes before adding other herbs in order to decrease its toxicity.

Precautions and contraindications

1. *Fu Zi* is contraindicated during pregnancy, or in the absence of deficiency-cold, damp-cold or Yin exuberance with Yang debilitation.
2. *Fu Zi* is incompatible with *Ban Xia* (Rhizoma Pinelliae Ternatae), *Gua Lou* (Fructus Trichosanthis), *Bei Mu* (Bulbus Fritillariae), *Bai Ji* (Rhizoma Bletillae Striatae) and *Bai Lian* (Radix Ampelopsis Japonicae), and antagonizes *Xi Jiao* (Cornu Rhinoceri).

Remarks This herb is extremely toxic; *Sheng Fu Zi* (Radix Lateralis Aconiti Carmichaeli Cruda), the raw herb, has a drastic effect and is normally only indicated for external use, whereas the processed herb, *Shu Fu Zi* (Radix Lateralis Aconiti Carmichaeli Conquita), is relatively mild. Clinically, *Fu Zi* should be decocted for at least two hours in order to decrease its toxicity when applying a large dosage (see note on *Legal status* above). Symptoms of a toxic overdose are generally manifested at an early stage as numbness of the lips and four limbs (see *Toxicity*). Traditionally, *Gan Cao* (Radix Glycyrrhizae) and *Xi Jiao* (Cornu Rhinoceri) can be used to relieve the toxicity of *Fu Zi* (for *Xi Jiao*, see notes on legal status).

Comparison of functions See *Gan Jiang* (Rhizoma Zingiberis Officinalis), *Rou Gui* (Cortex Cinnamomi Cassiae) and *Ren Shen* (Radix Ginseng).

Toxicity *Fu Zi* contains several types of relatively toxic aconitine compounds, which particularly affect the heart. The toxicity of the aconine formed after hydrolysing aconitine is considerably less. Toxicity can vary widely depending on the area in which the plant is grown. Very large dosages of the crude alkaloids contained in *Fu Zi* caused general paralysis and respiratory arrest in a number of animals. Subcutaneous injection of 0.2-0.5mg/kg of aconitine in mice resulted in death, as did oral administration of 1.0-3.0mg/kg. Toxic side-effects in humans can occur with dosages of 15-30g or oral administration of 0.2mg of aconitine. Death can occur after intake of 2-4mg of aconitine. Symptoms of overdose occur within 30 minutes to two hours, generally manifesting initially as numbness of the mouth, tongue, lips and limbs, followed by nausea, vomiting, agitation and vexation, and arrhythmia. As the difference between toxic and lethal dosages is relatively narrow, it is essential never to exceed the maximum dosage. The toxicity of *Fu Zi* can be reduced in combinations with *Gan Jiang* (Rhizoma Zingiberis Officinalis) and *Gan Cao* (Radix Glycyrrhizae). *Fu Zi* should not be used at the same time as other medicines that stimulate the central nervous system or accelerate the heart rate.

Modern research

1. Decoctions and preparations of *Fu Zi* have a cardiotonic effect;[1-3] injections of preparations of the herb inhibited arrhythmia.[4]
2. Enlarges the cardiovascular and cerebral vessels, prevents coma.[5, 6]
3. Affects the nervous system, has a tranquillizing function and alleviates pain.[7, 8]
4. Strengthens the immune function.[9]

Combinations and applications

Functions	Combinations	Applications
Returning Yang and stemming counterflow	*Gan Jiang* (Rhizoma Zingiberis Officinalis) *Zhi Gan Cao* (Radix Glycyrrhizae Praeparata)	Yang collapse patterns, manifesting as general deficiency in enduring illnesses, debilitation of Yang Qi and internal exuberance of Yin cold, or as profuse sweating, vomiting and diarrhoea
	Ren Shen (Radix Ginseng) *Long Gu* (Os Draconis) *Mu Li* (Concha Ostreae)	Incessant, profuse sweating due to Yang debilitation with exterior deficiency
Warming the Spleen and Kidneys to reinforce Yang	*Shu Di Huang* (Radix Rehmanniae Glutinosae Conquita) *Rou Gui* (Cortex Cinnamomi Cassiae) *Shan Zhu Yu* (Fructus Corni Officinalis) *Lu Jiao Jiao* (Gelatinum Cornu Cervi)	Impotence and cold uterus, infertility and sterility, cold and pain in the lumbar region and knees and frequent urination at night due to debilitation of fire at the gate of vitality and insufficiency of Kidney Yang
	Dang Shen (Radix Codonopsitis Pilosulae) *Gan Jiang* (Rhizoma Zingiberis Officinalis) *Bai Zhu* (Rhizoma Atractylodis Macrocephalae) *Wu Zhu Yu* (Fructus Evodiae Rutaecarpae)	Fatigue with a yellow facial complexion, cold limbs, pain in the abdomen and desire for warmth, and watery diarrhoea with undigested food in the stool due to insufficiency of Spleen Yang
	Bai Zhu (Rhizoma Atractylodis Macrocephalae) *Fu Ling* (Sclerotium Poriae Cocos)	Oedema and inhibited urination due to Yang deficiency
	Yin Chen Hao (Herba Artemisiae Scopariae) *Bai Zhu* (Rhizoma Atractylodis Macrocephalae) *Gan Jiang* (Rhizoma Zingiberis Officinalis)	Yin-type jaundice due to internal obstruction of cold-damp and insufficiency of Spleen Yang
	Ma Huang (Herba Ephedrae) (see notes on legal status) *Xi Xin* (Herba cum Radice Asari)	Insufficiency of Kidney Yang concurrent with externally-contracted wind-cold accompanied by fever and a sunken pulse

	Ren Shen (Radix Ginseng) *Gui Zhi* (Ramulus Cinnamomi Cassiae)	Heart palpitations and chest Bi syndrome due to Heart Yang deficiency
	Hu Tao Ren (Semen Juglandis Regiae) *Wu Wei Zi* (Fructus Schisandrae) *Dong Chong Xia Cao* (Cordyceps Sinensis) *Ren Shen* (Radix Ginseng)	Coughing and wheezing, shortness of breath, and pale tongue and weak pulse due to Kidney Yang deficiency
	Da Huang (Radix et Rhizoma Rhei)	Pain in the abdomen and constipation due to Yang deficiency and full-cold accumulation and stagnation
	Shi Jue Ming (Concha Haliotidis) *Mu Li* (Concha Ostreae)	Headache due to Yang deficiency
Dissipating cold and alleviating pain	*Ju Hong* (Pars Rubra Epicarpii Citri Erythrocarpae) *Yu Jin* (Radix Curcumae)	Severe heart pain with cold limbs
	Gui Zhi (Ramulus Cinnamomi Cassiae) *Xi Xin* (Herba cum Radice Asari) *Wei Ling Xian* (Radix Clematidis) *Bai Zhu* (Rhizoma Atractylodis Macrocephalae)	Limb joint pain, stiffness and inhibited bending and stretching due to damp-cold Bi syndrome pain, with aggravation in cold weather
	Hu Lu Ba (Semen Trigonellae Foeni-graeci)	Cold and pain in the lower abdomen and lower limbs due to exuberant cold
	Ju He (Semen Citri Reticulatae) *Chuan Lian Zi* (Fructus Meliae Toosendan)	Cold Shan disorders

Appendix

Wu Tou 乌头 (Aconite mother root, Radix Aconiti)

Wu Tou has similar properties and functions to *Fu Zi*, although *Fu Zi* is used more frequently for warming and returning Yang, *Wu Tou* for cold pain patterns. *Wu Tou* is now divided into two types:

1. *Chuan Wu* 川乌 (Sichuan aconite mother root, Radix Aconiti Carmichaeli)

Chuan Wu is the dried parent root of *Aconitum carmichaeli* Debx., family Ranunculaceae. As with *Fu Zi*, *Chuan Wu* is restricted to external use only. The functions, indications, combinations and applications described below are included for information only, insofar as they refer to internal use. *Chuan Wu* is acrid and bitter in taste, hot in nature and extremely toxic. It enters the Heart, Liver and Spleen channels. *Chuan Wu* has the functions of dispelling wind and overcoming dampness, and warming the channels and alleviating pain. It is indicated for joint pain, inhibited bending and stretching, numbness of the hands and feet, hypertonicity and pain of the sinews and vessels, chest Bi syndrome and heart pain, cold Shan disorders, and headache due to wind. The common dosage is 3-9g in decoction, or 1-2g in powder and tincture. It should be decocted for 30-60 minutes before adding other herbs. *Chuan Wu* is incompatible with *Ban Xia* (Rhizoma Pinelliae Ternatae), *Gua Lou* (Fructus Trichosanthis), *Bei Mu* (Bulbus Fritillariae), *Bai Ji* (Rhizoma Bletillae Striatae) and *Bai Lian* (Radix Ampelopsis Japonicae), and antagonizes *Xi Jiao* (Cornu Rhinoceri). It is contraindicated during pregnancy.

2. *Cao Wu* 草乌 (Wild aconite root, Radix Aconiti Kusnezoffii)

Cao Wu is the dried tuberous root of *Aconitum kusnezoffii* Reichb., family Ranunculaceae. It is similar to *Chuan Wu* (Radix Aconiti Carmichaeli) in taste, nature, functions, indications, administration, and precautions and contraindications, but is even more toxic. As a result, *Cao Wu*, like *Fu Zi* and *Chuan Wu*, is restricted to external use only. The common dosage is 1.5–4.5g.

Gan Jiang 干姜 (Dried ginger, Rhizoma Zingiberis Officinalis)

Gan Jiang is the dried rhizome of *Zingiber officinale* (Willd.) Rosc., family Zingiberaceae.

Main ingredients *Gan Jiang* contains 2% of volatile oils (including zingiberene, zingiberol, camphene, phellandrene, shogaol, gingerol, zingiberone, borneol and citral), resin, starch and amino acids.

Properties Taste: acrid; nature: hot.

Channels entered Spleen, Stomach, Heart and Lung.

Functions and indications Warms the Middle Jiao and dissipates cold, warms the Lungs and transforms fluids, returns Yang and frees the vessels. It is indicated for Spleen and Stomach deficiency-cold, pain in the stomach and abdomen, diarrhoea, nausea and vomiting, cold-damp Phlegm-fluids, coughing and wheezing, scant urine and oedema due to insufficiency of Kidney Yang, and cold limbs.

Common dosage 3–10g.

Precautions and contraindications *Gan Jiang* is contraindicated during pregnancy, in cases of Yin deficiency with internal heat, and where there is frenetic movement of hot Blood.

Remarks *Pao Jiang* (Rhizoma Zingiberis Officinalis Praeparata) is *Gan Jiang* that has been quick-fried at high temperature until the outer surface turns black (see chapter 11).

Comparison of functions *Gan Jiang* (Rhizoma Zingiberis Officinalis) and *Fu Zi* (Radix Lateralis Aconiti Carmichaeli Praeparata) are both important herbs for warming the Middle Jiao, dissipating cold and treating cold limbs. Since *Gan Jiang* mainly enters the Spleen and Stomach channels, it is effective for warming the Middle Jiao and dissipating cold as well as for fortifying and moving Spleen Yang. Although not as strong as *Fu Zi* in terms of returning Yang and stemming counterflow, *Gan Jiang* can be used in combination with it for Yang collapse patterns and for attenuating its toxicity. *Fu Zi* is a key herb for Yang collapse and deficiency desertion and is very effective in treating debilitation of fire at the gate of vitality and in reinforcing Yang. Since *Fu Zi* can dissipate cold and alleviate pain, it can be used for various pain syndromes due to cold congealing.

For additional comparisons, see *Sheng Jiang* (Rhizoma Zingiberis Officinalis Recens) and *Wu Zhu Yu* (Fructus Evodiae Rutaecarpae).

Toxicity *Gan Jiang* is relatively non-toxic; the LD_{50} of an infusion of the herb corresponds to 33.5g/kg of the raw herb (*Sheng Jiang*).

Modern research

1. Slightly stimulates the gastrointestinal tract to increase intestinal tension.[10]
2. Acetic and aqueous extracts of *Gan Jiang* have an obvious effect in alleviating pain and inhibiting inflammation.[11]

Combinations and applications

Functions	Combinations	Applications
Warming the Middle Jiao and dissipating cold	*Dang Shen* (Radix Codonopsitis Pilosulae) *Huang Qi* (Radix Astragali seu Hedysari) *Bai Zhu* (Rhizoma Atractylodis Macrocephalae) *Bai Shao* (Radix Paeoniae Lactiflorae) *Gan Cao* (Radix Glycyrrhizae)	Spleen and Stomach deficiency-cold with diarrhoea and pain in the stomach and abdomen accompanied by a desire for warmth and pressure
	Huang Lian (Rhizoma Coptidis) *Ban Xia* (Rhizoma Pinelliae Ternatae) *Dang Shen* (Radix Codonopsitis Pilosulae)	Heat in the chest and cold in the stomach, vexation, oppression and discomfort in the chest, pain in the abdomen
	Gao Liang Jiang (Rhizoma Alpiniae Officinari)	Vomiting due to Stomach-cold
	Ban Xia (Rhizoma Pinelliae Ternatae) *Chen Pi* (Pericarpium Citri Reticulatae)	Vomiting due to damp-cold obstructing the Middle Jiao
	Bai Zhu (Rhizoma Atractylodis Macrocephalae) *Fu Ling* (Sclerotium Poriae Cocos) *Ze Xie* (Rhizoma Alismatis Orientalis) *Rou Gui* (Cortex Cinnamomi Cassiae)	Scant urine and oedema due to insufficiency of Kidney Yang
Warming the Lungs and transforming fluids	*Bai Jie Zi* (Semen Sinapis Albae) *Xi Xin* (Herba cum Radice Asari) *Ban Xia* (Rhizoma Pinelliae Ternatae) *Wu Wei Zi* (Fructus Schisandrae)	Cough due to Lung-cold with copious, clear, thin sputum accompanied by wheezing and dizziness
	Wu Zhu Yu (Fructus Evodiae Rutaecarpae) *Hou Po* (Cortex Magnoliae Officinalis) *Ban Xia* (Rhizoma Pinelliae Ternatae) *Bai Zhu* (Rhizoma Atractylodis Macrocephalae)	Retching and distension in the stomach due to cold congealing in the Stomach
Returning Yang and freeing the vessels	*Fu Zi* (Radix Lateralis Aconiti Carmichaeli Praeparata) (see notes on legal status) *Gan Cao* (Radix Glycyrrhizae)	Desertion patterns, a faint pulse verging on expiry and counterflow cold of the limbs due to Yang collapse

Rou Gui 肉桂 (Cassia bark, Cortex Cinnamomi Cassiae)

Rou Gui is the bark of *Cinnamomum cassia* Presl., family Lauraceae.

Main ingredients *Rou Gui* contains 1-2% of volatile oils (mainly cinnamaldehyde), cinnamyl alcohol, cinnamyl acetate, cinnamic acid, phenylpropyl acetate and tannin.

Properties Taste: acrid and sweet; nature: hot.
Channels entered Spleen, Kidney, Heart and Liver.
Functions and indications Supplements fire and reinforces Yang, dissipates cold and alleviates pain, and warms and frees the channels and vessels. It is indicated for insufficiency of Kidney Yang, oedema and inhibited urination due to Kidney Yang deficiency, cold limbs, cold and pain in the stomach and abdomen, infertility, menstrual block due to Yang deficiency, and non-healing abscesses and sores.
Common dosage 3-6g, or 12g for large dosages; 1-3g when taken orally as powder or pills. When used in a decoction, add towards the end of the decocting process.
Precautions and contraindications *Rou Gui* is contraindicated in cases of effulgent Yin deficiency-fire, interior full-heat, or bleeding due to the frenetic movement of hot Blood, and during pregnancy. It should not be used in combination with *Chi Shi Zhi* (Halloysitum Rubrum).

Comparison of functions

1. Both *Rou Gui* (Cortex Cinnamomi Cassiae) and *Fu Zi* (Radix Lateralis Aconiti Carmichaeli Praeparata) supplement fire and reinforce Yang, and dissipate cold and alleviate pain. They are important herbs for warming the interior and dissipating cold to treat cold and pain in the lumbar region and knees. They are often used together to accentuate their effect. *Rou Gui* is less powerful than *Fu Zi* in reinforcing Yang and dissipating cold. It can enter the Xue level to warm the channels and free the vessels, while treating debilitation of fire at the gate of vitality. *Fu Zi* has a powerful and rapid action and is therefore very effective for returning Yang and stemming counterflow. It is a key herb for Yang collapse, as it supplements original Yang.
2. *Rou Gui* (Cortex Cinnamomi Cassiae) and *Gui Zhi* (Ramulus Cinnamomi Cassiae) come from the same plant, respectively the bark and the branch. Both can warm and free the channels and vessels, and dissipate cold and alleviate pain; they are used to treat wind-cold-damp Bi syndrome, menstrual block and painful menstruation. However, *Rou Gui*, acrid in taste and hot in nature, can enter the interior and is an important herb for interior cold patterns, as it can warm Heart and Kidney Yang. *Gui Zhi* has a dispersing action and acts on the exterior; it is very effective in inducing sweating and dissipating cold as well as in warming the channels in the limbs.

Toxicity Normal dosages of *Rou Gui* are generally very safe. The LD_{50} for intravenous injection of cinnamaldehyde in mice is 132mg/kg; for intraperitoneal injection, it is 610mg/kg, and for oral administration, it is 2225mg/kg. Administration of 6-18g of cassia oil to dogs can result in death, but no deaths occurred after mice were given 120g/kg of an aqueous extract of *Rou Gui* via intragastric administration. Large overdosages of the herb in humans can lead to slight nausea and vomiting, dizziness, lower blood pressure, lack of balance, pain in the abdomen and diarrhoea, and in more severe cases, to convulsions and rapid breathing.

Modern research

1. Lowers blood pressure.[12]
2. Acetic and aqueous extracts of *Rou Gui* can inhibit ulcers and alleviate pain.[13]
3. The cassia oil contained in *Rou Gui* inhibits Aspergillus niger, Proteus vulgaris, Penicillium notatum and other bacteria.[14]

Combinations and applications

Functions	Combinations	Applications
Supplementing fire and reinforcing Yang	*Fu Zi* (Radix Lateralis Aconiti Carmichaeli Praeparata) (see notes on legal status) *Shu Di Huang* (Radix Rehmanniae Glutinosae Conquita) *Shan Zhu Yu* (Fructus Corni Officinalis)	Impotence and cold uterus, cold and pain in the lumbar region and knees, frequent and profuse urination at night, seminal emission and enuresis due to debilitation of fire at the gate of vitality and insufficiency of Kidney Yang
	Shu Di Huang (Radix Rehmanniae Glutinosae Conquita) *Tu Si Zi* (Semen Cuscutae) *Rou Cong Rong* (Herba Cistanches Deserticolae) *Ba Ji Tian* (Radix Morindae Officinalis) *Gou Qi Zi* (Fructus Lycii)	Impotence and seminal cold due to insufficiency of Kidney Yang
	Fu Zi (Radix Lateralis Aconiti Carmichaeli Praeparata) (see notes on legal status) *Gan Jiang* (Rhizoma Zingiberis Officinalis) *Ren Shen* (Radix Ginseng)	Yang Qi exterior deficiency, manifesting as counterflow cold of the limbs, vomiting and diarrhoea, pain in the abdomen and shivering, with a pale tongue and a sunken and slow pulse
	Dang Gui (Radix Angelicae Sinensis) *Shu Di Huang* (Radix Rehmanniae Glutinosae Conquita) *Chuan Xiong* (Rhizoma Ligustici Chuanxiong) *Xiang Fu* (Rhizoma Cyperi Rotundi)	Infertility due to Yang deficiency
	Shan Yao (Rhizoma Dioscoreae Oppositae) *Mu Dan Pi* (Cortex Moutan Radicis) *Fu Ling* (Sclerotium Poriae Cocos) *Ze Xie* (Rhizoma Alismatis Orientalis)	Oedema and inhibited urination due to Kidney Yang deficiency
Dissipating cold and alleviating pain	*Dang Gui* (Radix Angelicae Sinensis) *Chuan Xiong* (Rhizoma Ligustici Chuanxiong) *Xiao Hui Xiang* (Fructus Foeniculi Vulgaris)	Painful menstruation and menstrual block due to cold congealing and Blood stagnation with deficiency-cold in the Chong and Ren vessels
	Gan Jiang (Rhizoma Zingiberis Officinalis) *Bai Shao* (Radix Paeoniae Lactiflorae) *Wu Zhu Yu* (Fructus Evodiae Rutaecarpae) *Wu Yao* (Radix Linderae Strychnifoliae)	Cold and pain in the stomach and abdomen, cold hands and feet, and a sunken and slow pulse due to Yang deficiency of the Spleen and Kidneys
	Du Huo (Radix Angelicae Pubescentis) *Sang Ji Sheng* (Ramulus Loranthi) *Du Zhong* (Cortex Eucommiae Ulmoidis)	Wind-cold-damp Bi syndrome, pain in the lumbar region and knees, lack of strength in the legs and feet, fear of cold and liking for warmth with white tongue fur and a slow pulse due to Liver and Kidney deficiency

Warming and freeing the channels and vessels	*Shu Di Huang* (Radix Rehmanniae Glutinosae Conquita) *Lu Jiao Jiao* (Gelatinum Cornu Cervi) *Bai Jie Zi* (Semen Sinapis Albae)	Yin abscesses manifesting as swelling of the affected region with no change in colour or sensation of heat
	Huang Qi (Radix Astragali seu Hedysari) *Bai Zhu* (Rhizoma Atractylodis Macrocephalae) *Dang Gui* (Radix Angelicae Sinensis) *Chuan Xiong* (Rhizoma Ligustici Chuanxiong)	Non-healing abscesses and sores

Note: Small amounts of *Rou Gui* can be added to prescriptions for supplementing Qi and boosting the Blood in order to warm and move Yang Qi and stimulate the generation of Qi and Blood in patients with insufficiency of Qi and Blood as a result of general deficiency in enduring illnesses.

Wu Zhu Yu 吴茱萸 (Evodia fruit, Fructus Evodiae Rutaecarpae)

Wu Zhu Yu is the fruit of *Evodia rutaecarpa* (Juss.) Benth., *E. rutaecarpa* (Juss.) Benth. var. *officinalis* (Dode) Huang or *E. rutaecarpa* (Juss.) Benth. var. *bodinieri* (Dode) Huang, family Rutaceae.

Main ingredients *Wu Zhu Yu* contains 0.4% of volatile oils (including evoden, ocimene, myrcene, evodin and evodol), alkaloids (including evodiamine, rutaecarpine, wuchuyine, hydroxyevodiamine and evocarpine), gushuynic acid, evodinone, evogin and rutaevin.

Properties Taste: acrid and bitter; nature: hot; slightly toxic.

Channels entered Liver, Spleen, Stomach and Kidney.

Functions and indications Allows constrained Liver Qi to flow freely, bears counterflow Qi downwards and stops vomiting, warms the Middle Jiao, dissipates cold and alleviates pain, and dries dampness. It is indicated for reverting Yin headache, cold and pain in the stomach and abdomen, painful menstruation due to Yang deficiency, vomiting and acid vomiting, acid regurgitation and heartburn, early-morning diarrhoea, and eczema.

Common dosage 3-10g; appropriate dosage for external application.

Precautions and contraindications

1. As *Wu Zhu Yu* is acrid, hot and extremely dry in nature, it easily damages Qi and stirs fire. It should not be used over a long period or in large dosages.
2. *Wu Zhu Yu* is contraindicated in cases of Yin deficiency with heat signs and should be used with caution during pregnancy.

Comparison of functions Both *Wu Zhu Yu* (Fructus Evodiae Rutaecarpae) and *Gan Jiang* (Rhizoma Zingiberis Officinalis) can warm the Middle Jiao, dissipate cold and alleviate pain. However, *Wu Zhu Yu* enters the Liver channel and acts on the Middle and Lower Jiao. It is an important herb for warming and dissipating cold stagnation in the Liver channel, bearing counterflow Qi downwards and drying dampness. *Gan Jiang* acts on the Upper and Middle Jiao and is a key herb for warming the Middle Jiao and dissipating cold. Other functions include returning Yang and freeing the vessels, and warming the Lungs to transform fluids.

Toxicity The toxicity of evoxine, an alkaloid extracted from another type of *Wu Zhu Yu* (*Evodia xanthoxyolides* F. Muell) is relatively low, with an LD_{50} for subcutaneous and intravenous injection in mice of 705mg/kg and 135mg/kg respectively.

Large dosages of *Wu Zhu Yu* can stimulate the central nervous system and lead to visual disturbances. The main symptoms of overdose include vomiting, pain in the abdomen, diarrhoea, higher blood pressure, hallucinations, hair loss and spontaneous abortion. There have been very few clinical reports of overdose, with only one report of oral administration of 30g of the herb causing toxic side-effects.

Modern research

1. The small intestine is stimulated by a low-concentration decoction of the herb and inhibited by a highly-concentrated decoction.[15, 16]
2. Inhibits haematoblastic concentration.[17, 18]
3. Preparations of *Wu Zhu Yu* can raise body temperature.[19]

Combinations and applications

Functions	Combinations	Applications
Allowing constrained Liver Qi to flow freely, bearing counterflow Qi downwards and stopping vomiting	*Chai Hu* (Radix Bupleuri) *Yu Jin* (Radix Curcumae) *Chuan Lian Zi* (Fructus Meliae Toosendan) *Dai Zhe Shi* (Haematitum)	Liver-Stomach disharmony, vomiting and acid vomiting, distension in the stomach and abdomen, belching
	Huang Lian (Rhizoma Coptidis) *Zhu Ru* (Caulis Bambusae in Taeniis) *Gua Lou* (Fructus Trichosanthis)	Vomiting and acid regurgitation, dry mouth and pain in the hypochondrium due to Liver depression transforming into fire and Liver-Stomach disharmony
	Dang Shen (Radix Codonopsitis Pilosulae) *Sheng Jiang* (Rhizoma Zingiberis Officinalis Recens) *Da Zao* (Fructus Ziziphi Jujubae)	Reverting Yin headache or vomiting due to Stomach-cold
Warming the Middle Jiao, dissipating cold and alleviating pain	*Sheng Jiang* (Rhizoma Zingiberis Officinalis Recens) *Ban Xia* (Rhizoma Pinelliae Ternatae) *Sha Ren* (Fructus Amomi) *Gao Liang Jiang* (Rhizoma Alpiniae Officinari)	Cold and pain in the stomach and abdomen, vomiting and acid regurgitation due to deficiency-cold in the Middle Jiao
	Chuan Xiong (Rhizoma Ligustici Chuanxiong) *Xiang Fu* (Rhizoma Cyperi Rotundi) *Xiao Hui Xiang* (Fructus Foeniculi Vulgaris) *Ai Ye* (Folium Artemisiae Argyi)	Painful menstruation due to cold with scant, dark blood
	Wu Yao (Radix Linderae Strychnifoliae) *Qing Pi* (Pericarpium Citri Reticulatae Viride) *Rou Gui* (Cortex Cinnamomi Cassiae) *Li Zhi He* (Semen Litchi Chinensis)	Cold Shan disorders, pain in the testicles

	Bu Gu Zhi (Fructus Psoraleae Corylifoliae) *Wu Wei Zi* (Fructus Schisandrae) *Rou Dou Kou* (Semen Myristicae Fragrantis)	Early-morning diarrhoea due to Yang deficiency of the Spleen and Kidneys
	Mu Gua (Fructus Chaenomelis)	Leg Qi pain with distension in the abdomen
Drying dampness (external use)	*Hai Piao Xiao* (Os Sepiae seu Sepiellae) *Liu Huang* (Sulphur)	Eczema

Note: *Wu Zhu Yu* can be ground into a powder and mixed with vinegar for application to the soles of the feet to guide fire downwards and treat mouth sores, mouth Gan and sore throat.

Hua Jiao 花椒 (Chinese prickly ash, Pericarpium Zanthoxyli)

Hua Jiao (also known as *Chuan Jiao*) is the dried pericarp of the ripe fruit of *Zanthoxylum schinifolium* Sieb. et Zucc. or *Z. bungeanum* Maxim., family Rutaceae.

Main ingredients

1. *Zanthoxylum bungeanum* contains volatile oils, including limonene, citronellal and citronellol xanthoxylin. The husk of the fruit also contains the volatile oils kokusaginine, skimmianine, haplopine and herniarin.
2. *Zanthoxylum schinifolium* (also known as *Qing Jiao*) contains volatile oils including estragol, methylchavicol, geraniol and bergapten. The husk of the fruit contains bergapten, the bark of the root contains skimmianine and berberine.

Properties Taste: acrid; nature: hot; slightly toxic.

Channels entered Spleen, Stomach and Kidney.

Functions and indications Warms the Middle Jiao, dissipates cold and dries dampness, kills worms and alleviates pain. It is indicated for Spleen and Stomach deficiency-cold, cold and pain in the stomach and abdomen with vomiting and diarrhoea, and pain in the abdomen and vomiting due to roundworm.

Common dosage 2-5g; appropriate dosage for external application.

Precautions and contraindications

1. *Hua Jiao* is contraindicated for patients with effulgent Yin deficiency-fire.
2. *Hua Jiao* should be used with caution during pregnancy.

Remarks *Hua Jiao* acts on the Middle Jiao and is frequently used for warming the Middle Jiao to alleviate pain. It is very effective for pain in the abdomen due to deficiency-cold or full-cold patterns.

Toxicity The minimum lethal dose for intravenous injection of *Hua Jiao* in rabbits is 50mg/kg; the LD_{50} for intraperitoneal or intravenous injection in mice of the water-soluble alkaloids contained in *Hua Jiao* is 19.85mg/kg and 3.61mg/kg respectively. The main cause of toxic symptoms is overdosage, which can produce such side-effects as nausea, vomiting, dry mouth and dizziness, and in more severe cases, convulsions, coma and respiratory difficulties. Dosage must therefore be carefully controlled.

Modern research

1. Aqueous preparations of *Hua Jiao* can have a significant inhibitory effect on gastric ulcers.[20]
2. Concentrated decoctions of *Hua Jiao* inhibited such bacteria as α- and β-haemolytic streptococci, staphylococci, pneumococci and Pseudomonas aeruginosa *in vitro*.[21]
3. Can strengthen the immune function.[22]
4. Aqueous and acetic extracts inhibit inflammation.[23]
5. Has significant pain-relieving effects.[20]
6. Can calm wheezing.[24]

Combinations and applications

Functions	Combinations	Applications
Warming the Middle Jiao, dissipating cold and drying dampness	*Gan Jiang* (Rhizoma Zingiberis Officinalis) *Ren Shen* (Radix Ginseng) *Yi Tang* (Saccharum Granorum)	Cold and pain in the stomach and abdomen, vomiting and lack of appetite due to Spleen and Stomach deficiency-cold
	Fu Zi (Radix Lateralis Aconiti Carmichaeli Praeparata) (see notes on legal status) *Gan Jiang* (Rhizoma Zingiberis Officinalis)	Pain in the abdomen and dysentery due to enduring cold
	Fu Zi (Radix Lateralis Aconiti Carmichaeli Praeparata) (see notes on legal status) *Ban Xia* (Rhizoma Pinelliae Ternatae)	Cold and pain in the stomach radiating to the back
	Cang Zhu (Rhizoma Atractylodis) *Sha Ren* (Fructus Amomi) *Cao Dou Kou* (Semen Alpiniae Katsumadai)	Pain in the abdomen, vomiting and diarrhoea due to cold-damp encumbering the Middle Jiao
Killing worms and alleviating pain	*Wu Mei* (Fructus Pruni Mume) *Gan Jiang* (Rhizoma Zingiberis Officinalis) *Huang Bai* (Cortex Phellodendri)	Pain in the abdomen due to worm accumulation, vomiting of roundworm with vexation and oppression

Note: *Hua Jiao* is often combined with *Ku Shen* (Radix Sophorae Flavescentis), *Di Fu Zi* (Fructus Kochiae Scopariae), *Huang Bai* (Cortex Phellodendri) and *She Chuang Zi* (Fructus Cnidii Monnieri) as an external wash for itchy skin due to eczema and for pudendal itch.

Appendix

Jiao Mu 椒目 (Chinese prickly ash seed, Semen Zanthoxyli)

Jiao Mu is the seed of *Hua Jiao*. Bitter in taste and cold in nature, it enters the Spleen and Bladder channels. The dosage is 2-5g. *Jiao Mu* has the functions of promoting the movement of water, dispersing swelling and calming wheezing; it is indicated for oedema with distension and fullness, drum-like abdominal distension, water-fluids invading the Lungs, and coughing and wheezing. It can be used with *Ting Li Zi* (Semen Lepidii seu Descurainiae), *Fang Ji* (Radix Stephaniae Tetrandrae) and *Da Huang* (Radix et Rhizoma Rhei) to treat fullness in the abdomen and retention of water in the Intestines (for *Fang Ji*, see notes on legal status).

Xiao Hui Xiang 小茴香 (Common fennel seed, Fructus Foeniculi Vulgaris)

Xiao Hui Xiang is the dried fruit of *Foeniculum vulgare* Mill., family Umbelliferae.

Main ingredients *Xiao Hui Xiang* contains 3-6% of volatile oils (including anethole, limonene, fenchone, estragole, terpinene, α-pinene and myrcene), sabinene, anethole, anise aldehyde, petroselinic acid, oleic acid, linoleic acid, palmitic acid, arachidic acid, behenic acid, sitosterol and stigmasterol.

Properties Taste: acrid; nature: warm.

Channels entered Liver, Kidney, Spleen and Stomach.

Functions and indications Dissipates cold and alleviates pain, regulates Qi and harmonizes the Stomach. It is indicated for cold and pain in the lower abdomen, cold Shan disorders, unilateral sagging of the testicles with distension and pain, pain in the lumbar region due to Kidney deficiency, and painful menstruation due to cold.

Common dosage 3-8g; or appropriate dosage for external application.

Precautions and contraindication *Xiao Hui Xiang* should be used with caution in cases of heat patterns or effulgent Yin deficiency-fire.

Remarks *Xiao Hui Xiang* acts on the Middle and Lower Jiao and is highly effective in dissipating cold in the Liver and Kidney channels. Its functions of warming the interior, dissipating cold and regulating Qi allow it to be used for cold congealing and Qi stagnation in the Middle and Lower Jiao.

Toxicity Alcoholic extracts of the fruit of *Xiao Hui Xiang* administered to mice did not result in any significant changes in comparison with a control group in terms of appearance, blood, sperm, weight or internal organs either in acute toxicity tests, where up to 3g/kg was given within 24 hours, or long-term toxicity tests, where 100mg/kg a day was given for 90 days. There has been one report of a patient having an allergic reaction to the smell of *Xiao Hui Xiang*.

Modern research

1. The anethole contained in *Xiao Hui Xiang* has a curare-like effect on the central nervous system.[25]
2. Promotes movement in the gastrointestinal tract and regulates the gastrointestinal function.[25]

Combinations and applications

Functions	Combinations	Applications
Dissipating cold and alleviating pain, regulating Qi and harmonizing the Stomach	*Chen Xiang* (Lignum Aquilariae Resinatum) *Chuan Lian Zi* (Fructus Meliae Toosendan) *Wu Yao* (Radix Linderae Strychnifoliae)	Cold Shan disorders manifesting as distension and pain in the lower abdomen and testicles
	Ju He (Semen Citri Reticulatae) *Shan Zha* (Fructus Crataegi)	Unilateral sagging of the testicles and distension and pain due to depression and stagnation of Liver Qi
	Wu Zhu Yu (Fructus Evodiae Rutaecarpae) *Rou Gui* (Cortex Cinnamomi Cassiae) *Gan Jiang* (Rhizoma Zingiberis Officinalis)	Cold and pain in the lower abdomen due to cold in the Liver channel
	Gao Liang Jiang (Rhizoma Alpiniae Officinari) *Xiang Fu* (Rhizoma Cyperi Rotundi)	Distension and pain in the stomach and abdomen due to Stomach-cold-induced Qi stagnation
	Rou Gui (Cortex Cinnamomi Cassiae) *Ai Ye* (Folium Artemisiae Argyi) *Yan Hu Suo* (Rhizoma Corydalis Yanhusuo)	Painful menstruation due to cold
	Zhi Ke (Fructus Citri Aurantii)	Pain in the hypochondrium

Functions	Combinations	Applications
	Rou Gui (Cortex Cinnamomi Cassiae) *Bu Gu Zhi* (Fructus Psoraleae Corylifoliae) *Gou Ji* (Rhizoma Cibotii Barometz) (see notes on legal status)	Pain in the lumbar region with aversion to cold due to Kidney deficiency

Note: *Xiao Hui Xiang* can be fried until hot and wrapped in a cloth before applying the package to the lower abdomen to alleviate pain due to cold.

Ding Xiang 丁香
(Cloves, Flos Caryophylli)

Ding Xiang is the dried flower-bud of *Eugenia caryophyllata* Thunb., family Myrtaceae.

Main ingredients *Ding Xiang* contains 16-19% of volatile oils (mainly eugenol, caryophyllene and acetyl eugenol) and small amounts of methyl-n-amylketone, chavicol, benzaldehyde, oleanolic acid, rhamnetin and kaempferol.

Properties Taste: acrid; nature: warm.

Channels entered Spleen, Stomach and Kidney.

Functions and indications Warms the Middle Jiao and bears counterflow Qi downwards, warms the Kidneys and reinforces Yang, and alleviates pain. It is indicated for vomiting due to Stomach-cold, hiccups due to deficiency-cold, reduced appetite, diarrhoea, pain in the lower abdomen, impotence and a feeling of cold in the genitalia due to Kidney deficiency.

Common dosage 2-5g.

Precautions and contraindications

1. *Ding Xiang* is contraindicated in cases of heat patterns or internal heat due to Yin deficiency.
2. *Ding Xiang* antagonizes *Yu Jin* (Radix Curcumae).

Toxicity The LD_{50} for intraperitoneal injection in mice of a decoction of *Ding Xiang* is 1.8g/kg, that for intragastric administration of the volatile oils contained in the herb is 1.6g/kg. The main cause of toxic side-effects is overdosage of *Ding Xiang* or the volatile oils it contains. Symptoms appearing in animals included inhibited respiration, trance, numbness of the rear limbs, vomiting, urinary incontinence and blood in the urine. There are no reports of normal dosage leading to toxic symptoms in humans.

Modern research

1. Has an anaesthetic function.[26]
2. Abates fever and alleviates pain, inhibits inflammation.[27, 28]
3. A steep of *Ding Xiang* can increase the secretion of gastric liquids and the activity of pepsins.[29]
4. Inhibits pathogenic dermatophytes and kills the larvae of Toxocara canis.[30]

Combinations and applications

Functions	Combinations	Applications
Warming the Middle Jiao and bearing counterflow Qi downwards, warming the Kidneys and reinforcing Yang, alleviating pain	*Shi Di* (Calyx Diospyri Kaki) *Dang Shen* (Radix Codonopsitis Pilosulae) *Sheng Jiang* (Rhizoma Zingiberis Officinalis Recens)	Hiccups due to deficiency-cold, cold and pain in the stomach
	Ban Xia (Rhizoma Pinelliae Ternatae) *Sheng Jiang* (Rhizoma Zingiberis Officinalis Recens)	Vomiting due to Stomach-cold

	Sha Ren (Fructus Amomi) *Bai Zhu* (Rhizoma Atractylodis Macrocephalae)	Vomiting, diarrhoea and reduced appetite due to Spleen and Stomach deficiency–cold
	Fu Zi (Radix Lateralis Aconiti Carmichaeli Praeparata) (see notes on legal status) *Chuan Lian Zi* (Fructus Meliae Toosendan) *Xiao Hui Xiang* (Fructus Foeniculi Vulgaris)	Cold Shan disorders in the lower abdomen
	Ba Ji Tian (Radix Morindae Officinalis)	Impotence or cold uterus due to Kidney deficiency

Gao Liang Jiang 高良姜 (Lesser galangal rhizome, Rhizoma Alpiniae Officinari)

Gao Liang Jiang is the dried rhizome of *Alpinia officinarum* Hance, family Zingiberaceae.

Main ingredients *Gao Liang Jiang* contains 0.5-1.5% of volatile oils (including cineole, methyl cinnamate, eugenol, pinene, cadinene and galangol), galangin, kaempferide, kaempferol, quercetin, isorhamnetin, galangin-3-methylether and quercetin-3-methylether.

Properties Taste: acrid; nature: hot.

Channels entered Spleen and Stomach.

Functions and indications Warms the Middle Jiao and dissipates cold, moves Qi and alleviates pain. It is indicated for cold and pain in the stomach and abdomen, vomiting, and cold Shan disorders.

Common dosage 3-10g.

Precautions and contraindications *Gao Liang Jiang* is contraindicated in cases of Yin deficiency with heat signs.

Remarks *Gao Liang Jiang* is used for stubborn cold patterns and is similar in function to *Fu Zi* (Radix Lateralis Aconiti Carmichaeli Praeparata) and *Rou Gui* (Cortex Cinnamomi Cassiae). It is therefore particularly used for severe cold patterns in the Middle Jiao.

Toxicity The LD_{50} for intragastric administration in mice of an acetic extract of *Gao Liang Jiang* is 4.2 ± 0.4ml/kg.

Modern research

1. A non-diluted solution of a decoction of *Gao Liang Jiang* inhibited Bacillus anthracis, α- and β-haemolytic streptococci, Corynebacterium diphtheriae, pneumococci and Staphylococcus aureus in laboratory tests.[31]
2. Aqueous extracts of *Gao Liang Jiang* alleviated pain and had an obvious effect in inhibiting inflammation.[32]
3. Inhibits ulcers, soothes the gallbladder and inhibits movement in the gastrointestinal tract.[33]

Combinations and applications

Functions	Combinations	Applications
Warming the Middle Jiao and dissipating cold, moving Qi and alleviating pain	*Xiang Fu* (Rhizoma Cyperi Rotundi)	Distension and pain in the stomach and abdomen due to Stomach-cold-induced Liver depression
	Pao Jiang (Rhizoma Zingiberis Officinalis Praeparata)	Cold and pain in the stomach and abdomen due to Stomach-cold

Sheng Jiang (Rhizoma Zingiberis Officinalis Recens) *Ban Xia* (Rhizoma Pinelliae Ternatae)	Vomiting due to Stomach-cold
Dang Shen (Radix Codonopsitis Pilosulae) *Fu Ling* (Sclerotium Poriae Cocos) *Bai Zhu* (Rhizoma Atractylodis Macrocephalae)	Vomiting due to deficiency-cold
Rou Gui (Cortex Cinnamomi Cassiae) *Gan Jiang* (Rhizoma Zingiberis Officinalis) *Wu Zhu Yu* (Fructus Evodiae Rutaecarpae)	Cold and pain in the lower abdomen
Xiao Hui Xiang (Fructus Foeniculi Vulgaris) *Wu Yao* (Radix Linderae Strychnifoliae)	Cold Shan disorders due to cold congealing and Qi stagnation

Modern research references

1. Zhou Yuanpeng et al., *Zhong Xi Yi Jie He Za Zhi* [Journal of Integrated TCM and Western Medicine] 4, 1 (1984): 48.
2. Shi Shan et al., *Zhong Yi Za Zhi* [Journal of Traditional Chinese Medicine] 12 (1981): 59.
3. Ibid., 9 (1980): 67.
4. Zhu Boqing et al., *Zhong Xi Yi Jie He Za Zhi* [Journal of Integrated TCM and Western Medicine] 5, 4 (1985): 219.
5. Mou Yuqing et al., *Shou Yi Ke Ji Za Zhi* [Journal of Veterinary Medicine Science and Technology] 9 (1983): 8; 4 (1985): 256.
6. Kuang Ankun et al., *Zhong Xi Yi Jie He Za Zhi* [Journal of Integrated TCM and Western Medicine] 4, 12 (1984): 732; 6, 6 (1986): 353.
7. Zheng Ping et al., *Zhong Guo Yao Li Xue Bao* [Chinese Journal of Pharmacology] 9, 6 (1988): 481.
8. H. Hikino et al., *J Pharm Soc Jap* 99 (1979): 252.
9. Zheng Jiaju et al., *Zhong Cheng Yao Yan Jiu* [Chinese Medicinal Preparation Research] 12 (1981): 28.
10. He Xingdong et al., *Lin Chuang Zhong Yao Shou Ce* [Clinical Handbook of Chinese Materia Medica] (Beijing: People's Medical Publishing House, 1998), 144.
11. Lei Zaiquan and Zhang Tingmo, *Zhong Hua Lin Chuang Zhong Yao Xue* [Chinese Clinical Materia Medica] (Beijing: People's Medical Publishing House, 1998), 924.
12. Kuang Ankun et al., *Zhong Xi Yi Jie He Za Zhi* [Journal of Integrated TCM and Western Medicine] 8, 3 (1988): 164.
13. Zhu Ziping et al., *Zhong Guo Zhong Yao Za Zhi* [Journal of Chinese Materia Medica] 18, 9 (1993): 553.
14. Zhang Ziyang et al., *Zhong Guo Zhong Yao Za Zhi* 15, 2 (1990): 31.
15. Zhang Mingfa et al., *Zhong Yi Za Zhi* [Journal of Traditional Chinese Medicine] 25 (1984): 943.
16. Zhang Mingfa et al., *Zhong Yi Yao Xue Bao* [Journal of Traditional Chinese Medicine and Materia Medica] 3 (1988): 260.
17. Xu Qingyuan et al., *Xi Bei Yao Xue Za Zhi* [Northwest Journal of Pharmacology] 5, 2 (1990): 9.
18. Lu Enwu et al., *Zhong Xi Yi Jie He Za Zhi* [Journal of Integrated TCM and Western Medicine] 1 (1981): 101.
19. Zhang Mingfa et al., *Ji Chu Yi Xue Yu Lin Chuang* [Foundations of Medicine and Clinical Application] 12 (1992): 151.
20. Zhang Mingfa et al., *Zhong Guo Zhong Yao Za Zhi* [Journal of Chinese Materia Medica] 16 (1991): 493.
21. Lan Zhongfen et al., *Lan Zhou Yi Xue Yuan Xue Bao* [Journal of Lanzhou Medical College] 15, 1 (1989): 1.
22. Duan Jingyun et al., *Zhong Xi Yi Jie He Za Zhi* [Journal of Integrated TCM and Western Medicine] 9 (special volume) (1989): 111.
23. Yan Yingju et al., *Qing Hai Yi Xue Yuan Xue Bao* [Journal of Qinghai Medical College] 2 (1979): 25.
24. Pu Peiying et al., *Nan Jing Tie Dao Yi Xue Yuan Xue Bao* [Journal of Nanjing Railway Medical College] 9, 1 (1990): 23.
25. He Xingdong et al., *Lin Chuang Zhong Yao Shou Ce*, 153.
26. P. Brodin et al., *Archives of Oral Biology* 19 (1984): 61.
27. J. Feng et al., *Neuropharmacology* 26 (1987): 1775.

28. R.J. Safford et al., *British Journal of Dermatology* 123 (1990): 959.
29. Li Zailiu et al., *Zhong Yi Za Zhi* [Journal of Traditional Chinese Medicine] 21 (1980): 148.
30. Zhou Honghui, *Zhong Yao Cai* [Chinese Materia Medica] 13, 10 (1990): 46.
31. Jiangsu New Medical College, *Zhong Yao Da Ci Dian* [Dictionary of Chinese Materia Medica], volume 2 (Shanghai: Shanghai People's Publishing House, 1977), 1907.
32. Duan Jingyun et al., *Zhong Xi Yi Jie He Za Zhi* [Journal of Integrated TCM and Western Medicine] 9 (special volume) (1989): 111.
33. Wang Zhijun, *Sheng Li Ke Xue Jin Zhan* [Developments in Physiological Science] 15, 1 (1984): 5.

Chapter 8

Herbs for regulating Qi 理气药

Herbs for regulating Qi

Herbs for regulating Qi are mostly acrid in taste and warm in nature and are generally aromatic in flavour. They can be used to regulate the movement of Qi and are hence mainly employed for Qi stagnation patterns. They have the functions of moving Qi to alleviate pain, soothing the Liver and relieving depression, regulating Qi and loosening the chest, breaking up Qi stagnation and dispersing accumulation, and bearing counterflow Qi downwards to stop vomiting, calm wheezing and stop hiccups.

Herbs for regulating Qi in the Spleen and Stomach are mainly used for Qi stagnation in the Spleen and Stomach, distension and fullness in the stomach and abdomen, oppression in the chest or upper abdomen, vomiting, hiccups and acid vomiting, and constipation or diarrhoea.

Herbs for soothing the Liver and regulating Qi are used for Liver depression and Qi stagnation, impairment of the Liver function, distension and fullness in the stomach, chest and abdomen, pain in the abdomen due to roundworm, distension and pain in the breasts, and disorders of the menstrual cycle.

Herbs for diffusing Lung Qi are used for Lung Qi stagnation, disorders of the diffusing and downward-bearing function of the Lungs, difficulty in breathing, fullness in the chest, or coughing and wheezing.

In addition, some herbs for regulating Qi can also transform Phlegm and harmonize the Spleen and Stomach; they can be used for food accumulation as well as for coughing and wheezing.

Clinically, herbs for regulating Qi can be used in combination with other herbs selected according to the nature of the syndrome involved, as described below:

1. Indigestion due to Qi stagnation of the Spleen and Stomach: in cases of food accumulation, use herbs for moving Qi, fortifying the Spleen and harmonizing the Stomach with herbs for dispersing food accumulation; in cases with Spleen and Stomach deficiency, use them with herbs for supplementing the Spleen and Stomach and boosting Qi; in cases of damp-heat in the Middle Jiao, use them with herbs for clearing heat and drying dampness; and in cases of damp-cold encumbering the Spleen, use them with herbs for warming the Middle Jiao and transforming dampness.
2. For disorders due to Liver depression and Qi stagnation, combinations with herbs for soothing the Liver and regulating Qi are as follows: in cases of insufficiency of Liver-Blood, combine with herbs for nourishing the Blood and emolliating the Liver; in cases with stagnation of damp-heat, combine with herbs for clearing damp-heat in the Liver and Gallbladder; in cases with stagnation of cold in the Liver channel, combine with herbs for warming the Liver channel and dissipating cold; and in cases of Blood stasis, combine with herbs for quickening the Blood and dispelling stasis.
3. Disorders due to stagnation of Lung Qi: in cases of invasion by external pathogenic factors, herbs for diffusing Lung Qi, regulating Qi and loosening the chest

should be used in combination with herbs for releasing the exterior; in cases with Phlegm-damp invading the Lungs, use them with herbs for drying and transforming dampness; in cases with Phlegm-heat invading the Lungs, use them with herbs for clearing heat and dispelling Phlegm; and in cases of Lung and Kidney deficiency, use them with herbs for supplementing and boosting the Kidneys and Lungs and with herbs for hosting Qi and calming wheezing.

Most herbs for regulating Qi are warm, acrid and dry, thus tending to consume Qi and damage Yin. These herbs should therefore be used with caution in cases of Qi and Yin deficiency.

Tab. 8 Herbs for regulating Qi

Herb	Functions	Indications
Chen Pi (Pericarpium Citri Reticulatae)	Regulating Qi and fortifying the Spleen, drying dampness and transforming Phlegm	Pain, distension and fullness in the chest, stomach and abdomen, poor appetite, vomiting and hiccups, cough with copious sputum
Zhi Shi (Fructus Immaturus Citri Aurantii)	Breaking up Qi stagnation and dispersing accumulation, transforming Phlegm and eliminating focal distension	Distension in the abdomen, nausea and vomiting, constipation, dysentery, belching, chest Bi syndrome
Mu Xiang (Radix Aucklandiae Lappae)	Moving Qi and alleviating pain, allowing constrained Liver Qi to flow freely and opening depression	Distension and pain in the stomach, vomiting, diarrhoea, abdominal urgency and tenesmus, cold Shan disorders, damp-heat jaundice
Xiang Fu (Rhizoma Cyperi Rotundi)	Regulating Qi and relieving depression, adjusting menstruation and alleviating pain	Distension and fullness in the stomach and abdomen, distension and pain in the hypochondrium due to binding depression of Liver Qi, cold Shan disorders, menstrual irregularities, distension and pain in the breasts due to Liver depression and Qi stagnation
Chen Xiang (Lignum Aquilariae Resinatum)	Moving Qi and alleviating pain, warming the Middle Jiao and stopping vomiting, warming the Kidneys and hosting Qi, calming wheezing	Distension and pain in the chest and abdomen, vomiting and hiccups, a cold feeling in the Stomach due to Yang deficiency, coughing and wheezing, premature ejaculation
Qing Pi (Pericarpium Citri Reticulatae Viride)	Soothing the Liver and regulating Qi, dispersing food accumulation and transforming stagnation, promoting the movement of Qi and Blood to break up stasis	Distension and pain in the stomach or hypochondrium, food accumulation, Shan disorders, pain in the breasts
Fo Shou (Fructus Citri Sarcodactylis)	Allowing constrained Liver Qi to flow freely, regulating Qi and alleviating pain, harmonizing the Middle Jiao and transforming stagnation, fortifying the Spleen and stopping vomiting, drying dampness and transforming Phlegm	Distension and pain in the chest and hypochondrium due to Liver depression and Qi stagnation, focal distension and fullness in the stomach, indigestion, belching, cough with copious sputum

Xiang Yuan (Fructus Citri Medicae seu Wilsonii)	Allowing constrained Liver Qi to flow freely, regulating Qi and alleviating pain, harmonizing the Middle Jiao, drying dampness and transforming Phlegm	Oppression in the chest, pain in the hypochondrium, distension and pain in the stomach, cough with copious sputum
Chuan Lian Zi (Fructus Meliae Toosendan)	Soothing the Liver and regulating Qi, draining fire and alleviating pain, killing worms	Pain in the hypochondrium, pain in the stomach and abdomen, Shan disorders, roundworm
Wu Yao (Radix Linderae Strychnifoliae)	Moving Qi and alleviating pain, warming the Kidneys and dissipating cold	Oppression in the chest, pain in the hypochondrium, distension and pain in the stomach and abdomen, cold Shan disorders, pain in the lower abdomen and testicles, urinary incontinence, frequent urination
Xie Bai (Bulbus Allii Macrostemi)	Freeing Yang and dissipating lumps, moving Qi and guiding out stagnation	Obstruction of Qi in the chest, mainly manifesting as pain in the chest radiating to the back; oppression in the chest, cough with copious thin sputum, diarrhoea and dysentery
Da Fu Pi (Pericarpium Arecae Catechu)	Causing Qi to descend and loosening the Middle Jiao, promoting the movement of water and dispersing swelling	Fullness and distension in the stomach and abdomen, leg Qi, oedema
Li Zhi He (Semen Litchi Chinensis)	Regulating Qi and alleviating pain, dispelling cold and dispersing stagnation	Shan disorder pain, swollen and painful testicles, pain in the stomach, premenstrual and postpartum pain in the abdomen
Mei Gui Hua (Flos Rosae Rugosae)	Allowing constrained Liver Qi to flow freely, moving Qi and relieving depression, and regulating Qi, harmonizing the Blood and dissipating stasis	Liver-Stomach disharmony, distension and pain in the chest and abdomen, menstrual irregularities, knocks and falls

Chen Pi 陈皮 (Tangerine peel, Pericarpium Citri Reticulatae)

Chen Pi is the peel of *Citrus reticulata* Blanco or its cultivars, family Rutaceae.

Main ingredients *Chen Pi* contains volatile oils (including α-thujene and limonene), nobiletin, hesperidin, neohesperidin, tangeridin, citromitin, synephrine, carotene, cryptoxanthin, inositol, vitamin B_1 and vitamin C.

Properties Taste: bitter and acrid; nature: warm.

Channels entered Spleen and Lung.

Functions and indications Regulates Qi and fortifies the Spleen, dries dampness and transforms Phlegm. It is indicated for pain, distension and fullness in the chest, stomach and abdomen, poor appetite, vomiting and hiccups, and cough with copious sputum.

Common dosage 3-10g.

Precautions and contraindications

1. *Chen Pi* is contraindicated in cases of internal full-heat or for dry cough without sputum resulting from Yin deficiency.
2. *Chen Pi* should be used with caution where the tongue is red.

Remarks Stir-fried *Chen Pi* is neutral in nature. It has a stronger effect than raw *Chen Pi* in fortifying the Spleen, warming the Middle Jiao, moving Qi and harmonizing the Stomach; it is normally used for dampness in the Middle Jiao. Charred *Chen Pi* does not have the function of moving Qi and is used for promoting contraction and stopping bleeding.

Comparison of functions See *Qing Pi* (Pericarpium Citri Reticulatae Viride), *Fo Shou* (Fructus Citri Sarcodactylis) and *Ban Xia* (Rhizoma Pinelliae Ternatae).

Toxicity Intragastric administration to mice of 3mg/kg of a 50% decoction of fresh *Chen Pi* did not lead to any acute toxic symptoms nor did continuous administration to a variety of animals of large dosages of decoctions of the dried herb. The LD_{50} for oral administration to mice of nobiletin is 0.78g/kg (results after 24 hours). There was one report in the early 1990s of death due to perforation of the digestive tract after oral administration of *Chen Pi* juice.

Modern research

1. Decoctions of *Chen Pi* and the volatile oils contained in the herb can inhibit contraction of the intestinal muscle, promote the secretion of digestive liquids, inhibit gastric ulcers, soothe the gallbladder and dissolve gallstones.[1]
2. Alcoholic extracts of *Chen Pi* and the nobiletin contained in the herb can expand the bronchus to calm wheezing.[1]
3. Decoctions and alcoholic extracts of *Chen Pi* can stimulate the heart and raise blood pressure.[1]

Combinations and applications

Functions	Combinations	Applications
Regulating Qi and fortifying the Spleen	*Mu Xiang* (Radix Aucklandiae Lappae) (see notes on legal status) *Sha Ren* (Fructus Amomi) *Zhi Ke* (Fructus Citri Aurantii) *Jiao San Xian* (scorch-fried combination of Fructus Crataegi, Massa Fermentata and Fructus Hordei Vulgaris Germinatus)	Distension and fullness in the stomach and abdomen and poor appetite due to Qi stagnation in the Spleen and Stomach

	Dang Shen (Radix Codonopsitis Pilosulae) *Bai Zhu* (Rhizoma Atractylodis Macrocephalae) *Fu Ling* (Sclerotium Poriae Cocos)	Abdominal pain that responds to pressure, indigestion and loose stool due to Qi stagnation and Spleen deficiency
	Sheng Jiang (Rhizoma Zingiberis Officinalis Recens) *Da Zao* (Fructus Ziziphi Jujubae)	Impaired harmonious downward-bearing of Stomach Qi, nausea and vomiting
	Zhu Ru (Caulis Bambusae in Taeniis) *Ban Xia* (Rhizoma Pinelliae Ternatae)	Distension in the abdomen and hiccups due to Stomach deficiency accompanied by heat signs
	Ren Shen (Radix Ginseng) *Sheng Jiang* (Rhizoma Zingiberis Officinalis Recens)	Vomiting due to deficiency-cold
	Bai Zhu (Rhizoma Atractylodis Macrocephalae) *Fang Feng* (Radix Ledebouriellae Divaricatae) *Bai Shao* (Radix Paeoniae Lactiflorae)	Pain in the abdomen, diarrhoea and rumbling intestines due to Liver Qi exploiting the Spleen
Drying dampness and transforming Phlegm	*Cang Zhu* (Rhizoma Atractylodis) *Hou Po* (Cortex Magnoliae Officinalis) *Ban Xia* (Rhizoma Pinelliae Ternatae) *Guang Huo Xiang* (Herba Pogostemi)	Damp-cold obstructing the Spleen and Stomach, manifesting as distension and pain in the stomach and abdomen, indigestion, fatigue, loose stool and a sticky feeling in the mouth with slimy tongue fur
	Ban Xia (Rhizoma Pinelliae Ternatae) *Fu Ling* (Sclerotium Poriae Cocos)	Cough due to damp-Phlegm
	Xing Ren (Semen Pruni Armeniacae) *Bai Zhu* (Rhizoma Atractylodis Macrocephalae) *Chao Lai Fu Zi* (Semen Raphani Sativi, stir-fried)	Damp cough with copious white sputum and oppression in the chest, accompanied by white, slimy tongue fur
	Zhi Shi (Fructus Immaturus Citri Aurantii) *Sheng Jiang* (Rhizoma Zingiberis Officinalis Recens)	Chest Bi syndrome due to Phlegm-damp

Note: *Chen Pi* is also used in herbal prescriptions with supplementing herbs, notably *Shu Di Huang* (Radix Rehmanniae Glutinosae Conquita), to safeguard Stomach Qi and prevent stagnation.

Appendix

Ju He 橘核 (Tangerine pip, Semen Citri Reticulatae)

Ju He is bitter in taste and neutral in nature, and enters the Liver channel. It regulates Qi, dissipates lumps and alleviates pain, and is indicated for pain in Shan disorders, distension and pain in the testicles and lumps in the breast. The dosage is 3-10g.

Ju Luo 橘络 (Tangerine pith, Retinervus Fructus Citri Reticulatae)

Ju Luo is sweet and bitter in taste and neutral in nature, and enters the Liver and Lung channels. It moves Qi and frees the network vessels, transforms Phlegm and stops coughing; it is used to treat pain in the chest and cough due to Phlegm stagnating in the channels and network vessels. The dosage is 3-5g.

Ju Ye 橘叶 (Tangerine leaf, Folium Citri Reticulatae)

Ju Ye is acrid and bitter in taste and neutral in nature, and enters the Liver channel. It allows constrained Liver Qi to flow freely, dissipates lumps and disperses swelling, and is indicated for pain in the hypochondrium, breast abscess and lumps in the breast. The dosage is 6-10g.

Ju Hong 橘红 (Red part of tangerine peel, Pars Rubra Epicarpii Citri Erythrocarpae)

Ju Hong is acrid and bitter in taste and warm in nature, and enters the Lung, Spleen and Stomach channels. It can dry dampness and transform Phlegm, and regulate Qi and loosen the Middle Jiao; it is used to treat cough due to damp-Phlegm or cold-Phlegm, and food accumulation, nausea and vomiting, and oppression in the chest. The dosage is 3-10g.

Zhi Shi 枳实
(Immature bitter orange fruit, Fructus Immaturus Citri Aurantii)

Zhi Shi is the immature fruit of *Citrus aurantium* L. and its cultivars or *C. sinensis* Osbeck, family Rutaceae.

Main ingredients *Zhi Shi* contains hesperidin, neohesperidin, rhoifolin, naringin, lonicerin, nobiletin, synephrine, noradrenaline and vitamin C.

Properties Taste: bitter and acrid; nature: slightly cold.

Channels entered Spleen, Stomach and Large Intestine.

Functions and indications Breaks up Qi stagnation and disperses accumulation, transforms Phlegm and eliminates focal distension. It is indicated for distension in the abdomen, nausea and vomiting, constipation, dysentery, belching, and chest Bi syndrome.

Common dosage 3-10g, or 30g for large dosages; appropriate dosage for external application.

Precautions and contraindications *Zhi Shi* is contraindicated in cases of loose stool due to Qi deficiency of the Spleen and Stomach without Qi stagnation, and during pregnancy.

Toxicity *Zhi Shi* has a low level of toxicity. No severe reaction was seen 30 minutes after intravenous injection in anaesthetized dogs of up to 2g/kg of the herb. The LD_{50} for intravenous injection of *Zhi Shi* in mice is 71.8 ± 6.5g/kg.

Modern research

1. Highly-concentrated decoctions of *Zhi Shi* can inhibit the intestinal smooth muscle, whereas lower concentrations can stimulate the intestines to strengthen peristalsis.[2, 3]
2. Contracts the blood vessels, raises blood pressure and strengthens myocardial contraction.[4, 5]
3. Promotes urination.[6]

Combinations and applications

Functions	Combinations	Applications
Breaking up Qi stagnation and dispersing accumulation	*Da Huang* (Radix et Rhizoma Rhei) *Mang Xiao* (Mirabilitum) *Huang Lian* (Rhizoma Coptidis)	Distension, fullness and pain in the stomach and abdomen with accumulation and stagnation of full-heat
	Da Huang (Radix et Rhizoma Rhei) *Hou Po* (Cortex Magnoliae Officinalis)	Constipation with binding of heat due to accumulation and stagnation in the Stomach and Intestines
	Huang Qin (Radix Scutellariae Baicalensis) *Mu Xiang* (Radix Aucklandiae Lappae) (see notes on legal status) *Da Huang* (Radix et Rhizoma Rhei) *Bai Shao* (Radix Paeoniae Lactiflorae)	Damp-heat stagnation causing pain in the abdomen, dysentery and diarrhoea accompanied by abdominal urgency and tenesmus
	Shen Qu (Massa Fermentata) *Mai Ya* (Fructus Hordei Vulgaris Germinatus) *Shan Zha* (Fructus Crataegi)	Belching with a foul odour due to the accumulation of food
Transforming Phlegm and eliminating focal distension	*Dan Nan Xing* (Pulvis Arisaematis cum Felle Bovis) *Huang Lian* (Rhizoma Coptidis) *Bai Zhu* (Rhizoma Atractylodis Macrocephalae) *Gou Teng* (Ramulus Uncariae cum Uncis)	Nausea and vomiting, dizziness and yellow, slimy tongue fur due to Phlegm-heat
	Gua Lou (Fructus Trichosanthis) *Gui Zhi* (Ramulus Cinnamomi Cassiae) *Xie Bai* (Bulbus Allii Macrostemi) *Hou Po* (Cortex Magnoliae Officinalis)	Chest Bi syndrome and Phlegm obstruction binding the chest due to non-arousal of chest Yang
	Bai Zhu (Rhizoma Atractylodis Macrocephalae)	Focal distension and fullness in the abdomen after eating
	Ban Xia Qu (Massa Fermentata Pinelliae) *Hou Po* (Cortex Magnoliae Officinalis)	Focal distension and fullness below the heart, no desire to eat
	Zhi Zi (Fructus Gardeniae Jasminoidis) *Dan Dou Chi* (Semen Sojae Praeparatum)	Focal distension and oppression below the heart, fever, taxation relapse in the aftermath of an illness

Appendix

Zhi Ke 枳壳 (Ripe bitter orange fruit, Fructus Citri Aurantii)

Zhi Ke (also known by its alternative pronunciation of *Zhi Qiao*) is the ripe fruit of *Citrus aurantium* L. (family Rutaceae); its functions are similar to but milder than those of the immature fruit. It mainly enters the Spleen and Stomach channels. *Zhi Ke* can regulate Qi and eliminate focal distension. It is normally used for distension and pain in the chest and hypochondrium, and focal distension and fullness in the stomach and abdomen. The dosage is 3-10g.

Mu Xiang 木香 (Aucklandia root, Radix Aucklandiae Lappae)

Mu Xiang is the root of *Aucklandia lappa* Decne., family Compositae.

Legal status *Mu Xiang* is a restricted substance listed in Appendix I of the Convention on International Trade in Endangered Species of Wild Fauna and Flora (CITES). All trade in the wild, non-cultivated variety of this herb is presently banned.

Main ingredients *Mu Xiang* contains 0.3-3% of volatile oils (including aplotaxene, α-ionone, β-selinene, costic acid, costol, α-costene, β-costene, costuslactone, dehydrocostuslactone, phellandrene and camphene), palmitic acid, linderic acid and amino acids.

Properties Taste: acrid and bitter; nature: warm.

Channels entered Spleen, Stomach, Gallbladder and Large Intestine.

Functions and indications Moves Qi and alleviates pain, allows constrained Liver Qi to flow freely and opens depression. It is indicated for distension and pain in the stomach, vomiting, diarrhoea, abdominal urgency and tenesmus, cold Shan disorders, and damp-heat jaundice.

Common dosage 3-10g, the maximum dosage is about 30g.

Precautions and contraindications The acrid, aromatic, warm and dry properties of *Mu Xiang* mean that it is contraindicated in cases of effulgent Yin deficiency-fire, dryness and heat in the Xue level, and insufficiency of body fluids.

Remarks Raw *Mu Xiang* should be selected for moving Qi and alleviating pain, whereas roasted *Mu Xiang* is used to fortify the Spleen to stop diarrhoea.

Comparison of functions See *Wu Yao* (Radix Linderae Strychnifoliae).

Toxicity In acute toxicity tests, the LD_{50} for intraperitoneal injection of costuslactone in rats was 300mg/kg. In laboratory tests on rats, the volatile oils contained in *Mu Xiang* were added to feed in the proportions of 1.77mg/kg for males and 2.17mg/kg for females; after 90 days of feeding, there was no significant change in terms of growth, blood, urine or the main organs when compared with a control group.

Modern research

1. The alkaloids contained in *Mu Xiang* have an obvious effect in relieving spasm of the bronchus and the smooth muscle of the small intestine.[7]
2. The volatile oils contained in *Mu Xiang* inhibit the heart, dilate the blood vessels and lower blood pressure.[8]
3. Very dilute preparations of the volatile oils contained in *Mu Xiang* inhibited the growth of streptococci and staphylococci, but had a much weaker effect on Escherichia coli and Corynebacterium diphtheriae.[8]

Combinations and applications

Functions	Combinations	Applications
Moving Qi and alleviating pain	*Bing Lang* (Semen Arecae Catechu) *Qing Pi* (Pericarpium Citri Reticulatae Viride) *Da Huang* (Radix et Rhizoma Rhei)	Full patterns of distension and pain in the stomach and abdomen due to Qi stagnation of the Spleen and Stomach accompanied by constipation, focal distension and fullness

	Huo Xiang (Herba Agastaches seu Pogostemi) *Zhu Ru* (Caulis Bambusae in Taeniis) *Ban Xia* (Rhizoma Pinelliae Ternatae) *Fu Ling* (Sclerotium Poriae Cocos)	Vomiting, pain in the abdomen and diarrhoea due to Qi stagnation in the Stomach and Intestines and non-transformation of dampness
	Zhi Ke (Fructus Citri Aurantii) *Chuan Lian Zi* (Fructus Meliae Toosendan) *Yan Hu Suo* (Rhizoma Corydalis Yanhusuo)	Distension and pain in the stomach and abdomen due to Qi stagnation
	Sha Ren (Fructus Amomi) *Zhi Shi* (Fructus Immaturus Citri Aurantii) *Bai Zhu* (Rhizoma Atractylodis Macrocephalae)	Low food intake due to Spleen deficiency accompanied by food accumulation and Qi stagnation
	Sha Ren (Fructus Amomi)	Focal distension and fullness in the stomach and abdomen
	Bing Lang (Semen Arecae Catechu) *Huang Lian* (Rhizoma Coptidis)	Abdominal urgency and tenesmus, purulent and bloody stool
	Lai Fu Zi (Semen Raphani Sativi)	Distension in the abdomen
	Xiao Hui Xiang (Fructus Foeniculi Vulgaris) *Chuan Lian Zi* (Fructus Meliae Toosendan)	Cold Shan disorders, unilateral sagging of the testicles, Qi pain in the Small Intestine
Allowing constrained Liver Qi to flow freely and opening depression	*Chai Hu* (Radix Bupleuri) *Yu Jin* (Radix Curcumae) *Zhi Ke* (Fructus Citri Aurantii) *Xiang Fu* (Rhizoma Cyperi Rotundi)	Distension and pain in the hypochondrium, a bitter taste in the mouth and yellow tongue fur due to constrained Liver Qi
	Yin Chen Hao (Herba Artemisiae Scopariae) *Da Huang* (Radix et Rhizoma Rhei) *Jin Qian Cao* (Herba Lysimachiae)	Damp-heat jaundice

Note: Since *Mu Xiang* can arouse the Spleen and reinforce the Stomach, it is often used in prescriptions with supplementing and boosting herbs to reduce their cloying and stagnating properties and aid in their absorption.

Xiang Fu 香附 (Nut-grass rhizome, Rhizoma Cyperi Rotundi)

Xiang Fu is the rhizome of *Cyperus rotundus* L., family Cyperaceae.

Main ingredients *Xiang Fu* contains cyperene, β-selinene, α-cyperone, β-cyperone, patchoulenone, cyperolone, cyperotundone, cyperol, isocyperol, limonene, camphene, alkaloids, cardiac glycosides, resin, glucose and fructose.

Properties Taste: acrid, slightly bitter and slightly sweet; nature: neutral.

Channels entered Liver and San Jiao.

Functions and indications Regulates Qi and relieves depression, adjusts menstruation and alleviates pain. It is indicated for distension and fullness in the stomach and abdomen, distension and pain in the hypochondrium due to binding depression of Liver Qi, cold Shan disorders, menstrual irregularities, and distension and pain in the breasts due to Liver depression and Qi stagnation.

Common dosage 6-12g; appropriate dosage as an external wash or external application in powder form.

Precautions and contraindications *Xiang Fu* is contraindicated in cases of Qi deficiency without stagnation, or Blood-heat due to Yin deficiency.

Remarks The nature of raw *Xiang Fu* is to move outwards; processed *Xiang Fu* enters the Liver and Kidney channels and is used for lower back and leg disorders; *Xiang Fu* mix-fried with alcohol can free the channels; *Xiang Fu* mix-fried with vinegar is good for dispersing accumulation; *Xiang Fu* mix-fried with ginger juice can transform Phlegm-fluids; and charred *Xiang Fu* is mainly used for uterine bleeding and profuse menstruation.

Comparison of functions See *Wu Yao* (Radix Linderae Strychnifoliae) and *Mu Hu Die* (Semen Oroxyli Indici).

Toxicity *Xiang Fu* has a low level of toxicity. Rats were able to tolerate feeding with a mixture containing up to 25% of the herb, but when the proportion was increased to 30-50%, growth was inhibited. In acute toxicity tests, the LD_{50} for intraperitoneal injection in mice of alcoholic extracts of *Xiang Fu* was in the region of 1500mg/kg.

Modern research

1. Has an inhibitory effect on both pregnant and non-pregnant uteri in animals.[9]
2. The volatile oils contained in *Xiang Fu* have an oestrogen-like function.[9]
3. Alleviates pain and has a tranquillizing effect.[9]
4. The volatile oils contained in *Xiang Fu* inhibited Staphylococcus aureus *in vitro*, but were not effective against other bacteria.[7]

Combinations and applications

Functions	Combinations	Applications
Regulating Qi and relieving depression	*Chai Hu* (Radix Bupleuri) *Yu Jin* (Radix Curcumae) *Bai Shao* (Radix Paeoniae Lactiflorae) *Qing Pi* (Pericarpium Citri Reticulatae Viride)	Distension and fullness in the stomach and abdomen and distension and pain in the hypochondrium due to binding depression of Liver Qi
	Gao Liang Jiang (Rhizoma Alpiniae Officinari)	Pain in the stomach with Liver depression invading the Stomach due to cold congealing and Qi stagnation
	Ban Xia (Rhizoma Pinelliae Ternatae) *Fu Ling* (Sclerotium Poriae Cocos) *Ju Hong* (Pars Rubra Epicarpii Citri Erythrocarpae)	Nausea and vomiting, copious sputum, poor appetite and white, slimy tongue fur due to Phlegm depression
	Mu Xiang (Radix Aucklandiae Lappae) (see notes on legal status) *Fo Shou* (Fructus Citri Sarcodactylis)	Distension and pain in the hypochondrium, stomach and abdomen due to hyperactive Liver Qi invading the Stomach
	Chao Bing Lang (Semen Arecae Catechu, stir-fried) *Jiao Shen Qu* (Massa Fermentata, scorch-fried) *Chao Mai Ya* (Fructus Hordei Vulgaris Germinatus, stir-fried)	Food depression manifesting as focal distension and fullness in the stomach, belching with a foul odour and acid vomiting
	Cang Zhu (Rhizoma Atractylodis) *Bai Zhu* (Rhizoma Atractylodis Macrocephalae) *Zhu Ling* (Sclerotium Polypori Umbellati) *Ze Xie* (Rhizoma Alismatis Orientalis)	Oppression in the chest and reduced food intake, loose stool, slimy tongue fur, and mild oedema due to damp depression

	Zhi Zi (Fructus Gardeniae Jasminoidis) *Huang Qin* (Radix Scutellariae Baicalensis) *Chuan Lian Zi* (Fructus Meliae Toosendan)	Bitter taste in the mouth, vexation, red tongue and yellow urine due to fire depression
	Xiao Hui Xiang (Fructus Foeniculi Vulgaris) *Wu Yao* (Radix Linderae Strychnifoliae)	Pain in the abdomen due to cold Shan disorders
Adjusting menstruation and alleviating pain	*Chuan Xiong* (Rhizoma Ligustici Chuanxiong) *Hong Hua* (Flos Carthami Tinctorii)	Menstrual block and a dark purple tongue due to Blood stasis
	Chai Hu (Radix Bupleuri) *Yu Jin* (Radix Curcumae) *Chuan Xiong* (Rhizoma Ligustici Chuanxiong)	Menstrual irregularities, painful menstruation, distension and pain in the breasts due to Liver depression and Qi stagnation
	Dang Shen (Radix Codonopsitis Pilosulae) *Shu Di Huang* (Radix Rehmanniae Glutinosae Conquita) *Dang Gui* (Radix Angelicae Sinensis) *Chuan Xiong* (Rhizoma Ligustici Chuanxiong)	Profuse, light-coloured menstruation and latent pain in the lower abdomen due to Qi and Blood deficiency

Chen Xiang 沉香 (Chinese eaglewood, Lignum Aquilariae Resinatum)

Chen Xiang is the resinous wood of *Aquilaria sinensis* (Lour.) Gilg., family Thymelaeaceae.

Main ingredients *Chen Xiang* contains baimuxinic acid, baimuxinal, α-garospirol, baimuxinol, dehydrobaimuxinol, isobaimuxinol, anisic acid, benzylacetone and sinenofuranol.

Properties Taste: acrid and bitter; nature: warm.

Channels entered Spleen, Stomach and Kidney.

Functions and indications Moves Qi and alleviates pain, warms the Middle Jiao and stops vomiting, warms the Kidneys and hosts Qi, and calms wheezing. It is indicated for distension and pain in the chest and abdomen, vomiting and hiccups, a cold feeling in the Stomach due to Yang deficiency, coughing and wheezing, and premature ejaculation.

Common dosage 1-1.5g in powder form for oral intake.

Precautions and contraindications *Chen Xiang* should be used with caution in cases of effulgent Yin deficiency-fire and Qi deficiency fall.

Remarks *Chen Xiang* is very good at moving Qi to alleviate pain. It can also bear Stomach Qi downwards to stop vomiting and can warm the Kidneys to host Qi and calm wheezing, and is therefore mainly used for vomiting due to cold and wheezing due to Kidney deficiency.

Toxicity There have been a number of reports of allergic reaction to *Chen Xiang*; for instance, one case was reported of an allergic skin rash during high-temperature frying of the herb.

Modern research

1. The volatile oils contained in *Chen Xiang* counteract asthenia and alleviate pain.[10]
2. Decoctions of *Chen Xiang* had a strong inhibitory effect on Mycobacterium tuberculosis and Shigella shigae.[10]
3. Calms wheezing and has a tranquillizing effect.[10]

Combinations and applications

Functions	Combinations	Applications
Moving Qi and alleviating pain	*Wu Yao* (Radix Linderae Strychnifoliae) *Mu Xiang* (Radix Aucklandiae Lappae) (see notes on legal status) *Bing Lang* (Semen Arecae Catechu)	Distension and pain in the chest and abdomen due to cold congealing and Qi stagnation
Warming the Middle Jiao and stopping vomiting	*Ding Xiang* (Flos Caryophylli) *Bai Dou Kou* (Fructus Amomi Kravanh) *Shi Di* (Calyx Diospyri Kaki)	Vomiting and hiccups due to Spleen and Stomach deficiency-cold
Warming the Kidneys and hosting Qi, calming wheezing	*Fu Zi* (Radix Lateralis Aconiti Carmichaeli Praeparata) (see notes on legal status) *Rou Gui* (Cortex Cinnamomi Cassiae) *Bu Gu Zhi* (Fructus Psoraleae Corylifoliae)	Deficiency wheezing due to inability of the Kidneys to host Qi with deficiency-cold of the lower origin
	Su Zi (Fructus Perillae Frutescentis) *Qian Hu* (Radix Peucedani) *Hou Po* (Cortex Magnoliae Officinalis) *Chen Pi* (Pericarpium Citri Reticulatae) *Ban Xia* (Rhizoma Pinelliae Ternatae)	Coughing and wheezing due to Phlegm-fluids with exuberance above and deficiency below
	Rou Cong Rong (Herba Cistanches Deserticolae) *Dang Gui* (Radix Angelicae Sinensis) *Zhi Ke* (Fructus Citri Aurantii)	Constipation due to deficiency-cold with Qi stagnation in the Stomach and Intestines
	Yang Qi Shi (Actinolitum) *Bu Gu Zhi* (Fructus Psoraleae Corylifoliae) *Fu Zi* (Radix Lateralis Aconiti Carmichaeli Praeparata) (see notes on legal status)	Premature ejaculation due to seminal cold

Qing Pi 青皮
(Green tangerine peel, Pericarpium Citri Reticulatae Viride)

Qing Pi is the dried green epicarp or fruit of *Citrus reticulata* Blanco, family Rutaceae.

Main ingredients *Qing Pi* contains volatile oils (including α-thujene and limonene), nobiletin, hesperidin, neohesperidin, tangeridin, citromitin, synephrine, carotene, cryptoxanthin, inositol, amino acids, vitamin B_1 and vitamin C.

Properties Taste: bitter and acrid; nature: warm.

Channels entered Liver, Gallbladder and Stomach.

Functions and indications Soothes the Liver and regulates Qi, disperses food accumulation and transforms stagnation, and promotes the movement of Qi and Blood to break up stasis. It is indicated for distension and pain in the stomach or hypochondrium, food accumulation, Shan disorders, and pain in the breasts.

Common dosage 3-10g.

Precautions and contraindications As *Qing Pi* tends to consume Qi, it should be used with caution in cases of Qi deficiency.

Comparison of functions Both *Qing Pi* (Pericarpium Citri Reticulatae Viride) and *Chen Pi* (Pericarpium Citri Reticulatae) can regulate Qi and transform stagnation to treat Qi stagnation patterns. *Chen Pi* is warm but not drastic in nature and has a relatively moderate effect in moving Qi; it is often used for Qi stagnation in the Spleen and Stomach. As it is light in quality, it floats upwards and, since it enters the Lung channel, it can also dry dampness and transform Phlegm to treat cough due to damp-Phlegm. *Qing Pi* is more drastic in nature and has a stronger effect in moving Qi; it can disperse constrained Liver Qi and break up Qi, as well as dispersing food accumulation and alleviating pain. It is mainly used for Liver depression patterns.

In *Ru Men Shi Qin* [Matters Relating to the Confucian Gate], Zhang Zihe says: '*Chen Pi* is upward-bearing and floating and enters the Spleen and Lung channels; it treats disorders in the upper part of the body and governs freeing. *Qing Pi* is sinking and downward-bearing and enters the Liver and Gallbladder channels; it treats disorders in the lower part of the body and governs draining.'

For an additional comparison, see *Xiang Yuan* (Fructus Citri Medicae seu Wilsonii).

Modern research

1. Relieves spasm through direct inhibition of the intestinal smooth muscle.[11]
2. The volatile oils contained in *Qing Pi* expel sputum.[12]
3. Affects the cardiovascular system, raises blood pressure and stimulates the heart.[13, 14]

Combinations and applications

Functions	Combinations	Applications
Soothing the Liver and regulating Qi	*Chai Hu* (Radix Bupleuri) *Yu Jin* (Radix Curcumae) *Xiang Fu* (Rhizoma Cyperi Rotundi)	Distension and pain in the chest and hypochondrium or Shan disorder pain due to Liver depression and Qi stagnation
	Chai Hu (Radix Bupleuri) *Zhi Ke* (Fructus Citri Aurantii) *Bai Shao* (Radix Paeoniae Lactiflorae)	Distension and pain in the chest and hypochondrium
	Wu Yao (Radix Linderae Strychnifoliae) *Xiao Hui Xiang* (Fructus Foeniculi Vulgaris)	Shan disorder pain
	Gua Lou (Fructus Trichosanthis) *Pu Gong Ying* (Herba Taraxaci cum Radice)	Distension and pain in the breasts, breast abscess
	Zhe Bei Mu (Bulbus Fritillariae Thunbergii) *Chuan Shan Jia* (Squama Manitis Pentadactylae) (see notes on legal status) *Xia Ku Cao* (Spica Prunellae Vulgaris)	Lumps in the breast due to Qi stagnation and binding of Phlegm

Dispersing food accumulation and transforming stagnation	*Shen Qu* (Massa Fermentata) *Shan Zha* (Fructus Crataegi) *Mai Ya* (Fructus Hordei Vulgaris Germinatus)	Distension and pain in the stomach and abdomen due to food accumulation and Qi stagnation
Promoting the movement of Qi and Blood to break up stasis	*San Leng* (Rhizoma Sparganii Stoloniferi) *Yu Jin* (Radix Curcumae) *E Zhu* (Rhizoma Curcumae)	Enlargement of the liver and/or spleen due to Qi stagnation and Blood stasis

Fo Shou 佛手
(Finger citron fruit or Buddha's hand, Fructus Citri Sarcodactylis)

Fo Shou is the fruit of *Citrus medica* L. var. *sarcodactylis* Swingle, family Rutaceae.

Main ingredients The skin of the fruit contains volatile oils; the fruit itself contains bergapten, limettin, hesperidin and diosmin.

Properties Taste: acrid and bitter; nature: warm.

Channels entered Liver, Spleen, Stomach and Lung.

Functions and indications Allows constrained Liver Qi to flow freely, regulates Qi and alleviates pain, harmonizes the Middle Jiao and transforms stagnation, fortifies the Spleen and stops vomiting, dries dampness and transforms Phlegm. It is indicated for distension and pain in the chest and hypochondrium due to Liver depression and Qi stagnation, focal distension and fullness in the stomach, indigestion, belching, and cough with copious sputum.

Common dosage 3-10g.

Comparison of functions Both *Fo Shou* (Fructus Citri Sarcodactylis) and *Chen Pi* (Pericarpium Citri Reticulatae) can dry dampness and transform Phlegm, but *Fo Shou* has a more moderate effect than *Chen Pi*, which tends to be bitter and dry. *Fo Shou* is extremely effective in allowing constrained Liver Qi to flow freely. Since it has similar functions to *Chen Pi*, the two herbs are often used in combination or as a substitute for one another.

For an additional comparison, see *Xiang Yuan* (Fructus Citri Medicae seu Wilsonii).

Toxicity The LD_{50} for intragastric administration to mice of the limettin contained in *Fo Shou* is 3.95g/kg.

Modern research

1. Decoctions of *Fo Shou* can calm wheezing and expel sputum.[15]
2. Injecting cats with *Fo Shou* had a certain effect in inhibiting the heart and lowering high blood pressure.[16]

Combinations and applications

Functions	Combinations	Applications
Allowing constrained Liver Qi to flow freely, regulating Qi and alleviating pain	*Xiang Fu* (Rhizoma Cyperi Rotundi) *Yu Jin* (Radix Curcumae) *Chai Hu* (Radix Bupleuri)	Distension and pain in the chest and hypochondrium due to Liver depression and Qi stagnation, focal distension and fullness in the stomach due to Liver-Stomach disharmony

Harmonizing the Middle Jiao and transforming stagnation	*Mu Xiang* (Radix Aucklandiae Lappae) (see notes on legal status) *Zhi Ke* (Fructus Citri Aurantii)	Focal distension and pain in the chest due to Qi stagnation caused by Phlegm-fluids collecting internally
	Chen Pi (Pericarpium Citri Reticulatae) *Mu Xiang* (Radix Aucklandiae Lappae) (see notes on legal status)	Distension, fullness, belching and acid regurgitation due to Qi stagnation of the Spleen and Stomach
Fortifying the Spleen and stopping vomiting	*Sha Ren* (Fructus Amomi) *Ban Xia* (Rhizoma Pinelliae Ternatae)	Indigestion, reduced appetite, belching and vomiting
Drying dampness and transforming Phlegm	*Si Gua Luo* (Fasciculus Vascularis Luffae) *Yu Jin* (Radix Curcumae) *Gua Lou Pi* (Pericarpium Trichosanthis) *Chen Pi* (Pericarpium Citri Reticulatae)	Enduring cough with copious sputum, pain in the chest

Appendix

Fo Shou Hua 佛手花 (Finger citron flower, Flos Citri Sarcodactylis)

Fo Shou Hua is the flower and bud of *Fo Shou*. Its taste, nature and functions are similar to *Fo Shou*, but its action is milder. Dosage is generally 3-6g.

Xiang Yuan 香橼 (Citron fruit, Fructus Citri Medicae seu Wilsonii)

Xiang Yuan is the fruit of *Citrus medica* L. or *C. wilsonii* Tanaka, family Rutaceae.

Main ingredients *Xiang Yuan* contains limonene, citral, linalyl acetate, geranyl acetate, phellandrene, limettin, citronin, hesperidin, β-sitosterol, carotene, palmitic acid, succinic acid, pectin and citrusin.

Properties Taste: acrid, slightly bitter and sour; nature: warm.

Channels entered Liver, Spleen and Lung.

Functions and indications Allows constrained Liver Qi to flow freely, regulates Qi and alleviates pain, harmonizes the Middle Jiao, dries dampness and transforms Phlegm. It is indicated for oppression in the chest, pain in the hypochondrium, distension and pain in the stomach, and cough with copious sputum.

Common dosage 3-10g.

Comparison of functions

1. Both *Xiang Yuan* (Fructus Citri Medicae seu Wilsonii) and *Qing Pi* (Pericarpium Citri Reticulatae Viride) can soothe the Liver and regulate Qi. *Xiang Yuan* frees the Liver channel and breaks up Qi stagnation of the Spleen and Stomach and is used for Liver depression and Qi stagnation patterns. However, it is more moderate in function than *Qing Pi*, which is stronger and bitterer. *Qing Pi* is also effective in dispersing food accumulation.
2. *Xiang Yuan* (Fructus Citri Medicae seu Wilsonii) and *Fo Shou* (Fructus Citri Sarcodactylis) have similar functions in allowing constrained Liver Qi to flow freely, regulating Qi and harmonizing the Middle Jiao, and drying dampness and transforming Phlegm. They are often used together to accentuate each other's effect. *Xiang Yuan* is more effective in transforming Phlegm, whereas *Fo Shou* is better at regulating Qi.

Modern research Inhibits inflammation and has an anti-viral function.[17]

Combinations and applications

Functions	Combinations	Applications
Allowing constrained Liver Qi to flow freely, regulating Qi and alleviating pain, harmonizing the Middle Jiao	*Gua Lou Pi* (Pericarpium Trichosanthis) *Yu Jin* (Radix Curcumae) *Xiang Fu* (Rhizoma Cyperi Rotundi)	Oppression in the chest and pain in the hypochondrium due to Liver depression and Qi stagnation
	Chai Hu (Radix Bupleuri) *Yu Jin* (Radix Curcumae) *Fo Shou* (Fructus Citri Sarcodactylis)	Distension and pain in the chest and hypochondrium due to Liver depression
	Mu Xiang (Radix Aucklandiae Lappae) (see notes on legal status) *Chuan Lian Zi* (Fructus Meliae Toosendan) *Wu Zhu Yu* (Fructus Evodiae Rutaecarpae)	Distension and pain in the stomach, lack of appetite and vomiting due to Qi stagnation of the Spleen and Stomach
	Huang Lian (Rhizoma Coptidis)	A bitter taste in the mouth and acid regurgitation
Drying dampness and transforming Phlegm	*Ban Xia* (Rhizoma Pinelliae Ternatae) *Fu Ling* (Sclerotium Poriae Cocos) *Sheng Jiang* (Rhizoma Zingiberis Officinalis Recens)	Oppression in the chest and cough with copious sputum due to Phlegm-damp obstruction

Chuan Lian Zi 川楝子
(Sichuan chinaberry, Fructus Meliae Toosendan)

Chuan Lian Zi is the dried ripe fruit of *Melia toosendan* Sieb. et Zucc., family Meliaceae.

Main ingredients *Chuan Lian Zi* contains toosendanin, mergsine, melianone, melialactone and meliamol.

Properties Taste: bitter; nature: cold; slightly toxic.

Channels entered Liver, Stomach, Small Intestine and Bladder.

Functions and indications Soothes the Liver and regulates Qi, drains fire and alleviates pain, and kills worms. It is indicated for pain in the hypochondrium, pain in the stomach and abdomen, Shan disorders, and roundworm.

Common dosage 3-10g; appropriate dosage for external application.

Precautions and contraindications

1. *Chuan Lian Zi* is contraindicated in cases of Spleen and Stomach deficiency-cold because of its bitter taste and cold nature.
2. Since *Chuan Lian Zi* is slightly toxic, dosage should not be exceeded, nor should the herb be administered over a long period.

Comparison of functions See *Ku Lian Pi* (Cortex Meliae Radicis).

Toxicity The main toxic ingredients of *Chuan Lian Zi* have been identified as toosendanin and melianone. The LD_{50} for intravenous injection and oral administration to mice of toosendanin is 14.6 ± 0.9mg/kg and 244.3 ± 44.0mg/kg respectively. *Chuan Lian Zi* can excite the gastrointestinal tract and harm the liver. Symptoms of mild overdose include dizziness, headache, somnolence, nausea and vomiting, and pain in the abdomen; in more severe cases, there may be hepatitis, internal haemorrhage and mental impairment. Severe side-effects from the use of *Chuan Lian Zi* in the clinic are rare, but toxic symptoms have been reported through overdosage of the related plant, *Ku Lian Pi* (*Melia azedarach* L.), which is sometimes used as a substitute.

Modern research

1. Non-diluted solutions of the alcoholic extract of *Chuan Lian Zi* can inhibit pathogenic fungi.[18]
2. Inhibits the respiratory system and may induce respiratory failure.[19]

Combinations and applications

Functions	Combinations	Applications
Soothing the Liver and regulating Qi, draining fire and alleviating pain	*Yan Hu Suo* (Rhizoma Corydalis Yanhusuo)	Distension and pain in the hypochondrium, pain in the stomach and abdomen and Shan disorders due to Liver depression and Qi stagnation or Liver-Stomach disharmony
	Chai Hu (Radix Bupleuri) *Yu Jin* (Radix Curcumae) *Xiang Fu* (Rhizoma Cyperi Rotundi)	Pain in the hypochondrium due to Liver depression and Qi stagnation
	Mu Xiang (Radix Aucklandiae Lappae) (see notes on legal status) *Gan Song* (Rhizoma Nardostachydis)	Distension and pain in the stomach and abdomen due to Liver depression and Qi stagnation
	Wu Zhu Yu (Fructus Evodiae Rutaecarpae) *Xiao Hui Xiang* (Fructus Foeniculi Vulgaris) *Li Zhi He* (Semen Litchi Chinensis)	Shan disorders and pain in the testicles due to cold congealing in the Liver channel
Killing worms	*Bing Lang* (Semen Arecae Catechu) *Shi Jun Zi* (Fructus Quisqualis Indicae)	Pain in the abdomen due to worm accumulation
	Wu Mei (Fructus Pruni Mume) *Hua Jiao* (Pericarpium Zanthoxyli)	Roundworm

Note: *Chuan Lian Zi* can also be used to treat tinea. Roast the herb until it turns brown and grind it into a powder. Then mix the powder with sesame oil, *Ma You* (Oleum Sesami), and apply the paste locally after washing the affected region with warm, salty water.

Wu Yao 乌药 (Lindera root, Radix Linderae Strychnifoliae)

Wu Yao is the dried tuberous root of *Lindera strychnifolia* (Sieb. et Zucc.) Villar, family Lauraceae.

Main ingredients *Wu Yao* contains linderol, linderane, linderene, linderol ester, linderic acid, isolinderalactone, neolinderalactone, linderoxide, isolinderoxide and laurolitsine.

Properties Taste: acrid; nature: warm.

Channels entered Spleen, Lung, Kidney and Bladder.

Functions and indications Moves Qi and alleviates pain, warms the Kidneys and dissipates cold. It is indicated for oppression in the chest, pain in the hypochondrium, distension and pain in the stomach and abdomen, cold Shan disorders, pain in the lower abdomen and testicles, urinary incontinence, and frequent urination.

Common dosage 3-10g.

Precautions and contraindications *Wu Yao* is contraindicated in cases of internal heat due to Yin deficiency, and for Qi deficiency without stagnation.

Comparison of functions *Wu Yao* (Radix Linderae Strychnifoliae), *Mu Xiang* (Radix Aucklandiae Lappae) and *Xiang Fu* (Rhizoma Cyperi Rotundi) can all move Qi and alleviate pain to treat abdominal pain due to Qi stagnation. *Mu Xiang* is warm, dry, aromatic and harsh, and can bear upwards and downwards to free the San Jiao and the Qi level. It is particularly effective in moving Qi stagnation of the Stomach and Intestines to treat distension and pain in the stomach and abdomen and diarrhoea with abdominal urgency and tenesmus. *Xiang Fu* is neutral and harmonizing and tends to allow constrained Liver Qi to flow freely and relieve depression, adjust menstruation and alleviate pain; it is often used for pain in the hypochondrium due to Liver depression, and for menstrual irregularities or painful menstruation. *Wu Yao* has strong warming and dissipating properties and is good at dissipating cold and moving Qi to alleviate pain. It is often used for pain in the chest and abdomen due to cold congealing and Qi stagnation. As it warms the Kidneys and reduces urination, it is good for treating frequent urination and enuresis due to deficiency-cold of the Bladder.

Modern research

1. Stimulates the intestinal smooth muscle.[20]
2. Stops bleeding.[21]
3. Decoctions of the leaves of fresh *Wu Yao* inhibited various common bacteria *in vitro*.[22]

Combinations and applications

Functions	Combinations	Applications
Moving Qi and alleviating pain	*Xie Bai* (Bulbus Allii Macrostemi) *Gua Lou Pi* (Pericarpium Trichosanthis) *Yu Jin* (Radix Curcumae) *Yan Hu Suo* (Rhizoma Corydalis Yanhusuo)	Oppression in the chest and pain in the hypochondrium due to cold congealing and Qi stagnation
	Mu Xiang (Radix Aucklandiae Lappae) (see notes on legal status) *Wu Zhu Yu* (Fructus Evodiae Rutaecarpae) *Zhi Ke* (Fructus Citri Aurantii)	Distension and pain in the stomach and abdomen
	Xiang Fu (Rhizoma Cyperi Rotundi) *Dang Gui* (Radix Angelicae Sinensis) *Mu Xiang* (Radix Aucklandiae Lappae) (see notes on legal status)	Pain in the abdomen during menstruation due to Qi stagnation and Blood stasis
	Xiao Hui Xiang (Fructus Foeniculi Vulgaris) *Mu Xiang* (Radix Aucklandiae Lappae) (see notes on legal status) *Qing Pi* (Pericarpium Citri Reticulatae Viride)	Cold Shan disorders and pain in the lower abdomen and testicles
Warming the Kidneys and dissipating cold	*Yi Zhi Ren* (Fructus Alpiniae Oxyphyllae) *Shan Yao* (Rhizoma Dioscoreae Oppositae)	Frequent urination and enuresis in children due to deficiency-cold of the Bladder and insufficiency of Kidney Yang

Xie Bai 薤白 (Chinese chive, Bulbus Allii Macrostemi)

Xie Bai is the dried bulb of *Allium macrostemon* Bge., family Liliaceae.

Main ingredients *Xie Bai* contains alliin, methylalliin, scorodose, and linoleic, palmitic and oleic acids.

Properties Taste: acrid and bitter; nature: warm.

Channels entered Lung, Stomach and Large Intestine.

Functions and indications Frees Yang and dissipates lumps, moves Qi and guides out stagnation. It is indicated for obstruction of Qi in the chest, mainly manifesting as pain in the chest radiating to the back; and for oppression in the chest, cough with copious thin sputum, and diarrhoea and dysentery.

Common dosage 5-10g.

Precautions and contraindications *Xie Bai* is contraindicated in cases of Qi deficiency without stagnation and also for food accumulation due to Stomach deficiency; avoid using with patients who dislike the garlicky smell.

Remarks *Xie Bai* promotes the movement of Yang Qi in the chest and dissipates cold-damp. It is an important herb for chest Bi syndrome. In addition, as it can move Qi to guide out stagnation in the Stomach and Intestines, it is used to treat diarrhoea and dysentery with abdominal urgency and tenesmus.

Modern research

1. Decoctions of *Xie Bai* inhibited Shigella shigae and Staphylococcus aureus *in vitro*.[23]
2. Reduces the level of blood lipids and prevents atherosclerosis.[24]
3. Inhibits haematoblastic concentration.[25]

Combinations and applications

Functions	Combinations	Applications
Freeing Yang and dissipating lumps	*Gui Zhi* (Ramulus Cinnamomi Cassiae) *Gua Lou* (Fructus Trichosanthis) *Dan Shen* (Radix Salviae Miltiorrhizae)	Pain and oppression in the chest due to obstruction of chest Yang, especially if it worsens in cold conditions
	Bai Jie Zi (Semen Sinapis Albae) *Ban Xia* (Rhizoma Pinelliae Ternatae) *Chen Pi* (Pericarpium Citri Reticulatae)	Cough with copious thin sputum and oppression in the chest due to Phlegm-fluids
	Tao Ren (Semen Persicae) *Hong Hua* (Flos Carthami Tinctorii) *Dan Shen* (Radix Salviae Miltiorrhizae)	Chest Bi syndrome with Blood stasis
Moving Qi and guiding out stagnation	*Chai Hu* (Radix Bupleuri) *Bai Shao* (Radix Paeoniae Lactiflorae) *Zhi Ke* (Fructus Citri Aurantii)	Diarrhoea and dysentery with purulent and bloody stool, and abdominal urgency and tenesmus due to stagnation of Stomach Qi
	Huang Bai (Cortex Phellodendri) *Qin Pi* (Cortex Fraxini)	Diarrhoea and dysentery with abdominal urgency and tenesmus due to damp-heat

Da Fu Pi 大腹皮
(Shell of areca nut, Pericarpium Arecae Catechu)

Da Fu Pi is the dried husk or peel of *Areca catechu* L., family Palmae.

Legal status In the UK, *Da Fu Pi* can only be sold in premises which are registered pharmacies and by or under the supervision of a pharmacist.

Main ingredients *Da Fu Pi* contains arecoline, arecaidine and α-catechin.

Properties Taste: acrid; nature: slightly warm.

Channels entered Spleen, Stomach, Large Intestine and Small Intestine.

Functions and indications Causes Qi to descend and loosens the Middle Jiao, promotes the movement of water and disperses swelling. It is indicated for fullness and distension in the stomach and abdomen, leg Qi, and oedema.

Common dosage 3-10g.

Precautions and contraindications *Da Fu Pi* should be used with caution for Qi deficiency and for patients with a weak constitution.

Comparison of functions *Da Fu Pi* (Pericarpium Arecae Catechu) and *Bing Lang* (Semen Arecae Catechu) come from the same plant. They have the functions of moving Qi and promoting the movement of water. *Bing Lang* is very effective for expelling worms and is a key herb for killing tapeworm; it can also move Qi and disperse stagnation. It is more effective than *Da Fu Pi* in promoting the movement of water and eliminating dampness. *Da Fu Pi* is relatively moderate in moving Qi and promoting the movement of water, but it is good at loosening the Middle Jiao and causing Qi to descend. *Bing Lang* is used for severe cases of Qi stagnation and collection of water and dampness; *Da Fu Pi* is used for milder cases.

Toxicity The use of *Da Fu Pi* does not generally result in toxic side-effects, although one case of allergic reaction has been reported. A patient with no history of allergy to the herb suffered from oppression in the chest, nausea, flusteredness, itchy skin, vexation and agitation, and restlessness after taking a prescription containing *Da Fu Pi*.

Modern research Stimulates the parasympathetic nervous system, excites the gastrointestinal tract and promotes the secretion of digestive juices.[26]

Combinations and applications

Functions	Combinations	Applications
Causing Qi to descend and loosening the Middle Jiao, promoting the movement of water and dispersing swelling	*Huo Xiang* (Herba Agastaches seu Pogostemi) *Pei Lan* (Herba Eupatorii Fortunei) *Hou Po* (Cortex Magnoliae Officinalis)	Distension and fullness in the stomach and abdomen, difficult defecation, and a sticky sensation in the mouth due to Qi stagnation and damp obstruction
	Fu Ling Pi (Cortex Poriae Cocos) *Bai Zhu* (Rhizoma Atractylodis Macrocephalae) *Che Qian Zi* (Semen Plantaginis)	Oedema, distension of the abdomen and scant urine due to Qi stagnation and water-damp
	Mu Gua (Fructus Chaenomelis) *Zi Su Ye* (Folium Perillae Frutescentis)	Puffy swelling in leg Qi
	Cao Dou Kou (Semen Alpiniae Katsumadai) *Fu Zi* (Radix Lateralis Aconiti Carmichaeli Praeparata) (see notes on legal status) *Gan Jiang* (Rhizoma Zingiberis Officinalis) *Fu Ling* (Sclerotium Poriae Cocos)	Oedema and scant urine due to cirrhosis of the liver or heart failure

Li Zhi He 荔枝核
(Lychee seed, Semen Litchi Chinensis)

Li Zhi He is the dried ripe seed of *Litchi chinensis* Sonn., family Sapindaceae.

Main ingredients *Li Zhi He* contains saponins and α-methylenecyclopropyl glycine; the fruit contains folic acid.

Properties Taste: sweet and astringent; nature: warm.

Channels entered Liver and Stomach.

Functions and indications Regulates Qi and alleviates pain, dispels cold and disperses stagnation. It is indicated for Shan disorder pain, swollen and painful testicles, pain in the stomach, and premenstrual and postpartum pain in the abdomen.

Common dosage 10-15g.

Precautions and contraindications *Li Zhi He* is contraindicated for cases without damp-cold and Qi stagnation.

Remarks *Li Zhi He* disperses Qi stagnation and dispels cold pathogenic factors by virtue of entering the Liver channel. As a result, it is effective for treating pain due to Liver depression and Qi stagnation or cold obstructing the Liver channel.

Toxicity No deaths had occurred among mice three days after being given 20g/kg of *Li Zhi He* via intragastric administration.

Modern research Lowers the blood sugar level.[27]

Combinations and applications

Functions	Combinations	Applications
Regulating Qi and alleviating pain, dispelling cold and dispersing stagnation	*Xiao Hui Xiang* (Fructus Foeniculi Vulgaris) *Wu Zhu Yu* (Fructus Evodiae Rutaecarpae) *Ju He* (Semen Citri Reticulatae)	Shan disorder pain and swollen and painful testicles due to cold congealing and Qi stagnation
	Long Dan Cao (Radix Gentianae Scabrae) *Chuan Lian Zi* (Fructus Meliae Toosendan)	Swollen and painful testicles with red and swollen scrotum due to damp-heat pouring down into the Liver channel
	Mu Xiang (Radix Aucklandiae Lappae) (see notes on legal status)	Enduring pain in the stomach due to Liver depression and Qi stagnation
	Xiang Fu (Rhizoma Cyperi Rotundi)	Premenstrual and postpartum pain in the abdomen due to Qi stagnation and Blood stasis

Mei Gui Hua 玫瑰花
(Chinese rose flower, Flos Rosae Rugosae)

Mei Gui Hua is the flower bud of *Rosa rugosa* Thunb., family Rosaceae.

Main ingredients *Mei Gui Hua* contains volatile oils including citronellol, geraniol, linalool, nerol and eugenol.

Properties Taste: sweet and slightly bitter; nature: warm.

Channels entered Liver and Spleen.

Functions and indications Allows constrained Liver Qi to flow freely, moves Qi and relieves depression, and regulates Qi, harmonizes the Blood and dissipates stasis. It is indicated for Liver-Stomach disharmony, distension and pain in the chest and abdomen, menstrual irregularities, and knocks and falls.

Common dosage 1.5-6g; or as an infusion.

Combinations and applications

Functions	Combinations	Applications
Allowing constrained Liver Qi to flow freely, moving Qi and relieving depression	*Fo Shou* (Fructus Citri Sarcodactylis) *Xiang Fu* (Rhizoma Cyperi Rotundi) *Sha Ren* (Fructus Amomi)	Distension and pain in the chest and abdomen due to Liver depression invading the Stomach, vomiting and reduced appetite
Regulating Qi, harmonizing the Blood and dissipating stasis	*Dang Gui* (Radix Angelicae Sinensis) *Chuan Xiong* (Rhizoma Ligustici Chuanxiong) *Bai Shao* (Radix Paeoniae Lactiflorae) *Ze Lan* (Herba Lycopi Lucidi)	Menstrual irregularities due to Liver depression and Qi stagnation, premenstrual distension and pain in the breasts
	Ji Xue Teng (Caulis Spatholobi) *Yan Hu Suo* (Rhizoma Corydalis Yanhusuo) *Chi Shao* (Radix Paeoniae Rubra)	Knocks and falls with stasis-induced swelling and pain

Modern research references

1. He Xingdong et al., *Lin Chuang Zhong Yao Shou Ce* [Clinical Handbook of Chinese Materia Medica] (Beijing: People's Medical Publishing House, 1998), 156.
2. Zhu Enming, *Zhong Hua Yi Xue Za Zhi* [Chinese Journal of Medicine] 42, 10 (1956): 946.
3. Xu Guansu et al., *An Hui Zhong Yi Xue Yuan Xue Bao* [Journal of Anhui College of Traditional Chinese Medicine] 3 (1989): 75.
4. Chen Xiu et al., *Yao Xue Xue Bao* [Pharmacology Journal] 15, 2 (1980): 71.
5. Jia Hongjun et al., *Ke Xue Tong Bao* [Science Bulletin] 25, 11 (1980): 522.
6. Chen Xiu, *Collection of Abstracts of Papers from the First Pharmacological Congress*, 1979, 41.
7. Lei Zaiquan and Zhang Tingmo, *Zhong Hua Lin Chuang Yao Li Xue* [Chinese Clinical Materia Medica] (Beijing: People's Medical Publishing House, 1998), 975.
8. He Xingdong et al., *Lin Chuang Zhong Yao Shou Ce*, 161.
9. Ibid., 162.
10. Ibid., 163.
11. Zhongshan Medical College et al., *Pharmacology* (Beijing: People's Medical Publishing House, 1979), 478.
12. Wang Junmo et al., *Zhong Cao Yao* [Journal of Chinese Herbs] 12, 6 (1981): 20.
13. Li Yikui et al., *Zhong Cao Yao* 14, 8 (1983): 22.
14. Wang Junmo et al., *Zhong Cao Yao*, 11, 4 (1980): 168; 11, 11 (1980): 501.
15. Wang Benxian, *Xin Bian Zhong Yao Xue Ci Dian* [New Dictionary of Chinese Materia Medica] (Tianjin: Tianjin Science and Technology Publishing House, 1996), 621.
16. Zhang Haigen et al., Research on Pharmacology of *Fo Shou*, *Digest of Material from the First National Conference on Pharmacology of the Central Nervous System*, 1986: 124, 359, 361.
17. Chinese Herbal Information Centre of the State Pharmaceutical Administrative Bureau, *Zhong Cao Yao You Xiao Cheng Fen Shou Ce* [Handbook of Active Ingredients of Chinese Medicinal Herbs] (Beijing: People's Medical Publishing House, 1983), 561.
18. Lei Zaiquan and Zhang Tingmo, *Zhong Hua Lin Chuang Yao Li Xue*, 999.
19. He Xingdong et al., *Lin Chuang Zhong Yao Shou Ce*, 164.
20. Xu Guansu et al., *An Hui Zhong Yi Xue Yuan Xue Bao* [Journal of Anhui College of Traditional Chinese Medicine] 3 (1989): 75.
21. Tianjin Nankai Hospital, *Tian Jin Yi Xue Tong Xun* [Tianjin Medical Newsletter] 8 (1971): 1.
22. Health and Epidemic Prevention Station of Hunan Province, *Wei Sheng Fang Yi Tong Xun* [Health and Epidemic Prevention Newsletter] 1 (1974): 112.

23. He Xingdong et al., *Lin Chuang Zhong Yao Shou Ce*, 167.
24. Zhao Jingbo et al., *Zhong Hua Yi Xue Za Zhi* [Chinese Journal of Medicine] 66, 3 (1986): 145.
25. Jiang Mantao et al., *Bai Qiu En Yi Ke Da Xue Xue Bao* [Journal of Bethune Medical University] 10, 6 (1984): 609.
26. Ding Xuemin et al., *Chang Yong Zhong Yi Fang Yao Shou Ce* [Handbook of Commonly-Used Chinese Herbs and Prescriptions] (Changsha: Hunan Science and Technology Publishing House, 1982), 71.
27. Wang Benxian, *Xin Bian Zhong Yao Xue Ci Dian*, 834.

Chapter 9

Herbs for dispersing food accumulation

消食药

Herbs for dispersing food accumulation

Most of the herbs for dispersing food accumulation are sweet and warm or sweet and neutral and enter the Spleen and Stomach channels. They can disperse food and guide out stagnation, fortify the Spleen and harmonize the Stomach, and increase the appetite. These herbs are mainly used for food accumulation, indigestion, a bloated feeling in the stomach, reduced appetite, belching with a foul odour, acid vomiting, nausea and vomiting, and irregular stool.

Clinically, herbs for dispersing food accumulation can be used in combination with other herbs selected in accordance with the nature of the accompanying pattern:

1. in cases of Spleen and Stomach deficiency, use them with herbs for fortifying the Spleen and harmonizing the Stomach;
2. for heat originating from food accumulation, use them with heat-clearing herbs that are bitter and cold;
3. for food accumulation with inhibited Qi dynamic, use them with herbs for regulating Qi;
4. for deficiency-cold of the Middle Jiao, use them with herbs for warming the Middle Jiao and fortifying the Spleen;
5. for indigestion due to cold and damp obstruction, use them with aromatic herbs for transforming dampness;
6. for food accumulation combined with constipation, use them with downward-draining herbs.

The desired effect cannot usually be achieved where herbs for dispersing food accumulation are used on their own.

Tab. 9 Herbs for dispersing food accumulation

Herb	Functions	Indications
Shan Zha (Fructus Crataegi)	Dispersing food and transforming accumulation, quickening the Blood and dissipating stasis	Indigestion, food accumulation, fullness in the stomach and abdomen, milk accumulation in infants due to improper feeding, diarrhoea and dysentery, postpartum pain in the abdomen due to Blood stasis, persistent flow of lochia, Shan disorders with unilateral sagging of the testicles
Shen Qu (Massa Fermentata)	Dispersing food accumulation, harmonizing the Stomach and fortifying the Spleen	Food accumulation, milk accumulation in infants, distension and fullness in the stomach and abdomen, vomiting and diarrhoea, indigestion
Mai Ya (Fructus Hordei Vulgaris Germinatus)	Dispersing food accumulation and harmonizing the Stomach, soothing the Liver, terminating lactation	Food accumulation, indigestion, distension and pain in the hypochondrium and stomach, belching, reduced appetite, swollen and painful breasts
Dao Ya (Fructus Oryzae Sativae Germinatus)	Fortifying the Spleen, increasing the appetite, dispersing food accumulation and harmonizing the Stomach	Indigestion, pain in the abdomen, reduced appetite due to Spleen deficiency
Lai Fu Zi (Semen Raphani Sativi)	Dispersing food and transforming accumulation, causing Qi to descend and transforming Phlegm	Food accumulation and indigestion, Qi stagnation in the Middle Jiao, distension and fullness in the stomach and abdomen, putrid belching and acid vomiting, diarrhoea
Ji Nei Jin (Endothelium Corneum Gigeriae Galli)	Fortifying the Spleen and harmonizing the Stomach, dispersing food and transforming accumulation, securing the Essence and reducing urine, stopping seminal emission, softening hardness and dispersing stones	Indigestion, distension and fullness in the stomach and abdomen, diarrhoea, Gan accumulation, urinary incontinence, gallstones and stones in the urinary system

Shan Zha 山楂 (Hawthorn fruit, Fructus Crataegi)

Shan Zha is the fruit of *Crataegus pinnatifida* Bge. var. *major* N. E. Br., *C. pinnatifida* Bge. or *C. cuneata* Sieb. et Zucc., family Rosaceae.

Main ingredients *Shan Zha* contains crataegolic, chlorogenic, ursolic, oleanolic and malic acids, quercetin, vitexin, hyperin, epicatechin, sitosterol, vanillic aldehyde, carotene and glycosides.

Properties Taste: sour and sweet; nature: slightly warm.

Channels entered Spleen, Stomach and Liver.

Functions and indications Disperses food and transforms accumulation, quickens the Blood and dissipates stasis. It is indicated for indigestion, food accumulation, fullness in the stomach and abdomen, milk accumulation in infants due to improper feeding, diarrhoea and dysentery, postpartum pain in the abdomen due to Blood stasis, persistent flow of lochia, and Shan disorders with unilateral sagging of the testicles.

Common dosage 10-15g, or 30g for large dosages; appropriate dosage for external application.

Precautions and contraindications *Shan Zha* should be used with caution in cases of Spleen and Stomach deficiency without food accumulation and stagnation.

Remarks Raw *Shan Zha* is used to increase the appetite and disperse food accumulation as well as to dissipate stasis by quickening the Blood; *Shan Zha* stir-fried until it darkens in colour can disperse food accumulation; charred *Shan Zha* can stop diarrhoea and disperse food accumulation. The cores of *Shan Zha* are normally used for treating Shan disorders.

Comparison of functions See *Mai Ya* (Fructus Hordei Vulgaris Germinatus) and *Lai Fu Zi* (Semen Raphani Sativi).

Toxicity Preparations of *Shan Zha* and its extracts have a very low level of toxicity and there have been no reports of long-term usage having any adverse effects.

Modern research

1. Promotes the secretion of digestive juices and regulates the gastrointestinal function to facilitate digestion.[1]
2. Strengthens the heart.[2]
3. Dilates blood vessels and lowers blood pressure.[2]
4. Inhibits cholesterin compounds.[3]
5. Increases the volume of blood flow in the coronary arteries.[2, 4]

Combinations and applications

Functions	Combinations	Applications
Dispersing food and transforming accumulation	*Ji Nei Jin* (Endothelium Corneum Gigeriae Galli) *Shen Qu* (Massa Fermentata) *Mai Ya* (Fructus Hordei Vulgaris Germinatus) *Jiao Bing Lang* (Semen Arecae Catechu, scorch-fried)	Meat-type food accumulation, distension in the abdomen and belching
	Chao Lai Fu Zi (Semen Raphani Sativi, stir-fried) *Chao Mai Ya* (Fructus Hordei Vulgaris Germinatus, stir-fried) *Mu Xiang* (Radix Aucklandiae Lappae) (see notes on legal status)	Food accumulation with abdominal pain in infants, diarrhoea with smelly stool, reduced food intake, slimy tongue fur

	Qing Pi (Pericarpium Citri Reticulatae Viride) *Zhi Shi* (Fructus Immaturus Citri Aurantii) *E Zhu* (Rhizoma Curcumae)	Relatively severe distension, fullness and pain in the abdomen due to food accumulation and Qi stagnation
	Shan Yao (Rhizoma Dioscoreae Oppositae) *Bai Zhu* (Rhizoma Atractylodis Macrocephalae) *Chen Pi* (Pericarpium Citri Reticulatae) *Shen Qu* (Massa Fermentata)	Stagnation of undigested food due to Spleen deficiency
	Mu Xiang (Radix Aucklandiae Lappae) (see notes on legal status) *Bing Lang* (Semen Arecae Catechu) *Zhi Ke* (Fructus Citri Aurantii)	Diarrhoea and dysentery, pain in the abdomen
Quickening the Blood and dissipating stasis	*Dang Gui* (Radix Angelicae Sinensis) *Hong Hua* (Flos Carthami Tinctorii) *Chuan Xiong* (Rhizoma Ligustici Chuanxiong) *Yi Mu Cao* (Herba Leonuri Heterophylli)	Postpartum pain in the abdomen or painful menstruation due to Blood stasis, persistent flow of lochia
	Jue Ming Zi (Semen Cassiae) (with white sugar for oral intake as an infusion)	Hypertension
	Qing Pi (Pericarpium Citri Reticulatae Viride) *Chuan Lian Zi* (Fructus Meliae Toosendan)	Shan disorders with unilateral sagging of the testicles and a feeling of distension
	Wu Zhu Yu (Fructus Evodiae Rutaecarpae) *Xiao Hui Xiang* (Fructus Foeniculi Vulgaris)	Cold and pain in the lower abdomen

Shen Qu 神曲 (Medicated leaven, Massa Fermentata)

Shen Qu is a leavened preparation of a mixture of wheat flour, bran and a variety of herbs such as fresh *Qing Hao* (Herba Artemisiae Chinghao), fresh *Cang Er Zi* (Fructus Xanthii Sibirici), *Xing Ren* (Semen Pruni Armeniacae) and *Chi Xiao Dou* (Semen Phaseoli Calcarati).

Main ingredients *Shen Qu* contains yeast, volatile oils, glycosides, fatty oils and vitamin B.

Properties Taste: sweet and acrid; nature: warm.

Channels entered Spleen and Stomach.

Functions and indications Disperses food accumulation, harmonizes the Stomach and fortifies the Spleen. It is indicated for food accumulation, milk accumulation in infants, distension and fullness in the stomach and abdomen, vomiting and diarrhoea, and indigestion.

Common dosage 6–15g; or appropriate dosage of the powder for external application.

Precautions and contraindications *Shen Qu* should be used with caution for patients with Stomach-fire.

Remarks Scorch-fried *Shen Qu* has a stronger effect in dispersing food accumulation. In addition to its function of fortifying the Spleen and increasing the appetite, raw *Shen Qu* also has a dispersing action, so it is suitable for use in cases of food accumulation with fever due to cold.

Comparison of functions See *Mai Ya* (Fructus Hordei Vulgaris Germinatus).

Modern research *Shen Qu* contains microzymes and amylase that can promote digestion and stimulate the appetite.[5]

Combinations and applications

Functions	Combinations	Applications
Dispersing food accumulation, harmonizing the Stomach and fortifying the Spleen	*Mai Ya* (Fructus Hordei Vulgaris Germinatus) *Shan Zha* (Fructus Crataegi) *Chen Pi* (Pericarpium Citri Reticulatae) *Lai Fu Zi* (Semen Raphani Sativi)	Distension and fullness in the stomach and abdomen due to food accumulation, reduced appetite, rumbling intestines and diarrhoea
	Jiao Shan Zha (Fructus Crataegi, scorch-fried) *Bai Zhu* (Rhizoma Atractylodis Macrocephalae) *Ji Nei Jin* (Endothelium Corneum Gigeriae Galli) (prepared as a powder to be taken orally)	Milk accumulation in infants, diarrhoea, reduced appetite

Notes:
1. As *Shen Qu* is acrid and warm, it can also dissipate cold and release the exterior, and can therefore be used with other acrid, warm herbs for releasing the exterior to treat wind-cold exterior patterns.
2. *Shen Qu* may be added to pills containing minerals or shells to aid in their digestion.

Mai Ya 麦芽
(Barley sprout, Fructus Hordei Vulgaris Germinatus)

Mai Ya is the dried germinated ripe fruit of *Hordeum vulgare* L., family Gramineae.

Main ingredients *Mai Ya* contains amylase, invertase, maltose, dextrin, vitamin B, fats, phospholipids, hordenine and maltoxin.

Properties Taste: sweet; nature: neutral.

Channels entered Spleen, Stomach and Liver.

Functions and indications Disperses food accumulation and harmonizes the Stomach, soothes the Liver, and terminates lactation. It is indicated for food accumulation, indigestion, distension and pain in the hypochondrium and stomach, belching, reduced appetite, and swollen and painful breasts.

Common dosage 10–15g, or 30–120g for large dosages; appropriate dosage for external application.

Precautions and contraindications *Mai Ya* is contraindicated during lactation.

Remarks Raw *Mai Ya* is generally better for dispersing food accumulation and harmonizing the Stomach, whereas the stir-fried herb is more effective for terminating lactation and dispersing swelling.

Comparison of functions *Mai Ya* (Fructus Hordei Vulgaris Germinatus), *Shan Zha* (Fructus Crataegi) and *Shen Qu* (Massa Fermentata) can all disperse food accumulation. *Mai Ya* is better at dispersing rice, flour and potato accumulation and concurrently reinforcing Stomach Qi. *Shan Zha* is good for dispersing meat-type accumulation and focal distension, and also for moving Qi and quickening the Blood. *Shen Qu* is more effective in dispersing grain accumulation, while concurrently guiding out stagnation in order to aid in the digestion of mineral substances. The three herbs can be used together scorch-fried as *Jiao San Xian* to strengthen their functions of dispersing food accumulation and guiding out stagnation.

For an additional comparison, see *Gu Ya* (Fructus Setariae Italicae Germinatus).

Toxicity The main toxic ingredient in *Mai Ya* is maltoxin, which accounts for only 0.02–0.35% of the content of the herb. As maltoxin is not easily absorbed through oral intake, it is not significant in terms of toxicity.

Modern research

1. Promotes the secretion of gastric acids and pepsins.[5]
2. The vitamin B contained in *Mai Ya* promotes digestion.[5]
3. Lowers the blood sugar level.[5]

Combinations and applications

Functions	Combinations	Applications
Dispersing food accumulation and harmonizing the Stomach	*Shan Zha* (Fructus Crataegi) *Shen Qu* (Massa Fermentata) *Ji Nei Jin* (Endothelium Corneum Gigeriae Galli)	Food stagnation and indigestion due to rice, flour and potato accumulation
	Bai Zhu (Rhizoma Atractylodis Macrocephalae) *Chen Pi* (Pericarpium Citri Reticulatae) *Shen Qu* (Massa Fermentata)	Reduced appetite and a bloated feeling after eating due to Spleen deficiency
	Shen Qu (Massa Fermentata) *Ban Xia* (Rhizoma Pinelliae Ternatae) *Chao Lai Fu Zi* (Semen Raphani Sativi, stir-fried) *Chen Pi* (Pericarpium Citri Reticulatae)	Distension and fullness in the stomach and abdomen, food accumulation
Soothing the Liver	*Qing Pi* (Pericarpium Citri Reticulatae Viride) *Chuan Lian Zi* (Fructus Meliae Toosendan)	Distension and pain in the hypochondrium and stomach and belching due to constrained Liver Qi

Note: Decoctions of raw or stir-fried *Mai Ya* (or a combination of the raw and stir-fried herb) can be used for terminating lactation or treating distension and pain in the breasts.

Dao Ya 稻芽 (Rice sprout, Fructus Oryzae Sativae Germinatus)

Dao Ya is the dried germinated ripe fruit of *Oryza sativa* L., family Gramineae.

Main ingredients *Dao Ya* contains starch, proteins, fats, vitamin B and amylase.

Properties Taste: sweet; nature: neutral.

Channels entered Spleen and Stomach.

Functions and indications Fortifies the Spleen, increases the appetite, disperses food accumulation and harmonizes the Stomach. It is indicated for indigestion, pain in the abdomen, and reduced appetite due to Spleen deficiency.

Common dosage 10-15g, or 30g for large dosages.

Remarks Raw *Dao Ya* is used to harmonize the Middle Jiao, whereas the stir-fried herb is better for dispersing food accumulation.

Comparison of functions See *Gu Ya* (Fructus Setariae Italicae Germinatus) below.

Modern research The microzymes and amylase contained in *Dao Ya* promote digestion.[6]

Combinations and applications

Functions	Combinations	Applications
Fortifying the Spleen, increasing the appetite, dispersing food accumulation and harmonizing the Stomach	*Sha Ren* (Fructus Amomi) *Bai Zhu* (Rhizoma Atractylodis Macrocephalae) *Gan Cao* (Radix Glycyrrhizae)	Qi deficiency of the Spleen and Stomach, manifesting as poor appetite, no desire to eat or low food intake
	Shen Qu (Massa Fermentata) *Shan Zha* (Fructus Crataegi) *Bai Bian Dou* (Semen Dolichoris Lablab)	Pain in the abdomen and diarrhoea due to Spleen deficiency
	Dang Shen (Radix Codonopsitis Pilosulae) *Bai Zhu* (Rhizoma Atractylodis Macrocephalae) *Chen Pi* (Pericarpium Citri Reticulatae)	Reduced appetite due to Spleen deficiency

Appendix

Gu Ya 谷芽 (Millet sprout, Fructus Setariae Italicae Germinatus)

Gu Ya, the dried germinated ripe fruit of *Setaria italica* (L.) Beauv., family Gramineae, has the same properties, functions, indications, combinations and applications as *Dao Ya*. *Gu Ya* and *Dao Ya* have similar functions to *Mai Ya* (Fructus Hordei Vulgaris Germinatus) in dispersing and transforming food accumulation, fortifying the Spleen and increasing the appetite, but have a weaker effect. These herbs are used for food stagnation patterns with accumulation of rice, flour or potatoes and for reduced appetite due to Spleen deficiency; they are often combined to strengthen their effect.

Lai Fu Zi 莱菔子 (Radish seed, Semen Raphani Sativi)

Lai Fu Zi is the dried seed of *Raphanus sativus* L., family Cruciferae.

Main ingredients *Lai Fu Zi* contains erucic acid, linoleic acid, linolenic acid, glycerol sinapate, sinapine, raphanin and volatile oils.

Properties Taste: acrid and sweet; nature: neutral.

Channels entered Spleen, Stomach and Lung.

Functions and indications Disperses food and transforms accumulation, causes Qi to descend and transforms Phlegm. It is indicated for food accumulation and indigestion, Qi stagnation in the Middle Jiao, distension and fullness in the stomach and abdomen, putrid belching and acid vomiting, and diarrhoea.

Common dosage 6-10g.

Precautions and contraindications

1. As *Lai Fu Zi* tends to consume Qi, it should be used with caution in cases of Qi deficiency without food accumulation or Phlegm stagnation.
2. *Lai Fu Zi* should not be used in combination with *Ren Shen* (Radix Ginseng).

Comparison of functions *Lai Fu Zi* (Semen Raphani Sativi) and *Shan Zha* (Fructus Crataegi) are both very effective in dispersing food and transforming accumulation to treat food accumulation and stagnation patterns. *Shan Zha* is good at dispersing accumulation and transforming stagnation, and is used particularly for accumulation of meat and greasy and oily foods. *Lai Fu Zi* can also move Qi and ease distension while dispersing food and transforming accumulation. It is therefore good for treating food accumulation with Qi stagnation.

For additional comparisons, see *Bai Jie Zi* (Semen Sinapis Albae) and *Chang Shan* (Radix Dichroae Febrifugae).

Toxicity The LD_{50} for intraperitoneal injection in rats of aqueous extracts of *Lai Fu Zi* is 127.4 ± 3.7g/kg. Intragastric administration to rats of 100g/kg, 200g/kg and 400g/kg of liquid extracts of the herb on a daily basis for three weeks did not result in any significant changes to the animals' blood or to the functioning of the liver and kidneys and other main organs.

Modern research

1. Inhibits gastric diarrhoea and dysentery, strengthens intestinal contraction.[7]
2. The raphanin contained in *Lai Fu Zi* significantly inhibits the growth of staphylococci and Escherichia coli.[8]
3. Inhibits inflammation.[8]
4. Slows the heart rate.[8]

Combinations and applications

Functions	Combinations	Applications
Dispersing food and transforming accumulation, causing Qi to descend and transforming Phlegm	*Shan Zha* (Fructus Crataegi) *Shen Qu* (Massa Fermentata) *Chen Pi* (Pericarpium Citri Reticulatae)	Indigestion, distension and fullness in the stomach and abdomen, and acid vomiting due to Qi stagnation in the Middle Jiao
	Zhi Ke (Fructus Citri Aurantii) *Da Fu Pi* (Pericarpium Arecae Catechu)	Distension in the abdomen and constipation with slimy tongue fur due to dampness
	Huang Lian (Rhizoma Coptidis) *Huang Qin* (Radix Scutellariae Baicalensis) *Dai Zhe Shi* (Haematitum)	Nausea with bad breath due to food accumulation and Stomach-fire
	Bai Jie Zi (Semen Sinapis Albae) *Su Zi* (Fructus Perillae Frutescentis)	Coughing and wheezing with oppression in the chest due to Phlegm-saliva congestion

Ji Nei Jin 鸡内金
(Internal lining of chicken gizzard, Endothelium Corneum Gigeriae Galli)

Ji Nei Jin is the dried internal lining membrane of the gizzard of *Gallus gallus domesticus* Brisson, family Phasianidae.

Main ingredients *Ji Nei Jin* contains ventriculin, keratin, amino acids, bilatriene, and vitamins B_1 and B_2.

Properties Taste: sweet; nature: neutral.
Channels entered Spleen, Stomach, Small Intestine and Bladder.
Functions and indications Fortifies the Spleen and harmonizes the Stomach, disperses food and transforms accumulation, secures the Essence and reduces urine, stops seminal emission, softens hardness and disperses stones. It is indicated for indigestion, distension and fullness in the stomach and abdomen, diarrhoea, Gan accumulation, urinary incontinence, gallstones and stones in the urinary system.
Common dosage 3–10g; or 1.5–3g in powder form for oral intake.
Remarks *Ji Nei Jin* is more effective in treating indigestion in powder form rather than as a decoction.

Modern research

1. Promotes the secretion of gastric juices and strengthens gastric peristalsis.[9]
2. Decoctions of *Ji Nei Jin* accelerated the discharge of radiostrontium from the urine in laboratory experiments.[8]

Combinations and applications

Functions	Combinations	Applications
Fortifying the Spleen and harmonizing the Stomach, dispersing food and transforming accumulation	*Shen Qu* (Massa Fermentata) *Shan Zha* (Fructus Crataegi) *Mai Ya* (Fructus Hordei Vulgaris Germinatus) *Lai Fu Zi* (Semen Raphani Sativi)	Distension and fullness in the stomach and abdomen, indigestion
	Fu Ling (Sclerotium Poriae Cocos) *Bai Zhu* (Rhizoma Atractylodis Macrocephalae) *Gan Jiang* (Rhizoma Zingiberis Officinalis)	Reduced appetite due to Spleen and Stomach deficiency, diarrhoea due to non-transformation of food
	Dang Shen (Radix Codonopsitis Pilosulae) *Bai Zhu* (Rhizoma Atractylodis Macrocephalae) *Sha Ren* (Fructus Amomi)	Gan accumulation in children due to Spleen deficiency
	Shi Jun Zi (Fructus Quisqualis Indicae) *Lei Wan* (Sclerotium Omphaliae Lapidescens)	Worm infestation
Securing the Essence and reducing urine, stopping seminal emission	*Qian Shi* (Semen Euryales Ferocis) *Tu Si Zi* (Semen Cuscutae) *Lian Zi* (Semen Nelumbinis Nuciferae)	Seminal emission
	Sang Piao Xiao (Oötheca Mantidis) *Fu Pen Zi* (Fructus Rubi Chingii) *Yi Zhi Ren* (Fructus Alpiniae Oxyphyllae)	Frequent urination, urinary incontinence
Softening hardness and dispersing stones	*Hai Jin Sha* (Spora Lygodii Japonicae) *Jin Qian Cao* (Herba Lysimachiae)	Gallstones and stones in the urinary system

Note: *Ji Nei Jin* can be taken orally as a powder to treat food accumulation with bad breath in children.

Modern research references

1. Wang Yusheng et al., *Zhong Yao Yao Li Yu Ying Yong* [Pharmacology and Application of Chinese Materia Medica] (Beijing: People's Medical Publishing House, 1998), 105.
2. Guangxi No. 4 Pharmaceutical Factory et al., *Zhong Cao Yao Tong Xun* [Chinese Herbs Newsletter] 9 (1977): 30.
3. Chu Yanfang et al., *Zhong Cao Yao* [Journal of Chinese Herbs] 19, 1 (1988): 25.
4. Li Qunai, *Hu Nan Zhong Yi Za Zhi* [Hunan Journal of Traditional Chinese Medicine] 4 (1988): 33.
5. He Xingdong et al., *Lin Chuang Zhong Yao Shou Ce* [Clinical Handbook of Chinese Materia Medica] (Beijing: People's Medical Publishing House, 1998), 175.
6. Ibid., 176.
7. Lei Zaiquan and Zhang Tingmo, *Zhong Hua Lin Chuang Zhong Yao Xue* [Chinese Clinical Materia Medica] (Beijing: People's Medical Publishing House, 1998), 1017.
8. He Xingdong et al., *Lin Chuang Zhong Yao Shou Ce*, 177.
9. Lei Zaiquan and Zhang Tingmo, *Zhong Hua Lin Chuang Zhong Yao Xue*, 1015.

Chapter 10

Herbs for expelling worms

驱虫药

Herbs for expelling worms

Herbs which can expel or kill worms are mainly used for infestation of the gastrointestinal tract with roundworm, threadworm, tapeworm, hookworm and intestinal flukes. Clinically, the main manifestations include distension and pain in the abdomen, voracious appetite or no desire for food, a predilection for strange foods, white patches on the face, and anal itch. If the disease lasts for a prolonged period, it will manifest as a yellow facial complexion and emaciation. Some herbs for expelling worms can also be used to treat such diseases as bilharzia, filariasis and trichomoniasis.

Different worm infestations have different clinical manifestations. Hence, the combination of other compatible herbs with herbs for expelling worms will depend on the type of worm, the general condition of the patient and any complications involved:

1. for cold-type cases, use herbs for expelling worms in combination with herbs for warming the interior and dispelling cold;
2. for heat-type cases, use them with heat-clearing herbs with bitter and cold properties;
3. for cases with Spleen and Stomach deficiency, use them with herbs for fortifying the Spleen and harmonizing the Stomach;
4. for weak patients, apply treatment to supplement vital Qi before using herbs for expelling worms, or apply both of the methods at the same time.

Herbs for expelling worms should be taken before eating in order for the herbs to affect the worms directly. Purgatives may be taken at the same time to increase the effect. Where herbs for expelling worms are toxic, special attention must be paid to the dosage.

Tab. 10 Herbs for expelling worms

Herb	Functions	Indications
Shi Jun Zi (Fructus Quisqualis Indicae)	Killing worms, fortifying the Spleen and dispersing food accumulation	Pain in the abdomen due to worm infestation, Gan accumulation, infantile indigestion
Ku Lian Pi (Cortex Meliae Radicis)	Killing worms, drying dampness, alleviating itching and treating tinea	Roundworm, pinworm, hookworm, eczema, tinea capitis
Bing Lang (Semen Arecae Catechu)	Killing worms, dispersing food accumulation and guiding out stagnation, moving Qi and promoting the movement of water, dispersing Phlegm, interrupting malaria	Infestation by tapeworm and intestinal flukes, food accumulation with Qi stagnation, distension in the abdomen and constipation, dysentery, oedema, painful swelling in leg Qi, malaria
Nan Gua Zi (Semen Cucurbitae Moschatae)	Killing worms, freeing milk	Tapeworm, roundworm, insufficient lactation
He Cao Ya (Gemma Agrimoniae Pilosae)	Killing intestinal worms	Tapeworm
Lei Wan (Sclerotium Omphaliae Lapidescens)	Dispersing food accumulation and killing intestinal worms	Tapeworm, hookworm, roundworm, Gan accumulation
Fei Zi (Semen Torreyae Grandis)	Killing worms, freeing the bowels, moistening the Lungs	Roundworm, hookworm and tapeworm, constipation due to haemorrhoids, cough due to dry Lungs

Shi Jun Zi 使君子 (Rangoon creeper fruit, Fructus Quisqualis Indicae)

Shi Jun Zi is the ripe fruit of *Quisqualis indica* L., family Combretaceae.

Main ingredients *Shi Jun Zi* contains quisqualic acid, potassium quisqualate, sucrose, fructose, malic acid, citric acid, succinic acid, trigonelline and pyvidine.

Properties Taste: sweet; nature: warm.

Channels entered Spleen and Stomach.

Functions and indications Kills worms, fortifies the Spleen and disperses food accumulation. It is indicated for pain in the abdomen due to worm infestation, Gan accumulation, and infantile indigestion.

Common dosage 6-10g; the dosage for adults is 10-20 seeds per day and for children 1-1.5 seeds per day for each year of age, but never more than 20 seeds per day. Take on an empty stomach for 2-3 days. The stir-fried herb should be chewed well before swallowing.

Precautions and contraindications If *Shi Jun Zi* is taken in large amounts or with tea, it may give rise to such reactions as hiccups, dizziness and vomiting, pain in the abdomen, and diarrhoea; these reactions will disappear spontaneously after intake of the herb ceases. Strong infusions of *Shi Jun Zi* should be avoided.

Comparison of functions Both *Shi Jun Zi* (Fructus Quisqualis Indicae) and *Ku Lian Pi* (Cortex Meliae Radicis) can kill worms, being particularly suitable for expelling and killing roundworm. *Ku Lian Pi* is bitter, cold and toxic and is good for killing worms, especially roundworm. However, *Shi Jun Zi*, sweet and warm, works even better in this respect and is a key herb for killing roundworm. In addition, it can warm and boost the Spleen and Stomach and is effective in the treatment of Gan accumulation and in eliminating deficiency-heat. *Ku Lian Pi* can also clear damp-heat to treat tinea.

For an additional comparison, see *Fei Zi* (Semen Torreyae Grandis).

Toxicity *Shi Jun Zi* has a relatively low level of toxicity. The minimum lethal dosage for subcutaneous injection in mice of a water-soluble extract of the herb is 20g/kg. Single use of a *Shi Jun Zi* decoction in mice had extremely low toxicity, with an LD_{50} in excess of 4g/kg. The main toxic ingredient is potassium quisqualate, which caused epilepsy in laboratory tests on animals. Toxic side-effects in humans of *Shi Jun Zi* include hiccups, headache, nausea, vomiting, cold sweats and cold limbs, and in severe cases, convulsions, dyspnoea and lower blood pressure. The main causes of toxic reaction are intake of the raw herb or overdosage in a simple formula.

Modern research

1. The decoction and steep of *Shi Jun Zi* both expel roundworm.[1]
2. Expels pinworm.[1]
3. Inhibits dermal epiphytes.[2]

Combinations and applications

Functions	Combinations	Applications
Killing worms, fortifying the Spleen and dispersing food accumulation	*Ku Lian Pi* (Cortex Meliae Radicis) *Bing Lang* (Semen Arecae Catechu)	Pain in the abdomen due to roundworm
	Mu Xiang (Radix Aucklandiae Lappae) (see notes on legal status) *Bai Zhu* (Rhizoma Atractylodis Macrocephalae) *Mai Ya* (Fructus Hordei Vulgaris Germinatus) *Bing Lang* (Semen Arecae Catechu)	Gan accumulation, emaciation with distension in the abdomen, yellow facial complexion and dry hair

	Fei Zi (Semen Torreyae Grandis)	Hookworm
	Bai Bu (Radix Stemonae) *Da Huang* (Radix et Rhizoma Rhei)	Pinworm

Ku Lian Pi 苦楝皮 (Chinaberry bark, Cortex Meliae Radicis)

Ku Lian Pi is the stem bark and root cortex of *Melia azedarach* L. or *M. toosendan* Sieb. et Zucc., family Meliaceae.

Main ingredients *Ku Lian Pi* contains toosendanin, isotoosendanin, kulactone, kulolactone, kulinone, nimbolin A and B, fraxinellone, gedunin and meliantriol.

Properties Taste: bitter; nature: cold; toxic.

Channels entered Spleen, Stomach and Liver.

Functions and indications Kills worms, dries dampness, alleviates itching and treats tinea. It is indicated for roundworm, pinworm, hookworm, eczema, and tinea capitis.

Common dosage 6-15g, or double this dosage for the fresh herb; appropriate dosage for external application as a wash prepared from a decoction of *Ku Lian Pi*, local use of an alcoholic extract of the herb, or application of powdered *Ku Lian Pi* mixed with alcohol.

Precautions and contraindications The toxicity of *Ku Lian Pi* means that overdosage should be avoided and it should not be used for prolonged periods. This herb should be used with caution for patients with a weak constitution or in cases of Spleen and Stomach deficiency-cold; it is contraindicated for those with liver or kidney malfunction.

Comparison of functions Both *Ku Lian Pi* (Cortex Meliae Radicis) and *Chuan Lian Zi* (Fructus Meliae Toosendan) can kill worms and treat tinea. *Chuan Lian Zi* can also guide out heat from the Small Intestine and Bladder to conduct Heart-fire downwards, thus moving Qi and alleviating pain. It is an important herb for pain in the Heart and abdomen and treats abdominal pain due to worm accumulation by moving Qi to alleviate pain rather than by killing worms. *Ku Lian Pi* is very effective in killing worms, but its toxic effect is more obvious than that of *Chuan Lian Zi*.

For an additional comparison, see *Shi Jun Zi* (Fructus Quisqualis Indicae).

Toxicity The LD_{50} of the toosendanin contained in *Ku Lian Pi* given to mice by intraperitoneal injection, intravenous injection and subcutaneous injection is in the region of 14mg/kg; for subcutaneous injection in rats, it is 9.8mg/kg and for intravenous injection in rabbits, it is 4.2mg/kg. The minimum lethal dosage is 30-32mg/kg for dogs, but only 3-4mg/kg for cats. When 10mg/kg of *Ku Lian Pi* was given to dogs via intragastric administration, some of them developed symptoms of violent vomiting. Rats given 20-40mg/kg via intragastric administration developed oedema of the gastric mucosa, gastritis and ulcers. The main toxic ingredients of *Ku Lian Pi* are toosendanin and isotoosendanin, which can stimulate the gastrointestinal tract and damage the liver. Toxic side-effects include dizziness, headache, drowsiness, nausea, vomiting and pain in the abdomen, and in severe cases, respiratory arrest, nephritis, haemorrhage and loss of visual acuity. *Ku Lian Pi* is contraindicated or should be used with great caution during pregnancy, for patients with a weak constitution, anaemia, liver or kidney malfunction, pulmonary TB, ulcers or serious heart problems.

Modern research

1. Expels roundworm.[3]
2. Decoctions of *Ku Lian Pi* have an inhibitory effect on many kinds of pathogenic epiphytes, especially tinea capitis epiphytes.[3]

Combinations and applications

Functions	Combinations	Applications
Killing worms, drying dampness, alleviating itching and treating tinea	*Shi Liu Pi* (Pericarpium Punicae Granati) *Bing Lang* (Semen Arecae Catechu)	Roundworm and hookworm
	Wu Mei (Fructus Pruni Mume) *Ku Shen* (Radix Sophorae Flavescentis) *Bai Bu* (Radix Stemonae)	Pinworm
	Xiang Fu (Rhizoma Cyperi Rotundi) *Yu Jin* (Radix Curcumae) *Mu Xiang* (Radix Aucklandiae Lappae) (see notes on legal status)	Biliary ascariasis
	Zao Jiao (Fructus Gleditsiae Sinensis)	Eczema

Note: *Ku Lian Pi* can be prepared with alcohol for external use to treat tinea capitis, or with water for application as an external wash to stop itching.

Bing Lang 槟榔
(Areca seed, Semen Arecae Catechu)

Bing Lang is the ripe seed of *Areca catechu* L., family Palmae.

Legal status In the UK, *Bing Lang* can only be sold in premises which are registered pharmacies and by or under the supervision of a pharmacist.

Main ingredients *Bing Lang* contains alkaloids (mainly arecoline, but also arecaidine, guvacoline, guvacine and arecolidine); myristic, louric, palmitic, oleic, linoleic and stearic acids; areca red, proline, arginine and catechin.

Properties Taste: bitter and acrid; nature: warm.

Channels entered Stomach and Large Intestine.

Functions and indications Kills worms, disperses food accumulation and guides out stagnation, moves Qi and promotes the movement of water, disperses Phlegm, and interrupts malaria. It is indicated for various types of parasitic infestation in the intestinal tract such as tapeworm and intestinal flukes (Fasciolopsis), food accumulation with Qi stagnation, distension in the abdomen and constipation, dysentery, oedema, painful swelling in leg Qi, and malaria.

Common dosage 6-15g. If *Bing Lang* is used alone for treating tapeworm and Fasciolopsis, the dosage can be as much as 60-120g.

Precautions and contraindications

1. *Bing Lang* is contraindicated in cases of loose stool due to Spleen deficiency, and for Qi deficiency fall.
2. *Bing Lang* should be used with caution during pregnancy.

Remarks Raw *Bing Lang* can be used for killing worms; it is a key herb for killing tapeworm. Stir-fried *Bing Lang* can be used for food accumulation, while in its charred form it can stop bleeding and is used for treating bloody dysentery.

Comparison of functions See *Nan Gua Zi* (Semen Cucurbitae Moschatae), *He Cao Ya* (Gemma Agrimoniae Pilosae) and *Da Fu Pi* (Pericarpium Arecae Catechu).

Toxicity The LD_{50} for a decoction of *Bing Lang* given to mice via intragastric administration is 120 ± 24g/kg. *Bing Lang* has very low level of toxicity. The main causes of toxic side-effects are overdosage or administration to patients with a weak constitution who are allergic to the herb; in the latter instance, intake of just 30g of the decoction can trigger a severe reaction. Toxic symptoms include increased salivation, nausea, vomiting, pain in the abdomen, palpitations, rapid breathing, dizziness and stupor.

Modern research

1. Expels tapeworm, roundworm and pinworm, inhibits schistosomes.[1]
2. The steep of *Bing Lang* inhibits dermal epiphytes and is effective against influenza viruses.[1]

Combinations and applications

Functions	Combinations	Applications
Killing worms	*Nan Gua Zi* (Semen Cucurbitae Moschatae)	Tapeworm
	Ku Lian Pi (Cortex Meliae Radicis) *Shi Jun Zi* (Fructus Quisqualis Indicae)	Roundworm, pinworm
	Guan Zhong (Rhizoma Dryopteris Crassirhizomae) (see notes on legal status) *Bai Bu* (Radix Stemonae)	Threadworm
	Fei Zi (Semen Torreyae Grandis)	Hookworm
	Wu Mei (Fructus Pruni Mume) *Gan Cao* (Radix Glycyrrhizae)	Fasciolopsis
Dispersing food accumulation and guiding out stagnation	*Mu Xiang* (Radix Aucklandiae Lappae) (see notes on legal status) *Zhi Ke* (Fructus Citri Aurantii) *Huang Qin* (Radix Scutellariae Baicalensis) *Su Geng* (Caulis Perillae Frutescentis)	Food accumulation with Qi stagnation, distension and pain in the stomach and abdomen, diarrhoea and dysentery
	Hou Po (Cortex Magnoliae Officinalis) *Da Huang* (Radix et Rhizoma Rhei)	Distension and fullness in the abdomen and tenesmus due to food accumulation with Qi stagnation
	Ban Xia (Rhizoma Pinelliae Ternatae) *Sha Ren* (Fructus Amomi) *Mai Ya* (Fructus Hordei Vulgaris Germinatus)	Distension and pain in the abdomen due to Spleen and Stomach deficiency
Moving Qi and promoting the movement of water, dispersing Phlegm	*Ze Xie* (Rhizoma Alismatis Orientalis) *Mu Tong* (Caulis Mutong) (see notes on legal status) *Che Qian Zi* (Semen Plantaginis)	Oedema due to stagnation of water and dampness
	Mu Gua (Fructus Chaenomelis) *Chen Pi* (Pericarpium Citri Reticulatae) *Wu Zhu Yu* (Fructus Evodiae Rutaecarpae)	Swelling and pain in cold-damp leg Qi
	Wu Yao (Radix Linderae Strychnifoliae) *Mu Xiang* (Radix Aucklandiae Lappae) (see notes on legal status) *Chuan Lian Zi* (Fructus Meliae Toosendan)	Shan disorders due to Qi stagnation in the Small Intestine

	Ting Li Zi (Semen Lepidii seu Descurainiae)	Coughing and wheezing due to Phlegm-damp
Interrupting malaria	*Chang Shan* (Radix Dichroae Febrifugae) *Cao Guo* (Fructus Amomi Tsaoko) *Hou Po* (Cortex Magnoliae Officinalis)	Malaria

Nan Gua Zi 南瓜子 (Pumpkin seed, Semen Cucurbitae Moschatae)

Nan Gua Zi is the ripe seed of *Cucurbita moschata* Duch., family Cucurbitaceae.

Legal status *Nan Gua Zi* was listed in a document entitled *A Review of Restricted Herbal Ingredients* issued by the Medicines Control Agency (MCA) in the UK in September 2001 with a view to the possible imposition of restrictions on its use at a future date. A related plant, *Cucurbita maxima*, is controlled under Schedule 1 of the Medicines (Retail Sale or Supply of Herbal Remedies) Order 1977, which prohibits the sale or supply of herbal medicines in the UK containing this plant, except where sold in premises which are registered pharmacies and by or under the supervision of a pharmacist. The MCA considers that other species of *Cucurbita* (including *C. moschata*) may also present a risk to public health.

Main ingredients *Nan Gua Zi* contains cucurbitine, fatty oils, proteins, vitamins A, B_1, B_2 and C, and carotene.

Properties Taste: sweet; nature: neutral.

Channels entered Stomach and Large Intestine.

Functions and indications Kills worms and frees milk. It is indicated for tapeworm, roundworm and insufficient lactation.

Common dosage 30-60g, or 120g for large dosages.

Precautions and contraindications *Nan Gua Zi* is contraindicated in cases of distension in the abdomen with diarrhoea.

Comparison of functions Both *Nan Gua Zi* (Semen Cucurbitae Moschatae) and *Bing Lang* (Semen Arecae Catechu) can expel tapeworm, but the location of the effect is different. *Nan Gua Zi* can cause paralysis of the middle and end sections of the body of the worm, whereas *Bing Lang* can bring about paralysis of the head and immature part of the worm. The two herbs are used together to strengthen their effect (see below for the procedure to be employed). *Nan Gua Zi* is used specifically to kill worms, while *Bing Lang* can also move Qi and promote the movement of water.

For an additional comparison, see *He Cao Ya* (Gemma Agrimoniae Pilosae).

Toxicity The LD_{50} for cucurbitine perchlorate and hydrochlorate given to mice via intragastric administration is 1.25g/kg and 1.10g/kg respectively. *Nan Gua Zi* and the cucurbitine it contains caused temporary pathological damage to the liver, lungs, kidneys and duodenum of mice in experiments. The main causes of toxic symptoms in humans are overdosage and administration to patients with abnormal liver function.

Modern research

1. Expels threadworm and schistosomes.[4]
2. An injection of the herb raised blood pressure and deepened breathing in experiments.[5]

Combinations and applications

Functions	Combinations	Applications
Killing worms	*Bing Lang* (Semen Arecae Catechu)	Tapeworm
Freeing milk	Pound raw, peeled *Nan Gua Zi* into pieces for taking orally with water	Postpartum loss of breast milk

Note: *Nan Gua Zi* can be used for tapeworm and roundworm. Using it in combination with *Bing Lang* (Semen Arecae Catechu) can strengthen the effect in treating tapeworm. The procedure is as follows: first, grind *Nan Gua Zi* (with its shell) into a powder and take orally with cold water; two hours later, take a decoction of *Bing Lang* (60-120g); half an hour afterwards, take 15g of *Mang Xiao* (Mirabilitum) with cooled boiled water to dislodge and expel the worms by purgation.

He Cao Ya 鹤草芽 (Agrimony bud, Gemma Agrimoniae Pilosae)

He Cao Ya is the dried bud, with a short piece of rhizome attached, of *Agrimonia pilosa* Ledeb., family Rosaceae.

Main ingredients *He Cao Ya* contains agrimophol, agrimonolide, agrimonol, apigenin, isocoumarin glycosides and sitosterol.

Properties Taste: bitter and astringent; nature: cool.

Channels entered Liver, Large Intestine and Small Intestine.

Functions and indications Kills intestinal worms. It is indicated for tapeworm.

Common dosage 30-50g of powder for oral use with water; 0.5-0.8g per kg of body weight for children.

Precautions and contraindications Some patients may be affected by nausea, vomiting, diarrhoea, dizziness or sweating after administration of the herb.

Remarks *He Cao Ya* should be ground into a powder and taken on an empty stomach in the morning; the worms will generally be discharged five or six hours later.

Comparison of functions *He Cao Ya* (Gemma Agrimoniae Pilosae), *Bing Lang* (Semen Arecae Catechu) and *Nan Gua Zi* (Semen Cucurbitae Moschatae) are commonly used in the clinic to kill worms and are particularly effective against tapeworm. *He Cao Ye* can be used on its own to kill worms and also has effect of draining downwards; *Bing Lang* and *Nan Gua Zi* function better when used together to strengthen their effect in killing worms. *He Cao Ya* is more effective against adult worms.

Toxicity *He Cao Ya* is relatively non-toxic, but its main active ingredient for expelling worms, agrimophol, has a certain degree of toxicity. The LD_{50} for intragastric administration of agrimophol to mice is 435 ± 88mg/kg. The main cause of toxic side-effects (such as occasional nausea and vomiting, dizziness, diarrhoea and sweating) is overdosage of extracts of the herb and injection of agrimophol.

Modern research Expels worms, especially effective for threadworm and cysticercus tapeworm; directly kills schistosomes.[6]

Lei Wan 雷丸 (Omphalia, Sclerotium Omphaliae Lapidescens)

Lei Wan is the dried sclerotium of *Omphalia lapidescens* Schroet., family Polyporaceae.

Main ingredients *Lei Wan* contains hydrolytic protease.

Properties Taste: bitter; nature: cold; slightly toxic.

Channels entered Stomach and Large Intestine.

Functions and indications Disperses food accumulation and kills intestinal worms. It is indicated for tapeworm, hookworm, roundworm, and Gan accumulation.

Common dosage 6-15g in pills or powder. For tapeworm, take 12-18g of the powder with cooled boiled water three times a day after meals for three days.

Precautions and contraindications *Lei Wan* should be used with caution for patients with worm accumulation and Spleen and Stomach deficiency-cold.

Remarks The active ingredient in *Lei Wan* is easily destroyed by warmer temperatures (about 60°C) and an acid environment, so it should be used in pills and powder or with an alkaline solution to strengthen its effect.

Comparison of functions *Lei Wan* (Sclerotium Omphaliae Lapidescens), *Fu Ling* (Sclerotium Poriae Cocos) and *Zhu Ling* (Sclerotium Polypori Umbellati) are all materia medica derived from fungi; *Fu Ling* comes from pine trees, *Zhu Ling* from the Chinese sweetgum and *Lei Wan* from bamboo. All three herbs can promote the elimination of dampness. *Fu Ling*, which fortifies the Spleen and quiets the Spirit, is a high-grade product; *Zhu Ling*, which functions specifically for promoting the movement of water, is a medium-grade product; and *Lei Wan*, which functions specifically for dispersing accumulation and killing worms, is a low-grade product.

Toxicity The protease contained in *Lei Wan* had a certain toxic effect on rats, which after being given intraperitoneal injection and intramuscular injection of the herb, suffered from water accumulation in the abdomen, but did not die. Oral administration of the herb is comparatively safe, although some clinical reports mention occasional side-effects such as nausea or temporary discomfort in the upper abdomen.

Modern research

1. Expels threadworm and hookworm.[7]
2. A 10% concentrate of the decoction of *Lei Wan* is effective against external Trichomonas infections.[8]
3. Inhibits carcinoma.[9]
4. Inhibits inflammation and strengthens the immune function.[10, 11]

Combinations and applications

Functions	Combinations	Applications
Dispersing food accumulation and killing intestinal worms	*Bing Lang* (Semen Arecae Catechu) *Ku Lian Pi* (Cortex Meliae Radicis) *Wu Mei* (Fructus Pruni Mume)	Roundworm
	Bing Lang (Semen Arecae Catechu) *Nan Gua Zi* (Semen Cucurbitae Moschatae)	Tapeworm
	Fei Zi (Semen Torreyae Grandis) *Da Suan* (Bulbus Allii Sativi)	Hookworm
	Lu Hui (Herba Aloes) (see notes on legal status) *Huang Lian* (Rhizoma Coptidis)	Gan accumulation

Fei Zi 榧子
(Torreya nut, Semen Torreyae Grandis)

Fei Zi is the ripe seed of *Torreya grandis* Fort., family Taxaceae.

Main ingredients *Fei Zi* contains linoleic, stearic, oleic, palmitic, linolenic, lauric and myristic acids, gliadin, sterols, tannin, polysaccharides and volatile oils.

Properties Taste: sweet; nature: neutral.

Channels entered Lung, Stomach and Large Intestine.

Functions and indications Kills worms, frees the bowels, and moistens the Lungs. It is indicated for roundworm, hookworm and tapeworm, constipation due to haemorrhoids, and cough due to dry Lungs.

Common dosage 30-50g; remove the shell after stir-frying and chew 30-40 nuts a day on an empty stomach until no hookworms can be found in the stool. *Fei Zi* can be ground into a powder for decocting, but it is more effective in direct oral use. The nut can also be cooked with a broken shell.

Precautions and contraindications *Fei Zi* is not suitable for patients with diarrhoea.

Remarks *Fei Zi* is sweet in taste, neutral in nature and non-toxic. It is an important herb for killing worms, but does not damage Stomach Qi. It also has the effect of moistening the Intestines and freeing the bowels to promote the expulsion of worms without the need to add draining herbs.

Comparison of functions Both *Fei Zi* (Semen Torreyae Grandis) and *Shi Jun Zi* (Fructus Quisqualis Indicae) are sweet in taste and can expel and kill intestinal parasites, moisten dryness and lubricate the Intestines. These herbs do not require the addition of other draining herbs. *Fei Zi* is very effective in expelling tapeworm and hookworm; it can also moisten the Lungs to stop coughing and moisten the Intestines to treat haemorrhoids. *Shi Jun Zi* is better at expelling and eliminating roundworm, while it can also boost the Spleen and Stomach and treat Gan accumulation.

Toxicity This herb may occasionally cause slight dizziness.

Combinations and applications

Functions	Combinations	Applications
Killing worms	*Guan Zhong* (Rhizoma Dryopteris Crassirhizomae) (see notes on legal status) *Bing Lang* (Semen Arecae Catechu)	Hookworm
	Nan Gua Zi (Semen Cucurbitae Moschatae) *Bing Lang* (Semen Arecae Catechu)	Tapeworm
	Shi Jun Zi (Fructus Quisqualis Indicae) *Ku Lian Pi* (Cortex Meliae Radicis) *Wu Mei* (Fructus Pruni Mume)	Roundworm

Additional applications:

1. Chewing stir-fried *Fei Zi* on its own can be used to treat constipation due to haemorrhoids.
2. *Fei Zi* also has the function of moistening the Lungs and stopping coughing and is suitable for a slight cough due to dry Lungs. It is often combined with *Chuan Bei Mu* (Bulbus Fritillariae Cirrhosae), *Gua Lou Ren* (Semen Trichosanthis), *Zhi Sang Ye* (prepared Folium Mori Albae), *Sha Shen* (Radix Glehniae seu Adenophorae) and *Dang Gui* (Radix Angelicae Sinensis) to strengthen its effect in stopping coughing.

Modern research references

1. Lei Zaiquan and Zhang Tingmo, *Zhong Hua Lin Chuang Zhong Yao Xue* [Chinese Clinical Materia Medica] (Beijing: People's Medical Publishing House, 1998), 1036.
2. Cao Renlie et al., *Zhong Hua Pi Fu Ke Za Zhi* [Chinese Dermatology Journal] 4 (1957): 286.
3. He Xingdong et al., *Lin Chuang Zhong Yao Shou Ce* [Clinical Handbook of Chinese Materia Medica] (Beijing: People's Medical Publishing House, 1998), 181.
4. Lei Zaiquan and Zhang Tingmo, *Zhong Hua Lin Chuang Zhong Yao Xue*, 1045.
5. He Xingdong et al., *Lin Chuang Zhong Yao Shou Ce*, 182.
6. Ibid., 183.
7. Jing Houde, *Zhong Hua Xin Yi Xue Bao* [Chinese Journal of New Medicine] 2, 10 (1951): 753.
8. Pharmacological Teaching and Research Group of Henan Medical College, *He Nan Yi Xue Yuan Xue Bao* [Journal of Henan Medical College] 7 (1960): 23.
9. Yan Mingyu et al., *Wen Zhou Yi Xue Yuan Xue Bao* [Journal of Wenzhou Medical College] 23, 1 (1993): 10.
10. Wang Wenjie et al., *Yao Xue Xue Bao* [Pharmacology Journal] 24, 2 (1989): 151.
11. Cheng Guifang et al., *Zhong Guo Yi Xue Ke Xue Yuan Xue Bao* [Journal of Chinese Academy of Medical Science] 12, 1 (1990): 60.

Chapter 11

Herbs for stopping bleeding

止血药

Herbs for stopping bleeding

The herbs listed in this chapter stop internal and external bleeding. They are used to treat such conditions as vomiting of blood, coughing of blood, nosebleed, blood in the stool or urine, uterine bleeding, purpura, and bleeding due to internal and external injury. These herbs may also prevent excessive blood loss and subsequent failure of the circulatory system.

Herbs for stopping bleeding can be divided into four categories according to their functions:

1. herbs for cooling the Blood and stopping bleeding are mainly used for the frenetic movement of hot Blood where the blood has a fresh red colour; this condition is often accompanied by vexation and agitation, thirst, a red facial complexion, a red tongue and a slippery or rapid pulse;
2. herbs for transforming stasis and stopping bleeding are used for concurrent bleeding and stasis patterns where the blood is a dull purple colour or where there are stasis clots accompanied by local pain in a fixed location;
3. herbs for promoting contraction and stopping bleeding are used for incessant bleeding, fatigued Spirit and lack of strength with a pale tongue and a fine pulse, or for bleeding due to external injury;
4. herbs for warming the channels and stopping bleeding are used for bleeding due to deficiency-cold with pale-coloured blood, a sallow yellow facial complexion, a pale tongue, lack of strength, aversion to cold, cold limbs, and a fine or slow pulse.

Herbs for stopping bleeding are predominantly used for the secondary symptoms and signs of bleeding patterns. They are selected in accordance with the cause and specific symptoms of bleeding and may be combined with other herbs. They cannot be used non-specifically for all types of bleeding patterns.

Major combination categories for herbs for stopping bleeding are as follows:

i. for bleeding due to the frenetic movement of hot Blood, herbs for cooling the Blood and stopping bleeding should be combined with herbs for clearing heat and draining fire and with herbs for clearing heat and cooling the Blood;
ii. for bleeding caused by effulgent Yin deficiency-fire and by hyperactivity of Yang due to Yin deficiency, combine herbs for cooling the Blood and stopping bleeding with herbs for enriching Yin and subduing Yang and with herbs for enriching Yin and bearing fire downwards;
iii. for bleeding due to Blood stasis with internal obstruction, herbs for transforming stasis and stopping bleeding should be selected in combination with herbs for quickening the Blood and moving Qi;
iv. for bleeding due to deficiency-cold, select herbs for warming the channels and stopping bleeding or herbs for promoting contraction and stopping bleeding and combine them with herbs for boosting Qi, fortifying the Spleen and warming Yang;
v. for profuse bleeding or Qi deserting with the Blood, herbs for strongly supplementing original Qi should be administered immediately to boost Qi and

curtail desertion in accordance with the principle of 'supplement Qi when the Blood is exhausted'.

The following precautions should be borne in mind when applying herbs for stopping bleeding:

a. herbs with strong contraction-promoting properties should not be used in the initial stage of bleeding patterns, as this will result in Blood stasis;
b. herbs of a cold nature for stopping bleeding may cause Blood stasis and Qi stagnation; in cases of bleeding due to the frenetic movement of hot Blood with obvious Blood stasis, these herbs must not be used in a single, large dosage in the initial stage of the condition.

Tab. 11.1 Herbs for cooling the Blood and stopping bleeding

Herb	Functions	Indications
Da Ji (Herba seu Radix Cirsii Japonici)	Cooling the Blood and stopping bleeding, quickening the Blood and dispersing swelling	Vomiting of blood, coughing of blood and nosebleed due to the frenetic movement of hot Blood; uterine bleeding, blood Lin syndrome, sores
Xiao Ji (Herba Cephalanoploris seu Cirsii)	Cooling the Blood and stopping bleeding, relieving toxicity, dissipating stasis and dispersing abscesses	Bleeding patterns due to the frenetic movement of hot Blood, such as coughing of blood, vomiting of blood, nosebleed, blood in the urine and profuse uterine bleeding; abscesses and sores
Di Yu (Radix Sanguisorbae Officinalis)	Cooling the Blood and stopping bleeding, relieving toxicity and draining fire to close sores	Bleeding patterns due to Blood-heat in the Lower Jiao, such as blood in the urine, blood in the stool, haemorrhoids, uterine bleeding and bloody dysentery; eczema, abscesses, sores, burns and scalds
Ce Bai Ye (Cacumen Biotae Orientalis)	Cooling the Blood and stopping bleeding, dispelling Phlegm and stopping coughing	Various bleeding patterns, especially for bleeding due to the frenetic movement of hot Blood; also coughing and wheezing with sputum
Huai Hua (Flos Sophorae Japonicae)	Cooling the Blood and stopping bleeding, clearing Liver-fire	All types of bleeding patterns due to Blood-heat (particularly nosebleed, blood in the stool, haemorrhoidal bleeding and profuse uterine bleeding), headache, dizziness and full-pattern hypertension
Bai Mao Gen (Rhizoma Imperatae Cylindricae)	Cooling the Blood and stopping bleeding, clearing heat and promoting urination	Coughing of blood, nosebleed, vomiting of blood and blood in the urine due to the frenetic movement of hot Blood; blood Lin syndrome, heat Lin syndrome, inhibited urination, oedema, jaundice

Zhu Ma Gen (Radix Boehmeriae Niveae)	Cooling the Blood and stopping bleeding, clearing heat and promoting urination, quieting the foetus, clearing heat and relieving toxicity	Bleeding patterns due to Blood-heat, stirring foetus with or without uterine bleeding, dribbling urinary incontinence or inhibited urination due to damp-heat invading the Lower Jiao, sores due to heat toxins

Tab. 11.2 Herbs for transforming stasis and stopping bleeding

Herb	Functions	Indications
San Qi (Radix Notoginseng)	Stopping bleeding and dissipating Blood stasis, dispersing swelling and alleviating pain	Coughing of blood, vomiting of blood, nosebleed, blood in the stool, bloody dysentery, uterine bleeding, damp-heat dysentery, pain in the abdomen, tenesmus, swollen and painful abscesses, bleeding due to external injury
Qian Cao Gen (Radix Rubiae Cordifoliae)	Cooling the Blood and stopping bleeding, quickening the Blood and dispelling stasis, stopping coughing and dispelling Phlegm	Coughing of blood, vomiting of blood, nosebleed, blood in the urine, uterine bleeding, blood in the stool, menstrual block, swelling and pain due to external injury, cough
Pu Huang (Pollen Typhae)	Cooling the Blood and stopping bleeding, quickening the Blood and transforming stasis	Coughing of blood, nosebleed, vomiting of blood, blood in the stool, uterine bleeding, pain due to Blood stasis caused by knocks and falls, pain in the chest and abdomen, painful menstruation
Hua Rui Shi (Ophicalcitum)	Transforming Blood stasis and stopping bleeding	Coughing of blood, nosebleed, vomiting of blood, blood in the stool, uterine bleeding; and Blood dizziness, retention of placenta and eye screen due to postpartum Blood stasis
Jiang Xiang (Lignum Dalbergiae Odoriferae)	Transforming Blood stasis and stopping bleeding, quickening the Blood and alleviating pain, bearing counterflow Qi downwards and repelling turbidity	Coughing of blood, nosebleed, pain due to knocks and falls, pain in the chest and hypochondrium, angina pectoris

Tab. 11.3 Herbs for promoting contraction and stopping bleeding

Herb	Functions	Indications
Bai Ji (Rhizoma Bletillae Striatae)	Supplementing the Lungs, promoting contraction and stopping bleeding, dispersing swelling and generating flesh, closing sores	Coughing of blood, nosebleed, bleeding due to external injury or incised wounds, swelling and toxins of sores, chapped hands and feet

Xian He Cao (Herba Agrimoniae Pilosae)	Promoting contraction and stopping bleeding, stopping dysentery, killing worms	Coughing of blood, vomiting of blood, blood in the urine, blood in the stool, nosebleed, uterine bleeding, bleeding due to injury, diarrhoea and dysentery
Zi Zhu (Folium Callicarpae)	Promoting contraction and stopping bleeding, relieving toxicity and treating sores	Nosebleed, spitting of blood, vomiting of blood, blood in the urine and stool, uterine bleeding, bleeding gums, external injury, burns and scalds, abscesses and sores
Zong Lü Tan (Fibra Carbonisata Trachycarpi Stipulae)	Promoting astriction and stopping bleeding	Vomiting of blood, nosebleed, blood in the stool, blood in the urine, uterine bleeding, vaginal discharge
Ou Jie (Nodus Nelumbinis Nuciferae Rhizomatis)	Promoting contraction, dissipating Blood stasis and stopping bleeding	Vomiting of blood, coughing of blood, nosebleed, blood in the urine, blood in the stool, bloody dysentery, uterine bleeding

Tab. 11.4 Herbs for warming the channels and stopping bleeding

Herb	Functions	Indications
Pao Jiang (Rhizoma Zingiberis Officinalis Praeparata)	Warming the channels and stopping bleeding, warming the Middle Jiao and dispelling cold	Bleeding patterns due to deficiency-cold such as vomiting of blood, blood in the stool and uterine bleeding; and pain in the abdomen, diarrhoea and dysentery due to Spleen and Stomach deficiency-cold
Ai Ye (Folium Artemisiae Argyi)	Warming the channels and stopping bleeding, dissipating cold and alleviating pain, expelling damp-cold, quieting the foetus	Uterine bleeding, coughing of blood, nosebleed, vaginal discharge, stirring foetus, diarrhoea, eczema
Zao Xin Tu (Terra Flava Usta)	Warming the Middle Jiao and stopping bleeding, stopping diarrhoea, harmonizing the Stomach and stopping vomiting	Blood in the stool, vomiting of blood, nosebleed, uterine bleeding, vomiting, morning sickness, diarrhoea

HERBS FOR COOLING THE BLOOD AND STOPPING BLEEDING

Da Ji 大薊 (Japanese thistle, Herba seu Radix Cirsii Japonici)

Da Ji is the dried aerial parts or root of *Cirsium japonicum* DC., family Compositae.

Main ingredients *Da Ji* contains aplotaxene, cyperene, caryophyllene, thujopsene, α-amyrin, β-amyrin, taraxasteryl acetate, β-sitosterol, stigmasterol and inulin.

Properties Taste: sweet; nature: cool.

Channels entered Heart and Liver.

Functions and indications Cools the Blood and stops bleeding, quickens the Blood and disperses swelling. It is indicated for vomiting of blood, coughing of blood and nosebleed due to the frenetic movement of hot Blood; and for uterine bleeding, blood Lin syndrome, and sores.

Common dosage 10-15g, or up to 30g for large dosages; 30-60g when the fresh herb is used; appropriate dosage for external application.

Precautions and contraindications *Da Ji* is contraindicated in cases of Spleen and Stomach deficiency-cold.

Comparison of functions See *Xiao Ji* (Herba Cephalanoploris seu Cirsii).

Modern research

1. Lowers blood pressure.[1]
2. Very dilute decoctions of the root or whole plant of *Da Ji* inhibited the growth of Mycobacterium tuberculosis *in vitro*.[1]

Combinations and applications

Functions	Combinations	Applications
Cooling the Blood and stopping bleeding	*Pu Huang* (Pollen Typhae) *Mu Tong* (Caulis Mutong) (see notes on legal status) *Hua Shi* (Talcum)	Blood Lin syndrome, vomiting of blood, nosebleed, uterine bleeding
	Xiao Ji (Herba Cephalanoploris seu Cirsii) *Ce Bai Ye* (Cacumen Biotae Orientalis) *Bai Mao Gen* (Rhizoma Imperatae Cylindricae) *Qian Cao Gen* (Radix Rubiae Cordifoliae) (use with char-fried *Da Ji*)	Vomiting of blood, spitting of blood
Quickening the Blood and dispersing swelling	*Ru Xiang* (Gummi Olibanum) *Ming Fan* (Alumen)	Clove sores, swelling and infection due to external injury
	Mu Tong (Caulis Mutong) (see notes on legal status) *Ze Xie* (Rhizoma Alismatis Orientalis) *Hua Shi* (Talcum)	Damp-heat jaundice, oedema, inhibited urination

Notes:

1. The root or leaves of fresh *Da Ji* can be pounded into juice and used to treat vomiting of blood, nosebleed and uterine bleeding.
2. Since the root of *Da Ji* is effective in lowering blood pressure, this herb can be used with *Xia Ku Cao* (Spica Prunellae Vulgaris) and *Xi Xian Cao* (Herba Siegesbeckiae) to treat hypertension.

Xiao Ji 小蓟 (Field thistle, Herba Cephalanoploris seu Cirsii)

Xiao Ji is the whole herb of *Cephalanoplos segetum* (Bge.) Kitam. or *Cirsium setosum* (Willd.) MB., family Compositae.

Main ingredients *Xiao Ji* contains rutin, acacetin-7-rhamnoglucoside, taraxasterol, taraxasteryl acetate, caffeic acid, chlorogenic acid, protocatechualdehyde, β-sitosterol and stigmasterol.

Properties Taste: sweet; nature: cool.

Channels entered Heart and Liver.

Functions and indications Cools the Blood and stops bleeding, and relieves toxicity, dissipates stasis and disperses abscesses. It is indicated for bleeding patterns due to the frenetic movement of hot Blood, such as coughing of blood, vomiting of blood, nosebleed, blood in the urine and profuse uterine bleeding, as well as for abscesses and sores.

Common dosage 10–15g, or 30–60g of the fresh herb; appropriate dosage for external application.

Precautions and contraindications *Xiao Ji* is contraindicated in cases of Spleen and Stomach deficiency-cold.

Comparison of functions Both *Xiao Ji* (Herba Cephalanoploris seu Cirsii) and *Da Ji* (Herba seu Radix Cirsii Japonici) cool the Blood and stop bleeding to treat bleeding patterns due to the frenetic movement of hot Blood; they also disperse swelling to treat abscesses and sores due to heat toxins. *Xiao Ji* has a weaker effect in these functions than *Da Ji*. As *Xiao Ji* is good at promoting urination, it is primarily used for blood Lin syndrome and blood in the urine. *Da Ji* is more effective for dissipating Blood stasis and dispersing swelling.

Toxicity Intragastric administration to rats for two weeks of 80g/kg per day of decoctions of *Xiao Ji* did not produce any toxic side-effects. There have been reports of use of the herb leading to high temperature, dizziness, fatigue, vomiting, pain in the abdomen or insomnia, frequent urination and urticaria; symptoms generally disappeared within two weeks, although in more serious cases, intake of the herb was halted.

Modern research

1. The caffeic acid contained in *Xiao Ji* can reduce blood clotting and bleeding time.[2]
2. Inhibits inflammation.[2]
3. Decoctions of *Xiao Ji* strengthen the heart, raise blood pressure and excite the uterus.[3]

Combinations and applications

Functions	Combinations	Applications
Cooling the Blood and stopping bleeding	*Bai Mao Gen* (Rhizoma Imperatae Cylindricae) *Ce Bai Ye* (Cacumen Biotae Orientalis) *Zhi Zi* (Fructus Gardeniae Jasminoidis) *Qian Cao Gen* (Radix Rubiae Cordifoliae) *Mu Dan Pi* (Cortex Moutan Radicis)	Coughing of blood and vomiting of blood due to Blood-heat
	Sheng Di Huang (Radix Rehmanniae Glutinosae) *Hua Shi* (Talcum) *Mu Tong* (Caulis Mutong) (see notes on legal status) *Ou Jie* (Nodus Nelumbinis Nuciferae Rhizomatis)	Blood Lin syndrome and blood in the urine due to binding of heat in the Lower Jiao

Relieving toxicity, dissipating stasis and dispersing abscesses	*Huang Bai* (Cortex Phellodendri) *Bing Pian* (Borneolum) (powder for external use)	Swollen, hot and painful abscesses

Note: The stem and leaves of *Xiao Ji*, pounded to a paste, can be added to a decoction of *Bai Zhu* (Rhizoma Atractylodis Macrocephalae) and the juice of *Sheng Di Huang* (Radix Rehmanniae Glutinosae) to treat profuse uterine bleeding.

Di Yu 地榆
(Sanguisorba root, Radix Sanguisorbae Officinalis)

Di Yu is the root of *Sanguisorba officinalis* L. or *S. officinalis* L. var. *longifolia* (Bert.) Yu et Li, family Rosaceae.

Main ingredients *Di Yu* contains ziyu glycosides, betulinic acid, sanguisorbin, sanguisorbigenin, gallic acid and tannin.

Properties Taste: bitter and sour; nature: slightly cold.

Channels entered Liver, Stomach and Large Intestine.

Functions and indications Cools the Blood and stops bleeding, and relieves toxicity and drains fire to close sores. It is indicated for bleeding patterns due to Blood-heat in the Lower Jiao, such as blood in the urine, blood in the stool, haemorrhoids, uterine bleeding and bloody dysentery, as well as for eczema, abscesses, sores, burns and scalds.

Common dosage 10-15g; appropriate dosage for external application.

Precautions and contraindications *Di Yu* is contraindicated for bleeding patterns due to deficiency-cold and for external application where burns are extensive.

Remarks Since raw *Di Yu* is bitter and sour in taste and slightly cold in nature, it can be used to cool the Blood and relieve toxicity in order to treat abscesses and burns; the charred herb (*Di Yu Tan*, Radix Sanguisorbae Officinalis Carbonisata) is bitter, sour and astringent in taste and slightly cold, tending to neutral in nature, and is more effective for stopping bleeding.

Comparison of functions See *Huai Hua* (Flos Sophorae Japonicae), *Bai Ji* (Rhizoma Bletillae Striatae) and *Zong Lü Tan* (Fibra Carbonisata Trachycarpi Stipulae).

Toxicity The LD_{50} for intraperitoneal injection in mice of aqueous extracts of *Di Yu* is 1.6 ± 0.29g/kg; for alcoholic extracts, it is 2.17 ± 0.49g/kg. Toxic symptoms included reduced activity, lack of strength in the limbs, respiratory difficulty and convulsions. Mice fed 2.5g/kg of aqueous or alcoholic extracts of *Di Yu* orally for seven days continued to move freely and no deaths were recorded.

Modern research

1. Arrests bleeding.[4]
2. *Di Yu* inhibited various bacteria *in vitro*, including Staphylococcus aureus, Pseudomonas aeruginosa, haemolytic streptococci and Bacillus subtilis.[5]
3. Inhibits inflammation and decreases secretion in wounds and infections.[6]
4. Stops vomiting.[7]

Combinations and applications

Functions	Combinations	Applications
Cooling the Blood and stopping bleeding	*Sheng Di Huang* (Radix Rehmanniae Glutinosae) *Bai Shao* (Radix Paeoniae Lactiflorae) *Huang Qin* (Radix Scutellariae Baicalensis) *Huai Hua* (Flos Sophorae Japonicae)	Relatively severe blood in the stool due to Blood-heat in the Lower Jiao

	Huai Jiao (Fructus Sophorae Japonicae) *Fang Feng* (Radix Ledebouriellae Divaricatae) *Huang Qin* (Radix Scutellariae Baicalensis) *Zhi Ke* (Fructus Citri Aurantii)	Haemorrhoidal bleeding due to Blood-heat binding the Large Intestine
	Han Lian Cao (Herba Ecliptae Prostratae) *Da Ji* (Herba seu Radix Cirsii Japonici) *Xiao Ji* (Herba Cephalanoploris seu Cirsii)	Blood in the urine due to Blood-heat
	Huang Qin (Radix Scutellariae Baicalensis) *Bai Shao* (Radix Paeoniae Lactiflorae)	Bloody dysentery due to damp-heat
	Huang Lian (Rhizoma Coptidis) *Mu Xiang* (Radix Aucklandiae Lappae) (see notes on legal status) *Wu Mei* (Fructus Pruni Mume) *He Zi* (Fructus Terminaliae Chebulae)	Diarrhoea, bloody dysentery, protracted menstruation
	Sheng Di Huang (Radix Rehmanniae Glutinosae) *E Jiao* (Gelatinum Corii Asini) *Da Huang Tan* (Radix et Rhizoma Rhei Carbonisatae)	Uterine bleeding due to Blood-heat, accompanied by dry mouth and parched lips
Relieving toxicity and draining fire to close sores	*Huang Bai* (Cortex Phellodendri)	Eczema and skin ulcers due to damp-heat

Note: Powdered *Di Yu* mixed with sesame oil, *Ma You* (Oleum Sesami), can be used externally for the treatment of burns and scalds.

Ce Bai Ye 侧柏叶
(Chinese arborvitae twig and leaf, Cacumen Biotae Orientalis)

Ce Bai Ye is the leafy twig of *Biota orientalis* (L.) Endl., family Cupressaceae. This plant is also known as *Platycladus orientalis* (L.) Franco.

Main ingredients *Ce Bai Ye* contains thujene, thujone, fenchone, pinene, caryophyllene, aromadendrin, quercetin, myricetin, hinokiflavone, amentoflavone, quercitrin, tannin and vitamin C.

Properties Taste: bitter and astringent; nature: slightly cold.

Channels entered Lung, Liver and Large Intestine.

Functions and indications Cools the Blood and stops bleeding, dispels Phlegm and stops coughing. It is indicated for various bleeding patterns, especially for bleeding due to the frenetic movement of hot Blood, and also for coughing and wheezing with sputum.

Common dosage 10–15g; appropriate dosage for external application.

Toxicity The LD_{50} for intraperitoneal injection in mice of decoctions of *Ce Bai Ye* is 15.2g/kg. No deaths were recorded among mice within 72 hours of being given 60g/kg of a decoction of the herb via intragastric administration. Rats were given decoctions of the herb at a strength 20 and 40 times greater than those normally used in the clinic; after six weeks of daily intragastric administration, they showed no significant differences in comparison with a control group, except for a slight reduction in activity and appetite.

Modern research

1. Shortens bleeding periods.[8]
2. Expels sputum, stops coughing and calms wheezing.[9–11]
3. Decoctions of *Ce Bai Ye* inhibited Staphylococcus aureus, Shigella shigae, Salmonella typhi and β-haemolytic streptococci *in vitro*.[12]
4. Has a tranquillizing function.[12]

Combinations and applications

Functions	Combinations	Applications
Cooling the Blood and stopping bleeding	*Da Ji* (Herba seu Radix Cirsii Japonici) *Xiao Ji* (Herba Cephalanoploris seu Cirsii) *Bai Mao Gen* (Rhizoma Imperatae Cylindricae)	Coughing of blood and nosebleed due to the frenetic movement of hot Blood; also for blood in the urine and blood Lin syndrome
	He Ye (Folium Nelumbinis Nuciferae) *Sheng Di Huang* (Radix Rehmanniae Glutinosae) *Ai Ye* (Folium Artemisiae Argyi) (all these herbs and *Ce Bai Ye* are used fresh)	Vomiting of blood and nosebleed due to the frenetic movement of hot Blood
	Ai Ye (Folium Artemisiae Argyi) *Gan Jiang* (Rhizoma Zingiberis Officinalis)	Bleeding due to deficiency-cold
	Dang Shen (Radix Codonopsitis Pilosulae) *Dang Gui* (Radix Angelicae Sinensis) *Sheng Di Huang* (Radix Rehmanniae Glutinosae) *Xian He Cao* (Herba Agrimoniae Pilosae)	Uterine bleeding due to Qi and Blood deficiency
Dispelling Phlegm and stopping coughing	*Zi Su Ye* (Folium Perillae Frutescentis) *Xing Ren* (Semen Pruni Armeniacae) *Bai Mao Gen* (Rhizoma Imperatae Cylindricae) *Chuan Bei Mu* (Bulbus Fritillariae Cirrhosae)	Coughing and wheezing due to Lung-heat and Lung Qi ascending counterflow

Note: A powder of *Ce Bai Ye* can be used externally to treat bleeding due to injury, and burns and scalds.

Huai Hua 槐花
(Pagoda tree flower, Flos Sophorae Japonicae)

Huai Hua is the dried flower or flower-bud of *Sophora japonica* L., family Leguminosae.

Main ingredients *Huai Hua* contains rutin, sophorins, quercetin, betulin, sophoradiol, isorhamnetin and β-sitosterol.

Properties Taste: bitter; nature: slightly cold.

Channels entered Liver and Large Intestine.

Functions and indications Cools the Blood and stops bleeding, and clears Liver-fire. It is indicated for all types of bleeding patterns due to Blood-heat (particularly nosebleed, blood in the stool, haemorrhoidal bleeding and profuse uterine bleeding), headache, dizziness, and full-pattern hypertension.

Common dosage 10-15g.

Remarks Raw *Huai Hua* should be used for cooling the Blood, draining fire and lowering blood pressure, whereas the charred or stir-fried herb is better for stopping bleeding.

Comparison of functions Both *Huai Hua* (Flos Sophorae Japonicae) and *Di Yu* (Radix Sanguisorbae Officinalis) can cool the Blood and stop bleeding. They are mainly used to treat bleeding due to Blood-heat, especially for bleeding in the lower part of the body such as haemorrhoidal bleeding and blood in the stool. *Di Yu* is also effective in relieving toxicity and closing sores and is an important herb for external application in the treatment of burns, scalds and sores. *Huai Hua* can clear and drain fire in the Liver to treat red eyes, dizziness and headache due to Liver-fire.

Modern research

1. Improves protection of the capillaries and inhibits inflammation.[13]
2. Strengthens the heart and enlarges the coronary artery, lowers blood pressure.[13]
3. Reduces the level of blood lipids and relieves spasms.[14]

Combinations and applications

Functions	Combinations	Applications
Cooling the Blood and stopping bleeding	*Di Yu* (Radix Sanguisorbae Officinalis) *Ce Bai Ye* (Cacumen Biotae Orientalis) *Zhi Ke* (Fructus Citri Aurantii)	All types of bleeding patterns (e.g. blood in the stool, haemorrhoidal bleeding, spitting of blood, nosebleed, blood in the urine, and uterine bleeding) due to Blood-heat
	Huang Lian (Rhizoma Coptidis)	Blood in the stool and other types of bleeding patterns due to damp-heat in the Large Intestine
	Huang Qin (Radix Scutellariae Baicalensis) *Huo Ma Ren* (Semen Cannabis Sativae)	Haemorrhoidal bleeding accompanied by constipation due to Blood-heat in the Large Intestine
Clearing Liver-fire	*Xia Ku Cao* (Spica Prunellae Vulgaris) *Xi Xian Cao* (Herba Siegesbeckiae)	Full-pattern hypertension manifesting as headache, dizziness and red eyes due to Liver-fire flaming upwards

Appendix

Huai Jiao 槐角 (Pagoda tree fruit, Fructus Sophorae Japonicae)

Huai Jiao is the dried fruit of *Sophora japonica* L., family Leguminosae. Bitter in taste and cold in nature, it enters the Liver and Large Intestine channels. It has similar functions to *Huai Hua*; although *Huai Jiao* is stronger in terms of draining heat, it is not as effective in stopping bleeding. Since *Huai Jiao* can clear the Liver and drain fire while lowering blood pressure, it is used with *Huang Lian* (Rhizoma Coptidis), *Jue Ming Zi* (Semen Cassiae) and *Xia Ku Cao* (Spica Prunellae Vulgaris) to treat red eyes, headache, dizziness and hypertension due to Liver-fire flaming upwards. The common dosage is 10-15g. *Huai Jiao* is contraindicated in cases of Spleen and Stomach deficiency-cold and during pregnancy.

Bai Mao Gen 白茅根 (Cogon grass rhizome, Rhizoma Imperatae Cylindricae)

Bai Mao Gen is the rhizome of *Imperata cylindrica* (L.) Beauv. var. *major* (Nees) C. E. Hubb., family Gramineae.

Main ingredients *Bai Mao Gen* contains glucose, sucrose, fructose, xylose, citric acid, malic acid, oxalic acid, cylindrin, arundoin, coixol and fernenol.

Properties Taste: sweet; nature: cold.

Channels entered Lung, Stomach and Bladder.

Functions and indications Cools the Blood and stops bleeding, clears heat and promotes urination. It is indicated for coughing of blood, nosebleed, vomiting of blood and blood in the urine due to the frenetic movement of hot Blood; and for blood Lin syndrome, heat Lin syndrome, inhibited urination, oedema, and jaundice.

Common dosage 10-30g, or 30-60g of the fresh herb used alone.

Remarks Fresh *Bai Mao Gen* is more effective than the dried herb.

Comparison of functions Both *Bai Mao Gen* (Rhizoma Imperatae Cylindricae) and *Lu Gen* (Rhizoma Phragmitis Communis) can clear heat in the Lungs and Stomach and promote urination. They are used to treat cough due to Lung-heat, as well as for vexation, thirst and vomiting due to Stomach-heat and can be used together to accentuate each other's effect. *Bai Mao Gen* tends to enter the Xue level and so is especially effective for cooling the Blood and stopping bleeding. *Lu Gen* enters the Qi level and is better for clearing heat and generating body fluids.

Modern research

1. *Bai Mao Gen* in powder form has an obvious effect in stopping bleeding.[15]
2. Decoctions of *Bai Mao Gen* promote urination.[16]
3. Decoctions of *Bai Mao Gen* had a clear inhibitory effect *in vitro* against Shigella flexneri and Shigella sonnei, but had no effect on Shigella shigae.[17]

Combinations and applications

Functions	Combinations	Applications
Cooling the Blood and stopping bleeding	*Xian He Cao* (Herba Agrimoniae Pilosae) *Pu Huang* (Pollen Typhae) *Xiao Ji* (Herba Cephalanoploris seu Cirsii)	Nosebleed, coughing of blood or blood in the urine due to the frenetic movement of hot Blood
Clearing heat and promoting urination	*Che Qian Cao* (Herba Plantaginis) *Mu Tong* (Caulis Mutong) (see notes on legal status) *Jin Qian Cao* (Herba Lysimachiae)	Heat Lin syndrome and oedema, damp-heat jaundice and inhibited urination
	Ge Gen (Radix Puerariae)	Nausea and vomiting in febrile diseases
	Lu Gen (Rhizoma Phragmitis Communis)	Vexation and thirst in febrile diseases, nausea due to Stomach-heat, cough due to Lung-heat

Note: *Bai Mao Gen* can be used on its own for coughing of blood, vomiting of blood and nosebleed, either as a decoction or as juice from the fresh herb. Its therapeutic effect is enhanced when it is combined with other herbs for cooling the Blood and stopping bleeding.

Zhu Ma Gen 苎麻根 (Ragon grass root, Radix Boehmeriae Niveae)

Zhu Ma Gen is the root, stem and leaves of *Boehmeria nivea* (L.) Gaud, family Urticaceae.

Main ingredients *Zhu Ma Gen* contains caffeic acid.

Properties Taste: sweet; nature: cold.

Channels entered Heart and Liver.

Functions and indications Cools the Blood and stops bleeding, clears heat and promotes urination, quiets the foetus, and clears heat and relieves toxicity. It is indicated for bleeding patterns due to Blood-heat, stirring foetus with or without uterine bleeding, dribbling urinary incontinence or inhibited urination due to damp-heat invading the Lower Jiao, and sores due to heat toxins.

Common dosage 10-30g, or 30-60g for the fresh herb; appropriate dosage for external application.

Remarks As *Zhu Ma Gen* is cold, it is an important herb for cooling the Blood and stopping bleeding.

Modern research

1. Preparations of *Zhu Ma Gen* can stop bleeding.[18]
2. The caffeic acid contained in *Zhu Ma Gen* can shorten bleeding time, especially in cases of bleeding in the upper digestive tract.[18]

Combinations and applications

Functions	Combinations	Applications
Cooling the Blood and stopping bleeding	*Xiao Ji* (Herba Cephalanoploris seu Cirsii) *Pu Huang* (Pollen Typhae)	Coughing of blood, vomiting of blood, blood in the urine, uterine bleeding and purpura due to Blood-heat
Clearing heat and promoting urination	*Bai Mao Gen* (Rhizoma Imperatae Cylindricae) *Che Qian Cao* (Herba Plantaginis) *Bian Xu* (Herba Polygoni Avicularis)	Heat or blood Lin syndromes, nephritic oedema, oedema during pregnancy
Quieting the foetus	*Sheng Di Huang* (Radix Rehmanniae Glutinosae) *Dang Gui* (Radix Angelicae Sinensis) *E Jiao* (Gelatinum Corii Asini)	Uterine bleeding during pregnancy
	Huang Qin (Radix Scutellariae Baicalensis) *Xian Zhu Ru* (Caulis Bambusae in Taeniis, fresh)	Stirring foetus and blood in the stool
Clearing heat and relieving toxicity	*Jin Yin Hua* (Flos Lonicerae) *Ye Ju Hua* (Flos Chrysanthemi Indici)	Swelling and toxins of abscesses and sores, or measles with high fever and a dull rash

HERBS FOR TRANSFORMING STASIS AND STOPPING BLEEDING

San Qi 三七
(Notoginseng root, Radix Notoginseng)

San Qi is the root of *Panax notoginseng* (Burk.) F. H. Chen, family Araliaceae.

Main ingredients *San Qi* contains volatile oils (including cyperene, elemene, cadinene, caryophyllene, guaiene and cedrene), ginsenosides, notoginsenosides, gypenoside, dencichine, quercetin, β-sitosterol, stigmasterol, daucosterol and sanchinan A.

Properties Taste: sweet and slightly bitter; nature: warm.

Channels entered Liver and Stomach.

Functions and indications Stops bleeding and dissipates Blood stasis, disperses swelling and alleviates pain. It is indicated for coughing of blood, vomiting of blood, nosebleed, blood in the stool, bloody dysentery, uterine bleeding, damp-heat dysentery, pain in the abdomen, tenesmus, swollen and painful abscesses, and bleeding due to external injury.

Common dosage 3-10g; 1-3g of the powder for internal use; juice from the fresh herb or an appropriate dosage of the powder for external application.

Precautions and contraindications

1. *San Qi* is contraindicated during pregnancy.
2. *San Qi* should be used with caution in cases without Blood stasis.
3. In cases of nosebleed due to Blood deficiency or bleeding patterns due to the frenetic movement of hot Blood, *San Qi* should be used in combination with herbs for enriching Yin and herbs for cooling the Blood.

Remarks As *San Qi* is bitter and warm, it can dissipate Blood stasis, stop bleeding and quicken the Blood to alleviate pain. It is used for both interior and exterior bleeding patterns and is especially good for bleeding with Blood stasis. *San Qi* is an important herb for alleviating pain, dispersing swelling and treating bleeding due to external injury.

Toxicity The LD_{50} for intravenous and subcutaneous injection in mice of the notoginsenosides contained in *San Qi* is 447mg/kg and 1246mg/kg respectively. The LD_{50} for intraperitoneal injection in mice of aqueous extracts of *San Qi Hua* (Flos Notoginseng) is 1.2g/kg, which is 21–42 times the normal dosage in the clinic. A single oral administration of 1-1.5g of *San Qi* does not usually have any side-effects, although a few patients may suffer from nausea, frequent vomiting and bleeding; these symptoms generally diminish or disappear with continued administration. There have also been reports of allergic rashes caused by intake of *San Qi* pills.

Modern research

1. Stops bleeding.[19, 20]
2. Inhibits haematoblastic concentration and decreases blood viscosity.[21]
3. Enlarges the coronary artery, regulates the levels of blood sugar and blood lipids.[22]
4. Inhibits arrhythmia.[23]
5. Inhibits inflammation and alleviates pain.[24]

Combinations and applications

Functions	Combinations	Applications
Stopping bleeding and dissipating Blood stasis	*Ren Shen* (Radix Ginseng)	Nosebleed, a pale white facial complexion and fatigue due to Qi deficiency of the Spleen and Lungs, which thus fail to contain the Blood

	He Ye (Folium Nelumbinis Nuciferae) *Ce Bai Ye* (Cacumen Biotae Orientalis) *Ji Zi Huang* (raw egg yolk)	Vomiting of blood due to internal heat resulting in Yin deficiency causing the frenetic movement of hot Blood, with dry mouth and throat, and a fine and rapid pulse
	Hua Rui Shi (Ophicalcitum) *Xue Yu Tan* (Crinis Carbonisatus Hominis)	Coughing of blood, vomiting of blood and nosebleed due to Blood stasis
	Da Huang (Radix et Rhizoma Rhei) *Huang Lian* (Rhizoma Coptidis) *Huang Bai* (Cortex Phellodendri) *Chi Shao* (Radix Paeoniae Rubra) *Dang Gui* (Radix Angelicae Sinensis)	Damp-heat dysentery, bloody dysentery, pain in the abdomen, tenesmus, heat in the anus, short voidings of reddish urine, and yellow, slimy tongue fur due to damp-heat obstruction in the Intestines, Qi stagnation and Blood stasis
	Ren Shen (Radix Ginseng) *Ru Xiang* (Gummi Olibanum) *Jiang Xiang* (Lignum Dalbergiae Odoriferae) *Xue Jie* (Resina Draconis) *Wu Bei Zi* (Galla Rhois Chinensis)	Prepared as a powder for external application to the site of bleeding due to external injury
	Huai Hua (Flos Sophorae Japonicae) *Jing Jie Sui* (Spica Schizonepetae Tenuifoliae) *Zhi Ke* (Fructus Citri Aurantii) *Ce Bai Ye* (Cacumen Biotae Orientalis)	Fresh blood in the stool due to stagnation of pathogenic wind and exuberant heat toxins or damp toxins in the Blood of the Intestines and Stomach
	E Jiao (Gelatinum Corii Asini) *Shu Di Huang* (Radix Rehmanniae Glutinosae Conquita) *Bai Zhu* (Rhizoma Atractylodis Macrocephalae) *Huang Qin* (Radix Scutellariae Baicalensis) *Gan Cao* (Radix Glycyrrhizae) *Fu Zi* (Radix Lateralis Aconiti Carmichaeli Praeparata) (see notes on legal status)	Blood in the stool, profuse uterine bleeding with dull and pale blood, cold limbs, a pale tongue with white fur, and a sunken and forceless pulse due to insufficiency of Spleen Yang and Middle Jiao deficiency-cold, thus resulting in failure to contain the Blood
Dispersing swelling and alleviating pain	*Ru Xiang* (Gummi Olibanum) *Mo Yao* (Myrrha) *Xue Jie* (Resina Draconis) *Bing Pian* (Borneolum) *Mi Cu* (Acetum Oryzae, rice vinegar)	Prepared as a powder for external application topically for stasis, swelling and pain due to knocks and falls, or for swollen and painful abscesses

Qian Cao Gen 茜草根 (Madder root, Radix Rubiae Cordifoliae)

Qian Cao Gen is the root and rhizome of *Rubia cordifolia* L., family Rubiaceae.

Main ingredients *Qian Cao Gen* contains purpurin, alizarin, manjistin, pseudopurpurin, anthraquinones, rubilactone, glucosides, β-sitosterol and daucosterol.

Properties Taste: bitter; nature: cold.

Channel entered Liver.

Functions and indications Cools the Blood and stops bleeding, quickens the Blood and dispels stasis, stops coughing and dispels Phlegm. It is indicated for coughing of blood, vomiting of blood, nosebleed, blood in the urine, uterine bleeding, blood in the stool, menstrual block, swelling and pain due to external injury, and cough.

Common dosage 12-15g.

Precautions and contraindications

1. *Qian Cao Gen* should be used with caution in cases of Spleen and Stomach deficiency-cold.
2. In cases without Blood stasis, *Qian Cao Gen* should be stir-fried before use.

Remarks Stir-fried *Qian Cao Gen* has the function of cooling the Blood and stopping bleeding and is used for various bleeding patterns due to Blood-heat. Raw *Qian Cao Gen* quickens the Blood and dispels Blood stasis to stop bleeding and is effective for menstrual block due to Blood stasis. The charred herb (*Qian Cao Tan*) is sometimes considered as being most effective in stopping bleeding.

Toxicity No deaths occurred when 150g/kg of decoctions of raw *Qian Cao Gen* were given to mice via intragastric administration; however, when the dosage was increased to 175g/kg, two out of the eight mice in the experiment died. The LD_{50} for intraperitoneal injection in mice of aqueous extracts of *Qian Cao Gen* is 49.0 ± 3.3g/kg.

Modern research

1. Stops bleeding.[25, 26]
2. Aqueous extracts of *Qian Cao Gen* had a certain inhibitory effect on Staphylococcus aureus, Streptococcus pneumoniae, Haemophilus influenzae and various dermatophytes *in vitro*.[27]

Combinations and applications

Functions	Combinations	Applications
Cooling the Blood and stopping bleeding	*Da Ji* (Herba seu Radix Cirsii Japonici) *Xiao Ji* (Herba Cephalanoploris seu Cirsii) *Ce Bai Ye* (Cacumen Biotae Orientalis) *Zhi Zi* (Fructus Gardeniae Jasminoidis)	Coughing and vomiting of bright-coloured blood, accompanied by a string-like and rapid pulse due to exuberant fire in the Liver and Stomach damaging the Blood vessels and to the frenetic movement of hot Blood
	Ai Ye (Folium Artemisiae Argyi) *Wu Mei* (Fructus Pruni Mume) *Sheng Di Huang* (Radix Rehmanniae Glutinosae)	Nosebleed due to Blood-heat causing the frenetic movement of hot Blood
	Qing Dai (Indigo Naturalis) *Gua Lou Ren* (Semen Trichosanthis) *Zhi Zi* (Fructus Gardeniae Jasminoidis) *He Zi* (Fructus Terminaliae Chebulae) *Fu Hai Shi* (Os Costaziae seu Pumex)	Cough with bloody and thick sputum, vexation and thirst, constipation, yellow tongue fur and a string-like, rapid pulse due to Liver-fire scorching the Lungs
	Huang Qi (Radix Astragali seu Hedysari) *Bai Zhu* (Rhizoma Atractylodis Macrocephalae) *Shan Zhu Yu* (Fructus Corni Officinalis) *Long Gu* (Os Draconis)	Uterine bleeding due to Qi deficiency failing to ensure containment

	Huang Lian (Rhizoma Coptidis) *Sheng Ma* (Rhizoma Cimicifugae) *Bai Shao* (Radix Paeoniae Lactiflorae) *Di Yu* (Radix Sanguisorbae Officinalis)	Red and white dysentery and injury to the Blood vessels due to damp-heat brewing in and binding the Large Intestine
Quickening the Blood and dispelling stasis	*Dang Gui* (Radix Angelicae Sinensis) *Chi Shao* (Radix Paeoniae Rubra) *Xiang Fu* (Rhizoma Cyperi Rotundi) *Huang Jiu* (Vinum Aureum)	Menstrual block, a purple tongue with stasis marks and a rough pulse due to Blood stasis
	Chuan Xiong (Rhizoma Ligustici Chuanxiong) *Tao Ren* (Semen Persicae) *Hong Hua* (Flos Carthami Tinctorii) *Dang Gui* (Radix Angelicae Sinensis)	Pain due to knocks and falls and Blood stasis
	Ji Xue Teng (Caulis Spatholobi) *Hai Feng Teng* (Caulis Piperis Kadsurae) *Yan Hu Suo* (Rhizoma Corydalis Yanhusuo) *Huang Jiu* (Vinum Aureum)	Limb joint pain resulting from an invasion of wind-damp leading to obstruction of the channels and network vessels
Stopping coughing and dispelling Phlegm	*Chen Pi* (Pericarpium Citri Reticulatae) *Ban Xia* (Rhizoma Pinelliae Ternatae) *Gua Lou* (Fructus Trichosanthis) *Xing Ren* (Semen Pruni Armeniacae)	Cough with yellow and sticky sputum, yellow and slimy tongue fur, and a slippery, rapid pulse due to Phlegm-heat obstructing the Lungs

Pu Huang 蒲黄 (Cat-tail pollen, Pollen Typhae)

Pu Huang is the pollen of *Typha angustifolia* L., *T. orientalis* Presl. or other plants of the same genus, family Typhaceae.

Main ingredients *Pu Huang* contains naringenin, isorhamnetin, typhaneoside, kaempferol, rutinosides, β-sitosterol, pentacosane and amino acids (*T. angustifolia*).

Properties Taste: sweet; nature: neutral.

Channels entered Liver and Heart.

Functions and indications Cools the Blood and stops bleeding, quickens the Blood and transforms stasis. It is indicated for coughing of blood, nosebleed, vomiting of blood, blood in the stool, uterine bleeding, pain due to Blood stasis caused by knocks and falls, pain in the chest and abdomen, and painful menstruation.

Common dosage 5-10g, wrapped in a cloth and decocted; 3g for oral use in powder form; or appropriate dosage for external application.

Precautions and contraindications *Pu Huang* should be used with caution during pregnancy.

Remarks Char-fried *Pu Huang* is more effective for stopping bleeding, whereas the raw herb is employed for quickening the Blood and transforming stasis to alleviate pain.

Toxicity Intravenous injection in mice of 500mg/kg of alcoholic extracts of *Pu Huang* did not cause any fatalities. Oral administration of normal therapeutic dosages does not lead to any obvious side-effects. However, since *Pu Huang* can cause contraction of the uterus, it is not suitable for use during pregnancy.

Modern research

1. Significantly reduces the overall cholesterol level.[28]
2. Inhibits inflammation.[29]
3. Excites the uterus.[30]

Combinations and applications

Functions	Combinations	Applications
Cooling the Blood and stopping bleeding	*Da Ji* (Herba seu Radix Cirsii Japonici) *Xiao Ji* (Herba Cephalanoploris seu Cirsii) *Di Yu* (Radix Sanguisorbae Officinalis) *Huai Hua* (Flos Sophorae Japonicae)	Coughing of blood, nosebleed, vomiting of blood, blood in the stool, uterine bleeding, bleeding due to external injury
	Dong Kui Zi (Semen Malvae Verticillatae) *Sheng Di Huang* (Radix Rehmanniae Glutinosae)	Blood Lin syndrome due to severe heat in the Bladder
Quickening the Blood and transforming stasis	*Wu Ling Zhi* (Excrementum Trogopteri)	Pain in the chest and abdomen, painful menstruation and postpartum pain in the abdomen due to Blood stasis
	Rou Gui (Cortex Cinnamomi Cassiae) *Pao Jiang* (Rhizoma Zingiberis Officinalis Praeparata) *Dang Gui* (Radix Angelicae Sinensis) *Shu Di Huang* (Radix Rehmanniae Glutinosae Conquita)	Retention of lochia with persistent dribbling, cold and pain in the umbilical region

Hua Rui Shi 花蕊石 (Ophicalcite, Ophicalcitum)

Hua Rui Shi is a type of marble containing green serpentine.

Main ingredients *Hua Rui Shi* contains large amounts of calcium and magnesium carbonate, as well as small quantities of ferric salt and aluminates.

Properties Taste: sour and astringent; nature: neutral.

Channel entered Liver.

Functions and indications Transforms Blood stasis and stops bleeding. It is indicated for coughing of blood, nosebleed, vomiting of blood, blood in the stool and uterine bleeding; and for Blood dizziness, retention of placenta and eye screen due to postpartum Blood stasis.

Common dosage 8-15g, or 1-1.5g of the powder for internal use; appropriate dosage for external application.

Precautions and contraindications

1. *Hua Rui Shi* is contraindicated during pregnancy.
2. *Hua Rui Shi* should be used with caution in the absence of internal Blood stasis.

Remarks

1. Crude *Hua Rui Shi* is sour, astringent and neutral and has a strong effect in transforming Blood stasis and stopping bleeding. *Hua Rui Shi* is more astringent in its calcined form, when it has a greater effect in promoting contraction to stop bleeding; calcined *Hua Rui Shi* can be ground to a powder and used to treat bleeding due to external injury.
2. The nature of *Hua Rui Shi* is downward-bearing, so it is mostly used for bleeding patterns in the upper part of the body, such as coughing of blood and nosebleed.

Modern research Increases the content of calcium ions in the blood to stop bleeding.[31]

Combinations and applications

Functions	Combinations	Applications
Transforming Blood stasis and stopping bleeding	*San Qi* (Radix Notoginseng) *Xue Yu Tan* (Crinis Carbonisatus Hominis) *Qian Cao Gen* (Radix Rubiae Cordifoliae)	Coughing of blood, nosebleed, vomiting of blood, blood in the stool, uterine bleeding; and Blood dizziness, retention of placenta and eye screen due to postpartum Blood stasis
	Ru Xiang (Gummi Olibanum) *Mo Yao* (Myrrha) *Bai Zhi* (Radix Angelicae Dahuricae)	Swelling and pain due to Blood stasis after external injury
	Bai Ji (Rhizoma Bletillae Striatae) (see notes on legal status) *Hai Piao Xiao* (Os Sepiae seu Sepiellae) *Duan Mu Li* (Concha Ostreae, calcined) (prepared as a powder for external application)	Bleeding due to external injury

Jiang Xiang 降香 (Dalbergia heartwood, Lignum Dalbergiae Odoriferae)

Jiang Xiang is the dried heartwood of *Dalbergia odorifera* T. Chen, family Leguminosae.

Main ingredients *Jiang Xiang* contains volatile oils (including β-angelica lactone and geranylactone), flavones (including luteolin, formononetin and odoriflavone) and cinnamyl phenols.

Properties Taste: acrid; nature: warm.

Channels entered Liver, Spleen and Stomach.

Functions and indications Transforms Blood stasis and stops bleeding, quickens the Blood and alleviates pain, bears counterflow Qi downwards and repels turbidity. It is indicated for coughing of blood, nosebleed, pain due to knocks and falls, pain in the chest and hypochondrium, and angina pectoris.

Common dosage 3-6g, or 1-2g of powder for internal use with water; appropriate dosage for external application.

Precautions and contraindications *Jiang Xiang* is contraindicated in cases of Yin deficiency, and for bleeding due to Blood-heat without stasis.

Modern research

1. Inhibits blood clotting and embolism.[32]
2. Inhibits the central nervous system to act as a tranquillizer, effective against convulsions.[33]
3. Reduces the level of blood lipids.[34]

Combinations and applications

Functions	Combinations	Applications
Transforming Blood stasis and stopping bleeding, quickening the Blood and alleviating pain	*Mu Dan Pi* (Cortex Moutan Radicis) *Yu Jin* (Radix Curcumae)	Vomiting of blood or spitting of blood due to Blood stasis or Qi and fire ascending counterflow
	Chi Shao (Radix Paeoniae Rubra) *Hong Hua* (Flos Carthami Tinctorii) *Chuan Xiong* (Rhizoma Ligustici Chuanxiong) *Dan Shen* (Radix Salviae Miltiorrhizae)	Coronary heart disease, angina pectoris due to Blood stasis

	Yu Jin (Radix Curcumae) *Tao Ren* (Semen Persicae) *Si Gua Luo* (Fasciculus Vascularis Luffae)	Pain in the chest and hypochondrium due to Qi stagnation and Blood stasis
	Ru Xiang (Gummi Olibanum) *Mo Yao* (Myrrha)	Swelling and pain due to knocks and falls and Blood stasis
Bearing counterflow Qi downwards and repelling turbidity	*Huo Xiang* (Herba Agastaches seu Pogostemi) *Mu Xiang* (Radix Aucklandiae Lappae) (see notes on legal status)	Vomiting and pain in the abdomen due to internal obstruction of foul turbidity

HERBS FOR PROMOTING CONTRACTION AND STOPPING BLEEDING

Bai Ji 白及
(Bletilla rhizome, Rhizoma Bletillae Striatae)

Bai Ji is the rhizome of *Bletilla striata* (Thunb.) Reichb. f., family Orchidaceae.

Legal status *Bai Ji* is a restricted substance listed in Appendix II of the Convention on International Trade in Endangered Species of Wild Fauna and Flora (CITES). Appropriate import and export permits are required for trade in this herb.

Main ingredients *Bai Ji* contains phenanthrenes, volatile oils, bletilla mannan, starch and glucose.

Properties Taste: bitter, sweet and astringent; nature: slightly cold.

Channels entered Lung, Liver and Stomach.

Functions and indications Supplements the Lungs, promotes contraction and stops bleeding, disperses swelling and generates flesh, and closes sores. It is indicated for coughing of blood, nosebleed, bleeding due to external injury or incised wounds, swelling and toxins of sores, and chapped hands and feet.

Common dosage 3-10g, or 1.5-3g of the powder for internal use; appropriate dosage for external application.

Precautions and contraindications
1. *Bai Ji* is incompatible with *Wu Tou* (Radix Aconiti).
2. *Bai Ji* is contraindicated in cases of externally-contracted disorders with coughing of blood, in the initial stage of Lung abscess and where there is full-heat in the Lungs and Stomach.

Comparison of functions Both *Bai Ji* (Rhizoma Bletillae Striatae) and *Di Yu* (Radix Sanguisorbae Officinalis) can stop bleeding. *Di Yu* tends to treat bleeding in the Lower Jiao, whereas *Bai Ji* is more effective for bleeding in the Upper Jiao and is an important herb for promoting contraction and stopping bleeding.

Toxicity The LD_{50} for intraperitoneal injection in mice of decoctions of *Bai Ji* is 21.19g/kg. There was one report of a large intake of *Bai Ji* causing slight hepatitis and pyelonephritis.

Modern research
1. Stops local bleeding.[35]
2. Inhibits ulcers and can be used to treat gastric perforation.[35]
3. Acetic extracts of *Bai Ji* had a clear inhibitory effect on Staphylococcus aureus *in vitro*.[36]

Combinations and applications

Functions	Combinations	Applications
Supplementing the Lungs	*E Jiao* (Gelatinum Corii Asini) *Kuan Dong Hua* (Flos Tussilaginis Farfarae) *Zi Wan* (Radix Asteris Tatarici)	Lung Wei syndrome, cough with sputum, pain in the chest, emaciation, deficiency wheezing, and a sunken and forceless pulse due to deficiency taxation
Promoting contraction and stopping bleeding	*Pi Pa Ye* (Folium Eriobotryae Japonicae) *E Jiao* (Gelatinum Corii Asini) *Ou Jie* (Nodus Nelumbinis Nuciferae Rhizomatis) *Sheng Di Huang* (Radix Rehmanniae Glutinosae)	Coughing of blood, dry mouth and throat, and a red tongue with thin white fur due to deficiency-fire damaging the Lung channel leading to insufficiency of Lung Yin

	Bai Bu (Radix Stemonae) *Chuan Xin Lian* (Herba Andrographitis Paniculatae)	Pulmonary consumption with expectoration of blood
	Hai Piao Xiao (Os Sepiae seu Sepiellae)	Vomiting of blood, blood in the stool and pain in the stomach and abdomen due to Stomach-fire
	Duan Shi Gao (Gypsum Fibrosum Calcinatum) (prepared as a powder for external use)	Bleeding due to external injury
Dispersing swelling and generating flesh, closing sores	*Jin Yin Hua* (Flos Lonicerae) *Zhe Bei Mu* (Bulbus Fritillariae Thunbergii) *Tian Hua Fen* (Radix Trichosanthis) *Zao Jiao Ci* (Spina Gleditsiae Sinensis)	Swelling and toxins of red, hot and painful abscesses and sores due to stagnation of heat toxins
	Jin Yin Hua (Flos Lonicerae) *Jie Geng* (Radix Platycodi Grandiflori) *Sha Shen* (Radix Glehniae seu Adenophorae) *Gan Cao* (Radix Glycyrrhizae) *Xian Lu Gen* (Rhizoma Phragmitis Communis Recens)	Lung abscess in the recovery stage with gradual reduction in coughing of fishy-smelling sputum and blood
	Zhe Bei Mu (Bulbus Fritillariae Thunbergii) *Huang Lian* (Rhizoma Coptidis) *Qing Fen* (Calomelas) (see notes on legal status) (prepared as a powder for external use)	Scrofula with continual oozing of pus

Note: Powdered *Bai Ji* mixed with sesame oil, *Ma You* (Oleum Sesami), can be used externally for the treatment of chapped hands and feet.

Xian He Cao 仙鶴草 (Hairy vein agrimony, Herba Agrimoniae Pilosae)

Xian He Cao is the dried aerial parts of *Agrimonia pilosa* Ledeb., family Rosaceae.

Main ingredients *Xian He Cao* contains agrimonine, agrimols, luteolin glucosides, quercetin, cosmosiin, hyperin, rutin, catechin, ellagic acid, pimic acid, caffeic acid, agrimonolide, coumarin, osthole and agrimophol.

Properties Taste: bitter and astringent; nature: neutral.

Channels entered Lung, Liver and Spleen.

Functions and indications Promotes contraction and stops bleeding, stops dysentery, and kills worms. It is indicated for coughing of blood, vomiting of blood, blood in the urine, blood in the stool, nosebleed, uterine bleeding, bleeding due to injury, and diarrhoea and dysentery.

Common dosage 10-15g, or 30-60g in large dosages; appropriate dosage for external application.

Remarks

1. The whole plant is better for promoting contraction and stopping bleeding, supplementing deficiency and dispersing accumulation; both the whole plant and the root buds can be used to stop dysentery and kill worms, but the root buds are more effective in these functions.

2. *Xian He Cao* is used for bleeding due to cold, heat, deficiency or full patterns.

Toxicity Neither oral administration of decoctions of the whole herb nor intramuscular or intravenous injection of agrimonine in quantities of up to 30ml within a two-hour period caused any adverse effects or toxic symptoms. The LD_{50} for oral administration of agrimophol to mice is 599.8mg/kg. When solutions containing 50% ethyl alcohol or soya bean oil were given after administration of the agrimophol, the LD_{50} fell to 540.0mg/kg and 453.3mg/kg respectively. This indicates that oily food and alcohol should be avoided when taking *Xian He Cao* to expel worms.

Modern research

1. Promotes blood circulation and stops bleeding.[37]
2. Expels worms.[38–40]
3. Inhibits carcinoma.[41–43]
4. Inhibits inflammation and alleviates pain.[44]
5. Inhibits intestinal contraction.[44]
6. Strengthens the heart and lowers the blood sugar level.[44]

Combinations and applications

Functions	Combinations	Applications
Promoting contraction and stopping bleeding	*Ce Bai Ye* (Cacumen Biotae Orientalis) *Ou Jie* (Nodus Nelumbinis Nuciferae Rhizomatis) *Bai Mao Gen* (Rhizoma Imperatae Cylindricae) *Xian Di Huang* (Radix Rehmanniae Glutinosae Recens)	Coughing of blood, vomiting of blood and nosebleed due to Yin deficiency with internal heat
	Pu Huang (Pollen Typhae) *Bai Mao Gen* (Rhizoma Imperatae Cylindricae) *Da Ji* (Herba seu Radix Cirsii Japonici)	Blood in the stool
	Dan Shen (Radix Salviae Miltiorrhizae) *Huang Qi* (Radix Astragali seu Hedysari) *Shu Di Huang* (Radix Rehmanniae Glutinosae Conquita) *Pao Jiang* (Rhizoma Zingiberis Officinalis Praeparata)	Incessant uterine bleeding with a sallow yellow facial complexion, a pale tongue and a fine, weak pulse
Stopping dysentery	*Jin Yin Hua* (Flos Lonicerae) *Huang Qin Tan* (Radix Scutellariae Baicalensis Carbonisata) *Di Yu Tan* (Radix Sanguisorbae Officinalis Carbonisata)	Enduring diarrhoea and dysentery

Notes:

1. *Xian He Cao* can be used on its own in a condensed decoction as a wash to treat vaginitis and trichomoniasis.
2. *Xian He Cao* is also effective in large dosages for malaria and can be used externally for abscesses, sores, bleeding and frostbite.

Zi Zhu 紫珠
(Callicarpa leaf, Folium Callicarpae)

Zi Zhu is the leaf of *Callicarpa pedunculata* R. Br., *C. macrophylla* Vahl. or *C. nudiflora* Hook. et Arn., family Verbenaceae.

Main ingredients *Zi Zhu* contains flavones, tannin, resin, carbohydrates, hydroxyl compounds, magnesium, calcium, and ferric salts.

Properties Taste: bitter and astringent; nature: cool.

Channels entered Liver, Lung and Stomach.

Functions and indications Promotes contraction and stops bleeding, relieves toxicity and treats sores. It is indicated for nosebleed, spitting of blood, vomiting of blood, blood in the urine and stool, uterine bleeding, bleeding gums, external injury, burns and scalds, and abscesses and sores.

Common dosage 10–15g in oral decoction, 1.5–3g as a powder for oral intake; appropriate dosage for external application topically as a powder.

Remarks *Zi Zhu*, astringent in taste and entering the Liver, Lung and Stomach channels, is effective in promoting contraction and stopping bleeding. It is used for both internal and external bleeding and is especially effective in treating bleeding in the stomach. The bitter taste and cool nature of *Zi Zhu* enable it to drain fire, thus clearing heat and relieving toxicity and making it suitable for treating burns and sores.

Modern research

1. Can stop bleeding.[45]
2. Inhibits inflammation.[45]

Combinations and applications

Functions	Combinations	Applications
Promoting contraction and stopping bleeding	*Xian He Cao* (Herba Agrimoniae Pilosae) *Han Lian Cao* (Herba Ecliptae Prostratae) *Qian Cao Gen* (Radix Rubiae Cordifoliae) *Bai Ji* (Rhizoma Bletillae Striatae) (see notes on legal status)	Nosebleed, spitting of blood, vomiting of blood, blood in the urine and stool, uterine bleeding

Additional applications

1. *Zi Zhu* is often used on its own as a powder or decoction for a variety of bleeding patterns.
2. *Zi Zhu* can be mashed while fresh or ground into a powder for external application to treat bleeding due to external injury, and burns and scalds.
3. *Zi Zhu* can be used simultaneously internally and externally to treat abscesses and sores.

Zong Lü Tan 棕榈炭
(Carbonized palm petiole fibre, Fibra Carbonisata Trachycarpi Stipulae)

Zong Lü Tan is the charred fibre of the petioles of the palm *Trachycarpus fortunei* H. Wendl., family Palmae.

Main ingredients *Zong Lü Tan* contains cellulose, tannin and carbohydrates.

Properties Taste: bitter and astringent; nature: neutral.

Channels entered Lung, Liver and Large Intestine.

Functions and indications Promotes astriction and stops bleeding. It is indicated for vomiting of blood, nosebleed, blood in the stool, blood in the urine, uterine bleeding, and vaginal discharge.

Common dosage 3-10g, or 1-2g of powder for internal use with water.

Comparison of functions Both *Zong Lü Tan* (Fibra Carbonisata Trachycarpi Stipulae) and *Di Yu* (Radix Sanguisorbae Officinalis) can stop bleeding. *Di Yu* is more effective for bleeding due to Blood-heat, especially with damp-heat in the Lower Jiao, whereas *Zong Lü Tan* is used for bleeding without Blood stasis.

Modern research Pronounced effect in stopping bleeding, notably in bleeding without Blood stasis.[46]

Combinations and applications

Functions	Combinations	Applications
Promoting astriction and stopping bleeding	*Xue Yu Tan* (Crinis Carbonisatus Hominis) *Lian Fang* (Receptaculum Nelumbinis Nuciferae)	Nosebleed, expectoration of blood, blood in the stool, uterine bleeding and other bleeding patterns without Blood stasis
	Da Ji (Herba seu Radix Cirsii Japonici) *Xiao Ji* (Herba Cephalanoploris seu Cirsii) *Zhi Zi* (Fructus Gardeniae Jasminoidis) *Bai Mao Gen* (Rhizoma Imperatae Cylindricae)	Vomiting of blood, nosebleed and expectoration of blood due to the frenetic movement of hot Blood
	Huang Qi (Radix Astragali seu Hedysari) *Bai Zhu* (Rhizoma Atractylodis Macrocephalae) *Qian Cao Gen* (Radix Rubiae Cordifoliae) *Hai Piao Xiao* (Os Sepiae seu Sepiellae)	Uterine bleeding due to insecurity of the Chong and Ren vessels
	Pu Huang (Pollen Typhae)	Red and white vaginal discharge

Ou Jie 藕节
(Node of lotus rhizome, Nodus Nelumbinis Nuciferae Rhizomatis)

Ou Jie is the dried node of the rhizome of *Nelumbo nucifera* Gaertn., family Nymphaeaceae.

Main ingredients *Ou Jie* contains tannin, asparagine, starch and vitamin C.

Properties Taste: sweet and astringent; nature: neutral.

Channels entered Lung, Liver and Stomach.

Functions and indications Promotes contraction, dissipates Blood stasis and stops bleeding. It is indicated for vomiting of blood, coughing of blood, nosebleed, blood in the urine, blood in the stool, bloody dysentery, and uterine bleeding.

Common dosage 10-30g, or juice from 30-60g of the fresh herb for oral use.

Remarks Use raw *Ou Jie* to stop bleeding and dissipate Blood stasis, and the juice of the fresh herb to cool the Blood and stop bleeding. Both can be employed to treat sudden bleeding due to heat, but the fresh herb is more effective. Charred *Ou Jie* stops bleeding by promoting contraction and is used for chronic bleeding due to deficiency-cold.

Modern research Shortens bleeding time.[47]

Combinations and applications

Functions	Combinations	Applications
Promoting contraction, dissipating Blood stasis and stopping bleeding	*Bai Ji* (Rhizoma Bletillae Striatae) (see notes on legal status) *Ce Bai Ye* (Cacumen Biotae Orientalis)	Vomiting and coughing of blood
	Xiao Ji (Herba Cephalanoploris seu Cirsii) *Huai Hua* (Flos Sophorae Japonicae)	Vomiting of blood, coughing of blood, nosebleed, blood in the urine and blood in the stool due to heat
	E Jiao (Gelatinum Corii Asini) *Bai Ji* (Rhizoma Bletillae Striatae) (see notes on legal status) *Pi Pa Ye* (Folium Eriobotryae Japonicae)	Coughing and expectoration of blood due to injury to the Lungs
	Xue Yu Tan (Crinis Carbonisatus Hominis) *Bai Ji* (Rhizoma Bletillae Striatae) (see notes on legal status)	Chronic bleeding (ulcers of the digestive system, uterine bleeding, coughing of blood in Lung Wei syndrome)

HERBS FOR WARMING THE CHANNELS AND STOPPING BLEEDING

Pao Jiang 炮姜
(Prepared dried ginger, Rhizoma Zingiberis Officinalis Praeparata)

Pao Jiang is *Gan Jiang* (dried ginger, Rhizoma Zingiberis Officinalis) that has been quick-fried until the outer surface turns black. *Gan Jiang* is the rhizome of *Zingiber officinale* (Willd.) Rosc., family Zingiberaceae.

Main ingredients *Gan Jiang* contains 2% of volatile oils (including zingiberene, zingiberol, camphene, phellandrene, shogaol, gingerol, zingiberone, borneol and citral), resin, starch and amino acids.

Properties Taste: bitter and astringent; nature: warm.

Channels entered Spleen and Liver.

Functions and indications Warms the channels and stops bleeding, warms the Middle Jiao and dispels cold. It is indicated for bleeding patterns due to deficiency-cold such as vomiting of blood, blood in the stool and uterine bleeding, as well as for pain in the abdomen, diarrhoea and dysentery due to Spleen and Stomach deficiency-cold.

Common dosage 3-6g; appropriate dosage for external use.

Precautions and contraindications

1. *Pao Jiang* is contraindicated in cases of Yin deficiency with internal heat, and where there is frenetic movement of hot Blood.
2. *Pao Jiang* should be used with caution during pregnancy.

Comparison of functions See *Sheng Jiang* (Rhizoma Zingiberis Officinalis Recens).

Combinations and applications

Functions	Combinations	Applications
Warming the channels and stopping bleeding	*Dang Gui* (Radix Angelicae Sinensis) *E Jiao* (Gelatinum Corii Asini) *Chuan Xiong* (Rhizoma Ligustici Chuanxiong) *Pu Huang* (Pollen Typhae) *Ce Bai Ye* (Cacumen Biotae Orientalis)	Vomiting of blood or blood in the stool with cold limbs, a pale white tongue and a fine pulse due to insufficiency of Spleen Yang and Qi deficiency, thus resulting in failure to contain the Blood
	Gui Zhi (Ramulus Cinnamomi Cassiae) *Wu Zhu Yu* (Fructus Evodiae Rutaecarpae) *E Jiao* (Gelatinum Corii Asini) *Bai Shao* (Radix Paeoniae Lactiflorae) *Dang Shen* (Radix Codonopsitis Pilosulae) *Chuan Xiong* (Rhizoma Ligustici Chuanxiong)	Menstrual irregularities, uterine bleeding with dark-coloured blood, and cold and pain in the lower abdomen due to Blood stasis caused by deficiency-cold in the Ren and Chong vessels
	Dang Gui (Radix Angelicae Sinensis) *Chuan Xiong* (Rhizoma Ligustici Chuanxiong) *Tao Ren* (Semen Persicae) *Zhi Gan Cao* (Radix Glycyrrhizae Praeparata)	Retention of lochia and cold and pain in the lower abdomen due to Blood deficiency and cold congealing with postpartum Blood stasis

Warming the Middle Jiao and dispelling cold	*Zhi Gan Cao* (Radix Glycyrrhizae Praeparata) *Bai Zhu* (Rhizoma Atractylodis Macrocephalae) *Mu Xiang* (Radix Aucklandiae Lappae) (see notes on legal status)	Diarrhoea, distension and pain in the abdomen, and cold limbs due to deficiency-cold in the Middle Jiao, which thus fails to transport and transform
	Zhi Gan Cao (Radix Glycyrrhizae Praeparata) *Fu Ling* (Sclerotium Poriae Cocos)	Dizziness, vomiting, slimy tongue fur and a soggy, weak pulse due to deficiency-cold of the Spleen and Stomach, which thus fail to transport and transform

Note: A powder made from *Pao Jiang* stir-fried until the surface is black can be applied externally in the initial stage of abscesses.

Ai Ye 艾叶 (Mugwort leaf, Folium Artemisiae Argyi)

Ai Ye is the leaf of *Artemisia argyi* Levl. et Vant., family Compositae.

Main ingredients *Ai Ye* contains volatile oils (including α-phellandrene, camphene, α-cedrene, transcarveol, bornyl acetate, elemol, isoborneol, α-terpineol, β-caryophyllene, carvone and cadinene), α-amyrin, β-amyrin, friedelin, matricarin, eupatilin and β-sitosterol.

Properties Taste: bitter and acrid; nature: warm.

Channels entered Liver, Spleen and Kidney.

Functions and indications Warms the channels and stops bleeding, dissipates cold and alleviates pain, expels damp-cold, and quiets the foetus. It is indicated for uterine bleeding, coughing of blood, nosebleed, vaginal discharge, stirring foetus, diarrhoea, and eczema.

Common dosage 3-10g; appropriate dosage for external application.

Precautions and contraindications *Ai Ye* should be used with caution in cases of Blood-heat and Yin deficiency.

Remarks Char-fried *Ai Ye* is used to stop bleeding (stir-frying in vinegar can enhance the herb's function in promoting contraction and stopping bleeding). Raw *Ai Ye* can be used to dissipate cold and alleviate pain. After being pounded into floss, the herb is used for moxibustion.

Comparison of functions See *Zao Xin Tu* (Terra Flava Usta).

Toxicity The LD_{50} for intraperitoneal injection in mice of decoctions of *Ai Ye* is 23g/kg. Daily intragastric administration to rabbits for 30 days of 0.45ml of the oils contained in *Ai Ye* did not have any significant effect on the animals' weight, blood or heart, liver and kidney functions. The volatile oils contained in *Ai Ye* are its main active and toxic ingredient. Oral intake of these substances can stimulate the gastrointestinal tract. Toxic side-effects may occur after intake of a single dose of 20-30g of *Ai Ye*.

Modern research

1. Stops coughing and calms wheezing, expels sputum, inhibits allergy and has a tranquillizing function.[48, 49]
2. Slows the heart rate.[50]
3. *In vitro* experiments indicated that the smoke from burning *Ai Ye* was more effective than infusions or decoctions of the herb in inhibiting a variety of bacteria.[51]

Combinations and applications

Functions	Combinations	Applications
Warming the channels and stopping bleeding	*E Jiao* (Gelatinum Corii Asini) *Dang Gui* (Radix Angelicae Sinensis) *Shu Di Huang* (Radix Rehmanniae Glutinosae Conquita) *Bai Shao* (Radix Paeoniae Lactiflorae) *Chuan Xiong* (Rhizoma Ligustici Chuanxiong)	Uterine bleeding, profuse menstruation, constant dribbling urination, pain in the abdomen in women due to deficiency-cold of the Chong and Ren vessels
	Sheng Di Huang (Radix Rehmanniae Glutinosae) *Ce Bai Ye* (Cacumen Biotae Orientalis) *He Ye* (Folium Nelumbinis Nuciferae) (these herbs should be used fresh)	Coughing of blood, vomiting of blood and nosebleed due to the frenetic movement of hot Blood with a red tongue and a rapid pulse
Dissipating cold and alleviating pain, expelling damp-cold	*Xiang Fu* (Rhizoma Cyperi Rotundi) *Dang Gui* (Radix Angelicae Sinensis) *Wu Zhu Yu* (Fructus Evodiae Rutaecarpae) *Gui Zhi* (Ramulus Cinnamomi Cassiae) *Bai Shao* (Radix Paeoniae Lactiflorae)	Pain in the abdomen, menstrual irregularities and painful menstruation due to deficiency-cold in the Lower Jiao
	Bai Zhu (Rhizoma Atractylodis Macrocephalae) *Cang Zhu* (Rhizoma Atractylodis) *Dang Gui* (Radix Angelicae Sinensis) *Sha Ren* (Fructus Amomi)	Clear, thin, odourless and dribbling vaginal discharge, pain in the lower abdomen, fatigue, loose stool, a pale tongue with white fur, and a soggy and weak pulse due to damp-cold in the Lower Jiao
	Pao Jiang (Rhizoma Zingiberis Officinalis Praeparata)	Diarrhoea, dysentery and pain in the abdomen due to obstruction of damp-cold in the Middle Jiao
Quieting the foetus	*Huang Qi* (Radix Astragali seu Hedysari) *Dang Gui* (Radix Angelicae Sinensis) *Huang Jiu* (Vinum Aureum)	Stirring foetus and pain in the lumbar region due to deficiency-cold in the Lower Jiao

Notes:

1. *Ai Ye* may also be decocted with vinegar for an external wash to treat abscesses; or ground into a powder with *Ku Fan* (Alumen Praeparatum) and *Huang Bai* (Cortex Phellodendri) and then mixed with *Ma You* (Oleum Sesami, sesame oil) for external application to treat eczema and itchy skin.
2. After being pounded into floss, *Ai Ye* can be made into moxa sticks or cones for burning at acupuncture points to warm Qi and Blood and penetrate the channels and network vessels.

Zao Xin Tu 灶心土
(Oven earth, Terra Flava Usta)

Zao Xin Tu is the ashes found at bottom of the centre of a cooking stove in which wood or grass has been burned.

Main ingredients *Zao Xin Tu* contains silicic acid and aluminium, ferric, sodium, potassium and magnesium oxides.

Properties Taste: acrid; nature: warm.
Channels entered Spleen and Stomach.
Functions and indications Warms the Middle Jiao and stops bleeding, stops diarrhoea, harmonizes the Stomach and stops vomiting. It is indicated for blood in the stool, vomiting of blood, nosebleed, uterine bleeding, vomiting, morning sickness, and diarrhoea.
Common dosage 15-30g, wrapped in a cloth and decocted before the other ingredients. Alternatively, cook 60-120g of *Zao Xin Tu* and remove it before adding other herbs to the decoction.
Precautions and contraindications *Zao Xin Tu* is not suitable in cases of vomiting due to heat patterns and vomiting of blood due to Yin deficiency.

Comparison of functions Both *Zao Xin Tu* (Terra Flava Usta) and *Ai Ye* (Folium Artemisiae Argyi) are warm in nature and can stop bleeding due to deficiency-cold. *Zao Xin Tu* is good for warming the Spleen and Stomach to stop bleeding, as well as for harmonizing the Stomach and stopping vomiting and diarrhoea. *Ai Ye* warms the channels to stop bleeding so that it is good for bleeding due to deficiency-cold in the Lower Jiao, for menstrual disorders, and for cold and pain in the abdomen. Nowadays, *Zao Xin Tu* has become relatively scarce, so *Chi Shi Zhi* (Halloysitum Rubrum) is often used as a substitute for warming the channels and stopping bleeding.

Combinations and applications

Functions	Combinations	Applications
Warming the Middle Jiao and stopping bleeding	*Fu Zi* (Radix Lateralis Aconiti Carmichaeli Praeparata) (see notes on legal status) *Bai Zhu* (Rhizoma Atractylodis Macrocephalae) *Sheng Di Huang* (Radix Rehmanniae Glutinosae) *E Jiao* (Gelatinum Corii Asini) *Huang Qin* (Radix Scutellariae Baicalensis)	Blood in the stool due to Spleen and Stomach deficiency-cold caused by failure of the Spleen to control the Blood
	E Jiao (Gelatinum Corii Asini) *Can Sha* (Excrementum Bombycis Mori)	Uterine bleeding
Warming the Middle Jiao and stopping diarrhoea	*Fu Zi* (Radix Lateralis Aconiti Carmichaeli Praeparata) (see notes on legal status) *Gan Jiang* (Rhizoma Zingiberis Officinalis) *Bai Zhu* (Rhizoma Atractylodis Macrocephalae) *Wei Rou Dou Kou* (Semen Myristicae Fragrantis, roasted)	Enduring diarrhoea due to Spleen deficiency
Warming the Middle Jiao, harmonizing the Stomach and stopping vomiting	*Su Geng* (Caulis Perillae Frutescentis) *Sha Ren* (Fructus Amomi) *Zhu Ru* (Caulis Bambusae in Taeniis)	Morning sickness, vomiting and lack of appetite
	Ban Xia (Rhizoma Pinelliae Ternatae) *Gan Jiang* (Rhizoma Zingiberis Officinalis)	Vomiting due to Spleen and Stomach deficiency-cold

Modern research references

1. Lei Zaiquan and Zhang Tingmo, *Zhong Hua Lin Chuang Zhong Yao Xue* [Chinese Clinical Materia Medica] (Beijing: People's Medical Publishing House, 1998), 1182.
2. He Xingdong et al., *Lin Chuang Zhong Yao Shou Ce* [Clinical Handbook of Chinese Materia Medica] (Beijing: People's Medical Publishing House, 1998), 188.
3. Lei Zaiquan and Zhang Tingmo, *Zhong Hua Lin Chuang Zhong Yao Xue*, 1185.
4. Pharmacology Group of Shandong Institute of Chinese Medicine and Materia Medica, *Yao Xue Tong Bao* [Pharmacology Bulletin] 11, 12 (1965): 562.
5. Dong Dianshun et al., *Zhong Hua Yi Xue Za Zhi* [Chinese Journal of Medicine] 48, 4 (1962): 240.
6. Ye Jurong et al., *Fu Jian Yi Yao Za Zhi* [Fujian Journal of Medicine and Pharmacology] 7, 6 (1985): 34.
7. Zhou Jigui et al., *Tian Jin Yi Xue Za Zhi* [Tianjin Journal of Medicine] 2, 2 (1960): 131.
8. Yan Lingxiao, *Zhong Yao Cai* [Chinese Materia Medica] 12, 7 (1989): 22.
9. No. 4 Military Medical University Pharmacology Group for the Prevention and Treatment of Tracheitis, *Science and Technology Documents (No. 4 Military Medical University)* 5 (1973): 10.
10. Jiangsu Province Cacumen Biotae Orientalis (Ce Bai Ye) Research Group, *Clinical Experiment on Treating Chronic Tracheitis with Cacumen Biotae Orientalis* (1973).
11. Research Group on the Prevention and Treatment of Tracheitis, Pharmacology Institute of Zhejiang Academy for Health Research, *Collection of Science and Research Documents of Zhejiang Academy for Health Research* (1973), 175.
12. Ibid. (1972), 130.
13. Wang Yusheng et al., *Zhong Yao Yao Li Yu Ying Yong* [Pharmacology and Application of Chinese Materia Medica] (Beijing: People's Medical Publishing House, 1998), 1170–1.
14. Lei Zaiquan and Zhang Tingmo, *Zhong Hua Lin Chuang Zhong Yao Xue*, 1194.
15. Tianjin Nankai Hospital, *Tian Jin Yi Xue Tong Xun* [Tianjin Medical Newsletter] 8 (1971): 1.
16. Xi'an Medical College, *Abstract of Science and Technology Reform (Volume 1)* 1959, 210.
17. Wang Guisen, *Zhong Guo Nong Cun Yi Xue* [Chinese Rural Medicine] 1 (1983): 23.
18. Lei Zaiquan and Zhang Tingmo, *Zhong Hua Lin Chuang Zhong Yao Xue*, 1202.
19. Jiangsu New Medical College, *Zhong Yao Da Ci Dian* [Dictionary of Chinese Materia Medica (Volume 1)] (Shanghai: Shanghai Science and Technology Publishing House, 1977), 54.
20. Quan Hongxun et al., *He Nan Zhong Yi* [Henan Journal of Traditional Chinese Medicine] 10, 1 (1990): 41.
21. Pan Xinxin et al., *Zhong Guo Yao Li Xue Yu Du Li Xue Za Zhi* [Chinese Journal of Pharmacology and Toxicology] 7, 2 (1993): 141.
22. Zhang Baoheng, *Zhong Cao Yao* [Journal of Chinese Herbs] 15, 11 (1984): 34.
23. Liu Sai et al., *Zhong Guo Yao Li Xue Bao* [Chinese Journal of Pharmacology] 5, 2 (1984): 100.
24. Wang Yiling et al., *Zhong Xi Yi Jie He Za Zhi* [Journal of Integrated TCM and Western Medicine] 14, 1 (1994): 35.
25. Wang Suxian et al., *Shen Yang Yao Xue Yuan Xue Bao* [Journal of Shenyang Pharmacology College] 7, 4 (1990): 303.
26. Song Shanjun, *Xin Yi Xue* [New Journal of Medicine] 9, 2 (1978): 55.
27. Jiangsu New Medical College, *Zhong Yao Da Ci Dian* [Dictionary of Chinese Materia Medica (Volume 2)] (Shanghai: Shanghai Science and Technology Publishing House, 1977), 1567.
28. Guo Xinchang et al., *Shanghai Zhong Yi Yao Za Zhi* [Shanghai Journal of Traditional Chinese Medicine and Materia Medica] 10 (1985): 44.
29. Xu Li et al., *Shen Yang Yao Xue Yuan Xue Bao* [Journal of Shenyang Pharmacology College] 18 (1983): 24.
30. Pharmacology Group of Shandong Institute of Chinese Medicine and Materia Medica, *Research Documents on Chinese Medicine and Materia Medica (Shandong Institute of Chinese Medicine and Materia Medica)* 8 (1975): 69.
31. He Xingdong et al., *Lin Chuang Zhong Yao Shou Ce*, 201.
32. Tianjin Nankai Hospital, *Tian Jin Yi Xue Tong Xun* [Tianjin Medical Newsletter] 8 (1971): 1.
33. Zhang Lei et al., *Shang Hai Zhong Yi Yao Za Zhi* [Shanghai Journal of Traditional Chinese Medicine and Materia Medica] 12 (1987): 39.
34. Xiao Xingche et al., *Guo Wai Yi Xue - Zhong Yi Zhong Yao Fen Ce* [Foreign Medicine - TCM Fascicule] 8, 6 (1986): 376.
35. Lei Zaiquan and Zhang Tingmo, *Zhong Hua Lin Chuang Zhong Yao Xue*, 1233.
36. He Xingdong et al., *Lin Chuang Zhong Yao Shou Ce*, 195.
37. Chen Liangcheng et al., *Xin Jiang Zhong Yi Yao* [Xinjiang Journal of Traditional Chinese Medicine and Materia Medica] 3 (1988): 46.
38. Feng Yushu et al., *Zhong Cao Yao Tong Xun* [Chinese Herbs Newsletter] 1 (1978): 32.
39. Liu Deshan, *Zhong Hua Yi Xue Za Zhi* [Chinese Journal of Medicine] 62 (1982): 336.
40. Yao Runhua, *Yao Xue Xue Bao* [Pharmacology Journal] 19, 3 (1984): 228.

41. Tang Xide, *Zhong Yao Tong Bao* [Bulletin of Chinese Materia Medica] 6, 6 (1981): 34.
42. Pan Yisheng et al., *Yao Xue Tong Bao* [Pharmacology Bulletin] 18, 7 (1983): 434.
43. Lin Ping et al., *Guo Wai Yi Xue - Zhong Yi Zhong Yao Fen Ce* [Foreign Medicine - TCM Fascicule] 10, 5 (1988): 57.
44. He Xingdong et al., *Lin Chuang Zhong Yao Shou Ce*, 194.
45. Lei Zaiquan and Zhang Tingmo, *Zhong Hua Lin Chuang Zhong Yao Xue*, 1218.
46. He Xingdong et al., *Lin Chuang Zhong Yao Shou Ce*, 196.
47. Lei Zaiquan and Zhang Tingmo, *Zhong Hua Lin Chuang Zhong Yao Xue*, 1251.
48. Chen Jiqiang et al , *Yao Xue Xue Bao* [Pharmacology Journal] 20, 3 (1985): 161.
49. Bian Rulian et al., *Zhong Guo Yao Li Xue Bao* [Chinese Journal of Pharmacology] 3 (1987): 323.
50. Sun Jingyun et al., *Yao Xue Xue Bao* [Pharmacology Journal] 22, 3 (1987): 179.
51. Lei Zaiquan and Zhang Tingmo, *Zhong Hua Lin Chuang Zhong Yao Xue*, 1273.

Chapter 12

Herbs for quickening the Blood and dispelling stasis

活血祛瘀药

Herbs for quickening the Blood and dispelling stasis

Most of the herbs which quicken the Blood and dispel stasis are acrid in taste and warm in nature. They can free the Blood vessels, dispel or break up Blood stasis, regulate the menstrual cycle, alleviate pain and disperse accumulation. These herbs are used for disorders due to Blood stasis or irregularities in the movement of Blood. Examples of such conditions include menstrual block due to Blood stasis, painful menstruation, menstrual irregularities, pain in the abdomen due to retention of lochia, retention of placenta, abdominal masses, knocks and falls, sharp pain in the chest or hypochondrium due to Blood stasis obstructing the Blood vessels, dull pain due to abscesses and sores, and wind-cold-damp Bi syndrome.

When using herbs for quickening the Blood and dispelling stasis, particular attention must be paid to the condition of the patient and the type of Blood stasis; the herbs should then be selected and combined with other herbs on this basis. Particular categories of combination are listed below:

1. for stasis due to Qi deficiency, herbs for quickening the Blood and dispelling stasis should be combined with herbs for supplementing Qi, thus enhancing the effect of quickening the Blood and transforming stasis;
2. for stasis due to cold congealing, these herbs should be combined with herbs for dispelling internal cold so that the channels will be warmed and the cold dispelled;
3. for wind-cold-damp Bi syndrome, herbs to eliminate wind-damp should be added;
4. for abscesses and sores, herbs for breaking up Blood stasis, dispersing swelling and dispersing accumulation should be combined with herbs for clearing heat and relieving toxicity;
5. for abdominal masses, these herbs should be combined with herbs for softening hardness and dispersing accumulation;
6. for patients in severe pain, herbs for quickening the Blood and dispelling stasis should be combined with herbs for alleviating pain and regulating Qi;
7. for bleeding patterns due to Blood stasis, herbs for dispelling stasis should be combined with herbs for stopping bleeding;
8. where patients with a strong constitution are suffering from Blood stasis, use may be made of stronger herbs to quicken the Blood and break up stasis;
9. where patients with a weak constitution have been suffering from Blood stasis over a prolonged period, milder herbs to quicken the Blood and dispel stasis should be used, possibly in combination with supplementing herbs; this combination of herbs can be prepared as pills of low dosage and administered over a longer period of time in order to achieve a gradual curative effect.

Herbs for quickening the Blood and dispelling stasis have the function of promoting the movement of Blood; as a result, they are not suitable for cases of profuse menstruation or Blood deficiency without stasis.

Some of these herbs also have the function of inducing abortion and hastening delivery, so they should be used with extreme caution, if at all, during pregnancy.

Tab. 12.1 Herbs for quickening the Blood and alleviating pain

Herb	Functions	Indications
Chuan Xiong (Rhizoma Ligustici Chuanxiong)	Quickening the Blood and moving Qi, dispelling wind and alleviating pain	Menstrual irregularities, painful menstruation, menstrual block, postpartum pain in the abdomen, pain in the hypochondrium, numbness of the limbs, knocks and falls, non-ulcerating abscesses, headache, wind-damp Bi syndrome
Yan Hu Suo (Rhizoma Corydalis Yanhusuo)	Quickening the Blood and dissipating stasis, moving Qi and alleviating pain	Qi stagnation and Blood stasis, all types of pain patterns, painful menstruation, knocks and falls
Yu Jin (Radix Curcumae)	Quickening the Blood and alleviating pain, moving Qi and relieving depression, cooling the Blood and clearing the Heart, benefiting the Gallbladder and abating jaundice	Distension and pain in the chest and hypochondrium, menstrual irregularities, painful menstruation, abdominal masses, vomiting of blood, nosebleed, blood in the urine, clouded Spirit, damp-heat jaundice
Jiang Huang (Rhizoma Curcumae Longae)	Quickening the Blood and moving Qi, freeing the channels and alleviating pain	Pain in the chest and abdomen, menstrual block, pain in the upper limbs due to wind-damp
Ru Xiang (Gummi Olibanum)	Soothing the sinews, quickening the network vessels and alleviating pain, quickening the Blood and moving Qi, dispersing swelling and generating flesh	Pain in the stomach and abdomen, abscesses and sores, knocks and falls, wind-damp Bi syndrome, painful menstruation
Mo Yao (Myrrha)	Quickening the Blood and alleviating pain, dispersing swelling and generating flesh	Pain in the chest and abdomen, abdominal masses, menstrual block, abscesses and sores, knocks and falls
Wu Ling Zhi (Excrementum Trogopteri)	Quickening the Blood and alleviating pain, transforming stasis and stopping bleeding	Pain in the chest and abdomen, painful menstruation and menstrual block due to Blood stasis, retention of lochia

Tab. 12.2 Herbs for quickening the Blood and adjusting menstruation

Herb	Functions	Indications
Dan Shen (Radix Salviae Miltiorrhizae)	Quickening the Blood and dispelling stasis, cooling the Blood and dispersing abscesses, clearing the Heart and eliminating vexation	Menstrual irregularities, painful menstruation due to Blood stasis, menstrual block, pain in the chest, stomach and abdomen, abscesses and sores, breast abscess due to heat toxins, pain in the limbs, palpitations, insomnia

Hong Hua (Flos Carthami Tinctorii)	Quickening the Blood and freeing menstruation, dispelling Blood stasis and alleviating pain	Painful menstruation, menstrual block, postpartum pain in the abdomen, abdominal masses, knocks and falls, severe heart pain, bedsores
Tao Ren (Semen Persicae)	Quickening the Blood and dispelling stasis, moistening the Intestines and freeing the bowels, bearing counterflow Lung Qi downwards and stopping coughing	Painful menstruation, menstrual block, postpartum pain in the abdomen, abdominal masses due to Blood stasis, chest Bi syndrome, pain in the hypochondrium, knocks and falls, Lung abscess, Intestinal abscess, Intestinal dryness with constipation, cough
Yi Mu Cao (Herba Leonuri Heterophylli)	Quickening the Blood and dispelling stasis, promoting urination and dispersing swelling, clearing heat and relieving toxicity	Menstrual irregularities, painful menstruation, postpartum pain in the abdomen, knocks and falls, oedema, sores
Niu Xi (Radix Achyranthis Bidentatae)	Quickening the Blood and dispelling stasis, supplementing the Liver and Kidneys, strengthening the sinews and bones, promoting urination and freeing Lin syndrome, guiding the downward movement of Blood	Menstrual irregularities, painful menstruation, menstrual block, postpartum pain in the abdomen, knocks and falls, limpness and aching in the lumbar region and knees, Wei syndrome of the lower limbs, Lin syndrome, blood in the urine, vomiting of blood
Ji Xue Teng (Caulis Spatholobi)	Quickening and supplementing the Blood, soothing the sinews and quickening the network vessels	Menstrual irregularities, menstrual block with pain in the abdomen, aching in the lumbar region and knees, numbness of the limbs, wind-damp Bi syndrome, knocks and falls
Wang Bu Liu Xing (Semen Vaccariae Segetalis)	Quickening the Blood and transforming stasis, causing milk to descend and dispersing swelling	Menstrual block, stoppage of breast milk, swelling and pain due to knocks and falls
Ze Lan (Herba Lycopi Lucidi)	Quickening the Blood and transforming stasis, promoting urination and dispersing swelling	Painful menstruation, menstrual block, postpartum pain in the abdomen due to Blood stasis, pain due to Blood stasis after knocks and falls, oedema

Tab. 12.3 *Herbs for quickening the Blood and treating injuries*

Herb	Functions	Indications
Su Mu (Lignum Sappan)	Quickening the Blood, dispelling stasis and freeing menstruation, dispersing swelling and alleviating pain	Painful menstruation, menstrual block, postpartum pain in the abdomen due to Blood stasis, abscesses and sores, knocks and falls
Gu Sui Bu (Rhizoma Drynariae)	Supplementing the Kidneys and joining the sinews and bones, quickening the Blood and alleviating pain	Pain in the lumbar region due to Kidney deficiency, damage to the sinews and bones, fractures

Liu Ji Nu (Herba Artemisiae Anomalae)	Breaking up Blood stasis and freeing menstruation, dissipating stasis and alleviating pain, dispersing food and transforming accumulation	Menstrual block, distension and pain in the chest and abdomen due to postpartum Blood stasis, indigestion, distension and fullness in the stomach, knocks and falls

Tab. 12.4 Herbs for breaking up Blood stasis and dispersing abdominal masses

Herb	Functions	Indications
E Zhu (Rhizoma Curcumae)	Breaking up Blood stasis and moving Qi, dispersing accumulation and alleviating pain	Menstrual block, abdominal masses due to Qi stagnation and Blood stasis, pain in the abdomen due to food accumulation
San Leng (Rhizoma Sparganii Stoloniferi)	Breaking up Blood stasis and moving Qi, dispersing food accumulation and alleviating pain	Menstrual block, pain in the chest and abdomen, postpartum abdominal masses, pain in the abdomen due to food accumulation
Shui Zhi (Hirudo seu Whitmania)	Breaking up and expelling Blood stasis, freeing menstruation	Abdominal masses, menstrual block due to Blood stasis, knocks and falls
Tu Bie Chong (Eupolyphaga seu Steleophaga)	Breaking up and expelling Blood stasis, joining the sinews and bones, alleviating pain	Abdominal masses and accumulations, menstrual block due to Blood stagnation, postpartum pain in the abdomen due to Blood stasis, knocks and falls, fractures
Chuan Shan Jia (Squama Manitis Pentadactylae)	Quickening the Blood and dispersing abdominal masses, freeing menstruation and causing milk to descend, expelling wind-damp from the channels, dispersing swelling and expelling pus	Abdominal masses, menstrual block due to Blood stasis, stoppage of breast milk, wind-damp Bi syndrome, inhibited bending and stretching, abscesses, scrofula

HERBS FOR QUICKENING THE BLOOD AND ALLEVIATING PAIN

Chuan Xiong 川芎 (Sichuan lovage rhizome, Rhizoma Ligustici Chuanxiong)

Chuan Xiong is the rhizome of *Ligusticum chuanxiong* Hort., family Umbelliferae.

Main ingredients *Chuan Xiong* contains cnidium lactone, chuanxingol, tetramethyl-pyrazine, ferulic acid, sedanoic acid, methyl phenylacetate, vanillin, β-sitosterol and vitamin A.

Properties Taste: acrid; nature: warm.

Channels entered Liver, Gallbladder and Pericardium.

Functions and indications Quickens the Blood and moves Qi, dispels wind and alleviates pain. It is indicated for menstrual irregularities, painful menstruation, menstrual block, postpartum pain in the abdomen, pain in the hypochondrium, numbness of the limbs, knocks and falls, non-ulcerating abscesses, headache, and wind-damp Bi syndrome.

Common dosage 3-10g, or 1-1.5g in powdered form for internal use with water.

Precautions and contraindications

1. *Chuan Xiong* is contraindicated in cases of effulgent Yin deficiency-fire and hyperactivity of Yang due to Yin deficiency.
2. *Chuan Xiong* should be used with caution during pregnancy and in cases of profuse menstruation and other bleeding patterns.

Remarks *Chuan Xiong*, with its properties of quickening the Blood and moving Qi, is considered as the best Qi-regulating herb among herbs for quickening the Blood. It has an upward-bearing action towards the head to alleviate headache and a downward-bearing action towards the sea of Blood to regulate menstruation. It is an important herb for quickening the Blood, dispelling wind and alleviating headache.

Toxicity The LD_{50} for intraperitoneal injection in mice of preparations of *Chuan Xiong* is 65.86g/kg, that for intravenous injection is 239mg/kg. There was no significant change in the weight, liver and kidney function and histopathology of mice after being given 5mg/kg or 10mg/kg per day of *Chuan Xiong* for four weeks. The use of *Chuan Xiong* does not generally produce toxic side-effects. Clinical reports indicate that overdosage may cause nausea, vomiting, oppression in the chest, itchy skin and maculopapular eruptions; a few female patients experienced advanced or profuse menstruation. One report mentioned pain in the abdomen and blood in the urine one hour after taking *Chuan Xiong*.

Modern research

1. Enlarges the coronary artery and has an evident effect in relieving angina.[1, 2]
2. Inhibits haematoblastic concentration.[3]
3. Relieves spasm of the intestinal smooth muscle, inhibits intestinal and uterine contractions.[4–6]
4. Has a tranquillizing function.[4]
5. Inhibited Pseudomonas aeruginosa, Shigella sonnei, Salmonella typhi and other bacteria *in vitro*.[4]

Combinations and applications

Functions	Combinations	Applications
Quickening the Blood and moving Qi	*Dang Gui* (Radix Angelicae Sinensis) *Chi Shao* (Radix Paeoniae Rubra) *Xiang Fu* (Rhizoma Cyperi Rotundi) *Chong Wei Zi* (Semen Leonuri Heterophylli)	Menstrual irregularities or painful menstruation with blood clots due to Qi stagnation and Blood stasis, accompanied by a rough pulse

	E Jiao (Gelatinum Corii Asini) *Ai Ye* (Folium Artemisiae Argyi) *Dang Gui* (Radix Angelicae Sinensis) *Gan Cao* (Radix Glycyrrhizae) *Bai Shao* (Radix Paeoniae Lactiflorae) *Shu Di Huang* (Radix Rehmanniae Glutinosae Conquita)	Uterine bleeding, profuse menstruation, continuous dribbling discharge or blood in the stool during pregnancy with pain in the abdomen due to deficiency of and damage to the Chong and Ren vessels
	Tao Ren (Semen Persicae) *Pao Jiang* (Rhizoma Zingiberis Officinalis Praeparata) *Dang Gui* (Radix Angelicae Sinensis) *Gan Cao* (Radix Glycyrrhizae)	Retention of lochia with cold and pain in the lower abdomen due to obstruction of Blood and Blood stasis with dampness
	Chai Hu (Radix Bupleuri) *Xiang Fu* (Rhizoma Cyperi Rotundi) *Da Huang* (Radix et Rhizoma Rhei) *Chuan Shan Jia* (Squama Manitis Pentadactylae) (see notes on legal status)	Pain in the hypochondrium due to Liver depression and Qi stagnation
	Xue Jie (Resina Draconis) *Ru Xiang* (Gummi Olibanum) *Mo Yao* (Myrrha) *Hong Hua* (Flos Carthami Tinctorii)	Local redness, swelling and pain due to knocks and falls, numbness of the limbs due to Qi and Blood obstruction
	Huang Qi (Radix Astragali seu Hedysari) *Dang Gui* (Radix Angelicae Sinensis) *Zao Jiao Ci* (Spina Gleditsiae Sinensis)	Non-ulcerating abscesses and sores where Qi deficiency inhibits the drawing of toxins
Dispelling wind and alleviating pain	*Jing Jie* (Herba Schizonepetae Tenuifoliae) *Bai Zhi* (Radix Angelicae Dahuricae) *Qiang Huo* (Rhizoma et Radix Notopterygii) *Xi Xin* (Herba cum Radice Asari) *Fang Feng* (Radix Ledebouriellae Divaricatae) *Gan Cao* (Radix Glycyrrhizae)	Headache, dizziness, nasal congestion and a floating pulse due to externally-contracted wind-cold
	Ju Hua (Flos Chrysanthemi Morifolii) *Shi Gao* (Gypsum Fibrosum)	Wind-heat headache
	Tian Ma (Rhizoma Gastrodiae Elatae) (see notes on legal status) *Lü Cha* (green tea)	Headache and dizziness due to ascendant hyperactivity of Liver Yang
	Sang Zhi (Ramulus Mori Albae) *Hai Feng Teng* (Caulis Piperis Kadsurae) *Du Huo* (Radix Angelicae Pubescentis) *Qiang Huo* (Rhizoma et Radix Notopterygii)	Bi syndrome, limpness and aching of the limbs, inhibited bending and stretching and hypertonicity of the sinews and vessels due to an invasion of wind-cold-damp
	Chi Shao (Radix Paeoniae Rubra) *Hong Hua* (Flos Carthami Tinctorii) *Bai Zhi* (Radix Angelicae Dahuricae) *Dan Shen* (Radix Salviae Miltiorrhizae)	Headache with stabbing pain, becoming worse at night, a purple tongue and a rough pulse due to obstruction caused by Blood stasis

	Dang Gui (Radix Angelicae Sinensis) *Shu Di Huang* (Radix Rehmanniae Glutinosae Conquita) *Bai Shao* (Radix Paeoniae Lactiflorae) *Ju Hua* (Flos Chrysanthemi Morifolii)	Headache with a fine and rough pulse due to deficiency of Blood, which fails to nourish the clear orifices

Note: *Chuan Xiong* may also be used in the treatment of angina pectoris and ischaemic cerebral diseases.

Yan Hu Suo 延胡索 (Corydalis tuber, Rhizoma Corydalis Yanhusuo)

Yan Hu Suo is the stem tuber of *Corydalis yanhusuo* W. T. Wang, family Papaveraceae.

Main ingredients *Yan Hu Suo* contains a large number of alkaloids, including d-corydaline, dl-tetrahydropalmatine, protopine, l- and dl-tetrahydrocoptisine, corybulbine, corydalis H to L, coptisine, corydalmine and columbamine.

Properties Taste: acrid and bitter; nature: warm.

Channels entered Heart, Liver and Spleen.

Functions and indications Quickens the Blood and dissipates stasis, moves Qi and alleviates pain. It is indicated for Qi stagnation and Blood stasis, all types of pain patterns, painful menstruation, and knocks and falls.

Common dosage 5-10g, or 1.5-3g in powdered form for internal use.

Precautions and contraindications

1. *Yan Hu Suo* is contraindicated during pregnancy.
2. *Yan Hu Suo* should be used with caution in cases of advanced menstruation or disorders due to Blood-heat.

Remarks

1. Stir-frying with vinegar strengthens the pain-alleviating qualities of the herb.
2. *Yan Hu Suo* is an important herb for alleviating pain and can be used for pain due to Qi stagnation and Blood stasis in any part of the body.

Toxicity The LD_{50} for oral administration to mice of alcoholic preparations of *Yan Hu Suo* is 100±4.53g/kg. Tetrahydropalmatine (corydalis B) has few side-effects on humans and no significant effect on the liver and kidney functions, blood pressure or heart rate. Therapeutic dosages may lead to dizziness and weakness, or occasionally to nausea. Since *Yan Hu Suo* is a comparatively strong medicinal when used on its own, special attention should be paid to dosage, form of dosage and combination.

Modern research

1. Has a clear effect in alleviating pain; also has tranquillizing and hypnotic functions.[7]
2. Increases the volume of coronary blood supply and nutritional blood supply to the myocardium, inhibits cardiac contractions and is effective against arrhythmia.[7]
3. Inhibits gastric secretion to counteract artificially-induced gastric ulcers.[8]
4. Lowers blood pressure, reduces the level of blood lipids and influences the endocrine function.[8]
5. Small dosages of *Yan Hu Suo* excite the uterus, whereas large dosages inhibit it.[7]

Combinations and applications

Functions	Combinations	Applications
Quickening the Blood and dissipating stasis, moving Qi and alleviating pain	*Chuan Lian Zi* (Fructus Meliae Toosendan)	Pain in the heart due to exuberant heat, or pain in the stomach and abdomen with a red tongue and yellow fur and a rapid pulse due to Liver depression and Qi stagnation leading to Liver-fire

Xiao Hui Xiang (Fructus Foeniculi Vulgaris) *Ju He* (Semen Citri Reticulatae) *Qing Pi* (Pericarpium Citri Reticulatae Viride)	Cold Shan disorders and pain in the lower abdomen with a string-like and tight pulse due to cold congealing in the Liver channel and leading to Qi stagnation and Blood stasis
Hong Hua (Flos Carthami Tinctorii) *Dan Shen* (Radix Salviae Miltiorrhizae) *Yi Mu Cao* (Herba Leonuri Heterophylli) *Chuan Lian Zi* (Fructus Meliae Toosendan)	Painful menstruation with oppression in the chest, menstrual blood with clots and a string-like, rough pulse due to Qi stagnation and Blood stasis
Yu Jin (Radix Curcumae) *Wu Yao* (Radix Linderae Strychnifoliae) *Xie Bai* (Bulbus Allii Macrostemi) *Gua Lou* (Fructus Trichosanthis)	Pain in the chest and hypochondrium with a string-like pulse due to stasis in the Liver channel
Gui Zhi (Ramulus Cinnamomi Cassiae) *Dang Gui* (Radix Angelicae Sinensis) *Chi Shao* (Radix Paeoniae Rubra) *Qiang Huo* (Rhizoma et Radix Notopterygii) *Di Long* (Lumbricus)	Generalized pain and pain in the joints due to wind-damp obstructing the channels and network vessels
Chuan Xiong (Rhizoma Ligustici Chuanxiong) *Dang Gui* (Radix Angelicae Sinensis) *Ru Xiang* (Gummi Olibanum) *Mo Yao* (Myrrha)	Pain due to knocks and falls

Yu Jin 郁金
(Turmeric root tuber, Radix Curcumae)

Yu Jin is the tuberous root of *Curcuma aromatica* Salisb., *C. zedoaria* (Berg.) Rosc., *C. longa* L. or *C. kwangsiensis* S. G. Lee et C. F. Liang, family Zingiberaceae.

Main ingredients *Yu Jin* contains d-camphene, d-camphor, curcumin, demethoxycurcumin, bis-demethoxycurcumin, turmerone, ar-turmerone, carvone, phellandrene, starch and fatty oils.

Properties Taste: acrid and bitter; nature: cold.

Channels entered Heart, Liver, Lung and Gallbladder.

Functions and indications Quickens the Blood and alleviates pain, moves Qi and relieves depression, cools the Blood and clears the Heart, benefits the Gallbladder and abates jaundice. It is indicated for distension and pain in the chest and hypochondrium, menstrual irregularities, painful menstruation, abdominal masses, vomiting of blood, nosebleed, blood in the urine, clouded Spirit, and damp-heat jaundice.

Common dosage 6-12g; appropriate dosage for external application.

Precautions and contraindications

1. *Yu Jin* is contraindicated in cases of bleeding due to Yin deficiency or in cases without Qi stagnation and Blood stasis.
2. The herb is also contraindicated during pregnancy.
3. *Yu Jin* antagonizes *Ding Xiang* (Flos Caryophylli).

Remarks There are two major varieties of *Yu Jin*. *Guang Yu Jin* is grown in Sichuan and is bright yellow in colour; it tends to move Qi and relieve depression. *Chuan Yu Jin* is grown in Zhejiang and is dull grey in colour; it tends to quicken the Blood and transform stasis.

Comparison of functions See *Jiang Huang* (Rhizoma Curcumae Longae).

Modern research

1. Reduces the level of blood fats, counteracts arteriosclerosis.[9]
2. The volatile oils contained in *Yu Jin* protect the liver and soothe the gallbladder.[10, 11]
3. Inhibits ulcers.[12]
4. Alleviates pain.[13]
5. Induces abortion.[14]

Combinations and applications

Functions	Combinations	Applications
Quickening the Blood and alleviating pain, moving Qi and relieving depression	*Chai Hu* (Radix Bupleuri) *Xiang Fu* (Rhizoma Cyperi Rotundi *Zhi Ke* (Fructus Citri Aurantii) *Dan Shen* (Radix Salviae Miltiorrhizae)	Distension and pain in the chest, hypochondrium and abdomen with a purple tongue and a string-like and rough pulse due to Liver depression and Qi stagnation leading to Blood stasis
	Dang Gui (Radix Angelicae Sinensis) *Bai Shao* (Radix Paeoniae Lactiflorae) *Chai Hu* (Radix Bupleuri) *Xiang Fu* (Rhizoma Cyperi Rotundi) *Yan Hu Suo* (Rhizoma Corydalis Yanhusuo)	Menstrual irregularities, painful menstruation, oppression in the chest and frequent sighing, with a string-like and rapid pulse due to Liver depression with heat
Cooling the Blood and clearing the Heart	*Zhu Li* (Succus Bambusae) *Zhi Zi* (Fructus Gardeniae Jasminoidis) *Lian Qiao* (Fructus Forsythiae Suspensae)	Focal distension and oppression in the chest and stomach, unclear Spirit and Mind with slimy tongue fur and a slippery pulse in damp-warm diseases due to turbid damp obstructing the clear orifices
	Sheng Di Huang (Radix Rehmanniae Glutinosae) *Mu Dan Pi* (Cortex Moutan Radicis) *Niu Xi* (Radix Achyranthis Bidentatae)	Nosebleed, vomiting of blood, blood in the urine, oppression in the chest and pain in the hypochondrium due to Liver depression transforming into fire to cause the frenetic movement of Blood
	Ming Fan (Alumen)	Epilepsy, and mania and withdrawal due to Phlegm Qi blocking the orifices of the Heart
Benefiting the Gallbladder and abating jaundice	*Yin Chen Hao* (Herba Artemisiae Scopariae) *Zhi Zi* (Fructus Gardeniae Jasminoidis) *Jin Qian Cao* (Herba Lysimachiae) *Gan Cao* (Radix Glycyrrhizae)	Jaundice or gallstones due to damp-heat obstructing the Middle Jiao, causing the Liver to fail in its dissipating and circulating function

Note: *Yu Jin* can be ground into a powder and mixed with water for external application in the treatment of haemorrhoids.

Jiang Huang 姜黄 (Turmeric rhizome, Rhizoma Curcumae Longae)

Jiang Huang is the dried rhizome of *Curcuma longa* L., family Zingiberaceae.

Main ingredients *Jiang Huang* contains curcumin, demethoxycurcumin, bisdemethoxycurcumin, turmerone, zingiberene and phellandrene.

Properties Taste: acrid and bitter; nature: warm.

Channels entered Liver, Spleen and Stomach.

Functions and indications Quickens the Blood and moves Qi, frees the channels and alleviates pain. It is indicated for pain in the chest and abdomen, menstrual block, and pain in the upper limbs due to wind-damp.

Common dosage 5-10g; appropriate dosage mixed into a paste with *Ma You* (Oleum Sesami) for external application.

Precautions and contraindications *Jiang Huang* has a comparatively strong effect in quickening the Blood and moving Qi; it should therefore not be used for patients with pain due to deficiency-cold in order to avoid a worsening of the deficiency pattern.

Comparison of functions *Jiang Huang* (Rhizoma Curcumae Longae) and *Yu Jin* (Radix Curcumae) have similar functions. They can originate from the same plant, *Yu Jin* being the root and *Jiang Huang* the rhizome of *Curcuma longa* L. Both herbs can quicken the Blood and move Qi to alleviate pain and can be used for pain in the chest, hypochondrium and abdomen due to Blood stasis and Qi stagnation. *Jiang Huang* is warm in nature and is very effective in breaking up stasis and freeing the channels to treat pain in the upper limbs due to wind-damp, swollen and painful sores, and toothache. *Yu Jin* is cold in nature and is more powerful for soothing the Liver to relieve depression by moving Qi; it can also cool the Blood and stop bleeding, and benefit the Gallbladder and abate jaundice.

Toxicity Mice were fed 40-100g of an alcoholic solution of raw *Jiang Huang* via intragastric administration; no death had been observed after three days. Rats were given 5g/kg, 2g/kg and 0.5g/kg of extracts of *Jiang Huang* mixed with feed; no abnormality in weight, food intake or activity was seen after 30 days. The LD_{50} for curcumin fed to mice via intragastric administration is in excess of 2g/kg.

Modern research

1. Reduces the level of blood lipids.[15]
2. Inhibits inflammation.[16]

Combinations and applications

Functions	Combinations	Applications
Quickening the Blood and moving Qi, freeing the channels and alleviating pain	*Dang Gui* (Radix Angelicae Sinensis) *Yan Hu Suo* (Rhizoma Corydalis Yanhusuo) *Bai Shao* (Radix Paeoniae Lactiflorae) *Hong Hua* (Flos Carthami Tinctorii)	Pain the hypochondrium due to Liver depression and Qi stagnation, pain in the abdomen due to Liver depression and Blood stasis
	Dan Shen (Radix Salviae Miltiorrhizae) *E Zhu* (Rhizoma Curcumae)	Menstrual block and abdominal masses due to Blood stasis
	Bai Shao (Radix Paeoniae Lactiflorae) *Dang Gui* (Radix Angelicae Sinensis) *Hong Hua* (Flos Carthami Tinctorii)	Postpartum pain in the abdomen

Qiang Huo (Rhizoma et Radix Notopterygii) *Hai Tong Pi* (Cortex Erythrinae) *Dang Gui* (Radix Angelicae Sinensis) *Bai Shao* (Radix Paeoniae Lactiflorae)	Pain in the upper limbs (especially the shoulders) due to wind-damp
Da Huang (Radix et Rhizoma Rhei) *Bai Zhi* (Radix Angelicae Dahuricae) *Tian Nan Xing* (Rhizoma Arisaematis) *Tian Hua Fen* (Radix Trichosanthis) (ground into a powder for external application)	The initial stage of abscesses and sores with local redness, swelling, heat and pain

Note: *Jiang Huang* can be ground into a powder with *Xi Xin* (Herba cum Radice Asari) and *Bai Zhi* (Radix Angelicae Dahuricae) and rubbed into the affected location to treat severe toothache.

Ru Xiang 乳香
(Frankincense, Gummi Olibanum)

Ru Xiang is the gum resin obtained from *Boswellia carterii* Birdw. and other related species, family Burseraceae.

Main ingredients *Ru Xiang* contains resin (including boswellic acids and olibanoresene), gums (including arabic acid and bassorin), picric acid, pinene, α-phellandrene and verbanone.

Properties Taste: acrid and bitter; nature: warm.

Channels entered Heart, Liver and Spleen.

Functions and indications Soothes the sinews, quickens the network vessels and alleviates pain, quickens the Blood and moves Qi, disperses swelling and generates flesh. It is indicated for pain in the stomach and abdomen, abscesses and sores, knocks and falls, wind-damp Bi syndrome, and painful menstruation.

Common dosage 3-10g; appropriate dosage for external application.

Precautions and contraindications *Ru Xiang* is contraindicated during pregnancy and in the absence of Blood stasis. In cases of Stomach deficiency, the dosage should be reduced to avoid inducing nausea and vomiting.

Comparison of functions See *Mo Yao* (Myrrha).

Toxicity *Ru Xiang* has a strong stimulative effect on the stomach and can cause vomiting, pain in the abdomen, diarrhoea and rumbling intestines. It can also cause allergic reactions such as stomach discomfort, lack of strength, fever, disturbed sleep, general skin flush, itchy rashes, vexation and agitation, redness and swelling of the ears and muscular twitch. This herb should therefore not be used during pregnancy and in cases of ulcerated abscesses, and should be used with great caution for patients with Stomach deficiency.

Modern research

1. Dilates blood vessels and diminishes external resistance in order to lower blood pressure and improve microcirculation.[17]
2. Decreases blood viscosity.[17]
3. Alleviates pain and reduces inflammation.[18]

Combinations and applications

Functions	Combinations	Applications
Soothing the sinews, quickening the network vessels and alleviating pain, quickening the Blood and moving Qi	*Mo Yao* (Myrrha) *Wu Ling Zhi* (Excrementum Trogopteri) *Cao Wu* (Radix Aconiti Kusnezoffii) (see notes on legal status)	Pain in the stomach and abdomen due to cold congealing and Blood stasis

	Mo Yao (Myrrha) *Dang Gui* (Radix Angelicae Sinensis) *Dan Shen* (Radix Salviae Miltiorrhizae)	Pain in the chest and abdomen, pain in the limbs and abdominal masses due to Qi stagnation and Blood stasis
	Dang Gui (Radix Angelicae Sinensis) *Chuan Xiong* (Rhizoma Ligustici Chuanxiong) *Xiang Fu* (Rhizoma Cyperi Rotundi)	Painful menstruation, menstrual block
	Mo Yao (Myrrha) *Di Long* (Lumbricus) *Chuan Wu* (Radix Aconiti Carmichaeli) (see notes on legal status) *Dan Nan Xing* (Pulvis Arisaematis cum Felle Bovis)	Wind-damp Bi syndrome, hemiplegia due to wind-stroke, pain in the limbs and hypertonicity of the sinews and vessels
	Mo Yao (Myrrha) *Xue Jie* (Resina Draconis) *Hong Hua* (Flos Carthami Tinctorii)	Swelling and pain due to stasis caused by knocks and falls
Dispersing swelling and generating flesh	*Mo Yao* (Myrrha) *Zao Jiao Ci* (Spina Gleditsiae Sinensis) *Jin Yin Hua* (Flos Lonicerae) *Tian Hua Fen* (Radix Trichosanthis)	Swelling and pain in the initial stage of abscesses and clove sores
	Mo Yao (Myrrha) *She Xiang* (Secretio Moschi) (see notes on legal status) *Xiong Huang* (Realgar) (see notes on legal status)	Hard, painful abscesses, sores and scrofula

Note: *Ru Xiang* can be prepared with *Mo Yao* (Myrrha) as a powder for external use to treat non-closure of open sores.

Mo Yao 没药 (Myrrh, Myrrha)

Mo Yao is a gum resin obtained from the stem of *Commiphora myrrha* Engl., family Burseraceae, and other related species.

Main ingredients *Mo Yao* contains commiphoric acid, heerabomyrrhols, formic acid, acetic acid, volatile oils (including cumin aldehyde, eugenol, limonene, pinene, dipentene, cinnamic aldehyde and m-cresol), catechol, resin and gum.

Properties Taste: bitter; nature: neutral.

Channels entered Heart, Liver and Spleen.

Functions and indications Quickens the Blood and alleviates pain, disperses swelling and generates flesh. It is indicated for pain in the chest and abdomen, abdominal masses, menstrual block, abscesses and sores, and knocks and falls.

Common dosage 3-10g; appropriate dosage for external application.

Precautions and contraindications

1. *Mo Yao* is contraindicated during pregnancy.
2. This herb should be used with caution in cases of Spleen and Stomach deficiency.

Comparison of functions Both *Mo Yao* (Myrrha) and *Ru Xiang* (Gummi Olibanum) can quicken the Blood and alleviate pain, and disperse swelling and generate flesh. They are used to treat menstrual block, painful menstruation and pain in the chest and abdomen due to Blood stasis as well as for knocks and falls, abscesses and clove sores, and non-ulcerating sores. Both herbs are commonly used for external injury and are often combined to accentuate each other's effect. In such instances, their dosage should be reduced. *Ru Xiang* tends to quicken the Blood and move Qi to treat Blood stasis and Qi stagnation, whereas *Mo Yao* is good at dissipating stasis and alleviating pain and is used more often for obstruction and stagnation due to Blood stasis. *Ru Xiang* is also effective in soothing the sinews and is good for wind-damp Bi syndrome and for inhibited bending and stretching.

Toxicity *Mo Yao* has a comparatively strong local stimulative effect. Intake of the unprocessed or improperly processed herb can cause vexation and oppression in the chest, disturbed sleep, vomiting, pain in the abdomen and diarrhoea. The processed herb may also cause general discomfort, facial flushes, general rashes, itchy skin, and puffy swelling of the eyes, face and lower limbs. This herb should therefore not be used during pregnancy and should be used with caution in cases of Stomach deficiency.

Modern research

1. Increases myocardial oxygen consumption, improves microcirculation, decreases blood viscosity and inhibits haematoblastic concentration.[19]
2. Reduces the level of blood lipids, alleviates pain and inhibits inflammation.[20]

Combinations and applications

Functions	Combinations	Applications
Quickening the Blood and alleviating pain	*Yan Hu Suo* (Rhizoma Corydalis Yanhusuo) *Xiang Fu* (Rhizoma Cyperi Rotundi)	Pain in the chest and abdomen and abdominal masses due to Qi stagnation and Blood stasis
	Hong Hua (Flos Carthami Tinctorii) *Dang Gui* (Radix Angelicae Sinensis)	Painful menstruation, menstrual block
	Ru Xiang (Gummi Olibanum) *Niu Xi* (Radix Achyranthis Bidentatae)	Pain in the chest and hypochondrium
Dispersing swelling and generating flesh	*Ru Xiang* (Gummi Olibanum) *Bai Zhi* (Radix Angelicae Dahuricae) *Chi Shao* (Radix Paeoniae Rubra)	Swollen and painful abscesses and sores, and non-closure of open sores

Wu Ling Zhi 五灵脂 (Flying squirrel faeces, Excrementum Trogopteri)

Wu Ling Zhi is the dried faeces of *Trogopterus xanthipes* Milne-Edwards, family Petauristidae.

Main ingredients *Wu Ling Zhi* contains resin, gum, urea, uric acid, ursolic acid, allantoin and vitamin A.

Properties Taste: bitter and sweet; nature: warm.

Channels entered Liver and Spleen.

Functions and indications Quickens the Blood and alleviates pain, transforms stasis and stops bleeding. It is indicated for pain in the chest and abdomen, painful menstruation and menstrual block due to Blood stasis, and retention of lochia.

Common dosage 3-10g, decocted in a cloth wrapping or used in pills and powder; appropriate dosage for external application.

Precautions and contraindications

1. *Wu Ling Zhi* should be used with caution during pregnancy.
2. *Wu Ling Zhi* antagonizes *Ren Shen* (Radix Ginseng).

Remarks *Wu Ling Zhi* is an important materia medica for pain due to Blood stasis, and is commonly used in gynaecological diseases. Stir-fried *Wu Ling Zhi* is effective in stopping bleeding, especially bleeding with Blood stasis.

Toxicity The LD_{50} for intraperitoneal injection of preparations of *Wu Ling Zhi* in mice is 42.60g/kg.

Modern research

1. Increases the volume of blood flow and decreases blood viscosity, inhibits haematoblastic concentration, is effective against embolisms, dilates the blood vessels and improves microcirculation.[21]
2. Alleviates pain and relieves convulsions.[22]

Combinations and applications

Functions	Combinations	Applications
Quickening the Blood and alleviating pain	*Pu Huang* (Pollen Typhae)	Menstrual block, painful menstruation, menstrual irregularities, and pain in the chest and abdomen due to Blood stasis
	Yan Hu Suo (Rhizoma Corydalis Yanhusuo) *Ru Xiang* (Gummi Olibanum) *Mo Yao* (Myrrha)	Pain below the heart due to Qi stagnation and Blood stasis
	Ru Xiang (Gummi Olibanum) *Mo Yao* (Myrrha) *Hong Hua* (Flos Carthami Tinctorii)	External injury
Transforming stasis and stopping bleeding	*Dang Gui* (Radix Angelicae Sinensis) *San Qi* (Radix Notoginseng) *Qian Cao Tan* (Radix Rubiae Cordifoliae Carbonisata) *Sheng Di Huang* (Radix Rehmanniae Glutinosae) *Mu Dan Pi* (Cortex Moutan Radicis) *E Jiao* (Gelatinum Corii Asini)	Uterine bleeding with Blood stasis

Note: *Wu Ling Zhi* can also be used internally or externally for treating snake, centipede and scorpion bites.

HERBS FOR QUICKENING THE BLOOD AND ADJUSTING MENSTRUATION

Dan Shen 丹参 (Red sage root, Radix Salviae Miltiorrhizae)

Dan Shen is the root and rhizome of *Salvia miltiorrhiza* Bge., family Labiatae.

Main ingredients *Dan Shen* contains tanshinone I, II_A and II_B, cryptotanshinone, miltirone, tanshinol I and II, nortanshinone, tanshilactone, salviol, protocatechuic acid, protocatechuic aldehyde, baicalin, ursolic acid, daucosterol and vitamin E.

Properties Taste: bitter; nature: slightly cold.

Channels entered Heart, Pericardium and Liver.

Functions and indications Quickens the Blood and dispels stasis, cools the Blood and disperses abscesses, clears the Heart and eliminates vexation. It is indicated for menstrual irregularities, painful menstruation due to Blood stasis, menstrual block, pain in the chest, stomach and abdomen, abscesses and sores, breast abscess due to heat toxins, pain in the limbs, palpitations, and insomnia.

Common dosage 5-15g; the maximum dosage for quickening or cooling the Blood is about 30g.

Precautions and contraindications

1. *Dan Shen* should be used with caution in cases without Blood stasis.
2. This herb is incompatible with *Li Lu* (Radix et Rhizoma Veratri).

Remarks *Dan Shen* fried in wine is more effective for quickening the Blood and dispelling stasis.

Comparison of functions See *Yi Mu Cao* (Herba Leonuri Heterophylli).

Toxicity The LD_{50} for intraperitoneal injection of *Dan Shen* in mice is 36.7 ± 3.8g/kg; that for *Dan Shen* compound formulae is 61.5 ± 5.3g/kg. Intraperitoneal injection of 2.4g/kg of preparations of *Dan Shen* in rabbits produced no toxic effects after 14 days. Since *Dan Shen* may cause secretion of the digestive juices, ingestion may lead to dry throat, nausea and vomiting. Prolonged use may result in pain in the stomach, reduced appetite or allergic reaction. This herb should therefore not be used for women with profuse menstruation or for patients with a tendency to bleed easily. It should also not be taken at the same time as milk or soya beans.

Modern research

1. Increases the volume of coronary blood flow and promotes blood circulation.[23, 24]
2. Inhibits haematoblastic concentration and decreases plasma viscosity, is effective against embolisms.[25, 26]
3. Inhibits inflammation.[27]
4. Protects the functions of the liver and promotes the regeneration of tissue.[28]
5. Inhibits atherosclerosis and carcinoma.[29, 30]
6. Strengthens the immune function.[31]
7. Inhibits ulcers.[32, 33]

Combinations and applications

Functions	Combinations	Applications
Quickening the Blood and dispelling stasis	*Yi Mu Cao* (Herba Leonuri Heterophylli) *Tao Ren* (Semen Persicae) *Hong Hua* (Flos Carthami Tinctorii)	Advanced menstruation of irregular quantity, vexation and agitation due to stasis caused by Blood-heat
	Xiang Fu (Rhizoma Cyperi Rotundi) *Yi Mu Cao* (Herba Leonuri Heterophylli)	Irregular and scant menstruation, postpartum pain in the abdomen, and painful menstruation with a rough pulse due to Blood stasis

	Tan Xiang (Lignum Santali Albi) *Sha Ren* (Fructus Amomi)	Pain in the chest, abdomen and stomach, and reduced food intake due to Qi stagnation and Blood stasis binding together in the Middle Jiao
	San Leng (Rhizoma Sparganii Stoloniferi) *E Zhu* (Rhizoma Curcumae) *Ze Lan* (Herba Lycopi Lucidi) *Bie Jia* (Carapax Amydae Sinensis) (see notes on legal status)	Focal distension and masses in the hypochondrium, soot-black facial complexion with a dull, purple tongue and a string-like, rough pulse due to prolonged stasis
	Chi Shao (Radix Paeoniae Rubra) *Sang Zhi* (Ramulus Mori Albae) *Qin Jiao* (Radix Gentianae Macrophyllae)	Bi syndrome due to wind, damp or heat obstructing the channels and network vessels, with red and swollen joints and yellow and slimy tongue fur
	Chuan Xiong (Rhizoma Ligustici Chuanxiong) *Dang Gui* (Radix Angelicae Sinensis) *Hong Hua* (Flos Carthami Tinctorii) *Mo Yao* (Myrrha)	Blood stasis and pain due to knocks and falls
Cooling the Blood and dispersing abscesses	*Ru Xiang* (Gummi Olibanum) *Jin Yin Hua* (Flos Lonicerae) *Lian Qiao* (Fructus Forsythiae Suspensae)	Breast abscess due to stagnation of heat toxins
	Huang Qi (Radix Astragali seu Hedysari) *Bai Shao* (Radix Paeoniae Lactiflorae) *Ru Xiang* (Gummi Olibanum)	Non-closure of open sores
Clearing the Heart and eliminating vexation	*Sheng Di Huang* (Radix Rehmanniae Glutinosae) *Xuan Shen* (Radix Scrophulariae Ningpoensis) *Dan Zhu Ye* (Herba Lophatheri Gracilis) *Jin Yin Hua* (Flos Lonicerae)	High fever, delirious speech, vexation and insomnia with a crimson tongue and a fine, rapid pulse due to heat invading the Ying and Xue levels in warm-febrile diseases
	Wu Wei Zi (Fructus Schisandrae) *Ye Jiao Teng* (Caulis Polygoni Multiflori) *Yuan Zhi* (Radix Polygalae)	Vexation, palpitations and insomnia due to Blood deficiency and Blood failing to nourish the Heart

Hong Hua 红花 (Safflower, Flos Carthami Tinctorii)

Hong Hua is the tubular corolla of *Carthamus tinctorius* L., family Compositae.

Main ingredients *Hong Hua* contains carthamin, carthamone, neocarthamin, dihydroflavones and palmitic, myristic, lauric, arachidic, stearic, oleic, linoleic and linolenic acids.

Properties Taste: acrid; nature: warm.

Channels entered Heart and Liver.

Functions and indications Quickens the Blood and frees menstruation, dispels Blood stasis and alleviates pain. It is indicated for painful menstruation, menstrual block, postpartum pain in the abdomen, abdominal masses, knocks and falls, severe heart pain, and bedsores.

Common dosage 3-10g; appropriate dosage for external application.

Precautions and contraindications *Hong Hua* is contraindicated during pregnancy.

Comparison of herbs See *Tao Ren* (Semen Persicae).

Toxicity Intraperitoneal injection of 1.0g/kg of *Hong Hua* in mice produced no toxic reaction, whereas injection of 1.2g/kg produced a slight reaction. No deaths occurred until injection of 2.0g/kg. The LD_{50} is 2.4 ± 0.35g/kg. When the dosage was increased to 7g/kg, all mice died. *Hong Hua* stimulates the gastrointestinal tract and uterus and excites the nervous system. Toxic dosages can cause such allergic reactions as abdominal discomfort and pain, diarrhoea or even haemorrhage of the gastrointestinal tract. In some women, menstrual flow increased after taking the herb. The majority of cases of reported side-effects resulted from improper use or overdosage.

Modern research

1. Slightly stimulates the heart, decreases resistance in the coronary artery, increases the volume of nutritional blood flow to the myocardium.[34]
2. Inhibits haematoblastic concentration, dilates the blood vessels.[34]
3. Decoctions of *Hong Hua* excite the uterus, especially the pregnant uterus.[35]

Combinations and applications

Functions	Combinations	Applications
Quickening the Blood and freeing menstruation, dispelling Blood stasis and alleviating pain	*Tao Ren* (Semen Persicae) *Chi Shao* (Radix Paeoniae Rubra) *San Leng* (Rhizoma Sparganii Stoloniferi) *Niu Xi* (Radix Achyranthis Bidentatae)	Menstrual block, oppression in the chest and vexation due to Blood stasis
	Chi Shao (Radix Paeoniae Rubra) *Yan Hu Suo* (Rhizoma Corydalis Yanhusuo) *Xiang Fu* (Rhizoma Cyperi Rotundi)	Painful menstruation
	Dang Gui (Radix Angelicae Sinensis) *Chuan Xiong* (Rhizoma Ligustici Chuanxiong) *Gan Jiang* (Rhizoma Zingiberis Officinalis) *Huang Jiu* (Vinum Aureum)	Retention of placenta with pain in the lower abdomen along with oppression in the chest and rapid breathing due to postpartum Blood stasis
	San Leng (Rhizoma Sparganii Stoloniferi) *E Zhu* (Rhizoma Curcumae)	Abdominal masses
	Sheng Di Huang (Radix Rehmanniae Glutinosae) *Tao Ren* (Semen Persicae) *Chi Shao* (Radix Paeoniae Rubra) *Chuan Xiong* (Rhizoma Ligustici Chuanxiong) *Yan Hu Suo* (Rhizoma Corydalis Yanhusuo) *Sha Ren* (Fructus Amomi) *Tan Xiang* (Lignum Santali Albi)	Severe heart pain with sweating, stifling oppression in the chest and a string-like pulse due to Blood stasis in the Heart channel

	Ru Xiang (Gummi Olibanum) *Mo Yao* (Myrrha) *Xue Jie* (Resina Draconis)	Joint pain, Blood stasis and pain due to knocks and falls
	Da Qing Ye (Folium Isatidis seu Baphicacanthi) *Zi Cao* (Radix Arnebiae seu Lithospermi) *Dang Gui* (Radix Angelicae Sinensis)	Maculopapular eruption with a dull, purple rash and fever, a dull, purple tongue and a fine, rapid pulse due to Blood stagnation caused by heat depression

Note: *Hong Hua* wine is effective in the treatment of bedsores.

Tao Ren 桃仁
(Peach kernel, Semen Persicae)

Tao Ren is the seed of *Prunus persica* (L.) Batsch or *P. davidiana* (Carr.) Franch., family Rosaceae.

Main ingredients *Tao Ren* contains glycerols, aspartic acid, threonine, serin, glutamic acid, glycine, alanine, amygdalin, emulsin, allantoinase, glycerols, prunin and kaempferol.

Properties Taste: bitter; nature: neutral.

Channels entered Heart, Liver, Lung and Large Intestine.

Functions and indications Quickens the Blood and dispels stasis, moistens the Intestines and frees the bowels, bears counterflow Lung Qi downwards and stops coughing. It is indicated for painful menstruation, menstrual block, postpartum pain in the abdomen, abdominal masses due to Blood stasis, chest Bi syndrome, pain in the hypochondrium, knocks and falls, Lung abscess, Intestinal abscess, Intestinal dryness with constipation, and cough.

Common dosage 6-10g; should be broken up before being decocted.

Precautions and contraindications *Tao Ren* is contraindicated during pregnancy.

Comparison of functions Both *Tao Ren* (Semen Persicae) and *Hong Hua* (Flos Carthami Tinctorii) can quicken the Blood and adjust menstruation, and dispel stasis to alleviate pain. They are used to treat menstrual block due to Blood stasis, painful menstruation, pain in the abdomen due to postpartum stasis, and abdominal masses. They are commonly used for gynaecological conditions, often being employed in combination to accentuate each other's effect. *Hong Hua* is acrid and dissipating and warms the channels. It has a more powerful effect in dispelling stasis to treat Blood stasis due to cold congealing; it is also used for maculopapular eruptions with a dull rash. *Tao Ren*, bitter and draining, is effective at breaking up stasis, with the result that it is often used for severe Blood stasis. It can also disperse abscesses and expel pus, moisten the Intestines to free the bowels, and stop coughing and calm wheezing.

Toxicity The LD_{50} for intraperitoneal injection in mice of a *Tao Ren* decoction is 222.5 ± 7.5g/kg. Long-term administration of *Tao Ren* to rats did not result in any toxic effects on heart, liver, kidney or stomach pathology. Exceeding the recommended intake in the clinic may lead to dizziness, headache, vomiting, palpitations, vexation and agitation, and in extreme cases to unclear Spirit and Mind and convulsions. It is also reported that contact with *Tao Ren* caused an allergic reaction in certain patients.

Modern research

1. Regulates blood circulation, dilates the blood vessels, inhibits blood clotting and embolisms.[36]
2. Inhibits inflammation, stops coughing.[37]
3. Inhibits allergy, alleviates pain.[37]

Combinations and applications

Functions	Combinations	Applications
Quickening the Blood and dispelling stasis	*Dang Gui* (Radix Angelicae Sinensis) *Hong Hua* (Flos Carthami Tinctorii) *Chuan Xiong* (Rhizoma Ligustici Chuanxiong) *Yan Hu Suo* (Rhizoma Corydalis Yanhusuo) *San Leng* (Rhizoma Sparganii Stoloniferi) *E Zhu* (Rhizoma Curcumae)	Painful menstruation, menstrual block, pain in the lower abdomen and vexation due to Blood stasis, with a dull, purple tongue and a rough pulse
	Pao Jiang (Rhizoma Zingiberis Officinalis Praeparata) *Chuan Xiong* (Rhizoma Ligustici Chuanxiong) *Dang Gui* (Radix Angelicae Sinensis)	Postpartum pain in the abdomen due to Blood stasis
	Da Huang (Radix et Rhizoma Rhei) *Chuan Shan Jia* (Squama Manitis Pentadactylae) (see notes on legal status) *Hong Hua* (Flos Carthami Tinctorii) *Mo Yao* (Myrrha)	Swelling and pain due to knocks and falls
	Da Huang (Radix et Rhizoma Rhei) *Mu Dan Pi* (Cortex Moutan Radicis) *Mang Xiao* (Mirabilitum)	Intestinal abscess due to pathogenic heat stagnation causing putrid flesh
	Dong Gua Zi (Semen Benincasae Hispidae) *Xian Lu Gen* (Rhizoma Phragmitis Communis Recens) *Yi Yi Ren* (Semen Coicis Lachrymajobi)	Lung abscess due to stagnation of pathogenic heat
	Bai Shao (Radix Paeoniae Lactiflorae) *Gui Zhi* (Ramulus Cinnamomi Cassiae) *Fu Ling* (Sclerotium Poriae Cocos) *Mu Dan Pi* (Cortex Moutan Radicis)	Abdominal masses and uterine bleeding due to Blood stasis
	Xiang Fu (Rhizoma Cyperi Rotundi) *Yu Jin* (Radix Curcumae) *Hong Hua* (Flos Carthami Tinctorii) *Xie Bai* (Bulbus Allii Macrostemi) *Gua Lou* (Fructus Trichosanthis)	Chest Bi syndrome, palpitations and shortness of breath with a dull, purple tongue and lips, and a slow and moderate, fine and rough pulse
	Mu Dan Pi (Cortex Moutan Radicis) *Dang Gui* (Radix Angelicae Sinensis) *Chi Shao* (Radix Paeoniae Rubra) *E Jiao* (Gelatinum Corii Asini) *Hua Shi* (Talcum)	Blood in the urine due to pathogenic heat in the Xue level
Moistening the Intestines and freeing the bowels	*Huo Ma Ren* (Fructus Cannabis Sativae) *Gua Lou Ren* (Semen Trichosanthis) *Bai Zi Ren* (Semen Biotae Orientalis)	Intestinal dryness with constipation and abdominal distension in elderly men due to Yin deficiency

Bearing counterflow Lung Qi downwards and stopping coughing	*Xing Ren* (Semen Pruni Armeniacae) *Ban Xia* (Rhizoma Pinelliae Ternatae) *Chen Pi* (Pericarpium Citri Reticulatae) *Fu Ling* (Sclerotium Poriae Cocos) *Gan Cao* (Radix Glycyrrhizae)	Cough, focal distension and fullness in the chest and diaphragm and irregular stool due to non-diffusion of Lung Qi

Yi Mu Cao 益母草 (Motherwort, Herba Leonuri Heterophylli)

Yi Mu Cao is the whole herb of *Leonurus heterophyllus* Sweet, family Labiatae.

Main ingredients *Yi Mu Cao* contains leonurine, stachydrine, leonuridine, linolenic acid, oleic acid, lauric acid, benzoic acid, rutin, fumaric acid, arginine, amyrin, stigmasterol and sitosterol.

Properties Taste: acrid and bitter; nature: slightly cold.

Channels entered Heart, Liver and Bladder.

Functions and indications Quickens the Blood and dispels stasis, promotes urination and disperses swelling, clears heat and relieves toxicity. It is indicated for menstrual irregularities, painful menstruation, postpartum pain in the abdomen, knocks and falls, oedema, and sores.

Common dosage 10–15g, with a maximum dosage of about 30g; appropriate dosage of the fresh herb for external application.

Precautions and contraindications

1. *Yi Mu Cao* should be used with caution in cases of Blood deficiency without Blood stasis.
2. *Yi Mu Cao* is contraindicated during pregnancy.

Comparison of functions Both *Yi Mu Cao* (Herba Leonuri Heterophylli) and *Dan Shen* (Radix Salviae Miltiorrhizae) are slightly cold herbs that can quicken the Blood to treat menstrual disorders, in particular patterns due to Blood stasis with heat. *Dan Shen* is more effective for quickening the Blood and can also be used for abscesses and sores due to heat toxins, and for high fever with delirious speech. *Yi Mu Cao* is more effective for gynaecological conditions and can also be used for inhibited urination and oedema.

For an additional comparison, see *Ze Lan* (Herba Lycopi Lucidi).

Toxicity Adult mice fed a powder containing 50% of *Yi Mu Cao* for 80 days showed no toxic side-effects or changes in procreative ability. Subcutaneous injection in rabbits of 30mg/kg per day for two days of the alkaloids contained in *Yi Mu Cao* did not affect food intake, stool or weight. The LD_{50} for intravenous injection in mice of the alkaloids contained in *Yi Mu Cao* is 572mg/kg. The main symptoms of overdosage in humans include general lack of strength, pain and limpness, and paralysis of the lower limbs, and in severe cases, sweating, a reduction in blood pressure or even deficiency desertion. Toxic dosages during pregnancy may cause abortion.

Modern research

1. Has an effect on the cardiovascular system and enlarges the coronary artery.[38, 39]
2. Inhibits haematoblastic concentration and the formation of embolisms.[40]
3. Stimulates the respiratory system.[39]
4. Has a curare-like action on the neuromuscular system.[38]

Combinations and applications

Functions	Combinations	Applications
Quickening the Blood and dispelling stasis	*Chuan Xiong* (Rhizoma Ligustici Chuanxiong) *Dang Gui* (Radix Angelicae Sinensis) *Chi Shao* (Radix Paeoniae Rubra) *Yan Hu Suo* (Rhizoma Corydalis Yanhusuo)	Menstrual irregularities, scant menstruation, pain in the lower abdomen and a string-like and rough pulse due to Blood stasis
	Dang Gui (Radix Angelicae Sinensis) *Tao Ren* (Semen Persicae) *Zhi Gan Cao* (Radix Glycyrrhizae Praeparata) *Huang Jiu* (Vinum Aureum)	Retention of lochia, vexation and agitation, and oppression in the chest due to postpartum Blood stasis
	Ru Xiang (Gummi Olibanum) *Mo Yao* (Myrrha) *Gua Lou Gen* (Radix Trichosanthis)	Swelling and pain due to knocks and falls
Promoting urination and dispersing swelling	*Bai Mao Gen* (Rhizoma Imperatae Cylindricae) *Fu Ling* (Sclerotium Poriae Cocos) *Sheng Di Huang* (Radix Rehmanniae Glutinosae) *Ze Xie* (Rhizoma Alismatis Orientalis)	Inhibited urination and oedema due to the Bladder failing to transform Qi
	Dang Gui (Radix Angelicae Sinensis) *Jin Qian Cao* (Herba Lysimachiae) *Bai Mao Gen* (Rhizoma Imperatae Cylindricae)	Blood in the urine with a red tongue and a fine and rapid pulse due to heat damaging the Blood vessels
Clearing heat and relieving toxicity	*Pu Gong Ying* (Herba Taraxaci cum Radice) *Ye Ju Hua* (Flos Chrysanthemi Indici)	Breast abscess
	Jin Yin Hua (Flos Lonicerae) *Lian Qiao* (Fructus Forsythiae Suspensae) *Da Qing Ye* (Folium Isatidis seu Baphicacanthi) *Shan Dou Gen* (Radix Sophorae Tonkinensis)	Sore throat, fever, chills and cough due to heat toxins

Note: Fresh *Yi Mu Cao* can be used in treating the swelling and toxins of sores as well as for itching.

Niu Xi 牛膝 (Achyranthes root, Radix Achyranthis Bidentatae)

Niu Xi is usually divided into *Huai Niu Xi*, which is the root of *Achyranthes bidentata* Blume, family Amaranthaceae, and *Chuan Niu Xi* (Radix Cyathulae Officinalis), which is the root of *Cyathula officinalis* Kuan, also family Amaranthaceae.

Main ingredients *Huai Niu Xi* contains ecdysterone, inokosterone, rubrosterone, oleanolic acid, triterpene saponins and sylvite; *Chuan Niu Xi* contains isocyasterone, sengosterone, cyasterone, amarasterone A, B and rubrosterone.

Properties Taste: bitter and sour; nature: neutral.

Channels entered Liver and Kidney.

Functions and indications Quickens the Blood and dispels stasis, supplements the Liver and Kidneys, strengthens the sinews and bones, promotes urination and frees Lin syndrome, and guides the downward movement of Blood. It is indicated for menstrual irregularities, painful menstruation, menstrual block, postpartum pain in the abdomen, knocks and falls, limpness and aching in the lumbar region and knees, Wei syndrome of the lower limbs, Lin syndrome, blood in the urine, and vomiting of blood.

Common dosage 6-15g.

Precautions and contraindications

1. *Niu Xi* is contraindicated during pregnancy and in cases of profuse menstruation.
2. *Niu Xi* should be used with caution in cases of seminal emission due to Kidney deficiency and diarrhoea due to Spleen deficiency.

Remarks

1. Raw *Niu Xi* quickens the Blood and dispels stasis; *Niu Xi* mix-fried with wine is good for supplementing the Liver and Kidneys and strengthening the sinews and bones.
2. *Chuan Niu Xi* has similar functions to *Huai Niu Xi,* but is more effective in quickening the Blood and dispelling stasis, whereas *Huai Niu Xi* is better for supplementing the Liver and Kidneys and strengthening the sinews and bones.

Toxicity The LD_{50} for intraperitoneal injection in mice of inokosterone is 7.8g/kg. A decoction of *Niu Xi* given to mice via intragastric administration for 30 days did not result in any abnormality in blood, liver and kidney functions, weight or activity.

Modern research

1. Excites the uterus.[41]
2. Decoctions of *Niu Xi* inhibit the heart and lower blood pressure.[41]
3. Inhibits inflammation, alleviates pain and promotes urination.[42]

Combinations and applications

Functions	Combinations	Applications
Quickening the Blood and dispelling stasis	*Dang Gui* (Radix Angelicae Sinensis) *Hong Hua* (Flos Carthami Tinctorii) *Tao Ren* (Semen Persicae) *Yan Hu Suo* (Rhizoma Corydalis Yanhusuo)	Menstrual irregularities, painful menstruation, menstrual block, a dull, purple tongue with stasis marks and a rough pulse due to Blood stasis
	Chuan Xiong (Rhizoma Ligustici Chuanxiong) *Tao Ren* (Semen Persicae) *Pao Jiang* (Rhizoma Zingiberis Officinalis Praeparata) *Gan Cao* (Radix Glycyrrhizae)	Retention of placenta with pain in the lower abdomen
	Xu Duan (Radix Dipsaci) *Dang Gui* (Radix Angelicae Sinensis) *Chuan Xiong* (Rhizoma Ligustici Chuanxiong) *Ru Xiang* (Gummi Olibanum)	Pain in the lumbar region, knees and feet due to knocks and falls leading to Blood stasis

Supplementing the Liver and Kidneys, strengthening the sinews and bones	*Shu Di Huang* (Radix Rehmanniae Glutinosae Conquita) *Du Zhong* (Cortex Eucommiae Ulmoidis) *Xu Duan* (Radix Dipsaci) *Sang Ji Sheng* (Ramulus Loranthi) *Mu Gua* (Fructus Chaenomelis)	Limpness and aching in the lumbar region and knees and lack of strength in the lower limbs due to insufficiency of the Liver and Kidneys
	Cang Zhu (Rhizoma Atractylodis) *Huang Bai* (Cortex Phellodendri) *Yi Yi Ren* (Semen Coicis Lachrymajobi)	Limpness and aching in the lumbar region, knees and joints, leg Qi with oedema, and yellow, slimy tongue fur and a slippery, rapid pulse due to damp-heat pouring down
	Mu Gua (Fructus Chaenomelis) *Fang Ji* (Radix Stephaniae Tetrandrae) (see notes on legal status) *Du Huo* (Radix Angelicae Pubescentis) *Bi Xie* (Rhizoma Dioscoreae)	Bi syndrome pain or pain in the lower limb joints due to wind-damp invading the channels
Promoting urination and freeing Lin syndrome	*Qu Mai* (Herba Dianthi) *Dang Gui* (Radix Angelicae Sinensis) *Tong Cao* (Medulla Tetrapanacis Papyriferi) *Hua Shi* (Talcum)	Lin syndrome, inhibited urination or blood in the urine, dryness and pain in the uterus, a red tongue and a rapid pulse due to damp-heat pouring down or pathogenic heat invading the network vessels
Guiding the downward movement of Blood	*Zhi Zi* (Fructus Gardeniae Jasminoidis) *Xiao Ji* (Herba Cephalanoploris seu Cirsii) *Bai Mao Gen* (Rhizoma Imperatae Cylindricae)	Nosebleed and vomiting of blood with a red tongue and a string-like, rapid pulse due to exuberant fire in the Liver and Stomach causing the frenetic movement of hot Blood
	Zhi Mu (Rhizoma Anemarrhenae Asphodeloidis) *Shi Gao* (Gypsum Fibrosum) *Shu Di Huang* (Radix Rehmanniae Glutinosae Conquita) *Mai Men Dong* (Radix Ophiopogonis Japonici)	Toothache, mouth sores, vexation and thirst, with a red and dry tongue and yellow and dry fur due to Liver-fire flaming upwards caused by Yin deficiency of the Liver and Kidneys
	Dai Zhe Shi (Haematitum) *Long Gu* (Os Draconis) *Mu Li* (Concha Ostreae) *Bai Shao* (Radix Paeoniae Lactiflorae)	Headache, dizziness, tinnitus, vexation and Heart-heat, and a string-like, long and forceful pulse due to ascendant hyperactivity of Liver Yang and Liver-wind stirring internally
	Chuan Xiong (Rhizoma Ligustici Chuanxiong) *Gui Ban* (Plastrum Testudinis) (see notes on legal status) *Dang Gui* (Radix Angelicae Sinensis)	Difficult labour

Ji Xue Teng 鸡血藤 (Spatholobus stem, Caulis Spatholobi)

Ji Xue Teng is the dried stem of *Spatholobus suberectus* Dunn., family Leguminosae.

Main ingredients *Ji Xue Teng* contains formonetin, ononin, prunetin, daidzein, afromosin, licochalcone A, 2,4,3,4-tetrahydroxychalcone, protocatechuic acid, β-sitosterol, daucosterol, campesterol, stigmasterol and milletol.

Properties Taste: bitter and sweet; nature: warm.

Channels entered Heart, Liver and Spleen.

Functions and indications Quickens and supplements the Blood, soothes the sinews and quickens the network vessels. It is indicated for menstrual irregularities, menstrual block with pain in the abdomen, aching in the lumbar region and knees, numbness of the limbs, wind-damp Bi syndrome, and knocks and falls.

Common dosage 10-15g, or 30g for large dosages.

Comparison of functions Both *Ji Xue Teng* (Caulis Spatholobi) and *Dang Gui* (Radix Angelicae Sinensis) can quicken and supplement the Blood to alleviate pain; they can be used to treat disorders due to Blood stasis and Blood deficiency. *Ji Xue Teng* is very effective for quickening the Blood and freeing menstruation and is generally used for pain due to obstruction of the channels and network vessels. *Dang Gui* is more effective for supplementing the Blood and adjusting menstruation and is more commonly used for menstrual irregularities caused by Blood stasis or Blood deficiency.

Toxicity The LD_{50} for intraperitoneal injection in mice of preparations of *Ji Xue Teng* is 101.5g/kg. Intravenous injection in dogs of 4.25g/kg of *Ji Xue Teng* caused death.

Modern research

1. Strengthens the rhythm of uterine contraction.[43]
2. Has tranquillizing and hypnotic functions.[44]
3. The steep of *Ji Xue Teng* inhibits carcinoma.[45]
4. Inhibits inflammation.[45]
5. Raises the haemoglobin level.[43]

Combinations and applications

Functions	Combinations	Applications
Quickening and supplementing the Blood	*Dang Gui* (Radix Angelicae Sinensis) *Shu Di Huang* (Radix Rehmanniae Glutinosae Conquita) *Bai Shao* (Radix Paeoniae Lactiflorae) *Chuan Xiong* (Rhizoma Ligustici Chuanxiong)	Menstrual block, painful menstruation or menstrual irregularities due to Blood deficiency and Blood stasis
Soothing the sinews and quickening the network vessels	*Qiang Huo* (Rhizoma et Radix Notopterygii) *Du Huo* (Radix Angelicae Pubescentis) *Wei Ling Xian* (Radix Clematidis)	Bi syndrome and numbness of the limbs due to wind-damp
	Chuan Xiong (Rhizoma Ligustici Chuanxiong) *Chi Shao* (Radix Paeoniae Rubra)	Numbness and hemiplegia due to wind-stroke
	Di Long (Lumbricus) *Tao Ren* (Semen Persicae) *Da Huang* (Radix et Rhizoma Rhei) *Chuan Shan Jia* (Squama Manitis Pentadactylae) (see notes on legal status)	Swelling and pain due to knocks and falls

Wang Bu Liu Xing 王不留行 (Vaccaria seed, Semen Vaccariae Segetalis)

Wang Bu Liu Xing is the dried seed of *Vaccaria segetalis* (Neck.) Garcke, family Caryophyllaceae.

Main ingredients *Wang Bu Liu Xing* contains vacsegoside, gypsogenin, d-glucose, l-arabinose, d-xylose, l-fucose, l-rhamnose and sapxanthone.

Properties Taste: bitter; nature: neutral.

Channels entered Liver and Stomach.

Functions and indications Quickens the Blood and transforms stasis, causes milk to descend and disperses swelling. It is indicated for menstrual block, stoppage of breast milk, and swelling and pain due to knocks and falls.

Common dosage 6-10g.

Precautions and contraindications *Wang Bu Liu Xing* should be used with caution during pregnancy.

Toxicity One case has been reported of photo-contact dermatitis after ingestion of *Wang Bu Liu Xing*, manifesting as oedema-like inflammation of the face, eyes and hands.

Modern research

1. Has a clear effect on the contraction function of the uterus in rats, induced abortion in the early stages of pregnancy.[46]
2. Alleviates pain.[47]

Combinations and applications

Functions	Combinations	Applications
Quickening the Blood and transforming stasis	*Dang Gui* (Radix Angelicae Sinensis) *Chuan Xiong* (Rhizoma Ligustici Chuanxiong) *Hong Hua* (Flos Carthami Tinctorii)	Menstrual block and painful menstruation due to Blood stasis
	Ru Xiang (Gummi Olibanum) *Mo Yao* (Myrrha) *Hong Hua* (Flos Carthami Tinctorii) *Xu Duan* (Radix Dipsaci)	Swelling and pain due to knocks and falls
Causing milk to descend and dispersing swelling	*Chuan Shan Jia* (Squama Manitis Pentadactylae) (see notes on legal status) *Tong Cao* (Medulla Tetrapanacis Papyriferi) *Dan Shen* (Radix Salviae Miltiorrhizae)	Stoppage of breast milk with distension and pain in the breasts due to Qi stagnation
	Huang Qi (Radix Astragali seu Hedysari) *Dang Gui* (Radix Angelicae Sinensis)	Stoppage of breast milk due to insufficiency of Qi and Blood
	Gua Lou (Fructus Trichosanthis) *Xia Ku Cao* (Spica Prunellae Vulgaris) *Pu Gong Ying* (Herba Taraxaci cum Radice)	Swollen and painful breast abscess

Ze Lan 泽兰 (Bugleweed, Herba Lycopi Lucidi)

Ze Lan is the whole herb of *Lycopus lucidus* Turcz. or *L. lucidus* Turcz. var. *hirtus* Regel, family Labiatae.

Main ingredients *Ze Lan* contains 0.2-0.4% of volatile oils (including hexanal, α-thujene, α-pinene, β-pinene, sabinene and myrcene), saccharides, triterpenes, flavones and saponins.

Properties Taste: bitter and acrid; nature: slightly warm.

Channels entered Liver and Spleen.

Functions and indications Quickens the Blood and transforms stasis, promotes urination and disperses swelling. It is indicated for painful menstruation, menstrual block, postpartum pain in the abdomen due to Blood stasis, pain due to Blood stasis after knocks and falls, and oedema.

Common dosage 10-15g.

Precautions and contraindications *Ze Lan* should be used with caution in cases of Blood deficiency and in the absence of Blood stasis.

Comparison of functions Both *Ze Lan* (Herba Lycopi Lucidi) and *Yi Mu Cao* (Herba Leonuri Heterophylli) have the effect of quickening the Blood and dispelling stasis, treating menstrual disorders, and promoting urination and dispersing swelling. They are important herbs for gynaecological conditions. *Yi Mu Cao*, which is slightly cold, is more suitable for Blood stasis patterns with heat and is used more frequently in the clinic than *Ze Lan*. It has a stronger effect than *Ze Lan* in terms of quickening the Blood and dispelling stasis, promoting urination, and clearing heat and relieving toxicity. *Ze Lan* transforms Blood stasis without damaging vital Qi. It has a comparatively moderate effect in terms of quickening the Blood, dispersing abscesses and sores, and promoting urination.

Modern research

1. Increases the volume of blood flow, decreases blood viscosity and fibrinogen content.[48]
2. Clearly improves microcirculation.[49]

Combinations and applications

Functions	Combinations	Applications
Quickening the Blood and transforming stasis	*Dang Gui* (Radix Angelicae Sinensis) *Chi Shao* (Radix Paeoniae Rubra) *Dan Shen* (Radix Salviae Miltiorrhizae) *Yi Mu Cao* (Herba Leonuri Heterophylli)	Blood stasis leading to painful menstruation, menstrual block, menstrual irregularities, abdominal masses or postpartum pain in the abdomen
	Dang Gui (Radix Angelicae Sinensis) *Bai Shao* (Radix Paeoniae Lactiflorae) *Sheng Di Huang* (Radix Rehmanniae Glutinosae)	Postpartum retention of lochia, pain in the abdomen due to Blood stasis
	Chi Shao (Radix Paeoniae Rubra) *Chuan Xiong* (Rhizoma Ligustici Chuanxiong) *Ru Xiang* (Gummi Olibanum) *Tao Ren* (Semen Persicae) *Hong Hua* (Flos Carthami Tinctorii)	Swelling and pain due to knocks and falls
	Dan Shen (Radix Salviae Miltiorrhizae) *Yu Jin* (Radix Curcumae) *Bai Ji Li* (Fructus Tribuli Terrestris)	Pain in the chest and abdomen

	Jin Yin Hua (Flos Lonicerae) *Lian Qiao* (Fructus Forsythiae Suspensae) *Chi Shao* (Radix Paeoniae Rubra)	The initial stage of abscesses and sores
Promoting urination and dispersing swelling	*Fang Ji* (Radix Stephaniae Tetrandrae) (see notes on legal status) *Fu Ling* (Sclerotium Poriae Cocos) *Yi Mu Cao* (Herba Leonuri Heterophylli) *Che Qian Zi* (Semen Plantaginis)	Inhibited urination or oedema (especially postpartum oedema)

HERBS FOR QUICKENING THE BLOOD AND TREATING INJURIES

Su Mu 苏木
(Sappan wood, Lignum Sappan)

Su Mu is the heartwood of *Caesalpinia sappan* L., family Leguminosae.

Main ingredients *Su Mu* contains brasilin, brasilein, quercetin, rhamnetin, palmitic acid, stearic acid, linoleic acid, oleic acid, β-sitosterol, octacosanol, taraxerol, d-α-phellandrene and ocimene.

Properties Taste: sweet and salty; nature: neutral.

Channels entered Heart, Liver and Spleen.

Functions and indications Quickens the Blood, dispels stasis and frees menstruation, disperses swelling and alleviates pain. It is indicated for painful menstruation, menstrual block, postpartum pain in the abdomen due to Blood stasis, abscesses and sores, and knocks and falls.

Common dosage 3-10g.

Precautions and contraindications *Su Mu* is contraindicated in cases of profuse menstruation and during pregnancy.

Toxicity The LD_{50} for intraperitoneal injection in mice of an aqueous extract of *Su Mu* is 18.9ml/kg.

Modern research

1. Inhibits inflammation.[50]
2. Inhibits haematoblastic concentration.[51]
3. Decoctions of *Su Mu* have a tranquillizing function and inhibit convulsions.[52]
4. The steep of *Su Mu* inhibits carcinoma.[53]

Combinations and applications

Functions	Combinations	Applications
Quickening the Blood, dispelling stasis and freeing menstruation	*Dang Gui* (Radix Angelicae Sinensis) *Chi Shao* (Radix Paeoniae Rubra) *Hong Hua* (Flos Carthami Tinctorii)	Painful menstruation, menstrual block or postpartum pain in the abdomen due to Blood stasis
	Ru Xiang (Gummi Olibanum) *Mo Yao* (Myrrha) *Xue Jie* (Resina Draconis)	Knocks and falls, damage to the sinews and bones, swelling and pain due to Blood stasis
Dispersing swelling and alleviating pain	*Jin Yin Hua* (Flos Lonicerae) *Lian Qiao* (Fructus Forsythiae Suspensae) *Bai Zhi* (Radix Angelicae Dahuricae)	Swollen and painful abscesses and sores

Gu Sui Bu 骨碎补
(Drynaria rhizome, Rhizoma Drynariae)

Gu Sui Bu is the dried rhizome of *Drynaria fortunei* (Kunze) J. Sm. or *D. baronii* (Christ) Diels, family Polypodiaceae.

Main ingredients *Gu Sui Bu* contains starch, glucose and naringin.

Properties Taste: bitter; nature: warm.

Channels entered Liver and Kidney.

Functions and indications Supplements the Kidneys and joins the sinews and bones, quickens the Blood and alleviates pain. It is indicated for pain in the lumbar region due to Kidney deficiency, damage to the sinews and bones, and fractures.

Common dosage 10-20g; appropriate dosage for external application.

Precautions and contraindications *Gu Sui Bu* is contraindicated in cases of Yin deficiency with internal heat, or in the absence of Blood stasis.

Toxicity It is reported that large dosages (100g per day or 250g in two days) led to such effects as dry mouth, excessive talking, a sensation of fear, palpitations and oppression in the chest, and rapid changes in mood.

Modern research

1. Has a clear effect on blood lipids and atherosclerosis.[54-56]
2. Improves myocardial contraction.[57]
3. Decoctions of *Gu Sui Bu* have a therapeutic effect on arthritis.[58]

Combinations and applications

Functions	Combinations	Applications
Supplementing the Kidneys and joining the sinews and bones	*Sang Ji Sheng* (Ramulus Loranthi) *Du Huo* (Radix Angelicae Pubescentis) *Du Zhong* (Cortex Eucommiae Ulmoidis) *Xi Xin* (Herba cum Radice Asari) *Shu Di Huang* (Radix Rehmanniae Glutinosae Conquita) *Ze Xie* (Rhizoma Alismatis Orientalis)	Pain in the lumbar region, limpness of the legs, pain in the heel and tinnitus due to Kidney deficiency
	Rou Gui (Cortex Cinnamomi Cassiae) *Niu Xi* (Radix Achyranthis Bidentatae) *Bing Lang* (Semen Arecae Catechu) *Bu Gu Zhi* (Fructus Psoraleae Corylifoliae)	Pain in the lumbar region due to Kidney deficiency, weakness of the bones and limpness of the legs
	Shu Di Huang (Radix Rehmanniae Glutinosae Conquita) *Shan Zhu Yu* (Fructus Corni Officinalis) *Fu Ling* (Sclerotium Poriae Cocos) *Mu Dan Pi* (Cortex Moutan Radicis) *Ze Xie* (Rhizoma Alismatis Orientalis)	Tinnitus and deafness due to Kidney deficiency, toothache and loose teeth with unbearable pain
Quickening the Blood and alleviating pain	*Xu Duan* (Radix Dipsaci) *Zi Ran Tong* (Pyritum) *Ru Xiang* (Gummi Olibanum)	Pain due to Blood stasis, fractures, damage to the sinews, and swelling due to knocks and falls

Note: *Gu Sui Bu* can be placed in a pig's kidney and roasted to treat enduring diarrhoea due to Kidney deficiency.

Liu Ji Nu 刘寄奴 (Artemisia, Herba Artemisiae Anomalae)

Liu Ji Nu is the whole herb of *Artemisia anomala* S. Moore, family Compositae.

Main ingredients *Liu Ji Nu* contains volatile oils, including benzine.

Properties Taste: bitter; nature: warm.

Channels entered Heart and Spleen.

Functions and indications Breaks up Blood stasis and frees menstruation, dissipates stasis and alleviates pain, disperses food and transforms accumulation. It is indicated for menstrual block, distension and pain in the chest and abdomen due to postpartum Blood stasis, indigestion, distension and fullness in the stomach, and knocks and falls.

Common dosage 3-10g; appropriate dosage for external application.

Precautions and contraindications Since *Liu Ji Nu* can break up Blood stasis and free menstruation, it is contraindicated during pregnancy.

Remarks A powder of *Liu Ji Nu* can be used locally to stop bleeding due to knocks and falls. Since the herb has a fragrant flavour, it also has the function of dispersing food accumulation and can be used to treat pain in the stomach and abdomen due to food accumulation either on its own or in combination with other herbs for dispersing food accumulation.

Modern research

1. Slows the heart rate, lowers blood pressure, decreases oxygen consumption in the cardiac muscle, dilates the blood vessels and improves microcirculation.[51]
2. Decreases blood viscosity, inhibits haematoblastic concentration and inhibits the formation of embolisms.[51]
3. Protects the functions of the liver.[51]
4. A decoction of *Liu Ji Nu* inhibited Shigella sonnei and Shigella flexneri *in vitro*.[59]

Combinations and applications

Functions	Combinations	Applications
Breaking up Blood stasis and freeing menstruation	*Dang Gui* (Radix Angelicae Sinensis) *Hong Hua* (Flos Carthami Tinctorii) *Chi Shao* (Radix Paeoniae Rubra)	Menstrual block or postpartum pain in the abdomen due to Blood stasis
	Chai Hu (Radix Bupleuri) *Xiang Fu* (Rhizoma Cyperi Rotundi) *Si Gua Luo* (Fasciculus Vascularis Luffae)	Distension and pain in the chest, stoppage of breast milk
Dissipating stasis and alleviating pain	*Gu Sui Bu* (Rhizoma Drynariae) *Yan Hu Suo* (Rhizoma Corydalis Yanhusuo)	Swelling and pain due to knocks and falls or fractures
Dispersing food and transforming accumulation	*Bai Zhu* (Rhizoma Atractylodis Macrocephalae) *Zhi Ke* (Fructus Citri Aurantii) *Qing Pi* (Pericarpium Citri Reticulatae Viride)	Indigestion, distension and fullness in the stomach and abdomen

HERBS FOR BREAKING UP BLOOD STASIS AND DISPERSING ABDOMINAL MASSES

E Zhu 莪术 (Zedoary rhizome, Rhizoma Curcumae)

E Zhu is the rhizome of *Curcuma zedoaria* (Berg.) Rosc., *C. aromatica* Salisb. or *C. kwangsiensis* S. G. Lee et C. F. Liang, family Zingiberaceae.

Main ingredients *E Zhu* contains curcumol, procurcumol, zederone, curcumenol, curculone, curcumin, limonene, arturmenene, zingiberene and turmerone.

Properties Taste: acrid and bitter; nature: warm.

Channels entered Liver and Spleen.

Functions and indications Breaks up Blood stasis and moves Qi, disperses accumulation and alleviates pain. It is indicated for menstrual block, abdominal masses due to Qi stagnation and Blood stasis, and pain in the abdomen due to food accumulation.

Common dosage 3-10g; *E Zhu* may be processed with vinegar to strengthen its functions of breaking up Blood stasis and alleviating pain.

Precautions and contraindications *E Zhu* is contraindicated during pregnancy and for patients with profuse menstruation.

Comparison of functions See *San Leng* (Rhizoma Sparganii Stoloniferi).

Toxicity The LD_{50} for intraperitoneal and intramuscular injection in mice of a solution containing 1% of the oil from *E Zhu* is 819.8mg/kg and 789.1 mg/kg respectively. Clinical reports indicated dizziness, nausea, facial flushes, difficulty in breathing and oppression in the chest in some patients after taking the herb.

Modern research

1. Inhibits carcinoma.[60]
2. Induces abortion in the early stages of pregnancy.[61]
3. The volatile oils contained in *E Zhu* inhibited the growth *in vitro* of Staphylococcus aureus, Salmonella typhi and Escherichia coli.[62]

Combinations and applications

Functions	Combinations	Applications
Breaking up Blood stasis and moving Qi	*Dan Shen* (Radix Salviae Miltiorrhizae) *San Leng* (Rhizoma Sparganii Stoloniferi) *Niu Xi* (Radix Achyranthis Bidentatae) *Chuan Xiong* (Rhizoma Ligustici Chuanxiong)	Blood stasis resulting in menstrual block, pain in the lower abdomen, vexation and agitation, stasis marks on the tongue and a string-like and rough pulse
	San Leng (Rhizoma Sparganii Stoloniferi) *Dang Gui* (Radix Angelicae Sinensis) *Xiang Fu* (Rhizoma Cyperi Rotundi)	Prolonged stasis and obstruction leading to abdominal masses and focal distension in the hypochondrium
Dispersing accumulation and alleviating pain	*San Leng* (Rhizoma Sparganii Stoloniferi) *Mu Xiang* (Radix Aucklandiae Lappae) (see notes on legal status) *Shan Zha* (Fructus Crataegi)	Distension and pain in the stomach and abdomen with thick, slimy tongue fur due to food accumulation

	Bai Zhu (Rhizoma Atractylodis Macrocephalae) *Dang Shen* (Radix Codonopsitis Pilosulae) *Mai Ya* (Fructus Hordei Vulgaris Germinatus) *Shan Zha* (Fructus Crataegi) *Sha Ren* (Fructus Amomi)	Distension and fullness accompanied by pain in the stomach and abdomen with thick, slimy tongue fur due to food accumulation caused by Spleen and Stomach deficiency

San Leng 三棱 (Burreed tuber, Rhizoma Sparganii Stoloniferi)

San Leng is the tuber of *Sparganium stoloniferum* Buch.-Ham., family Sparganiaceae.

Main ingredients *San Leng* contains volatile oils and starch.

Properties Taste: bitter and acrid; nature: neutral.

Channels entered Liver and Spleen.

Functions and indications Breaks up Blood stasis and moves Qi, disperses food accumulation and alleviates pain. It is indicated for menstrual block, pain in the chest and abdomen, postpartum abdominal masses, and pain in the abdomen due to food accumulation.

Common dosage 3-10g; processing *San Leng* with vinegar can strengthen its function in alleviating pain.

Precautions and contraindications

1. *San Leng* is contraindicated during pregnancy and in cases of profuse menstruation.
2. This herb is also contraindicated in cases of Qi deficiency, menstrual block due to drying up of blood, and for patients with a weak constitution.
3. *San Leng* antagonizes *Ya Xiao* (Mirabilitum Equidens).

Comparison of functions Both *San Leng* (Rhizoma Sparganii Stoloniferi) and *E Zhu* (Rhizoma Curcumae) have the function of breaking up the Blood and expelling stasis. They can disperse food accumulation and move Qi to alleviate pain and are often used together for abdominal masses, menstrual block due to Blood stasis, and pain in the stomach or abdomen due to food accumulation. *San Leng* tends to enter the Xue level and is more effective than *E Zhu* in terms of breaking up Blood stasis and quickening the Blood. *E Zhu* tends to enter the Qi level and is more effective than *San Leng* in terms of moving Qi and dispersing accumulation.

Toxicity A decoction of 280g/kg of *San Leng* was given to mice by intragastric administration. Activity was reduced after administration and the mice lay still initially, but they recovered on the second day; there were no deaths. The LD_{50} for intraperitoneal injection in mice of *San Leng* is 233.9± 9.9g/kg.

Modern research

1. Increases the volume of blood flow and decreases blood viscosity.[63, 64]
2. Inhibits inflammation and alleviates pain.[64]

Combinations and applications

Functions	Combinations	Applications
Breaking up Blood stasis and moving Qi	*E Zhu* (Rhizoma Curcumae) *Dang Gui* (Radix Angelicae Sinensis) *Tao Ren* (Semen Persicae)	Blood stasis resulting in menstrual block with pain in the abdomen, oppression in the chest and vexation, with a dull tongue and rough pulse

	Mu Xiang (Radix Aucklandiae Lappae) (see notes on legal status) *Xiao Hui Xiang* (Fructus Foeniculi Vulgaris)	Postpartum abdominal masses and pain in the lower abdomen due to Blood stasis
Dispersing food accumulation and alleviating pain	*Qing Pi* (Pericarpium Citri Reticulatae Viride) *Mai Ya* (Fructus Hordei Vulgaris Germinatus) *E Zhu* (Rhizoma Curcumae)	Distension and pain due to food accumulation and Qi stagnation
	Dang Shen (Radix Codonopsitis Pilosulae) *Mai Ya* (Fructus Hordei Vulgaris Germinatus) *Chen Pi* (Pericarpium Citri Reticulatae) *Sha Ren* (Fructus Amomi) *Bai Zhu* (Rhizoma Atractylodis Macrocephalae)	Food stagnation in the Middle Jiao and distension, fullness and pain in the abdomen due to deficiency of the Spleen and Stomach, which thus fail to transport and transform food and water

Shui Zhi 水蛭 (Leech, Hirudo seu Whitmania)

Shui Zhi is the dried body of *Hirudo nipponica* Whitman, *Whitmania pigra* (Whitman) or *W. acranulata* (Whitman), family Hirudinidae.

Main ingredients *Shui Zhi* contains proteins, hirudin, heparin and antithrombotin.

Properties Taste: salty and bitter; nature: neutral; slightly toxic.

Channel entered Liver.

Functions and indications Breaks up and expels Blood stasis, and frees menstruation. It is indicated for abdominal masses, menstrual block due to Blood stasis, and knocks and falls.

Common dosage 3-6g; or 0.3-0.5g in powder form for internal use.

Precautions and contraindications *Shui Zhi* is contraindicated for patients with a weak constitution, in cases without internal Blood stasis, during pregnancy or in cases of profuse menstruation.

Comparison of functions See *Tu Bie Chong* (Eupolyphaga seu Steleophaga).

Toxicity The LD_{50} for subcutaneous injection in mice of a decoction of *Shui Zhi* is 15.42 ± 2.04g/kg. There were no obvious toxic side-effects after intravenous or subcutaneous injection of hirudin; blood pressure, heartbeat and respiratory rate were unchanged.

Modern research

1. Increases the volume of blood flow, decreases blood viscosity, inhibits haematoblastic concentration.[65–67]
2. Inhibits blood clotting and the formation of embolisms.[68–70]
3. Inhibits inflammation.[68]
4. Induces abortion.[70]

Combinations and applications

Functions	Combinations	Applications
Breaking up and expelling Blood stasis, freeing menstruation	*Tao Ren* (Semen Persicae) *Da Huang* (Radix et Rhizoma Rhei)	Inhibited menstrual flow, and fullness and urgency in the bladder in men due to Blood stasis in the Lower Jiao

Ren Shen (Radix Ginseng) *Dang Gui* (Radix Angelicae Sinensis) *Shu Di Huang* (Radix Rehmanniae Glutinosae Conquita)	Abdominal masses and menstrual block due to Blood stasis in deficiency patterns
San Leng (Rhizoma Sparganii Stoloniferi) *Su Mu* (Lignum Sappan) *Tao Ren* (Semen Persicae)	Abdominal masses and pain in the lower abdomen, accompanied by a dull, purple tongue with stasis marks and a rough pulse resulting from prolonged Qi stagnation and Blood stasis
Da Huang (Radix et Rhizoma Rhei) *Qian Niu Zi* (Semen Pharbitidis) *Huang Jiu* (Vinum Aureum)	Pain in the chest and abdomen caused by knocks and falls; inhibited bowel movement and urination due to Blood stasis caused by internal injury

Tu Bie Chong 土鳖虫 (Wingless cockroach, Eupolyphaga seu Steleophaga)

Tu Bie Chong is the dried body of the mature female of *Eupolyphaga sinensis* Walk. or *Steleophaga plancyi* (Bol.), family Corydiidae.

Main ingredients *Tu Bie Chong* contains glycerin ethers, uracil, allantoin, amino acids, trace elements and alkaloids.

Properties Taste: salty; nature: cold; slightly toxic.

Channel entered Liver.

Functions and indications Breaks up and expels Blood stasis, joins the sinews and bones, and alleviates pain. It is indicated for abdominal masses and accumulations, menstrual block due to Blood stagnation, postpartum pain in the abdomen due to Blood stasis, knocks and falls, and fractures.

Common dosage 3-10g as an oral decoction; 1-1.5g when ground to a powder.

Precautions and contraindications *Tu Bie Chong* is contraindicated during pregnancy.

Comparison of functions Both *Tu Bie Chong* (Eupolyphaga seu Steleophaga) and *Shui Zhi* (Hirudo seu Whitmania) have a potent effect in breaking up and expelling Blood stasis and both are slightly toxic. *Shui Zhi* has the more drastic, longer-lasting effect in breaking up and expelling Blood stasis, dispersing masses and freeing menstruation. It is very effective in the treatment of menstrual block due to Blood stasis, abdominal masses, and injury due to knocks and falls. *Tu Bie Chong* is milder in action, but functions very well in promoting the healing of fractures.

Toxicity The LD_{50} for intraperitoneal injection in mice of the alkaloid extract of *Tu Bie Chong* (TAE_{S2}) is 136.45 ± 7.98mg/kg. After injection, the mice began to tremble and shake; most died within 10-20 minutes.

Modern research

1. Has a significant effect in inhibiting thrombosis.[71]
2. Inhibits oxygen deficiency.[72]
3. Reduces the level of blood lipids.[73]

Combinations and applications

Functions	Combinations	Applications
Breaking up and expelling Blood stasis, joining the sinews and bones, alleviating pain	*Da Huang* (Radix et Rhizoma Rhei) *Tao Ren* (Semen Persicae)	Menstrual block due to Blood stasis, postpartum pain in the abdomen due to Blood stasis and stagnation
	Da Huang (Radix et Rhizoma Rhei) *Tao Ren* (Semen Persicae) *Bie Jia* (Carapax Amydae Sinensis) (see notes on legal status) *Mu Dan Pi* (Cortex Moutan Radicis)	Abdominal masses and accumulations due to Blood stasis
	Gu Sui Bu (Rhizoma Drynariae) *Zi Ran Tong* (Pyritum) *Ru Xiang* (Gummi Olibanum)	Blood stasis, swelling and pain due to knocks and falls, fractures

Note: *Tu Bie Chong* can be stone-baked and ground into a powder to treat acute sprain of the lumbar region.

Chuan Shan Jia 穿山甲
(Pangolin scales, Squama Manitis Pentadactylae)

Chuan Shan Jia is the scales of the pangolin, *Manis pentadactyla* L., family Manidae.

Legal status *Chuan Shan Jia* is a restricted substance listed in Appendix II of the Convention on International Trade in Endangered Species of Wild Fauna and Flora (CITES). Appropriate import and export permits are required for trade in this materia medica.

Main ingredients *Chuan Shan Jia* contains stearic acid, volatile oils, amino acids and alkaloids.

Properties Taste: salty; nature: slightly cold.

Channels entered Liver and Stomach.

Functions and indications Quickens the Blood and disperses abdominal masses, frees menstruation and causes milk to descend, expels wind-damp from the channels, disperses swelling and expels pus. It is indicated for abdominal masses, menstrual block due to Blood stasis, stoppage of breast milk, wind-damp Bi syndrome, inhibited bending and stretching, abscesses, and scrofula.

Common dosage 3-10g, or 1-2g of the powder for oral use.

Precautions and contraindications *Chuan Shan Jia* is contraindicated during pregnancy and where abscesses have already ulcerated.

Remarks *Chuan Shan Jia* is more effective in powder form than in decoction.

Modern research

1. Decreases blood viscosity, prolongs blood clotting time, and increases the white blood cell count.[74]
2. The steep of *Chuan Shan Jia* inhibits inflammation.[75]
3. Improves the ability to endure oxygen deprivation.[75]

Combinations and applications

Functions	Combinations	Applications
Quickening the Blood and dispersing abdominal masses, freeing menstruation and causing milk to descend	*Wang Bu Liu Xing* (Semen Vaccariae Segetalis) *Tong Cao* (Medulla Tetrapanacis Papyriferi) *Dang Gui* (Radix Angelicae Sinensis)	Stoppage of breast milk
	San Leng (Rhizoma Sparganii Stoloniferi) *E Zhu* (Rhizoma Curcumae)	Abdominal masses due to Blood stasis
	Dang Gui (Radix Angelicae Sinensis) *Hong Hua* (Flos Carthami Tinctorii) *Bie Jia* (Carapax Amydae Sinensis) (see notes on legal status) *Chuan Xiong* (Rhizoma Ligustici Chuanxiong)	Menstrual block
Expelling wind-damp from the channels	*Dang Gui* (Radix Angelicae Sinensis) *Chuan Xiong* (Rhizoma Ligustici Chuanxiong) *Qiang Huo* (Rhizoma et Radix Notopterygii)	Bi syndrome, rigidity of the limbs and limb pain due to wind-damp
Dispersing swelling and expelling pus	*Chi Shao* (Radix Paeoniae Rubra) *Ru Xiang* (Gummi Olibanum) *Jin Yin Hua* (Flos Lonicerae)	The initial stage of abscesses and sores
	Huang Qi (Radix Astragali seu Hedysari) *Dang Gui* (Radix Angelicae Sinensis)	Non-ulcerating sores with pus
	Chuan Xiong (Rhizoma Ligustici Chuanxiong) *Huang Qi* (Radix Astragali seu Hedysari) *Zao Jiao Ci* (Spina Gleditsiae Sinensis)	Suppurative abscesses
	Xia Ku Cao (Spica Prunellae Vulgaris) *Hai Zao* (Herba Sargassi) *Mu Li* (Concha Ostreae)	Scrofula, goitre

Modern research references

1. Beijing Pharmacology Industry Institute, *Bei Jing Yi Yao Gong Ye* [Beijing Medical and Pharmacology Industry] 4 (1975): 22.
2. Ibid., 27.
3. Chinese Academy of Traditional Chinese Medicine Xiyuan Hospital Pharmacology Group, *Zhong Yi Xue Yan Jiu Can Kao* [Journal of Chinese Medicine Research] 8 (1975): 37.
4. Lei Zaiquan and Zhang Tingmo, *Zhong Hua Lin Chuang Zhong Yao Xue* [Chinese Clinical Materia Medica] (Beijing: People's Medical Publishing House, 1998), 1053.
5. Jiangsu New Medical College, *Zhong Yao Da Ci Dian* [Dictionary of Chinese Materia Medica], volume 1 (Shanghai: Shanghai People's Publishing House, 1977), 220.
6. Zhang Gongshou et al., *Tong Ji Yi Ke Da Xue Xue Bao* [Journal of Tongji Medical University] 18, 6 (1989): 412.

7. Lei Zaiquan and Zhang Tingmo, *Zhong Hua Lin Chuang Zhong Yao Xue*, 1059.
8. He Xingdong et al., *Lin Chuang Zhong Yao Shou Ce* [Clinical Handbook of Chinese Materia Medica] (Beijing: People's Medical Publishing House, 1998), 209.
9. Dai Kemin, *Chang Yong Zhong Yao Yao Li Yu Ying Yong* [Pharmacology and Application of Commonly-Used Chinese Materia Medica] (Nanjing: Jiangsu Science and Technology Publishing House, 1980), 77.
10. Editorial Group of Zhongshan Medical College, *Clinical Application of Chinese Materia Medica* (Guangzhou: Guangdong People's Publishing House, 1985), 181.
11. Liu Baolin et al, *Zhong Yao Tong Bao* [Bulletin of Chinese Materia Medica] 13, 1 (1988): 46.
12. Li Chengzhang et al., *Zhong Yao Tong Bao* 12, 6 (1987): 32.
13. Liang Denian, *Zhong Yi Yao Xue Bao* [Journal of Traditional Chinese Medicine and Materia Medica] 1 (1987): 40.
14. S.K. Gray, *Planta Medica* 26, 3 (1974): 225.
15. Xu Shibo et al., *Zhong Cao Yao* [Journal of Chinese Herbs] 22, 3 (1991): 141.
16. Wang Yusheng, *Zhong Yao Yao Li Yu Ying Yong* [Pharmacology and Application of Chinese Materia Medica] (Beijing: People's Medical Publishing House, 1983), 864.
17. He Xingdong et al., *Lin Chuang Zhong Yao Shou Ce*, 207.
18. Lei Zaiquan and Zhang Tingmo, *Zhong Hua Lin Chuang Zhong Yao Xue*, 1071.
19. He Xingdong et al., *Lin Chuang Zhong Yao Shou Ce*, 208.
20. Lei Zaiquan and Zhang Tingmo, *Zhong Hua Lin Chuang Zhong Yao Xue*, 1074.
21. He Xingdong et al., *Lin Chuang Zhong Yao Shou Ce*, 220.
22. Lei Zaiquan and Zhang Tingmo, *Zhong Hua Lin Chuang Zhong Yao Xue*, 1269.
23. Sang Guowei et al., *Zhe Jiang Yi Xue* [Zhejiang Journal of Medicine] 1, 1 (1979): 25.
24. Xue Quanfu, *Zhong Hua Yi Xue Za Zhi* [Chinese Journal of Medicine] 66, 6 (1986): 334.
25. Luan Zhihe et al., *Shan Dong Yi Yao* [Shandong Medical Journal] 28, 12 (1988): 1.
26. Song Jiannan et al., *Zhong Yao Tong Bao* [Bulletin of Chinese Materia Medica] 9, 4 (1984): 38.
27. Liu Ping et al., *Zhong Yao Yao Li Yu Lin Chuang* [Pharmacology and Clinical Application of Chinese Materia Medica] 9, 3 (1993): 13.
28. Han Dewu et al., *Lin Chuang Gan Dan Bing Za Zhi* [Journal of Clinical Hepatology] 4, 3 (1988): 38.
29. Mou Yongfang et al., *Zhong Hua Lao Nian Bing Xue Za Zhi* [Chinese Journal of Geriatrics] 6, 4 (1987): 256.
30. Ying Rongduo, *Zhong Yi Za Zhi* [Journal of Traditional Chinese Medicine] 5 (1988): 60.
31. Sun Jiemin et al., *Zhong Yi Yao Yan Jiu* [Traditional Chinese Medicine and Materia Medica Research] 3 (1991): 50.
32. Li Hequan et al., *Zhong Guo Yi Ke Da Xue Xue Bao* [Journal of Chinese Medical University] 17, 2 (1988): 113.
33. Wang Guozhong et al., *Zhong Guo Yi Ke Da Xue Xue Bao* 23, 4 (1994): 311.
34. He Xingdong et al., *Lin Chuang Zhong Yao Shou Ce*, 219.
35. Lei Zaiquan and Zhang Tingmo, *Zhong Hua Lin Chuang Zhong Yao Xue*, 1112.
36. He Xingdong et al., *Lin Chuang Zhong Yao Shou Ce*, 218.
37. Lei Zaiquan and Zhang Tingmo, *Zhong Hua Lin Chuang Zhong Yao Xue*, 1122
38. Zhu Yeqing, *Guo Wai Yi Xue – Yao Xue Fen Ce* [Foreign Medicine – Pharmacology Fascicule] 2 (1979): 120.
39. Zhang Chenfu et al., *Zhong Xi Yi Jie He Za Zhi* [Journal of Integrated TCM and Western Medicine] 4, 10 (1984): 638.
40. Jia Yunsheng et al., *Shang Hai Zhong Yi Yao Za Zhi* [Shanghai Journal of Traditional Chinese Medicine and Materia Medica] 8 (1983): 45.
41. He Xingdong et al., *Lin Chuang Zhong Yao Shou Ce*, 221.
42. Lei Zaiquan and Zhang Tingmo, *Zhong Hua Lin Chuang Zhong Yao Xue*, 1126.
43. Editorial Group, *Quan Guo Zhong Cao Yao Hui Bian* [National Collection of Chinese Herbs] (Beijing: People's Medical Publishing House, 1975), 426.
44. Lei Zaiquan and Zhang Tingmo, *Zhong Hua Lin Chuang Zhong Yao Xue*, 1134.
45. He Xingdong et al., *Lin Chuang Zhong Yao Shou Ce*, 217.
46. Ibid., 228.
47. Lei Zaiquan and Zhang Tingmo, *Zhong Hua Lin Chuang Zhong Yao Xue*, 1141.
48. Ibid., 1138.
49. He Xingdong et al., *Lin Chuang Zhong Yao Shou Ce*, 226.
50. Lei Zaiquan and Zhang Tingmo, *Zhong Hua Lin Chuang Zhong Yao Xue*, 1083.
51. He Xingdong et al., *Lin Chuang Zhong Yao Shou Ce*, 229.
52. Ren Liansheng et al., *Zhong Guo Zhong Yao Za Zhi* [Journal of Chinese Materia Medica] 15, 5 (1990): 50.
53. Ma Junying et al., *Tian Jin Yi Yao* [Tianjin Journal of Medicine and Pharmacology] 18, 1 (1990): 41.
54. Wang Weixin et al., *Zhong Yi Za Zhi* [Journal of Traditional Chinese Medicine] 21, 12 (1980): 65.
55. Wang Aoge et al., *Zhong Yi Za Zhi* 22, 7 (1981): 69.
56. Wang Aoge et al., *Zhong Guo Yao Li Tong Xun* [Chinese Pharmacology Newsletter] 1 (1985): 36.
57. Ibid., 3-4 (1984): 166.
58. Zhao Xianghong et al., *Zhong Yao Tong Bao* [Bulletin of Chinese Materia Medica] 12, 10 (1987): 41.
59. Lei Zaiquan and Zhang Tingmo, *Zhong Hua Lin Chuang Zhong Yao Xue*, 1151.
60. Shi Jihui, *Zhong Yao Tong Bao* [Bulletin of Chinese Materia Medica] 6, 6 (1981): 32.

61. Health Board of Sichuan Province, *Sichuan Province Family Planning Technology Congress Documents*, 2 (1980): 191.
62. Qiu Mingming, *Guang Xi Yi Yao Tong Xun* [Guangxi Medicine and Pharmacology Newsletter] 1 (1988): 37.
63. Gao Yingdou et al., *Shan Xi Yi Xue Yuan Xue Bao* [Journal of Shanxi College of Medicine] 1 (1982): 12.
64. Shanxi College of Medicine, *Zhong Hua Yi Xue Za Zhi* [Chinese Journal of Medicine] 55, 6 (1975): 408.
65. A.H. Sutor et al., *CA* 93 (1981): 191153g.
66. F. Markwardt, *Nouv Rev Fr Hematol* 30 (1988): 161.
67. P. Walsmann, *Pharmazie* 43 (1988): 737.
68. Lu Wenhai et al., *Zhong Yao Cai* [Chinese Materia Medica] 17, 12 (1994): 21.
69. A. Ishikawa et al., *Thromb Res* 19, 3 (1980): 351.
70. Zhou Shiqing et al., *Zhong Cao Yao* [Journal of Chinese Herbs] 15, 3 (1984): 18.
71. Tong Li et al., *Zhong Yao Yao Li Yu Lin Chuang* [Pharmacology and Clinical Application of Chinese Materia Medica] 7, 7 (1991): 4.
72. Yang Yaofang et al., *Zhong Cao Yao* [Journal of Chinese Herbs] 20, 6 (1989): 20.
73. Wang Wei et al., *Zhong Guo Zhong Yao Za Zhi* [Journal of Chinese Materia Medica] 16, 5 (1991): 299.
74. Lei Zaiquan and Zhang Tingmo, *Zhong Hua Lin Chuang Zhong Yao Xue*, 1174.
75. He Xingdong et al., *Lin Chuang Zhong Yao Shou Ce*, 222.

Chapter 13

Herbs for transforming Phlegm, stopping coughing and calming wheezing

化痰止咳平喘药

Herbs for transforming Phlegm, stopping coughing and calming wheezing

Cough and Phlegm originate mainly from the Lungs, and they are closely linked in their pathogenesis. There is Phlegm when a patient coughs, whereas Phlegm itself leads to cough. In terms of function, herbs for transforming Phlegm can stop coughing and calm wheezing and herbs for stopping coughing and calming wheezing can transform Phlegm. In clinical practice they are always combined, so they are known collectively as herbs for transforming Phlegm, stopping coughing and calming wheezing.

Herbs for transforming Phlegm are mainly used for cough with copious sputum, difficult expectoration, wheezing due to Phlegm-fluids, and other diseases for which Phlegm is at the origin, such as epilepsy, spasms, goitre, scrofula, streaming Yin abscesses and Phlegm collapse in wind-stroke. In addition, herbs for stopping coughing and calming wheezing can be used for cases of chronic cough and taxation disorders.

Cough and Phlegm may be caused by external factors or internal damage, in which case herbs for transforming Phlegm, stopping coughing and calming wheezing may be selected in combination with other herbs according to the specific pathogenesis of the condition and the identification of patterns according to the six factors: interior-exterior, hot-cold and deficient-full. Particular categories of combination are listed below:

1. where coughing is due to external factors, herbs for releasing the exterior should be added to the prescription;
2. in cases of Lung-heat and fire depression, add herbs for clearing the Lungs and bearing fire downwards;
3. in cases of cold pathogenic factors depressing the Lungs, add herbs for warming the Lungs and dissipating cold;
4. where Spleen deficiency generates Phlegm, add herbs for fortifying the Spleen and drying dampness;
5. in cases of coughing and wheezing due to Lung deficiency, add herbs for supplementing the Lungs and boosting Qi;
6. in cases of wheezing due to Kidney deficiency, add herbs for supplementing the Kidneys and hosting Qi;
7. for cough in consumption or taxation disorders, supplementing herbs should be added;
8. in cases of cough due to damage to the Lungs caused by dry-heat, herbs for clearing heat from the Lungs and moistening dryness should be added;
9. for cough due to damp-cold, herbs for warming the interior and drying dampness should be added.

Strong herbs for transforming Phlegm are not suitable in cases of cough with coughing of blood, as they might induce bleeding.

HERBS FOR TRANSFORMING PHLEGM

Herbs for transforming Phlegm can be divided into two types – herbs that warm and transform Phlegm-cold and herbs that clear and transform Phlegm-heat:

1. Herbs for warming and transforming Phlegm-cold are generally warm in nature. Their function is to warm the Lungs and dissipate cold, dry dampness and dispel Phlegm. They can be used to treat diseases due to Phlegm-cold and Phlegm-damp as well as swollen abscesses and sores due to cold and damp attacking the Lung and Spleen channels. In clinical practice, they are usually combined with herbs for warming the interior and dispelling cold and herbs for drying dampness.

   Herbs for warming and transforming Phlegm-cold are extremely warm and dry in nature, so they should be used with great caution in cases of cough due to Phlegm-heat, cough due to Yin deficiency and subsequent dryness, or in cases with a medical history of coughing of blood or vomiting of blood.
2. Herbs for clearing and transforming Phlegm-heat are cold (or slightly cold) in nature. Their function is to clear heat, dry dampness and dispel Phlegm. They can be used for cough with copious sticky or thick yellow sputum, difficult expectoration caused by the accumulation of Phlegm-heat in the Lungs, and irregularity in the movement of Qi. These herbs may also be used for such conditions as epilepsy, convulsions, collapse, wind-stroke, scrofula, goitre and tumours due to Phlegm-heat.

   In clinical practice, these herbs are used in combination with herbs for clearing heat in cases of cough due to Phlegm-heat; with herbs for nourishing Yin and moistening the Lungs in cases of cough due to Yin deficiency and subsequent dryness of the Lungs; with herbs for clearing heat, herbs for regulating Liver Qi and herbs for quieting the Spirit in cases of seizures, convulsions and collapse; and with herbs for softening hardness and dissipating lumps in cases of scrofula, goitre and tumours.

   As these herbs are cold in nature and tend to damage Yang and reinforce dampness, they are contraindicated in cases of Phlegm-cold and Phlegm-damp or for patients with Spleen and Stomach deficiency.

Tab. 13.1(a) Herbs for warming and transforming Phlegm-cold

Herb	Functions	Indications
Ban Xia (Rhizoma Pinelliae Ternatae)	Drying dampness and transforming Phlegm, bearing counterflow Qi downwards and stopping vomiting, dispersing focal distension and dissipating lumps	Coughing and wheezing with copious sputum, nausea and vomiting, focal distension and oppression in the chest and stomach due to binding of Phlegm-heat, headache, dizziness, insomnia, goitre
Tian Nan Xing (Rhizoma Arisaematis)	Drying dampness and transforming Phlegm, dispelling wind and alleviating tetany, dispersing swelling and dissipating lumps	Cough with stubborn sputum, dizziness due to wind-Phlegm, wind-stroke due to congestion of Phlegm, facial paralysis, hemiplegia, sudden collapse, convulsions, tetanus, sore throat, scrofula, abscesses, sores and boils

Bai Fu Zi (Rhizoma Typhonii Gigantei)	Drying dampness and transforming Phlegm, dispelling wind and alleviating tetany, relieving toxicity and dissipating lumps	Facial paralysis due to exuberance of wind-Phlegm, tetanus, migraine and headache, poisonous snake bites, scrofula and Phlegm nodes
Jie Geng (Radix Platycodi Grandiflori)	Opening up and diffusing Lung Qi, dispelling Phlegm and benefiting the throat, expelling pus and dispersing abscesses	Cough due to externally-contracted wind-cold and wind-heat, sore throat and hoarse voice, Lung abscess, focal distension and oppression in the chest
Bai Jie Zi (Semen Sinapis Albae)	Warming the Lungs and transforming Phlegm, promoting the movement of Qi and dissipating lumps, freeing the network vessels and alleviating pain	Cough due to Phlegm-fluids obstructing the chest and hypochondrium, distension and pain in the chest and hypochondrium, Bi syndrome of the limbs, Yin abscesses, swelling and pain caused by knocks and falls
Zao Jiao (Fructus Gleditsiae Sinensis)	Dispelling Phlegm and opening the orifices, dissipating lumps and dispersing swelling, freeing the bowels	Wind-stroke with clenched jaw, sudden stupor, cough with difficult expectoration due to Phlegm obstruction, oppression in the chest and coughing and wheezing due to stubborn Phlegm, swollen abscesses and sores, dry stool
Xuan Fu Hua (Flos Inulae)	Dispersing Phlegm and moving water, bearing Qi downwards and stopping vomiting	Coughing and wheezing with copious sputum, focal distension and oppression in the chest and diaphragm, belching, vomiting
Bai Qian (Radix et Rhizoma Cynanchi Stauntonii)	Clearing the Lungs and bearing Qi downwards, dispelling Phlegm and stopping coughing	Wheezing with fullness in the chest due to congestion of Qi in the Lungs, cough with copious sputum

Tab. 13.1(b) Herbs for clearing and transforming Phlegm-heat

Herb	Functions	Indications
Chuan Bei Mu (Bulbus Fritillariae Cirrhosae)	Moistening the Lungs, transforming Phlegm and stopping coughing, clearing heat and dissipating lumps	Enduring cough due to Lung deficiency, fulminant coughing and wheezing, Lung Wei syndrome, scrofula, Phlegm nodes, sore throat
Zhe Bei Mu (Bulbus Fritillariae Thunbergii)	Clearing heat and transforming Phlegm, dissipating lumps and relieving toxicity	Cough due to wind-heat or Phlegm-fire, Lung abscess, sore throat, scrofula, sores
Gua Lou (Fructus Trichosanthis)	Clearing the Lungs and transforming Phlegm, promoting the movement of Qi and loosening the chest, lubricating the Intestines and freeing the bowels, dissipating lumps and dispersing abscesses	Coughing and wheezing due to Lung-heat, pain in the chest, coughing of blood, wasting and thirsting, constipation, abscesses

Qian Hu (Radix Peucedani)	Bearing counterflow Lung Qi downwards and dispelling Phlegm, diffusing and dissipating wind-heat	Cough due to Lung-heat with copious sticky sputum, oppression in the chest, difficulty in spitting sputum due to wind-heat obstructing the Lungs
Zhu Ru (Caulis Bambusae in Taeniis)	Clearing heat and transforming Phlegm, eliminating vexation and stopping vomiting	Cough due to Phlegm-heat, vexation and insomnia, vomiting due to Stomach-heat, morning sickness
Tian Zhu Huang (Concretio Silicea Bambusae)	Clearing heat and transforming Phlegm, clearing the Heart and settling fright	Cough due to Phlegm-heat, convulsions and spasms, delirious speech, wind-stroke, child fright wind
Zhu Li (Succus Bambusae)	Clearing heat and dislodging Phlegm, settling fright and benefiting the orifices	Cough due to Phlegm-heat with thick sputum, Phlegm-heat obstructing the clear orifices
Fu Hai Shi (Os Costaziae seu Pumex)	Clearing the Lungs and transforming Phlegm, softening hardness and dissipating lumps, dispersing stones and freeing Lin syndrome	Cough due to Phlegm-heat, cough with thick and sticky sputum and difficult expectoration, scrofula, Phlegm nodes, Lin syndrome
Hai Ge Ke (Concha Meretricis seu Cyclinae)	Clearing the Lungs and dispersing Phlegm, softening hardness and dissipating lumps, promoting the movement of water and dispersing swelling	Coughing and wheezing due to Lung-heat with thick sputum that is difficult to expectorate, goitre, scrofula, puffy swelling, inhibited urination
Hai Zao (Herba Sargassi)	Dispersing Phlegm and softening hardness, promoting the movement of water and dispersing swelling	Goitre, scrofula, Wei syndrome, swollen and painful testicles, oedema and puffy swelling
Kun Bu (Thallus Laminariae seu Eckloniae)	Dispersing Phlegm and softening hardness, promoting the movement of water and dispersing swelling	Scrofula, goitre, oedema, Wei syndrome, leg Qi
Pang Da Hai (Semen Sterculiae Lychnophorae)	Clearing the Lungs and diffusing Lung Qi, benefiting the throat, clearing the Intestines and freeing the bowels	Cough due to Phlegm-heat, sore throat and hoarse voice; and headache, toothache and constipation due to heat binding in the Stomach and Intestines
Huang Yao Zi (Rhizoma Dioscoreae Bulbiferae)	Dissipating lumps and dispersing goitre, clearing heat and relieving toxicity, cooling the Blood and stopping bleeding, stopping coughing and calming wheezing	Goitre and scrofula, swelling and toxins of sores, poisonous snake bites, bleeding due to Blood-heat, whooping cough

HERBS FOR WARMING AND TRANSFORMING PHLEGM-COLD

Ban Xia 半夏 (Pinellia tuber, Rhizoma Pinelliae Ternatae)

Ban Xia is the tuber of *Pinellia ternata* (Thunb.) Breit., family Araceae.

Legal status *Ban Xia* was listed in a document entitled *A Review of Restricted Herbal Ingredients* issued by the Medicines Control Agency (MCA) in the UK in September 2001 with a view to the possible imposition of restrictions on its use at a future date. The unprocessed rhizome is controlled in Hong Kong and the MCA is considering imposing strict quality control requirements for UK use (see also *Remarks* below).

Main ingredients *Ban Xia* contains β-sitosterol, choline, daucosterol, nicotine, coniine, protoanemonin, l-ephedrine, homogentisic acid, volatile oils, saponins and calcium oxalate.

Properties Taste: acrid; nature: warm; toxic.

Channels entered Spleen, Stomach and Lung.

Functions and indications Dries dampness and transforms Phlegm, bears counterflow Qi downwards and stops vomiting, disperses focal distension and dissipates lumps. It is indicated for coughing and wheezing with copious sputum, nausea and vomiting, focal distension and oppression in the chest and stomach due to binding of Phlegm-heat, headache, dizziness, insomnia, and goitre.

Common dosage 5-10g; or appropriate dosage of the powdered herb mixed with egg white for external application.

Precautions and contraindications

1. *Ban Xia* is incompatible with *Wu Tou* (Radix Aconiti).
2. Since *Ban Xia* is warm and dry, it is contraindicated for all bleeding patterns, for dry cough due to Yin deficiency and for thirst due to damage to body fluids.

Remarks

1. Raw *Ban Xia* is toxic and is only used externally for boils, abscesses and sores. In the clinic, the processed herb *Fa Ban Xia* (Rhizoma Pinelliae Ternatae Praeparata) is prescribed for internal use (in prescriptions, *Ban Xia* is assumed to mean *Fa Ban Xia*). It is better for drying dampness to fortify the Spleen and is used for cough with copious sputum. The purified herb, *Qing Ban Xia* (Rhizoma Pinelliae Ternatae Depurata), disperses focal distension and harmonizes the Stomach, dries dampness and transforms Phlegm; it is used for treating patterns of focal distension and fullness in the chest and stomach. *Ban Xia* processed with ginger (*Jiang Ban Xia*) is good for bearing counterflow Qi downwards and stopping nausea and vomiting.
2. *Ban Xia* can dry dampness in the Spleen and bear counterflow Stomach Qi downwards. Since the Spleen is fortified by the elimination of dampness, Phlegm will be transformed. As the Stomach is harmonized by bearing ascending counterflow Qi downwards, distension and vomiting will be relieved.

Comparison of functions Both *Ban Xia* (Rhizoma Pinelliae Ternatae) and *Chen Pi* (Pericarpium Citri Reticulatae) have the functions of drying dampness to transform Phlegm and stop vomiting. However, *Ban Xia* is more powerful in this function and is also used for dispersing focal distension and dissipating lumps. *Chen Pi* is better at regulating Qi to harmonize the Middle Jiao (thus fortifying the Spleen and harmonizing the Stomach) and is used for Qi stagnation in the Spleen and Stomach.

For additional comparisons, see *Tian Nan Xing* (Rhizoma Arisaematis), *Xuan Fu Hua* (Flos Inulae), *Chuan Bei Mu* (Bulbus Fritillariae Cirrhosae), *Zhu Ru* (Caulis Bambusae in Taeniis) and *Pi Pa Ye* (Folium Eriobotryae Japonicae).

Toxicity The LD_{50} for intraperitoneal injection in mice of extracts of raw *Ban Xia* is approximately 325mg/kg, that for suspensions of raw *Ban Xia* fed to mice via intragastric administration is 42.7g/kg. Raw *Ban Xia* is more toxic than *Jiang Ban Xia*, which in turn is more toxic than decoctions of the herb and preparations of *Ban Xia* with alum. Internal administration of 30-90g is toxic. Clinical manifestations of overdosage or prolonged administration of raw *Ban Xia* include a bitter taste in the mouth, abundant saliva, inability to enunciate clearly, headache, dizziness, nausea and vomiting, watery diarrhoea, palpitations and lack of strength; in severe cases, there may be difficulty in breathing and a reduction in blood pressure.

Modern research

1. The alkaloids contained in *Ban Xia* stop coughing.[1]
2. The raw herb can induce vomiting.[2]
3. The proteins contained in *Ban Xia* can inhibit uterine contractions.[3-5]
4. Regulates the gastrointestinal function and inhibits the secretion of gastric juices.[6]
5. Lowers intra-ocular pressure.[7]
6. Inhibits arrhythmia.[8, 9]

Combinations and applications

Functions	Combinations	Applications
Drying dampness and transforming Phlegm	*Chen Pi* (Pericarpium Citri Reticulatae) *Fu Ling* (Sclerotium Poriae Cocos) *Gan Cao* (Radix Glycyrrhizae)	Cough with copious sputum, fullness and oppression in the chest and diaphragm, white and moist tongue fur and a slippery pulse due to damp obstruction caused by deficiency of the Spleen, which thus fails in its transportation and transformation function
	Huang Qin (Radix Scutellariae Baicalensis) *Zhi Mu* (Rhizoma Anemarrhenae Asphodeloidis) *Gua Lou* (Fructus Trichosanthis)	Cough with yellow and sticky sputum, oppression in the chest, yellow and slimy tongue fur and a rapid, slippery pulse due to pathogenic damp continually transforming into heat
	Fang Feng (Radix Ledebouriellae Divaricatae) *Gan Cao* (Radix Glycyrrhizae) *Sheng Jiang* (Rhizoma Zingiberis Officinalis Recens)	Dizziness, copious sputum, slimy tongue fur and a string-like and slippery pulse due to obstruction of Phlegm-damp in the Middle Jiao and clear Yang failing to rise
	Tian Ma (Rhizoma Gastrodiae Elatae) (see notes on legal status) *Bai Zhu* (Rhizoma Atractylodis Macrocephalae) *Man Jing Zi* (Fructus Viticis)	Dizziness due to wind-Phlegm, headache due to Phlegm collapse, distension and oppression in the chest and diaphragm
	Gan Jiang (Rhizoma Zingiberis Officinalis) *Gui Zhi* (Ramulus Cinnamomi Cassiae) *Xi Xin* (Herba cum Radice Asari)	Coughing and wheezing with spitting of clear, thin sputum due to cold fluids invading the Lungs

Bearing counterflow Qi downwards and stopping vomiting	*Ren Shen* (Radix Ginseng) *Bai Mi* (white honey)	Nausea and vomiting due to Spleen and Stomach deficiency and Stomach Qi counterflow
	Gan Jiang (Rhizoma Zingiberis Officinalis) *Ren Shen* (Radix Ginseng) *Su Geng* (Caulis Perillae Frutescentis)	Morning sickness
	Huang Lian (Rhizoma Coptidis) *Zhu Ru* (Caulis Bambusae in Taeniis) *Chen Pi* (Pericarpium Citri Reticulatae)	Vomiting and bad breath, with yellow, slimy tongue fur and a rapid, slippery pulse due to Stomach-heat and Stomach Qi counterflow
	Zhu Ru (Caulis Bambusae in Taeniis) *Zhi Shi* (Fructus Immaturus Citri Aurantii) *Chen Pi* (Pericarpium Citri Reticulatae)	Deficiency vexation and insomnia due to Gallbladder-heat invading the Lungs
Dispersing focal distension and dissipating lumps	*Zi Su Ye* (Folium Perillae Frutescentis) *Hou Po* (Cortex Magnoliae Officinalis) *Fu Ling* (Sclerotium Poriae Cocos)	Plum-pit Qi (globus hystericus), oppression in the chest and a string-like and slippery pulse due to binding depression of Phlegm and Qi
	Huang Lian (Rhizoma Coptidis) *Gua Lou Ren* (Semen Trichosanthis)	Yellow and greasy sputum, focal distension and oppression in the chest and stomach due to Phlegm-heat binding in the chest
	Kun Bu (Thallus Laminariae seu Ecloniae) *Hai Zao* (Herba Sargassi) *Zhe Bei Mu* (Bulbus Fritillariae Thunbergii)	Phlegm nodes and goitre due to Qi stagnation

Note: For external use, powdered *Ban Xia* can be mixed with egg white to treat abscesses and breast abscesses; or mixed with powdered *Hai Piao Xiao* (Os Sepiae seu Sepiellae) to stop bleeding due to external injury.

Tian Nan Xing 天南星
(Jack-in-the-pulpit tuber, Rhizoma Arisaematis)

Tian Nan Xing is the tuber of *Arisaema consanguineum* Schott, *A. amurense* Maxim. or *A. heterophyllum* Bl., family Araceae.

Legal status *Tian Nan Xing* was listed in a document entitled *A Review of Restricted Herbal Ingredients* issued by the Medicines Control Agency (MCA) in the UK in September 2001 with a view to the possible imposition of restrictions on its use at a future date. The unprocessed rhizome is controlled in Hong Kong and the MCA is considering imposing strict quality control requirements for processing before use in the UK.

Main ingredients *Tian Nan Xing* contains alkaloids, triterpene saponins, d-mannitol, benzoic acid, palmitic acid and β-sitosterol. The toxic nature of the herb comes from the alkaloids it contains.

Properties Taste: bitter and acrid; nature: warm; toxic.

Channels entered Lung, Liver and Spleen.

Functions and indications Dries dampness and transforms Phlegm, dispels wind and alleviates tetany, disperses swelling and dissipates lumps. It is indicated for cough with stubborn sputum, dizziness due to wind-Phlegm, wind-stroke due to congestion of Phlegm, facial paralysis, hemiplegia, sudden collapse, convulsions, tetanus, sore throat, scrofula, and abscesses, sores and boils.

Common dosage For the prepared herb, *Zhi Nan Xing* (Rhizoma Arisaematis Praeparata): 5-10g; for raw *Tian Nan Xing*: 0.3-1g taken in pills; appropriate dosage for external application.

Precautions and contraindications

1. Since *Tian Nan Xing* is dry, dissipating and toxic, it is easy for it to damage Yin liquids; it is therefore contraindicated for dry cough due to Yin deficiency, in cases of extreme heat generating wind, and during pregnancy.
2. Raw *Tian Nan Xing* is generally contraindicated for internal use.

Comparison of functions Both *Tian Nan Xing* (Rhizoma Arisaematis) and *Ban Xia* (Rhizoma Pinelliae Ternatae) can dry dampness and transform Phlegm. They are key herbs for this purpose and are often used together for cold and damp Phlegm patterns. Both herbs can transform Phlegm, but *Tian Nan Xing* acts in the channels and network vessels, while *Ban Xia* regulates the Spleen and Stomach. *Ban Xia* is acrid and dissipating, and specifically fortifies the Spleen and harmonizes the Stomach to dispel Phlegm-damp and stop coughing. *Tian Nan Xing* is stronger than *Ban Xia* in terms of its acrid and dissipating properties and is also warmer and drier. It specifically enters the channels and network vessels to dispel wind and settle fright and can eliminate wind-Phlegm in the channels and network vessels. *Ban Xia* is often used for Phlegm-damp, whereas *Tian Nan Xing* is employed more often for wind-Phlegm.

For an additional comparison, see *Bai Fu Zi* (Rhizoma Typhonii Gigantei).

Toxicity The LD_{50} for intraperitoneal injection in mice of *Tian Nan Xing* is 13.5g/kg. The toxic amount of the fresh herb is 15g for adults, 10g for children. If raw *Tian Nan Xing* is eaten, toxic effects include itching, burning and numbness of the mouth and throat, a painful and swollen tongue, unclear speech, loss of taste, difficulty in opening the mouth and abundant saliva. In severe cases, numbness of the limbs, coma, shortness of breath or convulsions may occur. As a result, only processed *Tian Nan Xing* should generally be used internally.

Modern research

1. Expels sputum.[10]
2. Has a tranquillizing function, inhibits convulsions and alleviates pain.[11]
3. Inhibits carcinoma.[12]
4. Inhibits the heart and decreases cardiac contractions.[13]

Combinations and applications

Functions	Combinations	Applications
Drying dampness and transforming Phlegm	*Chen Pi* (Pericarpium Citri Reticulatae) *Ban Xia* (Rhizoma Pinelliae Ternatae) *Fu Ling* (Sclerotium Poriae Cocos) *Zhi Shi* (Fructus Immaturus Citri Aurantii)	Cough with stubborn sputum, oppression in the chest and slimy tongue fur due to Phlegm-damp obstructing the Lungs
	Huang Qin (Radix Scutellariae Baicalensis) *Gua Lou* (Fructus Trichosanthis) *Chen Pi* (Pericarpium Citri Reticulatae)	Cough, yellow and thick sputum, thirst and vexation, with yellow, slimy tongue fur and a rapid, slippery pulse due to Lung-heat
	Ban Xia (Rhizoma Pinelliae Ternatae) *Rou Gui* (Cortex Cinnamomi Cassiae)	Cough due to cold-Phlegm with clear, thin, white sputum

Dispelling wind and alleviating tetany	*Ban Xia* (Rhizoma Pinelliae Ternatae) *Bai Fu Zi* (Rhizoma Typhonii Gigantei) *Chuan Wu* (Radix Aconiti Carmichaeli) (see notes on legal status)	Numbness of the hands and feet, hemiplegia, facial paralysis and a string-like and slippery pulse due to wind-Phlegm stagnating in the channels and network vessels
	Sheng Jiang (Rhizoma Zingiberis Officinalis Recens) *Ren Shen* (Radix Ginseng) *Shi Chang Pu* (Rhizoma Acori Graminei)	Sudden collapse, foaming at the mouth, and spasms of the hands and feet due to internal obstruction of wind-Phlegm
	Zi Su Ye (Folium Perillae Frutescentis) *Sheng Jiang* (Rhizoma Zingiberis Officinalis Recens) *Xiong Zhu Dan Zhi* (Bilis Suis, male pig bile)	Wind-stroke, clenched jaw preventing speech
	Ban Xia (Rhizoma Pinelliae Ternatae) *Tian Ma* (Rhizoma Gastrodiae Elatae) (see notes on legal status) *Bai Zhu* (Rhizoma Atractylodis Macrocephalae) *Ju Hong* (Pars Rubra Epicarpii Citri Erythrocarpae) *Fu Ling* (Sclerotium Poriae Cocos)	Dizziness, headache, focal distension and oppression in the chest and diaphragm, white, slimy tongue fur and a slippery pulse due to wind-Phlegm
Dispersing swelling and dissipating lumps	*Jiang Can* (Bombyx Batryticatus) *Huang Qin* (Radix Scutellariae Baicalensis) *Lian Qiao* (Fructus Forsythiae Suspensae) *She Gan* (Rhizoma Belamcandae Chinensis)	Sore and swollen throat, hoarse voice, thirst and a reduced level of body fluids, accompanied by a red tongue with dry, yellow fur and a slippery, rapid pulse due to congestion and stagnation of heat toxins

Note: Mixing *Tian Nan Xing* in powder form with vinegar for external application is effective in the treatment of abscesses, sores, boils and scrofula.

Appendix

Dan Nan Xing 胆南星 (Arisaema powder with bovine bile, Pulvis Arisaematis cum Felle Bovis)

Dan Nan Xing is prepared by mixing a powder of *Tian Nan Xing* with bovine bile. Bitter in taste and cool in nature, *Dan Nan Xing* enters the Lung, Liver and Spleen channels. It has the functions of clearing heat and transforming Phlegm, and extinguishing wind and settling fright, and is used in the treatment of convulsions, child fright wind, wind-stroke, mania, and other disorders due to Phlegm-heat. The common dosage is 2-5g. For a comparison of functions, see *Tian Zhu Huang* (Concretio Silicea Bambusae).

Bai Fu Zi 白附子 (Typhoneum rhizome, Rhizoma Typhonii Gigantei)

Bai Fu Zi is the dried rhizome of *Typhonium giganteum* Engl., family Araceae.

Legal status *Bai Fu Zi* was listed in a document entitled *A Review of Restricted Herbal Ingredients* issued by the Medicines Control Agency (MCA) in the UK in September 2001 with a view to the possible imposition of restrictions on its use at a future date. The unprocessed rhizome of this herb is controlled in Hong Kong and the MCA is considering the introduction of strict quality control requirements for processing before use in the UK.

Main ingredients *Bai Fu Zi* contains calcium oxalate, choline, uracil, succinic acid, tyrosine, valine, palmitic acid, linoleic acid, oleic acid, β-sitosterol and saponins.

Properties Taste: acrid and sweet; nature: warm; toxic.

Channels entered Spleen, Stomach and Liver.

Functions and indications Dries dampness and transforms Phlegm, dispels wind and alleviates tetany, relieves toxicity and dissipates lumps. It is indicated for facial paralysis due to exuberance of wind-Phlegm, tetanus, migraine and headache, poisonous snake bites, and scrofula and Phlegm nodes.

Common dosage 3-5g of the processed herb; after boiling the fresh herb down to a paste, appropriate dosage for external application to wounds.

Precautions and contraindications

1. *Bai Fu Zi* is contraindicated in cases of dry heat due to Yin deficiency and during pregnancy.
2. The raw herb is not normally taken orally.

Comparison of functions

1. Both *Bai Fu Zi* (Rhizoma Typhonii Gigantei) and *Tian Nan Xing* (Rhizoma Arisaematis) dry dampness to transform Phlegm and dispel wind to alleviate tetany; they are important herbs in the treatment of wind-Phlegm patterns and are often used together. They can also both be used externally to relieve toxicity and dissipate lumps. *Bai Fu Zi* is upward-bearing in nature and tends to work upwards, thus being more effective for wind-Phlegm patterns in the head and face such as facial paralysis and migraine. *Tian Nan Xing* is more powerful in drying dampness to transform Phlegm and dispelling wind to alleviate tetany; it is mainly used for wind-Phlegm in the channels as well as for damp or cold Phlegm or cough with stubborn sputum. With its ability to dispel wind-Phlegm, it is effective in treating wind-stroke, convulsions and tetanus.
2. Both *Bai Fu Zi* (Rhizoma Typhonii Gigantei) and *Quan Xie* (Buthus Martensi) can dispel wind and alleviate tetany; they are often used together for facial paralysis due to wind-stroke and for tetanus. *Bai Fu Zi* is acrid, sweet, warm, very dry, and toxic. It enters the Stomach channel and is good for eliminating cold-damp to transform Phlegm and for dispelling pathogenic wind to alleviate tetany; it is used to treat wind-Phlegm patterns. Since *Bai Fu Zi* is upward-bearing and dissipating, it is very good for raising Qi to treat pathogenic wind affecting the head and face, and for treating facial paralysis, headache and dizziness due to wind-Phlegm. *Quan Xie* is acrid and toxic and mainly enters the Liver channel; it works powerfully in extinguishing wind and settling tetany and is very effective for spasm and convulsion patterns. As *Quan Xie* is neutral in nature, it can be used in combinations for both cold and heat patterns. It can also attack toxins and dissipate lumps, free the network vessels and alleviate pain, and is frequently used for hemilateral or ambilateral headache, limb joint Bi syndrome pain, and scrofula, Phlegm nodes and toxic sores.

Toxicity The daily toxic adult dosage of raw *Bai Fu Zi* is 15-30g; daily intake of 45g of the raw herb may cause death. Raw *Bai Fu Zi* is toxic and irritates the mouth and alimentary canal, manifesting with such symptoms as numbness of the mouth and tongue, general sweating, thirst, palpitations and agitation, and in severe cases, vomiting and diarrhoea, a purple face and pain when breathing. As a result, the raw herb should not be used internally.

Modern research

1. Has a tranquillizing effect.[14]
2. Inhibits Mycobacterium tuberculosis.[15]

Combinations and applications

Functions	Combinations	Applications
Drying dampness and transforming Phlegm, dispelling wind and alleviating tetany	*Tian Nan Xing* (Rhizoma Arisaematis) *Ban Xia* (Rhizoma Pinelliae Ternatae) *Chuan Wu* (Radix Aconiti Carmichaeli) (see notes on legal status)	Hemiplegia or facial paralysis due to exuberance of wind-Phlegm
	Quan Xie (Buthus Martensi) *Jiang Can* (Bombyx Batryticatus)	Facial paralysis due to wind-Phlegm obstructing the channels
	Tian Ma (Rhizoma Gastrodiae Elatae) (see notes on legal status) *Fang Feng* (Radix Ledebouriellae Divaricatae) *Tian Nan Xing* (Rhizoma Arisaematis)	Tetanus, tightly-contracted lips, rigid body
	Tian Nan Xing (Rhizoma Arisaematis) *Tian Ma* (Rhizoma Gastrodiae Elatae) (see notes on legal status) *Jiang Can* (Bombyx Batryticatus)	Dizziness and headache due to wind-Phlegm invading upwards
	Bai Zhi (Radix Angelicae Dahuricae) *Chuan Xiong* (Rhizoma Ligustici Chuanxiong)	Migraine due to ascending wind-Phlegm
	Ma Huang (Herba Ephedrae) (see notes on legal status) *Chuan Wu* (Radix Aconiti Carmichaeli) (see notes on legal status) *Quan Xie* (Buthus Martensi)	Migraine radiating to the eyes due to wind-cold lodging in the head

Notes: *Bai Fu Zi* also has the function of relieving toxicity and dissipating lumps:

1. It can be used to treat knocks and falls and the swelling and toxins of abscesses by topical application on its own or in combination with *Tian Nan Xing* (Rhizoma Arisaematis), *Sheng Chuan Wu* (Radix Aconiti Carmichaeli Cruda) and *Sheng Cao Wu* (Radix Aconiti Kusnezoffii Cruda) either for topical application or oral intake (*Chuan Wu* and *Cao Wu* cannot be used internally in the UK – see notes on legal status).
2. *Bai Fu Zi* can be ground with *Xiong Huang* (Realgar) to treat poisonous snake bites (for *Xiong Huang*, see notes on legal status).
3. Fresh, raw *Bai Fu Zi* can be crushed for topical application to treat scrofula and Phlegm nodes.

Jie Geng 桔梗 (Platycodon root, Radix Platycodi Grandiflori)

Jie Geng is the root of *Platycodon grandiflorum* (Jacq.) A. DC., family Campanulaceae.

Main ingredients *Jie Geng* contains platycodin, platycodigenin, platycogenic acids, phytosterol, α-spinasterol and inulin.

Properties Taste: bitter and acrid; nature: neutral.

Channel entered Lung.

Functions and indications Opens up and diffuses Lung Qi, dispels Phlegm and benefits the throat, expels pus and disperses abscesses. It is indicated for cough due to externally-contracted wind-cold and wind-heat, sore throat and hoarse voice, Lung abscess, and focal distension and oppression in the chest.

Common dosage 3-10g.

Precautions and contraindications *Jie Geng* is contraindicated in cases with coughing of blood or effulgent Yin deficiency-fire.

Comparison of functions See *Bai Qian* (Radix et Rhizoma Cynanchi Stauntonii) and *Xing Ren* (Semen Pruni Armeniacae).

Modern research

1. Stops coughing and expels sputum.[16, 17]
2. Inhibits inflammation and strengthens the immune function.[16]
3. Inhibits gastric secretion and counteracts ulcers of the digestive system.[17]
4. Has a tranquillizing function, alleviates pain, abates fever, and reduces the levels of blood sugar and blood lipids.[18]

Combinations and applications

Functions	Combinations	Applications
Opening up and diffusing Lung Qi, dispelling Phlegm and benefiting the throat	*Xing Ren* (Semen Pruni Armeniacae) *Zi Su Ye* (Folium Perillae Frutescentis) *Chen Pi* (Pericarpium Citri Reticulatae) *Qian Hu* (Radix Peucedani)	Cough with copious, clear sputum, chills, absence of sweating, and a slight headache, with white tongue fur and a string-like and tight pulse due to wind-cold
	Sang Ye (Folium Mori Albae) *Sha Shen* (Radix Glehniae seu Adenophorae) *Zhe Bei Mu* (Bulbus Fritillariae Thunbergii) *Xing Ren* (Semen Pruni Armeniacae)	Cough with sparse and greasy sputum, headache, generalized fever, thirst and a red tongue with thin, white, dry fur due to externally-contracted wind-heat
	Zhi Ke (Fructus Citri Aurantii) *Gua Lou Pi* (Pericarpium Trichosanthis)	Focal distension and oppression in the chest and vexation due to Qi stagnation and Phlegm obstruction
	Bo He (Herba Menthae Haplocalycis) *Niu Bang Zi* (Fructus Arctii Lappae) *Chan Tui* (Periostracum Cicadae) *Jin Yin Hua* (Flos Lonicerae)	Cough, sore throat, hoarse voice, slight fever, redness of the tip and side margins of the tongue and a rapid and floating pulse due to wind-heat
	Sheng Di Huang (Radix Rehmanniae Glutinosae) *Xuan Shen* (Radix Scrophulariae Ningpoensis) *Mai Men Dong* (Radix Ophiopogonis Japonici)	Cough with loss of voice, and dry mouth and throat due to deficiency-fire flaming upwards and Yin depletion of the Liver and Kidneys

Expelling pus and dispersing abscesses	*Gan Cao* (Radix Glycyrrhizae) *Yu Xing Cao* (Herba Houttuyniae Cordatae) *Zhe Bei Mu* (Bulbus Fritillariae Thunbergii) *Dong Gua Ren* (Semen Benincasae Hispidae) *Yi Yi Ren* (Semen Coicis Lachrymajobi)	Lung abscess with pain in the chest, coughing of blood and yellow sputum

Bai Jie Zi 白芥子 (White mustard seed, Semen Sinapis Albae)

Bai Jie Zi is the dried, ripe seed of *Sinapis alba* L., family Cruciferae.

Main ingredients *Bai Jie Zi* contains sinapine, sinalbin, myrosin and vitamin A.

Properties Taste: acrid; nature: warm.

Channel entered Lung.

Functions and indications Warms the Lungs and transforms Phlegm, promotes the movement of Qi and dissipates lumps, frees the network vessels and alleviates pain. It is indicated for cough due to Phlegm-fluids obstructing the chest and hypochondrium, distension and pain in the chest and hypochondrium, Bi syndrome of the limbs, Yin abscesses, and swelling and pain caused by knocks and falls.

Common dosage 3-10g; or appropriate dosage of the herb when mixed with vinegar for external application.

Precautions and contraindications

1. The acrid, warm and dissipating properties of *Bai Jie Zi* mean that it consumes Qi and damages Yin; it is therefore contraindicated in cases of effulgent Yin deficiency-fire or dry cough due to Lung deficiency.
2. External application of *Bai Jie Zi* may induce blisters, so it is contraindicated for patients with skin allergies.
3. Overdosage may cause diarrhoea.

Comparison of functions Both *Bai Jie Zi* (Semen Sinapis Albae) and *Lai Fu Zi* (Semen Raphani Sativi) can transform Phlegm. *Bai Jie Zi* can dispel cold-Phlegm and dissipate cold lumps. It is better for warming the Lungs to dislodge Phlegm and for transforming Phlegm between the skin and the membranes to promote the movement of Qi. It is also used for limb joint pain due to Phlegm-damp. *Lai Fu Zi* regulates Qi and harmonizes the Middle Jiao; it transforms Phlegm by moving Qi. It treats Phlegm and food stagnation in the Lungs, Stomach and Large Intestine and is effective for both cold-Phlegm and heat-Phlegm.

For an additional comparison, see *Su Zi* (Fructus Perillae Frutescentis).

Modern research

1. Stops coughing and expels sputum.[19]
2. Inhibits the thyroid function.[20]
3. Stimulates the skin.[21]

Combinations and applications

Functions	Combinations	Applications
Warming the Lungs and transforming Phlegm	*Su Zi* (Fructus Perillae Frutescentis) *Lai Fu Zi* (Semen Raphani Sativi)	Oppression in the chest, coughing and wheezing with copious, clear, white sputum due to cold-Phlegm obstructing the Lungs

	Jing Da Ji (Radix Euphorbiae Pekinensis) *Gan Sui* (Radix Euphorbiae Kansui)	Cough, slight pain in the chest and hypochondrium, and sticky and thick sputum due to Phlegm-fluids collecting and stagnating in the hypochondrium
Promoting the movement of Qi and dissipating lumps	*Mu Xiang* (Radix Aucklandiae Lappae) (see notes on legal status) *Mo Yao* (Myrrha)	Numbness of the limbs and limb joint pain due to Phlegm-damp obstructing the channels and network vessels
Freeing the network vessels and alleviating pain	*Lu Jiao Jiao* (Gelatinum Cornu Cervi) *Rou Gui* (Cortex Cinnamomi Cassiae) *Shu Di Huang* (Radix Rehmanniae Glutinosae Conquita)	External use for Yin abscesses and streaming sores and for Bi syndrome obstruction due to cold-Phlegm

Zao Jiao 皂角
(Chinese honey locust fruit, Fructus Gleditsiae Sinensis)

Zao Jiao is the dried ripe fruit of *Gleditsia sinensis* Lam., family Leguminosae.

Main ingredients *Zao Jiao* contains triterpene saponins (including gledigenin, gledinin and gleditsia saponin C), tannin, polysaccharides, ceryl alcohol, nonacosane, stigmasterol and sitosterol; the spike of the plant contains fustin and fusetin.

Properties Taste: acrid and salty; nature: warm; slightly toxic.

Channels entered Lung and Large Intestine.

Functions and indications Dispels Phlegm and opens the orifices, dissipates lumps and disperses swelling, and frees the bowels. It is indicated for wind-stroke with clenched jaw, sudden stupor, cough with difficult expectoration due to Phlegm obstruction, oppression in the chest and coughing and wheezing due to stubborn Phlegm, swollen abscesses and sores, and dry stool.

Common dosage 1.5-5g in an oral decoction; after stone-baking and grinding into a powder, 0.6-1.5g each time; appropriate dosage for external application.

Precautions and contraindications

1. It is important not to exceed the recommended oral dosage, as overdosage of *Zao Jiao* can cause vomiting and diarrhoea.
2. Since *Zao Jiao* has strong dissipating, acrid, mobile and penetrating characteristics, it is contraindicated during pregnancy, for patients with Qi deficiency and Yin depletion or in cases of coughing of blood.

Remarks *Zao Jiao* is very warm in nature and has strong dissipating properties; it is very effective in dispelling Phlegm, being particularly suitable for dispersing and expelling stubborn Phlegm. Its acrid, mobile and penetrating properties also enable it to be used to open the orifices to treat wind-stroke and similar conditions. As a nasal insufflation, it can induce sneezing to bring about recovery of consciousness.

Modern research

1. Inhibited Bacterium coli, Shigella sonnei, Proteus vulgaris, Salmonella typhi and Pseudomonas aeruginosa *in vitro*.[22]
2. Expels sputum.[23]
3. Kills worms.[24]

Combinations and applications

Functions	Combinations	Applications
Dispelling Phlegm and opening the orifices	*Xi Xin* (Herba cum Radice Asari) *Bo He* (Herba Menthae Haplocalycis) *Xiong Huang* (Realgar) (see notes on legal status) (ground into a powder and insufflated into the nose to cause sneezing)	Wind-stroke and Phlegm collapse, sudden collapse and loss of consciousness with clenched jaw
	Ming Fan (Alumen) (ground into a powder to swallow with warm water)	Wind-stroke and clouded Spirit, throat Bi syndrome due to Phlegm obstruction
	Bo He (Herba Menthae Haplocalycis) *Huo Xiang* (Herba Agastaches seu Pogostemi) *Guan Zhong* (Rhizoma Dryopteris Crassirhizomae) (see notes on legal status)	Stupor due to summerheat-stroke, clenched jaw, pain in the abdomen, vomiting and diarrhoea
	Ban Xia (Rhizoma Pinelliae Ternatae) *Ming Fan* (Alumen) *Shi Bing* (Fructus Kaki Exsiccatus) (pounded to a pulp and made into pills with *Zao Jiao* boiled to a paste)	Oppression in the chest with cough, difficult expectoration of sticky sputum
	Mi Tuo Seng (Lithargyrum) (see notes on legal status) *Cang Er Zi* (Fructus Xanthii Sibirici)	Epilepsy due to pathogenic wind
Dissipating lumps and dispersing swelling	*Ku Shen* (Radix Sophorae Flavescentis) *Bai Zhi* (Radix Angelicae Dahuricae) *Qi She* (Agkistrodon)	Itching due to hard, swollen abscesses and sores
Freeing the bowels	*Xi Xin* (Herba cum Radice Asari) *Feng Mi* (Mel)	Prepared as an anal suppository to promote the expulsion of dry stool
	Zhi Ke (Fructus Citri Aurantii) *Huo Ma Ren* (Semen Cannabis Sativae) *Xing Ren* (Semen Pruni Armeniacae)	Dry stool

Note: *Zao Jiao* can be boiled to a paste on its own or pounded to a pulp with vinegar for application to swollen sores (before ulceration).

Appendix

Zao Jiao Ci 皂角刺 (Spine of Chinese honey locust fruit, Spina Gleditsiae Sinensis)

Zao Jiao Ci is the spine of *Gleditsia sinensis* Lam. Acrid in taste and warm in nature, it enters the Liver and Stomach channels. Dosage is 3-10g in decoction, or an appropriate amount for external application. *Zao Jiao Ci* has the functions of drawing out toxins and expelling pus, and quickening the Blood and dispersing abscesses. It is frequently used to disperse the swelling of sores in the initial stage or to expel pus once it has formed in the sores. *Zao Jiao Ci* can also expel wind and kill worms and is used to treat leprosy, scabies and tinea. It is contraindicated where abscesses have already opened.

Xuan Fu Hua 旋复花 (Inula flower, Flos Inulae)

Xuan Fu Hua is the dried capitulum of *Inula japonica* Thunb. or *I. britannica* L., family Compositae.

Main ingredients *Xuan Fu Hua* contains britannin, inulicin, inulin, quercetin, isoquercetin, caffeic acid, chlorogenic acid, taraxasterol and inula britannica sterols (A, B, C).

Properties Taste: bitter, acrid and salty; nature: slightly warm.

Channels entered Lung, Spleen, Stomach and Large Intestine.

Functions and indications Disperses Phlegm and moves water, bears Qi downwards and stops vomiting. It is indicated for coughing and wheezing with copious sputum, focal distension and oppression in the chest and diaphragm, belching, and vomiting.

Common dosage 3-10g, wrapped in a piece of cloth for decoction.

Precautions and contraindications *Xuan Fu Hua* is contraindicated for dry cough due to Yin deficiency or loose stool due to Qi deficiency.

Comparison of functions Both *Xuan Fu Hua* (Flos Inulae) and *Ban Xia* (Rhizoma Pinelliae Ternatae) can transform Phlegm and dissipate binding, bear counterflow Qi downwards and stop vomiting. They are often used together to treat coughing and wheezing due to Phlegm-fluids, and retching and belching. The bitter taste of *Xuan Fu Hua* makes it suitable for bearing counterflow Qi downwards and moving water, while its salty taste enables it to soften and transform Phlegm. It is used for copious, sticky sputum that is difficult to expectorate, for belching due to Qi deficiency of the Spleen and Stomach, and for focal distension and oppression in the chest. *Ban Xia* regulates the Spleen and Stomach to transform Phlegm; it fortifies the Spleen and harmonizes the Stomach to dispel Phlegm-damp and stop coughing, and is especially effective for treating cough with copious sputum or clear, thin sputum.

For an additional comparison, see *Dai Zhe Shi* (Haematitum).

Modern research

1. Decoctions of *Xuan Fu Hua* and the flavones contained in the herb stop coughing and calm wheezing.[25]
2. A decoction of *Xuan Fu Hua* clearly inhibited such bacteria as Staphylococcus aureus, Bacillus anthracis and Shigella flexneri *in vitro*.[26]

Combinations and applications

Functions	Combinations	Applications
Dispersing Phlegm and moving water	*Bing Lang* (Semen Arecae Catechu) *Sang Bai Pi* (Cortex Mori Albae Radicis) *Ting Li Zi* (Semen Lepidii seu Descurainiae)	Focal distension and oppression in the chest, wheezing and shortness of breath due to Phlegm obstructing the chest
	Ban Xia (Rhizoma Pinelliae Ternatae) *Sheng Jiang* (Rhizoma Zingiberis Officinalis Recens) *Xi Xin* (Herba cum Radice Asari)	Coughing and wheezing due to cold-Phlegm accompanied by exterior patterns
	Sang Bai Pi (Cortex Mori Albae Radicis) *Da Huang* (Radix et Rhizoma Rhei) *Jie Geng* (Radix Platycodi Grandiflori)	Full-type coughing and wheezing due to Phlegm-heat

Bearing Qi downwards and stopping vomiting	*Ban Xia* (Rhizoma Pinelliae Ternatae) *Dai Zhe Shi* (Haematitum) *Sheng Jiang* (Rhizoma Zingiberis Officinalis Recens)	Vomiting and belching due to Qi deficiency of the Spleen and Stomach and ascendant counterflow of Phlegm-damp
	Ban Xia (Rhizoma Pinelliae Ternatae) *Bai Zhu* (Rhizoma Atractylodis Macrocephalae) *Ju Hong* (Pars Rubra Epicarpii Citri Erythrocarpae)	Vomiting and dizziness due to Phlegm-fluids collecting and stagnating in the Stomach

Bai Qian 白前
(Willow-leaf swallowwort rhizome, Radix et Rhizoma Cynanchi Stauntonii)

Bai Qian is the dried rhizome and root of *Cynanchum stauntonii* (Decne.) Schltr. ex Lévl. or *C. glaucescens* (Decne.) Hand.-Mazz., family Asclepiadaceae.

Main ingredients *Bai Qian* contains triterpene saponins and glucosides.

Properties Taste: acrid and sweet; nature: slightly warm.

Channel entered Lung.

Functions and indications Clears the Lungs and bears Qi downwards, dispels Phlegm and stops coughing. It is indicated for wheezing with fullness in the chest due to congestion of Qi in the Lungs and for cough with copious sputum.

Common dosage 3-10g.

Precautions and contraindications *Bai Qian* is contraindicated in cases of deficiency wheezing due to Lung and Kidney deficiency.

Comparison of functions *Bai Qian* (Radix et Rhizoma Cynanchi Stauntonii) and *Jie Geng* (Radix Platycodi Grandiflori) are both effective in dispelling Phlegm. *Bai Qian* mainly bears Qi downwards to treat Phlegm rale in the throat and rapid wheezing due to counterflow and fullness in the chest and diaphragm in Lung Qi congestion patterns. *Jie Geng* diffuses Lung Qi and can be used for cough due to wind-heat or wind-cold as well as for oppression in the chest and sore throat. The two herbs are often used together for cough with copious sputum due to Lung Qi failing to diffuse and bear downwards and for fullness and oppression in the chest and diaphragm.

For an additional comparison, see *Qian Hu* (Radix Peucedani).

Modern research

1. Expels sputum.[27]
2. Inhibits leukaemia cells.[28]

Combinations and applications

Functions	Combinations	Applications
Clearing the Lungs and bearing Qi downwards, dispelling Phlegm and stopping coughing	*Jie Geng* (Radix Platycodi Grandiflori) *Ban Xia* (Rhizoma Pinelliae Ternatae) *Xing Ren* (Semen Pruni Armeniacae)	Cough, rapid wheezing, focal distension and fullness in the chest and stomach due to Phlegm-damp
	Sang Bai Pi (Cortex Mori Albae Radicis) *Huang Qin* (Radix Scutellariae Baicalensis)	Cough with thick sputum due to Phlegm-heat congesting the Lungs
	Zi Wan (Radix Asteris Tatarici) *Ban Xia* (Rhizoma Pinelliae Ternatae)	Cough, counterflow Qi and rapid wheezing due to Phlegm-damp congesting the Lungs

Chen Pi (Pericarpium Citri Reticulatae) *Jing Jie* (Herba Schizonepetae Tenuifoliae) *Jie Geng* (Radix Platycodi Grandiflori)	Persistent cough due to externally contracted wind-cold
Zi Wan (Radix Asteris Tatarici) *Jing Da Ji* (Radix Euphorbiae Pekinensis)	Full-type cough with Phlegm rale in the throat and oedema
Bai Bu (Radix Stemonae)	Cough with scant sputum, coughing of blood in pulmonary consumption

HERBS FOR CLEARING AND TRANSFORMING PHLEGM-HEAT

Chuan Bei Mu 川贝母 (Sichuan fritillary bulb, Bulbus Fritillariae Cirrhosae)

Chuan Bei Mu is the bulb of *Fritillaria cirrhosa* D. Don, *F. unibracteata* Hsiao et K. C. Hsia, *F. przewalskii* Maxim. or *F. delavayi* Franch., family Liliaceae.

Main ingredients *Chuan Bei Mu* contains fritimine, chinpeimine, beilupeimine, fritiminine, sonpeimine, sipeimine, minpeimine and minpeiminine.

Properties Taste: bitter and sweet; nature: slightly cold.

Channels entered Lung and Heart.

Functions and indications Moistens the Lungs, transforms Phlegm and stops coughing, clears heat and dissipates lumps. It is indicated for enduring cough due to Lung deficiency, fulminant coughing and wheezing, Lung Wei syndrome, scrofula, Phlegm nodes, and sore throat.

Common dosage 3-10g, or 1-1.5g as a powder for internal use.

Precautions and contraindications

1. *Chuan Bei Mu* is incompatible with *Wu Tou* (Radix Aconiti).
2. *Chuan Bei Mu* is contraindicated in cases of Spleen and Stomach deficiency-cold and damp-Phlegm.

Comparison of functions *Bei Mu* – both *Chuan Bei Mu* (Bulbus Fritillariae Cirrhosae) and *Zhe Bei Mu* (Bulbus Fritillariae Thunbergii) – and *Ban Xia* (Rhizoma Pinelliae Ternatae) are key herbs for transforming Phlegm and stopping coughing. However, *Ban Xia* is acrid and warm and is able to dry dampness to transform Phlegm through acting on the Spleen and Stomach. *Bei Mu* is bitter and slightly cold and can clear heat to transform Phlegm, acting specifically on the Lungs. It is most effective for Phlegm-heat and dry Phlegm.

For an additional comparison, see *Zhe Bei Mu* (Bulbus Fritillariae Thunbergii).

Modern research

1. The alkaloids contained in *Chuan Bei Mu* stop coughing and expel sputum.[29]
2. Raises the blood sugar level and excites the uterus.[30]

Combinations and applications

Functions	Combinations	Applications
Moistening the Lungs, transforming Phlegm and stopping coughing	*Sha Shen* (Radix Glehniae seu Adenophorae) *Mai Men Dong* (Radix Ophiopogonis Japonici) *Tian Men Dong* (Radix Asparagi Cochinchinensis)	Enduring cough with scant sputum, dry throat, shortness of breath and a fine, weak pulse due to Lung deficiency
	Ma Huang (Herba Ephedrae) (see notes on legal status) *Kuan Dong Hua* (Flos Tussilaginis Farfarae) *Xing Ren* (Semen Pruni Armeniacae) *Gan Cao* (Radix Glycyrrhizae)	Cough, chills, aching head and body and a floating pulse due to externally-contracted pathogenic cold

	Jie Geng (Radix Platycodi Grandiflori) *Zi Wan* (Radix Asteris Tatarici) *Gan Cao* (Radix Glycyrrhizae) *Xing Ren* (Semen Pruni Armeniacae)	Fulminant coughing and wheezing due to an invasion of cold, possibly developing into Lung Wei syndrome or taxation cough
	Tian Zhu Huang (Concretio Silicea Bambusae) *Peng Sha* (Borax) *Zhi Pa Ye* (Folium Eriobotryae Japonicae Praeparatum)	Lung abscess or Lung Wei syndrome
Clearing heat and dissipating lumps	*Zao Jiao Zi* (Semen Gleditsiae Sinensis) *Xuan Shen* (Radix Scrophulariae Ningpoensis)	Scrofula and Phlegm nodes without pain or itching
	Jie Geng (Radix Platycodi Grandiflori) *Shan Dou Gen* (Radix Sophorae Tonkinensis) *Gan Cao* (Radix Glycyrrhizae) *Jing Jie* (Herba Schizonepetae Tenuifoliae) *Bo He* (Herba Menthae Haplocalycis)	Sore throat, fever and a rapid pulse

Note: *Chuan Bei Mu* can be combined with *Mu Li* (Concha Ostreae) and *Zhi Mu* (Rhizoma Anemarrhenae Asphodeloidis) and taken orally with soup made from pig's knuckle to treat scant breast milk.

Zhe Bei Mu 浙贝母 (Zhejiang fritillary bulb, Bulbus Fritillariae Thunbergii)

Zhe Bei Mu is the bulb of *Fritillaria thunbergii* Miq., family Liliaceae.

Main ingredients *Zhe Bei Mu* contains peimine, peiminine, zhebeinine, peimisine, peimiphine, peimidine, peimitidine, propeimine and peiminoside.

Properties Taste: bitter; nature: cold.

Channels entered Lung and Heart.

Functions and indications Clears heat and transforms Phlegm, dissipates lumps and relieves toxicity. It is indicated for cough due to wind-heat or Phlegm-fire, Lung abscess, sore throat, scrofula, and sores.

Common dosage 3-10g, or 1-1.5g as a powder for internal use.

Precautions and contraindications

1. *Zhe Bei Mu* is incompatible with *Wu Tou* (Radix Aconiti).
2. *Zhe Bei Mu* is contraindicated in cases of damp-Phlegm and Spleen and Stomach deficiency-cold.

Comparison of functions Both *Zhe Bei Mu* (Bulbus Fritillariae Thunbergii) and *Chuan Bei Mu* (Bulbus Fritillariae Cirrhosae) can transform Phlegm to stop coughing, clear heat and dissipate lumps. *Chuan Bei Mu* is sweet and lubricating and functions well in moistening the Lungs to transform Phlegm. It is used for enduring cough with scant sputum and dry throat due to Lung deficiency. *Zhe Bei Mu* is colder than *Chuan Bei Mu* and is better for clearing heat and dissipating lumps. It is mostly used for cough with thick, yellow sputum due to wind-heat or Phlegm-fire and for scrofula and sores.

For an additional comparison, see *Chuan Bei Mu* (Bulbus Fritillariae Cirrhosae).

Modern research

1. Clearly relieves coughing through its effect on the central nervous system, calms wheezing.[17, 30]
2. Expels sputum.[30]
3. Excites the uterus and contracts the intestinal muscles.[30]

Combinations and applications

Functions	Combinations	Applications
Clearing heat and transforming Phlegm	*Zhi Mu* (Rhizoma Anemarrhenae Asphodeloidis) *Sang Ye* (Folium Mori Albae) *Xing Ren* (Semen Pruni Armeniacae) *Zi Su Ye* (Folium Perillae Frutescentis)	Common cold, cough, sore throat, redness of the tip and side margins of the tongue, and a rapid and floating pulse
	Sang Ye (Folium Mori Albae) *Niu Bang Zi* (Fructus Arctii Lappae) *Qian Hu* (Radix Peucedani) *Xing Ren* (Semen Pruni Armeniacae)	Cough, oppression in the chest and thick, yellow sputum due to depression of Phlegm-fire in the Lungs, accompanied by a red tongue with yellow fur, and a rapid and slippery pulse
Dissipating lumps and relieving toxicity	*Mu Li* (Concha Ostreae) *Xuan Shen* (Radix Scrophulariae Ningpoensis)	Scrofula or Phlegm nodes without pain or itching
	Pu Gong Ying (Herba Taraxaci cum Radice) *Lian Qiao* (Fructus Forsythiae Suspensae) *Tian Hua Fen* (Radix Trichosanthis)	Breast abscess, the initial stage of abscesses and sores with local redness, swelling, heat and pain
	Yu Xing Cao (Herba Houttuyniae Cordatae) *Xian Lu Gen* (Rhizoma Phragmitis Communis Recens) *Dong Gua Ren* (Semen Benincasae Hispidae)	Lung abscess
	Xia Ku Cao (Spica Prunellae Vulgaris) *Hai Zao* (Herba Sargassi) *Kun Bu* (Thallus Laminariae seu Eckloniae) *E Zhu* (Rhizoma Curcumae)	Goitre at the initial stage with unbroken, hard swelling

Gua Lou 栝蒌 (Trichosanthes fruit, Fructus Trichosanthis)

Gua Lou is the fruit of *Trichosanthes kirilowii* Maxim. or *T. rosthornii* Harms, family Cucurbitaceae.

Legal status *Gua Lou* was listed in a document entitled *A Review of Restricted Herbal Ingredients* issued by the Medicines Control Agency (MCA) in the UK in September 2001 with a view to the possible imposition of restrictions on its use at a future date. The MCA is concerned that *T. kirilowii* is used to induce abortions in China and is therefore suggesting that use of this herb may require medical supervision.

Main ingredients *Gua Lou* contains triterpene saponins, organic acids, resin, saccharides and pigments. *Gua Lou Pi* contains nonanoic, capric, lauric, myristic, palmitic, linoleic, linolenic and stearic acids. *Gua Lou Ren* contains fatty oils (including trichosanthic acid), campesterol, sitosterol, stigmasterol and vanillic acid.

Properties Taste: sweet; nature: cold.

Channels entered Lung, Stomach and Large Intestine.

Functions and indications Clears the Lungs and transforms Phlegm, promotes the movement of Qi and loosens the chest, lubricates the Intestines and frees the bowels, dissipates lumps and disperses abscesses. It is indicated for coughing and wheezing due to Lung-heat, pain in the chest, coughing of blood, wasting and thirsting, constipation, and abscesses.

Common dosage The whole fruit: 10-20g; the husk of the fruit: 6-12g; the seeds of the fruit: 10-15g.

Precautions and contraindications

1. *Gua Lou* is incompatible with *Wu Tou* (Radix Aconiti).
2. *Gua Lou* is contraindicated for loose stool due to Spleen and Stomach deficiency-cold, and in cases of cold-Phlegm or damp-Phlegm.

Remarks *Gua Lou Pi* (Pericarpium Trichosanthis), the husk of the fruit, is especially good at clearing Lung-heat, transforming Phlegm, promoting the movement of Qi and loosening the chest. It is indicated for cough and chest Bi syndrome due to Lung-heat. *Gua Lou Ren* (Semen Trichosanthis), the seed of the fruit, is good for moistening the Lungs and lubricating the Intestines, transforming Phlegm and freeing the bowels. It is indicated for coughing and wheezing accompanied by constipation due to Phlegm-heat. *Quan Gua Lou*, the whole fruit, possesses the functions of both *Gua Lou Pi* and *Gua Lou Ren*; it is good for treating chest Bi syndrome, and oppression and pain in the chest and diaphragm.

Comparison of functions See *Fu Hai Shi* (Os Costaziae seu Pumex).

Toxicity The toxicity of injections of *Gua Lou* is extremely low. The LD_{50} for intraperitoneal injection in mice of *Gua Lou* is 363 ± 33g/kg; that for intravenous injection is 306 ± 22g/kg. No obvious toxic reaction was observed in long-term toxicity tests involving daily intravenous injection in dogs of 30g/kg of the herb for 21 days.

Modern research

1. The aminophenols contained in *Gua Lou* can expel sputum.[31]
2. Enlarges the coronary artery.[32]
3. A decoction of *Gua Lou Pi* can inhibit such bacteria as Staphylococcus aureus, Streptococcus pneumoniae and Nocardia asteroides.[29, 33]

Combinations and applications

Functions	Combinations	Applications
Clearing the Lungs and transforming Phlegm	*Zhe Bei Mu* (Bulbus Fritillariae Thunbergii) *Zhi Mu* (Rhizoma Anemarrhenae Asphodeloidis) *Huang Qin* (Radix Scutellariae Baicalensis)	Coughing and wheezing due to Lung-heat with thick, yellow sputum, oppression in the chest and vexation, accompanied by yellow, slimy tongue fur and a rapid, slippery pulse
	Zhe Bei Mu (Bulbus Fritillariae Thunbergii) *Tian Hua Fen* (Radix Trichosanthis) *Jie Geng* (Radix Platycodi Grandiflori)	Cough with yellow sputum that is difficult to expectorate and a sore, dry throat due to dry-heat injuring the Lungs
	Xing Ren (Semen Pruni Armeniacae) *Lai Fu Zi* (Semen Raphani Sativi)	Infantile coughing and wheezing with sputum due to Lung-heat
Promoting the movement of Qi and loosening the chest	*Huang Lian* (Rhizoma Coptidis) *Fa Ban Xia* (Rhizoma Pinelliae Ternatae Praeparata)	Focal distension and fullness in the chest and hypochondrium due to Phlegm and heat binding in the chest

	Xie Bai (Bulbus Allii Macrostemi) *Fa Ban Xia* (Rhizoma Pinelliae Ternatae Praeparata) *Bai Jiu* (Granorum Spiritus Incolor)	Chest Bi syndrome, manifesting as pain in the chest radiating to the back, difficulty in sleeping and a sunken, tight pulse
	Huang Jiu (Vinum Aureum) *Ming Fan* (Alumen)	Wasting and thirsting and vexation due to heat disturbing the Spirit
	Wu Mei (Fructus Pruni Mume) *Xing Ren* (Semen Pruni Armeniacae)	Lung Wei syndrome, coughing of blood
Lubricating the Intestines and freeing the bowels	*Huo Ma Ren* (Semen Cannabis Sativae) *Yu Li Ren* (Semen Pruni) *Zhi Ke* (Fructus Citri Aurantii)	Intestinal dryness with constipation, thirst
Dissipating lumps and dispersing abscesses	*Gan Cao* (Radix Glycyrrhizae) *Dang Gui* (Radix Angelicae Sinensis) *Ru Xiang* (Gummi Olibanum) *Mo Yao* (Myrrha)	Initial stage of breast abscess with redness, swelling, heat and pain due to congestion and stagnation of heat toxins
	Bai Jiang Cao (Herba Patriniae cum Radice) *Hong Teng* (Caulis Sargentodoxae Cuneatae) *Yi Yi Ren* (Semen Coicis Lachrymajobi)	Swollen and painful Intestinal abscess due to depression binding of fire toxins and heat accumulation in the Stomach and Intestines

Qian Hu 前胡 (Hogfennel root, Radix Peucedani)

Qian Hu is the dried root of *Peucedanum praeruptorum* Dunn or *P. decursivum* (Miq.) Maxim., family Umbelliferae.

Main ingredients *Qian Hu* contains umbelliferone, scopolin, skimmin, nodakenin, nodakenetin, decursin, decursidin, praeruptorins, volatile oils (including limonene), spongesterol, β-sitosterol and mannitol.

Properties Taste: bitter and acrid; nature: slightly cold.

Channel entered Lung.

Functions and indications Bears counterflow Lung Qi downwards and dispels Phlegm, and diffuses and dissipates wind-heat. It is indicated for cough due to Lung-heat with copious sticky sputum, oppression in the chest, and difficulty in spitting sputum due to wind-heat obstructing the Lungs.

Common dosage 6-10g.

Precautions and contraindications *Qian Hu* is contraindicated for cough due to Yin deficiency.

Comparison of functions

1. *Qian Hu* (Radix Peucedani) and *Bai Qian* (Radix et Rhizoma Cynanchi Stauntonii) are important herbs for bearing counterflow Qi downwards and dispelling Phlegm. They can be used together for cough with copious sputum and wheezing due to counterflow Lung Qi. However, *Qian Hu* is mainly used for cough due to Lung-heat or Phlegm-heat, whereas *Bai Qian* is better for cold cough or heat cough.
2. *Qian Hu* (Radix Peucedani) and *Chai Hu* (Radix Bupleuri) are traditionally known as the 'two *Hu*'s'. *Qian Hu* mainly enters the Lung channel to bear Qi downwards and dispel Phlegm. *Chai Hu* mainly enters the Liver and Gallbladder channels to uplift Yang Qi and disperse half-exterior, half-interior pathogenic factors.

In cases of cold-heat complex patterns with concurrent cough, ascending counterflow Qi and oppression in the chest, these two herbs can be used together to accentuate each other's effect, as in the *Jing Fang Bai Du San* (Schizonepeta and Ledebouriella Toxicity-Vanquishing Powder) formula.

Modern research

1. Expels sputum.[34]
2. Enlarges the coronary artery.[35, 36]
3. Inhibits bacillary dysentery.[37]

Combinations and applications

Functions	Combinations	Applications
Bearing counterflow Lung Qi downwards and dispelling Phlegm	*Sang Bai Pi* (Cortex Mori Albae Radicis) *Xing Ren* (Semen Pruni Armeniacae) *Zhe Bei Mu* (Bulbus Fritillariae Thunbergii)	Cough with yellow sputum and oppression in the chest due to Lung-heat
	Ban Xia (Rhizoma Pinelliae Ternatae) *Fu Ling* (Sclerotium Poriae Cocos) *Chen Pi* (Pericarpium Citri Reticulatae)	Cough due to damp-Phlegm with copious sputum and rapid breathing
Diffusing and dissipating wind-heat	*Niu Bang Zi* (Fructus Arctii Lappae) *Bo He* (Herba Menthae Haplocalycis) *Jie Geng* (Radix Platycodi Grandiflori)	Cough, headache and sore throat due to externally-contracted wind-heat
	Bai Qian (Radix et Rhizoma Cynanchi Stauntonii) *Bo He* (Herba Menthae Haplocalycis) *Sang Ye* (Folium Mori Albae)	Cough with copious sputum due to externally-contracted wind-heat
	Bai Qian (Radix et Rhizoma Cynanchi Stauntonii)	Impaired functioning of the Lungs due to externally-contracted wind-heat
	Ren Shen (Radix Ginseng) *Zi Su Ye* (Folium Perillae Frutescentis) *Ban Xia* (Rhizoma Pinelliae Ternatae)	Wind-cold-type common cold, cough with copious sputum, oppression in the chest

Zhu Ru 竹茹 (Bamboo shavings, Caulis Bambusae in Taeniis)

Zhu Ru is the culm shavings of *Bambusa breviflora* Munro, *Sinocalamus beecheyanus* (Munro) McClure var. *pubescens* P. F. Li or *Phyllostachys nigra* (Lodd.) Munro var. *henonis* Stapf, family Gramineae.

Main ingredients *Zhu Ru* contains alkaloids, tannins, saponins and amino acids.

Properties Taste: sweet; nature: slightly cold.

Channels entered Lung, Stomach and Gallbladder.

Functions and indications Clears heat and transforms Phlegm, eliminates vexation and stops vomiting. It is indicated for cough due to Phlegm-heat, vexation and insomnia, vomiting due to Stomach-heat, and morning sickness.

Common dosage 6-10g.

Precautions and contraindications Contraindicated in cases of vomiting due to Stomach-cold or cold food accumulation.

Remarks Raw *Zhu Ru* is more effective for clearing heat and transforming Phlegm; use *Zhu Ru* processed with ginger juice for bearing counterflow Qi downwards and stopping vomiting.

Comparison of functions Both *Zhu Ru* (Caulis Bambusae in Taeniis) and *Ban Xia* (Rhizoma Pinelliae Ternatae) have the functions of transforming Phlegm and stopping vomiting. They can be used for depression binding of Phlegm-heat due to Gallbladder deficiency, manifesting as vexation, oppression, disquiet and vomiting. They are often used together to strengthen their effect in transforming Phlegm, stopping vomiting and eliminating vexation. *Zhu Ru*, slightly cold and moistening, tends to clear Lung-heat to transform Phlegm and to clear Stomach-heat to stop vomiting. It can also open depression and eliminate vexation and is particularly suitable for oppression and vexation due to depression binding of Phlegm and heat. *Ban Xia*, which is acrid, warm and dry, tends to treat vomiting due to cold-Phlegm, Phlegm-damp and Phlegm-fluids. Since it opens with acridity and bears downward with bitterness, it can also dissipate lumps and disperse focal distension. It is particularly suitable for Phlegm-damp collecting below the Heart, manifesting as focal distension, oppression and discomfort, and inability to keep food down.

For an additional comparison, see *Zhu Li* (Succus Bambusae).

Modern research

1. A powder of *Zhu Ru* inhibited Staphylococcus albus, Escherichia coli and Salmonella typhi *in vitro*.[38]
2. Raises the blood sugar level and increases the discharge of chloride in the urine.[39]
3. Stops coughing, dissolves sputum and stops vomiting.[40]

Combinations and applications

Functions	Combinations	Applications
Clearing heat and transforming Phlegm	*Chen Pi* (Pericarpium Citri Reticulatae) *Fu Ling* (Sclerotium Poriae Cocos) *Ban Xia* (Rhizoma Pinelliae Ternatae) *Zhi Shi* (Fructus Immaturus Citri Aurantii)	Oppression in the chest, copious sputum, vexation, insomnia, palpitations, and a rapid and slippery pulse due to Phlegm-fire harassing the Lungs and Heart
	Huang Qin (Radix Scutellariae Baicalensis) *Gua Lou* (Fructus Trichosanthis) *Zhe Bei Mu* (Bulbus Fritillariae Thunbergii) *Qian Hu* (Radix Peucedani)	Cough with thick, yellow sputum, oppression in the chest, yellow and slimy tongue fur, and a rapid and slippery pulse due to pathogenic heat congesting the Lungs
Eliminating vexation and stopping vomiting	*Ban Xia* (Rhizoma Pinelliae Ternatae) *Fu Ling* (Sclerotium Poriae Cocos) *Chen Pi* (Pericarpium Citri Reticulatae) *Gan Cao* (Radix Glycyrrhizae)	Vexation and insomnia due to deficiency of Qi and Blood after a severe illness
	Huang Lian (Rhizoma Coptidis) *Ban Xia* (Rhizoma Pinelliae Ternatae) *Chen Pi* (Pericarpium Citri Reticulatae)	Oppression in the chest, vexation, vomiting and hiccups due to heat and Phlegm binding together
	Fu Ling (Sclerotium Poriae Cocos) *Ban Xia* (Rhizoma Pinelliae Ternatae) *Sheng Jiang* (Rhizoma Zingiberis Officinalis Recens)	Morning sickness, nausea and poor appetite during pregnancy

Functions	Combinations	Applications
	Mai Men Dong (Radix Ophiopogonis Japonici) *Fu Xiao Mai* (Fructus Tritici Aestivi Levis) *Gan Cao* (Radix Glycyrrhizae) *Da Zao* (Fructus Ziziphi Jujubae) *Sheng Jiang* (Rhizoma Zingiberis Officinalis Recens)	Vexation and agitation, headache and shortness of breath due to postpartum deficiency of Qi and Blood
	Wu Mei (Fructus Pruni Mume) *Gan Cao* (Radix Glycyrrhizae)	Summerheat-heat with vexation and incessant thirst

Tian Zhu Huang 天竺黄 (Tabasheer, Concretio Silicea Bambusae)

Tian Zhu Huang is the dried secretion found in the stem of *Bambusa textilis* McClure or *Schizostachyum chinense* Rendle, family Gramineae.

Main ingredients *Tian Zhu Huang* contains potassium hydroxide, silicon, aluminium oxide and ferric oxide.

Properties Taste: sweet; nature: cold.

Channels entered Heart, Liver and Gallbladder.

Functions and indications Clears heat and transforms Phlegm, clears the Heart and settles fright. It is indicated for cough due to Phlegm-heat, convulsions and spasms, delirious speech, wind-stroke, and child fright wind.

Common dosage 3-6g, or 0.6-1g as a powder for oral use.

Comparison of functions Both *Tian Zhu Huang* (Concretio Silicea Bambusae) and *Dan Nan Xing* (Pulvis Arisaematis cum Felle Bovis) can clear heat, transform Phlegm and settle fright. They can treat fever, hasty wheezing, coma and convulsions in children due to Phlegm-heat blocking the Lungs. They are often used together to accentuate each other's effect. *Tian Zhu Huang* is more effective for settling fright and stopping convulsions, whereas *Dan Nan Xing* is better for clearing heat and transforming Phlegm.

For an additional comparison, see *Zhu Li* (Succus Bambusae).

Modern research

1. Obstructs the conduction of electricity in the nerve trunk to alleviate pain.[41]
2. Inhibits pathogenic and suppurative bacteria in the intestines.[42]

Combinations and applications

Functions	Combinations	Applications
Clearing heat and transforming Phlegm	*Huang Lian* (Rhizoma Coptidis) *Jiang Can* (Bombyx Batryticatus)	Vexation, shortness of breath and oppression in the chest due to full Phlegm-heat
	Ban Xia (Rhizoma Pinelliae Ternatae)	Cough with sputum that is difficult to expectorate and pain in the chest
	Dan Nan Xing (Pulvis Arisaematis cum Felle Bovis) *Shi Chang Pu* (Rhizoma Acori Graminei) *Tian Ma* (Rhizoma Gastrodiae Elatae) (see notes on legal status) *Quan Xie* (Buthus Martensi)	Wind-stroke, facial paralysis

Clearing the Heart and settling fright	*Dan Zhu Ye* (Herba Lophatheri Gracilis) *Gou Teng* (Ramulus Uncariae cum Uncis) *Jiang Can* (Bombyx Batryticatus)	Night crying in infants, child fright wind due to Phlegm-heat, convulsions of the limbs
	Chan Tui (Periostracum Cicadae) *Jiang Can* (Bombyx Batryticatus) *Zhi Zi* (Fructus Gardeniae Jasminoidis) *Gan Cao* (Radix Glycyrrhizae) *Yu Jin* (Radix Curcumae)	Child fright wind
	Dan Nan Xing (Pulvis Arisaematis cum Felle Bovis) *Zhu Sha* (Cinnabaris) (see notes on legal status) *Jiang Can* (Bombyx Batryticatus)	Convulsions, delirious speech and spasms due to Phlegm-heat

Zhu Li 竹沥
(Dried bamboo sap, Succus Bambusae)

Zhu Li is baked bamboo sap from fresh *Bambusa breviflora* Munro, *Sinocalamus beecheyanus* (Munro) McClure var. *pubescens* P. F. Li or *Phyllostachys nigra* (Lodd.) Munro var. *henonis* Stapf, family Gramineae.

Properties Taste: sweet; nature: cold.

Channels entered Heart, Lung and Stomach.

Functions and indications Clears heat and dislodges Phlegm, settles fright and benefits the orifices. It is indicated for cough due to Phlegm-heat with thick sputum and for Phlegm-heat obstructing the clear orifices.

Common dosage 15-30ml, to which ginger juice is added.

Precautions and contraindications *Zhu Li* is contraindicated in cases of cold cough or for patients with loose stool due to Spleen deficiency, since the cold nature of the herb damages the Stomach and lubricates the Intestines.

Comparison of functions *Zhu Li* (Succus Bambusae), *Zhu Ru* (Caulis Bambusae in Taeniis) and *Tian Zhu Huang* (Concretio Silicea Bambusae), all of which originate from bamboo, are sweet in taste and cold in nature. They can transform Phlegm (particularly Phlegm-heat) and treat coughing and wheezing due to Phlegm-heat as well as being used for wind-stroke and Phlegm collapse and for child fright convulsions due to Phlegm-heat. *Zhu Li* works best when taken with ginger juice, whereas *Tian Zhu Huang* is best taken as powder. *Tian Zhu Huang* is harmonizing and moderating in property and is good at clearing heat from the Heart and settling fright. *Zhu Ru* is more effective for clearing Phlegm-heat from the Lungs and Stomach and for eliminating vexation. *Zhu Li* is extremely slippery in nature and is more effective in freeing the network vessels and tracking Phlegm. It can lubricate and moisten, thus being appropriate for freeing the orifices by dislodging Phlegm.

Combinations and applications

Functions	Combinations	Applications
Clearing heat and dislodging Phlegm	*Ban Xia* (Rhizoma Pinelliae Ternatae) *Chen Pi* (Pericarpium Citri Reticulatae) *Huang Qin* (Radix Scutellariae Baicalensis)	Cough due to Phlegm-heat with thick sputum that is difficult to expectorate or cough due to stubborn Phlegm binding together

	Tian Zhu Huang (Concretio Silicea Bambusae) *Sang Bai Pi* (Cortex Mori Albae Radicis) *Xing Ren* (Semen Pruni Armeniacae)	Wheezing and panting due to Phlegm-fire congesting the chest and diaphragm
Settling fright and benefiting the orifices	*Tian Nan Xing* (Rhizoma Arisaematis) *Ban Xia* (Rhizoma Pinelliae Ternatae) *Zhi Shi* (Fructus Immaturus Citri Aurantii)	Wind-stroke with loss of speech, hemiplegia
	Qing Meng Shi (Lapis Chloriti) *Da Huang* (Radix et Rhizoma Rhei) *Chen Xiang* (Lignum Aquilariae Resinatum)	Mania and withdrawal and fright epilepsy due to Phlegm-heat retention

Note: *Zhu Li* can also be used alone to treat Phlegm-heat obstructing the clear orifices, wind-stroke with clenched jaw, and loss of consciousness. In addition, this herb is also frequently used for encephalitis B, epidemic cerebrospinal meningitis with high fever, Phlegm confounding the Heart orifices, and vomiting.

Fu Hai Shi 浮海石 (Costazia bone or pumice, Os Costaziae seu Pumex)

The name *Fu Hai Shi* refers to two materia medica of different origin:

1. the dried bones of *Costazia aculeata* Canu et Bassler or *C. costazii* Audouin, family Poripidae (also known as *Shi Hua*);
2. porous volcanic rock, generally able to float on water, hence its name in Chinese (also known as *Fu Shi*).

Main ingredients *Shi Hua* contains calcium carbonate and small amounts of magnesium, iron and acid-insoluble materials. *Fu Shi* contains aluminium, potassium and sodium silicates, and silicon dioxide.

Properties Taste: salty; nature: cold.

Channel entered Lung.

Functions and indications Clears the Lungs and transforms Phlegm, softens hardness and dissipates lumps, disperses stones and frees Lin syndrome. It is indicated for cough due to Phlegm-heat, cough with thick and sticky sputum and difficult expectoration, scrofula, Phlegm nodes, and Lin syndrome.

Common dosage 6-10g; broken up and wrapped in a cloth for decoction before other ingredients: often used in pills and powders.

Precautions and contraindications *Fu Hai Shi* is contraindicated in cases of cough due to deficiency-cold.

Comparison of functions Both *Fu Hai Shi* (Os Costaziae seu Pumex) and *Gua Lou* (Fructus Trichosanthis) can clear Lung-heat to transform Phlegm in order to treat oppression in the chest, sticky sputum and difficult expectoration. *Fu Hai Shi* is salty in taste and cold in nature, and is therefore good at dispersing hard Phlegm, accumulated masses, scrofula and Phlegm nodes, and at clearing heat. It can also clear the upper part of the body and free the lower part to promote urination and free Lin syndrome. Although *Gua Lou* is also cold in nature, it is sweet in taste and possesses moistening and downward-bearing properties. It is therefore good for promoting the movement of Qi and loosening the chest and is effective in guiding Phlegm-heat out downwards. It is often used for depression binding of Phlegm-heat, inhibited Qi dynamic, and fullness and oppression in the chest and hypochondrium. It also has the functions of lubricating the Intestines and moistening the stool, and dispersing swelling and treating abscesses.

For an additional comparison, see *Hai Ge Ke* (Concha Meretricis seu Cyclinae).

Combinations and applications

Functions	Combinations	Applications
Clearing the Lungs and transforming Phlegm	*Dan Nan Xing* (Pulvis Arisaematis cum Felle Bovis) *Chuan Bei Mu* (Bulbus Fritillariae Cirrhosae) *Bai Jie Zi* (Semen Sinapis Albae)	Cough due to Phlegm-heat with yellow, thick and sticky sputum and difficult expectoration
	Gua Lou Ren (Semen Trichosanthis) *Zhi Zi* (Fructus Gardeniae Jasminoidis) *Qing Dai* (Indigo Naturalis)	Enduring cough with blood-streaked sputum due to Lung-heat and Liver-fire scorching the Lungs
	Bo He (Herba Menthae Haplocalycis) *Xing Ren* (Semen Pruni Armeniacae) *Bai Bu* (Radix Stemonae)	Wind-Phlegm transforming into dryness, coughing and wheezing due to Phlegm
Softening hardness and dissipating lumps	*Mu Li* (Concha Ostreae) *Zhe Bei Mu* (Bulbus Fritillariae Thunbergii) *Hai Zao* (Herba Sargassi) *Kun Bu* (Thallus Laminariae seu Eckloniae)	Scrofula and Phlegm nodes due to depression binding of Phlegm-fire
Dispersing stones and freeing Lin syndrome	*Gan Cao* (Radix Glycyrrhizae) (taken as a decoction with *Fu Hai Shi* ground into a powder)	Sand, stone and blood Lin syndromes

Hai Ge Ke 海蛤壳 (Clam shell, Concha Meretricis seu Cyclinae)

Hai Ge Ke is the shell of *Meretrix meretrix* L. or *Cyclina sinensis* Gmelin, family Veneridae.

Main ingredients *Hai Ge Ke* contains calcium carbonate and conchiolin.

Properties Taste: bitter and salty; nature: cold.

Channels entered Lung and Stomach.

Functions and indications Clears the Lungs and disperses Phlegm, softens hardness and dissipates lumps, promotes the movement of water and disperses swelling. It is indicated for coughing and wheezing due to Lung-heat with thick sputum that is difficult to expectorate, goitre, scrofula, puffy swelling, and inhibited urination.

Common dosage 10-15g, made into a powder and wrapped in a cloth for decocting; 1-3g in pills or powders; appropriate dosage for external application.

Precautions and contraindications *Hai Ge Ke* is contraindicated in cases of cold due to Lung deficiency or insufficiency of Yang in the Middle Jiao.

Comparison of functions *Hai Ge Ke* (Concha Meretricis seu Cyclinae), *Fu Hai Shi* (Os Costaziae seu Pumex), *Kun Bu* (Thallus Laminariae seu Eckloniae) and *Hai Zao* (Herba Sargassi) are all derived from marine substances and are salty in taste and cold in nature. They all have the functions of dispersing Phlegm, softening hardness and promoting the movement of water. *Hai Ge Ke* and *Fu Hai Shi* are more effective for clearing heat and dispersing or transforming Phlegm; with their attribution to the Lung channel, they are often used for coughing and wheezing due to Phlegm-heat and for cough with thick sputum and difficult expectoration. *Hai Ge Ke* is indicated for cough with pain in the chest due to Phlegm-fire, whereas *Fu Hai Shi* can be used for cough due to wind-Phlegm transforming into dryness. Entering the Liver channel, *Kun Bu* and *Hai Zao* have a more powerful effect in softening hardness and dissipating lumps as well as being able to promote the movement of water and disperse swelling. In the clinic, they are often used together to treat goitre and scrofula. *Kun Bu* is generally more effective than *Hai Zao*.

Combinations and applications

Functions	Combinations	Applications
Clearing the Lungs and dispersing Phlegm	*Pi Pa Ye* (Folium Eriobotryae Japonicae) *Xing Ren* (Semen Pruni Armeniacae) *Sang Bai Pi* (Cortex Mori Albae Radicis)	Coughing and wheezing with thick, yellow sputum and difficult expectoration due to Lung-fire tending towards exuberance
	Fu Hai Shi (Os Costaziae seu Pumex)	Coughing and wheezing due to Phlegm-heat
	Qing Dai (Indigo Naturalis)	Pain in the chest and hypochondrium and coughing of blood due to depression binding of Phlegm-fire damaging the network vessels of the Lungs
Softening hardness and dissipating lumps	*Hai Zao* (Herba Sargassi) *Kun Bu* (Thallus Laminariae seu Eckloniae) *Wa Leng Zi* (Concha Arcae)	Goitre, scrofula and Phlegm nodes due to congealing of Phlegm-fire
Promoting the movement of water and dispersing swelling	*Ze Xie* (Rhizoma Alismatis Orientalis) *Fang Ji* (Radix Stephaniae Tetrandrae) (see notes on legal status) *Lai Fu Zi* (Semen Raphani Sativi)	Coughing and wheezing, rapid breathing, generalized oedema with distension and fullness due to water and dampness collecting and stagnating
	Gan Sui (Radix Euphorbiae Kansui) *Yu Li Ren* (Semen Pruni) *Sang Bai Pi* (Cortex Mori Albae Radicis)	Severe generalized oedema
	Fang Ji (Radix Stephaniae Tetrandrae) (see notes on legal status) *Ting Li Zi* (Semen Lepidii seu Descurainiae) *Yu Li Ren* (Semen Pruni)	Drum distension and ascites with inhibited urination

Notes:

1. The calcined form of *Hai Ge Ke* can control acidity and alleviate pain to treat pain in the stomach with acid regurgitation.
2. When ground into a powder, *Hai Ge Ke* can be applied externally to promote the contraction of open sores.
3. Mixed with oil, *Hai Ge Ke* can also be used externally to treat scalds and eczema.

Hai Zao 海藻 (Seaweed, Herba Sargassi)

Hai Zao is the dried alga of *Sargassum pallidum* (Turn.) C. Ag. or *S. fusiforme* (Harv.) Setch., family Sargassaceae.

Main ingredients *Hai Zao* contains alginic acid, iodine, potassium, mannitol, sargassan and mucoproteins.

Properties Taste: bitter and salty; nature: cold.

Channels entered Liver, Stomach and Kidney.

Functions and indications Disperses Phlegm and softens hardness, promotes the movement of water and disperses swelling. It is indicated for goitre, scrofula, Wei syndrome, swollen and painful testicles, oedema and puffy swelling.

Common dosage 10–15g.

Precautions and contraindications *Hai Zao* is incompatible with *Gan Cao* (Radix Glycyrrhizae).

Comparison of functions See *Hai Ge Ke* (Concha Meretricis seu Cyclinae).

Toxicity There was no obvious effect on the formation, growth and development of the foetus in pregnant rats exposed to alginic acid for 6–15 days.

Modern research

1. Since *Hai Zao* contains iodine, it can rectify thyroid deficiency caused by lack of iodine.[43]
2. Stops bleeding and lowers blood pressure.[43]
3. An aqueous extract of *Hai Zao* inhibited certain pathogenic fungi *in vitro*.[43]
4. Reduces the level of blood lipids and reduces weight, but does not cause insomnia.[44]
5. Inhibits carcinoma and endotoxins.[45, 46]

Combinations and applications

Functions	Combinations	Applications
Dispersing Phlegm and softening hardness	*Kun Bu* (Thallus Laminariae seu Eckloniae) *Zhe Bei Mu* (Bulbus Fritillariae Thunbergii) *Qing Pi* (Pericarpium Citri Reticulatae Viride)	Goitre
	Xia Ku Cao (Spica Prunellae Vulgaris) *Xuan Shen* (Radix Scrophulariae Ningpoensis) *Lian Qiao* (Fructus Forsythiae Suspensae)	Scrofula
	Kun Bu (Thallus Laminariae seu Eckloniae) *Mu Li* (Concha Ostreae)	Shan disorders, swollen and painful testicles
Promoting the movement of water and dispersing swelling	*Fu Ling* (Sclerotium Poriae Cocos) *Da Fu Pi* (Pericarpium Arecae Catechu)	Wei syndrome of the lower limbs, oedema and puffy swelling

Kun Bu 昆布
(Laminaria, Thallus Laminariae seu Ecklonlae)

Kun Bu is the dried thallus of *Laminaria japonica* Aresch., family Laminariaceae, or *Ecklonia kurome* Okam., family Alariaceae.

Main ingredients *Kun Bu* contains potassium iodide, laminarin, laminine, alginic acid, iodine, mannitol, carotene, riboflavin, thiamine and nicotinic acid (*Laminaria*); iodine, bromine, calcium and arginic acid (*Ecklonia*).

Properties Taste: salty; nature: cold.

Channels entered Liver, Stomach and Kidney.

Functions and indications Disperses Phlegm and softens hardness, promotes the movement of water and disperses swelling. It is indicated for scrofula, goitre, oedema, Wei syndrome, and leg Qi.

Common dosage 10-15g.

Precautions and contraindications *Kun Bu* is contraindicated for diarrhoea due to Spleen deficiency.

Comparison of functions See *Hai Ge Ke* (Concha Meretricis seu Cyclinae).

Modern research

1. Reduces the level of blood lipids.[47]
2. A laminine extract from *Kun Bu* can lower blood pressure.[48, 49]
3. Lowers the blood sugar level.[50]
4. Inhibits carcinoma.[51]

Combinations and applications

Functions	Combinations	Applications
Dispersing Phlegm and softening hardness	*Hai Zao* (Herba Sargassi) *Hai Ge Ke* (Concha Meretricis seu Cyclinae)	Goitre and scrofula
Promoting the movement of water and dispersing swelling	*Fang Ji* (Radix Stephaniae Tetrandrae) (see notes on legal status) *Mu Tong* (Caulis Mutong) (see notes on legal status) *Fu Ling* (Sclerotium Poriae Cocos)	Wei syndrome of the lower limbs, oedema and puffy swelling

Pang Da Hai 胖大海
(Boat-fruited sterculia seed, Semen Sterculiae Lychnophorae)

Pang Da Hai is the dried seed of *Sterculia lychnophora* Hance, family Sterculiaceae.

Main ingredients *Pang Da Hai* contains bassorin, galactose and arabinose.

Properties Taste: sweet; nature: cold.

Channels entered Lung and Large Intestine.

Functions and indications Clears the Lungs and diffuses Lung Qi, benefits the throat, clears the Intestines and frees the bowels. It is indicated for cough due to Phlegm-heat, sore throat and hoarse voice; and for headache, toothache and constipation due to heat binding in the Stomach and Intestines.

Common dosage 3-5 pieces, or half dosage as a powder.

Remarks *Pang Da Hai* can be used on its own as an infusion or in a decoction. It is commonly employed for throat conditions. In addition, it can be used for constipation due to heat in the Intestines; however, its action in freeing the bowels is relatively weak and the herb is only appropriate for mild cases. It should be combined with herbs for clearing heat and downward-draining herbs in more severe cases.

Toxicity In an acute toxicity test, *Pang Da Hai* seeds given to rabbits caused difficulty in breathing and loss of balance. The LD_{50} for *Pang Da Hai* fed to mice via intragastric administration is 12.96g/kg.

Modern research

1. The steep of *Pang Da Hai* induces diarrhoea.[52]
2. Inhibits inflammation, relieves convulsions and alleviates pain.[53]
3. The seed and peel of *Pang Da Hai* promote urination.[53]

Combinations and applications

Functions	Combinations	Applications
Clearing the Lungs and diffusing Lung Qi, benefiting the throat	*Jie Geng* (Radix Platycodi Grandiflori) *Chan Tui* (Periostracum Cicadae)	Hoarse voice due to Lung-heat and cough due to Phlegm-heat
	Xuan Shen (Radix Scrophulariae Ningpoensis) *Qing Guo* (Fructus Canarii Albi)	Sore throat, hoarse voice and dry throat due to effulgent Yin deficiency-fire
Clearing the Intestines and freeing the bowels	*Gua Lou Ren* (Semen Trichosanthis) *Zhi Ke* (Fructus Citri Aurantii) *Yu Li Ren* (Semen Pruni)	Constipation with headache, red eyes, toothache and slight fever due to heat in the Intestines

Huang Yao Zi 黄药子 (Air potato yam, Rhizoma Dioscoreae Bulbiferae)

Huang Yao Zi is the dried rhizome of *Dioscorea bulbifera* L., family Dioscoreacae.

Main ingredients *Huang Yao Zi* contains sucrose, starch, tannin and small amounts of diosgenin and diosbulbins B and C.

Properties Taste: bitter; nature: cold.

Channels entered Lung and Liver.

Functions and indications Dissipates lumps and disperses goitre, clears heat and relieves toxicity, cools the Blood and stops bleeding, stops coughing and calms wheezing. It is indicated for goitre and scrofula, swelling and toxins of sores, poisonous snake bites, bleeding due to Blood-heat, and whooping cough.

Common dosage 10-15g.

Precautions and contraindications *Huang Yao Zi* should be used with caution for patients with Spleen and Stomach deficiency or disorders of the Liver.

Toxicity Large dosages of *Huang Yao Zi* or administration over a long period can cause alimentary canal reaction (manifesting as vomiting, diarrhoea and pain in the abdomen) and damage the functioning of the liver.

Modern research

1. Inhibits the intestinal smooth muscle.[54]
2. Aqueous extracts of *Huang Yao Zi* inhibited Trichophyton schoenleinii and other dermatophytes *in vitro*.[55]

Combinations and applications

Functions	Combinations	Applications
Dissipating lumps and dispersing goitre	*Hai Zao* (Herba Sargassi) *Mu Li* (Concha Ostreae) *Tu Bei Mu* (Tuber Bolbostemmatis)	Goitre and scrofula due to congealing of Phlegm-fire
Clearing heat and relieving toxicity	*Hai Zao* (Herba Sargassi) *Kun Bu* (Thallus Laminariae seu Eckloniae) *Bai Hua She She Cao* (Herba Hedyotidis Diffusae) *Yi Yi Ren* (Semen Coicis Lachrymajobi) *Shan Ci Gu* (Pseudobulbus Shancigu)	Various tumours, including those in the oesophagus, lungs, liver, stomach and rectum
Cooling the Blood and stopping bleeding	*Pu Huang* (Pollen Typhae) *Zong Lü Tan* (Fibra Carbonisata Trachycarpi Stipulae)	Vomiting of blood, coughing of blood and nosebleed due to Blood-heat

Notes:

1. *Huang Yao Zi* can be used externally on its own or with other herbs for relieving toxicity to treat poisonous snake bites.
2. According to clinical reports, *Huang Yao Zi* can also be used with sugar candy (*Bing Tang*, Saccharon Crystallinum) to treat whooping cough.

HERBS FOR STOPPING COUGHING AND CALMING WHEEZING

Most herbs for stopping coughing and calming wheezing have the function of diffusing Lung Qi and transforming Phlegm, moistening the Lungs and stopping coughing, and bearing counterflow Lung Qi downwards and calming wheezing. They are also used for coughing and wheezing due to Lung Qi deficiency.

The manifestations and pathogenesis of coughing and wheezing are comparatively complex. Differentiation must be made between externally-contracted conditions and conditions due to internal damage, and among cold, heat, deficiency and full patterns. Externally-contracted coughing and wheezing can be attributed to overwhelming by the six excesses, for example by wind-cold, wind-heat, or dry-heat invading the Lungs. Internal damage may be caused by diet, taxation damage, emotional disturbances or enduring illnesses. Coughing and wheezing may also be found in full patterns, manifesting as damp-Phlegm, cold-Phlegm, heat-Phlegm or dry Phlegm obstructing the Lungs and impairing them in their diffusing and downward-bearing functions. In deficiency patterns, coughing and wheezing may be caused by depletion and consumption of Lung Yin, deficiency-fire scorching the Lungs or Lung and Kidney deficiency.

The pathogenesis and symptoms of cough can thus be differentiated by the identification of patterns according to the six factors: invasion by external pathogenic factors, internal damage, cold, heat, deficiency and fullness.

Appropriate herbs for stopping coughing and calming wheezing must therefore be selected and combined in accordance with this differentiation; they should not be used alone. For cough due to Yin deficiency and subsequent Lung-heat, herbs for stopping coughing and calming wheezing should be combined with herbs for clearing Lung-heat and supplementing Yin; for cough due to exterior wind-heat, they should be combined with herbs for clearing heat and acrid, cool herbs for releasing the exterior; and for cough with copious sputum, they should be combined with herbs for transforming Phlegm. These combinations of herbs will treat the root and manifestation of the disorder simultaneously.

Even though patients may have a cough, herbs of a warm nature and herbs for promoting contraction are contraindicated at the initial stage of measles or for patients with skin rashes due to invasion by external pathogenic factors, as these herbs enhance the dispersion of measles and aggravate skin rashes, thus exacerbating the condition.

Tab. 13.2 Herbs for stopping coughing and calming wheezing

Herb	Functions	Indications
Xing Ren (Semen Pruni Armeniacae)	Stopping coughing and calming wheezing, moistening the Intestines and freeing the bowels	Coughing and wheezing, sore throat and constipation
Su Zi (Fructus Perillae Frutescentis)	Bearing Qi downwards and dispersing Phlegm, stopping coughing and calming wheezing, moistening the Intestines and freeing the bowels	Coughing and wheezing with copious sputum, constipation
Bai Bu (Radix Stemonae)	Moistening the Lungs and stopping coughing, exterminating lice and killing worms	Recent or enduring cough, whooping cough, threadworm, body and head lice

Sang Bai Pi (Cortex Mori Albae Radicis)	Draining the Lungs and calming wheezing, promoting the movement of water and dispersing swelling	Coughing and wheezing due to Lung-heat, cough with copious sputum, oedema, leg Qi, inhibited urination
Ting Li Zi (Semen Lepidii seu Descurainiae)	Draining the Lungs and calming wheezing, moving water and dispersing swelling	Wheezing, cough with copious sputum, oedema, inhibited urination
Zi Wan (Radix Asteris Tatarici)	Moistening the Lungs and causing Qi to descend, transforming Phlegm and stopping coughing	Cough due to counterflow Qi, difficult expectoration, enduring cough, coughing of blood
Kuan Dong Hua (Flos Tussilaginis Farfarae)	Moistening the Lungs and causing Qi to descend, stopping coughing and transforming Phlegm	Various types of cough
Ma Dou Ling (Fructus Aristolochiae)	Clearing the Lungs and transforming Phlegm, stopping coughing and calming wheezing, clearing the Intestines and dispersing haemorrhoids	Coughing and wheezing due to Lung-heat, coughing of blood, loss of voice, swelling and pain from haemorrhoids
Pi Pa Ye (Folium Eriobotryae Japonicae)	Clearing the Lungs, transforming Phlegm and stopping coughing, harmonizing the Stomach, bearing counterflow Qi downwards and stopping vomiting	Coughing and wheezing due to Lung-heat, coughing of blood, nausea and vomiting due to Stomach-heat
Ai Di Cha (Herba Ardisiae Japonicae)	Stopping coughing and dispelling Phlegm, clearing damp-heat and abating jaundice, promoting the movement of water and percolating dampness, quickening the Blood and transforming stasis, freeing menstruation and alleviating pain	Coughing and wheezing with copious sputum, damp-heat jaundice, oedema, knocks and falls, wind-damp Bi syndrome pain, menstrual block with pain in the abdomen
Bai Guo (Semen Ginkgo Bilobae)	Constraining the Lungs and stabilizing wheezing, stopping vaginal discharge and reducing urine	Cough with copious sputum, wheezing, vaginal discharge, urinary turbidity, frequent urination
Yang Jin Hua (Flos Daturae)	Stopping coughing and calming wheezing, alleviating pain, relieving tetany	Coughing and wheezing due to cold-Phlegm with little or no sputum, cold and pain in the stomach and abdomen, wind-damp Bi syndrome pain, convulsions and spasms

Xing Ren 杏仁 (Apricot kernel, Semen Pruni Armeniacae)

Xing Ren is the mature seed of *Prunus armeniaca* L. var. *ansu* Maxim, *P. armeniaca* L., *P. mandshurica* (Maxim.) Koehne or *P. sibirica* L., family Rosaceae.

Main ingredients *Xing Ren* contains 50% of fatty oils (including oleic, linoleic, palmitic, stearic and linolenic acids), as well as amygdalin, amygdalase and prunase. Hydrolysing amygdalin generates benzaldehyde and hydrocyanic acid, which is toxic.

Properties Taste: bitter; nature: slightly warm; slightly toxic.

Channels entered Lung and Large Intestine.

Functions and indications Stops coughing and calms wheezing, moistens the Intestines and frees the bowels. It is indicated for coughing and wheezing, sore throat and constipation.

Common dosage 3-10g, decocted for a short time only.

Precautions and contraindications

1. As *Xing Ren* is slightly toxic, large dosages should be avoided, especially when treating infants.
2. Contraindicated in cases of weak constitution and profuse sweating.

Remarks *Ku Xing Ren* (Semen Pruni Armeniacae Amarum), or bitter apricot kernel, is normally used for this herb.

Comparison of functions

1. Both *Xing Ren* (Semen Pruni Armeniacae) and *Ma Huang* (Herba Ephedrae) enter the Lung channel and are effective in stopping coughing and calming wheezing. *Ma Huang* can diffuse Lung Qi to calm wheezing, whereas *Xing Ren* can bear counterflow Lung Qi downwards to stop coughing and calm wheezing and to dispel wind-heat from the Lungs. The two herbs are often used together, since one is diffusing and the other downward-bearing. In addition, *Ma Huang* can also promote urination and disperse swelling, while *Xing Ren* can moisten the Large Intestine to treat dryness in the Intestines.
2. *Xing Ren* (Semen Pruni Armeniacae) and *Jie Geng* (Radix Platycodi Grandiflori) both enter the Qi level and the Lung channel; they are used for various types of coughing and wheezing. However, *Xing Ren* has a downward-bearing function and acts against counterflow Lung Qi to stop coughing and calm wheezing, whereas *Jie Geng* has an upward-bearing function and promotes the movement of Lung Qi to dispel Phlegm and treat sore throat. When used in combination, they are very effective for cough with wheezing due to externally-contracted pathogenic factors or Phlegm obstruction of the Lungs.
3. For an additional comparison, see *Su Zi* (Fructus Perillae Frutescentis).

Toxicity The LD_{50} for intravenous injection of amygdalin in mice or rats is 25g/kg; for intraperitoneal injection, it is 8g/kg; and for oral administration, it is 0.6g/kg. Oral administration of 55 pieces (the equivalent of about 60g) of *Ku Xing Ren*, containing 1.8g of amygdalin, can cause death in humans. The main symptoms of toxic reaction include a bitter taste in the mouth, dizziness, nausea, vomiting, pain in the abdomen, diarrhoea, agitation, vexation and restlessness, palpitations, and weakness of the limbs, and in severe cases, oppression in the chest, difficulty in breathing, loss of consciousness, a reduction in blood pressure and even coma. *Ku Xing Ren* should therefore not be used raw and overdosage must be avoided.

Modern research

1. Inhibits the respiratory centre to stop coughing and calm wheezing.[56]
2. Affects digestion by inhibiting the activity of pepsins.[53]
3. Reduces the level of blood fats.[57]
4. Inhibits inflammation and alleviates pain.[58]
5. Inhibits carcinoma.[59]

Combinations and applications

Functions	Combinations	Applications
Stopping coughing and calming wheezing	*Ju Hua* (Flos Chrysanthemi Morifolii) *Sang Ye* (Folium Mori Albae) *Lian Qiao* (Fructus Forsythiae Suspensae)	Cough due to externally-contracted wind-heat with generalized fever, redness of the tip and side margins of the tongue, a thin tongue with yellow fur, and a rapid, floating pulse
	Sang Ye (Folium Mori Albae) *Ju Hua* (Flos Chrysanthemi Morifolii) *Jie Geng* (Radix Platycodi Grandiflori)	Cough due to wind-heat with thick, yellow sputum
	Chuan Bei Mu (Bulbus Fritillariae Cirrhosae) *Sha Shen* (Radix Glehniae seu Adenophorae) *Mai Men Dong* (Radix Ophiopogonis Japonici) *Sang Ye* (Folium Mori Albae)	Dry cough, scant and sticky sputum, a thin, dry tongue and a rapid pulse due to dry-heat damaging the Lungs
	Shi Gao (Gypsum Fibrosum) *Ma Huang* (Herba Ephedrae) (see notes on legal status) *Gan Cao* (Radix Glycyrrhizae)	Coughing and wheezing, generalized fever, yellow tongue fur and a rapid, slippery pulse due to stagnation of heat in the Lungs and counterflow Lung Qi
	Gui Zhi (Ramulus Cinnamomi Cassiae) (prepared as a powder for retention in the mouth)	Sore throat, cough with sputum, mouth sores
Moistening the Intestines and freeing the bowels	*Huo Ma Ren* (Semen Cannabis Sativae) *Dang Gui* (Radix Angelicae Sinensis) *Zhi Ke* (Fructus Citri Aurantii) *Tao Ren* (Semen Persicae)	Intestinal dryness with constipation

Su Zi 苏子
(Perilla fruit, Fructus Perillae Frutescentis)

Su Zi is the mature fruit of *Perilla frutescens* (L.) Britt., family Labiatae.

Main ingredients *Su Zi* contains fatty oils, vitamin B_1 and amino acids.

Properties Taste: acrid; nature: warm.

Channels entered Lung and Large Intestine.

Functions and indications Bears Qi downwards and disperses Phlegm, stops coughing and calms wheezing, moistens the Intestines and frees the bowels. It is indicated for coughing and wheezing with copious sputum, and for constipation.

Common dosage 5-10g.

Precautions and contraindications *Su Zi* should be used with caution in cases of wheezing due to Yin deficiency and loose stool due to Spleen deficiency.

Comparison of functions

1. Both *Su Zi* (Fructus Perillae Frutescentis) and *Bai Jie Zi* (Semen Sinapis Albae) can treat coughing and wheezing due to cold-Phlegm; they are frequently used in combination. *Su Zi* is good at bearing Qi downwards to disperse Phlegm and calm wheezing in order to treat coughing and wheezing due to cold-Phlegm congesting the

Lungs. *Bai Jie Zi* is more effective in warming the Lungs and promoting the movement of Qi to disperse Phlegm in order to treat Phlegm lodged between the skin and membranes.

2. Both *Su Zi* (Fructus Perillae Frutescentis) and *Xing Ren* (Semen Pruni Armeniacae) can stop coughing and calm wheezing, and moisten the Intestines and free the bowels. *Xing Ren* can bear counterflow Lung Qi downwards and dispel wind in the Lung channel to stop coughing and calm wheezing and is therefore used for various types of coughing and wheezing. On the other hand, *Su Zi* bears counterflow Lung Qi downwards and disperses Phlegm to stop coughing and calm wheezing and is mainly used for cold cough and wheezing due to obstruction of Phlegm in the Lungs and counterflow Qi.

Modern research Promotes gastrointestinal movement and can be used to cure roundworm.[60]

Combinations and applications

Functions	Combinations	Applications
Bearing Qi downwards and dispersing Phlegm, stopping coughing and calming wheezing	*Bai Jie Zi* (Semen Sinapis Albae) *Lai Fu Zi* (Semen Raphani Sativi)	Coughing and wheezing with copious sputum and focal distension in the chest, low food intake, difficulty in digestion, a white tongue with slimy fur, and a slippery pulse due to obstruction of Phlegm and stagnation of Lung Qi
	Chen Pi (Pericarpium Citri Reticulatae) *Hou Po* (Cortex Magnoliae Officinalis) *Ban Xia* (Rhizoma Pinelliae Ternatae)	Full pattern in the Upper Jiao and deficiency pattern in the Lower Jiao, manifesting as fullness and oppression in the chest and diaphragm, wheezing, coughing and shortness of breath due to cold-Phlegm congesting the Lungs
	Bai Guo (Semen Ginkgo Bilobae) *Ma Huang* (Herba Ephedrae) (see notes on legal status) *Kuan Dong Hua* (Flos Tussilaginis Farfarae) *Xing Ren* (Semen Pruni Armeniacae)	Wheezing due to internal retention of Phlegm-heat and externally-contracted wind-cold
	Xing Ren (Semen Pruni Armeniacae) *Bai Mi* (white honey)	Enduring cough in infants with sputum producing a whistling sound in the throat
Moistening the Intestines and freeing the bowels	*Huo Ma Ren* (Semen Cannabis Sativae) *Gua Lou Ren* (Semen Trichosanthis) *Xing Ren* (Semen Pruni Armeniacae)	Intestinal dryness with constipation in the elderly

Bai Bu 百部
(Stemona root, Radix Stemonae)

Bai Bu is the tuberous root of *Stemona sessilifolia* (Miq.) Franch. et Sav., *S. japonica* (Bl.) Miq. or *S. tuberosa* Lour., family Stemonaceae.

Main ingredients All types of *Bai Bu* contain alkaloids. The root of *Zhi Li Bai Bu* (*S. sessilifolia*) contains stemonine, protostemonine, stemonidine, isostemonidine, tuberostemonine, hodorine and sessilistemonine; the root of *Dui Ye Bai Bu* (*S. tuberosa*) contains stemonine, tuberostemonine, isotuberostemonine, stenine and stemonitine; and the root of *Man Sheng Bai Bu* (*S. japonica*) contains stemonine, protostemonine, stemonidine, isostemonidine, paipunine, stemoninine, neostemonine and stemodiol.

Properties Taste: sweet and bitter; nature: neutral.

Channel entered Lung.

Functions and indications Moistens the Lungs and stops coughing, exterminates lice and kills worms. It is indicated for recent or enduring cough, whooping cough, threadworm, and body and head lice.

Common dosage 5-10g; appropriate dosage for external application.

Precautions and contraindications Since *Bai Bu* can damage the Stomach and lubricate the Intestines, it is contraindicated in cases of loose stool due to Spleen deficiency.

Comparison of functions Both *Bai Bu* (Radix Stemonae) and *Bai He* (Bulbus Lilii) enter the Lung channel and can moisten the Lungs to stop coughing. They can be used for damage to Yin and dryness of the Lungs, enduring cough, and cough with scant sputum or without sputum. *Bai He* can enrich Yin and moisten the Lungs to stop coughing. It concurrently enters the Heart channel to clear heat from the Heart and quiet the Spirit; it is also used for lily disease due to deficiency vexation and sleeplessness. *Bai Bu* can moisten the Lungs and bear counterflow Qi downwards to stop coughing. It tends to be sweet and moistening and is used for recent and enduring cough in cold, heat, deficiency or full patterns; it can also kill worms.

Modern research

1. The alkaloids contained in *Bai Bu* stop coughing and expel sputum.[61]
2. The steep of *Bai Bu* kills parasites, especially head lice.[62]
3. Inhibits influenza viruses, Mycobacterium tuberculosis and Streptococcus pneumoniae.[61-63]

Combinations and applications

Functions	Combinations	Applications
Moistening the Lungs and stopping coughing	*Jing Jie* (Herba Schizonepetae Tenuifoliae) *Jie Geng* (Radix Platycodi Grandiflori) *Zi Wan* (Radix Asteris Tatarici) *Chen Pi* (Pericarpium Citri Reticulatae)	Cough, itchy throat, slight fever and chills and a thin tongue with white fur due to wind-cold invading the Lungs
	Sha Shen (Radix Glehniae seu Adenophorae) *Chuan Bei Mu* (Bulbus Fritillariae Cirrhosae) *Bai Qian* (Radix et Rhizoma Cynanchi Stauntonii)	Whooping cough due to Yin deficiency and Lung-heat
	Sheng Di Huang (Radix Rehmanniae Glutinosae) *Mai Men Dong* (Radix Ophiopogonis Japonici) *Bai Shao* (Radix Paeoniae Lactiflorae) *Dang Gui* (Radix Angelicae Sinensis) *Chuan Bei Mu* (Bulbus Fritillariae Cirrhosae) *Xuan Shen* (Radix Scrophulariae Ningpoensis)	Yin deficiency of the Lungs and Kidneys with deficiency-fire flaming upwards, manifesting as coughing and wheezing, blood-streaked sputum, heat in the palms and soles, a red tongue with thin fur, and a fine, rapid pulse

Notes:

1. An enteroclysm prepared with *Bai Bu* is effective against threadworm.
2. The juice of the fresh herb is indicated for external use for erysipelas, dermatitis, tinea corporis and mosquito bites.
3. A decoction of *Bai Bu* can be used as a wash to treat body and head lice.

Sang Bai Pi 桑白皮 (White mulberry root bark, Cortex Mori Albae Radicis)

Sang Bai Pi is the root bark of *Morus alba* L., family Moraceae.

Main ingredients *Sang Bai Pi* contains flavone derivatives (including mulberrin, morusin, mulberrochromene, cyclomulberrin and cyclomulberrochromene), betulinic acid, amyrins, volatile oils, palmitic acid, resinotannol, sitosterol and glucose.

Properties Taste: sweet; nature: cold.

Channel entered Lung.

Functions and indications Drains the Lungs and calms wheezing, promotes the movement of water and disperses swelling. It is indicated for coughing and wheezing due to Lung-heat, cough with copious sputum, oedema, leg Qi, and inhibited urination.

Common dosage 10-15g.

Precautions and contraindications *Sang Bai Pi* cannot be used on its own to treat cough due to wind-cold or cough due to Lung Qi deficiency.

Remarks Raw *Sang Bai Pi* is used to drain the Lungs and promote the movement of water, whereas the herb mix-fried with honey is better for moistening the Lungs and stopping coughing.

Comparison of functions *Sang Bai Pi* (Cortex Mori Albae Radicis), *Sang Ye* (Folium Mori Albae), *Sang Zhi* (Ramulus Mori Albae) and *Sang Shen* (Fructus Mori Albae) are respectively the root bark, leaf, twig and fruit of *Morus alba* L. However, their functions and effects differ. *Sang Bai Pi* drains Lung-fire to move Phlegm and water and is commonly used for coughing and wheezing due to Lung-heat and for oedema with distension and fullness. *Sang Ye* dissipates wind-heat in the Lung channel and can clear heat from the Liver and brighten the eyes; it is often used for cough due to dry-heat damaging the Lungs. *Sang Zhi* can dispel wind, free the channels and treat Bi syndrome, particularly wind-damp Bi syndrome. *Sang Shen* is good for supplementing the Blood and enriching Liver and Kidney Yin to blacken the hair and brighten the eyes.

For an additional comparison, see *Ting Li Zi* (Semen Lepidii seu Descurainiae).

Modern research

1. Decoctions of *Sang Bai Pi* can promote urination and induce diarrhoea.[64]
2. Has a tranquillizing function and alleviates pain.[64]
3. The steep of *Sang Bai Pi* stops coughing.[65]
4. Inhibits haematoblastic concentration.[65]

Combinations and applications

Functions	Combinations	Applications
Draining the Lungs and calming wheezing	*Di Gu Pi* (Cortex Lycii Radicis) *Zhi Gan Cao* (Radix Glycyrrhizae Praeparata) *Jing Mi* (Oryza Sativa)	Hasty breathing and cough, fever, a red tongue with yellow fur and a fine, rapid pulse due to Lung Qi failing to bear downwards as a result of pathogenic heat lying in the Lungs
	Ma Huang (Herba Ephedrae) (see notes on legal status) *Gui Zhi* (Ramulus Cinnamomi Cassiae) *Xing Ren* (Semen Pruni Armeniacae) *Xi Xin* (Herba cum Radice Asari) *Gan Jiang* (Rhizoma Zingiberis Officinalis)	Distension and fullness in the chest and hypochondrium, hasty breathing and cough due to water-fluids collecting in the Lungs

Promoting the movement of water and dispersing swelling	*Da Fu Pi* (Pericarpium Arecae Catechu) *Fu Ling Pi* (Cortex Poriae Cocos) *Sheng Jiang Pi* (Cortex Zingiberis Officinalis Recens)	Generalized oedema, heavy limbs, distension of the abdomen, counterflow Qi and inhibited urination due to Spleen deficiency and obstruction of body fluids
	Dong Gua Ren (Semen Benincasae Hispidae) *Ting Li Zi* (Semen Lepidii seu Descurainiae)	Inhibited urination, facial oedema
	Gou Qi Zi (Fructus Lycii)	Wasting and thirsting

Ting Li Zi 葶苈子 (Lepidium or descurainia seed, Semen Lepidii seu Descurainiae)

Ting Li Zi is the mature seed of *Lepidium apetalum* Willd. or *Descurainia sophia* (L.) Webb ex Prantl., family Cruciferae.

Main ingredients *Bei Ting Li Zi* (*Lepidium*) contains sinigrin, fatty oils, proteins and carbohydrates; *Nan Ting Li Zi* (*Descurainia*) contains cardiac glycosides (including strophanthidine, evomonoside, helveticoside and evobioside), benzyl isothiocyanate, allyl isothiocyanate, and linolenic, linoleic, oleic, palmitic and stearic acids.

Properties Taste: acrid and bitter; nature: extremely cold.

Channels entered Lung and Bladder.

Functions and indications Drains the Lungs and calms wheezing, moves water and disperses swelling. It is indicated for wheezing, cough with copious sputum, oedema, and inhibited urination.

Common dosage 3-10g.

Precautions and contraindications *Ting Li Zi* should be used with caution in cases of cough due to Lung deficiency and oedema due to Spleen deficiency.

Comparison of functions Both *Ting Li Zi* (Semen Lepidii seu Descurainiae) and *Sang Bai Pi* (Cortex Mori Albae Radicis) drain heat from the Lungs and calm wheezing, and promote the movement of water and disperse swelling. They are often used together to treat coughing and wheezing and full-type oedema. However, *Ting Li Zi* is more effective in eliminating Phlegm to treat coughing and wheezing due to Phlegm accumulation in the Lungs, whereas *Sang Bai Pi* is better for draining heat from the Lungs to treat coughing and wheezing due to Lung-heat.

Modern research

1. Strengthens cardiac contraction, slows the heart rate, inhibits arrhythmia.[66]
2. The benzyl isothiocyanate contained in *Ting Li Zi* inhibits various saccharomycete fungi.[67]
3. Calms wheezing, has a tranquillizing function and promotes urination.[68]

Combinations and applications

Functions	Combinations	Applications
Draining the Lungs and calming wheezing	*Da Zao* (Fructus Ziziphi Jujubae)	Cough with copious sputum due to Phlegm-saliva congesting the Lungs, inability to lie down due to counterflow Qi, puffy swelling of the face and eyes, generalized oedema

	Zhi Mu (Rhizoma Anemarrhenae Asphodeloidis) *Chuan Bei Mu* (Bulbus Fritillariae Cirrhosae) *Da Zao* (Fructus Ziziphi Jujubae)	Coughing and wheezing due to stagnation of Lung Qi
	Ban Xia (Rhizoma Pinelliae Ternatae) *Sheng Jiang* (Rhizoma Zingiberis Officinalis Recens)	Phlegm-saliva congestion, coughing and wheezing due to counterflow Qi
Moving water and dispersing swelling	*Xing Ren* (Semen Pruni Armeniacae) *Da Huang* (Radix et Rhizoma Rhei) *Mang Xiao* (Mirabilitum)	Fullness, oppression and pain below the heart and in the abdomen, shortness of breath, vexation, stiff neck, and a sunken, tight pulse
	Fang Ji (Radix Stephaniae Tetrandrae) (see notes on legal status) *Jiao Mu* (Semen Zanthoxyli) *Da Huang* (Radix et Rhizoma Rhei)	Inhibited urination and defecation with a gurgling sound due to water entering the Intestines and fluids lingering in the Intestines and Stomach
	Qian Niu Zi (Semen Pharbitidis) *Jiao Mu* (Semen Zanthoxyli) *Yu Li Ren* (Semen Pruni)	Oedema with distension and fullness and inhibited urination due to water-Qi not moving and impairment of the diffusing and downward-bearing functions of the Lungs

Note: In recent years, *Ting Li Zi* has been used in combination with *Lai Fu Zi* (Semen Raphani Sativi), *Fu Zi* (Radix Lateralis Aconiti Carmichaeli Praeparata) and *Huang Qi* (Radix Astragali seu Hedysari) for oedema, wheezing and fullness in cases of heart failure or pulmonary heart disease (for *Fu Zi*, see notes on legal status).

Zi Wan 紫菀 (Purple aster root, Radix Asteris Tatarici)

Zi Wan is the root and rhizome of *Aster tataricus* L. f., family Compositae.

Main ingredients *Zi Wan* contains astersaponins, shionone, quercetin, friedelin, epifriedelinol, shionosides, asterin, astins, volatile oils (including lachnophyllol and anethole), aromatic acids and hydrocarbons.

Properties Taste: bitter and sweet; nature: slightly warm.

Channel entered Lung.

Functions and indications Moistens the Lungs and causes Qi to descend, transforms Phlegm and stops coughing. It is indicated for cough due to counterflow Qi, difficult expectoration, enduring cough, and coughing of blood.

Common dosage 5-10g.

Remarks

1. Raw *Zi Wan* should be used for externally-contracted fulminant cough, whereas the herb mix-fried with honey is better for enduring cough due to Lung deficiency.
2. *Zi Wan* is an important herb for transforming Phlegm and stopping coughing and can be used to treat all types of cough, whether recent or enduring, due to heat or cold, or in deficiency or full patterns. Nevertheless, *Zi Wan* is most effective for cough due to externally-contracted wind-cold.

Comparison of functions See *Kuan Dong Hua* (Flos Tussilaginis Farfarae).

Modern research

1. Decoctions of *Zi Wan* can expel sputum and stop coughing.[69, 70]
2. A decoction of the herb inhibited various bacteria *in vitro*, including Escherichia coli, Shigella sonnei, Salmonella typhi and Pseudomonas aeruginosa.[71]
3. Inhibits carcinoma.[71]
4. Promotes urination.[69]

Combinations and applications

Functions	Combinations	Applications
Moistening the Lungs and causing Qi to descend, transforming Phlegm and stopping coughing	*Jie Geng* (Radix Platycodi Grandiflori) *Jing Jie* (Herba Schizonepetae Tenuifoliae) *Chen Pi* (Pericarpium Citri Reticulatae) *Bai Bu* (Radix Stemonae)	Cough with copious sputum due to externally-contracted wind-cold
	Huang Qin (Radix Scutellariae Baicalensis) *Zhe Bei Mu* (Bulbus Fritillariae Thunbergii) *Gua Lou* (Fructus Trichosanthis)	Cough due to Lung-heat with thick and yellow sputum
	Tian Men Dong (Radix Asparagi Cochinchinensis) *Zhi Mu* (Rhizoma Anemarrhenae Asphodeloidis) *Chuan Bei Mu* (Bulbus Fritillariae Cirrhosae) *E Jiao* (Gelatinum Corii Asini)	Enduring cough and coughing of blood due to Yin deficiency
	Kuan Dong Hua (Flos Tussilaginis Farfarae) *Bai Bu* (Radix Stemonae) *Wu Mei* (Fructus Pruni Mume)	Enduring, persistent cough due to Lung-cold
	E Jiao (Gelatinum Corii Asini) *Wu Wei Zi* (Fructus Schisandrae) *Chuan Bei Mu* (Bulbus Fritillariae Cirrhosae)	Pulmonary consumption cough with blood-streaked sputum

Kuan Dong Hua 款冬花 (Coltsfoot flower, Flos Tussilaginis Farfarae)

Kuan Dong Hua is the dried flower-bud of *Tussilago farfara* L., family Compositae.

Main ingredients *Kuan Dong Hua* contains rutin, quercetin, hyperin, tussilagone, tussilagin, faradiol, phytosterol, taraxanthin, tannin, ferulic acid and caffeic acid.

Properties Taste: acrid; nature: warm.

Channel entered Lung.

Functions and indications Moistens the Lungs and causes Qi to descend, stops coughing and transforms Phlegm. It is indicated for various types of cough.

Common dosage 5-10g.

Remarks The raw herb is used for externally-contracted fulminant cough, whereas *Kuan Dong Hua* mix-fried with honey is better for enduring cough due to internal damage.

Comparison of functions Both *Kuan Dong Hua* (Flos Tussilaginis Farfarae) and *Zi Wan* (Radix Asteris Tatarici) have the effect of warming and moistening Lung Qi to stop coughing and transform Phlegm. *Kuan Dong Hua* is better at stopping coughing, whereas *Zi Wan* is more effective in transforming Phlegm. *Kuan Dong Hua* is more suitable for cough due to heat damaging the Lungs, *Zi Wan* for cough due to externally-contracted wind-cold. The two herbs are often processed with honey to treat a variety of coughs with copious sputum.

Modern research

1. Stops coughing and calms wheezing, expels sputum.[60, 70]
2. Benefits breathing, increases external resistance and raises blood pressure.[72]
3. Inhibits haematoblastic concentration.[60]
4. Stimulates the central nervous system and inhibits intestinal muscular contraction, relieves convulsions.[72]

Combinations and applications

Functions	Combinations	Applications
Moistening the Lungs and causing Qi to descend, stopping coughing and transforming Phlegm	*Bai He* (Bulbus Lilii)	Enduring cough with blood-streaked sputum due to Yin deficiency
	Zi Wan (Radix Asteris Tatarici)	Persistent cough due to pathogenic heat damaging the Lungs
	Xing Ren (Semen Pruni Armeniacae) *Zhi Mu* (Rhizoma Anemarrhenae Asphodeloidis) *Zhe Bei Mu* (Bulbus Fritillariae Thunbergii) *Sang Bai Pi* (Cortex Mori Albae Radicis)	Fulminant cough with copious sputum due to dry-heat damaging the Lungs
	Ma Huang (Herba Ephedrae) (see notes on legal status) *Zi Wan* (Radix Asteris Tatarici) *Xi Xin* (Herba cum Radice Asari) *Gan Jiang* (Rhizoma Zingiberis Officinalis)	Cough with sputum, shortness of breath and pain in the chest due to cold fluids
	Yi Yi Ren (Semen Coicis Lachrymajobi) *Gan Cao* (Radix Glycyrrhizae) *Jie Geng* (Radix Platycodi Grandiflori)	Lung abscess, cough with smelly sputum, chills, dry mouth and throat, rapid pulse

Ma Dou Ling 马兜铃
(Aristolochia fruit, Fructus Aristolochiae)

Ma Dou Ling is the dried capsule of *Aristolochia contorta* Bge. or *A. debilis* Sieb. et Zucc., family Aristolochiaceae.

Legal status At the time of publication, the Medicines (*Aristolochia* and Mu Tong etc.) (Prohibition) Order 2001 renders illegal in the UK the sale, supply and importation of unlicensed medicines for human use containing or presented as containing this herb. The prohibition of the use of this herb has been implemented as a result of the toxic nature of various aristolochia plants.

Main ingredients *Ma Dou Ling* contains aristolochic acid, aristolochine, aristolochinic acid and magnoflorine.

Properties Taste: bitter and slightly acrid; nature: cold.

Channels entered Lung and Large Intestine.

Functions and indications Clears the Lungs and transforms Phlegm, stops coughing and calms wheezing, clears the Intestines and disperses haemorrhoids. It is indicated for coughing and wheezing due to Lung-heat, coughing of blood, loss of voice, and swelling and pain from haemorrhoids.

Common dosage 3-10g.

Precautions and contraindications

1. Since *Ma Dou Ling* is acrid and cold, it can easily damage Stomach Qi; it is therefore contraindicated in all cases of loose stool due to Spleen deficiency and cough due to deficiency-cold.
2. A large dosage of *Ma Dou Ling* may induce vomiting.

Remarks Raw *Ma Dou Ling* is used for cough due to Lung-heat, whereas the herb mix-fried with honey is better for enduring cough due to Lung deficiency.

Toxicity For information on the toxic effects of aristolochic acid, reference should be made to the toxicity section of *Mu Tong* (see Chapter 6).

Modern research

1. Expands the bronchus and expels sputum.[73]
2. Lowers blood pressure, strengthens the immune function, and promotes the production of blood.[34, 73]
3. An aqueous extract of *Ma Dou Ling* inhibited Trichophyton schoenleinii and other dermatophytes *in vitro*.[34, 73]
4. Overdosage can result in blood in the urine and difficulty in breathing.[74]

Combinations and applications

Functions	Combinations	Applications
Clearing the Lungs and transforming Phlegm, stopping coughing and calming wheezing	*Huang Qin* (Radix Scutellariae Baicalensis) *Sang Bai Pi* (Cortex Mori Albae Radicis) *Xing Ren* (Semen Pruni Armeniacae)	Cough with copious, sticky sputum and pain in the chest due to Lung-heat
	Xing Ren (Semen Pruni Armeniacae) *E Jiao* (Gelatinum Corii Asini) *Niu Bang Zi* (Fructus Arctii Lappae)	Enduring cough with dry mouth and sparse sputum or blood-streaked sputum due to exuberant Yin deficiency-fire in the Liver channel, with a red tongue and thin tongue body
Clearing the Intestines and dispersing haemorrhoids	*Jin Yin Hua* (Flos Lonicerae) *Huai Hua* (Flos Sophorae Japonicae) *Xiao Ji* (Herba Cephalanoploris seu Cirsii)	Bleeding, pain and swelling due to haemorrhoids

Note: In addition, *Ma Dou Ling* can be used with *Huang Qin* (Radix Scutellariae Baicalensis), *Xia Ku Cao* (Spica Prunellae Vulgaris) and *Gou Teng* (Ramulus Uncariae cum Uncis) to treat hypertension manifesting as dizziness, headache and red face due to ascendant hyperactivity of Liver Yang.

Pi Pa Ye 枇杷叶 (Loquat leaf, Folium Eriobotryae Japonicae)

Pi Pa Ye is the dried leaf of *Eriobotrya japonica* (Thunb.) Lindl., family Rosaceae.

Main ingredients *Pi Pa Ye* contains tormentic acid, ursolic acid, oleanolic acid, nerolidol, farnesol, amygdalin, caryophyllin, tannin, and vitamins B_1 and C.

Properties Taste: bitter; nature: slightly cold.

Channels entered Lung and Stomach.

Functions and indications Clears the Lungs, transforms Phlegm and stops coughing, harmonizes the Stomach, bears counterflow Qi downwards and stops vomiting. It is indicated for coughing and wheezing due to Lung-heat, coughing of blood, and nausea and vomiting due to Stomach-heat.

Common dosage 10-15g.

Precautions and contraindications *Pi Pa Ye* is contraindicated in cases of coughing and wheezing due to Lung-cold and vomiting due to Stomach-cold.

Remarks Raw *Pi Pa Ye* is used to stop vomiting, whereas the mix-fried herb is better for stopping coughing.

Comparison of functions Although both *Pi Pa Ye* (Folium Eriobotryae Japonicae) and *Ban Xia* (Rhizoma Pinelliae Ternatae) can treat disorders in the Lung and Stomach channels, they are of a different nature. *Pi Pa Ye*, cold and moist, is mainly used to clear and bear heat downwards in the Lung and Stomach channels, whereas *Ban Xia*, warm and dry, is used to dry dampness and transform Phlegm. When treating disorders in the Lungs, *Pi Pa Ye* works by clearing and bearing Lung-heat downwards to stop coughing and transform Phlegm; it is often used for Phlegm-heat and for cough due to dryness in the Lungs. By contrast, when treating these disorders, *Ban Xia* works by fortifying the Spleen and drying dampness to transform Phlegm; it is often used for Phlegm-damp and cold-Phlegm patterns. When used for disorders in the Stomach, *Pi Pa Ye* clears and bears Stomach-heat downwards to treat vomiting and thirst due to heat, whereas *Ban Xia* transforms Phlegm-fluids to harmonize the Stomach and stop vomiting. It is more often used for nausea and vomiting due to Phlegm-damp invading the Stomach.

Modern research

1. The laetrile contained in *Pi Pa Ye* stops coughing, calms wheezing and expels sputum.[75]
2. Inhibits microzymes in the digestive tract.[73]
3. Inhibits carcinoma.[76]

Combinations and applications

Functions	Combinations	Applications
Clearing the Lungs, transforming Phlegm and stopping coughing	*Nan Sha Shen* (Radix Adenophorae) *Sang Bai Pi* (Cortex Mori Albae Radicis) *Bai Mao Gen* (Rhizoma Imperatae Cylindricae)	Cough, dry throat and coughing of blood due to dry-heat
	Qian Hu (Radix Peucedani) *Sang Ye* (Folium Mori Albae)	Cough due to wind-heat
	Sang Bai Pi (Cortex Mori Albae Radicis) *Huang Lian* (Rhizoma Coptidis) *Huang Bai* (Cortex Phellodendri) *Ren Shen* (Radix Ginseng) *Gan Cao* (Radix Glycyrrhizae)	Cough with yellow sputum, dry mouth and a bitter taste in the mouth due to Lung-heat

	Dan Zhu Ye (Herba Lophatheri Gracilis)	Hoarse voice
Harmonizing the Stomach, bearing counterflow Qi downwards and stopping vomiting	*Chen Pi* (Pericarpium Citri Reticulatae) *Ban Xia* (Rhizoma Pinelliae Ternatae) *Zhu Ru* (Caulis Bambusae in Taeniis) *Lu Gen* (Rhizoma Phragmitis Communis) *Mai Men Dong* (Radix Ophiopogonis Japonici)	Nausea, vomiting, and vexation and dry mouth due to Stomach-heat
	Ren Shen (Radix Ginseng) *Fu Ling* (Sclerotium Poriae Cocos) *Sheng Jiang* (Rhizoma Zingiberis Officinalis Recens)	Nausea and vomiting and focal distension in the chest due to ascendant counterflow of Stomach Qi caused by Qi deficiency

Ai Di Cha 矮地茶
(Japanese ardisia, Herba Ardisiae Japonicae)

Ai Di Cha is the whole plant of *Ardisia japonica* (Hornst.) Bl., family Myrsinaceae.

Main ingredients *Ai Di Cha* contains bergenin, ilexol, quercitrin, myricitrin, 2-hydroxyphenylacetic acid, tannin and volatile oils.

Properties Taste: acrid and bitter; nature: neutral.

Channels entered Lung and Liver.

Functions and indications Stops coughing and dispels Phlegm, clears damp-heat and abates jaundice, promotes the movement of water and percolates dampness, quickens the Blood and transforms stasis, frees menstruation and alleviates pain. It is indicated for coughing and wheezing with copious sputum, damp-heat jaundice, oedema, knocks and falls, wind-damp Bi syndrome pain, and menstrual block with pain in the abdomen.

Common dosage 10-30g.

Remarks Since *Ai Di Cha* is neutral in nature, it can be used for coughing and wheezing due both to Lung-heat and cold-Phlegm.

Modern research

1. Stops coughing, expels sputum and calms wheezing.[77]
2. A decoction of *Ai Di Cha* inhibited Staphylococcus aureus in laboratory tests.[78]

Combinations and applications

Functions	Combinations	Applications
Stopping coughing and dispelling Phlegm	*Pi Pa Ye* (Folium Eriobotryae Japonicae) *Ye Ju Hua* (Flos Chrysanthemi Indici) *Gan Cao* (Radix Glycyrrhizae)	Cough with copious sputum due to Lung-heat
	Ma Huang (Herba Ephedrae) (see notes on legal status) *Xi Xin* (Herba cum Radice Asari)	Cough due to cold-Phlegm
	Bai Bu (Radix Stemonae) *Sang Bai Pi* (Cortex Mori Albae Radicis) *Bai Ji* (Rhizoma Bletillae Striatae)	Cough with blood-streaked sputum due to pulmonary consumption

Clearing damp-heat and abating jaundice	*Yin Chen Hao* (Herba Artemisiae Scopariae) *Zhi Zi* (Fructus Gardeniae Jasminoidis) *Hu Zhang* (Radix et Rhizoma Polygoni Cuspidati)	Damp-heat jaundice
Promoting the movement of water and percolating dampness	*Fu Ling* (Sclerotium Poriae Cocos) *Ze Xie* (Rhizoma Alismatis Orientalis) *Che Qian Zi* (Semen Plantaginis)	Puffy swelling of the face and eyes and inhibited urination due to water and dampness collecting internally
Quickening the Blood and transforming stasis, freeing menstruation and alleviating pain	*Su Mu* (Lignum Sappan) *Dang Gui* (Radix Angelicae Sinensis) *Hong Hua* (Flos Carthami Tinctorii)	Knocks and falls with swelling and pain at the site of the injury
	Wei Ling Xian (Radix Clematidis) *Fang Ji* (Radix Stephaniae Tetrandrae) (see notes on legal status)	Wind-damp Bi syndrome pain, numbness of the joints, inhibited bending and stretching
	Yi Mu Cao (Herba Leonuri Heterophylli) *Chuan Xiong* (Rhizoma Ligustici Chuanxiong) *Dang Gui* (Radix Angelicae Sinensis)	Menstrual block with pain in the abdomen

Bai Guo 白果
(Ginkgo nut, Semen Ginkgo Bilobae)

Bai Guo is the dried ripe seed of *Ginkgo biloba* L., family Ginkgoaceae.

Legal status *Bai Guo* was listed in a document entitled *A Review of Restricted Herbal Ingredients* issued by the Medicines Control Agency (MCA) in the UK in September 2001 with a view to the possible imposition of restrictions on its use at a future date. The MCA is concerned that the seed contains a substance (4-O-methylpyridoxine) that can cause severe allergic reactions and convulsions.

Main ingredients *Bai Guo* contains flavone compounds (including kaempferol, quercetin, isorhamnetin, rutin and bilobetin), ginkgolic acid, hydroginkgolic acid, gingkolinic acid, ginkgol, bilobol, ginnol and gibberellin.

Properties Taste: sweet, bitter and astringent; nature: neutral; slightly toxic.

Channel entered Lung.

Functions and indications Constrains the Lungs and stabilizes wheezing, stops vaginal discharge and reduces urine. It is indicated for cough with copious sputum, wheezing, vaginal discharge, urinary turbidity, and frequent urination.

Common dosage 6–10g.

Precautions and contraindications

1. Raw *Bai Guo* is slightly toxic, so this herb should not be used raw in large dosages.
2. *Bai Guo* should be used with caution for cough with sticky sputum and difficult expectoration.

Toxicity The LD_{50} for intraperitoneal injection in mice of an extract of the outer husk of the seed of *Bai Guo* is 5.02 ± 0.31g/kg. Raw *Bai Guo* is comparatively toxic, the green plumule being the most toxic part. The toxic elements of *Bai Guo* are soluble and are reduced by heating. The ingestion of raw *Bai Guo* can result in irritation of the gastrointestinal tract; after absorption, the toxins can affect the nervous system. Toxic quantities vary from 7 to 150 seeds for children and from 40 to 300 seeds for adults. Symptoms of toxic reaction are similar to those for *Xing Ren*.

Modern research Preparations of *Bai Guo* inhibited staphylococci, streptococci, Corynebacterium diphtheriae, Escherichia coli and Bacillus anthracis *in vitro*.[34, 79]

Combinations and applications

Functions	Combinations	Applications
Constraining the Lungs and stabilizing wheezing	*Ma Huang* (Herba Ephedrae) (see notes on legal status) *Gan Cao* (Radix Glycyrrhizae)	Wheezing with productive cough and sputum
	Sang Bai Pi (Cortex Mori Albae Radicis) *Huang Qin* (Radix Scutellariae Baicalensis)	Cough with copious sputum and hasty breathing due to Lung-heat
	He Zi (Fructus Terminaliae Chebulae)	Enduring cough or night cough due to Yin deficiency
Stopping vaginal discharge and reducing urine	*Lian Zi* (Semen Nelumbinis Nuciferae) *Hu Jiao* (Fructus Piperis Nigri)	Vaginal discharge due to Yang deficiency in the Lower Jiao
	Qian Shi (Semen Euryales Ferocis) *Huang Bai* (Cortex Phellodendri)	Yellow and smelly vaginal discharge due to damp-heat
	Bi Xie (Rhizoma Dioscoreae) *Yi Zhi Ren* (Fructus Alpiniae Oxyphyllae)	Urinary turbidity

Yang Jin Hua 洋金花
(Datura flower, Flos Daturae)

Yang Jin Hua is the dried flower of *Datura metel L.*, family Solanaceae.

Legal status *Yang Jin Hua* was listed in a document entitled *A Review of Restricted Herbal Ingredients* issued by the Medicines Control Agency (MCA) in the UK in September 2001 with a view to the possible imposition of restrictions on its use at a future date. The MCA is concerned that a related plant, *Datura stramonium*, listed in Schedule II of The Medicines (Retail Sale or Supply of Herbal Remedies) Order 1977, is subject to dosage restrictions and can only be sold through registered pharmacies.

Main ingredients *Yang Jin Hua* contains tropine, scopolamine, hyoscyamine, atropine and datumetine.

Properties Taste: acrid; nature: warm; extremely toxic.

Channels entered Heart, Lung and Spleen.

Functions and indications Stops coughing and calms wheezing, alleviates pain, and relieves tetany. It is indicated for coughing and wheezing due to cold-Phlegm with little or no sputum, cold and pain in the stomach and abdomen, wind-damp Bi syndrome pain, and convulsions and spasms.

Common dosage 0.3-0.6g, in powder form for oral use; no more than 1.5g per day when added to cigarettes; appropriate dosage for external application.

Precautions and contraindications *Yang Jin Hua* is extremely toxic and the dosage should be strictly controlled to avoid poisoning. This herb is contraindicated in cases of externally-contracted cough and cough due to Phlegm-heat and for patients with glaucoma or hypertension; it should be used with caution for patients with heart problems or a weak constitution, and during pregnancy. Since *Yang Jin Hua* inhibits sweating, it should not be used for unreleased exterior patterns.

Remarks *Yang Jin Hua* has a relatively drastic action and is effective for coughing and wheezing, being used principally for cough with little or no sputum or for cold coughing and wheezing. Since it strongly alleviates pain, it can be used as the principal constituent of an anaesthetic.

Toxicity The minimum lethal dosage for intravenous injection in dogs of the alkaloids contained in *Yang Jin Hua* is 75-80mg/kg. Overdosage can cause dry mouth, dry skin, hoarse voice, tachycardia, reddening of the skin, headache and dizziness, and in severe cases, convulsions and coma.

Modern research

1. Alleviates pain.[80]
2. Inhibits convulsion of the trachea smooth muscle and inhibits glandular secretion.[81, 82]

Combinations and applications

Functions	Combinations	Applications
Stopping coughing and calming wheezing	*Dan Nan Xing* (Pulvis Arisaematis cum Felle Bovis) *Wu Wei Zi* (Fructus Schisandrae) *Ma Huang* (Herba Ephedrae) (see notes on legal status)	Coughing and wheezing, enduring and persistent cough due to the Lungs failing to diffuse and bear downwards
Alleviating pain	*Cao Wu* (Radix Aconiti Kusnezoffii) (see notes on legal status) *Chuan Xiong* (Rhizoma Ligustici Chuanxiong) *Fang Ji* (Radix Stephaniae Tetrandrae) (see notes on legal status)	Wind-damp Bi syndrome pain, knocks and falls (used externally as an anaesthetic)
Relieving tetany	*Quan Xie* (Buthus Martensi) *Tian Ma* (Rhizoma Gastrodiae Elatae) (see notes on legal status) *Tian Nan Xing* (Rhizoma Arisaematis)	Spasms and convulsions, epilepsy and fright wind

Additional applications:

1. *Yang Jin Hua* can be ground into a powder and mixed with an equal amount of leaf tobacco for smoking as a cigarette to treat coughing and wheezing due to cold-Phlegm with little or no sputum.
2. *Yang Jin Hua* can be taken orally for cold and pain in the stomach and abdomen.
3. An external wash of *Yang Jin Hua* can treat wind-damp Bi syndrome and knocks and falls.

Modern research references

1. Zou Jilong et al., *Shan Dong Zhong Yi Xue Yuan Xue Bao* [Journal of Shandong College of Traditional Chinese Medicine] 16, 1 (1992): 54.
2. Yan Shouye et al., *Zhong Cao Yao* [Journal of Chinese Herbs] 19, 8 (1988): 37.
3. Xiong Sufang et al., *Bei Jing Zhong Yi Za Zhi* [Beijing Journal of Traditional Chinese Medicine] 6 (1987): 51.
4. Tao Zongjin et al., *Sheng Li Xue Bao* [Physiology Journal] 35, 1 (1983): 107.
5. Xia Linna et al., *Shang Hai Di Yi Yi Xue Yuan Xue Bao* [Journal of Shanghai No. 1 Medical College] 13, 3 (1985): 193.
6. Liu Shouyi et al., *Zhong Yao Yao Li Yu Lin Chuang* [Pharmacology and Clinical Application of Chinese Materia Medica] 9, 3 (1993): 27.
7. Clinic 4 of Houzi 236 Unit, *Health Research* 3 (1972): 18.
8. Teng Shouzhi et al., *Zhong Hua Xin Xue Guan Bing Za Zhi* [Chinese Journal of Cardiology] 11, 2 (1983): 34.
9. Liu Jiling et al., *Cheng Du Zhong Yi Xue Yuan Xue Bao* [Journal of Chengdu College of TCM] 12, 2 (1989): 105.
10. Pharmacology Institute of the Chinese Academy of Science, *Zhong Yao Zhi* [Chinese Materia Medica Records], volume 2 (Beijing: People's Medical Publishing House, 1982), 32.
11. Xue Guohua et al., *Xi An Yi Xue Yuan Xue Bao* [Journal of Xi'an Medical College] 5 (1985): 22.
12. Xiao Zhixiong et al., *Si Chuan Da Xue Xue Bao* [Journal of Sichuan University] 1 (1985): 92.
13. Wang Yixiong et al., *Zhong Guo Yao Li Tong Bao* [Chinese Bulletin of Pharmacology] 7, 5 (1986): 435.

14. Chan Dongming et al., *Zhong Yao Tong Bao* [Bulletin of Chinese Materia Medica] 4 (1981): 23.
15. Wang Caixia et al., *He Bei Zhong Yi* [Hebei Journal of Traditional Chinese Medicine] 12, 2 (1990): 5.
16. He Xingdong et al., *Lin Chuang Zhong Yao Shou Ce* [Clinical Handbook of Chinese Materia Medica] (Beijing: People's Medical Publishing House, 1998), 237.
17. Ding Xuemin et al., *Chang Yong Zhong Yi Fang Yao Shou Ce* [Handbook of Commonly-Used Chinese Herbs and Prescriptions] (Changsha: Hunan Science and Technology Publishing House, 1982), 33.
18. Lei Zaiquan and Zhang Tingmo, *Zhong Hua Lin Chuang Zhong Yao Xue* [Chinese Clinical Materia Medica] (Beijing: People's Medical Publishing House, 1998), 1320.
19. He Xingdong et al., *Lin Chuang Zhong Yao Shou Ce*, 235.
20. Pharmacological Group of Xi'an Medical College, *Shan Xi Xin Yi Yao* [Shaanxi New Medical Journal] 3 (1975): 51.
21. Lei Zaiquan and Zhang Tingmo, *Zhong Hua Lin Chuang Zhong Yao Xue*, 1303.
22. Jia Yuyin et al., *Zhong Yao Tong Bao* [Bulletin of Chinese Materia Medica] 12, 11 (1987): 35.
23. Gao Yingdou et al., *Zhong Hua Yi Xue Za Zhi* [Chinese Journal of Medicine] 5 (1954): 331.
24. Zhou Bangjing et al., *Zhe Jiang Zhong Yi Za Zhi* [Zhejiang Journal of Traditional Chinese Medicine] 11, 12 (1980): 286.
25. Pharmacology Group of the Second Military Medical University, *Preparation of the extract of inula flower and pharmacological experiments performed* (1972).
26. P. Azoulay et al., *Pharm Acta Helv* 6, 12 (1986): 345.
27. Lei Zaiquan and Zhang Tingmo, *Zhong Hua Lin Chuang Zhong Yao Xue*, 1309.
28. He Xingdong et al., *Lin Chuang Zhong Yao Shou Ce*, 238.
29. Lei Zaiquan and Zhang Tingmo, *Zhong Hua Lin Chuang Zhong Yao Xue*, 1322.
30. He Xingdong et al., *Lin Chuang Zhong Yao Shou Ce*, 240.
31. Xi Zhaoqing et al., *Shan Xi Zhong Yi* [Shaanxi Journal of Traditional Chinese Medicine] 11, 3 (1990): 108.
32. Ling Hong et al., *Hu Bei Yi Xue Yuan Xue Bao* [Journal of Hubei Medical College] 92, 2 (1988): 138.
33. Pierre Casellas et al., *Eur Biochem* 176, 3 (1988): 581.
34. Lei Zaiquan and Zhang Tingmo, *Zhong Hua Lin Chuang Zhong Yao Xue*, 1330.
35. Wu Xin et al., *Zhong Guo Yao Li Xue Bao* [Chinese Journal of Pharmacology] 11, 3 (1990): 235.
36. Wu Xin et al., *Zhong Guo Yao Li Xue Yu Du Li Xue Za Zhi* [Chinese Journal of Pharmacology and Toxicology] 4, 2 (1990): 104.
37. He Fanzhong, *Jiang Su Zhong Yi Za Zhi* [Jiangsu Journal of Traditional Chinese Medicine] 8 (1981): 358.
38. Ding Xuemin et al., *Chang Yong Zhong Yi Fang Yao Shou Ce*, 330.
39. He Xingdong et al., *Lin Chuang Zhong Yao Shou Ce*, 242.
40. Lei Zaiquan and Zhang Tingmo, *Zhong Hua Lin Chuang Zhong Yao Xue*, 1336.
41. Zhu Liqing et al., *Zhong Cao Yao* [Journal of Chinese Herbs] 21, 1 (1990): 22.
42. He Xingdong et al., *Lin Chuang Zhong Yao Shou Ce*, 241.
43. Ibid., 245.
44. Lei Zaiquan and Zhang Tingmo, *Zhong Hua Lin Chuang Zhong Yao Xue*, 1356.
45. Zhang Helin et al., *Zhong Guo Hai Yang Yao Wu* [Chinese Marine Materia Medica] 7, 4 (1988): 18.
46. Ji Ningbin et al., *Zhong Guo Hai Yang Yao Wu* 13, 2 (1994): 20.
47. Zhang Rongrui et al., *Nan Jing Zhong Yi Xue Yuan Xue Bao* [Journal of Nanjing College of Traditional Chinese Medicine] 4 (1988): 57.
48. Hou Yuli, *Zhong Cao Yao* [Journal of Chinese Herbs] 15, 12 (1984): 19.
49. Sun Shixi et al., *Zhong Guo Hai Yang Yao Wu* [Chinese Marine Materia Medica] 8, 1 (1989): 56.
50. Zhao Xuezeng et al., *Zhong Guo Yao Li Tong Bao* [Chinese Bulletin of Pharmacology] 9, 3 (1993): 221.
51. Deng Huaichun et al., *Zhong Cao Yao* [Journal of Chinese Herbs] 18, 2 (1987): 15.
52. Lei Zaiquan and Zhang Tingmo, *Zhong Hua Lin Chuang Zhong Yao Xue*, 627.
53. He Xingdong et al., *Lin Chuang Zhong Yao Shou Ce*, 247.
54. Wang Benxian, *Xin Bian Zhong Yao Xue Ci Dian* [New Dictionary of Chinese Materia Medica] (Tianjin: Tianjin Science and Technology Publishing House, 1996), 1087.
55. Ma Qingjun et al., *Chang Yong Zhong Yao Xian Dai Yan Jiu Yu Lin Chuang* [Current Research and Clinical Application of Commonly-Used Chinese Materia Medica] (Tianjin: Tianjin Science and Technology Translation Publishing House, 1995), 464.
56. Liu Bingkun et al., *Zhong Guo Yi Xue Za Zhi* [China Medical Journal] 67, 7 (1987): 408.
57. Chen Shuimu, *Modern Application of Medicine* 8, 3 (1991): 44.
58. Nagamoto Tensei et al., *Sheng Yao Xue Za Zhi* [Journal of Raw Herbs] 42, 1 (1988): 81.
59. Xue Wanli, *Xin Yao Yu Lin Chuang* [New Drugs and Clinical Applications] 3, 5 (1984): 37.
60. He Xingdong et al., *Lin Chuang Zhong Yao Shou Ce*, 251.
61. Lei Zaiquan and Zhang Tingmo, *Zhong Hua Lin Chuang Zhong Yao Xue*, 1369.
62. He Xingdong et al., *Lin Chuang Zhong Yao Shou Ce*, 249.

63. Ding Xuemin et al., *Chang Yong Zhong Yi Fang Yao Shou Ce*, 40.
64. Lei Zaiquan and Zhang Tingmo, *Zhong Hua Lin Chuang Zhong Yao Xue*, 1378.
65. He Xingdong et al., *Lin Chuang Zhong Yao Shou Ce*, 252.
66. Lei Zaiquan and Zhang Tingmo, *Zhong Hua Lin Chuang Zhong Yao Xue*, 1334.
67. He Xingdong et al., *Lin Chuang Zhong Yao Shou Ce*, 253.
68. Ding Xuemin et al., *Chang Yong Zhong Yi Fang Yao Shou Ce*, 35.
69. He Xingdong et al., *Lin Chuang Zhong Yao Shou Ce*, 250.
70. Ding Xuemin et al., *Chang Yong Zhong Yi Fang Yao Shou Ce,* 39.
71. Lei Zaiquan and Zhang Tingmo, *Zhong Hua Lin Chuang Zhong Yao Xue*, 1305.
72. Ibid., 1371.
73. He Xingdong et al., *Lin Chuang Zhong Yao Shou Ce*, 254.
74. Lei Zaiquan and Zhang Tingmo, *Zhong Hua Lin Chuang Zhong Yao Xue*, 1375.
75. Editorial Group of Sichuan Chinese Herbal Records, *Sichuan Chinese Herbal Records*, volume 1 (Chengdu: Sichuan People's Publishing House, 1980), 144.
76. Lei Zaiquan and Zhang Tingmo, *Zhong Hua Lin Chuang Zhong Yao Xue*, 1381.
77. Yan Zhenghua, *Zhong Yao Xue* [Chinese Materia Medica] (Beijing: People's Medical Publishing House, 1991), 562.
78. Wu Baojie, *Zhong Cao Yao Yao Li Xue* [Pharmacology of Chinese Herbs] (Beijing: People's Medical Publishing House, 1983), 178.
79. He Xingdong et al., *Lin Chuang Zhong Yao Shou Ce*, 256.
80. Pian Chunpu et al., *Zhong Ma Tong Xun* [Chinese Anaesthetics Newsletter] 3-4 (1978): 6.
81. Bao Tou Medical School Pharmacology Teaching Group, *Bao Tou Yi Xue* [Bao Tou Journal of Medicine] 4 (1977): 61.
82. Bethune International Peace Hospital, *Zhong Xi Yi Jie He Ci Liao* [Papers on Integrated TCM and Western Medicine] 14 (1975): 4.

Chapter 14

Substances for quieting the Spirit

安神药

Substances for quieting the Spirit

Herbs and other substances for quieting the Spirit function mainly as tranquillizing agents and are used to treat disorders of disquieted Heart and Spirit.

These substances can be divided into two categories depending on their nature – substances that settle fright and quiet the Spirit and herbs that nourish the Heart and quiet the Spirit. Most of the substances in the first category are minerals, fossils or shells that are heavy in weight and have a downward-bearing action. Many of the herbs in the second category are seeds which are sweet and moist in nature and have an enriching and nourishing action.

Substances for quieting the Spirit are mainly used to treat vexation and agitation, palpitations, insomnia, child fright wind, mania and withdrawal, and depression patterns, where these are caused by deficiency of Heart-Blood, insufficiency of Heart Qi, or Heart-fire or Liver-fire flaming upwards.

Although these substances can be used to treat disorders of disquieted Heart and Spirit, they cannot deal with any other accompanying pathogenic factors on their own. Hence, they should be used in combination with other herbs according to the principle of treating the root (*běn*) and the manifestation (*biāo*) of the disorder simultaneously. These combinations are listed below:

1. in cases due to full-heat, substances for quieting the Spirit should be used with herbs for clearing heat and draining fire;
2. in cases due to ascendant hyperactivity of Liver Yang, select herbs for calming the Liver and subduing Yang alongside substances for quieting the Spirit;
3. in cases due to deficiency of Blood and Yin deficiency of the Heart and Liver, these substances should be combined with herbs for nourishing Yin and supplementing the Blood;
4. in cases due to internal damage to the seven emotions, these substances should be used with herbs for allowing constrained Liver Qi to flow freely;
5. for mania and withdrawal and fright wind, substances for quieting the Spirit are often combined with herbs for opening the orifices and transforming Phlegm, or with herbs for calming the Liver and extinguishing wind.

SUBSTANCES FOR SETTLING FRIGHT AND QUIETING THE SPIRIT

Most of the substances used to settle fright and quiet the Spirit are heavy in weight and originate from minerals, fossils or shells. They are mainly used for palpitations, insomnia, vexation and agitation, as well as for mania and withdrawal caused by Heart-fire or Liver-fire flaming upwards or by exuberant Yang Qi. In cases of fire flaming upwards, these substances should be combined with herbs for clearing heat and draining fire; in cases of ascendant hyperactivity of Liver Yang, they should be used with herbs for calming the Liver and subduing Yang.

Since most of these substances are cold or slightly cold in nature and heavy in weight, it is easy for them to damage Stomach Qi and cause indigestion. As a result, they should be used with herbs for nourishing the Stomach and fortifying the Spleen in order to prevent damage to Stomach Qi.

Tab. 14.1 Substances for settling fright and quieting the Spirit

Herb	Functions	Indications
Zhu Sha (Cinnabaris)	Settling the Heart and quieting the Spirit, clearing heat and relieving toxicity	Palpitations, insomnia, mania and withdrawal, dizziness, swelling and toxins of sores, sore throat, mouth sores
Ci Shi (Magnetitum)	Calming the Liver and subduing Yang, settling fright and quieting the Spirit, sharpening the hearing and brightening the eyes, hosting Qi and stabilizing wheezing	Dizziness, tinnitus and deafness, palpitations, insomnia, disquieted Heart and Spirit, wheezing due to Kidney deficiency
Long Gu (Os Draconis)	Settling fright and quieting the Spirit, calming the Liver and subduing Yang, promoting contraction and securing astriction, stopping vaginal discharge and seminal emission	Mania and withdrawal, fright epilepsy, palpitations, forgetfulness, insomnia, spontaneous sweating and night sweating, seminal emission, urinary turbidity, uterine bleeding, vaginal discharge, diarrhoea, dysentery, non-closure of open sores
Hu Po (Succinum)	Settling fright and quieting the Spirit, quickening the Blood and dissipating stasis, promoting urination and freeing Lin syndrome	Fright wind and epilepsy, insomnia, and heat, blood and stone Lin syndromes

Zhu Sha 朱砂
(Cinnabar, Cinnabaris)

Zhu Sha is a red mineral ore crystallizing in the hexagonal system.

Legal status The use of this materia medica is illegal in the UK as a result of its toxic nature.

Main ingredients *Zhu Sha* contains up to 96% of mercuric sulphide (HgS) as well as small amounts of lead, barium, magnesium, iron, zinc and ferric oxide.

Properties Taste: sweet; nature: slightly cold; toxic.

Channel entered Heart.

Functions and indications Settles the Heart and quiets the Spirit, clears heat and relieves toxicity. It is indicated for palpitations, insomnia, mania and withdrawal, dizziness, swelling and toxins of sores, sore throat, and mouth sores.

Common dosage 0.3-1g, prepared as powder or pills for oral use, or decocted with other herbs; appropriate dosage for external application.

Precautions and contraindications

1. *Zhu Sha* must not be used internally in large dosages or for a prolonged period in order to avoid giving rise to toxic side-effects.
2. *Zhu Sha* should be used with caution in cases with abnormal functioning of the liver and kidneys.
3. In order to avoid releasing the mercury in *Zhu Sha*, it must not be calcined.

Comparison of functions See *Ci Shi* (Magnetitum) and *Hu Po* (Succinum).

Toxicity The LD_{5C} for intravenous injection in mice of *Zhu Sha* in medicinal form is 12.1g/kg. Acute toxicity tests on mice fed a 9.5g/kg suspended solution of *Zhu Sha* containing 3% starch via intragastric administration resulted in no deaths from toxic causes. *Zhu Sha* contains inorganic mercury compounds. Where high concentrations of mercury build up in the body, the central nervous system may be damaged. Prolonged use and overdosage can result in such toxic effects as vomiting of bloody mucus, pain in the abdomen, purulent and bloody urine, and trembling of the muscles; in severe cases, manifestations can include oliguria or ischuria, oedema, coma and convulsions, a reduction in blood pressure and renal failure resulting in death. Strict control of dosage and length of administration is extremely important.

Modern research

1. Has tranquillizing and anti-convulsion functions.[1]
2. Inhibits such bacteria as Streptococcus pyogenes, Pseudomonas pyocyanea and Staphylococcus aureus.[2]
3. External use of *Zhu Sha* kills parasites.[2]
4. The high concentration of mercury from overdosage of *Zhu Sha* can inhibit the activity of polyenzymes and damage the central nervous system (see *Toxicity*).[2]

Combinations and applications

Functions	Combinations	Applications
Settling the Heart and quieting the Spirit	*Sheng Di Huang* (Radix Rehmanniae Glutinosae) *Huang Lian* (Rhizoma Coptidis) *Dang Gui* (Radix Angelicae Sinensis) *Zhi Gan Cao* (Radix Glycyrrhizae Praeparata)	Vexation and agitation, fearful throbbing, a sensation of heat in the chest, insomnia, profuse dreaming, a red tongue and a fine, rapid pulse due to Heart-fire flaming upwards and damaging Yin-Blood
	Suan Zao Ren (Semen Ziziphi Spinosae) *Ru Xiang* (Gummi Olibanum) *Huang Jiu* (Vinum Aureum)	Mania and withdrawal, manic ravings and frenetic movement, sudden loss of consciousness, foaming at the mouth due to pathogenic wind

	Ci Shi (Magnetitum) *Shen Qu* (Massa Fermentata) (prepared as pills for oral use)	Palpitations, insomnia, tinnitus and deafness, blurred vision, and epilepsy due to non-interaction of the Heart and Kidneys
	Cooked inside a pig's heart	Palpitations, fearful throbbing and seminal emission due to fright or Heart deficiency
Clearing heat and relieving toxicity (external use)	*Bing Pian* (Borneolum) *Peng Sha* (Borax)	Sore throat and mouth and tongue sores due to stagnation of heat toxins
	Xiong Huang (Realgar) (see notes on legal status)	Swelling and toxins of sores

Ci Shi 磁石
(Magnetite, Magnetitum)

Ci Shi is the ore of natural magnetite, a black mineral form of iron oxide crystallizing in the cubic system.

Main ingredients *Ci Shi* contains ferrosoferric oxide Fe_3O_4 (also known as tri-iron tetroxide), manganese and magnesium.

Properties Taste: acrid and salty; nature: cold.

Channels entered Liver, Heart and Kidney.

Functions and indications Calms the Liver and subdues Yang, settles fright and quiets the Spirit, sharpens the hearing and brightens the eyes, hosts Qi and stabilizes wheezing. It is indicated for dizziness, tinnitus and deafness, palpitations, insomnia, disquieted Heart and Spirit, and wheezing due to Kidney deficiency.

Common dosage 10-30g (crush and decoct before other ingredients); or 1-3g prepared as powder or pills for oral use.

Precautions and contraindications

1. Dosages as powder or pills should be restricted to the above amounts as *Ci Shi* is difficult to digest.
2. *Ci Shi* should be used with caution for patients with Spleen and Stomach deficiency.

Remarks Crude *Ci Shi* is used for settling fright, quieting the Spirit, calming the Liver and subduing Yang; *Ci Shi* dipped in vinegar and calcined is better for sharpening the hearing, brightening the eyes, hosting Qi and stabilizing wheezing.

Comparison of functions Both *Ci Shi* (Magnetitum) and *Zhu Sha* (Cinnabaris) are heavy and cold and enter the Heart channel; they are commonly used as heavy settlers for quieting the Spirit (for *Zhu Sha*, see notes on legal status). However, *Ci Shi* boosts Kidney Yin and subdues Liver Yang and is often used for disquieted Heart and Spirit, vexation and agitation, palpitations, insomnia, dizziness and headache due to Kidney deficiency and Liver-fire harassing the Heart. It can also sharpen the hearing and brighten the eyes to treat tinnitus and deafness and blurred vision, and can host Qi and stabilize wheezing to treat insufficiency of the Liver and Kidneys and asthma due to Kidney deficiency. *Zhu Sha* quiets the Spirit through settling and clearing the Heart and is good at treating exuberant fire in the Heart, manifesting as disquieted Heart and Spirit, vexation and heat in the chest, and palpitations and insomnia. It can also relieve toxicity and treat sores.

For an additional comparison, see *Dai Zhe Shi* (Haematitum).

Modern research Enriches the blood, especially in cases of anaemia due to iron deficiency.[3]

Combinations and applications

Functions	Combinations	Applications
Calming the Liver and subduing Yang, settling fright and quieting the Spirit	*Zhu Sha* (Cinnabaris) (see notes on legal status) *Shen Qu* (Massa Fermentata)	Disquieted Heart and Spirit, fright palpitations, insomnia and epilepsy due to the Spirit failing to keep to its abode, irregular breathing due to fright, or Liver-fire flaming upwards to harass the Heart and Spirit due to Kidney deficiency and Liver effulgence
	Sheng Di Huang (Radix Rehmanniae Glutinosae) *Shi Jue Ming* (Concha Haliotidis) *Bai Shao* (Radix Paeoniae Lactiflorae)	Palpitations, insomnia, vexation, agitation and dizziness due to ascendant hyperactivity of Liver Yang caused by Yin deficiency
Sharpening the hearing and brightening the eyes	*Shu Di Huang* (Radix Rehmanniae Glutinosae Conquita) *Shan Yao* (Rhizoma Dioscoreae Oppositae) *Wu Wei Zi* (Fructus Schisandrae)	Tinnitus and deafness, blurred vision, and a sunken, fine pulse due to Yin deficiency of the Liver and Kidneys
Hosting Qi and stabilizing wheezing	*Hu Tao Ren* (Semen Juglandis Regiae) *Wu Wei Zi* (Fructus Schisandrae) *Dai Zhe Shi* (Haematitum) *Ren Shen* (Radix Ginseng)	Deficiency wheezing, emaciation, weak voice, limpness and aching in the lumbar region and legs and a sunken, weak pulse due to inability of the Kidneys to host Qi

Long Gu 龙骨
(Dragon bone, Os Draconis)

Long Gu is the skeletal fossil of ancient mammals such as *Stegodon orientalis* and *Rhinoceros sinensis*.

Main ingredients *Long Gu* contains calcium carbonate, calcium phosphate, sodium, potassium and titanium.

Properties Taste: sweet and astringent; nature: slightly cold.

Channels entered Heart, Liver and Kidney.

Functions and indications Settles fright and quiets the Spirit, calms the Liver and subdues Yang, promotes contraction and secures astriction, and stops vaginal discharge and seminal emission. It is indicated for mania and withdrawal, fright epilepsy, palpitations, forgetfulness, insomnia, spontaneous sweating and night sweating, seminal emission, urinary turbidity, uterine bleeding, vaginal discharge, diarrhoea, dysentery, and non-closure of open sores.

Common dosage 15-30g, decocted for 20 minutes alone before adding other substances; appropriate dosage for external application.

Precautions and contraindications *Long Gu* should be used with caution in cases of damp-heat or stagnation patterns.

Remarks Raw *Long Gu* is good for calming the Liver and subduing Yang and is indicated for dizziness, vexation and agitation, fright wind, mania and withdrawal, and other disorders of disquieted Heart and Spirit. The calcined material, *Duan Long Gu* (Os Draconis Calcinatum), is effective in promoting contraction to prevent the discharge of body fluids; it is suitable for seminal emission, vaginal discharge, sweating due to deficiency of defensive Qi, profuse bleeding and non-closure of open sores.

Comparison of functions See *Mu Li* (Concha Ostreae).

Toxicity Two cases of allergic reaction during the processing of powdered *Long Gu* have been reported; symptoms included itching of exposed skin areas, red rashes and local swelling. It is also reported that a decoction of *Long Gu* caused one case of arrhythmia.

Modern research Decreases the permeability of blood vessels, promotes blood clotting and inhibits the stimulation of skeletal muscles.[4]

Combinations and applications

Functions	Combinations	Applications
Settling fright and quieting the Spirit	*Hu Po* (Succinum) *Sheng Di Huang* (Radix Rehmanniae Glutinosae) *Gou Teng* (Ramulus Uncariae cum Uncis) *Su He Xiang* (Styrax Liquidus) *Dan Nan Xing* (Pulvis Arisaematis cum Felle Bovis)	Wind epilepsy, mania and withdrawal, convulsions, and vexation and agitation in adults and children
	Zhu Sha (Cinnabaris) (see notes on legal status) *Yuan Zhi* (Radix Polygalae) *Suan Zao Ren* (Semen Ziziphi Spinosae) *Dang Gui* (Radix Angelicae Sinensis)	Vexation and agitation, palpitations, fearful throbbing, insomnia and profuse dreaming due to Heart deficiency
	Fu Ling (Sclerotium Poriae Cocos) *Ren Shen* (Radix Ginseng) *Lian Zi* (Semen Nelumbinis Nuciferae) *Mai Men Dong* (Radix Ophiopogonis Japonici)	Restless sleep, insomnia
Calming the Liver and subduing Yang	*Niu Xi* (Radix Achyranthis Bidentatae) *Gui Ban* (Plastrum Testudinis) (see notes on legal status) *Bai Shao* (Radix Paeoniae Lactiflorae) *Chuan Lian Zi* (Fructus Meliae Toosendan) *Mu Li* (Concha Ostreae)	Dizziness, vexation and agitation, Heart-heat and belching due to Liver-wind stirring internally caused by ascendant hyperactivity of Liver Yang
	Shan Yao (Rhizoma Dioscoreae Oppositae) *Dai Zhe Shi* (Haematitum) *Mu Li* (Concha Ostreae) *Bai Shao* (Radix Paeoniae Lactiflorae) *Bai Zi Ren* (Semen Biotae Orientalis)	Dizziness, tinnitus, a distending sensation in the eyes, palpitations, forgetfulness, and a string-like, long and forceful pulse due to ascendant hyperactivity of Liver Yang
Promoting contraction and securing astriction	*Ma Huang Gen* (Radix Ephedrae)	Postpartum spontaneous sweating
	Mu Li (Concha Ostreae) *Fu Xiao Mai* (Fructus Tritici Aestivi Levis) *Wu Wei Zi* (Fructus Schisandrae) *Sheng Di Huang* (Radix Rehmanniae Glutinosae) *Huang Qi* (Radix Astragali seu Hedysari)	Spontaneous sweating due to exterior deficiency, night sweating due to Yin deficiency

	Sang Piao Xiao (Oötheca Mantidis) *Gui Ban* (Plastrum Testudinis) (see notes on legal status) *Fu Shen* (Sclerotium Poriae Cocos cum Ligno Hospite)	Frequent urination and urinary incontinence due to Heart and Kidney deficiency
	Zi Su Ye (Folium Perillae Frutescentis) *Mu Gua* (Fructus Chaenomelis)	Diarrhoea due to Spleen deficiency
	Huang Qi (Radix Astragali seu Hedysari) *Hai Piao Xiao* (Os Sepiae seu Sepiellae) *Wu Wei Zi* (Fructus Schisandrae)	Uterine bleeding and vaginal discharge due to insecurity of the Chong and Ren vessels and Qi deficiency, resulting in failure of the containment function
	He Zi (Fructus Terminaliae Chebulae) *Zhu Ma Gen* (Radix Boehmeriae Niveae)	Bleeding due to incised wounds
Stopping vaginal discharge and seminal emission	*Mu Li* (Concha Ostreae) *Sha Yuan Zi* (Semen Astragali Complanati) *Qian Shi* (Semen Euryales Ferocis) *Bai Ji Li* (Fructus Tribuli Terrestris)	Seminal emission due to Kidney deficiency
	Dang Gui (Radix Angelicae Sinensis) *Xiang Fu* (Rhizoma Cyperi Rotundi) *Zong Lü Tan* (Fibra Carbonisata Trachycarpi Stipulae)	Profuse menstruation due to insufficiency of the Spleen and Kidneys
	Mu Li (Concha Ostreae) *Hai Piao Xiao* (Os Sepiae seu Sepiellae) *Shan Yao* (Rhizoma Dioscoreae Oppositae)	Vaginal discharge (with or without blood) due to deficiency of the Spleen, which thus fails to secure and contain

Note: In addition, external use of the powder prepared from *Duan Long Gu* (Os Draconis Calcinatum) is effective against damp sores, ulcerating sores, non-healing sores, papules and itchy skin.

Hu Po 琥珀 (Amber, Succinum)

Hu Po is a yellowish or brownish fossil resin exuded by certain trees and plants.

Main ingredients *Hu Po* contains succoxyabietic acid, succinoabietinolic acid, succinosilvic acid, succinoresinol, succinoabietinol and succinic acid.

Properties Taste: sweet; nature: neutral.

Channels entered Heart, Liver and Bladder.

Functions and indications Settles fright and quiets the Spirit, quickens the Blood and dissipates stasis, promotes urination and frees Lin syndrome. It is indicated for fright wind and epilepsy, insomnia, and heat, blood and stone Lin syndromes.

Common dosage 1.5-3g of the powder for oral use; *Hu Po* is not suitable for decoction.

Comparison of functions Both *Hu Po* (Succinum) and *Zhu Sha* (Cinnabaris) enter the Heart channel and have the functions of settling fright and quieting the Spirit (for *Zhu Sha*, see notes on legal status). They are used for palpitations, insomnia, profuse dreaming, forgetfulness, fright wind and epilepsy. Both substances should be ground into powder or pills to be taken and neither should be calcined. *Zhu Sha* is slightly cold in nature and clears heat, so that is more suitable for disquieted Heart and Spirit due to the flaming upwards of Heart-fire. It can also clear heat and relieve toxicity to treat sores due to heat toxins and sore and swollen throat. *Hu Po* is neutral in nature and has the additional functions of quickening the Blood and dissipating stasis to treat a variety of menstrual disorders and Lin syndromes.

Modern research

1. Has a tranquillizing function, inhibits convulsions, and lowers body temperature.[5]
2. Promotes urination and stimulates blood circulation.[6]

Combinations and applications

Functions	Combinations	Applications
Settling fright and quieting the Spirit	*Zhu Sha* (Cinnabaris) (see notes on legal status) *Suan Zao Ren* (Semen Ziziphi Spinosae) *Ye Jiao Teng* (Caulis Polygoni Multiflori) *Fu Shen* (Sclerotium Poriae Cocos cum Ligno Hospite) *Yuan Zhi* (Radix Polygalae)	Palpitations, insomnia, profuse dreaming
	Zhu Sha (Cinnabaris) (see notes on legal status) *Tian Nan Xing* (Rhizoma Arisaematis) *Quan Xie* (Buthus Martensi)	Fright wind and epilepsy
	Tian Zhu Huang (Concretio Silicea Bambusae) *Fu Ling* (Sclerotium Poriae Cocos) *Dan Nan Xing* (Pulvis Arisaematis cum Felle Bovis)	Child fright wind
Quickening the Blood and dissipating stasis	*Dang Gui* (Radix Angelicae Sinensis) *Wu Yao* (Radix Linderae Strychnifoliae) *E Zhu* (Rhizoma Curcumae)	Menstrual block due to Qi stagnation and Blood obstruction, swelling and pain due to external injury
	San Qi (Radix Notoginseng)	Pain in the heart and chest Bi syndrome due to Heart-Blood stasis obstruction
Promoting urination and freeing Lin syndrome	*Jin Qian Cao* (Herba Lysimachiae) *Hai Jin Sha* (Spora Lygodii Japonici) *Mu Tong* (Caulis Mutong) (see notes on legal status) *Bian Xu* (Herba Polygoni Avicularis)	Heat Lin syndrome, stone Lin syndrome

Note: Used on its own, *Hu Po* is effective for blood Lin syndrome, and swelling of the scrotum or vulva.

HERBS FOR NOURISHING THE HEART AND QUIETING THE SPIRIT

Unlike the substances in the previous section, the medicinals in this section for nourishing the Heart and quieting the Spirit all originate from plants. They have the functions of nourishing the Heart and Liver, enriching Yin and supplementing the Blood, and quieting the Spirit. They are mainly used for disquieted Heart and Spirit, palpitations, fearful throbbing, insomnia, deficiency vexation, profuse dreaming, forgetfulness and spontaneous sweating, where these conditions are due to insufficiency of Yin and Blood, failure to nourish the Heart, Heart and Spleen deficiency, and non-interaction of the Heart and Kidneys. In order to increase their effect, herbs for nourishing the Heart and quieting the Spirit are usually combined with herbs for supplementing the Blood, herbs for supplementing Yin or substances for settling the Heart and quieting the Spirit.

Some of the herbs for nourishing the Heart and quieting the Spirit are seeds containing oils or fats, which means that they are not suitable in cases of full-fire or for patients with loose stool due to Qi deficiency.

Tab. 14.2 Herbs for nourishing the Heart and quieting the Spirit

Herb	Functions	Indications
Suan Zao Ren (Semen Ziziphi Spinosae)	Nourishing the Heart and boosting the Liver, quieting the Spirit, constraining sweating	Deficiency vexation, insomnia, palpitations, thirst, spontaneous sweating, night sweating
Yuan Zhi (Radix Polygalae)	Quieting the Heart and Spirit, sharpening the wits, dispelling Phlegm and opening the orifices, dispersing abscesses and dissipating swelling	Palpitations, insomnia, forgetfulness, profuse dreaming, cough with copious sputum, abscesses, sores and swellings
Bai Zi Ren (Semen Biotae Orientalis)	Nourishing the Heart and quieting the Spirit, moistening the Intestines and freeing the bowels, constraining Yin and stopping sweating	Deficiency vexation, insomnia, palpitations, night sweating due to Yin deficiency, Intestinal dryness with constipation
He Huan Pi (Cortex Albizziae Julibrissin)	Quieting the Spirit and relieving depression, nourishing the Heart, quickening the Blood and dispersing swelling	Disquieted Heart and Spirit, insomnia and forgetfulness due to damage to the seven emotions, vexation and agitation, anxiety, Lung abscess, abscesses and sores, knocks and falls
Ye Jiao Teng (Caulis Polygoni Multiflori)	Nourishing the Heart and quieting the Spirit, dispelling wind and freeing the channels	Disquieted Heart and Spirit, insomnia, profuse dreaming, generalized pain due to Blood deficiency, wind-damp Bi syndrome, itchy papules

Suan Zao Ren 酸枣仁 (Spiny jujube seed, Semen Ziziphi Spinosae)

Suan Zao Ren is the mature seed of *Ziziphus jujuba* Mill. var. *spinosa* (Bunge) Hu ex H. F. Chou, family Rhamnaceae.

Main ingredients *Suan Zao Ren* contains jujubosides, jujubogenin, ebelin lactone, triterpenes (including betulin and betulic acid), fatty oils, proteins and vitamin C.

Properties Taste: sweet and sour; nature: neutral.

Channels entered Heart, Liver and Gallbladder.

Functions and indications Nourishes the Heart and boosts the Liver, quiets the Spirit, and constrains sweating. It is indicated for deficiency vexation, insomnia, palpitations, thirst, spontaneous sweating, and night sweating.

Common dosage 10-20g, or 1.5-3g of the powder for oral use with water before going to bed.

Precautions and contraindications *Suan Zao Ren* should be used with caution in cases of depression-fire due to full-heat pathogenic factors, or in cases with severe diarrhoea.

Remarks Use dry-fried *Suan Zao Ren* for cold-type insomnia due to Gallbladder deficiency patterns; use raw *Suan Zao Ren* for heat-type somnolence due to Gallbladder full patterns.

Comparison of functions See *Bai Zi Ren* (Semen Biotae Orientalis).

Toxicity Mice fed a decoction of *Suan Zao Ren* in a proportion of 50g/kg presented no toxic symptoms. The LD_{50} of intraperitoneal injection in mice of a decoction of *Suan Zao Ren* is 14.3 ± 2.0g/kg. Reports of allergic reaction to decoctions are extremely rare.

Modern research

1. Has a hypnotic effect.[7]
2. Significantly inhibits the central nervous system in order to perform a tranquillizing function, alleviate pain and lower body temperature.[8]
3. Inhibits arrhythmia, lowers blood pressure and reduces the level of blood fats.[9]
4. Strengthens the immune function.[10]
5. Inhibits carcinoma.[11]

Combinations and applications

Functions	Combinations	Applications
Nourishing the Heart and boosting the Liver, quieting the Spirit	*Bai Shao* (Radix Paeoniae Lactiflorae) *He Shou Wu* (Radix Polygoni Multiflori) *Dang Gui* (Radix Angelicae Sinensis)	Palpitations, fearful throbbing, insomnia, forgetfulness and a fine pulse due to Yin and Blood deficiency of the Heart and Liver
	Zhi Mu (Rhizoma Anemarrhenae Asphodeloidis) *Fu Ling* (Sclerotium Poriae Cocos)	Insomnia, palpitations, night sweating and a fine, rapid pulse due to Liver deficiency with heat
	Xuan Shen (Radix Scrophulariae Ningpoensis) *Bai Zi Ren* (Semen Biotae Orientalis) *Sheng Di Huang* (Radix Rehmanniae Glutinosae) *Mai Men Dong* (Radix Ophiopogonis Japonici)	Vexation, insomnia, palpitations, forgetfulness, dry mouth and throat, a red tongue with scant fur and a sunken, fine and rapid pulse due to hyperactivity of Yang caused by Yin deficiency and insufficiency of the Heart and Kidneys
Constraining sweating	*Ren Shen* (Radix Ginseng) *Fu Ling* (Sclerotium Poriae Cocos)	Spontaneous sweating due to Qi deficiency
	Wu Wei Zi (Fructus Schisandrae) *Shan Zhu Yu* (Fructus Corni Officinalis)	Night sweating due to insufficiency of Yin and Blood

Yuan Zhi 远志 (Polygala root, Radix Polygalae)

Yuan Zhi is the root of *Polygala tenuifolia* Willd. or *P. sibirica* L., family Polygalaceae.

Main ingredients *Yuan Zhi* contains onjisaponins, tenuifolin, tenuigenins, polygalitol, tenuidine, xanthones, fatty oils and resin.

Properties Taste: acrid and bitter; nature: slightly warm.

Channels entered Lung and Heart.

Functions and indications Quiets the Heart and Spirit, sharpens the wits, dispels Phlegm and opens the orifices, disperses abscesses and dissipates swelling. It is indicated for palpitations, insomnia, forgetfulness, profuse dreaming, cough with copious sputum, and abscesses, sores and swellings.

Common dosage 3-10g; appropriate dosage for external application.

Precautions and contraindications Since *Yuan Zhi* stimulates the lining of the stomach, it should be used with caution in cases of full-heat or exuberant internal Phlegm-fire and for patients suffering from gastric ulcers or gastritis.

Remarks Raw *Yuan Zhi* is very effective in dispelling Phlegm and opening the orifices and is often used to treat patterns of Phlegm obstructing the orifices of the Heart. The dry nature of processed *Yuan Zhi* allows it to moderate and harmonize; it is better for quieting the Heart and Spirit and is used to treat disquieted Heart and Spirit, insomnia and forgetfulness. *Yuan Zhi* processed with honey has the function of transforming Phlegm and stopping coughing and is frequently used for cough with copious sputum.

Comparison of functions See *Shi Chang Pu* (Rhizoma Acori Graminei).

Toxicity The LD_{50} of the root bark of *Yuan Zhi* fed to mice via intragastric administration is 10.03 ± 1.98g/kg, that of the whole root is 16.95 ± 2.01g/kg.

Modern research

1. Has a tranquillizing function and relieves convulsions.[12]
2. Expels sputum.[13]
3. Excites the uterus.[13]
4. The polygalitol contained in *Yuan Zhi* inhibited Gram-positive bacteria, Shigella shigae, Salmonella typhi and Mycobacterium tuberculosis *in vitro*.[13]

Combinations and applications

Functions	Combinations	Applications
Quieting the Heart and Spirit, sharpening the wits	*Zhu Sha* (Cinnabaris) (see notes on legal status) *Long Chi* (Dens Draconis)	Disquieted Heart and Spirit and palpitations due to Heart deficiency
	Shi Chang Pu (Rhizoma Acori Graminei) *Ren Shen* (Radix Ginseng) *Dang Gui* (Radix Angelicae Sinensis)	Insomnia or forgetfulness due to insufficiency of Heart-Blood
	Fu Ling (Sclerotium Poriae Cocos) *Sheng Di Huang* (Radix Rehmanniae Glutinosae) *Xuan Shen* (Radix Scrophulariae Ningpoensis) *Mai Men Dong* (Radix Ophiopogonis Japonici) *Suan Zao Ren* (Semen Ziziphi Spinosae)	Insufficiency of the Heart and Kidneys, Yin depletion and Blood deficiency causing the Heart to be deprived of nourishment and manifesting as insomnia, palpitations, dream emission and forgetfulness, accompanied by a red tongue with thin fur and a fine, rapid pulse

Dispelling Phlegm and opening the orifices	*Xing Ren* (Semen Pruni Armeniacae) *Jie Geng* (Radix Platycodi Grandiflori) *Sha Shen* (Radix Glehniae seu Adenophorae) *Gan Cao* (Radix Glycyrrhizae)	Cough with copious sputum and difficult expectoration due to dry pathogenic factors damaging the Lungs
	Yu Jin (Radix Curcumae) *Shi Chang Pu* (Rhizoma Acori Graminei) *Ming Fan* (Alumen)	Fright epilepsy and Essence-Spirit trance due to Phlegm confusing the orifices of the Heart

Note: In addition, a powder of *Yuan Zhi* can be mixed with *Huang Jiu* (Vinum Aureum) and used orally or applied externally for abscesses, sores, sore throat and breast abscesses. This powder also has the function of dispersing stagnated Liver Qi and can be used with *Shi Chang Pu* (Rhizoma Acori Graminei) for enduring pain in the chest due to Qi stagnation.

Bai Zi Ren 柏子仁 (Chinese arborvitae seed, Semen Biotae Orientalis)

Bai Zi Ren is the dried seed of *Biota orientalis* (L.) Endl., family Cupressaceae. This plant is also known as *Platycladus orientalis* (L.) Franco.

Main ingredients *Bai Zi Ren* contains fatty oils, volatile oils and saponins.

Properties Taste: sweet; nature: neutral.

Channels entered Heart, Kidney and Large Intestine.

Functions and indications Nourishes the Heart and quiets the Spirit, moistens the Intestines and frees the bowels, constrains Yin and stops sweating. It is indicated for deficiency vexation, insomnia, palpitations, night sweating due to Yin deficiency, and Intestinal dryness with constipation.

Common dosage 10-18g.

Precautions and contraindications *Bai Zi Ren* should be used with caution in cases of loose stool or copious sputum.

Comparison of functions Both *Bai Zi Ren* (Semen Biotae Orientalis) and *Suan Zao Ren* (Semen Ziziphi Spinosae) are sweet and neutral and enter the Heart channel to nourish the Heart and quiet the Spirit. They are used to treat palpitations, fearful throbbing, insomnia and forgetfulness due to Yin and Blood deficiency and the Heart and Spirit being deprived of nourishment. They are often used in combination to enhance their effect. *Bai Zi Ren* is effective in nourishing the Heart to quiet the Spirit and is mainly used for insomnia and palpitations due to the Blood failing to nourish the Heart. Being oily and moist, it can also moisten the Intestines and free the bowels to treat Intestinal dryness with constipation. *Suan Zao Ren* has a stronger effect in quieting the Spirit. As it can nourish Heart Yin and Liver-Blood, it is mainly used for insomnia and palpitations due to Yin and Blood deficiency of the Heart and Liver. Being sour, it is also able to promote contraction to stop sweating and is often used for spontaneous sweating and night sweating.

Modern research

1. Slows the heart rate and has a tranquillizing function.[14]
2. The oils contained in *Bai Zi Ren* induce diarrhoea.[15]

Combinations and applications

Functions	Combinations	Applications
Nourishing the Heart and quieting the Spirit	*Ren Shen* (Radix Ginseng) *Wu Wei Zi* (Fructus Schisandrae) *Bai Zhu* (Rhizoma Atractylodis Macrocephalae)	Palpitations, fearful throbbing, deficiency vexation, insomnia, dizziness and forgetfulness due to the Heart and Spirit being deprived of nourishment as a result of insufficiency of Heart Yin and deficiency of Heart-Blood
	Fu Shen (Sclerotium Poriae Cocos cum Ligno Hospite) *Suan Zao Ren* (Semen Ziziphi Spinosae) *Wu Wei Zi* (Fructus Schisandrae)	Palpitations and insomnia due to the Blood failing to nourish the Heart
	Sheng Di Huang (Radix Rehmanniae Glutinosae) *Xuan Shen* (Radix Scrophulariae Ningpoensis) *Suan Zao Ren* (Semen Ziziphi Spinosae)	Palpitations, forgetfulness and dry mouth due to Yin deficiency of the Heart and Kidneys
Moistening the Intestines and freeing the bowels	*Yu Li Ren* (Semen Pruni) *Xing Ren* (Semen Pruni Armeniacae) *Tao Ren* (Semen Persicae)	Intestinal dryness with constipation in the elderly or postpartum due to Yin deficiency and Blood depletion
Constraining Yin and stopping sweating	*Ren Shen* (Radix Ginseng) *Wu Wei Zi* (Fructus Schisandrae) *Mu Li* (Concha Ostreae)	Night sweating and palpitations due to Yin deficiency

He Huan Pi 合欢皮
(Albizzia bark, Cortex Albizziae Julibrissin)

He Huan Pi is the dried bark of *Albizzia julibrissin* Durazz., family Leguminosae.

Main ingredients *He Huan Pi* contains tannin, saponins and glucosides.

Properties Taste: sweet; nature: neutral.

Channels entered Heart and Liver.

Functions and indications Quiets the Spirit and relieves depression, nourishes the Heart, quickens the Blood and disperses swelling. It is indicated for disquieted Heart and Spirit, insomnia and forgetfulness due to damage to the seven emotions, vexation and agitation, anxiety, Lung abscess, abscesses and sores, and knocks and falls.

Common dosage 10-15g.

Remarks *He Huan Pi* is very mild in its effects and requires administration over a prolonged period.

Modern research

1. Has a tranquillizing function, relieves insomnia and alleviates pain.[12]
2. Has a pronounced effect in expelling parasites and inducing urination.[16]
3. Induced labour in animal experiments.[16]

Combinations and applications

Functions	Combinations	Applications
Quieting the Spirit and relieving depression, nourishing the Heart	*Suan Zao Ren* (Semen Ziziphi Spinosae) *Bai Zi Ren* (Semen Biotae Orientalis) *Bai Shao* (Radix Paeoniae Lactiflorae) *Ye Jiao Teng* (Caulis Polygoni Multiflori)	Deficiency vexation, depression and agitation, insomnia and forgetfulness due to damage to the seven emotions
Quickening the Blood and dispersing swelling	*Dang Gui* (Radix Angelicae Sinensis) *Chuan Xiong* (Rhizoma Ligustici Chuanxiong)	Knocks and falls, fractures, swelling and pain due to Blood stasis
	Yu Xing Cao (Herba Houttuyniae Cordatae) *Dong Gua Zi* (Semen Benincasae Hispidae) *Tao Ren* (Semen Persicae) *Lu Gen* (Rhizoma Phragmitis Communis)	Lung abscess with pain in the chest and coughing and spitting of pus and blood
	Pu Gong Ying (Herba Taraxaci cum Radice) *Zi Hua Di Ding* (Herba Violae Yedoensitis) *Lian Qiao* (Fructus Forsythiae Suspensae) *Ye Ju Hua* (Flos Chrysanthemi Indici)	Swelling and toxins of abscesses and sores

Ye Jiao Teng 夜交藤 (Fleece-flower stem, Caulis Polygoni Multiflori)

Ye Jiao Teng is the dried stem of *Polygonum multiflorum* Thunb., family Polygonaceae.

Main ingredients *Ye Jiao Teng* contains emodin, chrysophanol, physcion, emodin-6-methylether, emodin glucoside and β-sitosterol.

Properties Taste: sweet; nature: neutral.

Channels entered Heart and Liver.

Functions and indications Nourishes the Heart and quiets the Spirit, dispels wind and frees the channels. It is indicated for disquieted Heart and Spirit, insomnia, profuse dreaming, generalized pain due to Blood deficiency, wind-damp Bi syndrome, and itchy papules.

Common dosage 15-30g, or 60g for mental illness; appropriate dosage for external application as a wash for the affected area.

Toxicity Two cases of allergic reaction caused by the decoction of formulae containing *Ye Jiao Teng* have been reported. Once *Ye Jiao Teng* was removed from the formulae, the allergy symptoms disappeared.

Modern research Possesses sedative and hypnotic functions.[17]

Combinations and applications

Functions	Combinations	Applications
Nourishing the Heart and quieting the Spirit	*Bai Zi Ren* (Semen Biotae Orientalis) *Suan Zao Ren* (Semen Ziziphi Spinosae) *He Huan Pi* (Cortex Albizziae Julibrissin)	Insomnia, profuse dreaming, palpitations, fearful throbbing and dizziness due to Yin and Blood deficiency
	Ji Xue Teng (Caulis Spatholobi) *Dang Gui* (Radix Angelicae Sinensis) *Chuan Xiong* (Rhizoma Ligustici Chuanxiong)	Generalized pain due to Blood deficiency
	He Huan Hua (Flos Albizziae Julibrissin)	Palpitations and depression due to stagnation of Heart Qi
Dispelling wind and freeing the channels	*Qiang Huo* (Rhizoma et Radix Notopterygii) *Du Huo* (Radix Angelicae Pubescentis) *Sang Ji Sheng* (Ramulus Loranthi) *Qin Jiao* (Radix Gentianae Macrophyllae)	Wind-damp Bi syndrome pain, inhibited bending and stretching

Note: *Ye Jiao Teng* can be used as an external wash on its own or in combination with *Chan Tui* (Periostracum Cicadae), *Fu Ping* (Herba Spirodelae Polyrrhizae), *Di Fu Zi* (Fructus Kochiae Scopariae) and *She Chuang Zi* (Fructus Cnidii Monnieri) to treat itchy skin due to wind papules or scabies and tinea.

Modern research references

1. He Xingdong et al., *Lin Chuang Zhong Yao Shou Ce* [Clinical Handbook of Chinese Materia Medica] (Beijing: People's Medical Publishing House, 1998), 259.
2. Lei Zaiquan and Zhang Tingmo, *Zhong Hua Lin Chuang Zhong Yao Xue* [Chinese Clinical Materia Medica] (Beijing: People's Medical Publishing House, 1998), 1534.
3. He Xingdong et al., *Lin Chuang Zhong Yao Shou Ce*, 260.
4. Lei Zaiquan and Zhang Tingmo, *Zhong Hua Lin Chuang Zhong Yao Xue*, 1414.
5. Ibid., 1539.
6. He Xingdong et al., *Lin Chuang Zhong Yao Shou Ce*, 261.
7. Chai Tianwan et al., *Yao Xue Za Zhi* [Journal of Pharmacology] 4 (1975): 465.
8. Pharmacology Group of Shandong Institute of Medicine and Materia Medica, *Research Documents on Traditional Chinese Medicine and Materia Medica (Shandong Institute of Medicine and Materia Medica)* 8 (1975): 35.
9. Xu Shunrao et al., *Zhong Cao Yao* [Journal of Chinese Herbs] 18, 2 (1987): 18.
10. Lang Xingcai et al., *Zhong Yao Tong Bao* [Bulletin of Chinese Materia Medica] 13, 11 (1988): 43.
11. Wang Qinglian et al., *Xi An Yi Xue Yuan Xue Bao* [Journal of Xi'an Medical College] 16, 3 (1995): 295.
12. He Xingdong et al., *Lin Chuang Zhong Yao Shou Ce*, 264.
13. Lei Zaiquan and Zhang Tingmo, *Zhong Hua Lin Chuang Zhong Yao Xue*, 1520.
14. He Xingdong et al., *Lin Chuang Zhong Yao Shou Ce*, 263.
15. Lei Zaiquan and Zhang Tingmo, *Zhong Hua Lin Chuang Zhong Yao Xue*, 1503.
16. Ding Xuemin et al., *Chang Yong Zhong Yi Fang Yao Shou Ce* [Handbook of Commonly-Used Chinese Herbs and Prescriptions] (Changsha: Hunan Science and Technology Publishing House, 1982), 98.
17. Yang Junye et al., *Hua Xi Yi Ke Da Xue Xue Bao* [Journal of Huaxi Medical University] 2, 2 (1990): 175.

Chapter 15

Substances for calming the Liver and extinguishing wind

平肝息风药

Substances for calming the Liver and extinguishing wind

Substances for calming the Liver and extinguishing wind include herbs and other substances which have the functions of cooling Liver-Blood to extinguish the internal stirring of Liver-wind, calming the Liver, subduing Liver Yang and alleviating tetany. They are used for spasms and convulsions due to high fever, and fright epilepsy; or for ascendant hyperactivity of Liver Yang and an upward attack of Liver-wind manifesting as dizziness, headache with a feeling of heat and distension in the head, red face, facial paralysis, or even sudden loss of consciousness or hemiplegia. The animal and insect substances included in this category can also be used for stubborn Bi syndrome and numbness of the limbs.

The combinations of these substances with other herbs depend on the nature of the pathogenic factors involved:

1. in cases of Yin deficiency and Yang exuberance, use these substances with herbs for enriching and nourishing Kidney Yin;
2. for Liver-fire flaming upwards, use them with herbs for clearing and draining Liver-fire; with concurrent disquieted Heart and Spirit, insomnia and profuse dreaming, add herbs for quieting the Spirit;
3. for Liver-wind stirring internally due to Liver Yang transforming wind, combine substances for extinguishing wind and alleviating tetany with substances for calming the Liver and subduing Yang;
4. for Liver-wind stirring internally due to extreme heat generating wind, use substances for calming the Liver and extinguishing wind with herbs for clearing heat, draining fire and relieving toxicity;
5. for Liver-wind stirring internally due to Yin deficiency and Blood depletion, use these substances with herbs for supplementing Yin and nourishing the Blood;
6. in cases of chronic fright due to Spleen deficiency, use them with herbs for supplementing Qi and fortifying the Spleen; with concurrent pathogenic Phlegm, add herbs for dispelling Phlegm.

The wind pattern changes fast. Pathogenic wind and fire are related to each other and can easily cause Phlegm obstruction of the Upper Jiao, leading to fright epilepsy. In these cases, first wake the patient from unconsciousness by dispelling Phlegm, and then give the appropriate treatment according to TCM differentiation. Additionally, patients suffering from convulsions and collapse due to dizziness usually have symptoms of palpitations and insomnia, so substances for quieting the Spirit are often combined with substances for calming the Liver and extinguishing wind.

The substances in this chapter have different natures and functions, so differentiation should be made between them in the clinic. Materia medica such as *Ling Yang Jiao* (Cornu Antelopis) and *Gou Teng* (Ramulus Uncariae cum Uncis) are cool or cold in nature, and so can extinguish Liver-heat. They are suitable for child fright epilepsy and convulsions due to exuberant heat in the Liver channel. However, these cool or cold substances are not appropriate for convulsions due to Spleen deficiency. Other substances such as *Quan Xie* (Buthus Martensi) and *Wu Gong* (Scolopendra Subspinipes) are warm or neutral and dry and are especially good at alleviating tetany. However, they should be used with caution in cases of Blood deficiency.

The mineral and shell materials in this chapter should be broken into pieces before decocting and then decocted for a prolonged period to ensure effective performance.

Tab. 15.1 Substances for calming the Liver and subduing Yang

Herb	Functions	Indications
Shi Jue Ming (Concha Haliotidis)	Calming the Liver and subduing Yang, clearing the Liver and brightening the eyes	Headache and dizziness due to ascendant hyperactivity of Liver Yang, blurred vision, red, sore and swollen eyes due to Liver-fire flaming upwards
Mu Li (Concha Ostreae)	Calming the Liver and subduing Yang, softening hardness and dissipating lumps, promoting contraction and securing astriction	Dizziness, palpitations, insomnia, convulsions, scrofula, spontaneous sweating, night sweating, seminal emission, uterine bleeding, vaginal discharge, pain in the stomach
Dai Zhe Shi (Haematitum)	Calming the Liver and subduing Yang, strongly bearing counterflow Qi downwards, cooling the Blood and stopping bleeding	Dizziness and headache due to ascendant hyperactivity of Liver Yang, hiccups, vomiting, wheezing, nosebleed, vomiting of blood, uterine bleeding
Zhen Zhu (Margarita)	Settling fright and quieting the Spirit, clearing the Liver and eliminating eye screen, promoting contraction and generating flesh	Palpitations, fearful throbbing, disquieted Heart and Spirit, epilepsy, convulsions, red, sore and swollen eyes, eye screen, non-closure of open sores
Zhen Zhu Mu (Concha Margaritifera)	Calming the Liver and subduing Yang, clearing the Heart and quieting the Spirit, clearing the Liver and brightening the eyes	Mania and withdrawal, fright epilepsy, dizziness, tinnitus, palpitations, insomnia, blurred vision, red, sore and swollen eyes, coughing of blood, nosebleed
Bai Ji Li (Fructus Tribuli Terrestris)	Calming the Liver, subduing Yang and allowing constrained Liver Qi to flow freely, dispelling wind and alleviating itching, dispelling wind-heat and brightening the eyes	Headache, dizziness, distension and pain in the chest and hypochondrium, stoppage of breast milk, red eyes with profuse lacrimation, itchy skin

Tab. 15.2 Substances for extinguishing wind and alleviating tetany

Herb	Functions	Indications
Ling Yang Jiao (Cornu Antelopis)	Calming the Liver and extinguishing wind, clearing heat and relieving toxicity, clearing the Liver and brightening the eyes	Fright epilepsy, delirious speech, convulsions, dizziness due to ascendant hyperactivity of Liver Yang, vexation and agitation, high fever in warm-febrile diseases, red eyes and headache due to Liver-fire flaming upwards

Niu Huang (Calculus Bovis)	Clearing the Heart, opening the orifices and dispelling Phlegm, extinguishing wind and alleviating tetany, clearing heat and relieving toxicity	Fright epilepsy, clouded Spirit and delirious speech, mania, child fright wind, sore throat, painful and swollen gums, mouth and tongue sores, and boils, abscesses and sores
Gou Teng (Ramulus Uncariae cum Uncis)	Extinguishing wind and alleviating tetany, clearing heat and calming the Liver	Fright epilepsy and convulsions due to Liver-wind stirring internally, dizziness and headache, hypertension due to ascendant hyperactivity of Liver Yang
Tian Ma (Rhizoma Gastrodiae Elatae)	Calming the Liver and subduing Yang, extinguishing wind and alleviating tetany, dispelling wind-damp and alleviating Bi syndrome pain	Fright wind, dizziness, headache, opisthotonos, convulsions, numbness of the limbs, wind-damp Bi syndrome
Di Long (Lumbricus)	Extinguishing wind and alleviating tetany, clearing heat and settling fright, calming wheezing, promoting urination, freeing the channels and quickening the network vessels	Dizziness, headache and red eyes, epilepsy and convulsions, coughing and wheezing, oedema, inhibited urination, hemiplegia, numbness of the limbs, inhibited bending and stretching
Quan Xie (Buthus Martensi)	Extinguishing wind and settling tetany, freeing the network vessels and alleviating pain, attacking toxins and dissipating lumps	Spasms and convulsions, child fright wind, facial paralysis, wind-stroke, hemiplegia, tetanus, migraine, wind-damp Bi syndrome, scrofula and Phlegm nodes, sores
Wu Gong (Scolopendra Subspinipes)	Extinguishing wind and alleviating tetany, attacking toxins and dissipating lumps, freeing the network vessels and alleviating pain	Spasms and convulsions, acute and chronic child fright wind, tetanus, opisthotonos, severe intermittent headache, sores
Jiang Can (Bombyx Batryticatus)	Extinguishing wind and alleviating tetany, dispelling wind and alleviating pain, transforming Phlegm and dissipating lumps	Fright epilepsy, convulsions, child fright wind, facial paralysis, headache, red eyes, sore throat, scrofula, wind papules

SUBSTANCES FOR CALMING THE LIVER AND SUBDUING YANG

Shi Jue Ming 石决明 (Abalone shell, Concha Haliotidis)

Shi Jue Ming is the shell of *Haliotis diversicolor* Reeve, *H. gigantea discus* Reeve, *H. ovina* Gmelin, *H. ruber* (Leach), *H. asinina* L. or *H. laevigata* (Donovan), family Haliotidae.

Main ingredients *Shi Jue Ming* contains at least 90% of calcium carbonate as well as small amounts of magnesium, iron, silicates, phosphates and chlorides.

Properties Taste: salty; nature: cold.

Channel entered Liver.

Functions and indications Calms the Liver and subdues Yang, clears the Liver and brightens the eyes. It is indicated for headache and dizziness due to ascendant hyperactivity of Liver Yang, blurred vision, and red, sore and swollen eyes due to Liver-fire flaming upwards.

Common dosage 10–30g, decocted before adding other substances.

Precautions and contraindications According to some sources, including the herb classic *Ben Cao Jing Shu* [Classical Commentary on the Materia Medica], *Shi Jue Ming* antagonizes *Xuan Fu Hua* (Flos Inulae).

Remarks Crude *Shi Jue Ming* is used to calm the Liver and subdue Yang, whereas calcined *Shi Jue Ming* is used as a topical application for the eyes or as a laryngeal insufflation.

Comparison of functions Both *Shi Jue Ming* (Concha Haliotidis) and *Jue Ming Zi* (Semen Cassiae) have the functions of clearing the Liver and brightening the eyes and are used to treat red, sore and swollen eyes due to Liver-fire flaming upwards and other eye disorders due to Liver-heat. *Shi Jue Ming* is heavy and cold; it enters the Liver channel and the Xue level to cool and settle the Liver and enrich and nourish Liver Yin. It can be used to treat dizziness, headache and tinnitus due to ascendant hyperactivity of Liver Yang and aversion to light, dim vision, clear-eye blindness (glaucoma) and other eye disorders due to Blood deficiency and Liver-heat. *Jue Ming Zi* is bitter and cool; it tends to clear and drain Liver-fire to brighten the eyes, but it can also moisten the Intestines and free the bowels. It is used to treat red, sore and swollen eyes and headache due to full-fire in the Liver channel, as well as dry stool and constipation.

For an additional comparison, see *Zhen Zhu Mu* (Concha Margaritifera).

Modern research

1. Abates fever, has a tranquillizing function and lowers blood pressure.[1]
2. Inhibits infection and has an immunosuppressive function.[2]

Combinations and applications

Functions	Combinations	Applications
Calming the Liver and subduing Yang	*Tian Ma* (Rhizoma Gastrodiae Elatae) (see notes on legal status) *Gou Teng* (Ramulus Uncariae cum Uncis) *Niu Xi* (Radix Achyranthis Bidentatae) *Zhi Zi* (Fructus Gardeniae Jasminoidis)	Headache, dizziness, tinnitus and blurred vision, a red tongue and a string-like and rapid pulse due to ascendant hyperactivity of Liver Yang and Liver-wind stirring internally

	Xia Ku Cao (Spica Prunellae Vulgaris) *Huang Qin* (Radix Scutellariae Baicalensis) *Ju Hua* (Flos Chrysanthemi Morifolii)	Dizziness, headache, vexation and agitation and insomnia due to ascendant hyperactivity of Liver Yang with heat signs
	Bai Shao (Radix Paeoniae Lactiflorae) *Sheng Di Huang* (Radix Rehmanniae Glutinosae) *Mu Li* (Concha Ostreae)	Dizziness, headache, belching and vexation due to ascendant hyperactivity of Liver Yang caused by Yin deficiency of the Liver and Kidneys
Clearing the Liver and brightening the eyes	*Shu Di Huang* (Radix Rehmanniae Glutinosae Conquita) *Tu Si Zi* (Semen Cuscutae) *Dang Gui* (Radix Angelicae Sinensis)	Blurred vision due to deficiency of Liver-Blood
	Ju Hua (Flos Chrysanthemi Morifolii) *Jue Ming Zi* (Semen Cassiae) *Xia Ku Cao* (Spica Prunellae Vulgaris)	Red, sore and swollen eyes due to Liver-fire flaming upwards
	Hai Jin Sha (Spora Lygodii Japonici) *Gan Cao* (Radix Glycyrrhizae) *Ju Hua* (Flos Chrysanthemi Morifolii)	Aversion to light due to wind-heat attacking upwards
	Cang Zhu (Rhizoma Atractylodis) *Zhu Gan* (pig's liver)	Clear-eye blindness (glaucoma) and night blindness due to deficiency of the Liver, which fails to nourish the eyes

Mu Li 牡蛎 (Oyster shell, Concha Ostreae)

Mu Li is the shell of *Ostrea gigas* Thunb., *O. talienwhanensis* Crosse or *O. rivularis* Gould, family Ostreidae.

Main ingredients *Mu Li* contains approximately 90% of calcium carbonate as well as small quantities of magnesium, iron, phosphates, silicates, sulphates and chlorides.

Properties Taste: salty and astringent; nature: slightly cold.

Channels entered Liver and Kidney.

Functions and indications Calms the Liver and subdues Yang, softens hardness and dissipates lumps, promotes contraction and secures astriction. It is indicated for dizziness, palpitations, insomnia, convulsions, scrofula, spontaneous sweating, night sweating, seminal emission, uterine bleeding, vaginal discharge, and pain in the stomach.

Common dosage 15-30g, decocted before adding other substances.

Precautions and contraindications *Mu Li* should be used with caution in cases of cold in deficiency patterns.

Remarks Crude *Mu Li* is good for calming the Liver and subduing Yang and for softening hardness and dissipating lumps, whereas calcined *Mu Li* is better for promoting contraction and securing astriction and for controlling acidity and alleviating pain.

Comparison of functions Both *Mu Li* (Concha Ostreae) and *Long Gu* (Os Draconis) are heavy, astringent substances. They can calm the Liver and subdue hyperactivity of Liver Yang as well as being able to secure astriction; they can be used together for palpitations and insomnia due to disquieted Heart and Spirit, for dizziness, vexation, agitation and irascibility due to ascendant hyperactivity of Liver Yang caused by Yin deficiency, and for vaginal discharge and sweating. *Long Gu* mainly enters the Heart channel and is an important materia medica for treating vexation, palpitations and insomnia as a result of its powerful effect in quieting the Spirit. It is more effective than *Mu Li* in promoting contraction and securing astriction, but not as good for softening hardness and dissipating lumps. *Mu Li* mainly enters the Liver channel and achieves good results in calming the Liver and subduing Yang. Since it can soften hardness and dissipate lumps, it is used to treat scrofula, Phlegm nodes and abdominal masses.

Modern research

1. Strengthens the immune function, promotes macrophage activity.[3]
2. Regulates gastric acid, inhibits ulcers and neuromuscular stimulation.[4]

Combinations and applications

Functions	Combinations	Applications
Calming the Liver and subduing Yang	*Bai Shao* (Radix Paeoniae Lactiflorae) *Long Gu* (Os Draconis) *Gui Ban* (Plastrum Testudinis) (see notes on legal status) *Ju Hua* (Flos Chrysanthemi Morifolii) *Gou Qi Zi* (Fructus Lycii) *He Shou Wu* (Radix Polygoni Multiflori)	Dizziness, palpitations and insomnia, vexation and agitation, and tinnitus due to ascendant hyperactivity of Liver Yang caused by Yin deficiency
	Sheng Di Huang (Radix Rehmanniae Glutinosae) *Bie Jia* (Carapax Amydae Sinensis) (see notes on legal status) *Gui Ban* (Plastrum Testudinis) (see notes on legal status)	Convulsion of the limbs, heat in the palms and soles, dry mouth and tongue, and a large, deficient pulse due to damage to Yin leading to Liver-wind stirring internally during prolonged febrile diseases
Softening hardness and dissipating lumps	*Xuan Shen* (Radix Scrophulariae Ningpoensis) *Zhe Bei Mu* (Bulbus Fritillariae Thunbergii)	Scrofula and Phlegm nodes due to depression binding of Phlegm-fire
	San Leng (Rhizoma Sparganii Stoloniferi) *E Zhu* (Rhizoma Curcumae) *Bie Jia* (Carapax Amydae Sinensis) (see notes on legal status)	Abdominal masses and accumulations due to Qi stagnation and Blood stasis
	Bie Jia (Carapax Amydae Sinensis) (see notes on legal status) *Ze Lan* (Herba Lycopi Lucidi) *San Leng* (Rhizoma Sparganii Stoloniferi) *E Zhu* (Rhizoma Curcumae) *Dan Shen* (Radix Salviae Miltiorrhizae)	Goitre due to prolonged Qi stagnation and Blood stasis
Promoting contraction and securing astriction	*Huang Qi* (Radix Astragali seu Hedysari) *Fu Xiao Mai* (Fructus Tritici Aestivi Levis) *Ma Huang Gen* (Radix Ephedrae)	Spontaneous sweating and night sweating, emaciation, shortness of breath, vexation and fatigue in deficiency patterns

Qian Shi (Semen Euryales Ferocis) *Lian Xu* (Stamen Nelumbinis Nuciferae) *Sha Yuan Zi* (Semen Astragali Complanati) *Bai Ji Li* (Fructus Tribuli Terrestris)	Seminal emission, limpness and aching in the lumbar region and knees and lack of strength in the lower limbs due to deficiency of the Kidneys, which thus fail to secure the Essence
Sang Piao Xiao (Oötheca Mantidis) *Jin Ying Zi* (Fructus Rosae Laevigatae) *Yi Zhi Ren* (Fructus Alpiniae Oxyphyllae) *Long Gu* (Os Draconis)	Enuresis, frequent urination
Shan Yao (Rhizoma Dioscoreae Oppositae) *Duan Long Gu* (Os Draconis Calcinatum) *Hai Piao Xiao* (Os Sepiae seu Sepiellae)	Uterine bleeding and vaginal discharge due to Spleen deficiency
Gua Lou Gen (Radix Trichosanthis)	Lily disease (see *Bai He*, Bulbus Lilii)

Note: In its calcined form, *Mu Li* can be used for pain in the stomach, acid regurgitation and vomiting.

Dai Zhe Shi 代赭石 (Haematite, Haematitum)

Dai Zhe Shi is the ore of haematite, the mineral form of iron (III) oxide Fe_2O_3.

Main ingredients *Dai Zhe Shi* contains up to 60% of iron (III) oxide and smaller amounts of cadmium, cobalt, chromium, copper, manganese, nickel and magnesium.

Properties Taste: bitter; nature: cold.

Channels entered Liver and Heart.

Functions and indications Calms the Liver and subdues Yang, strongly bears counterflow Qi downwards, cools the Blood and stops bleeding. It is indicated for dizziness and headache due to ascendant hyperactivity of Liver Yang, hiccups, vomiting, wheezing, nosebleed, vomiting of blood, and uterine bleeding.

Common dosage 10-30g, decocted before other ingredients; appropriate dosage for external application.

Precautions and contraindications *Dai Zhe Shi* should be used with caution during pregnancy and in cases of Yin-type jaundice due to Yang deficiency.

Remarks Crude *Dai Zhe Shi* is used to calm the Liver and bear counterflow Qi downwards, whereas calcined *Dai Zhe Shi* is better for stopping bleeding.

Comparison of functions

1. *Dai Zhe Shi* (Haematitum) and *Ci Shi* (Magnetitum) are iron ores, being cold and heavy. Both mineral substances can calm the Liver, subdue Yang, bear counterflow Qi downwards and stabilize wheezing to treat dizziness due to hyperactivity of Liver Yang and dyspnoea due to Qi counterflow. *Dai Zhe Shi* mainly enters the Liver channel to calm the Liver and subdue Yang and cool the Blood and stop bleeding. It is effective for bearing counterflow Lung and Stomach Qi downwards to stop vomiting, hiccups and belching. *Ci Shi* enters the Kidney channel to boost Kidney Yin to settle floating Yang, host Qi and stabilize wheezing, and settle fright and quiet the Spirit. It is very effective for dizziness, blurred vision, deafness and tinnitus due to Kidney deficiency and Essence depletion, wheezing due to Kidney deficiency, and palpitations and insomnia.
2. *Dai Zhe Shi* (Haematitum) and *Xuan Fu Hua* (Flos Inulae) can bear counterflow Lung and Stomach

Qi downwards to stop vomiting and belching and stabilize wheezing. They are often used together to bear counterflow Qi downwards. *Dai Zhe Shi* is a mineral product, effective in calming the Liver and subduing Yang, clearing the Liver and bearing fire downwards, and cooling the Blood and stopping bleeding. Although *Xuan Fu Hua* is a plant, it specifically bears counterflow Qi downwards and disperses Phlegm-fire; it is frequently used for hasty breathing due to Phlegm obstruction, focal distension in the chest due to binding of Phlegm, and distension and fullness due to collection of fluids.

Toxicity Some reports indicate that *Dai Zhe Shi* contains one part per 100,000 of arsenic salts. Long-term administration of small quantities of *Dai Zhe Shi* to animals produced symptoms similar to arsenic poisoning. Oral administration of 2g per day to mice resulted in all animals dying within seven days; 5g per day given to rabbits resulted in all animals dying within 14 days. Symptoms of toxicity included lethargic movement, muscular weakness, convulsions with subsequent paralysis, and respiratory arrest.

Modern research

1. Astringes the gastrointestinal wall, stimulates the mucous membrane and promotes the production of blood cells.[5]
2. Prolonged use of *Dai Zhe Shi* may result in arsenic poisoning (see *Toxicity* above).[6]

Combinations and applications

Functions	Combinations	Applications
Calming the Liver and subduing Yang	*Bai Shao* (Radix Paeoniae Lactiflorae) *Mu Li* (Concha Ostreae) *Gui Ban* (Plastrum Testudinis) (see notes on legal status) *Niu Xi* (Radix Achyranthis Bidentatae)	Dizziness, red face, vexation and agitation with a string-like, long and forceful pulse due to ascendant hyperactivity of Liver Yang and Liver-wind stirring internally
	Sheng Di Huang (Radix Rehmanniae Glutinosae) *Bai Shao* (Radix Paeoniae Lactiflorae) *Bai Zi Ren* (Semen Biotae Orientalis) *Long Gu* (Os Draconis)	Dizziness, vertigo, palpitations, forgetfulness, profuse dreaming, insomnia and a string-like pulse due to ascendant hyperactivity of Liver Yang
Strongly bearing counterflow Qi downwards	*Ban Xia* (Rhizoma Pinelliae Ternatae) *Sheng Jiang* (Rhizoma Zingiberis Officinalis Recens) *Xuan Fu Hua* (Flos Inulae)	Hiccups and vomiting with white and slimy tongue fur and a string-like, deficient pulse due to deficiency and ascending counterflow of Stomach Qi and internal obstruction of turbid Phlegm
	Shan Zhu Yu (Fructus Corni Officinalis) *Dang Shen* (Radix Codonopsitis Pilosulae) *Gan Cao* (Radix Glycyrrhizae)	Wheezing with a sunken and weak pulse due to Lung and Kidney deficiency
	Chen Pi (Pericarpium Citri Reticulatae) *Tao Ren* (Semen Persicae) *Gui Zhi* (Ramulus Cinnamomi Cassiae) *Wu Zhu Yu* (Fructus Evodiae Rutaecarpae)	Full patterns with dyspnoea and hiccups due to counterflow Qi surging upwards and obstruction of the respiratory tract
Cooling the Blood and stopping bleeding	*Zhu Ru* (Caulis Bambusae in Taeniis) *Bai Shao* (Radix Paeoniae Lactiflorae) *Niu Bang Zi* (Fructus Arctii Lappae)	Vomiting of blood and nosebleed due to the frenetic movement of hot Blood

Wu Ling Zhi (Excrementum Trogopteri) *Yu Yu Liang* (Limonitum) *Chi Shi Zhi* (Halloysitum Rubrum)	Enduring uterine bleeding with dizziness
Sheng Di Huang (Radix Rehmanniae Glutinosae)	Miscarriage, persistent bleeding

Note: In addition, *Dai Zhe Shi* can be prepared with *Qing Dai* (Indigo Naturalis), *Hua Shi* (Talcum) and *Jing Jie* (Herba Schizonepetae Tenuifoliae) and mixed with honey and water for internal and external use to treat erysipelas.

Zhen Zhu 珍珠 (Pearl, Margarita)

Zhen Zhu is the pearl formed through stimulation of the bivalves *Pteria martensii* (Dunker), family Pteriidae, and *Hyriopsis cumingii* (Lea) and *Cristaria plicata* (Leach), family Unionidae.

Main ingredients *Zhen Zhu* contains calcium carbonate, threonine, leucine, methionine, alanine, glycine, glutamic acid and aspartic acid.

Properties Taste: sweet and salty; nature: cold.

Channels entered Heart and Liver.

Functions and indications Settles fright and quiets the Spirit, clears the Liver and eliminates eye screen, promotes contraction and generates flesh. It is indicated for palpitations, fearful throbbing, disquieted Heart and Spirit, epilepsy, convulsions, red, sore and swollen eyes, eye screen, and non-closure of open sores.

Common dosage 0.3-1g in pills or powder; appropriate dosage for external application as a powder, eye drops or laryngeal insufflation.

Precautions and contraindications *Zhen Zhu* is usually made into pills or very fine powder, otherwise it may damage the Zang-Fu organs.

Comparison of functions Both *Zhen Zhu* (Margarita) and *Zhen Zhu Mu* (Concha Margaritifera) are cold, heavy, sinking and downward-bearing. They have the functions of settling fright and quieting the Spirit, clearing the Liver and brightening the eyes to eliminate eye screen, and closing open sores. They can treat palpitations and insomnia, disquieted Heart and Spirit, red, sore and swollen eyes and eye screen due to Liver-fire attacking upwards, and damp, ulcerating sores. *Zhen Zhu* tends to settle fright and quiet the Spirit and is often used for treating palpitations and insomnia, disquieted Heart and Spirit, convulsions, and epilepsy. It is good for closing sores, absorbing dampness and generating flesh. *Zhen Zhu Mu* tends to calm the Liver and subdue Yang and is often used to treat dizziness due to hyperactivity of Liver Yang and Liver-fire attacking upwards. It is not as effective in quieting the Spirit and closing sores as *Zhen Zhu* and does not have the function of generating flesh.

Combinations and applications

Functions	Combinations	Applications
Settling fright and quieting the Spirit	*Zhu Sha* (Cinnabaris) (see notes on legal status) *Hu Po* (Succinum) *Tian Nan Xing* (Rhizoma Arisaematis)	Palpitations, epilepsy

	Niu Huang (Calculus Bovis) *Dan Nan Xing* (Pulvis Arisaematis cum Felle Bovis) *Tian Zhu Huang* (Concretio Silicea Bambusae)	Acute convulsions due to Phlegm-heat, clouded Spirit due to high fever, spasms and convulsions, opisthotonos
	Zhu Sha (Cinnabaris) (see notes on legal status) *Niu Huang* (Calculus Bovis) *Huang Lian* (Rhizoma Coptidis)	Child fright epilepsy, fear and disquiet, convulsions with protrusion of the tongue
	Feng Mi (Mel)	Palpitations and insomnia, forgetfulness, neurasthenia
Clearing the Liver and eliminating eye screen	*Qing Xiang Zi* (Semen Celosiae Argenteae) *Ju Hua* (Flos Chrysanthemi Morifolii) *Shi Jue Ming* (Concha Haliotidis)	Dry, sore and red eyes and eye screen due to wind-heat in the Liver channel or Liver-heat attacking upwards
	Hu Po (Succinum) *Bing Pian* (Borneolum) (for external use as topical eye medication)	Eye screen
Promoting contraction and generating flesh	*Lu Gan Shi* (Calamina) *Xue Jie* (Resina Draconis) (ground into a fine powder)	Non-closure of open sores

Zhen Zhu Mu 珍珠母 (Mother-of-pearl, Concha Margaritifera)

Zhen Zhu Mu is the pearly layer of the shell of *Pteria martensii* (Dunker), family Pteriidae, and *Hyriopsis cumingii* (Lea) and *Cristaria plicata* (Leach), family Unionidae.

Main ingredients *Zhen Zhu Mu* contains conchiolin, calcium carbonate, calcium oxide, small amounts of magnesium, iron, silicates, sulphates and phosphates, and amino acids.

Properties Taste: salty; nature: cold.

Channels entered Liver and Heart.

Functions and indications Calms the Liver and subdues Yang, clears the Heart and quiets the Spirit, clears the Liver and brightens the eyes. It is indicated for mania and withdrawal, fright epilepsy, dizziness, tinnitus, palpitations, insomnia, blurred vision, red, sore and swollen eyes, coughing of blood, and nosebleed.

Common dosage 10-30g, decocted before other ingredients; appropriate dosage for external application.

Precautions and contraindications *Zhen Zhu Mu* should be used with caution in cases of Spleen and Stomach deficiency-cold and during pregnancy.

Remarks *Zhen Zhu Mu* should be decocted for 30 minutes before adding other substances.

Comparison of functions Both *Zhen Zhu Mu* (Concha Margaritifera) and *Shi Jue Ming* (Concha Haliotidis) enter the Liver channel and can cool and settle the Liver and subdue Yang to treat dizziness and headache, tinnitus, and red, sore and swollen eyes due to heat in the Liver channel and ascendant hyperactivity of Liver Yang. The difference between the substances is that *Zhen Zhu Mu* also enters the Heart channel and has the functions of clearing the Heart and quieting the Spirit to treat insomnia, vexation and agitation, and disquieted Heart and Spirit. *Shi Jue Ming* is more effective in clearing the Liver and subduing Yang and it can also enrich and nourish Liver Yin. It is therefore used to treat aversion to light, blurred vision and clear-eye blindness (glaucoma) due to Blood deficiency and Liver-heat, as well as for dizziness and tinnitus due to Yin deficiency and ascendant hyperactivity of Liver Yang.

For an additional comparison, see *Zhen Zhu* (Margarita).

Toxicity *Zhen Zhu Mu* has a very low level of toxicity. Intraperitoneal injection in mice of 450mg/kg of a powder of *Zhen Zhu Mu* did not result in any side-effects. The LD_{50} of a powder of *Zhen Zhu Mu* fed to rats via intragastric administration is 21.5g/kg.

Modern research Protects the liver, brightens the eyes, inhibits ulcers and allergies.[7]

Combinations and applications

Functions	Combinations	Applications
Calming the Liver and subduing Yang	*Bai Shao* (Radix Paeoniae Lactiflorae) *Sheng Di Huang* (Radix Rehmanniae Glutinosae) *Long Chi* (Dens Draconis)	Dizziness, tinnitus, vexation and agitation, and insomnia due to ascendant hyperactivity of Liver Yang
Clearing the Heart and quieting the Spirit	*Zhu Sha* (Cinnabaris) (see notes on legal status) *Ci Shi* (Magnetitum)	Mania and withdrawal, fright epilepsy
	Zhu Sha (Cinnabaris) (see notes on legal status) *Long Gu* (Os Draconis) *Hu Po* (Succinum)	Palpitations, insomnia, disquieted Heart and Spirit
Clearing the Liver and brightening the eyes	*Ju Hua* (Flos Chrysanthemi Morifolii) *Qian Li Guang* (Herba Senecionis Scandentis) *Che Qian Zi* (Semen Plantaginis) *Jue Ming Zi* (Semen Cassiae)	Red, sore and swollen eyes and aversion to light due to wind-fire in the Liver channel
	Cang Zhu (Rhizoma Atractylodis) *Zhu Gan* (pig's liver)	Blurred vision and night blindness due to Liver deficiency

Note: In addition, external application of a powder of *Zhen Zhu Mu* can dry dampness to treat damp abscesses and itchy skin.

Bai Ji Li 白蒺藜
(Tribulus fruit, Fructus Tribuli Terrestris)

Bai Ji Li is the dried fruit of *Tribulus terrestris* L., family Zygophyllaceae.

Main ingredients *Bai Ji Li* contains kaempferol, tribuloside, harman, harmol, furostanol, spirostanol, tannin, resins and sylvite.

Properties Taste: acrid and bitter; nature: warm.

Channel entered Liver.

Functions and indications Calms the Liver, subdues Yang and allows constrained Liver Qi to flow freely, dispels wind and alleviates itching, dispels wind-heat and brightens the eyes. It is indicated for headache, dizziness, distension and pain in the chest and hypochondrium, stoppage of breast milk, red eyes with profuse lacrimation, and itchy skin.

Common dosage 6-10g.

Precautions and contraindications *Bai Ji Li* should be used with caution in cases of Blood and Qi deficiency, and during pregnancy.

Remarks As *Bai Ji Li* acts in the Liver channel, not only can it calm the Liver and subdue the ascendant hyperactivity of Liver Yang, it can also soothe the Liver and promote the movement of Qi.

Comparison of functions Both *Bai Ji Li* (Fructus Tribuli Terrestris) and *Sha Yuan Zi* (Semen Astragali Complanati) enter the Liver channel and can brighten the eyes. However, *Bai Ji Li* is bitter and acrid and is effective for calming the Liver and dispelling wind-heat to brighten the eyes; it is mainly used for full patterns due to ascendant hyperactivity of Liver Yang, Liver Qi depression or wind-heat in the Liver channel. *Sha Yuan Zi* is sweet and warm, and enters the Kidney channel as well as the Liver channel. It can supplement the Liver and brighten the eyes to treat eye disorders due to insufficiency of the Liver and Kidneys.

Modern research

1. The steep of *Bai Ji Li* lowers blood pressure.[8]
2. Promotes urination.[9]
3. The alkaloids contained in *Bai Ji Li* inhibit intestinal muscular contraction.[9]

Combinations and applications

Functions	Combinations	Applications
Calming the Liver, subduing Yang and allowing constrained Liver Qi to flow freely	*Ju Hua* (Flos Chrysanthemi Morifolii) *Bai Shao* (Radix Paeoniae Lactiflorae) *Man Jing Zi* (Fructus Viticis) *Gou Teng* (Ramulus Uncariae cum Uncis) *Zhen Zhu Mu* (Concha Margaritifera)	Headache and dizziness due to ascendant hyperactivity of Liver Yang
	Chai Hu (Radix Bupleuri) *Qing Pi* (Pericarpium Citri Reticulatae Viride) *Xiang Fu* (Rhizoma Cyperi Rotundi)	Distension and pain in the chest and hypochondrium and stoppage of breast milk due to depression binding of Liver Qi
Dispelling wind and alleviating itching	*Dang Gui* (Radix Angelicae Sinensis) *Jing Jie* (Herba Schizonepetae Tenuifoliae) *Fang Feng* (Radix Ledebouriellae Divaricatae) *Chan Tui* (Periostracum Cicadae) *Di Fu Zi* (Fructus Kochiae Scopariae)	Wind papules with itchy skin due to an invasion of wind
Dispelling wind-heat and brightening the eyes	*Ju Hua* (Flos Chrysanthemi Morifolii) *Lian Qiao* (Fructus Forsythiae Suspensae) *Jue Ming Zi* (Semen Cassiae) *Man Jing Zi* (Fructus Viticis)	Red eyes with profuse lacrimation due to wind-heat

SUBSTANCES FOR EXTINGUISHING WIND AND ALLEVIATING TETANY

Ling Yang Jiao 羚羊角 (Antelope horn, Cornu Antelopis)

Ling Yang Jiao is the horn of *Saiga tatarica* L., family Bovidae.

Legal status *Ling Yang Jiao* is a restricted substance listed in Appendix II of the Convention on International Trade in Endangered Species of Wild Fauna and Flora (CITES). Appropriate import and export permits are required for trade in this materia medica.

Main ingredients *Ling Yang Jiao* contains keratin, phosphatide, calcium phosphate, cholesterol, vitamin A and insoluble inorganic salts.

Properties Taste: salty; nature: cold.

Channels entered Liver and Heart.

Functions and indications Calms the Liver and extinguishes wind, clears heat and relieves toxicity, clears the Liver and brightens the eyes. It is indicated for fright epilepsy, delirious speech, convulsions, dizziness due to ascendant hyperactivity of Liver Yang, vexation and agitation, high fever in warm-febrile diseases, and red eyes and headache due to Liver-fire flaming upwards.

Common dosage 1-3g, decocted on its own for at least two hours; or 0.3-0.5g of powder for oral use directly or mixed with water.

Remarks *Shan Yang Jiao* (Cornu Naemorhedi), or the horn of the goat *Naemorhedus goral* Hardwicke, family Bovidae, can be used clinically instead of *Ling Yang Jiao*. Salty and cold, its effects are similar to but weaker than those of *Ling Yang Jiao*, so the dosage should be increased to 10-15g.

Comparison of functions See *Niu Huang* (Calculus Bovis) and *Gou Teng* (Ramulus Uncariae cum Uncis).

Toxicity Acute toxicity tests on mice involving administration of 2g/kg of a 10% *Ling Yang Jiao* decoction for seven days resulted in no marked changes apart from a slowdown in weight increase.

Modern research

1. Has a tranquillizing function and relieves convulsions.[2]
2. Abates fever and lowers blood pressure.[2]
3. Decoctions of *Ling Yang Jiao* stimulate the smooth muscle of both the intestine and the uterus, whereas its hydrolysed liquid inhibits the smooth muscle of the intestine only.[10]

Combinations and applications

Functions	Combinations	Applications
Calming the Liver and extinguishing wind	*Gou Teng* (Ramulus Uncariae cum Uncis) *Ju Hua* (Flos Chrysanthemi Morifolii) *Sheng Di Huang* (Radix Rehmanniae Glutinosae)	High fever and convulsions of the limbs due to exuberant heat in the Liver channel in patterns of extreme heat stirring wind in warm-febrile diseases
	Deng Xin Cao (Medulla Junci Effusi) *Gan Cao* (Radix Glycyrrhizae)	Palpitations, vexation and agitation, fright and delirious speech, and a rapid, racing pulse due to internal exuberance of pathogenic heat
	Shi Jue Ming (Concha Haliotidis) *Ju Hua* (Flos Chrysanthemi Morifolii) *Gou Teng* (Ramulus Uncariae cum Uncis)	Dizziness and vertigo due to ascendant hyperactivity of Liver Yang

	Fang Feng (Radix Ledebouriellae Divaricatae) *Du Huo* (Radix Angelicae Pubescentis) *Fu Shen* (Sclerotium Poriae Cocos cum Ligno Hospite) *Suan Zao Ren* (Semen Ziziphi Spinosae) *Chuan Xiong* (Rhizoma Ligustici Chuanxiong) *Dang Gui* (Radix Angelicae Sinensis)	Eclampsia (convulsions during pregnancy)
	Huang Qin (Radix Scutellariae Baicalensis) *Shui Niu Jiao* (Cornu Bubali) *Gan Cao* (Radix Glycyrrhizae) *Fu Shen* (Sclerotium Poriae Cocos cum Ligno Hospite)	Fever due to fright, night crying in infants
Clearing heat and relieving toxicity	*Shi Gao* (Gypsum Fibrosum) *Shui Niu Jiao* (Cornu Bubali) *Han Shui Shi* (Calcitum)	High fever, vexation and agitation, clouded Spirit and delirious speech, convulsions and thirst due to pathogenic heat invading the Pericardium in warm-febrile diseases
	Jin Yin Hua (Flos Lonicerae) *Huang Qi* (Radix Astragali seu Hedysari)	Swelling and pain throughout the body due to persistence of toxins after chicken pox
	Huang Qin (Radix Scutellariae Baicalensis) *Zhi Zi* (Fructus Gardeniae Jasminoidis) *Sheng Ma* (Rhizoma Cimicifugae) *Zhi Ke* (Fructus Citri Aurantii)	Vexation and agitation, distension in the chest and diaphragm, red eyes and insomnia due to externally-contracted pathogenic heat
Clearing the Liver and brightening the eyes	*Ju Hua* (Flos Chrysanthemi Morifolii) *Huang Qin* (Radix Scutellariae Baicalensis) *Shi Jue Ming* (Concha Haliotidis) *Long Dan Cao* (Radix Gentianae Scabrae)	Red eyes and headache due to Liver-fire flaming upwards

Niu Huang 牛黄
(Cow bezoar, Calculus Bovis)

Niu Huang includes both natural *Niu Huang* (*Tian Ran Niu Huang*) and artificial *Niu Huang* (*Ren Gong Niu Huang*). Natural *Niu Huang* is the stones found in the gallbladder or biliary ducts of *Bos taurus domesticus* Gmelin, family Bovidae; artificial *Niu Huang* is abstracted and processed from cattle or pig bile.

Main ingredients *Niu Huang* contains cholic acid, deoxycholic acid, cholesterol, bilirubin, ergosterol, vitamin D, sodium, calcium, magnesium, copper, phosphorus, zinc, carotene and a number of amino acids including alanine and glycine.

Properties Taste: bitter and sweet; nature: cool.

Channels entered Liver and Heart.

Functions and indications Clears the Heart, opens the orifices and dispels Phlegm, extinguishes wind and alleviates tetany, clears heat and relieves toxicity. It is indicated for fright epilepsy, clouded Spirit and delirious speech, mania, child fright wind, sore throat, painful and swollen gums, mouth and tongue sores, and boils, abscesses and sores.

Common dosage 0.15-0.45g for oral use in pills or powder.

Precautions and contraindications

1. *Niu Huang* is contraindicated for patterns not involving full-heat.
2. *Niu Huang* should be used with caution during pregnancy.

Comparison of functions Both *Niu Huang* (Calculus Bovis) and *Ling Yang Jiao* (Cornu Antelopis) enter the Liver and Heart channels; they can extinguish wind and alleviate tetany as well as being able to clear heat and relieve toxicity. They are used for extreme heat stirring wind in warm-febrile diseases, high fever in child acute fright wind, clouded Spirit and delirious speech, spasms and convulsions, and dizziness and red, sore and swollen eyes due to Liver-fire attacking upwards. *Ling Yang Jiao* acts more effectively on the Liver to extinguish Liver-wind, clear Liver-fire and calm Liver Yang to treat high fever due to Liver-wind stirring internally, spasms and convulsions, and eye disorders due to Liver-fire. *Niu Huang* acts more effectively on the Heart to clear Heart-heat, open the orifices, arouse the Spirit and transform Phlegm. It has the stronger effect in relieving toxicity and is therefore used for heat invading the Pericardium, wind-stroke and fright wind, and also for high fever, clouded Spirit and delirious speech due to Phlegm-heat blocking the orifices of the Heart.

Toxicity The LD_{50} for intraperitoneal injection in mice of cholic acid is 1.52g/kg, that for intravenous injection of deoxycholic acid is 0.15g/kg. Intraperitoneal injection in mice of 0.6g/kg per day of natural *Niu Huang* for six days caused no reduction in weight. In the 1980s, reports began to appear of allergic reactions caused by overdosage and prolonged use of medicines containing *Niu Huang*.

Modern research

1. Has a tranquillizing function and relieves convulsions.[11, 12]
2. Abates fever and inhibits inflammation.[11, 12]
3. Strengthens the heart and lowers blood pressure.[12]
4. The deoxycholic acid contained in *Niu Huang* inhibited such pathogenic micro-organisms as Staphylococcus aureus and various streptococci in laboratory experiments.[13]
5. Strengthens the immune function.[14]

Combinations and applications

Functions	Combinations	Applications
Clearing the Heart, opening the orifices and dispelling Phlegm, extinguishing wind and alleviating tetany	*Shui Niu Jiao* (Cornu Bubali) *Yu Jin* (Radix Curcumae) *She Xiang* (Secretio Moschi) (see notes on legal status) *Huang Lian* (Rhizoma Coptidis) *Zhu Sha* (Cinnabaris) (see notes on legal status)	High fever, vexation and agitation, clouded Spirit and delirious speech, stiff tongue, convulsion of the limbs, wind-stroke or child fright wind due to Phlegm-heat blocking the orifices of the Heart or pathogenic heat invading the Pericardium in warm diseases
	Yu Jin (Radix Curcumae) *Gan Cao* (Radix Glycyrrhizae) *Zhu Sha* (Cinnabaris) (see notes on legal status) *Mu Dan Pi* (Cortex Moutan Radicis)	Mania in women due to heat invading the Blood chamber
	Qian Niu Zi (Semen Pharbitidis) *Zhu Sha* (Cinnabaris) (see notes on legal status)	Wind-stroke and loss of consciousness, collapse due to exuberant Phlegm and Qi block, child fright wind

	Dan Nan Xing (Pulvis Arisaematis cum Felle Bovis) *Jiang Can* (Bombyx Batryticatus) *Tian Zhu Huang* (Concretio Silicea Bambusae)	Child fright wind due to Phlegm-heat
Clearing heat and relieving toxicity	*Feng Mi* (Mel)	Foetal heat and jaundice after birth
	She Xiang (Secretio Moschi) (see notes on legal status) *Ru Xiang* (Gummi Olibanum) *Mo Yao* (Myrrha)	Scrofula, Phlegm nodes, breast abscess, Lung abscess, Intestinal abscess
	Mang Xiao (Mirabilitum) *Sheng Ma* (Rhizoma Cimicifugae) *Zhi Zi* (Fructus Gardeniae Jasminoidis) *Gan Cao* (Radix Glycyrrhizae) *Bai Shao* (Radix Paeoniae Lactiflorae)	Sore throat and mouth and tongue sores due to Phlegm-heat
	Zhen Zhu (Margarita) (as a fine powder for laryngeal insufflation)	Sore and swollen throat
	Gan Cao (Radix Glycyrrhizae) *Jin Yin Hua* (Flos Lonicerae)	Boils, abscesses and sores
	Huang Lian (Rhizoma Coptidis) *Shi Gao* (Gypsum Fibrosum) *Ju Hua* (Flos Chrysanthemi Morifolii)	Dizziness, red, sore and swollen eyes, generalized fever, thirst

Gou Teng 钩藤
(Uncaria stem and thorns, Ramulus Uncariae cum Uncis)

Gou Teng is the hook-bearing stem and branch of *Uncaria rhynchophylla* (Miq.) Jacks., *U. macrophylla* Wall., *U. hirsuta* Havil., *U. sinensis* (Oliv.) Havil. or *U. sessilifructus* Roxb., family Rubiaceae.

Main ingredients *Gou Teng* contains rhynchophylline, isorhynchophylline, corynoxeine, isocorynoxeine, corynantheine, hirsutine, corynoxine, hyperin and trifolin.

Properties Taste: sweet; nature: slightly cold.

Channels entered Liver and Pericardium.

Functions and indications Extinguishes wind and alleviates tetany, clears heat and calms the Liver. It is indicated for fright epilepsy and convulsions due to Liver-wind stirring internally, dizziness and headache, and hypertension due to ascendant hyperactivity of Liver Yang.

Common dosage 10-15g; should not be decocted for a long time (a maximum of 20 minutes).

Precautions and contraindications *Gou Teng* should be used with caution in cases of wind-heat and full-heat.

Comparison of functions

1. *Gou Teng* (Ramulus Uncariae cum Uncis) and *Ling Yang Jiao* (Cornu Antelopis) have similar functions in extinguishing Liver-wind, calming Liver Yang and clearing Liver-fire and are often used together to treat fright epilepsy and convulsions due to Liver-wind stirring internally, dizziness due to hyperactivity of Liver Yang, and red eyes and headache. *Ling Yang Jiao* is cold and salty and has the stronger effect in extinguishing Liver-wind, calming Liver Yang

and clearing Liver-fire. It has a powerful function in alleviating spasms and convulsions and is particularly good for wind patterns with extreme heat. *Gou Teng*, slightly cold in nature and moderate in effect, is weaker in clearing heat from the Liver and Pericardium. It is effective for extinguishing internal wind and alleviating tetany, especially for wind patterns due to full-heat. It can also dissipate wind-heat to treat headache and red eyes due to externally-contracted wind-heat.

2. Both *Gou Teng* (Ramulus Uncariae cum Uncis) and *Ju Hua* (Flos Chrysanthemi Morifolii) can calm Liver Yang, clear Liver-fire and dissipate wind-heat. They are often combined to treat dizziness due to hyperactivity of Liver Yang and Liver-fire attacking upwards and for headache and red eyes due to externally-contracted wind-heat. *Gou Teng* is better for extinguishing wind and alleviating tetany, whereas *Ju Hua* is more effective in dispersing wind and draining heat.
3. For an additional comparison, see *Tian Ma* (Rhizoma Gastrodiae Elatae).

Toxicity The LD_{50} for intraperitoneal injection in mice of a decoction of *Gou Teng* is 29.0 ± 0.8g/kg; for intraperitoneal injection of rhynchophylline, it is 162.3mg/kg. Rabbits fed 5g/kg (2.5 times the normal dosage) of a decoction of *Gou Teng* twice a day for ten days exhibited no toxic reaction.

Modern research

1. Lowers blood pressure.[15]
2. Has a tranquillizing function and relieves convulsions.[15]
3. Inhibits arrhythmia.[16]

Combinations and applications

Functions	Combinations	Applications
Extinguishing wind and alleviating tetany	*Tian Ma* (Rhizoma Gastrodiae Elatae) (see notes on legal status) *Shi Jue Ming* (Concha Haliotidis) *Quan Xie* (Buthus Martensi) *Niu Xi* (Radix Achyranthis Bidentatae)	Fright epilepsy, convulsions, hemiplegia, with a red tongue and a string-like pulse due to Liver-wind stirring internally
	Ling Yang Jiao (Cornu Antelopis) (see notes on legal status) *Ju Hua* (Flos Chrysanthemi Morifolii) *Long Dan Cao* (Radix Gentianae Scabrae) *Zhi Zi* (Fructus Gardeniae Jasminoidis)	Fright epilepsy, convulsions, high fever, headache, vexation and agitation, with a red tongue and a string-like and rapid pulse due to exuberant heat stirring wind
Clearing heat and calming the Liver	*Huang Qin* (Radix Scutellariae Baicalensis) *Xia Ku Cao* (Spica Prunellae Vulgaris) *Zhi Zi* (Fructus Gardeniae Jasminoidis)	Distension in the head and headache due to heat in the Liver channel
	Shi Jue Ming (Concha Haliotidis) *Ju Hua* (Flos Chrysanthemi Morifolii) *Gou Qi Zi* (Fructus Lycii) *Sheng Di Huang* (Radix Rehmanniae Glutinosae)	Dizziness and vertigo due to ascendant hyperactivity of Liver Yang caused by Yin deficiency

	Bo He (Herba Menthae Haplocalycis) *Chan Tui* (Periostracum Cicadae) *Jing Jie* (Herba Schizonepetae Tenuifoliae) *Ju Hua* (Flos Chrysanthemi Morifolii) *Zi Cao* (Radix Arnebiae seu Lithospermi) *Niu Bang Zi* (Fructus Arctii Lappae)	Headache and red eyes due to externally-contracted wind-heat

Notes:

1. A decoction of *Gou Teng* and fresh *He Shou Wu* (Radix Polygoni Multiflori) is effective in treating facial paralysis.
2. *Gou Teng* can also be used in combination with *Xia Ku Cao* (Spica Prunellae Vulgaris), *Ju Hua* (Flos Chrysanthemi Morifolii), *Sang Ye* (Folium Mori Albae) and *Shi Jue Ming* (Concha Haliotidis) to treat hypertension due to ascendant hyperactivity of Liver Yang.

Tian Ma 天麻 (Gastrodia tuber, Rhizoma Gastrodiae Elatae)

Tian Ma is the tuber of *Gastrodia elata* Bl., family Orchidaceae.

Legal status *Tian Ma* is a restricted substance listed in Appendix II of the Convention on International Trade in Endangered Species of Wild Fauna and Flora (CITES). Appropriate import and export permits are required for trade in this materia medica.

Main ingredients *Tian Ma* contains gastrodin, β-sitosterol, citric acid, palmitic acid, succinic acid, vanillyl alcohol, vanillin, amino acids and small amounts of alkaloids.

Properties Taste: sweet; nature: neutral.

Channel entered Liver.

Functions and indications Calms the Liver and subdues Yang, extinguishes wind and alleviates tetany, dispels wind-damp and alleviates Bi syndrome pain. It is indicated for fright wind, dizziness, headache, opisthotonos, convulsions, numbness of the limbs, and wind-damp Bi syndrome.

Common dosage 3-10g; or 1-1.5g as a powder for oral use with water or a herbal decoction.

Comparison of functions Both *Tian Ma* (Rhizoma Gastrodiae Elatae) and *Gou Teng* (Ramulus Uncariae cum Uncis) can subdue hyperactivity of Liver Yang, extinguish wind and alleviate tetany. They can be used together to enhance each other's effect in treating convulsions and spasms, dizziness, and headache. *Tian Ma* is sweet, neutral and nourishing, but it is not as powerful in clearing heat as *Gou Teng*. However, it is very effective in calming the Liver and extinguishing wind to treat convulsions due to Liver-wind, dizziness and many types of headache. *Gou Teng* is sweet and slightly cold and clears Liver-heat; it is used to clear heat and extinguish wind to treat extreme heat generating wind or headache and dizziness due to Liver-heat.

Toxicity The LD_{50} for intraperitoneal injection in mice of an extract of *Tian Ma* is 51.4-61.4g/kg. Intraperitoneal injection in rabbits of 12g/kg of an aqueous extract of raw *Tian Ma* resulted in slower reactions within 30 minutes; after five hours, the heart beat had reached 300 per minute, and most of the animals died within 48 hours. *Tian Ma* has low toxicity and no side-effects have been reported in clinical use. However, there was one report of dizziness, fever and fainting after cooking 80g of *Tian Ma* with chicken.

Modern research

1. Has a tranquillizing function and relieves convulsions.[17, 18]
2. Effective anaesthetic function without causing addiction.[19]

3. Increases the volume of coronary and cerebral blood supply, dilates external blood vessels and lowers blood pressure.[20, 21]
4. Inhibits inflammation and strengthens the immune function.[22]

Combinations and applications

Functions	Combinations	Applications
Calming the Liver and subduing Yang	*Gou Teng* (Ramulus Uncariae cum Uncis) *Niu Xi* (Radix Achyranthis Bidentatae) *Shi Jue Ming* (Concha Haliotidis) *Fu Shen* (Sclerotium Poriae Cocos cum Ligno Hospite)	Dizziness, headache, insomnia, with a red tongue and a string-like, rapid pulse due to ascendant hyperactivity of Liver Yang
	Bai Zhu (Rhizoma Atractylodis Macrocephalae) *Ban Xia* (Rhizoma Pinelliae Ternatae) *Fu Ling* (Sclerotium Poriae Cocos)	Headache, dizziness, focal distension and oppression in the chest and diaphragm, with white and slimy tongue fur and a rapid, slippery pulse due to wind-Phlegm attacking upwards
	Chuan Xiong (Rhizoma Ligustici Chuanxiong) *Jing Jie Sui* (Spica Schizonepetae Tenuifoliae) *Ban Xia* (Rhizoma Pinelliae Ternatae) *Gui Zhi* (Ramulus Cinnamomi Cassiae)	Headache and migraine with dizziness due to an invasion of wind
Extinguishing wind and alleviating tetany	*Ren Shen* (Radix Ginseng) *Jiang Can* (Bombyx Batryticatus) *Bai Zhu* (Rhizoma Atractylodis Macrocephalae)	Chronic child fright wind due to Spleen deficiency leading to generation of damp-Phlegm and Liver-wind stirring internally
	Ling Yang Jiao (Cornu Antelopis) (see notes on legal status) *Gou Teng* (Ramulus Uncariae cum Uncis) *Quan Xie* (Buthus Martensi)	Acute child fright wind due to high fever leading to Liver-wind stirring internally
	Dan Nan Xing (Pulvis Arisaematis cum Felle Bovis) *Bai Fu Zi* (Rhizoma Typhonii Gigantei) *Fang Feng* (Radix Ledebouriellae Divaricatae)	Spasms and convulsions, opisthotonos due to tetanus
Dispelling wind-damp and alleviating Bi syndrome pain	*Di Yu* (Radix Sanguisorbae Officinalis) *Mo Yao* (Myrrha) *Wu Tou* (Radix Aconiti) (see notes on legal status) *Xuan Shen* (Radix Scrophulariae Ningpoensis) *She Xiang* (Secretio Moschi) (see notes on legal status)	Aching sinews and bones, a sensation of heaviness in the lumbar region and legs, and inhibited bending and stretching due to wind-stroke

	Qin Jiao (Radix Gentianae Macrophyllae) *Qiang Huo* (Rhizoma et Radix Notopterygii) *Sang Ji Sheng* (Ramulus Loranthi) *Niu Xi* (Radix Achyranthis Bidentatae)	Wind-damp Bi syndrome pain, numbness or paralysis of the limbs

Di Long 地龙 (Earthworm, Lumbricus)

Di Long is the dried body of *Pheretima aspergillum* Perrier or *Allolobophora caliginosa* (Savigny) *trapezoides* (Ant. Deges), family Megascolecidae.

Main ingredients *Di Long* contains lumbrofebrin, lumbritin, terrestro lumbrolysin, xanthine, hypoxanthine, adenine, guanine, choline, fatty acids, amino acids, cholesterol and phospholipids.

Properties Taste: salty; nature: cold.

Channels entered Liver, Spleen, Lung and Bladder.

Functions and indications Extinguishes wind and alleviates tetany, clears heat and settles fright, calms wheezing, promotes urination, frees the channels and quickens the network vessels. It is indicated for dizziness, headache and red eyes, epilepsy and convulsions, coughing and wheezing, oedema, inhibited urination, hemiplegia, numbness of the limbs, and inhibited bending and stretching.

Common dosage 5-15g dried or 10-20g fresh; 1-2g as a powder for oral use; appropriate dosage for external application.

Comparison of functions See *Quan Xie* (Buthus Martensi).

Toxicity The LD_{50} for intraperitoneal injection of *Di Long* in mice is 95-115g/kg. Liquid preparations of 25g/kg of fresh *Di Long* fed to mice via intragastric administration once a day for 14 days caused no toxic symptoms or deaths. Overdosage in humans can result in such toxic side-effects as headache, dizziness, pain in the abdomen, palpitations and, in more severe cases, respiratory difficulties.

Modern research

1. Has a tranquillizing function and relieves convulsions.[23]
2. Relieves asthma.[24]
3. Abates fever.[25]
4. Inhibits the formation of thrombi.[26]
5. Inhibits arrhythmia.[27]

Combinations and applications

Functions	Combinations	Applications
Extinguishing wind and alleviating tetany, clearing heat and settling fright	*Gou Teng* (Ramulus Uncariae cum Uncis) *Jiang Can* (Bombyx Batryticatus) *Chong Lou* (Rhizoma Paridis) *Zhu Sha* (Cinnabaris) (see notes on legal status)	Headache, dizziness, red eyes, convulsions or fright epilepsy due to Liver-wind
	Gou Teng (Ramulus Uncariae cum Uncis) *Shi Gao* (Gypsum Fibrosum) *Chong Lou* (Rhizoma Paridis) *Quan Xie* (Buthus Martensi)	Convulsions, high fever, fright epilepsy

	Xia Ku Cao (Spica Prunellae Vulgaris) *Shi Jue Ming* (Concha Haliotidis)	Hypertension due to ascendant hyperactivity of Liver Yang
Calming wheezing	*Shi Gao* (Gypsum Fibrosum) *Ma Huang* (Herba Ephedrae) (see notes on legal status) *Xing Ren* (Semen Pruni Armeniacae) *Zhi Mu* (Rhizoma Anemarrhenae Asphodeloidis)	Coughing and wheezing with yellow and sticky sputum due to Lung-heat
Promoting urination	*Che Qian Zi* (Semen Plantaginis) *Mu Tong* (Caulis Mutong) (see notes on legal status) *Hua Shi* (Talcum)	Inhibited urination due to binding of heat in the Bladder
Freeing the channels and quickening the network vessels	*Sang Zhi* (Ramulus Mori Albae) *Ren Dong Teng* (Caulis Lonicerae Japonicae) *Luo Shi Teng* (Caulis Trachelospermi Jasminoidis) *Yi Yi Ren* (Semen Coicis Lachrymajobi)	Heat Bi syndrome with red, swollen and painful joints
	Chuan Wu (Radix Aconiti Carmichaeli) (see notes on legal status) *Cao Wu* (Radix Aconiti Kusnezoffii) (see notes on legal status) *Dan Nan Xing* (Pulvis Arisaematis cum Felle Bovis) *Ru Xiang* (Gummi Olibanum) *Mo Yao* (Myrrha)	Stubborn wind-damp Bi syndrome pain with numb and extremely painful limb joints and inhibited bending and stretching
	Chi Shao (Radix Paeoniae Rubra) *Chuan Xiong* (Rhizoma Ligustici Chuanxiong) *Dang Gui* (Radix Angelicae Sinensis) *Huang Qi* (Radix Astragali seu Hedysari)	Sequelae of wind-stroke, hemiplegia due to Qi deficiency and Blood stagnation

Notes:

1. *Di Long* can be used on its own to treat clouded Spirit, delirious speech, spasms, convulsions and child fright wind due to extreme heat generating wind.
2. A paste made from chopped fresh *Di Long* and white sugar is effective in external application for acute mumps, chronic sores on the legs, and scalds.

Quan Xie 全蝎 (Scorpion, Buthus Martensi)

Quan Xie is the dried body of *Buthus martensi* Karsch, family Buthidae.

Main ingredients *Quan Xie* contains buthotoxin (also known as katsutoxin), betaine, trimethylamine, sterols, taurine, lecithin and ammonium salts.

Properties Taste: salty and acrid; nature: neutral; toxic.

Channel entered Liver.

Functions and indications Extinguishes wind and settles tetany, frees the network vessels and alleviates pain, attacks toxins and dissipates lumps.

It is indicated for spasms and convulsions, child fright wind, facial paralysis, wind-stroke, hemiplegia, tetanus, migraine, wind-damp Bi syndrome, scrofula and Phlegm nodes, and sores.

Common dosage 2-5g, or 0.6-1g of powder for oral use; appropriate dosage for external application.

Precautions and contraindications

1. As this substance is toxic, overdosage must be avoided.
2. *Quan Xie* should be used with caution in cases of internal wind patterns due to Blood deficiency, and during pregnancy.

Comparison of functions *Quan Xie* (Buthus Martensi), *Wu Gong* (Scolopendra Subspinipes) and *Di Long* (Lumbricus) can all extinguish wind and alleviate tetany, and free the channels and quicken the network vessels; they are commonly used for the treatment of spasms and convulsions due to Liver-wind stirring internally. *Di Long* is cold, so it has the strongest effect in clearing heat and is often used for clouded Spirit and convulsions due to extreme heat generating wind, and for fever with acute child fright wind. *Quan Xie* and *Wu Gong* are acrid and have a more mobile and penetrating effect; they can extinguish internal wind and dispel external wind to alleviate tetany and are suitable for treating spasms and convulsions from a variety of causes.

These three substances are also often used to treat wind-damp Bi syndrome pain, and numbness and paralysis of the limbs. *Di Long* frees the channels and quickens the network vessels to alleviate pain; it can treat hemiplegia due to Qi deficiency and Blood stagnation, inhibited bending and stretching, and heat Bi syndrome with red, swollen and painful joints. *Quan Xie* and *Wu Gong* can free the network vessels and dispel wind to treat stubborn wind-damp Bi syndrome, stubborn headache and facial paralysis due to wind in the channels and network vessels. For further comparison of these two materia medica, see *Wu Gong* (Scolopendra Subspinipes).

For additional comparisons, see *Jiang Can* (Bombyx Batryticatus) and *Bai Fu Zi* (Rhizoma Typhonii Gigantei).

Toxicity The tail of *Quan Xie* is six times as toxic as the body of the insect. The LD_{50} for intravenous injection in mice of an aqueous solution of *Quan Xie* is 6.15g/kg for the body and 0.88g/kg for the tail. The LD_{50} for intraperitoneal injection of buthotoxin is just 0.48mg/kg. The toxic dosage of *Quan Xie* for adults is 30-60g with an incubation period of one to four hours. The main symptoms are headache, dizziness, high blood pressure, palpitations, inhibited urination, vexation, agitation and restlessness. In more serious cases, blood pressure will suddenly drop, breathing will become difficult and the patient may fall into a coma.

Modern research

1. Has a tranquillizing function, relieves convulsions and alleviates pain.[28]
2. The toxins contained in *Quan Xie* can cause respiratory arrest, spasms, salivation, an increase in blood pressure, or, in the most extreme cases, death (see *Toxicity* above).[29]

Combinations and applications

Functions	Combinations	Applications
Extinguishing wind and settling tetany, freeing the network vessels and alleviating pain	*Wu Gong* (Scolopendra Subspinipes)	Acute spasms and convulsions due to heat
	Dang Shen (Radix Codonopsitis Pilosulae) *Bai Zhu* (Rhizoma Atractylodis Macrocephalae) *Tian Ma* (Rhizoma Gastrodiae Elatae) (see notes on legal status)	Chronic child fright wind due to Spleen deficiency

	Wu Gong (Scolopendra Subspinipes) *Tian Nan Xing* (Rhizoma Arisaematis) *Chan Tui* (Periostracum Cicadae)	Tetanus, spasms and convulsions, opisthotonos
	Tian Ma (Rhizoma Gastrodiae Elatae) (see notes on legal status) *Wu Gong* (Scolopendra Subspinipes) *Gou Teng* (Ramulus Uncariae cum Uncis) *Jiang Can* (Bombyx Batryticatus)	Headache or migraine due to wind-fire in the Liver channel
	Jiang Can (Bombyx Batryticatus) *Bai Fu Zi* (Rhizoma Typhonii Gigantei)	Facial paralysis, sluggish tongue and inhibited speech due to wind-stroke
	Wu Shao She (Zaocys Dhumnades) *Di Long* (Lumbricus) *Bai Shao* (Radix Paeoniae Lactiflorae) *Qiang Huo* (Rhizoma et Radix Notopterygii) *Du Huo* (Radix Angelicae Pubescentis)	Wind-damp Bi syndrome pain
Attacking toxins and dissipating lumps	*Zhi Zi* (Fructus Gardeniae Jasminoidis) *Pu Gong Ying* (Herba Taraxaci cum Radice)	Swelling and toxins of sores
	Xia Ku Cao (Spica Prunellae Vulgaris) *Mu Li* (Concha Ostreae)	Scrofula and Phlegm nodes

Wu Gong 蜈蚣
(Centipede, Scolopendra Subspinipes)

Wu Gong is the dried body of the centipede *Scolopendra subspinipes mutilans* L. Koch., family Scolopendridae.

Main ingredients *Wu Gong* contains histamine, formic acid, cholesterol, amino acids and fatty acids.

Properties Taste: acrid; nature: warm; toxic.

Channel entered Liver.

Functions and indications Extinguishes wind and alleviates tetany, attacks toxins and dissipates lumps, frees the network vessels and alleviates pain. It is indicated for spasms and convulsions, acute and chronic child fright wind, tetanus, opisthotonos, severe intermittent headache, and sores.

Common dosage 1-3g, or 0.6-1g as a powder for oral use; appropriate dosage for external use by mixing the powder with sesame oil and applying to the affected area.

Precautions and contraindications

1. The toxicity of this substance means that it must not be used in large dosages.
2. *Wu Gong* is contraindicated during pregnancy.

Comparison of functions Both *Wu Gong* (Scolopendra Subspinipes) and *Quan Xie* (Buthus Martensi) can extinguish wind and alleviate tetany, attack toxins and dissipate lumps, and free the network vessels to alleviate pain. They are often combined to accentuate each other's effect. *Quan Xie*, neutral in nature, is less effective than *Wu Gong* in terms of extinguishing wind, alleviating tetany, attacking toxins and dissipating lumps. It is used more often for convulsions caused by wind due to full-heat or Spleen deficiency. *Wu Gong* is warm and dry and is more effective in extinguishing wind and alleviating tetany, especially for more serious conditions. In relation to these functions, *Quan Xie* is better for frequent convulsions and for tremors of the hands and feet, whereas *Wu Gong* is more effective for treating opisthotonos, rigidity of the limbs, and spasms. Generally speaking, *Quan Xie* is used more often internally, *Wu Gong* externally.

For an additional comparison, see *Jiang Can* (Bombyx Batryticatus).

Toxicity The LD_{50} for intraperitoneal injection in mice of *Wu Gong* toxins is 22.5mg/kg. Mice given five times the maximum adult dosage of *Wu Gong* daily for 30 days experienced no changes in weight, haemochrome or internal organs. Frequent use of *Wu Gong* in treatment may result in some patients experiencing a feeling of scorching heat with distension of the head, dizziness and facial flushes. Symptoms of overdosage include nausea and vomiting, pain in the abdomen, diarrhoea, general lack of strength, palpitations, respiratory difficulties, a reduction in body temperature and lower blood pressure. Overdosage of *Wu Gong* can also cause an allergic reaction.

Modern research

1. Relieves convulsions.[30]
2. Inhibits inflammation and alleviates pain.[31]
3. Lowers blood pressure.[32]
4. Inhibits carcinoma and pathogens.[30, 33]

Combinations and applications

Functions	Combinations	Applications
Extinguishing wind and alleviating tetany	*Quan Xie* (Buthus Martensi)	Spasms and convulsions
	Quan Xie (Buthus Martensi) *Gou Teng* (Ramulus Uncariae cum Uncis) *Zhu Sha* (Cinnabaris) (see notes on legal status) *Jiang Can* (Bombyx Batryticatus) *She Xiang* (Secretio Moschi) (see notes on legal status)	Acute spasms and convulsions of the hands and feet due to heat
	Tian Nan Xing (Rhizoma Arisaematis) *Fang Feng* (Radix Ledebouriellae Divaricatae)	Tetanus, opisthotonos
Attacking toxins and dissipating lumps	*Jin Yin Hua* (Flos Lonicerae) *Lian Qiao* (Fructus Forsythiae Suspensae)	Swelling and toxins of sores
	Da Huang (Radix et Rhizoma Rhei) *Huang Lian* (Rhizoma Coptidis) *Gan Cao* (Radix Glycyrrhizae)	Snake bite
	Xia Ku Cao (Spica Prunellae Vulgaris) *Mu Li* (Concha Ostreae)	Scrofula and Phlegm nodes
Freeing the network vessels and alleviating pain	*Tian Ma* (Rhizoma Gastrodiae Elatae) (see notes on legal status) *Quan Xie* (Buthus Martensi) *Jiang Can* (Bombyx Batryticatus) *Chuan Xiong* (Rhizoma Ligustici Chuanxiong)	Stubborn headache or migraine that is unresponsive to treatment, wind-damp Bi syndrome pain
	Fang Feng (Radix Ledebouriellae Divaricatae) *Du Huo* (Radix Angelicae Pubescentis) *Wei Ling Xian* (Radix Clematidis)	Wind-cold-damp Bi syndrome with severe, wandering pain

Note: For external application, grind *Wu Gong* into a powder with green tea leaves to treat ulcerating scrofula.

Jiang Can 僵蚕 (Stiff silkworm, Bombyx Batryticatus)

Jiang Can is the dried larva of the dead silkworm *Bombyx mori* L., family Bombycidae, stiffened due to infection by *Beauveria bassiana* (Bals.), family Moniliaceae.

Main ingredients *Jiang Can* contains lipids, proteins, bassianins, beauvericin and ammonium oxalate.

Properties Taste: salty and acrid; nature: neutral.

Channels entered Liver and Lung.

Functions and indications Extinguishes wind and alleviates tetany, dispels wind and alleviates pain, transforms Phlegm and dissipates lumps. It is indicated for fright epilepsy, convulsions, child fright wind, facial paralysis, headache, red eyes, sore throat, scrofula, and wind papules.

Common dosage 3-10g; 1-1.5g as a powder for oral use.

Remarks

1. This substance is normally stir-fried before use, but raw *Jiang Can* should be selected for dissipating wind-heat.
2. As *Jiang Can* enters the Liver channel, it can extinguish Liver-wind to alleviate tetany and is used for convulsions and epilepsy due to Liver-wind and Phlegm-heat. Since it also enters the Lung channel, it can dispel wind-heat in the Lungs and extinguish internal wind to alleviate pain, being used for headache, red eyes and sore throat due to wind-heat.

Comparison of functions *Jiang Can* (Bombyx Batryticatus), *Quan Xie* (Buthus Martensi) and *Wu Gong* (Scolopendra Subspinipes) are all used frequently to treat wind patterns. However, *Jiang Can* is not as effective in extinguishing wind as *Quan Xie* and *Wu Gong* and is therefore often used in the clinic in combination with *Quan Xie* to treat mild convulsions due to Liver-wind and with both *Quan Xie* and *Wu Gong* for severe convulsion patterns.

Modern research

1. The ammonium oxalate contained in *Jiang Can* has a tranquillizing function and relieves convulsions.[34]
2. The alcoholic extract of *Jiang Can* can inhibit carcinoma.[35]

Combinations and applications

Functions	Combinations	Applications
Extinguishing wind and alleviating tetany	*Chan Tui* (Periostracum Cicadae) *Ling Yang Jiao* (Cornu Antelopis) (see notes on legal status) *Gou Teng* (Ramulus Uncariae cum Uncis) *Ju Hua* (Flos Chrysanthemi Morifolii)	Convulsions due to high fever
	Tian Ma (Rhizoma Gastrodiae Elatae) (see notes on legal status) *Dan Nan Xing* (Pulvis Arisaematis cum Felle Bovis)	Fright epilepsy, facial paralysis, convulsions due to exuberant Phlegm-heat
	Dang Shen (Radix Codonopsitis Pilosulae) *Bai Zhu* (Rhizoma Atractylodis Macrocephalae) *Tian Ma* (Rhizoma Gastrodiae Elatae) (see notes on legal status)	Chronic fright, convulsions and enduring diarrhoea due to Spleen deficiency in children

	Quan Xie (Buthus Martensi) *Wu Gong* (Scolopendra Subspinipes) *Gou Teng* (Ramulus Uncariae cum Uncis) *Zhu Sha* (Cinnabaris) (see notes on legal status)	Tetanus, opisthotonos
	Quan Xie (Buthus Martensi) *Bai Fu Zi* (Rhizoma Typhonii Gigantei)	Facial paralysis due to wind in the channels and network vessels
Dispelling wind and alleviating pain	*Sang Ye* (Folium Mori Albae) *Mu Zei* (Herba Equiseti Hiemalis) *Jing Jie* (Herba Schizonepetae Tenuifoliae)	Headache and red eyes due to wind-heat
	Jing Jie (Herba Schizonepetae Tenuifoliae) *Fang Feng* (Radix Ledebouriellae Divaricatae) *Jie Geng* (Radix Platycodi Grandiflori) *Gan Cao* (Radix Glycyrrhizae)	Sore throat and hoarse voice due to wind-heat
	Chan Tui (Periostracum Cicadae) *Bo He* (Herba Menthae Haplocalycis)	Wind papules, itchy skin
Transforming Phlegm and dissipating lumps	*Jin Yin Hua* (Flos Lonicerae) *Lian Qiao* (Fructus Forsythiae Suspensae) *Ban Lan Gen* (Radix Isatidis seu Baphicacanthi) *Huang Qin* (Radix Scutellariae Baicalensis)	Mastitis, swelling of abscesses and clove sores
	Zhe Bei Mu (Bulbus Fritillariae Thunbergii) *Xia Ku Cao* (Spica Prunellae Vulgaris)	Scrofula and Phlegm nodes

Modern research references

1. Lei Zaiquan and Zhang Tingmo, *Zhong Hua Lin Chuang Zhong Yao Xue* [Chinese Clinical Materia Medica] (Beijing: People's Medical Publishing House, 1998), 1417.
2. He Xingdong et al., *Lin Chuang Zhong Yao Shou Ce* [Clinical Handbook of Chinese Materia Medica] (Beijing: People's Medical Publishing House, 1998), 266.
3. Ibid., 267.
4. Lei Zaiquan and Zhang Tingmo, *Zhong Hua Lin Chuang Zhong Yao Xue*, 1407.
5. Ibid., 1437.
6. Tianjin Medical College Pharmacology Teaching Research Group, *Zhong Hua Fang She Xue Za Zhi* [Chinese Radiology Journal] 8, 3 (1960): 203.
7. He Xingdong et al., *Lin Chuang Zhong Yao Shou Ce*, 269.
8. Lei Zaiquan and Zhang Tingmo, *Zhong Hua Lin Chuang Zhong Yao Xue*, 1444.
9. He Xingdong et al., *Lin Chuang Zhong Yao Shou Ce*, 273.
10. Lei Zaiquan and Zhang Tingmo, *Zhong Hua Lin Chuang Zhong Yao Xue*, 1451.
11. He Chunyang et al., *Zhong Cao Yao* [Journal of Chinese Herbs] 19, 5 (1988): 21.
12. Yuan Huinan et al., *Zhong Guo Zhong Yao Za Zhi* [Journal of Chinese Materia Medica] 16, 2 (1991): 105.
13. Jin Enyuan et al., *Zhong Cao Yao* [Journal of Chinese Herbs] 14, 12 (1983): 20.
14. Wu Tie et al., *Zhong Cao Yao* 15, 2 (1984): 30.
15. Qin Cailing et al., *Zhong Guo Zhong Yao Za Zhi* [Journal of Chinese Materia Medica] 19, 6 (1994): 371.
16. Sun Ansheng et al., *Guang Xi Yi Xue* [Guangxi Journal of Medicine] 5, 1 (1983): 6.
17. Liu Guoqing et al., *Zhong Cao Yao Tong Xun* [Chinese Herbs Newsletter] 5 (1974): 33.

18. Shao Jianping et al., *Zhong Guo Yao Xue Za Zhi* [Journal of Chinese Pharmacology] 24, 2 (1989): 163.
19. Chinese Society of Pharmacology, *Yao Li Xue Jin Zhan* [Development of Pharmacology] (Beijing: People's Medical Publishing House, 1982), 129.
20. Ren Shilan et al., *Zhong Cao Yao* [Journal of Chinese Herbs] 23, 6 (1992): 302.
21. Deng Shixian et al., *Yun Nan Yi Yao* [Yunnan Journal of Medicine and Pharmacology] 4 (1980): 48.
22. Yu Longshun et al., *Zhong Cao Yao* [Journal of Chinese Herbs] 20, 5 (1989): 19.
23. Miao Jin, *Zhe Jiang Zhong Yi Yao Za Zhi* [Zhejiang Journal of Traditional Chinese Medicine and Materia Medica] 19, 4 (1984): 188.
24. Hunan Industrial Institute of Medicine and Pharmaceuticals, *Zhong Cao Yao Tong Xun* [Chinese Herbs Newsletter] 10 (1974): 16.
25. Fu Junlu, *Shan Xi Zhong Yi* [Shaanxi Journal of Traditional Chinese Medicine] 3 (1989): 138.
26. Guo Fengtao, *Zhong Xi Yi Jie He Za Zhi* [Journal of Integrated TCM and Western Medicine] 7 (1988): 400.
27. Shen Qianshou et al., *Hu Nan Yi Yao Za Zhi* [Hunan Journal of Medicine and Pharmacology] 6 (1982): 68.
28. Liu Congming et al., *Shen Yang Yao Xue Yuan Xue Bao* [Journal of Shenyang Pharmacology College] 6, 2 (1989): 95.
29. Jiangsu New Medical College, *Zhong Yao Da Ci Dian* [Dictionary of Chinese Materia Medica] volume 1 (Shanghai: Shanghai People's Publishing House, 1977), 932.
30. Jiangsu New Medical College, *Zhong Yao Da Ci Dian* [Dictionary of Chinese Materia Medica] volume 2 (Shanghai: Shanghai People's Publishing House, 1986), 2473.
31. Wang Yufen et al., *Zhong Yao Yao Li Yu Lin Chuang* [Pharmacology and Clinical Application of Chinese Materia Medica], supplement to 8 (1992): 32.
32. Chen Changyu et al., *Zhong Yao Yao Li Yu Lin Chuang*, launch issue (1985): 124.
33. Wang Quan et al., *Zhong Yao Yao Li Yu Lin Chuang* 3 (1987): 127.
34. Beijing Pharmacology Institute, Chinese Academy of Medical Science, *Zhong Cao Yao Tong Xun* [Chinese Herbs Newsletter] 9, 12 (1978): 24.
35. Li Junde et al., *Zhong Cheng Yao* [Journal of Chinese Medicinal Preparations] 14, 2 (1992): 40.

Chapter 16

Aromatic herbs for opening the orifices

芳香开窍药

Aromatic herbs for opening the orifices

Herbs for opening the orifices are acrid, aromatic and dissipating, and enter the Heart channel. They have the functions of breaking block and freeing obstructed orifices, restoring consciousness, and arousing the brain and restoring the Spirit; they are used to treat heat invading the Pericardium in warm-febrile diseases and clouded Spirit and delirious speech due to obstruction of Phlegm turbidity, and for wind-stroke, fright wind, epilepsy and summerheat-stroke. As well as opening the orifices, some of these herbs can concurrently repel foulness and transform turbidity, quicken the Blood and move Qi, free the channels and alleviate pain, and transform dampness and relieve toxicity. They can be used to treat damp turbidity obstructing the Middle Jiao, cold, pain, fullness and oppression in the chest and stomach, pain due to Blood stasis and Qi stagnation, menstrual block, abdominal masses, reduced appetite, and abscesses and sores.

If the orifices of the Heart are blocked through clouding by pathogenic factors or confounding by Phlegm, the Spirit light is blocked internally, the Spirit becomes clouded and loss of consciousness or coma may occur.

Coma can be divided into two types:

1. The deficiency pattern of coma is also known as Tuo or desertion pattern (severe depletion of Yang Qi and separation of Yin and Yang). This pattern is caused by profuse perspiration, severe vomiting and loss of blood, or Blood and Qi deficiency due to ageing. It mainly manifests as open mouth, closed eyes, limp hands, urinary incontinence, profuse sweating, weak breath, cold limbs, and a faint, weak pulse. The treatment principle indicated is supplementing deficiency and rescuing Yang collapse. Aromatic herbs for opening the orifices are not suitable in such cases.
2. The full pattern of coma is also known as Bi or block pattern (a full wind-stroke pattern). It mainly manifests as clenched fists, clenched jaw and incontinence of urine and stool. Aromatic herbs for opening the orifices are applicable in these cases.

Block patterns can be divided into heat-type and cold-type according to their clinical manifestations:

i. Heat block patterns manifest as generalized heat with a red face, heavy breathing and vexation, yellow tongue fur and a rapid pulse. They are mainly caused by blockage of heat in the Pericardium or Phlegm-heat blocking the orifices. Heat block patterns should be treated by cold aromatic herbs for opening the orifices together with herbs for clearing heat, draining fire and relieving toxicity.

ii. Cold block patterns manifest as generalized cold, an ashen face, white tongue fur and a slow pulse. They are commonly seen with wind-stroke or sudden collapse caused by Phlegm blocking the orifices. Cold block patterns should be treated by warm aromatic herbs for opening the orifices together with herbs for warming the interior and dispelling cold.

Other combinations in block patterns should be selected as follows:

a. in cases of clouded Spirit with fright collapse and convulsions, add substances for calming the Liver, extinguishing wind and alleviating tetany;
b. in cases of vexation, agitation and disquiet, add herbs for quieting the Spirit and stabilizing fright;
c. where pain is the main symptom, add herbs for moving Qi or herbs for quickening the Blood and transforming stasis;
d. in cases of congestion of Phlegm turbidity, add herbs for transforming dampness and dispelling Phlegm.

Most of these herbs should be used in pill or powder form. They must not be decocted, otherwise the effective ingredients will volatilize. Since herbs for opening the orifices are aromatic, they should only be used temporarily for emergency and symptomatic treatment, as they consume vital Qi; they are contraindicated for desertion pattern. These herbs also induce abortion, so they are likewise contraindicated during pregnancy.

Tab. 16 Aromatic herbs for opening the orifices

Herb	Functions	Indications
She Xiang (Secretio Moschi)	Opening the orifices and arousing the Spirit, quickening the Blood, dissipating lumps and alleviating pain, hastening delivery	Clouded Spirit in block patterns, wind-stroke and Phlegm collapse, pathogenic heat invading the Pericardium in warm-febrile diseases, sudden collapse, fright wind, sudden pain in the chest and abdomen, abdominal masses, knocks and falls, sores, retention of dead foetus and placenta
Su He Xiang (Styrax Liquidus)	Opening the orifices and repelling foulness, alleviating pain	Cold block patterns, clouded Spirit, and cold, pain, fullness and oppression in the chest and abdomen
Bing Pian (Borneolum)	Opening the orifices and arousing the Spirit, clearing heat, dispersing swelling and alleviating pain	Wind-stroke and Phlegm collapse, clouded Spirit in warm-febrile diseases, stupor, sore throat, mouth sores, earache, abscesses and sores
Shi Chang Pu (Rhizoma Acori Graminei)	Aromatically opening the orifices and quieting the Spirit, transforming dampness and harmonizing the Middle Jiao, repelling foulness	Confused Spirit and Mind, epilepsy, mania and withdrawal, forgetfulness, tinnitus and deafness, distension and oppression in the chest and abdomen, diarrhoea with lack of hunger

She Xiang 麝香 (Musk, Secretio Moschi)

She Xiang is the secretion obtained from the musk gland of the mature male *Moschus berezovskii* Flerov, *M. sifanicus* Przewalski or *M. moschiferus* L., family Cervidae.

Legal status *She Xiang* is a restricted substance listed in Appendix I of the Convention on International Trade in Endangered Species of Wild Fauna and Flora (CITES). All trade in this materia medica is presently banned.

Main ingredients *She Xiang* contains muscone, normuscone, cholesterol and steroid hormones.

Properties Taste: acrid; nature: warm.

Channels entered Heart and Spleen.

Functions and indications Opens the orifices and arouses the Spirit, quickens the Blood, dissipates lumps and alleviates pain, and hastens delivery. It is indicated for clouded Spirit in block patterns, wind-stroke and Phlegm collapse, pathogenic heat invading the Pericardium in warm-febrile diseases, sudden collapse, fright wind, sudden pain in the chest and abdomen, abdominal masses, knocks and falls, sores, and retention of dead foetus and placenta.

Common dosage 0.06–0.1g, taken as pills or powder; appropriate dosage for external application as a plaster.

Precautions and contraindications *She Xiang* is contraindicated during pregnancy.

Comparison of functions See *Bing Pian* (Borneolum) and *Su He Xiang* (Styrax Liquidus).

Toxicity Both *She Xiang* and muscone have very low toxicity. There were no abnormal changes in terms of blood, weight, and liver and kidney function after 60mg/kg of *She Xiang* was fed to rats and 62mg/kg to rabbits for 15 days. The LD_{50} for intravenous injection of natural and artificial *She Xiang* in mice is 172mg/kg and 152mg/kg respectively.

Modern research

1. *She Xiang* has a benign function in stimulating and calming the central nervous system.[1]
2. Lowers blood pressure, relieves angina pectoris, inhibits haematoblastic concentration and inflammation.[2]
3. Excites the uterus and inhibits carcinoma.[3]

Combinations and applications

Functions	Combinations	Applications
Opening the orifices and arousing the Spirit	*Niu Huang* (Calculus Bovis) *Yu Jin* (Radix Curcumae) *Shui Niu Jiao* (Cornu Bubali) *Zhi Zi* (Fructus Gardeniae Jasminoidis)	High fever, vexation and agitation, clouded Spirit and delirious speech, stiff tongue and cold limbs due to pathogenic heat invading the Pericardium in warm-febrile diseases
	Han Shui Shi (Calcitum) *Shi Gao* (Gypsum Fibrosum) *Shui Niu Jiao* (Cornu Bubali) *Ling Yang Jiao* (Cornu Antelopis) (see notes on legal status)	High fever and child fright collapse associated with exuberant heat stirring wind
	Bing Pian (Borneolum) *An Xi Xiang* (Benzoinum) *Niu Huang* (Calculus Bovis) *Dai Mao* (Carapax Eretmochelydis) (see notes on legal status)	Summerheat-stroke, wind-stroke, or clouded Spirit and inability to speak, exuberant Phlegm and heavy breathing, generalized fever and agitation due to internal obstruction of Phlegm turbidity in warm diseases

	Ding Xiang (Flos Caryophylli) *Su He Xiang* (Styrax Liquidus) *Tan Xiang* (Lignum Santali Albi) *An Xi Xiang* (Benzoinum)	Sudden collapse and clenched jaw due to wind-stroke, loss of consciousness, pain in the abdomen, focal distension and fullness in the chest, nausea and diarrhoea in cold-damp or Phlegm turbidity patterns
	Chuan Bei Mu (Bulbus Fritillariae Cirrhosae) *Mu Xiang* (Radix Aucklandiae Lappae) (see notes on legal status) *Tian Zhu Huang* (Concretio Silicea Bambusae) *Jiang Can* (Bombyx Batryticatus) *Tian Ma* (Rhizoma Gastrodiae Elatae) (see notes on legal status)	Acute child fright wind, fever and wheezing, agitation, vomiting of milk and night crying in infants due to Phlegm-heat blocking the orifices of the Heart
Quickening the Blood, dissipating lumps and alleviating pain	*Tan Xiang* (Lignum Santali Albi) *Bing Pian* (Borneolum) *Mu Xiang* (Radix Aucklandiae Lappae) (see notes on legal status) *Tao Ren* (Semen Persicae)	Coronary heart disease, angina pectoris or myocardial infarction due to Qi stagnation and Blood stasis
	Ru Xiang (Gummi Olibanum) *Xiong Huang* (Realgar) (see notes on legal status) *Jin Yin Hua* (Flos Lonicerae)	Swelling and toxins of sores
	Tao Ren (Semen Persicae) *Hong Hua* (Flos Carthami Tinctorii) *Niu Xi* (Radix Achyranthis Bidentatae) *Gui Zhi* (Ramulus Cinnamomi Cassiae)	Menstrual block and pain in the lower abdomen in women due to Blood stasis
	San Leng (Rhizoma Sparganii Stoloniferi) *E Zhu* (Rhizoma Curcumae) *Mu Xiang* (Radix Aucklandiae Lappae) (see notes on legal status) *Zhi Ke* (Fructus Citri Aurantii)	Abdominal masses due to prolonged Qi stagnation and Blood stasis
	Xi Xin (Herba cum Radice Asari) *Bing Pian* (Borneolum) *Tian Nan Xing* (Rhizoma Arisaematis) *Mo Yao* (Myrrha)	Local swelling and pain due to knocks and falls and sprains
	Niu Huang (Calculus Bovis) *Bing Pian* (Borneolum) *Zhen Zhu* (Margarita)	Sore and swollen throat
Hastening delivery	*Rou Gui* (Cortex Cinnamomi Cassiae)	Retention of dead foetus, retention of placenta

Su He Xiang 苏合香
(Liquid storax, Styrax Liquidus)

Su He Xiang is the purified balsam obtained from the trunk of *Liquidambar orientalis* Mill., family Hamamelidaceae.

Main ingredients *Su He Xiang* contains styrene, storesinol, phenylpropyl cinnamate, cinnamic aldehyde, vanillin and oleanolic acid.

Properties Taste: sweet and acrid; nature: warm.

Channels entered Heart and Spleen.

Functions and indications Opens the orifices and repels foulness, and alleviates pain. It is indicated for cold block patterns, clouded Spirit, and cold, pain, fullness and oppression in the chest and abdomen.

Common dosage 0.3-1g in pill or powder form; not taken as a decoction.

Precautions and contraindications *Su He Xiang* is contraindicated in cases of high fever and collapse.

Comparison of functions Both *Su He Xiang* (Styrax Liquidus) and *She Xiang* (Secretio Moschi) are aromatic herbs that are acrid in taste and warm in nature (for *She Xiang*, see notes on legal status). They can open the orifices and arouse the Spirit and are often used in combination. *She Xiang* has a stronger effect than *Su He Xiang* for these functions and is frequently used in combinations for both cold block and heat block patterns. Although *Su He Xiang* has similar functions to *She Xiang* in opening the orifices and arousing the Spirit, its effect is weaker, and it is mainly used for wind-stroke, sudden collapse and cold block patterns. In addition, *She Xiang* can quicken the Blood, dissipate lumps and alleviate pain and is used in combination with herbs for quickening the Blood and dispelling stasis to treat menstrual block, abdominal masses, pain in the heart and abdomen, knocks and falls, and swollen abscesses and sores. *Su He Xiang* also repels foulness, transforms turbidity and alleviates pain, with the result that it is often used for fullness, oppression and sudden pain in the chest and abdomen.

Combinations and applications

Functions	Combinations	Applications
Opening the orifices and repelling foulness, alleviating pain	*She Xiang* (Secretio Moschi) (see notes on legal status) *Ding Xiang* (Flos Caryophylli) *An Xi Xiang* (Benzoinum)	Wind-stroke and Phlegm collapse with a cool body, ashen face, white tongue fur and a slow pulse (cold block patterns)
	Tan Xiang (Lignum Santali Albi) *Bing Pian* (Borneolum) *Ru Xiang* (Gummi Olibanum)	Angina pectoris

Bing Pian 冰片
(Borneol, Borneolum)

Bing Pian is the crystalline compound derived by distilling the tree trunk of the evergreen *Dryobalanops aromatica* Gaertn. f., family Dipterocarpaceae, or *Blumea balsamifera* DC., family Compositae. Synthetic borneol is made from turpentine oil or camphor.

Main ingredients Synthetic *Bing Pian* (Borneolum Syntheticum) contains borneol, isoborneol and camphor; *Ai Pian* (*Blumea*) contains l-borneol; *Mei Pian* (*Dryobalanops*) contains d-borneol, humulene, oleanolic acid and dryobalanone.

Properties Taste: acrid and bitter; nature: slightly cold.

Channels entered Heart, Spleen and Lung.

Functions and indications Opens the orifices and arouses the Spirit, clears heat, disperses swelling and alleviates pain. It is indicated for wind-stroke and Phlegm collapse, clouded Spirit in warm-febrile diseases, stupor, sore throat, mouth sores, earache, and abscesses and sores.

Common dosage 0.03-0.1g prepared as pills or powder; appropriate dosage for external application.

Precautions and contraindications

1. *Bing Pian* should be used with caution during pregnancy.
2. *Bing Pian* is contraindicated in cases of Qi and Blood deficiency.

Comparison of functions Both *Bing Pian* (Borneolum) and *She Xiang* (Secretio Moschi) can open the orifices and arouse the Spirit to treat clouded Spirit in warm-febrile diseases, wind-stroke and Phlegm collapse, blockage of the orifices and stupor. *She Xiang* is more effective than *Bing Pian* in terms of opening the orifices, quickening the Blood and dissipating lumps; it is therefore also used for treating menstrual block due to Blood stasis, abdominal masses, and pain in the heart and abdomen (for *She Xiang*, see notes on legal status). Since *Bing Pian* is slightly cold in nature, it is better at clearing heat and alleviating pain to treat disorders of the mouth, throat, ears and eyes. In addition, *Bing Pian* is often selected in prescriptions for external application for clearing heat and generating flesh, as it can strengthen the functions of dispersing swelling and alleviating pain.

Modern research

1. Alleviates pain and stops bleeding.[4]
2. Induces abortion.[4]
3. Both natural and synthetic *Bing Pian* inhibited various bacteria *in vitro*.[5]

Combinations and applications

Functions	Combinations	Applications
Opening the orifices and arousing the Spirit	*Niu Huang* (Calculus Bovis) *She Xiang* (Secretio Moschi) (see notes on legal status) *Shui Niu Jiao* (Cornu Bubali)	High fever, clouded Spirit and delirious speech, vexation and agitation due to heat invading the Pericardium in warm-febrile diseases, or high fever, stiff tongue and cold limbs due to wind-stroke
	Shui Niu Jiao (Cornu Bubali) *An Xi Xiang* (Benzoinum) *Hu Po* (Succinum) *She Xiang* (Secretio Moschi) (see notes on legal status)	Clouded Spirit and delirious speech, exuberant Phlegm and heavy breathing, generalized fever, vexation and agitation due to internal obstruction of Phlegm-heat
	Ding Xiang (Flos Caryophylli) *She Xiang* (Secretio Moschi) (see notes on legal status) *Su He Xiang* (Styrax Liquidus) *Mu Xiang* (Radix Aucklandiae Lappae) (see notes on legal status)	Fullness, pain and cold in the chest and abdomen, and sudden stupor due to an invasion of pathogenic factors and Phlegm obstruction
Clearing heat, dispersing swelling and alleviating pain	*Peng Sha* (Borax) *Xuan Ming Fen* (Mirabilitum Depuratum) *Zhu Sha* (Cinnabaris) (see notes on legal status) (for external use)	Sore and swollen throat, mouth and tongue sores

Deng Xin Cao (Medulla Junci Effusi) *Huang Bai* (Cortex Phellodendri) *Mai Men Dong* (Radix Ophiopogonis Japonici)	Wind-heat throat Bi syndrome
Niu Huang (Calculus Bovis) *Huang Qin* (Radix Scutellariae Baicalensis) *Da Huang* (Radix et Rhizoma Rhei) *Shi Gao* (Gypsum Fibrosum) *Gan Cao* (Radix Glycyrrhizae)	Warm-febrile diseases, toothache, earache, sores in the mouth and nose, and red, sore and swollen eyes
Ru Xiang (Gummi Olibanum) *Mo Yao* (Myrrha) *Niu Huang* (Calculus Bovis) (ground into a powder for external use)	Abscesses and sores, or knocks and falls, swelling and pain due to Blood stasis
Niu Huang (Calculus Bovis) *Zhen Zhu* (Margarita) *Lu Gan Shi* (Calamina)	Persistent non-closure of sores after ulceration

Shi Chang Pu 石菖蒲
(Grass-leaf sweetflag rhizome, Rhizoma Acori Graminei)

Shi Chang Pu is the dried rhizome of *Acorus gramineus* Soland., family Araceae.

Main ingredients *Shi Chang Pu* contains asarone, α-asarone, β-asarone, caryophyllene, α-humulene, sekishone, asaryl aldehyde, safrole, eugenol, thymol and myristic acid.

Properties Taste: acrid; nature: warm.

Channels entered Heart and Stomach.

Functions and indications Aromatically opens the orifices and quiets the Spirit, transforms dampness and harmonizes the Middle Jiao, and repels foulness. It is indicated for confused Spirit and Mind, epilepsy, mania and withdrawal, forgetfulness, tinnitus and deafness, distension and oppression in the chest and abdomen, and diarrhoea with lack of hunger.

Common dosage 5-8g, or double this dosage for the fresh herb; appropriate dosage for external application.

Comparison of functions Both *Shi Chang Pu* (Rhizoma Acori Graminei) and *Yuan Zhi* (Radix Polygalae) can dispel and eliminate Phlegm-damp. Not only can they open the orifices and quiet the Spirit, they can also sharpen the wits. They are used for confused Spirit and Mind due to Phlegm-damp turbidity clouding the clear orifices, and for disquieted Heart and Spirit, insomnia and forgetfulness. *Yuan Zhi* is better at dispelling Phlegm while stopping coughing and is commonly used for cough with copious sputum. *Shi Chang Pu* is better at transforming dampness while harmonizing the Stomach and is commonly used for damp turbidity obstructing the Middle Jiao and for distension and oppression in the chest and abdomen.

Modern research

1. Has a tranquillizing function and relieves convulsions.[6]
2. Attenuates gastrointestinal spasms.[7]
3. Decoctions of *Shi Chang Pu* and the volatile oils it contains can inhibit carcinoma.[8]
4. Reduces the level of blood lipids.[9]
5. The volatile oils and α-asarone contained in *Shi Chang Pu* expel sputum, stop coughing and calm wheezing.[10]

Combinations and applications

Functions	Combinations	Applications
Aromatically opening the orifices and quieting the Spirit	*Yu Jin* (Radix Curcumae) *Ban Xia* (Rhizoma Pinelliae Ternatae)	Confused Spirit and Mind due to Phlegm-damp clouding the clear orifices
	Fu Ling (Sclerotium Poriae Cocos) *Yuan Zhi* (Radix Polygalae) *Long Chi* (Dens Draconis)	Forgetfulness, tinnitus, deafness
	Tu Si Zi (Semen Cuscutae) *Nü Zhen Zi* (Fructus Ligustri Lucidi) *Han Lian Cao* (Herba Ecliptae Prostratae)	Tinnitus and deafness, dizziness and palpitations due to Heart and Kidney deficiency
	Niu Huang (Calculus Bovis) *Zhu Li* (Succus Bambusae)	Confused Spirit and Mind, mania or epilepsy due to Phlegm-heat clouding the Pericardium
Transforming dampness and harmonizing the Middle Jiao, repelling foulness	*Huo Xiang* (Herba Agastaches seu Pogostemi) *Bai Dou Kou* (Fructus Amomi Kravanh) *Yin Chen Hao* (Herba Artemisiae Scopariae) *Hou Po* (Cortex Magnoliae Officinalis)	Obstruction of damp turbidity in the Middle Jiao, manifesting as distension and oppression in the chest and abdomen, a bitter taste in the mouth and reduced appetite
	Ku Shi Lian Zi (Semen Caesalpiniae Minax) *Huang Lian* (Rhizoma Coptidis) *Chen Pi* (Pericarpium Citri Reticulatae)	Vomiting, frequent diarrhoea, lack of hunger

Note: *Shi Chang Pu* can also be used in combination with *Shan Dou Gen* (Radix Sophorae Tonkinensis), *Ma Bo* (Sclerotium Lasiosphaerae seu Calvatiae) and *She Gan* (Rhizoma Belamcandae Chinensis) to treat throat Bi syndrome and loss of voice.

Modern research references

1. Lei Zaiquan and Zhang Tingmo, *Zhong Hua Lin Chuang Zhong Yao Xue* [Chinese Clinical Materia Medica] (Beijing: People's Medical Publishing House, 1998), 1552.
2. He Xingdong et al., *Lin Chuang Zhong Yao Shou Ce* [Clinical Handbook of Chinese Materia Medica] (Beijing: People's Medical Publishing House, 1998), 281.
3. Ding Xuemin et al., *Chang Yong Zhong Yi Fang Yao Shou Ce* [Handbook of Commonly-Used Chinese Herbs and Prescriptions] (Changsha: Hunan Science and Technology Publishing House, 1982), 94.
4. He Xingdong et al., *Lin Chuang Zhong Yao Shou Ce*, 282.
5. Mou Jiawan, *Hua Xi Yao Xue Za Zhi* [Huaxi Pharmacology Journal] 4, 1 (1989): 335.
6. Xue Chengyi et al., *Zhong Guo Yi Yuan Yao Xue Za Zhi* [Chinese Journal of Hospital Pharmacology] 3, 8 (1983): 341.
7. Qiao Lixin, *Zhong Yi Yao Xue Bao* [Journal of Traditional Chinese Medicine and Materia Medica] 5, 7 (1991): 24.
8. Yin Chunnan et al., *Guang Zhou Yi Yao* [Guangzhou Journal of Medicine and Pharmacology] 3 (1981): 31.
9. Yuan Qisheng et al., *Zhong Cao Yao* [Journal of Chinese Herbs] 13, 9 (1982): 387.
10. Liu Guoqing et al., *Zhong Guo Yao Li Xue Bao* [Chinese Journal of Pharmacology] 4, 2 (1983): 95.

Chapter 17

Supplementing herbs 补益药

Supplementing herbs

Supplementing herbs, most of which are sweet in taste, can be used to supplement and boost vital Qi, strengthen the constitution to improve the body's ability to resist disease, relieve and aid recovery from taxation and deficiency patterns, or support vital Qi and dispel pathogenic factors. They can therefore help the body to recover from chronic disorders.

In clinical practice, these herbs must be carefully selected in accordance with the type of deficiency pattern involved. Deficiency patterns are generally divided into four types: Qi deficiency, treated with herbs for supplementing Qi; Yang deficiency, treated with herbs for supplementing Yang; Blood deficiency, treated with herbs for supplementing the Blood; and Yin deficiency, treated with herbs for supplementing Yin.

However, in the normal course of life, Yin, Yang, Qi and Blood depend on one another, and they always affect each other in conditions of deficiency and taxation. A worsening of Qi deficiency will result in Yang deficiency, and when patients have Yang deficiency, their Qi must be deficient as well. Hence, Qi deficiency and Yang deficiency signify a deterioration in the functioning of the body, which is why Yang deficiency generally occurs with Qi deficiency and vice versa. Therefore, herbs for supplementing Yang used in the treatment of Yang deficiency patterns are often supported by herbs for supplementing Qi.

Qi deficiency causes Blood deficiency due to the inability of Qi to generate transformation; Blood deficiency causes Qi deficiency due to an absence of source for generating transformation and the Blood being unable to transform Qi. Therefore, in the treatment of Blood deficiency, herbs selected for supplementing the Blood are combined with herbs for supplementing Qi in order to achieve transformation of Qi and generation of Blood. Although herbs for supplementing the Blood are used in combinations in the treatment of Qi deficiency patterns in order to generate sufficient Blood and Qi, in clinical practice, the emphasis is often placed on limiting the dosage of herbs for supplementing the Blood to be added to herbs for supplementing Qi, thus preventing herbs for supplementing the Blood from enriching stagnated Qi.

Both Qi and Yin deficiency often occur in the final stage of a febrile disease. Non-recovery from a chronic illness and consumption of Qi and Yin can cause deficiency of Qi and Yin. Herbs for supplementing Qi can boost Stomach Qi and generate body fluids, thus being of benefit in the treatment of Yin deficiency and depletion of body fluids. Herbs for enriching Yin can generate body fluids and moisten dryness, thus aiding body organs to recover their normal functions. Hence, herbs for supplementing Qi and herbs for supplementing Yin are commonly used together.

Yin deficiency and Blood deficiency signify insufficiency of the body's Essence, Blood and body fluids, which is why Yin deficiency usually combines with Blood deficiency and vice versa. Herbs for supplementing Yin and herbs for supplementing the Blood are commonly used together.

Herbs for supplementing Yin and herbs for supplementing Yang should be applied at the same time. Yin and Yang are interdependent and mutually transformable. Yang deficiency causes poor generation of transformation, resulting in Yin deficiency. Yin depletion causes a lack of source for enriching and nourishing and for generation of transformation; as a result, Qi is not transformed, leading to Yang deficiency. If Yang deficiency or Yin deficiency persists, this can lead to deficiency of both Yin and Yang. In this case, the use of herbs for supplementing Yin supports transformation of the source and benefits generation of Yang. The use of herbs for supplementing Yang reinforces Yang Qi, thus transforming Qi and benefiting the generation of Yin. Consequently, the use of herbs for enriching Yin with herbs for reinforcing Yang is considered as the best combination for eliminating dual Yin and Yang deficiency.

Different deficiency patterns often occur concurrently and attention should be paid to selecting appropriate herbs to accompany herbs for supplementing deficiency:

1. in cases of Yang deficiency generating internal cold, it is easy to attract an invasion of external cold, and herbs for supplementing Yang should therefore be used with herbs for warming the interior, thus dissipating cold;
2. in cases of Yin deficiency generating internal heat, there is often lingering deficiency-heat, and herbs for supplementing Yin should therefore be used with herbs for clearing deficiency-heat, thus enriching Yin and bearing fire downwards;
3. in cases of Yin deficiency with hyperactivity of Yang, herbs for subduing Yang should be added to herbs for enriching Yin, thus invigorating water to restrain fire;
4. in cases of Qi deficiency impairing transportation and transformation, Qi stagnation may also be produced; herbs for moving Qi can therefore be added to herbs for supplementing Qi;
5. in cases of insomnia and forgetfulness or disquieted Spirit and Mind due to Blood deficiency, herbs for quieting the Spirit should be added to herbs for nourishing the Blood.

Where supplementing herbs are used to support vital Qi and dispel pathogenic factors, the relationship between supporting vital Qi and dispelling the pathogenic factors must be clearly recognized, and supplementing herbs and herbs for eliminating pathogenic factors must be used appropriately. For patterns with deficiency of vital Qi and exuberant pathogenic factors, supplementing herbs should not be used early or on their own, thus avoiding locking pathogenic factors inside. If pathogenic factors have not been thoroughly dispelled and vital Qi is deficient, herbs for dispelling pathogenic factors should be added to supplementing herbs to support vital Qi and strengthen the supplementing effect.

The Spleen and Stomach should be considered first when prescribing supplementing herbs; only if the Spleen and Stomach are healthy can the effect of these herbs be exerted to the full.

The following aspects should be taken into account when using supplementing herbs to treat deficiency. For patients with a weak constitution and those suffering from chronic diseases, a small dosage of mild supplementing herbs should be prescribed; on the contrary, where there is a sudden collapse of Yin and Yang, use large dosages of supplementing herbs with a strong effect.

Most supplementing herbs are the root of plants and are generally greasy or oily in property, so they should be decocted for a relatively lengthy period.

HERBS FOR SUPPLEMENTING QI

Herbs for supplementing Qi include those herbs that can supplement or boost the Qi of the Zang-Fu organs and supplement vital Qi. They have the function of supplementing Spleen Qi, Lung Qi and Heart Qi in Qi deficiency patterns:

1. Spleen Qi deficiency patterns manifest as fatigued Spirit and lack of strength, limpness of the limbs, a sallow yellow facial complexion, indigestion, poor appetite, distension of the abdomen and loose stool; or middle Qi fall, pain in the abdomen, prolapse of the rectum or uterus, pain in the lumbar region, and puffy swelling. Herbs for supplementing Qi can fortify the Spleen and boost Qi; some of these herbs also have the function of bearing Yang upwards and raising middle Qi.
2. Lung Qi deficiency patterns are indicated by shortness of breath, wheezing after movement, laziness in speech, lack of strength, chills, spontaneous sweating, a haggard complexion, a pale tongue, and a weak and deficient pulse. Herbs for supplementing Qi can supplement and boost Lung Qi; some of these herbs can also moisten the Lungs and stop coughing.
3. Heart Qi deficiency manifests as insomnia and forgetfulness, palpitations, shortness of breath, distension or pain in the chest, a haggard complexion, a pale tongue with white fur, and a weak pulse. Herbs for supplementing Qi can supplement and boost Heart Qi; some of these herbs can also boost Qi and generate Blood in order to nourish the Heart and Spirit, boost the Heart and increase wisdom.

In clinical practice, when prescribing herbs for supplementing Qi, attention should be paid not only to the pattern of Qi deficiency involved, but also to the accompanying patterns in order to achieve the correct combination of herbs:

i. to treat patients with Qi deficiency accompanied by Yin deficiency, herbs for supplementing Qi should be prescribed in combination with herbs for supplementing Yin;
ii. to treat patients with Qi deficiency accompanied by Yang deficiency, herbs for supplementing Qi should be prescribed in combination with herbs for supplementing Yang in order to boost Qi and warm Yang;
iii. to treat patients with Qi deficiency accompanied by Blood deficiency, herbs for supplementing Qi should be prescribed in combination with herbs for supplementing the Blood;
iv. to treat patients with Qi deficiency accompanied by depletion of body fluids, herbs for supplementing Qi should be prescribed in combination with herbs for generating body fluids.

Since the relationship between Blood and Qi is very close, the generation and movement of Blood also depend on the normal functioning of Qi, so herbs for supplementing Qi are also used for Blood-deficiency patterns manifesting as blood loss, sweating and urinary incontinence.

Herbs for supplementing Qi are generally warm, sweet and greasy and may affect the appetite, so herbs for promoting the movement of Qi may be added where necessary.

Tab. 17.1 Herbs for supplementing Qi

Herb	Functions	Indications
Ren Shen (Radix Ginseng)	Strongly supplementing original Qi, supplementing the Spleen and boosting the Lungs, generating body fluids and allaying thirst, quieting the Spirit and increasing wisdom	Desertion patterns, reduced appetite and loose stool, fatigue and lack of strength, nausea and vomiting, coughing and wheezing due to Qi deficiency of the Lungs and Kidneys, spontaneous sweating, palpitations, forgetfulness, impotence, wasting and thirsting, uterine bleeding and other patterns caused by an insufficiency of Qi, Blood and body fluids
Dang Shen (Radix Codonopsitis Pilosulae)	Supplementing the Middle Jiao and boosting Qi, generating body fluids, nourishing the Blood, supporting vital Qi and dispelling pathogenic factors	Spleen and Stomach deficiency manifesting as insufficiency of middle Qi, reduced appetite and loose stool; coughing and wheezing, shortness of breath due to Lung Qi deficiency; palpitations and a sallow yellow facial complexion due to Qi and Blood deficiency; fatigue, thirst
Huang Qi (Radix Astragali seu Hedysari)	Supplementing Qi and bearing Yang upwards, boosting defensive Qi and securing the exterior, stopping sweating, promoting urination and reducing swelling, drawing out toxins and generating flesh	Enduring diarrhoea and dysentery, reduced appetite and reduced food intake, fatigue and lack of strength due to Spleen and Stomach deficiency, prolapse of the rectum, uterus or stomach, spontaneous sweating, night sweating, numbness of the limbs or Wei syndrome of the lower limbs due to Qi deficiency and Blood stasis, puffy swelling, non-healing sores and abscesses
Bai Zhu (Rhizoma Atractylodis Macrocephalae)	Supplementing Qi and fortifying the Spleen, drying dampness and promoting urination, securing the exterior and stopping sweating, quieting the foetus	Qi deficiency of the Spleen and Stomach, reduced appetite, fatigue, diarrhoea, distension and fullness in the chest and hypochondrium, oedema and inhibited urination due to Spleen deficiency, spontaneous sweating, stirring foetus
Gan Cao (Radix Glycyrrhizae)	Fortifying the Spleen and boosting Qi, clearing heat and relieving toxicity, dispelling Phlegm and stopping coughing, relaxing tension and alleviating pain, adjusting and harmonizing the nature of other herbs	Qi deficiency of the Spleen and Stomach, palpitations, sore and swollen throat, abscesses and sores, coughing and wheezing, spasms and pain in the stomach and abdomen, moderating the potency of other herbs
Shan Yao (Rhizoma Dioscoreae Oppositae)	Fortifying the Spleen and stopping diarrhoea, supplementing the Lungs and stopping coughing, supplementing Qi and nourishing Yin, supplementing the Kidneys, securing the Essence and stopping vaginal discharge	Enduring diarrhoea and dysentery due to Spleen deficiency, fatigue, enduring coughing and wheezing, wasting and thirsting, seminal emission, vaginal discharge, frequent urination

Bai Bian Dou (Semen Dolichoris Lablab)	Fortifying the Spleen and harmonizing the Middle Jiao, clearing summerheat and transforming dampness, relieving toxicity	Vomiting, diarrhoea and vaginal discharge due to Spleen deficiency, vomiting and diarrhoea due to pathogenic summerheat-damp
Xi Yang Shen (Radix Panacis Quinquefolii)	Supplementing Qi and nourishing Yin, generating body fluids, boosting the Lungs and clearing fire	Coughing and wheezing due to Lung Yin deficiency; vexation, thirst, shortness of breath and lack of strength due to Qi and Yin deficiency; dry mouth, blood in the stool
Tai Zi Shen (Radix Pseudostellariae Heterophyllae)	Boosting Qi and generating body fluids, fortifying the Spleen and moistening the Lungs	Fatigue and reduced appetite due to Spleen deficiency, sweating due to Qi deficiency, cough and shortness of breath due to damage to Qi and Yin, thirst due to loss of body fluids
Da Zao (Fructus Ziziphi Jujubae)	Supplementing the Spleen and boosting Qi, nourishing the Blood and quieting the Spirit, moderating and harmonizing the nature of other herbs	Spleen and Stomach deficiency, diarrhoea and reduced appetite, Blood deficiency patterns, emotional depression in women, moderating the drastic action of other herbs
Yi Tang (Saccharum Granorum)	Supplementing the Spleen and boosting Qi, relaxing tension and alleviating pain, moistening the Lungs and stopping coughing	Taxation fatigue damaging the Spleen, shortness of breath, lack of strength and reduced food intake, pain in the chest and abdomen, dry cough due to Lung deficiency

Ren Shen 人参 (Ginseng, Radix Ginseng)

Ren Shen is the root of *Panax ginseng* C. A. Mey., family Araliaceae.

Main ingredients *Ren Shen* contains ginsenosides (including protopanaxadiol, protopanaxatriol, panaxosides and oleanolic acid), panaxynol, panaxydol, α-panasinsene, β-farnesene, citric acid, linoleic acid, panax acid, vitamins B_1, B_2, B_{12} and C, nicotinic acid, folic acid, sterols and carbohydrates.

Properties Taste: sweet and slightly bitter; nature: slightly warm.

Channels entered Spleen and Lung.

Functions and indications Strongly supplements original Qi, supplements the Spleen and boosts the Lungs, generates body fluids and allays thirst, quiets the Spirit and increases wisdom. It is indicated for desertion patterns, reduced appetite and loose stool, fatigue and lack of strength, nausea and vomiting, coughing and wheezing due to Qi deficiency of the Lungs and Kidneys, spontaneous sweating, palpitations, forgetfulness, impotence, wasting and thirsting, and uterine bleeding and other patterns caused by an insufficiency of Qi, Blood and body fluids.

Common dosage 5-10g, initially decocted on its own over mild heat for at least one hour, with the liquid then being mixed with the decoction obtained from other herbs; or 1-2g of the powder for oral ingestion, 2-3 times a day. For deficiency desertion, a large dosage (15-30g) of *Ren Shen* can be decocted on its own to be taken orally in frequent small doses.

Precautions and contraindications

1. *Ren Shen* is incompatible with *Li Lu* (Radix et Rhizoma Veratri) and antagonizes *Wu Ling Zhi* (Excrementum Trogopteri).
2. *Ren Shen* is contraindicated in full patterns and heat patterns and in cases without deficiency of vital Qi.
3. It is not advisable to drink tea or eat vegetables of the turnip family after taking *Ren Shen*, as this will diminish the supplementing effect of the herb.

Remarks Old, wild *Ren Shen* (*Ye Shan Shen*) has the best quality, but the relative scarcity of its production makes it expensive. It is generally only used in treating the most severe conditions. Cultivated *Ren Shen* (*Yuan Shen*) has a milder effect, but is produced in relatively abundant quantities, so it is much less expensive, resulting in its common use for general deficiency patterns in clinical practice. Different cultivation processes lead to the effects also being slightly different. Red ginseng, or *Hong Shen* (Radix Ginseng Rubra), is better in quality than white ginseng, or *Bai Shen* (Radix Ginseng Alba). *Bai Shen*, in turn, is more effective than *Shen Xu* (ginseng rootlets). *Hong Shen* is warmer in nature and is used for Qi and Yang deficiency; sun-dried *Ren Shen* (*Sheng Shai Shen*) is cooler and is used for supplementing Qi and nourishing Yin; *Bai Shen* is used for insufficiency of Qi and Yin; and *Shen Xu* is generally used for depletion of Qi and damage to body fluids.

Comparison of functions *Ren Shen* (Radix Ginseng) and *Fu Zi* (Radix Lateralis Aconiti Carmichaeli Praeparata) are often used for severe deficiency desertion. *Fu Zi* is acrid and sweet in taste and extremely hot in nature; it can support Heart Yang, warm Spleen Yang and supplement Kidney Yang. It is often used to treat Yang collapse due to Yang Qi debilitation and internal exuberance of Yin Qi. *Ren Shen* is sweet and slightly warm; it can strongly supplement original Qi and boost Qi to stem desertion. It is often used to treat desertion patterns due to Qi deficiency with a faint pulse verging on expiry.

For additional comparisons, see *Dang Shen* (Radix Codonopsitis Pilosulae), *Huang Qi* (Radix Astragali seu Hedysari) and *Xi Yang Shen* (Radix Panacis Quinquefolii).

Toxicity The saponins contained in *Ren Shen* have a very low level of toxicity. The LD_{50} for intraperitoneal injection in mice of the stem and leaves of *Ren Shen* is 20.6g/kg. Humans given 100ml of a 3% tincture of *Ren Shen* felt slightly uneasy and excited. Such toxic reactions as itching, dizziness, headache, fever and haemorrhage appeared after ingestion of 200ml. One death was reported after one 500ml dose of the tincture.

Modern research

1. Improves the memory and benefits intelligence.[1-3]
2. Strengthens the heart, improves defences against cardiac ischaemia, dilates blood vessels.[4-7]
3. Promotes the production of blood by the marrow, prevents blood clotting.[8, 9]
4. Lowers the blood sugar level.[10]
5. Inhibits carcinoma.[11, 12]
6. Strengthens the endocrine function, inhibits the ageing process.[13-15]

Combinations and applications

Functions	Combinations	Applications
Strongly supplementing original Qi	Used on its own after preparation into a thick decoction	Desertion pattern, severe bleeding and vomiting, and all patterns caused by deficiency of original Qi accompanied by a faint pulse verging on expiry
	Fu Zi (Radix Lateralis Aconiti Carmichaeli Praeparata) (see notes on legal status)	Original Qi verging on desertion accompanied by sweating and cold limbs
Supplementing the Spleen and boosting the Lungs	*Fu Ling* (Sclerotium Poriae Cocos) *Bai Zhu* (Rhizoma Atractylodis Macrocephalae) *Zhi Gan Cao* (Radix Glycyrrhizae Praeparata)	Poor appetite, fatigued Spirit and lack of strength, distension and fullness in the stomach and abdomen, and vomiting and diarrhoea due to Qi deficiency of the Spleen and Stomach, which are thus impaired in their transportation and transformation functions
	Huang Qi (Radix Astragali seu Hedysari) *Sheng Ma* (Rhizoma Cimicifugae) *Chai Hu* (Radix Bupleuri)	Prolapse of the rectum and uterus due to middle Qi fall caused by extreme deficiency of Spleen Qi
	Fu Ling (Sclerotium Poriae Cocos) *Bai Zhu* (Rhizoma Atractylodis Macrocephalae) *Bai Bian Dou* (Semen Dolichoris Lablab)	Recurring diarrhoea due to Spleen deficiency with clear and thin stool
	Hu Tao Ren (Semen Juglandis Regiae) *Sheng Jiang* (Rhizoma Zingiberis Officinalis Recens)	Short and rapid breath, wheezing after movement and spontaneous sweating with a deficient pulse due to insufficiency of the Lungs and Kidneys
	Ge Jie (Gekko) *Chuan Bei Mu* (Bulbus Fritillariae Cirrhosae) *Sang Bai Pi* (Cortex Mori Albae Radicis) *Zhi Mu* (Rhizoma Anemarrhenae Asphodeloidis)	Deficiency patterns in the Lungs and Kidneys in enduring diseases accompanied by coughing and wheezing due to Lung-heat

	Fu Zi (Radix Lateralis Aconiti Carmichaeli Praeparata) (see notes on legal status) *Sheng Jiang* (Rhizoma Zingiberis Officinalis Recens)	Wheezing due to Yang deficiency, spontaneous sweating, shortness of breath, dizziness
Generating body fluids and allaying thirst	*Mai Men Dong* (Radix Ophiopogonis Japonici) *Wu Wei Zi* (Fructus Schisandrae)	Cough with scant sputum, hasty wheezing and spontaneous sweating, dryness of the throat and tongue and a weak pulse due to Qi and Yin deficiency
	Tian Hua Fen (Radix Trichosanthis) *Mai Men Dong* (Radix Ophiopogonis Japonici) *Shi Hu* (Herba Dendrobii) (see notes on legal status)	Thirst with a strong desire to drink in patients with a wasting and thirsting pattern
	Shi Gao (Gypsum Fibrosum) *Zhi Mu* (Rhizoma Anemarrhenae Asphodeloidis) *Gan Cao* (Radix Glycyrrhizae) *Jing Mi* (Oryza Sativa)	Vigorous fever, vexation, thirst, profuse sweating with a weak, floating, large and forceless pulse due to damage to Qi and Yin and exuberant heat in the Yangming channel
Quieting the Spirit and increasing wisdom	*Dang Gui* (Radix Angelicae Sinensis) *Suan Zao Ren* (Semen Ziziphi Spinosae) *Long Yan Rou* (Arillus Euphoriae Longanae) *Yuan Zhi* (Radix Polygalae)	Palpitations and fearful throbbing, forgetfulness, insomnia, profuse dreaming, fatigued body and reduced appetite with a fine and weak pulse due to damage to the Spleen and Heart caused by excessive thought and preoccupation
	Shi Chang Pu (Rhizoma Acori Graminei) *Yuan Zhi* (Radix Polygalae) *Fu Ling* (Sclerotium Poriae Cocos) *Zhu Sha* (Cinnabaris) (see notes on legal status)	Palpitations and fearful throbbing, fright and disquiet, profuse dreaming and moodiness due to insufficiency of Heart Qi

Notes: *Ren Shen* also has many other therapeutic functions:

1. when combined with *Dang Gui* (Radix Angelicae Sinensis), *Shu Di Huang* (Radix Rehmanniae Glutinosae Conquita), *Bai Shao* (Radix Paeoniae Lactiflorae) and other herbs for supplementing the Blood, it can boost Qi and generate Blood to treat patterns due to Blood deficiency;
2. when used with *Lu Rong* (Cornu Cervi Parvum), *Ba Ji Tian* (Radix Morindae Officinalis), *Zi He Che* (Placenta Hominis) or other herbs for supplementing Yang, it can boost Qi and invigorate Yang to treat impotence;
3. when used with *Gan Jiang* (Rhizoma Zingiberis Officinalis), *Gan Cao* (Radix Glycyrrhizae) and *Bai Zhu* (Rhizoma Atractylodis Macrocephalae), it can treat chest Bi syndrome and obstruction of Qi in the Heart due to binding of Qi in the chest resulting in fullness in the chest and pain in the hypochondrium;
4. it can be combined with herbs for releasing the exterior and herbs for dispersing food accumulation to treat weak patients with externally-contracted pathogenic factors, interior full patterns, and deficiency of vital Qi so that vital Qi is supported in dispelling pathogenic factors.

Dang Shen 党参 (Codonopsis root, Radix Codonopsitis Pilosulae)

Dang Shen is the root of *Codonopsis pilosula* (Franch.) Nannf., family Campanulaceae.

Main ingredients *Dang Shen* contains stigmasterol, α-spinasterol, inulin, fructose, choline, caproic acid, enanthic acid, pinene, saponins and alkaloids.

Properties Taste: sweet; nature: neutral.

Channels entered Spleen and Lung.

Functions and indications Supplements the Middle Jiao and boosts Qi, generates body fluids, nourishes the Blood, and supports vital Qi and dispels pathogenic factors. It is indicated for Spleen and Stomach deficiency manifesting as insufficiency of middle Qi, reduced appetite and loose stool; coughing and wheezing and shortness of breath due to Lung Qi deficiency; palpitations and a sallow yellow facial complexion due to Qi and Blood deficiency; fatigue and thirst.

Common dosage 10-30g.

Precautions and contraindications

1. *Dang Shen* is contraindicated in cases of Qi stagnation and exuberance of Liver-fire, and where there is exuberance of pathogenic factors without vital Qi deficiency.
2. *Dang Shen* is incompatible with *Li Lu* (Radix et Rhizoma Veratri).

Comparison of functions *Dang Shen* (Radix Codonopsitis Pilosulae) is similar to *Ren Shen* (Radix Ginseng) in its functions, but is less powerful. Although *Dang Shen* can supplement Spleen and Lung Qi, nourish the Blood and generate body fluids, and is used as a substitute for *Ren Shen* for many Qi deficiency patterns, it does not have the powerful effect that *Ren Shen* possesses in strongly supplementing original Qi. *Ren Shen* is also extremely effective in boosting Qi and generating the Blood, benefiting the Zang organs and stemming desertion. It is considered to be the most important herb for interior impairment due to deficiency or overwork and is used for all patterns due to depletion or deficiency of Qi or Blood or insufficiency of Yin fluids. *Dang Shen* can be used for mild and chronic disorders, whereas *Ren Shen* can be used for severe and acute cases.

For an additional comparison, see *Shan Yao* (Rhizoma Dioscoreae Oppositae).

Toxicity The LD_{50} for mice given a decoction of *Dang Shen* via intragastric administration is 240.3g/kg. Rats given a subcutaneous injection of 0.5g of *Dang Shen* for 13 days exhibited no toxic reaction. Generally speaking, clinical dosages of *Dang Shen* produce no adverse effect, but overdosage can result in arrhythmia, which corrects itself automatically once administration is halted.

Modern research

1. Strengthens the immune function.[16–18]
2. Increases adaptability to oxygen deficit and raises reaction capability.[16, 19, 20]
3. Inhibits ulcers and prevents damage to the gastric mucous membrane, inhibits gastric secretion, regulates gastrointestinal movement.[21-23]
4. Strengthens cardiac contractions and raises blood pressure, dilates external blood vessels, inhibits haematoblastic concentration and inhibits embolism.[24]
5. Improves the memory and benefits intelligence.[25]

Combinations and applications

Functions	Combinations	Applications
Supplementing the Middle Jiao and boosting Qi	*Bai Zhu* (Rhizoma Atractylodis Macrocephalae) *Fu Ling* (Sclerotium Poriae Cocos) *Gan Cao* (Radix Glycyrrhizae) *Chen Pi* (Pericarpium Citri Reticulatae)	Reduced appetite, loose stool, fatigue and lack of strength, a pale tongue with white fur and a deficient, weak and forceless pulse due to Spleen and Stomach deficiency
	Huang Qi (Radix Astragali seu Hedysari) *Bai Zhu* (Rhizoma Atractylodis Macrocephalae) *Shan Yao* (Rhizoma Dioscoreae Oppositae) *Sheng Ma* (Rhizoma Cimicifugae) *Zhi Gan Cao* (Radix Glycyrrhizae Praeparata)	Enduring diarrhoea and dysentery, prolapse of the rectum or uterus due to Qi deficiency of the Spleen and Stomach and middle Qi fall
	Wu Wei Zi (Fructus Schisandrae) *Huang Qi* (Radix Astragali seu Hedysari) *E Jiao* (Gelatinum Corii Asini)	Shortness of breath, coughing and wheezing and weak voice due to Lung Qi deficiency
	Fu Ling (Sclerotium Poriae Cocos) *Yi Yi Ren* (Semen Coicis Lachrymajobi) *Bai Zhu* (Rhizoma Atractylodis Macrocephalae) *Sha Ren* (Fructus Amomi) *Shan Yao* (Rhizoma Dioscoreae Oppositae)	Lack of strength, indigestion, vomiting or diarrhoea, discomfort and oppression in the chest and stomach, white and slimy tongue fur and a deficient, moderate pulse due to Spleen deficiency with dampness
Generating body fluids	*Mai Men Dong* (Radix Ophiopogonis Japonici) *Shi Hu* (Herba Dendrobii) (see notes on legal status) *Wu Wei Zi* (Fructus Schisandrae) *Yu Zhu* (Rhizoma Polygonati Odorati)	Shortness of breath and thirst due to febrile diseases damaging body fluids
Nourishing the Blood	*Dang Gui* (Radix Angelicae Sinensis) *Shu Di Huang* (Radix Rehmanniae Glutinosae Conquita) *Bai Shao* (Radix Paeoniae Lactiflorae)	A sallow yellow facial complexion, palpitations, dizziness and a weak, fine pulse due to Qi and Blood deficiency

Note: *Dang Shen* can also be used together with herbs for releasing the exterior and downward-draining herbs to treat invasion by external pathogenic factors or interior full patterns accompanied by vital Qi deficiency; in this way, vital Qi can be supported while dispelling pathogenic factors.

Huang Qi 黄芪
(Milk vetch or sweet vetch root, Radix Astragali seu Hedysari)

Huang Qi is the root of *Astragalus membranaceus* (Fisch.) Bge., *A. membranaceus* Bge. var. *mongholicus* (Bge.) Hsiao or *Hedysarum polybotrys* Hand.-Mazz., family Leguminosae. *Hedysarum polybotrys* is usually known as *Hong Qi*.

Main ingredients *Huang Qi* contains astragalosides, daucosterol, β-sitosterol, palmitic acid, astragalus saponins, kumatakenin, choline, betaine, folic acid, formononetin, calycosin, cycloastragenol and glucuronic acid.

Properties Taste: sweet; nature: slightly warm.
Channels entered Spleen and Lung.
Functions and indications Supplements Qi and bears Yang upwards, boosts defensive Qi and secures the exterior, stops sweating, promotes urination and reduces swelling, draws out toxins and generates flesh. It is indicated for enduring diarrhoea and dysentery, reduced appetite and reduced food intake, fatigue and lack of strength due to Spleen and Stomach deficiency, prolapse of the rectum, uterus or stomach, spontaneous sweating, night sweating, numbness of the limbs or Wei syndrome of the lower limbs due to Qi deficiency and Blood stasis, puffy swelling, and non-healing sores and abscesses.
Common dosage 10-15g, or 30-60g for large dosages (e.g. in the *Bu Yang Huan Wu Tang* [Yang-Supplementing Five-Returning Decoction] for hemiplegia).
Precautions and contraindications Since *Huang Qi* can supplement Qi and bear Yang upwards, it tends to reinforce fire and can stop sweating. As a result, it should not be used for exterior full patterns and exuberance of pathogenic factors, Qi stagnation and dampness obstruction, food accumulation, hyperactivity of Yang due to Yin deficiency, and abscesses at the initial stage or where there are full-heat toxins after their rupture.
Remarks Use *Huang Qi* mix-fried with honey for supplementing Qi and bearing Yang upwards; use raw *Huang Qi* for other applications.
Comparison of functions Both *Huang Qi* (Radix Astragali seu Hedysari) and *Ren Shen* (Radix Ginseng) are key herbs for supplementing Qi and are often combined to strengthen their effect. *Ren Shen* can strongly supplement original Qi, boost the Blood and generate body fluids, and quiet the Spirit and increase wisdom. It is a key herb for treating internal damage and Qi deficiency. Although *Huang Qi* is not as effective as *Ren Shen* in terms of supplementing original Qi, it is much better than *Ren Shen* at warming and bearing upwards. It can also secure the exterior and stop sweating, draw out toxins and generate flesh, and promote urination and reduce swelling; *Ren Shen* does not possess these functions. Since it can bear Yang upwards and raise the fall as well as being able to supplement Qi, *Huang Qi* is an important herb for Qi fall in the Middle Jiao.
Toxicity Amounts of 75g/kg and 100g/kg of *Huang Qi* administered orally to mice produced no adverse effects within 48 hours (by comparison, the normal oral dosage for humans for promoting urination is 0.2g/kg). The LD_{50} for intraperitoneal injection in mice of decoctions of the herb is 40g/kg. There are reports of very large dosages of *Huang Qi* causing severe limb pain and other reports of an injection of the herb at acupuncture points resulting in a mild toxic reaction.
Modern research
1. Strengthens the immune function.[26]
2. Strengthens the heart, dilates external blood vessels and the coronary artery.[27-29]
3. Inhibits haematoblastic concentration and promotes the generation, growth and maturing of blood cells.[27, 30]
4. Inhibited Shigella shigae, α- and β-haemolytic streptococci, Staphylococcus aureus, and influenza viruses *in vitro*.[31, 32]
5. Slows the ageing process by reducing free radicals.[31]
6. Inhibits gastric secretion and prevents gastric ulcers.[33]
7. Inhibits inflammation.[34]
8. Lowers the blood sugar level.[35]

Combinations and applications

Functions	Combinations	Applications
Supplementing Qi and bearing Yang upwards	*Ren Shen* (Radix Ginseng)	Reduced appetite, distension in the stomach after eating, fatigue and lack of strength and a sallow yellow facial complexion due to deficiency of the Spleen, which is thus impaired in its transportation function
	Ren Shen (Radix Ginseng) *Bai Zhu* (Rhizoma Atractylodis Macrocephalae) *Sheng Ma* (Rhizoma Cimicifugae) *Dang Gui* (Radix Angelicae Sinensis)	Enduring diarrhoea and dysentery, prolapse of the rectum, uterus or stomach due to Qi deficiency of the Spleen and Stomach and middle Qi fall
	Dang Gui (Radix Angelicae Sinensis) *Ren Shen* (Radix Ginseng) *Long Yan Rou* (Arillus Euphoriae Longanae) *Suan Zao Ren* (Semen Ziziphi Spinosae)	Blood in the stool, uterine bleeding, fatigued body and reduced appetite, a pale tongue with thin, white fur and a fine, weak pulse due to deficiency of Spleen Qi, which thus fails to contain the Blood
	Dang Gui (Radix Angelicae Sinensis)	Fever with red face, vexation and thirst and a desire for drink, with a surging, large, but deficient pulse, forceless under heavy pressure, due to deficiency of Qi and Blood and internal damage due to overstrain and overwork
	Rou Gui (Cortex Cinnamomi Cassiae) *Ren Shen* (Radix Ginseng) *Bai Zhu* (Rhizoma Atractylodis Macrocephalae) *Dang Gui* (Radix Angelicae Sinensis) *Chuan Xiong* (Rhizoma Ligustici Chuanxiong)	Coughing and wheezing, seminal emission, bleeding, uterine bleeding or menstrual irregularities due to deficiency of vital Qi
	Fu Zi (Radix Lateralis Aconiti Carmichaeli Praeparata) (see notes on legal status)	Aversion to cold and profuse sweating due to Yang exhaustion and Qi deficiency
	Gui Zhi (Ramulus Cinnamomi Cassiae) *Bai Shao* (Radix Paeoniae Lactiflorae) *Da Zao* (Fructus Ziziphi Jujubae)	Numbness of the limbs due to Qi deficiency and Blood stasis
	Fang Feng (Radix Ledebouriellae Divaricatae) *Qiang Huo* (Rhizoma et Radix Notopterygii) *Jiang Huang* (Rhizoma Curcumae Longae)	Pain in the upper limbs and shoulders due to an invasion of wind-cold-damp resulting in Yang Qi deficiency
	Chuan Xiong (Rhizoma Ligustici Chuanxiong) *Dang Gui* (Radix Angelicae Sinensis) *Tao Ren* (Semen Persicae) *Hong Hua* (Flos Carthami Tinctorii)	Hemiplegia due to wind-stroke, facial paralysis and Wei syndrome of the lower limbs due to Qi deficiency and Blood stasis with white tongue fur and a moderate pulse

Boosting defensive Qi and securing the exterior, stopping sweating	*Fu Xiao Mai* (Fructus Tritici Aestivi Levis) *Mu Li* (Concha Ostreae) *Ma Huang Gen* (Radix Ephedrae)	Spontaneous sweating, shortness of breath and lack of strength due to Lung Qi deficiency and defensive Qi failing to secure the exterior
	Sheng Di Huang (Radix Rehmanniae Glutinosae) *Huang Bai* (Cortex Phellodendri) *Huang Qin* (Radix Scutellariae Baicalensis) *Dang Gui* (Radix Angelicae Sinensis)	Fever, night sweating, dry mouth, vexation and dry stool accompanied by a red tongue and a fine, rapid pulse due to Yin deficiency with heat
	Fang Feng (Radix Ledebouriellae Divaricatae) *Bai Zhu* (Rhizoma Atractylodis Macrocephalae)	Aversion to wind, spontaneous sweating, pale complexion, a pale tongue with white fur and a floating, deficient and weak pulse due to exterior deficiency failing to secure defensive Yang
Promoting urination and reducing swelling	*Fang Ji* (Radix Stephaniae Tetrandrae) (see notes on legal status) *Bai Zhu* (Rhizoma Atractylodis Macrocephalae) *Sheng Jiang* (Rhizoma Zingiberis Officinalis Recens)	Puffy swelling and scant urine due to deficiency of Spleen Qi, which fails to transport and transform, resulting in water and dampness collecting
Drawing out toxins and generating flesh	*Chuan Shan Jia* (Squama Manitis Pentadactylae) (see notes on legal status) *Zao Jiao Ci* (Spina Gleditsiae Sinensis) *Dang Gui* (Radix Angelicae Sinensis)	Persistent, non-ulcerating abscesses with a deficient and weak pulse
	Ren Shen (Radix Ginseng) *Zhi Gan Cao* (Radix Glycyrrhizae Praeparata) *Wu Wei Zi* (Fructus Schisandrae) *Mu Li* (Concha Ostreae)	Non-healing sores due to deficiency of Qi and Blood

Note: In addition, *Huang Qi* can be used with *Fu Shen* (Sclerotium Poriae Cocos cum Ligno Hospite), *Gua Lou* (Fructus Trichosanthis), *Mai Men Dong* (Radix Ophiopogonis Japonici), *Gan Cao* (Radix Glycyrrhizae) and *Sheng Di Huang* (Radix Rehmanniae Glutinosae) for wasting and thirsting patterns.

Bai Zhu 白术 (White atractylodes rhizome, Rhizoma Atractylodis Macrocephalae)

Bai Zhu is the rhizome of *Atractylodes macrocephala* Koidz., family Compositae.

Main ingredients *Bai Zhu* contains 1.4% of volatile oils (notably atractylol, atractylon, butenolide A and B, and atractylenolide), sesquiterpenes and vitamin A.

Properties Taste: bitter and sweet; nature: warm.

Channels entered Spleen and Stomach.

Functions and indications Supplements Qi and fortifies the Spleen, dries dampness and promotes urination, secures the exterior and stops sweating, and quiets the foetus. It is indicated for Qi deficiency of the Spleen and Stomach, reduced appetite, fatigue, diarrhoea, distension and fullness in the chest and hypochondrium, oedema and inhibited urination due to Spleen deficiency, spontaneous sweating, and stirring foetus.

Common dosage 5-15g.

Precautions and contraindications

1. As *Bai Zhu* tends to dry dampness and damage Yin, it can only be used for dampness in the Middle Jiao. It should not be employed for internal heat due to Yin deficiency or vexation and thirst due to depletion and consumption of body fluids.
2. *Bai Zhu* should be used with caution for distension and oppression in the chest due to Qi stagnation.

Remarks Use stir-fried *Bai Zhu* for supplementing Qi and fortifying the Spleen, and for quieting the foetus; scorch-fried *Bai Zhu* is employed to fortify the Spleen and stop diarrhoea; and the raw herb should be used for drying dampness and promoting urination.

Comparison of functions Both *Bai Zhu* (Rhizoma Atractylodis Macrocephalae) and *Cang Zhu* (Rhizoma Atractylodis) can dry dampness and fortify the Spleen, being important herbs for treating dampness encumbering the Spleen and Stomach. Since *Bai Zhu* mainly fortifies the Middle Jiao and supplements Qi, it is used more often for deficiency patterns of Spleen weakness. *Cang Zhu* is an aromatic herb which overcomes dampness. It has a stronger effect than *Bai Zhu* in drying dampness and is mainly used for disorders due to damp obstruction in the Middle Jiao. *Bai Zhu* can also stop sweating, promote urination and quiet the foetus, whereas *Cang Zhu* has the additional functions of dissipating pathogenic factors and dispelling wind-damp.

For an additional comparison, see *Shan Yao* (Rhizoma Dioscoreae Oppositae).

Toxicity The LD_{50} for intraperitoneal injection in mice of a decoction of *Bai Zhu* is 13.3g/kg. Rats fed 0.5g/kg of a *Bai Zhu* decoction daily for 14 days via intragastric administration showed a reduction in the white blood cell count; when fed the decoction for two months, the rats exhibited signs of anaemia, but no changes were recorded in brain, heart or liver functions.

Modern research

1. Has a pronounced effect in increasing weight, improving endurance and strengthening the immune function.[36, 37]
2. Obvious function in inhibiting platelet aggregation.[38]
3. The volatile oils contained in *Bai Zhu* clearly inhibit carcinoma cells in the oesophagus.[39, 40]

Combinations and applications

Functions	Combinations	Applications
Supplementing Qi and fortifying the Spleen	*Ren Shen* (Radix Ginseng) *Fu Ling* (Sclerotium Poriae Cocos)	Fatigue and lack of strength, reduced appetite, loose stool, and distension and fullness in the stomach and abdomen due to deficiency of the Spleen and Stomach, which are thus impaired in their transportation and transformation functions
	Zhi Shi (Fructus Immaturus Citri Aurantii)	Focal distension and fullness in the stomach and abdomen and reduced appetite due to Spleen deficiency and Qi stagnation with food accumulation
	Gan Jiang (Rhizoma Zingiberis Officinalis) *Zhi Gan Cao* (Radix Glycyrrhizae Praeparata) *Dang Shen* (Radix Codonopsitis Pilosulae)	Cold and pain in the stomach and abdomen, diarrhoea due to Spleen and Stomach deficiency-cold, chronic fright in children, drooling at the mouth after illness

	Ban Xia (Rhizoma Pinelliae Ternatae) *Ding Xiang* (Flos Caryophylli) *Sheng Jiang* (Rhizoma Zingiberis Officinalis Recens)	Difficult intake of food by children as a result of Spleen deficiency due to enduring diarrhoea
Drying dampness and promoting urination	*Gui Zhi* (Ramulus Cinnamomi Cassiae) *Fu Ling* (Sclerotium Poriae Cocos) *Gan Cao* (Radix Glycyrrhizae)	Distension and fullness in the chest and hypochondrium due to insufficiency of Spleen Yang and internal exuberance of Phlegm-fluids, accompanied by dizziness, palpitations, shortness of breath, coughing, white and slippery tongue fur, and a string-like, slippery pulse
	Da Fu Pi (Pericarpium Arecae Catechu) *Fu Ling Pi* (Cortex Poriae Cocos) *Chen Pi* (Pericarpium Citri Reticulatae)	Oedema and inhibited urination due to Spleen deficiency resulting in flooding of water and dampness
	Fu Zi (Radix Lateralis Aconiti Carmichaeli Praeparata) (see notes on legal status) *Zhi Gan Cao* (Radix Glycyrrhizae Praeparata) *Sheng Jiang* (Rhizoma Zingiberis Officinalis Recens) *Da Zao* (Fructus Ziziphi Jujubae)	Vexation, generalized pain, inability to turn the body due to an invasion of wind-damp, with a floating, deficient and rough pulse
	Shan Yao (Rhizoma Dioscoreae Oppositae) *Cang Zhu* (Rhizoma Atractylodis) *Che Qian Zi* (Semen Plantaginis)	Thin, clear and profuse vaginal discharge due to damp turbidity pouring down in Spleen deficiency patterns
Securing the exterior and stopping sweating	*Fang Feng* (Radix Ledebouriellae Divaricatae) *Huang Qi* (Radix Astragali seu Hedysari)	Spontaneous sweating caused by insecurity of defensive Qi due to exterior deficiency
Quieting the foetus	*Du Zhong* (Cortex Eucommiae Ulmoidis) *Xu Duan* (Radix Dipsaci) *E Jiao* (Gelatinum Corii Asini)	Stirring foetus, insecurity of original Qi in cultivating the foetus, limpness in the lumbar region and pain in the abdomen due to insufficiency of the Spleen and Kidneys
	Dang Gui (Radix Angelicae Sinensis) *Bai Shao* (Radix Paeoniae Lactiflorae) *Shu Di Huang* (Radix Rehmanniae Glutinosae Conquita)	Stirring foetus, dizziness, palpitations, and a thin, weak pulse due to Blood deficiency and lack of nutrition for the Chong and Ren channels

Gan Cao 甘草
(Liquorice root, Radix Glycyrrhizae)

Gan Cao is the root and rhizome of *Glycyrrhiza uralensis* Fisch., *G. inflata* Bat. or *G. glabra* L., family Leguminosae.

Main ingredients *Gan Cao* contains glycyrrhizin, glycyrrhizic acid, glucuronic acid, glycyrrhetic acid, liquorice saponins, liquiritin, licoflavone, isolicoflavonol, liquiritigenin, formononetin, betulic acid, and urease and sucrase enzymes.

Properties Taste: sweet; nature: neutral.

Channels entered Heart, Lung, Spleen and Stomach.

Functions and indications Fortifies the Spleen and boosts Qi, clears heat and relieves toxicity, dispels Phlegm and stops coughing, relaxes tension and alleviates pain, and adjusts and harmonizes the nature of other herbs. It is indicated for Qi deficiency of the Spleen and Stomach, palpitations, sore and swollen throat, abscesses and sores, coughing and wheezing, spasms and pain in the stomach and abdomen, and for moderating the potency of other herbs.

Common dosage 3-10g, or 30g for large dosages; appropriate dosage for external application.

Precautions and contraindications

1. Since *Gan Cao* is sweet in taste and can reinforce dampness and cause fullness in the Middle Jiao, it is contraindicated in cases of distension and fullness in the chest and abdomen due to exuberant dampness, and for nausea and vomiting.
2. *Gan Cao* is incompatible with *Gan Sui* (Radix Euphorbiae Kansui), *Jing Da Ji* (Radix Euphorbiae Pekinensis), *Yuan Hua* (Flos Daphnes Genkwa) and *Hai Zao* (Herba Sargassi).
3. Long-term use of large dosages of *Gan Cao* can result in oedema, an increase in blood pressure, retention of sodium, a reduction in the blood potassium level, lack of strength in the limbs, spasms and numbness, dizziness, and headache. *Gan Cao* should therefore be used with caution for patients with these conditions.

Remarks Raw *Gan Cao* is used for clearing heat and relieving toxicity, moderating the potency of other herbs, relaxing tension and alleviating pain, and dispelling Phlegm and stopping coughing; the herb mix-fried with honey, *Zhi Gan Cao* (Radix Glycyrrhizae Praeparata), is generally used for boosting Qi and supplementing the Middle Jiao or for treating deficiency-cold patterns; the tips of the herb (*Gan Cao Shao*) are mainly used for Lin syndrome and painful urination.

Comparison of functions *Gan Cao* (Radix Glycyrrhizae), *Shan Yao* (Rhizoma Dioscoreae Oppositae) and *Bai Bian Dou* (Semen Dolichoris Lablab) are all harmonizing herbs and can fortify the Spleen and boost Qi. *Shan Yao* both supplements Qi and nourishes Yin and is a key herb for neutrally supplementing the Spleen, Lung and Kidney channels. It can also supplement the Kidneys and secure the Essence, and reduce urine and stop vaginal discharge. *Bai Bian Dou* can fortify the Spleen and transform dampness, supplementing the Spleen without being greasy and transforming dampness without causing dryness. It is particularly suitable for weak patients recovering from an illness and just beginning to take supplementing decoctions.

Gan Cao can boost Qi and fortify the Middle Jiao and is also able to clear heat and relieve toxicity; it is an important herb for moistening the Lungs to dispel Phlegm and stop coughing. However, as it acts on congested Qi with sweetness and can cause fullness in the Middle Jiao, it is not suitable for patients with exuberant dampness and distension and fullness in the chest and abdomen. In addition, *Gan Cao* can moderate the potency of other herbs and harmonize the action of herbs in a prescription formula; for this reason, it is known as *guo lao* (literally, head of state).

For an additional comparison, see *Da Zao* (Fructus Ziziphi Jujubae).

Toxicity The LD_{100} for subcutaneous injection in mice of an extract of *Gan Cao* is 3.6g/kg, with the cause of death identified as respiratory paralysis. A group of rabbits was fed 1g per day of an extract of *Gan Cao* for 40 days, resulting in a weight increase compared with that of the control group; after one week, the level of sodium in the blood had increased and there was slight atrophy of the adrenal gland (see also *Precautions and contraindications* above).

Modern research

1. Has a cortisone-like function, inhibits inflammation and allergic reactions, and promotes urination.[41]

2. Protects the functions of the liver and relieves spasms in the gastrointestinal tract.[41–43]
3. Inhibits the hepatitis virus and HIV.[44, 45]
4. Stops coughing and promotes bronchial secretion, thus encouraging the discharge of sputum.[46]
5. Reduces the level of blood lipids.[47, 48]
6. Inhibits carcinoma.[49]
7. The glycyrrhizic acid contained in *Gan Cao* inhibited Staphylococcus aureus, Mycobacterium tuberculosis, Escherichia coli, and amoebic protozoa and trichomonads *in vitro*.[50, 51]

Combinations and applications

Functions	Combinations	Applications
Fortifying the Spleen and boosting Qi	*Ren Shen* (Radix Ginseng) *Bai Zhu* (Rhizoma Atractylodis Macrocephalae) *Fu Ling* (Sclerotium Poriae Cocos)	Fatigue and lack of strength, low food intake and loose stool due to Qi deficiency of the Spleen and Stomach
	Ren Shen (Radix Ginseng) *Gui Zhi* (Ramulus Cinnamomi Cassiae) *Gan Jiang* (Rhizoma Zingiberis Officinalis) *E Jiao* (Gelatinum Corii Asini) *Sheng Di Huang* (Radix Rehmanniae Glutinosae) *Mai Men Dong* (Radix Ophiopogonis Japonici)	Palpitations, shortness of breath, spontaneous sweating and profuse sweating with a bound, intermittent pulse due to insufficiency of Heart Qi and devitalized Heart Yang
Clearing heat and relieving toxicity	*Jie Geng* (Radix Platycodi Grandiflori) *Shan Dou Gen* (Radix Sophorae Tonkinensis)	Red, sore and swollen throat due to heat toxins attacking the Upper Jiao
	Pu Gong Ying (Herba Taraxaci cum Radice) *Jin Yin Hua* (Flos Lonicerae) *Lian Qiao* (Fructus Forsythiae Suspensae) *Zi Hua Di Ding* (Herba Violae Yedoensitis)	Abscesses and sores, breast abscess due to exuberant heat toxins
	Lü Dou (Semen Phaseoli Radiati)	Relieving the toxicity of food and drug poisoning
Dispelling Phlegm and stopping coughing	*Jie Geng* (Radix Platycodi Grandiflori) *Niu Bang Zi* (Fructus Arctii Lappae) *Xing Ren* (Semen Pruni Armeniacae)	Cough due to an attack of wind-heat
	Ma Huang (Herba Ephedrae) (see notes on legal status) *Zi Wan* (Radix Asteris Tatarici)	Cough due to an attack of wind-cold
	Shi Gao (Gypsum Fibrosum) *Ma Huang* (Herba Ephedrae) (see notes on legal status) *Xing Ren* (Semen Pruni Armeniacae)	Coughing and wheezing due to Lung-heat

	Gua Lou (Fructus Trichosanthis) *Huang Qin* (Radix Scutellariae Baicalensis)	Cough due to Phlegm-heat
	Gan Jiang (Rhizoma Zingiberis Officinalis) *Xi Xin* (Herba cum Radice Asari)	Cough due to Phlegm-cold
	Bei Sha Shen (Radix Glehniae Littoralis) *Mai Men Dong* (Radix Ophiopogonis Japonici) *Yu Zhu* (Rhizoma Polygonati Odorati)	Cough due to Lung Yin deficiency
Relaxing tension and alleviating pain	*Bai Shao* (Radix Paeoniae Lactiflorae) *Da Zao* (Fructus Ziziphi Jujubae) *Yi Tang* (Saccharum Granorum)	Spasms and pain in the stomach and abdomen, spasms of the limbs due to depletion of Yin and Blood
	Feng Mi (Mel)	Intermittent pain in the stomach due to deficiency-cold in the Middle Jiao
	Sheng Di Huang (Radix Rehmanniae Glutinosae) *Mu Tong* (Caulis Mutong) (see notes on legal status)	Burning pain during urination due to damp-heat
Adjusting and harmonizing the nature of other herbs	*Fu Zi* (Radix Lateralis Aconiti Carmichaeli Praeparata) (see notes on legal status) *Gan Jiang* (Rhizoma Zingiberis Officinalis)	Moderates and harmonizes the hot and dry properties of these herbs to prevent damage to Yin
	Shi Gao (Gypsum Fibrosum) *Zhi Mu* (Rhizoma Anemarrhenae Asphodeloidis)	Moderates and harmonizes the cold nature of these substances to protect the Spleen and Stomach
	Da Huang (Radix et Rhizoma Rhei) *Mang Xiao* (Mirabilitum)	Moderates and harmonizes the offensive downward-draining function of these substances to reduce the rate of draining
	Ren Shen (Radix Ginseng) *Bai Zhu* (Rhizoma Atractylodis Macrocephalae) *Shu Di Huang* (Radix Rehmanniae Glutinosae Conquita) *Dang Gui* (Radix Angelicae Sinensis)	Moderates and harmonizes the supplementing power of these herbs to prolong their effect

Note: When used in combination with both warm and cold herbs, *Gan Cao* can adjust and harmonize the potency of both types.

Shan Yao 山药 (Chinese yam, Rhizoma Dioscoreae Oppositae)

Shan Yao is the dried rhizome of *Dioscorea opposita* Thunb., family Dioscoreaceae.

Main ingredients *Shan Yao* contains diosgenin, choline, saponins, starch, glycoproteins, mannan, phytic acid, allantoin, diastase enzymes, and vitamin C.

Properties Taste: sweet; nature: neutral.

Channels entered Spleen, Lung and Kidney.

Functions and indications Fortifies the Spleen and stops diarrhoea, supplements the Lungs and stops coughing, supplements Qi and nourishes Yin, and supplements the Kidneys, secures the Essence and stops vaginal discharge. It is indicated for enduring diarrhoea and dysentery due to Spleen deficiency, fatigue, enduring coughing and wheezing, wasting and thirsting, seminal emission, vaginal discharge, and frequent urination.

Common dosage 10-30g, or 60-250g in large dosages; 6-10g of powder for oral use.

Precautions and contraindications *Shan Yao* is contraindicated in cases with exuberant dampness in the Middle Jiao or for patients with accumulation or stagnation patterns.

Remarks

1. *Shan Yao* can be used on its own in large dosages as an infusion to treat wasting and thirsting and deficiency cough.
2. Raw *Shan Yao* is good for nourishing Yin, while the stir-fried herb fortifies the Spleen and stops diarrhoea.

Comparison of functions *Shan Yao* (Rhizoma Dioscoreae Oppositae), *Dang Shen* (Radix Codonopsitis Pilosulae) and *Bai Zhu* (Rhizoma Atractylodis Macrocephalae) can all supplement Qi and fortify the Spleen to treat Qi deficiency of the Spleen and Stomach. *Bai Zhu*, which enters the Spleen and Stomach channels, is a key herb for fortifying the Middle Jiao and boosting Qi. As it is bitter and warm, it can dry dampness and promote urination and is effective in treating Phlegm-fluid patterns and oedema. Since it can supplement Qi, it is also used for stopping sweating and quieting the foetus. *Dang Shen* is also good for supplementing the Middle Jiao and boosting Qi, and is more effective than *Shan Yao*; it can also generate body fluids and nourish the Blood. Although *Shan Yao* is not as powerful in supplementing Qi as *Bai Zhu* or *Dang Shen*, it can both supplement Lung and Spleen Qi and boost Lung and Kidney Yin. As it is astringent as well as neutral, *Shan Yao* is used to secure the Kidneys and astringe the Essence, functions that the other two herbs do not possess.

For additional comparisons, see *Gan Cao* (Radix Glycyrrhizae), *Bai Bian Dou* (Semen Dolichoris Lablab) and *Huang Jing* (Rhizoma Polygonati).

Modern research

1. Has a supplementing function, helps digestion.[52]
2. Decoctions of *Shan Yao* lower the blood sugar level and strengthen the immune function.[52]
3. Regulates gastrointestinal movement.[53]
4. Stops diarrhoea and expels sputum.[53]

Combinations and applications

Functions	Combinations	Applications
Fortifying the Spleen and stopping diarrhoea	*Dang Shen* (Radix Codonopsitis Pilosulae) *Bai Zhu* (Rhizoma Atractylodis Macrocephalae) *Bai Bian Dou* (Semen Dolichoris Lablab) *Lian Zi* (Semen Nelumbinis Nuciferae)	Reduced appetite and fatigued body, loose stool and enduring diarrhoea due to Spleen and Stomach deficiency
	Mai Ya (Fructus Hordei Vulgaris Germinatus) *Shen Qu* (Massa Fermentata) *Ji Nei Jin* (Endothelium Corneum Gigeriae Galli)	Food accumulation due to Spleen and Stomach deficiency with reduced appetite and distension in the stomach and abdomen

Supplementing the Lungs and stopping coughing	*Dang Shen* (Radix Codonopsitis Pilosulae) *Mai Men Dong* (Radix Ophiopogonis Japonici) *Wu Wei Zi* (Fructus Schisandrae)	Enduring coughing and wheezing due to Lung deficiency
	Shu Di Huang (Radix Rehmanniae Glutinosae Conquita) *Shan Zhu Yu* (Fructus Corni Officinalis) *Su Zi* (Fructus Perillae Frutescentis)	Deficiency wheezing due to Lung and Kidney deficiency
Supplementing Qi and nourishing Yin, supplementing the Kidneys, securing the Essence and stopping vaginal discharge	*Shu Di Huang* (Radix Rehmanniae Glutinosae Conquita) *Shan Zhu Yu* (Fructus Corni Officinalis) *Jin Ying Zi* (Fructus Rosae Laevigatae)	Limpness and aching in the lumbar region and knees, seminal emission, dizziness and blurred vision due to depletion and deficiency of Kidney Yin
	Yi Zhi Ren (Fructus Alpiniae Oxyphyllae) *Wu Yao* (Radix Linderae Strychnifoliae)	Seminal emission and frequent urination due to Bladder deficiency-cold
	Dang Shen (Radix Codonopsitis Pilosulae) *Che Qian Zi* (Semen Plantaginis) *Bai Zhu* (Rhizoma Atractylodis Macrocephalae) *Qian Shi* (Semen Euryales Ferocis) *Cang Zhu* (Rhizoma Atractylodis)	Thick, yellow vaginal discharge due to damp-heat pouring down in Spleen deficiency patterns
	Huang Bai (Cortex Phellodendri)	Vaginal discharge due to damp-heat
	Huang Qi (Radix Astragali seu Hedysari) *Tian Hua Fen* (Radix Trichosanthis) *Ge Gen* (Radix Puerariae)	Wasting and thirsting patterns due to Qi and Yin deficiency

Bai Bian Dou 白扁豆 (White hyacinth bean, Semen Dolichoris Lablab)

Bai Bian Dou is the dried ripe seed of *Dolichos lablab* L., family Leguminosae.

Main ingredients *Bai Bian Dou* contains proteins, fats, carbohydrates, calcium, phosphorus, iron, phytin, pantothenic acid and zinc.

Properties Taste: sweet; nature: slightly warm.

Channels entered Spleen and Stomach.

Functions and indications Fortifies the Spleen and harmonizes the Middle Jiao, clears summerheat and transforms dampness, and relieves toxicity. It is indicated for vomiting, diarrhoea and vaginal discharge due to Spleen deficiency, and vomiting and diarrhoea due to pathogenic summerheat-damp.

Common dosage 10-20g.

Remarks Use stir-fried *Bai Bian Dou* to fortify the Spleen and Stomach and stop diarrhoea; use the raw herb to clear summerheat and relieve toxicity.

Comparison of functions Both *Bai Bian Dou* (Semen Dolichoris Lablab) and *Shan Yao* (Rhizoma Dioscoreae Oppositae) can fortify the Spleen and boost Qi. *Shan Yao* can concurrently supplement Qi and nourish Yin to treat wasting and thirsting patterns and, with its astringent properties, it can secure the Kidneys and stop vaginal discharge. *Bai Bian Dou* does not have these functions. However, unlike *Shan Yao*, it is aromatic and can transform dampness, being an important herb for fortifying the Spleen and eliminating dampness; it can also clear summerheat and relieve toxicity, functions that *Shan Yao* does not possess.

For an additional comparison, see *Gan Cao* (Radix Glycyrrhizae).

Modern research

1. Inhibits enteroviruses.[54]
2. The steep of *Bai Bian Dou* strengthens the immune function.[55]

Combinations and applications

Functions	Combinations	Applications
Fortifying the Spleen and harmonizing the Middle Jiao	*Dang Shen* (Radix Codonopsitis Pilosulae) *Fu Ling* (Sclerotium Poriae Cocos) *Bai Zhu* (Rhizoma Atractylodis Macrocephalae) *Yi Yi Ren* (Semen Coicis Lachrymajobi) *Shan Yao* (Rhizoma Dioscoreae Oppositae)	Fatigued body and lack of strength, reduced appetite, loose stool or vomiting and diarrhoea with slimy tongue fur and a moderate pulse due to Spleen and Stomach deficiency with exuberant dampness
Clearing summerheat and transforming dampness	*Xiang Ru* (Herba Elsholtziae seu Moslae) *Hou Po* (Cortex Magnoliae Officinalis)	Oppression in the chest, vomiting and diarrhoea due to Spleen-Stomach disharmony and summerheat-damp damaging the Middle Jiao
Relieving toxicity	*Ge Hua* (Flos Puerariae) *Bai Dou Kou* (Fructus Amomi Kravanh) *Nan Sha Shen* (Radix Adenophorae)	Alcohol toxins

Note: Stir-fried ground *Bai Bian Dou* can be used to treat profuse, clear, thin white vaginal discharge due to damp turbidity pouring down as a result of Spleen deficiency with exuberant dampness.

Xi Yang Shen 西洋参
(American ginseng root, Radix Panacis Quinquefolii)

Xi Yang Shen is the dried root of *Panax quinquefolium* L., family Araliaceae.

Legal status *Xi Yang Shen* (in whole root form) is a restricted substance listed in Appendix II of the Convention on International Trade in Endangered Species of Wild Fauna and Flora (CITES). Appropriate import and export permits are required for trade in this materia medica.

Main ingredients *Xi Yang Shen* contains ginsenosides, volatile oils, holosides, fatty oils, amino acids and microelements.

Properties Taste: sweet and slightly bitter; nature: cold.

Channels entered Heart, Lung and Kidney.

Functions and indications Supplements Qi and nourishes Yin, generates body fluids, and boosts the Lungs and clears fire. It is indicated for coughing and wheezing due to Lung Yin deficiency; vexation, thirst, shortness of breath and lack of strength due to Qi and Yin deficiency; dry mouth, and blood in the stool.

Common dosage 3-6g, decocted separately.

Precautions and contraindications

1. The cold nature of *Xi Yang Shen* may damage Yang in the Middle Jiao and reinforce dampness; this herb is therefore contraindicated in cases with damp-cold obstructing the Middle Jiao.

2. *Xi Yang Shen* is incompatible with *Li Lu* (Radix et Rhizoma Veratri).

Remarks *Xi Yang Shen* must not be stir-fried in an iron vessel.

Comparison of functions Although both *Xi Yang Shen* (Radix Panacis Quinquefolii) and *Ren Shen* (Radix Ginseng) are very effective in supplementing Qi, *Ren Shen* has a stronger supplementing and boosting effect than *Xi Yang Shen*. It strongly supplements original Qi as well as supplementing the Spleen and boosting the Lungs, generating body fluids, and quieting the Spirit; it is the most important herb for the treatment of deficiency taxation and internal damage. However, it tends to be warm and is not suitable for deficiency taxation with internal fire and heat. In such cases, *Xi Yang Shen* can be used as a substitute. It is sweet, slightly bitter and cold and can nourish Yin in addition to supplementing Qi; it can also clear Lung-fire and generate body fluids and is an important herb for Qi and Yin deficiency patterns with fire.

For an additional comparison, see *Tai Zi Shen* (Radix Pseudostellariae Heterophyllae).

Toxicity The LD_{50} for intraperitoneal injection in mice of the saponins contained in *Xi Yang Shen* is 204mg/kg. Rats fed up to 200mg/kg per day for 90 days showed no appreciable change in weight in comparison with a control group and the white blood cell count, haemoglobin, zinc sulphate turbidity and thymol turbidity were all normal.

Modern research

1. *Xi Yang Shen* has similar functions to ginseng in stimulating and inhibiting the central nervous system.[56]
2. Inhibits arrhythmia.[57]
3. Strengthens the immune function.[58]
4. Inhibits carcinoma.[59, 60]

Combinations and applications

Functions	Combinations	Applications
Supplementing Qi and nourishing Yin, generating body fluids, boosting the Lungs and clearing fire	*Mai Men Dong* (Radix Ophiopogonis Japonici) *Zhi Mu* (Rhizoma Anemarrhenae Asphodeloidis) *E Jiao* (Gelatinum Corii Asini) *Zhe Bei Mu* (Bulbus Fritillariae Thunbergii)	Enduring cough with scant or blood-streaked sputum due to Yin deficiency of the Lungs and Kidneys
	Mai Men Dong (Radix Ophiopogonis Japonici) *Wu Wei Zi* (Fructus Schisandrae) *Sheng Di Huang* (Radix Rehmanniae Glutinosae) *Shi Hu* (Herba Dendrobii) (see notes on legal status)	Vexation, fatigue, shortness of breath and lack of strength, dry mouth and thirst due to Qi and Yin deficiency
	Tian Men Dong (Radix Asparagi Cochinchinensis) *Mai Men Dong* (Radix Ophiopogonis Japonici) *Zhi Mu* (Rhizoma Anemarrhenae Asphodeloidis) *Yu Zhu* (Rhizoma Polygonati Odorati)	Dry mouth due to deficiency of body fluids
	Long Yan Rou (Arillus Euphoriae Longanae) (steamed together)	Intestinal dryness and blood in the stool

Note: *Xi Yang Shen* can be used on its own to enrich Yin and generate body fluids.

Tai Zi Shen 太子参 (Pseudostellaria root, Radix Pseudostellariae Heterophyllae)

Tai Zi Shen is the dried tuberous root of *Pseudostellaria heterophylla* (Miq.) Pax ex Pax et Hoffm., family Caryophyllaceae.

Main ingredients *Tai Zi Shen* contains starch, polysaccharides, saponins, phenolic acid, palmitic acid, linoleic acid and heterophyllin.

Properties Taste: sweet and slightly bitter; nature: neutral.

Channels entered Spleen and Lung.

Functions and indications Boosts Qi and generates body fluids, fortifies the Spleen and moistens the Lungs. It is indicated for fatigue and reduced appetite due to Spleen deficiency, sweating due to Qi deficiency, cough and shortness of breath due to damage to Qi and Yin, and thirst due to loss of body fluids.

Common dosage 10-30g.

Remarks A decoction of *Tai Zi Shen* and *Yu Mi Xu* (Stylus Zeae Mays) can be used for acute and chronic hepatitis.

Comparison of functions Both *Tai Zi Shen* (Radix Pseudostellariae Heterophyllae) and *Xi Yang Shen* (Radix Panacis Quinquefolii) can supplement Qi, nourish Yin and generate body fluids to treat damage to Qi and Yin. *Xi Yang Shen* is cold and has a stronger effect than *Tai Zi Shen* in clearing fire. *Tai Zi Shen* is neutral and harmonizing and has a weaker effect than *Xi Yang Shen* in terms of supplementing Qi, boosting Yin and generating body fluids. As a result, it is particularly suitable for children or for patients with a weak constitution who cannot tolerate drastic supplementing herbs.

Modern research Strengthens the immune function and stimulates the metabolism.[61]

Combinations and applications

Functions	Combinations	Applications
Boosting Qi and generating body fluids, fortifying the Spleen and moistening the Lungs	*Shan Yao* (Rhizoma Dioscoreae Oppositae) *Bai Bian Dou* (Semen Dolichoris Lablab) *Gu Ya* (Fructus Setariae Italicae Germinatus)	Fatigue and reduced appetite due to insufficiency of Stomach Yin and deficiency of Spleen Qi in the aftermath of an illness
	Suan Zao Ren (Semen Ziziphi Spinosae) *Wu Wei Zi* (Fructus Schisandrae) *Huang Qi* (Radix Astragali seu Hedysari)	Spontaneous sweating, thirst and insomnia due to Qi deficiency
	Nan Sha Shen (Radix Adenophorae) *Mai Men Dong* (Radix Ophiopogonis Japonici) *Zhe Bei Mu* (Bulbus Fritillariae Thunbergii) *Sang Ye* (Folium Mori Albae)	Lung deficiency dry cough, shortness of breath and scant sputum due to damage to Qi and Yin as a result of dryness or heat pathogenic factors settling in the Lungs
	Shi Hu (Herba Dendrobii) (see notes on legal status) *Wu Wei Zi* (Fructus Schisandrae) *Tian Hua Fen* (Radix Trichosanthis) *Mai Men Dong* (Radix Ophiopogonis Japonici)	Thirst with a thin pulse and red tongue due to damage to body fluids and Qi deficiency in the final stage of febrile diseases

Da Zao 大枣
(Chinese date, Fructus Ziziphi Jujubae)

Da Zao is the dried ripe fruit of *Ziziphus jujuba* Mill., family Rhamnaceae.

Main ingredients *Da Zao* contains betulinic, oleanolic, malic and stearic acids, zizyphus saponins, vitamins B_2 and C, carotene, sitosterol, stigmasterol, calcium, phosphorus, iron, catechol and tannin.

Properties Taste: sweet; nature: warm.

Channels entered Spleen and Stomach.

Functions and indications Supplements the Spleen and boosts Qi, nourishes the Blood and quiets the Spirit, and moderates and harmonizes the nature of other herbs. It is indicated for Spleen and Stomach deficiency, diarrhoea and reduced appetite, Blood deficiency patterns, and emotional depression in women; and for moderating the drastic action of other herbs.

Common dosage 3-12 pieces, or 10-30g.

Precautions and contraindications As *Da Zao* can reinforce dampness and generate heat, it is contraindicated in cases of distension below the heart due to Phlegm-damp and for food accumulation, disorders due to intestinal worms, toothache, and cough due to Phlegm-heat.

Remarks *Da Zao* is often combined with *Sheng Jiang* (Rhizoma Zingiberis Officinalis Recens):

1. Used with herbs for releasing the exterior, they can adjust and harmonize the Ying and Wei levels.
2. Used with supplementing herbs, they can harmonize the Spleen and Stomach and boost the supplementing effect.

Comparison of functions Both *Da Zao* (Fructus Ziziphi Jujubae) and *Gan Cao* (Radix Glycyrrhizae) can supplement the Middle Jiao and boost Qi. They can also adjust and harmonize the nature of other herbs and are often combined to strengthen their effect. Unlike *Da Zao*, *Gan Cao* also has the functions of clearing heat and relieving toxicity, and dispelling Phlegm and stopping coughing. *Da Zao* has the additional functions of nourishing the Blood and quieting the Spirit and is used in particular for treating Blood deficiency with a sallow yellow facial complexion and for disquieted Heart and Spirit.

Toxicity Acute toxicity tests for 24 hours on animals and long-term toxicity tests lasting three months did not result in any changes in terms of external appearance or haematological function or in toxic effects on internal organs.

Modern research

1. Alcoholic extracts of *Da Zao* inhibit allergic reactions.[62]
2. Has a tranquillizing function, inhibits the production of carcinoma cells and strengthens the muscles.[62]
3. Lowers blood pressure.[63]

Combinations and applications

Functions	Combinations	Applications
Supplementing the Spleen and boosting Qi	*Dang Shen* (Radix Codonopsitis Pilosulae) *Bai Zhu* (Rhizoma Atractylodis Macrocephalae)	Fatigue, lack of strength, reduced appetite and loose stool due to Spleen and Stomach deficiency
	Bai Zhu (Rhizoma Atractylodis Macrocephalae) *Gan Jiang* (Rhizoma Zingiberis Officinalis) *Ji Nei Jin* (Endothelium Corneum Gigeriae Galli)	Reduced appetite and diarrhoea due to Yang deficiency in the Middle Jiao

Nourishing the Blood and quieting the Spirit	*Shu Di Huang* (Radix Rehmanniae Glutinosae Conquita) *Dang Gui* (Radix Angelicae Sinensis) *E Jiao* (Gelatinum Corii Asini) *Huang Qi* (Radix Astragali seu Hedysari)	Dizziness, a sallow yellow facial complexion, reduced menstruation or menstrual block due to Blood deficiency
	Gan Cao (Radix Glycyrrhizae) *Fu Xiao Mai* (Fructus Tritici Aestivi Levis)	Emotional depression in women, visceral agitation due to disquieted Heart and Spirit

Notes:

1. *Da Zao* can be used with drastic downward-draining herbs such as *Gan Sui* (Radix Euphorbiae Kansui), *Jing Da Ji* (Radix Euphorbiae Pekinensis) and *Yuan Hua* (Flos Daphnes Genkwa) to moderate their drastic action and prevent damage to the Stomach.
2. *Da Zao* can be used with *Ting Li Zi* (Semen Lepidii seu Descurainiae) to protect Lung Qi while draining the Lungs, moving water, causing Qi to descend and calming wheezing.

Yi Tang 饴糖
(Malt sugar, Saccharum Granorum)

Yi Tang is made by adding barley malt to rice flour, glutinous rice flour or wheat flour and cooking the mixture slowly over a low heat.

Main ingredients *Yi Yang* contains maltose and small amounts of proteins, fats and vitamin B.

Properties Taste: sweet; nature: warm.

Channels entered Spleen, Stomach and Lung.

Functions and indications Supplements the Spleen and boosts Qi, relaxes tension and alleviates pain, moistens the Lungs and stops coughing. It is indicated for taxation fatigue damaging the Spleen, shortness of breath, lack of strength and reduced food intake, pain in the chest and abdomen, and dry cough due to Lung deficiency.

Common dosage 30-60g, dissolved in a decoction strained two or three times; can also be prepared into an extract or pills.

Precautions and contraindications As *Yi Tang* can reinforce dampness and generate heat to cause fullness in the Middle Jiao, it is contraindicated in cases of damp-heat brewing internally, vomiting due to fullness in the Middle Jiao, cough due to Phlegm-heat, and infantile Gan accumulation.

Remarks *Yi Tang* is relatively weak in its actions and is therefore generally used as an auxiliary substance in combinations.

Comparison of functions Both *Yi Tang* (Saccharum Granorum) and *Feng Mi* (Mel) can supplement the Middle Jiao and relax tension, and moisten the Lungs and stop coughing. *Yi Tang* is warm in nature and is therefore more suitable for pain in the abdomen due to deficiency-cold. *Feng Mi* is neutral in nature and is therefore better for pain in the stomach and abdomen due to deficiency in the Middle Jiao. It is also effective in relieving toxicity and inhibits the toxic effects of *Wu Tou* (Radix Aconiti) and related herbs.

Combinations and applications

Functions	Combinations	Applications
Supplementing the Spleen and boosting Qi, relaxing tension and alleviating pain	*Gui Zhi* (Ramulus Cinnamomi Cassiae) *Bai Shao* (Radix Paeoniae Lactiflorae) *Zhi Gan Cao* (Radix Glycyrrhizae Praeparata)	Taxation fatigue damaging the Spleen, shortness of breath and lack of strength, reduced food intake, pain in the abdomen due to deficiency-cold

	Huang Qi (Radix Astragali seu Hedysari) (add to the above combination)	The above symptoms plus severe Qi deficiency
	Dang Gui (Radix Angelicae Sinensis) (add to the first combination above)	The above symptoms plus concurrent Blood deficiency
	Hua Jiao (Pericarpium Zanthoxyli) *Gan Jiang* (Rhizoma Zingiberis Officinalis) *Ren Shen* (Radix Ginseng)	Extreme cold and pain in the chest and abdomen due to internal exuberance of Yin cold and Yang deficiency in the Middle Jiao
Moistening the Lungs and stopping coughing	*Feng Mi* (Mel) *Bai Bu* (Radix Stemonae) *Xing Ren* (Semen Pruni Armeniacae)	Dry cough due to Lung deficiency

HERBS FOR SUPPLEMENTING YANG

Herbs for supplementing Yang include those herbs which can supplement Yang Qi and disperse or eliminate Yang deficiency patterns.

Yang deficiency patterns normally relate to deficiency of Heart Yang, Spleen Yang and Kidney Yang. Since Kidney Yang governs Yang Qi, mild exhaustion of Kidney Yang can result in Yang deficiency throughout the body. Kidney Yang deficiency, irrespective of the factor by which it is caused, can affect the functions of the Kidneys in storing the Essence, governing reproduction, warming the Zang-Fu organs, transforming Qi and governing water.

Herbs for supplementing Yang are generally warm in nature and sweet, salty or acrid in taste. Since sweetness has supplementing and boosting functions, salt can enter the Kidneys and acridity can support Yang and dissipate cold, this results in herbs for supplementing Yang having the functions of warming and supplementing Kidney Yang, reinforcing or invigorating Yang, securing the Essence, and strengthening the sinews and bones. These herbs are used for impotence, premature ejaculation, seminal emission, cold uterus and infertility, frequent urination and urinary incontinence due to Kidney Yang deficiency; for chills, fatigue, cold limbs, pain in the lumbar region and loose stool due to Yang deficiency of the Spleen and Kidneys; and for wheezing due to Kidney deficiency.

Herbs for supplementing Yang are combined with other herbs according to the patterns identified. They are used together with herbs for warming the interior for patients with Yang deficiency and interior cold; for patients with insufficiency of the Liver and Kidneys, they are combined with herbs for enriching and supplementing the Liver and Kidneys; for patients with diarrhoea due to Yang deficiency of the Spleen and Kidneys, they are used with herbs for warming and fortifying the Spleen and supplementing Qi; for wheezing due to Lung and Kidney deficiency, they are combined with herbs for supplementing Lung Qi; and for patients suffering from general weakness or in cases of deficiency taxation due to depletion of the Essence and Blood, they are used with herbs for supplementing the Essence and Blood.

As herbs for supplementing Yang are dry and warm in nature, they can damage Yin and reinforce fire. For this reason, they should not be used in cases of effulgent Yin deficiency-fire and for patients who have a bitter taste in the mouth or dry mouth and dry lips due to heat.

Tab. 17.2 Herbs for supplementing Yang

Herb	Functions	Indications
Lu Rong (Cornu Cervi Parvum)	Supplementing the Kidneys and reinforcing Yang, regulating the Chong and Ren vessels, boosting the Essence and Blood, strengthening the sinews and bones	Aversion to cold, cold limbs, impotence and premature ejaculation, infertility due to cold uterus, dizziness, tinnitus, uterine bleeding, vaginal discharge due to deficiency-cold of the Chong and Ren vessels, lack of strength in the sinews and bones due to insufficiency of the Essence and Blood
Yin Yang Huo (Herba Epimedii)	Supplementing the Kidneys and invigorating Yang, dispelling wind and eliminating dampness	Impotence due to insufficiency of Kidney Yang, frequent urination, hypertonicity of the sinews and bones, lack of strength in the lumbar region and knees, hemiplegia, wind-damp Bi syndrome pain, numbness of the limbs

Tu Si Zi (Semen Cuscutae)	Supplementing Kidney Yang and boosting Kidney Yin, securing the Essence and reducing urine, nourishing the Liver and brightening the eyes, fortifying the Spleen and stopping diarrhoea, quieting the foetus	Limpness and aching in the lumbar region and knees, impotence, seminal emission, frequent urination, vaginal discharge, blurred vision, diarrhoea due to Spleen and Kidney deficiency, wasting and thirsting due to Yin deficiency
Du Zhong (Cortex Eucommiae Ulmoidis)	Supplementing the Liver and Kidneys, strengthening the sinews and bones, quieting the foetus	Insufficiency of the Liver and Kidneys, lack of strength in the lumbar region and knees, impotence, frequent urination, habitual miscarriage, dizziness and headache
Xu Duan (Radix Dipsaci)	Supplementing the Liver and Kidneys, stopping bleeding and quieting the foetus, strengthening the sinews and bones, treating injuries and joining fractures	Pain in the lumbar region, weakness of the legs, uterine bleeding and vaginal discharge, knocks and falls, abscesses and sores
Ba Ji Tian (Radix Morindae Officinalis)	Supplementing the Kidneys and reinforcing Yang, strengthening the sinews and bones, dispelling wind and eliminating dampness	Impotence due to Kidney Yang deficiency, pain and cold in the lower abdomen, frequent urination, infertility due to cold uterus, wind-cold-damp Bi syndrôme, limpness and aching in the lumbar region and knees
Xian Mao (Rhizoma Curculiginis Orchioidis)	Warming the Kidneys and invigorating Yang, dispelling cold and eliminating dampness	Impotence, seminal cold, cold and aching in the lumbar region and knees, Wei syndrome of the sinews and bones, cold-damp Bi syndrome pain, frequent urination
Bu Gu Zhi (Fructus Psoraleae Corylifoliae)	Supplementing the Kidneys and invigorating Yang, securing the Essence and reducing urine, warming the Spleen and stopping diarrhoea, hosting Qi and calming wheezing	Cold and aching in the lumbar region and knees, impotence, seminal emission, urinary incontinence, frequent urination, diarrhoea due to Yang deficiency, coughing and wheezing due to deficiency-cold
Yi Zhi Ren (Fructus Alpiniae Oxyphyllae)	Warming the Kidneys, securing the Essence and reducing urine, warming the Spleen and stopping diarrhoea	Seminal emission, urinary incontinence, child bed-wetting, cold and pain in the abdomen, vomiting and diarrhoea, reduced appetite, excessive salivation
Rou Cong Rong (Herba Cistanches Deserticolae)	Supplementing the Kidneys and invigorating Yang, boosting the Essence and Blood, moistening the Intestines and freeing the bowels	Impotence, seminal emission and premature ejaculation due to insufficiency of Kidney Yang, cold and aching in the lumbar region and knees, lack of strength in the sinews and bones, constipation in the elderly, postpartum Blood deficiency
Suo Yang (Herba Cynomorii Songarici)	Supplementing the Kidneys and reinforcing Yang, moistening the Intestines and freeing the bowels	Impotence, seminal emission, sterility, limpness and aching in the lumbar region and knees, difficulty in movement, Intestinal dryness with constipation

Sha Yuan Zi (Semen Astragali Complanati)	Boosting the Kidneys and securing the Essence, supplementing the Liver and brightening the eyes	Liver and Kidney deficiency, limpness and aching in the lumbar region and knees, dizziness, tinnitus, blurred vision, seminal emission, premature ejaculation, frequent urination, enuresis, vaginal discharge
Jiu Cai Zi (Semen Allii Tuberosi)	Invigorating Yang and securing the Essence	Impotence, seminal emission and frequent urination due to Kidney deficiency
Dong Chong Xia Cao (Cordyceps Sinensis)	Supplementing the Lungs and boosting the Kidneys, transforming Phlegm and stopping coughing	Coughing and wheezing due to Lung and Kidney deficiency, spontaneous sweating and night sweating, lack of strength after illness, pain and aching in the lumbar region and knees due to Kidney deficiency, impotence and seminal emission
Ge Jie (Gekko)	Supplementing the Lungs and boosting the Kidneys, hosting Qi and stabilizing wheezing, reinforcing Kidney Yang and boosting the Essence and Blood	Deficiency wheezing and enduring cough, coughing of blood due to deficiency taxation, impotence and seminal emission, frequent urination
Hu Tao Ren (Semen Juglandis Regiae)	Supplementing the Kidneys and strengthening the lumbar region and knees, astringing the Essence and stopping seminal emission, moistening the Lungs, hosting Qi and stabilizing wheezing, moistening the Intestines and freeing the bowels	Coughing and wheezing due to Kidney deficiency, limpness and aching in the lumbar region and knees, seminal emission, frequent urination, Intestinal dryness with constipation
Hu Lu Ba (Semen Trigonellae Foeni-graeci)	Warming the Kidneys and reinforcing Yang, dissipating cold and alleviating pain	Cold Shan disorders, cold-damp leg Qi, cold and pain in the legs and knees or lumbar region, impotence, seminal cold
Zi He Che (Placenta Hominis)	Supplementing the Kidneys and boosting the Essence, nourishing the Blood and boosting Qi, supplementing the Lungs and calming wheezing	Insufficiency of Qi and Blood, emaciation, coughing and wheezing due to Lung deficiency, tidal fever due to steaming bone disorder, night sweating, seminal emission and impotence, infertility

Lu Rong 鹿茸 (Pilose antler of young deer, Cornu Cervi Parvum)

Lu Rong is the velvet of the young male *Cervus nippon* Temminck or *C. elaphus* L., family Cervidae.

Main ingredients *Lu Rong* contains pantocrine, oestrone, colloids, amino acids, calcium, magnesium and phosphorus.

Properties Taste: sweet and salty; nature: warm.

Channels entered Liver and Kidney.

Functions and indications Supplements the Kidneys and reinforces Yang, regulates the Chong and Ren vessels, boosts the Essence and Blood, and strengthens the sinews and bones. It is indicated for aversion to cold, cold limbs, impotence and premature ejaculation, infertility due to cold uterus, dizziness, tinnitus, uterine bleeding, vaginal discharge due to deficiency-cold of the Chong and Ren vessels, and lack of strength in the sinews and bones due to insufficiency of the Essence and Blood.

Common dosage 1-3g, pounded to pieces, three times a day, or taken as pills or powder.

Precautions and contraindications

1. *Lu Rong* is contraindicated for hyperactivity of Yang due to Yin deficiency, heat in the Xue level, exuberant Stomach-fire, Phlegm-heat in the Lungs, and externally-contracted febrile diseases.
2. Administration should start from small dosages and gradually increase; *Lu Rong* should not be used immediately in large dosages in case it causes upward bearing of Yang and stirring of wind with dizziness and vertigo, or stirring of Blood through damage to Yin.

Comparison of functions See *Rou Cong Rong* (Herba Cistanches Deserticolae).

Toxicity The LD_{50} for intravenous injection of pantocrine in rats is 18.3ml/kg; for intraperitoneal injection, it is 82ml/kg.

Modern research

1. Increases capacity to work, and improves sleep and appetite.[64]
2. Promotes the regeneration of blood.[65-67]
3. Strengthens the immune system.[68]
4. Has a sex hormone-like function.[69]

Combinations and applications

Functions	Combinations	Applications
Supplementing the Kidneys and reinforcing Yang	*Dang Gui* (Radix Angelicae Sinensis) *Ren Shen* (Radix Ginseng) *Gou Qi Zi* (Fructus Lycii) *Tu Si Zi* (Semen Cuscutae)	Limpness and aching in the lumbar region and knees, aversion to cold, cold limbs, impotence and premature ejaculation, infertility due to cold uterus, and frequent urination caused by the exhaustion of fire at the gate of vitality
	Fu Zi (Radix Lateralis Aconiti Carmichaeli Praeparata) (see notes on legal status) *Cao Guo* (Fructus Amomi Tsaoko) *Fu Ling* (Sclerotium Poriae Cocos) *Tu Si Zi* (Semen Cuscutae)	Oedema of the foot and generalized pain with white and slimy tongue fur due to deficiency of Kidney Yang, which thus fails to transform Qi and move water

Regulating the Chong and Ren vessels	*Hai Piao Xiao* (Os Sepiae seu Sepiellae) *Cao Guo* (Fructus Amomi Tsaoko) *Fu Ling* (Sclerotium Poriae Cocos) *Tu Si Zi* (Semen Cuscutae)	Insufficiency of the Liver and Kidneys and deficiency-cold of the Chong and Ren vessels, manifesting as incessant uterine bleeding, cold limbs, limpness and aching in the lumbar region and knees, and a sunken, fine pulse
	Gou Ji (Rhizoma Cibotii Barometz) (see notes on legal status) *Bai Lian* (Radix Ampelopsis Japonicae)	Profuse white vaginal discharge due to deficiency-cold of the Chong and Ren vessels
Boosting the Essence and Blood, strengthening the sinews and bones	*Dang Gui* (Radix Angelicae Sinensis) *Wu Mei* (Fructus Pruni Mume)	Severe deficiency of the Essence and Blood, manifesting as a soot-black complexion, tinnitus, thirst, dry mouth, pain in the lumbar region and lack of strength in the feet, and white urinary turbidity
	Shan Yao (Rhizoma Dioscoreae Oppositae) *Shan Zhu Yu* (Fructus Corni Officinalis) *Shu Di Huang* (Radix Rehmanniae Glutinosae Conquita) *Fu Ling* (Sclerotium Poriae Cocos)	Lack of strength in the sinews and bones, insufficient development of the bones in infants, slowness in walking and teething, non-closure of the fontanelle due to insufficiency of the Essence and Blood

Note: *Lu Rong* can also be used with *Rou Gui* (Cortex Cinnamomi Cassiae), *Shu Di Huang* (Radix Rehmanniae Glutinosae Conquita) and *Ma Huang* (Herba Ephedrae) for persistent non-ulcerating sores with thin, clear pus and for collapsed Yin abscesses and sores where the toxins cannot be drawn out as a result of Kidney deficiency and Essence depletion (for *Ma Huang*, see notes on legal status).

Appendix

Lu Jiao 鹿角 (Mature deer antler, Cornu Cervi)

Lu Jiao is the antler of *Cervus nippon* Temminck, *C. elaphus* L. or other kinds of adult male deer. It is salty in taste and warm in nature, and enters the Liver and Kidney channels. It can supplement the Kidneys and reinforce Yang and can be used as a substitute for *Lu Rong* (Cornu Cervi Parvum), but its effect is weaker. At the same time, it quickens the Blood to dispel stasis and also disperses swelling, and can be used for abscesses and sores, breast abscess, pain due to Blood stasis and other kinds of pain in the lumbar region and spine and in the sinews and bones. It can be taken orally or used topically. The dosage for oral use is 5-10g, either decocted or pounded to a powder. Use topically as juice or powder. *Lu Jiao* is contraindicated in cases of effulgent Yin deficiency-fire.

Lu Jiao Jiao 鹿角胶 (Mature deer antler glue, Gelatinum Cornu Cervi)

Lu Jiao Jiao is the glue-like substance made as a concentrate from a decoction of deer antler. It is sweet and salty in taste and warm in nature, and enters the Liver and Kidney channels. It can supplement the Liver and Kidneys, boost the Essence and Blood, and stop bleeding. It is indicated for bleeding patterns due to deficiency-cold caused by Kidney Yang insufficiency and depletion and deficiency of the Essence and Blood, manifesting as deficiency taxation, emaciation, vomiting, bleeding, uterine bleeding and blood in the urine, and also for unhealed Yin abscesses. The dosage should be 5-10g. *Lu Jiao Jiao* should be dissolved in boiling water or yellow wine (*Huang Jiu*, Vinum Aureum), or added to pills or powders. It is contra-indicated in cases of effulgent Yin deficiency-fire.

***Lu Jiao Shuang* 鹿角霜 (Degelatined mature deer antler, Cornu Cervi Degelatinatum)**
Lu Jiao Shuang is the residue left over after extracting *Lu Jiao Jiao* from *Lu Jiao*. Salty in taste and warm in nature, it enters the Liver and Kidney channels. It is effective for boosting the Kidneys and reinforcing Yang, although its effect is relatively weak; it also has an astringent function. It can be used for insufficiency of Kidney Yang, Spleen and Stomach deficiency-cold, vomiting and reduced appetite with loose stool, uterine bleeding, vaginal discharge due to deficiency, and cold in the uterus. It also has a topical application for injury, bleeding and non-healing abscesses. The dosage should be 10-15g, or an appropriate dosage for external application. *Lu Jiao Shuang* is contraindicated in cases of effulgent Yin deficiency-fire.

Yin Yang Huo 淫羊藿 (Epimedium, Herba Epimedii)

Yin Yang Huo is the whole herb of *Epimedium brevicornum* Maxim., *E. koreanum* Nakai or *E. sagittatum* (Sieb. et Zucc.) Maxim., family Berberidaceae.

Main ingredients *Yin Yang Huo* contains icariin, icarisides and epimedoside A (*E. brevicornum*); epimedins, epimedokoreanosides, epimedoside A and icariin (*E. koreanum*); icariin, icarisides, isoquercetin, hyperin, sagitattosides and icarisides (*E. sagittatum*); as well as ceryl alcohol, phytosterol, palmitic, stearic, oleic, linoleic and linolenic acids, bilobol, magnoflorin, glucose and fructose.

Properties Taste: acrid and sweet; nature: warm.

Channels entered Liver and Kidney.

Functions and indications Supplements the Kidneys and invigorates Yang, dispels wind and eliminates dampness. It is indicated for impotence due to insufficiency of Kidney Yang, frequent urination, hypertonicity of the sinews and bones, lack of strength in the lumbar region and knees, hemiplegia, wind-damp Bi syndrome pain, and numbness of the limbs.

Common dosage 10-15g, taken as a decoction; the herb can also be steeped in alcohol or processed into powder and pills.

Precautions and contraindications Since *Yin Yang Huo* is dry and harsh and can reinforce fire, it is contraindicated in cases of effulgent Yin deficiency-fire.

Comparison of functions See *Xian Mao* (Rhizoma Curculiginis Orchioidis).

Toxicity The LD_{50} for intraperitoneal injection in mice of an extract of *Yin Yang Huo* is 36g/kg.

Modern research

1. The polysaccharides contained in *Yin Yang Huo* can strengthen the immune function.[70]
2. The processed herb has a male hormone-like function, which can improve sexual ability.[71, 72]
3. Lowers blood pressure, inhibits coronary heart diseases.[73, 74]
4. Inhibits the effects of ageing.[75, 76]
5. Preparations of *Yin Yang Huo* clearly inhibited Staphylococcus albus, Staphylococcus aureus, the polio virus and enteroviruses *in vitro*.[77]
6. Stops coughing and calms wheezing, expels sputum.[78]
7. Has a tranquillizing function.[79]

Combinations and applications

Functions	Combinations	Applications
Supplementing the Kidneys and invigorating Yang	*Gou Qi Zi* (Fructus Lycii) *Xian Mao* (Rhizoma Curculiginis Orchioidis) *Shu Di Huang* (Radix Rehmanniae Glutinosae Conquita)	Lack of strength in the lumbar region and knees, frequent urination, impotence and premature ejaculation due to insufficiency of Kidney Yang
	Xian Mao (Rhizoma Curculiginis Orchioidis) *Dang Gui* (Radix Angelicae Sinensis) *Ba Ji Tian* (Radix Morindae Officinalis) *Huang Bai* (Cortex Phellodendri)	Menopausal hypertension or menstrual irregularities and dizziness resulting from the flaming upwards of fire due to deficiency of both Kidney Yin and Kidney Yang
Dispelling wind and eliminating dampness	*Gui Zhi* (Ramulus Cinnamomi Cassiae) *Wei Ling Xian* (Radix Clematidis) *Cang Er Zi* (Fructus Xanthii Sibirici)	Wind-damp Bi syndrome, limb joint pain, hypertonicity and numbness of the limbs
	Chuan Xiong (Rhizoma Ligustici Chuanxiong) *Ren Shen* (Radix Ginseng) *Dang Gui* (Radix Angelicae Sinensis) *Di Long* (Lumbricus)	Hemiplegia due to sequelae of wind-stroke, numbness of the skin

Note: In addition, *Yin Yang Huo* can be combined with *Gua Lou* (Fructus Trichosanthis) and green tea to treat dizziness and eye screen.

Tu Si Zi 菟丝子
(Dodder seed, Semen Cuscutae)

Tu Si Zi is the mature seed of *Cuscuta chinensis* Lam. or *C. japonica* Choisy, family Convolvulaceae.

Main ingredients *Tu Si Zi* contains quercetin, astragalin, hyperin, cholesterol, campesterol, β-sitosterol, stigmasterol, saccharides, alkaloids, anthraquinones, coumarins and vitamin A.

Properties Taste: acrid and sweet; nature: neutral.

Channels entered Liver and Kidney.

Functions and indications Supplements Kidney Yang and boosts Kidney Yin, secures the Essence and reduces urine, nourishes the Liver and brightens the eyes, fortifies the Spleen and stops diarrhoea, and quiets the foetus. It is indicated for limpness and aching in the lumbar region and knees, impotence, seminal emission, frequent urination, vaginal discharge, blurred vision, diarrhoea due to Spleen and Kidney deficiency, and wasting and thirsting due to Yin deficiency.

Common dosage 10-15g.

Precautions and contraindications Although *Tu Si Zi* is a neutral supplementing herb, it nevertheless has a tendency to supplement Yang, and should therefore not be used in cases of effulgent Yin deficiency-fire, dry stool and short voidings of reddish urine.

Comparison of functions See *Sha Yuan Zi* (Semen Astragali Complanati).

Toxicity The LD_{50} for subcutaneous injection in mice of an aqueous solution of *Tu Si Zi* is 2.465g/kg; daily feeding to rats via intragastric administration of 30-40g/kg of the steep or tincture of the herb for 70 days did not result in the appearance of any toxic symptoms.

Modern research

1. Increases immune activity.[80, 81]
2. Inhibits carcinoma by inhibiting DNA biological compounds in cancer cells.[82]
3. Inhibits the effects of ageing.[83]

Combinations and applications

Functions	Combinations	Applications
Supplementing Kidney Yang and boosting Kidney Yin, securing the Essence and reducing urine	*Wu Wei Zi* (Fructus Schisandrae) *Gou Qi Zi* (Fructus Lycii) *Fu Pen Zi* (Fructus Rubi Chingii)	Impotence, seminal emission or sterility due to Kidney Yang deficiency
	Du Zhong (Cortex Eucommiae Ulmoidis) *Shan Yao* (Rhizoma Dioscoreae Oppositae)	Aching in the lumbar region and knees due to insufficiency of Kidney Yang and deficiency of Kidney Yin, with a thin and sunken pulse
	Lian Zi (Semen Nelumbinis Nuciferae) *Fu Ling* (Sclerotium Poriae Cocos)	Seminal emission and white turbidity due to insecurity of the Kidneys and insufficiency of Kidney Qi
	Niu Xi (Radix Achyranthis Bidentatae) *Huang Jiu* (Vinum Aureum)	Cold and aching in the lumbar region and knees in men due to Kidney deficiency, possibly accompanied by numbness and lack of strength
	Wu Wei Zi (Fructus Schisandrae) *Sang Piao Xiao* (Oötheca Mantidis) *Lu Rong* (Cornu Cervi Parvum) *Mu Li* (Concha Ostreae)	Frequent urination or urinary incontinence due to Kidney Qi deficiency
Nourishing the Liver and brightening the eyes	*Ju Hua* (Flos Chrysanthemi Morifolii) *Shi Jue Ming* (Concha Haliotidis) *Shu Di Huang* (Radix Rehmanniae Glutinosae Conquita) *He Shou Wu* (Radix Polygoni Multiflori)	Blurred vision with a string-like, fine pulse due to Yin deficiency of the Liver and Kidneys
Fortifying the Spleen and stopping diarrhoea	*Dang Shen* (Radix Codonopsitis Pilosulae) *Bai Zhu* (Rhizoma Atractylodis Macrocephalae) *Huang Qi* (Radix Astragali seu Hedysari) *Mu Xiang* (Radix Aucklandiae Lappae) (see notes on legal status)	Loose stool, diarrhoea and reduced appetite due to Spleen and Kidney deficiency

Notes:

1. *Tu Si Zi* can be used with *E Jiao* (Gelatinum Corii Asini), *Sang Ji Sheng* (Ramulus Loranthi) and *Xu Duan* (Radix Dipsaci) to treat stirring foetus and foetal bleeding due to insufficiency of the Spleen and Kidneys.
2. *Tu Si Zi* can also be used on its own in powder or honey-coated pill form for wasting and thirsting patterns.

Du Zhong 杜仲 (Eucommia bark, Cortex Eucommiae Ulmoidis)

Du Zhong is the bark of *Eucommia ulmoides* Oliv., family Eucommiaceae.

Main ingredients *Du Zhong* contains gutta-percha, pinoresinols, syringaresinols, glucopyranosides, medioresinols, coniferin, eucommiol, eucommiosides, organic acids, glucose, fructose and kaempferol.

Properties Taste: sweet; nature: warm.

Channels entered Liver and Kidney.

Functions and indications Supplements the Liver and Kidneys, strengthens the sinews and bones, and quiets the foetus. It is indicated for insufficiency of the Liver and Kidneys, lack of strength in the lumbar region and knees, impotence, frequent urination, habitual miscarriage, and dizziness and headache.

Common dosage 10-15g.

Precautions and contraindications As *Du Zhong* has a warming and supplementing effect, it is contraindicated in cases of effulgent Yin deficiency-fire.

Remarks *Du Zhong* mix-fried in salt water is more effective than the raw herb.

Comparison of functions See *Xu Duan* (Radix Dipsaci).

Toxicity The LD_{50} for intravenous injection of preparations of raw *Du Zhong* is 574.1g/kg. Up to 12g/kg of a decoction of *Du Zhong* fed to rats via intragastric administration for 21 days did not cause any obvious difference in terms of weight and appearance in comparison with a control group.

Modern research

1. Lowers blood pressure, decreases the cholesterol level in serum.[84]
2. The steep of *Du Zhong* dilates the blood vessels and strengthens the immune function.[84]
3. Decoctions of *Du Zhong* benefit the adrenocortical function and inhibit inflammation.[85]
4. Has a tranquillizing function, alleviates pain, promotes urination and inhibits uterine contraction.[84, 85]

Combinations and applications

Functions	Combinations	Applications
Supplementing the Liver and Kidneys, strengthening the sinews and bones	*Hu Tao Ren* (Semen Juglandis Regiae) *Bu Gu Zhi* (Fructus Psoraleae Corylifoliae) *Tu Si Zi* (Semen Cuscutae)	Limpness and aching in the lumbar region and knees and lack of strength in the sinews due to improper nourishment of the sinews and insufficiency of the Liver and Kidneys
	Chuan Xiong (Rhizoma Ligustici Chuanxiong) *Fu Zi* (Radix Lateralis Aconiti Carmichaeli Praeparata) (see notes on legal status) *Gui Zhi* (Ramulus Cinnamomi Cassiae) *Sheng Jiang* (Rhizoma Zingiberis Officinalis Recens)	Yang deficiency in the aftermath of wind-stroke, hypertonicity of the sinews and vessels, cold and aching in the lumbar region and knees, lack of strength
	Yin Yang Huo (Herba Epimedii) *Bu Gu Zhi* (Fructus Psoraleae Corylifoliae) *Shan Zhu Yu* (Fructus Corni Officinalis) *Lian Xu* (Stamen Nelumbinis Nuciferae)	Impotence or frequent urination due to deficiency-cold of the Liver and Kidneys
	Xiao Hui Xiang (Fructus Foeniculi Vulgaris) *Che Qian Zi* (Semen Plantaginis) *Shan Zhu Yu* (Fructus Corni Officinalis)	Dribbling after urination or pudendal itch due to Kidney Yang deficiency

Quieting the foetus	*Shan Yao* (Rhizoma Dioscoreae Oppositae) *Xu Duan* (Radix Dipsaci) *Bai Zhu* (Rhizoma Atractylodis Macrocephalae) *E Jiao* (Gelatinum Corii Asini)	Insecurity of foetal origin, stirring foetus or habitual miscarriage due to insecurity of the Chong and Ren vessels and Liver and Kidney depletion

Note: In addition, *Du Zhong* can be used with *Huang Qin* (Radix Scutellariae Baicalensis), *Xia Ku Cao* (Spica Prunellae Vulgaris), *Shi Jue Ming* (Concha Haliotidis) and *Bai Shao* (Radix Paeoniae Lactiflorae) to treat Yin deficiency of the Liver and Kidneys and ascendant hyperactivity of Liver Yang, manifesting as dizziness and headache.

Xu Duan 续断
(Dipsacus root, Radix Dipsaci)

Xu Duan is the root of *Dipsacus asperoides* C. Y. Cheng et T. M. Ai or *D. japonicus* Miq., family Dipsacaceae.

Main ingredients *Xu Duan* contains alkaloids, volatile oils, triterpene saponins, gentianine, β-sitosterol, daucosterol and vitamin E.

Properties Taste: bitter, sweet and acrid; nature: slightly warm.

Channels entered Liver and Kidney.

Functions and indications Supplements the Liver and Kidneys, stops bleeding and quiets the foetus, strengthens the sinews and bones, treats injuries and joins fractures. It is indicated for pain in the lumbar region, weakness of the legs, uterine bleeding and vaginal discharge, knocks and falls, and abscesses and sores.

Common dosage 10-20g.

Precautions and contraindications According to *De Pei Ben Cao* [Materia Medica of Combinations]: '*Xu Duan* should not be used in the initial stage of dysentery, and it is forbidden for depression due to anger.'

Remarks Use the charred herb for uterine bleeding, *Xu Duan* mix-fried in brine for supplementing the Liver and Kidneys, and *Xu Duan* mix-fried in alcohol for stopping bleeding and treating injuries.

Comparison of functions *Xu Duan* (Radix Dipsaci), *Du Zhong* (Cortex Eucommiae Ulmoidis) and *Gou Ji* (Rhizoma Cibotii Barometz) can all supplement the Liver and Kidneys and strengthen the sinews and bones; they can be used to treat aching and pain in the lumbar region and knees and lack of strength in the sinews and bones due to insufficiency of the Liver and Kidneys (for *Gou Ji*, see notes on legal status). *Gou Ji* can also dispel wind-damp and is frequently used for Bi syndrome pain and lack of strength in the lumbar region and knees due to wind-cold-damp pathogenic factors and depletion and deficiency of the Liver and Kidneys. It has warming, supplementing, securing and astringing properties and can treat insecurity of Kidney Qi, enuresis and profuse white vaginal discharge.

Both *Du Zhong* and *Xu Duan* can supplement the Liver and Kidneys and quiet the foetus. They are often used together to treat pain in the lumbar region and weakness in the legs due to insufficiency of the Liver and Kidneys, and for stirring foetus. *Du Zhong* has the stronger supplementing and boosting function and is very effective in supplementing the Liver and Kidneys and strengthening the sinews and bones. *Xu Duan* can free the Blood vessels and join the sinews and bones and is used more often for foetal bleeding, stoppage of breast milk, abscesses and sores, and knocks and falls.

Modern research

1. Stops bleeding and drains pus, alleviates pain and promotes the regeneration of tissue.[86]
2. Promotes lactation and reduces vitamin E deficiency.[87]

Combinations and applications

Functions	Combinations	Applications
Supplementing the Liver and Kidneys, stopping bleeding and quieting the foetus	*Du Zhong* (Cortex Eucommiae Ulmoidis) *Niu Xi* (Radix Achyranthis Bidentatae) *Bu Gu Zhi* (Fructus Psoraleae Corylifoliae)	Pain in the lumbar region and weakness of the legs due to insufficiency of the Liver and Kidneys
	Yin Yang Huo (Herba Epimedii) *Niu Xi* (Radix Achyranthis Bidentatae) *Ba Ji Tian* (Radix Morindae Officinalis)	Aversion to cold and limb joint pain in elderly patients due to deficiency-cold of the Liver and Kidneys
	Chi Shi Zhi (Halloysitum Rubrum) *E Jiao* (Gelatinum Corii Asini) *Tu Si Zi* (Semen Cuscutae) *Shu Di Huang* (Radix Rehmanniae Glutinosae Conquita)	Profuse menstruation and incessant uterine bleeding due to insufficiency of the Liver and Kidneys and insecurity of the Chong and Ren vessels
	E Jiao (Gelatinum Corii Asini) *Sang Ji Sheng* (Ramulus Loranthi) *Tu Si Zi* (Semen Cuscutae)	Stirring foetus and uterine bleeding due to insufficiency of the Liver and Kidneys
Strengthening the sinews and bones, treating injuries and joining fractures	*Gu Sui Bu* (Rhizoma Drynariae) *Xue Jie* (Resina Draconis)	Wounds, fractures, knocks and falls
	Tao Ren (Semen Persicae) *Hong Hua* (Flos Carthami Tinctorii) *Chuan Shan Jia* (Squama Manitis Pentadactylae) (see notes on legal status) *Su Mu* (Lignum Sappan)	Knocks and falls, swelling and pain due to Blood stasis, fractured bones and ruptured sinews

Notes:

1. *Xu Duan* can be used with *Pu Gong Ying* (Herba Taraxaci cum Radice) to treat breast abscess.
2. *Xu Duan* can also be used with *Dang Gui* (Radix Angelicae Sinensis), *Chuan Shan Jia* (Squama Manitis Pentadactylae), *Chuan Xiong* (Rhizoma Ligustici Chuanxiong) and *Tian Hua Fen* (Radix Trichosanthis) for stoppage of breast milk (for *Chuan Shan Jia*, see notes on legal status).

Ba Ji Tian 巴戟天 (Morinda root, Radix Morindae Officinalis)

Ba Ji Tian is the dried root of *Morinda officinalis* How., family Rubiaceae.

Main ingredients *Ba Ji Tian* contains anthraquinones, saccharides, resin, vitamins, β-sitosterol, monotropein, asperuloside tetra-acetate and palmitic acid.

Properties Taste: acrid and sweet; nature: slightly warm.

Channels entered Liver and Kidney.

Functions and indications Supplements the Kidneys and reinforces Yang, strengthens the sinews and bones, and dispels wind and eliminates dampness. It is indicated for impotence due to Kidney Yang deficiency, pain and cold in the lower abdomen, frequent urination, infertility due to cold uterus, wind-cold-damp Bi syndrome, and limpness and aching in the lumbar region and knees.

Common dosage 10-15g.

Precautions and contraindications *Ba Ji Tian* is contraindicated in cases of effulgent Yin deficiency-fire or damp-heat.

Comparison of functions See *Xian Mao* (Rhizoma Curculiginis Orchioidis).

Toxicity A decoction of *Ba Ji Tian* given to animals in the proportion of 250g/kg did not result in any deaths.

Modern research

1. Promotes luteinization and ovulation.[88]
2. Promotes the production of adrenocortical hormones.[89]
3. Has a supplementing and strengthening function.[90]

Combinations and applications

Functions	Combinations	Applications
Supplementing the Kidneys and reinforcing Yang	*Rou Cong Rong* (Herba Cistanches Deserticolae) *Tu Si Zi* (Semen Cuscutae) *Fu Pen Zi* (Fructus Rubi Chingii)	Impotence, seminal emission, frequent urination, male sterility and cold and pain in the abdomen due to Kidney Yang deficiency
	Lu Jiao Jiao (Gelatinum Cornu Cervi) *Zi He Che* (Placenta Hominis) *Yin Yang Huo* (Herba Epimedii) *Dang Gui* (Radix Angelicae Sinensis) *Huang Qi* (Radix Astragali seu Hedysari)	Infertility due to cold uterus and deficiency of the Chong and Ren vessels
Strengthening the sinews and bones	*Du Zhong* (Cortex Eucommiae Ulmoidis) *Rou Cong Rong* (Herba Cistanches Deserticolae) *Bi Xie* (Rhizoma Dioscoreae) *Tu Si Zi* (Semen Cuscutae)	Lack of strength in the sinews and bones due to insufficiency of the Liver and Kidneys, difficulty in walking
	Yi Zhi Ren (Fructus Alpiniae Oxyphyllae) *Sang Piao Xiao* (Oötheca Mantidis) *Wu Yao* (Radix Linderae Strychnifoliae) *Tu Si Zi* (Semen Cuscutae)	Frequent urination and urinary incontinence due to Yang deficiency in the Lower Jiao
Dispelling wind and eliminating dampness	*Niu Xi* (Radix Achyranthis Bidentatae) *Du Huo* (Radix Angelicae Pubescentis) *Qiang Huo* (Rhizoma et Radix Notopterygii) *Xu Duan* (Radix Dipsaci) *Du Zhong* (Cortex Eucommiae Ulmoidis)	Bi syndrome, limb joint pain and lack of strength in the lumbar region and knees due to an invasion of wind-cold-damp and Liver and Kidney deficiency

Xian Mao 仙茅 (Curculigo rhizome, Rhizoma Curculiginis Orchioidis)

Xian Mao is the dried rhizome of *Curculigo orchioides* Gaertn., family Amaryllidaceae.

Main ingredients *Xian Mao* contains curculigenins, curculigosaponins, curculigol, curculigoside, orcinol glucoside, curculigine, corchioside, sterols and fats.

Properties Taste: acrid; nature: hot; toxic.

Channels entered Kidney, Liver and Spleen.

Functions and indications Warms the Kidneys and invigorates Yang, dispels cold and eliminates dampness. It is indicated for impotence, seminal cold, cold and aching in the lumbar region and knees, Wei syndrome of the sinews and bones, cold-damp Bi syndrome pain, and frequent urination.

Common dosage 3-10g, prepared as a decoction, pills or powder, or soaked in alcohol.

Precautions and contraindications

1. Since *Xian Mao* has similar functions to *Yin Yang Huo* (Herba Epimedii), it is also contraindicated in cases of effulgent Yin deficiency-fire.
2. The hot and dry properties of *Xian Mao* mean that it should not be used for prolonged periods.

Comparison of functions *Xian Mao* (Rhizoma Curculiginis Orchioidis), *Yin Yang Huo* (Herba Epimedii) and *Ba Ji Tian* (Radix Morindae Officinalis) can supplement the Kidneys and invigorate Yang, and dispel wind and eliminate dampness to treat insufficiency of Kidney Yang, impotence, cold uterus, and cold and aching in the lumbar region and knees due to Kidney deficiency accompanied by wind-damp. They are often used together to enhance their effect.

Xian Mao is acrid, hot, toxic, dry and drastic, and is very effective for dissipating cold-damp; it is a powerful herb for invigorating Yang and dissipating cold and has a stronger action than *Ba Ji Tian* and *Yin Yang Huo*. Prolonged use can cause parched lips and dry mouth and may damage Yin. *Ba Ji Tian* is acrid, sweet and slightly warm, but not dry. It can supplement without causing stagnation, while nourishing and boosting the Essence and Blood. It is often used for cold uterus, and cold and pain in the lower abdomen. *Yin Yang Huo* is acrid, sweet and warm. It is warmer and drier than *Ba Ji Tian* and is an important herb for supplementing Kidney Yang. It can be also used for hemiplegia, but tends to damage Yin and reinforce fire.

Toxicity *Xian Mao* has a relatively low level of toxicity. Mice were fed one dose of up to 150g/kg of curculigol via intragastric administration; no death had been reported seven days later. However, overdosage can cause palpitations and, in severe cases, paralysis with toxic side-effects on the cardiovascular system.

Modern research

1. The steep of *Xian Mao* strengthens the immune function.[91]
2. Has a tranquillizing function, relieves convulsions and inhibits inflammation.[92]
3. Has a male hormone-like function.[92]

Combinations and applications

Functions	Combinations	Applications
Warming the Kidneys and invigorating Yang, dispelling cold and eliminating dampness	*Yin Yang Huo* (Herba Epimedii) *Ba Ji Tian* (Radix Morindae Officinalis) *Wu Wei Zi* (Fructus Schisandrae) *Tu Si Zi* (Semen Cuscutae)	Cold and pain in the lumbar region, impotence, seminal cold and male sterility, frequent urination and urinary incontinence due to insufficiency of Kidney Yang and debilitation of fire at the gate of vitality

Ba Ji Tian (Radix Morindae Officinalis) *Du Zhong* (Cortex Eucommiae Ulmoidis) *Sang Ji Sheng* (Ramulus Loranthi) *Yin Yang Huo* (Herba Epimedii)	Insufficiency of the Liver and Kidneys, manifesting as aching and pain in the lumbar region and knees or Wei syndrome and limpness of the sinews and bones
Du Huo (Radix Angelicae Pubescentis) *Qiang Huo* (Rhizoma et Radix Notopterygii) *Chuan Wu* (Radix Aconiti Carmichaeli) (see notes on legal status)	Bi syndrome pain and hypertonicity of the sinews and bones in enduring illnesses due to cold-damp
Rou Dou Kou (Semen Myristicae Fragrantis) *Bu Gu Zhi* (Fructus Psoraleae Corylifoliae) *Wu Zhu Yu* (Fructus Evodiae Rutaecarpae)	Cold and pain in the stomach and abdomen, reduced appetite and diarrhoea due to Yang deficiency of the Spleen and Kidneys

Bu Gu Zhi 补骨脂 (Psoralea fruit, Fructus Psoraleae Corylifoliae)

Bu Gu Zhi is the dried fruit of *Psoralea corylifolia* L., family Leguminosae.

Legal status *Bu Gu Zhi* was listed in a document entitled *A Review of Restricted Herbal Ingredients* issued by the Medicines Control Agency (MCA) in the UK in September 2001 with a view to the possible imposition of restrictions on its use at a future date. As this herb contains psoralen, which can be an irritant, the MCA is considering introducing requirements for specialized medical expertise and standardized products.

Main ingredients *Bu Gu Zhi* contains psoralen, isopsoralen, psoralidin, isopsoralidin, bavachalcone, isobavachalcone, bavachromene, neobavachalcone, bavachin, bavachinin, isobavachin, corylin, bakachiol and psoraldehyde.

Properties Taste: acrid and bitter; nature: warm.

Channels entered Kidney and Spleen.

Functions and indications Supplements the Kidneys and invigorates Yang, secures the Essence and reduces urine, warms the Spleen and stops diarrhoea, hosts Qi and calms wheezing. It is indicated for cold and aching in the lumbar region and knees, impotence, seminal emission, urinary incontinence, frequent urination, diarrhoea due to Yang deficiency, and coughing and wheezing due to deficiency-cold.

Common dosage 5-10g.

Precautions and contraindications The warm and dry nature of *Bu Gu Zhi* means that it is not suitable for cases with Yin deficiency stirring fire, blood in the urine, and constipation.

Comparison of functions See *Yi Zhi Ren* (Fructus Alpiniae Oxyphyllae).

Toxicity Mice fed large quantities of bakachiol for up to four weeks suffered progressive damage to the kidneys. Large dosages of psoralen given to mice under conditions of ultraviolet radiation resulted in slight changes to the liver, reproductive organs and adrenal cortex.

Modern research

1. Stops bleeding.[93]
2. Strengthens the immune function.[94]
3. Inhibits carcinoma.[95-97]
4. Raises the white blood cell count.[98-100]

Combinations and applications

Functions	Combinations	Applications
Supplementing the Kidneys and invigorating Yang, securing the Essence and reducing urine	*Hu Tao Ren* (Semen Juglandis Regiae) *Du Zhong* (Cortex Eucommiae Ulmoidis)	Insufficiency of Kidney Yang, deficiency-cold of the Kidneys or Kidney deficiency, manifesting as pain in the lumbar region as severe as if it had been broken, difficulty in sitting down or standing up, inhibited bending backwards and forwards, and inability to turn to the side
	Tu Si Zi (Semen Cuscutae) *Hu Tao Ren* (Semen Juglandis Regiae) *Chen Xiang* (Lignum Aquilariae Resinatum)	Impotence, premature ejaculation and frequent urination due to Kidney Yang deficiency
Warming the Spleen and stopping diarrhoea	*Wu Zhu Yu* (Fructus Evodiae Rutaecarpae) *Rou Dou Kou* (Semen Myristicae Fragrantis) *Wu Wei Zi* (Fructus Schisandrae)	Enduring diarrhoea and daily early-morning diarrhoea due to Yang deficiency of the Spleen and Kidneys
Hosting Qi and calming wheezing	*Hu Tao Ren* (Semen Juglandis Regiae) *Feng Mi* (Mel)	Deficiency wheezing manifesting as rapid breathing at the slightest exertion and exhalation exceeding inhalation due to failure of the Kidneys to host Qi and depletion and consumption of Kidney Qi

Yi Zhi Ren 益智仁
(Bitter cardamom, Fructus Alpiniae Oxyphyllae)

Yi Zhi Ren is the dried mature fruit of *Alpinia oxyphylla* Miq., family Zingiberaceae.

Main ingredients *Yi Zhi Ren* contains yakuchinone A and B, and 0.7% of volatile oils (including cineol, zingiberene and zingiberol).

Properties Taste: acrid; nature: warm.

Channels entered Spleen and Kidney.

Functions and indications Warms the Kidneys, secures the Essence and reduces urine, warms the Spleen and stops diarrhoea. It is indicated for seminal emission, urinary incontinence, child bed-wetting, cold and pain in the abdomen, vomiting and diarrhoea, reduced appetite, and excessive salivation.

Common dosage 3-6g.

Precautions and contraindications Since *Yi Zhi Ren* is warm and dry and can damage Yin and reinforce fire, it is contraindicated in cases of effulgent Yin deficiency-fire, or for patients with seminal emission, frequent urination or uterine bleeding due to heat.

Comparison of functions Both *Yi Zhi Ren* (Fructus Alpiniae Oxyphyllae) and *Bu Gu Zhi* (Fructus Psoraleae Corylifoliae) can warm and supplement the Spleen and Kidneys, and secure the Essence and reduce urine to treat impotence, seminal emission and urinary incontinence due to insufficiency of Kidney Yang. *Yi Zhi Ren* has a stronger effect in warming the Middle Jiao and dissipating cold than in warming the Kidneys and is often used for pain in the abdomen due to cold in the Middle Jiao and for vomiting and reduced appetite. *Bu Gu Zhi* is good for supplementing the Kidneys and invigorating Yang and is often used for Kidney deficiency manifesting as pain in the lumbar region or aching, limpness and lack of strength.

Modern research Benefits the stomach, slightly inhibits urination, and reduces saliva secretion.[101]

Combinations and applications

Functions	Combinations	Applications
Warming the Kidneys, securing the Essence and reducing urine	*Jin Ying Zi* (Fructus Rosae Laevigatae) *Tu Si Zi* (Semen Cuscutae)	Seminal emission due to Kidney Qi deficiency
	Shan Yao (Rhizoma Dioscoreae Oppositae) *Wu Yao* (Radix Linderae Strychnifoliae)	Frequent urination (day or night), urinary incontinence
	Bai Zhu (Rhizoma Atractylodis Macrocephalae) *Fu Ling* (Sclerotium Poriae Cocos)	Child bed-wetting, urinary turbidity
Warming the Spleen and stopping diarrhoea	*Dang Shen* (Radix Codonopsitis Pilosulae) *Bai Zhu* (Rhizoma Atractylodis Macrocephalae) *Zhi Gan Cao* (Radix Glycyrrhizae Praeparata) *Gan Jiang* (Rhizoma Zingiberis Officinalis)	Cold and pain in the abdomen, vomiting, diarrhoea, reduced appetite
	Dang Shen (Radix Codonopsitis Pilosulae) *Fu Ling* (Sclerotium Poriae Cocos) *Che Qian Zi* (Semen Plantaginis)	Excessive salivation due to Yang deficiency in the Middle Jiao

Rou Cong Rong 肉苁蓉 (Desert-living cistanche, Herba Cistanches Deserticolae)

Rou Cong Rong is the dried fleshy stem of *Cistanche deserticola* Y. C. Ma, family Orobanchaceae.

Main ingredients *Rou Cong Rong* contains alkaloids, orobanchin, daucosterol, β-sitosterol, succinic acid, betaine and glucose.

Properties Taste: sweet and salty; nature: warm.

Channels entered Kidney and Large Intestine.

Functions and indications Supplements the Kidneys and invigorates Yang, boosts the Essence and Blood, moistens the Intestines and frees the bowels. It is indicated for impotence, seminal emission and premature ejaculation due to insufficiency of Kidney Yang, cold and aching in the lumbar region and knees, lack of strength in the sinews and bones, constipation in the elderly, and post-partum Blood deficiency.

Common dosage 10-20g, or double this dosage for severe cases.

Precautions and contraindications *Rou Cong Rong* is contraindicated in cases of effulgent Yin deficiency-fire or loose stool with diarrhoea, or in cases of dry stool due to full-heat in the Stomach and Large Intestine.

Comparison of functions Both *Rou Cong Rong* (Herba Cistanches Deserticolae) and *Lu Rong* (Cornu Cervi Parvum) can supplement the Kidneys, reinforce Yang and boost the Essence and Blood. Being warm, dry and very strong, *Lu Rong* is a key materia medica for supplementing Kidney Yin and Kidney Yang, but should not be used unless there is severe deficiency. *Rou Cong Rong* is warm, but not dry, and has a moderate effect in supplementing the Kidneys and invigorating Yang. Effective for nourishing and strengthening the body, it is used for disorders due to Kidney deficiency and Essence depletion.

For an additional combination, see *Suo Yang* (Herba Cynomorii Songarici).

Modern research

1. Regulates the endocrine function, benefits the metabolism and strengthens the body.[102]
2. Strengthens the immune function.[102]
3. Inhibits inflammation.[102]
4. Stimulates peristalsis, inhibits the absorption of water in the intestines and promotes the passage of stool.[102]

Combinations and applications

Functions	Combinations	Applications
Supplementing the Kidneys and invigorating Yang, boosting the Essence and Blood	*Bu Gu Zhi* (Fructus Psoraleae Corylifoliae) *Xu Duan* (Radix Dipsaci)	Cold and aching in the lumbar region and knees, lack of strength in the sinews and bones
	Tu Si Zi (Semen Cuscutae) *Wu Wei Zi* (Fructus Schisandrae) *Shu Di Huang* (Radix Rehmanniae Glutinosae Conquita)	Impotence, premature ejaculation, seminal emission, cold uterus and persistent inability to conceive due to depletion and deficiency of the Essence and Blood and insufficiency of Kidney Yang
	Zi He Che (Placenta Hominis) *Lu Rong* (Cornu Cervi Parvum) *Dang Gui* (Radix Angelicae Sinensis) *Shu Di Huang* (Radix Rehmanniae Glutinosae Conquita)	Infertility due to cold uterus
Moistening the Intestines and freeing the bowels	*Chen Xiang* (Lignum Aquilariae Resinatum) *Huo Ma Ren* (Semen Cannabis Sativae) *Zhi Ke* (Fructus Citri Aurantii) *Dang Gui* (Radix Angelicae Sinensis)	Constipation and profuse sweating in the elderly and those with a weak constitution, postpartum Blood deficiency and insufficiency of body fluids

Suo Yang 锁阳 (Cynomorium stem, Herba Cynomorii Songarici)

Suo Yang is the dried fleshy stem of *Cynomorium songaricum* Rupr., family Cynomoriaceae.

Main ingredients *Suo Yang* contains anthocyanin, catechin, triterpene saponins, ursolic acid, tannin, proline and glucose.

Properties Taste: sweet; nature: warm.

Channels entered Liver, Kidney and Large Intestine.

Functions and indications Supplements the Kidneys and reinforces Yang, moistens the Intestines and frees the bowels. It is indicated for impotence, seminal emission, sterility, limpness and aching in the lumbar region and knees, difficulty in movement, and Intestinal dryness with constipation.

Common dosage 10-15g; up to 30g when used alone.

Precautions and contraindications *Suo Yang* is contraindicated for hyperactivity of Yang due to Yin deficiency, diarrhoea due to Spleen deficiency, and constipation due to full-heat.

Comparison of functions Both *Suo Yang* (Herba Cynomorii Songarici) and *Rou Cong Rong* (Herba Cistanches Deserticolae) can supplement the Kidneys and reinforce Yang, moisten the Intestines and free the bowels. They are used to treat insufficiency of Kidney Yang, impotence, infertility due to cold uterus, cold and aching in the lumbar region and knees, and Intestinal dryness with constipation due to scant body fluids and Blood depletion. *Suo Yang* is often used in combination with or as a substitute for *Rou Cong Rong*, although it is less effective in its moistening effect. *Suo Yang* also enters the Liver and Kidney channels to strengthen the sinews and bones, moisten dryness and nourish the sinews. It is often used for insufficiency of the Liver and Kidneys manifesting as limpness and aching in the lumbar region and knees, slow movement due to soft bones, weakness in the feet and lack of strength. *Rou Cong Rong* is moderate but persistent in supplementing and boosting Kidney Yang; it supplements without drying. It concurrently boosts the Essence and Blood and is often used for insufficiency of Kidney Yang and depletion of the Essence and Blood.

Combinations and applications

Functions	Combinations	Applications
Supplementing the Kidneys and reinforcing Yang	*Shu Di Huang* (Radix Rehmanniae Glutinosae Conquita) *Gui Ban* (Plastrum Testudinis) (see notes on legal status) *Niu Xi* (Radix Achyranthis Bidentatae)	Limpness and aching in the lumbar region and knees, lack of strength in the sinews and bones, and difficulty in walking due to insufficiency of the Liver and Kidneys
	Sang Piao Xiao (Oötheca Mantidis) *Long Gu* (Os Draconis)	Impotence and seminal emission
	Rou Cong Rong (Herba Cistanches Deserticolae)	Impotence, seminal emission, seminal cold and sterility due to insufficiency of Kidney Yang
Moistening the Intestines and freeing the bowels	*Huo Ma Ren* (Semen Cannabis Sativae) *Dang Gui* (Radix Angelicae Sinensis)	Intestinal dryness with difficult defecation due to Blood deficiency and depletion of body fluids

Sha Yuan Zi 沙苑子
(Flat-stem milkvetch seed, Semen Astragali Complanati)

Sha Yuan Zi is the seed of *Astragalus complanatus* R. Br., family Leguminosae.

Main ingredients *Sha Yuan Zi* contains complanatuside, astragalin, myricetin, kaempferide, neocomplanoside, myricomplanoside, ononin, triterpene glucosides, β-sitosterol, amino acids and fatty acids.

Properties Taste: sweet; nature: warm.

Channels entered Liver and Kidney.

Functions and indications Boosts the Kidneys and secures the Essence, supplements the Liver and brightens the eyes. It is indicated for Liver and Kidney deficiency, limpness and aching in the lumbar region and knees, dizziness, tinnitus, blurred vision, seminal emission, premature ejaculation, frequent urination, enuresis, and vaginal discharge.

Common dosage 10-20g.

Precautions and contraindications *Sha Yuan Zi* is contraindicated in cases of effulgent Yin deficiency-fire and inhibited urination.

Comparison of functions Both *Sha Yuan Zi* (Semen Astragali Complanati) and *Tu Si Zi* (Semen Cuscutae) can supplement Yang and boost the Kidneys, secure the Essence and reduce urine, and nourish the Liver to brighten the eyes. They are used to treat insufficiency of the Liver and Kidneys, limpness and aching in the lumbar region and knees, impotence and seminal emission, enuresis and frequent urination, white vaginal discharge and white turbidity.

Sha Yuan Zi is sweet, warm and astringent and is often used for seminal emission and enuresis, vaginal discharge and white turbidity. It is an important herb for supplementing Yin and Yang of the Liver and Kidneys and for stopping discharge. *Tu Si Zi* is acrid, sweet and neutral, neither warm nor dry; it can supplement Yang and boost Yin. It is an important herb for neutrally supplementing the Liver, Kidneys and Spleen and is very effective for nourishing and strengthening the body. It can be used to treat disorders due to deficiency of the Liver and Kidneys and to supplement Spleen Qi to stop diarrhoea.

For an additional comparison, see *Bai Ji Li* (Fructus Tribuli Terrestris).

Toxicity The LD_{50} for a pure decoction of *Sha Yuan Zi* fed to mice via intragastric administration is 37.75g/kg. Wistar rats given preparations of up to 5g/kg of *Sha Yuan Zi* via intragastric administration daily for 60 days showed no marked pathological changes.

Modern research

1. Lowers blood pressure, slows the heart rate, improves cerebral blood circulation.[103, 104]
2. Decreases blood viscosity and increases the volume of blood flow.[105]
3. Inhibits inflammation.[106]
4. Alleviates pain and relieves convulsions.[107]

Combinations and applications

Functions	Combinations	Applications
Boosting the Kidneys and securing the Essence	*Shu Di Huang* (Radix Rehmanniae Glutinosae Conquita) *Shan Yao* (Rhizoma Dioscoreae Oppositae) *Shan Zhu Yu* (Fructus Corni Officinalis)	Limpness and aching in the lumbar region and knees, and dizziness and tinnitus due to Liver and Kidney deficiency
	Du Zhong (Cortex Eucommiae Ulmoidis) *Xu Duan* (Radix Dipsaci) *Hu Tao Ren* (Semen Juglandis Regiae)	Pain in the lumbar region due to Kidney depletion, deficiency-cold of the lower origin
	Long Gu (Os Draconis) *Mu Li* (Concha Ostreae) *Qian Shi* (Semen Euryales Ferocis) *Lian Xu* (Stamen Nelumbinis Nuciferae)	Seminal emission, premature ejaculation, frequent urination, enuresis or vaginal discharge due to Kidney deficiency

Supplementing the Liver and brightening the eyes	*Gou Qi Zi* (Fructus Lycii) *Tu Si Zi* (Semen Cuscutae) *Ju Hua* (Flos Chrysanthemi Morifolii)	Dizziness, blurred vision and dry eyes due to insufficiency of the Liver and Kidneys

Jiu Cai Zi 韭菜子 (Chinese leek seed, Semen Allii Tuberosi)

Jiu Cai Zi is the dried seed of *Allium tuberosum* Rottler, family Liliaceae.

Main ingredients *Jiu Cai Zi* contains alkaloids and saponins.

Properties Taste: acrid and sweet; nature: warm.

Channels entered Liver and Kidney.

Functions and indications Invigorates Yang and secures the Essence. It is indicated for impotence, seminal emission and frequent urination due to Kidney deficiency.

Common dosage 5-10g.

Precautions and contraindications *Jiu Cai Zi* is contraindicated in cases of effulgent Yin deficiency-fire.

Toxicity The LD_{50} for intravenous injection in mice of *Jiu Cai Zi* is 60mg/kg, that for subcutaneous injection is 120mg/kg.

Modern research

1. Supplements the spleen.[108]
2. Inhibits many types of Gram-positive and Gram-negative bacteria.[108]

Combinations and applications

Functions	Combinations	Applications
Invigorating Yang and securing the Essence	*Jiu Xiang Chong* (Aspongopus) *Bu Gu Zhi* (Fructus Psoraleae Corylifoliae) *Jin Ying Zi* (Fructus Rosae Laevigatae)	Impotence, seminal emission and frequent urination due to Kidney deficiency
	Bu Gu Zhi (Fructus Psoraleae Corylifoliae) *Long Gu* (Os Draconis) *Yi Zhi Ren* (Fructus Alpiniae Oxyphyllae)	Impotence, seminal emission and enuresis due to deficiency-cold of the lower origin and deficiency of Kidney Yang

Dong Chong Xia Cao 冬虫夏草 (Chinese caterpillar fungus, Cordyceps Sinensis)

Dong Chong Xia Cao is the whole dried fungus of *Cordyceps sinensis* (Berk.) Sacc., family Clavicipitaceae, and the carcass of the larva of *Hepialus armoricarus* Oberthur, family Hepialidae, from which it grows.

Main ingredients *Dong Chong Xia Cao* contains cordycepic acid, d-mannitol, cordycepin, uridine, adenine, vitamin B_{12}, oleic, linoleic, linolenic, palmitic and stearic acids, ergosterol, β-sitosterol and amino acids.

Properties Taste: sweet; nature: warm.

Channels entered Kidney and Lung.

Functions and indications Supplements the Lungs and boosts the Kidneys, transforms Phlegm and stops coughing. It is indicated for coughing and wheezing due to Lung and Kidney deficiency, spontaneous sweating and night sweating, lack of strength after illness, pain and aching in the lumbar region and knees due to Kidney deficiency, and impotence and seminal emission.

Common dosage 5-10g, or 1.5-3g as a powder for oral use, or 15-30g for stewing with chicken, duck or pork.

Precautions and contraindications *Dong Chong Xia Cao* should be used with caution in exterior patterns and should not be used on its own in cases of effulgent Yin deficiency-fire.

Remarks Since *Dong Chong Xia Cao* enters the Kidney and Lung channels, it is very effective in supplementing the Kidneys and boosting the Lungs to stop coughing and calm wheezing. With its ability to supplement both Yin and Yang, *Dong Chong Xia Cao* has a strong effect in nourishing and strengthening the body and is used for deficiency patterns and weakness.

Comparison of functions See *Ge Jie* (Gekko).

Toxicity The LD_{50} for intraperitoneal and subcutaneous injection in mice of an aqueous extract of *Dong Chong Xia Cao* is 27.8g/kg and 18.23g/kg respectively. *Dong Chong Xia Cao* has a low level of toxicity. There was one instance of death 72 hours after oral administration to mice of 100g of the substance. Another group of mice was fed 10g/kg of a suspension of *Dong Chong Xia Cao* powder daily for five days; there was no death within a ten-day observation period.

Modern research

1. Strengthens the immune function.[109]
2. The steep of *Dong Chong Xia Cao* inhibits arrhythmia, myocardial ischaemia and oxygen deficiency.[110, 111]
3. Lowers blood pressure.[112]
4. Calms wheezing and expels sputum.[113, 114]
5. Inhibits carcinoma.[115-118]
6. The cordycepic acid contained in *Dong Chong Xia Cao* inhibited staphylococci, streptococci, Bacillus anthracis and other bacteria in laboratory tests.[119, 120]

Combinations and applications

Functions	Combinations	Applications
Supplementing the Lungs and boosting the Kidneys	*Tu Si Zi* (Semen Cuscutae) *Rou Cong Rong* (Herba Cistanches Deserticolae) *Ba Ji Tian* (Radix Morindae Officinalis)	Impotence, seminal emission and aching and pain in the lumbar region and knees due to depletion and deficiency of the Essence and Blood and insufficiency of Kidney Yang
	Huang Qi (Radix Astragali seu Hedysari) *Hu Tao Ren* (Semen Juglandis Regiae)	Coughing and wheezing, shortness of breath, reduced appetite and fatigue due to Lung and Kidney deficiency
	E Jiao (Gelatinum Corii Asini) *Mai Men Dong* (Radix Ophiopogonis Japonici) *Wu Wei Zi* (Fructus Schisandrae)	Cough with blood-streaked sputum, spontaneous sweating, or postpartum weak constitution due to insufficiency of Qi and Yin
	Sha Shen (Radix Glehniae seu Adenophorae) *E Jiao* (Gelatinum Corii Asini) *Chuan Bei Mu* (Bulbus Fritillariae Cirrhosae) *San Qi* (Radix Notoginseng) *Bai Bu* (Radix Stemonae)	Taxation cough with coughing of blood due to Yang deficiency of the Lungs and Kidneys

Transforming Phlegm and stopping coughing	*Chuan Bei Mu* (Bulbus Fritillariae Cirrhosae) *Zhi Mu* (Rhizoma Anemarrhenae Asphodeloidis)	Enduring cough and deficiency wheezing with sticky sputum or coughing of blood

Note: *Dong Chong Xia Cao* can be stewed with chicken, duck, fish or pork to treat general deficiency after illness, manifesting as spontaneous sweating and aversion to cold, dizziness, anaemia and scant body fluids, and a tendency to be affected by wind-cold.

Ge Jie 蛤蚧
(Gecko, Gekko)

Ge Jie is the dried body with viscera removed of *Gekko gecko* L., family Gekkonidae.

Main ingredients The flesh of *Ge Jie* contains carnosine, choline, carnitine, guanine, proteins and fats; the sloughed skin contains keratin.

Properties Taste: salty; nature: neutral.

Channels entered Lung and Kidney.

Functions and indications Supplements the Lungs and boosts the Kidneys, hosts Qi and stabilizes wheezing, reinforces Kidney Yang and boosts the Essence and Blood. It is indicated for deficiency wheezing and enduring cough, coughing of blood due to deficiency taxation, impotence and seminal emission, and frequent urination.

Common dosage 3-7g in decoction; 1-2g taken orally as a powder, three times a day; alternatively, steep one or two pieces in 500 ml of white alcohol and drink 25-50 ml of the medicinal wine every day.

Precautions and contraindications *Ge Jie* is contraindicated for coughing and wheezing due to full-heat or externally-contracted wind-cold.

Comparison of functions Both *Ge Jie* (Gekko) and *Dong Chong Xia Cao* (Cordyceps Sinensis) can supplement the Lungs and boost the Kidneys. They are effective for stopping coughing and calming wheezing as well as for nourishing and strengthening the body. *Ge Jie* is an important materia medica for hosting Qi to stabilize wheezing due to deficiency or overwork and for reinforcing Yang to treat impotence and seminal emission due to Kidney Yang deficiency. *Dong Chong Xia Cao* is very effective in supplementing both Yin and Yang, and can nourish and strengthen the body when taken with food; it can also stop bleeding and transform Phlegm.

For an additional comparison, see *Hu Tao Ren* (Semen Juglandis Regiae).

Toxicity *Ge Jie* has a low level of toxicity. The LD_{50} for intraperitoneal injection in mice of extracts of the liposoluble constituents of *Ge Jie* is 5.24g/kg. There was no toxic reaction in animals after administration of 25-200 times the normal quantity of the brains and eyes of *Ge Jie*.

Modern research

1. Alcoholic extracts of *Ge Jie* induced oestrus in mice; preparations of *Ge Jie* had an androgen-like effect on mice.[121]
2. Has a non-specific effect in strengthening the immune function.[122]
3. Inhibits inflammation.[123]
4. Lowers the blood sugar level.[124]

Combinations and applications

Functions	Combinations	Applications
Supplementing the Lungs and boosting the Kidneys, hosting Qi and stabilizing wheezing	*Ren Shen* (Radix Ginseng) *Wu Wei Zi* (Fructus Schisandrae) *Bu Gu Zhi* (Fructus Psoraleae Corylifoliae)	Deficiency wheezing patterns with difficulty in speaking and rapid wheezing on exertion due to failure of the Kidneys to host Qi and deficiency of the Lungs and Kidneys
	Xing Ren (Semen Pruni Armeniacae) *Chuan Bei Mu* (Bulbus Fritillariae Cirrhosae) *Zi Wan* (Radix Asteris Tatarici)	Coughing of blood due to deficiency taxation
Reinforcing Kidney Yang and boosting the Essence and Blood	*Ren Shen* (Radix Ginseng) *Lu Rong* (Cornu Cervi Parvum) *Yin Yang Huo* (Herba Epimedii)	Impotence, seminal emission and frequent urination due to Kidney Yang deficiency and depletion of the Essence and Blood

Hu Tao Ren 胡桃仁 (Walnut kernel, Semen Juglandis Regiae)

Hu Tao Ren is the nut of *Juglans regia* L., family Juglandaceae. This herb is also known as *Hu Tao*, *Hu Tao Rou*, *He Tao* and *He Tao Ren*.

Main ingredients *Hu Tao Ren* contains linoleic acid, linolenic acid, oleic acid, proteins, carbohydrates, calcium, phosphorus, iron, carotene and ovoflavin.

Properties Taste: sweet; nature: warm.

Channels entered Kidney, Lung and Large Intestine.

Functions and indications Supplements the Kidneys and strengthens the lumbar region and knees, astringes the Essence and stops seminal emission, moistens the Lungs, hosts Qi and stabilizes wheezing, moistens the Intestines and frees the bowels. It is indicated for coughing and wheezing due to Kidney deficiency, limpness and aching in the lumbar region and knees, seminal emission, frequent urination, and Intestinal dryness with constipation.

Common dosage 10-30g; can be used as a decoction or as pills, powder or extract.

Precautions and contraindications *Hu Tao Ren* is contraindicated in cases of effulgent Yin deficiency-fire, cough due to Phlegm-heat, and loose stool.

Remarks

1. Peeled *Hu Tao Ren* is used for moistening the Intestines and freeing the bowels, whereas the peel is left on when moistening the Lungs to calm wheezing.
2. The moderate qualities of *Hu Tao Ren* make it suitable for treating constipation in the elderly and deficiency wheezing.

Comparison of functions Both *Hu Tao Ren* (Semen Juglandis Regiae) and *Ge Jie* (Gekko) can supplement the Lungs and boost the Kidneys to stop coughing and stabilize wheezing. They can be used for wheezing due to Lung and Kidney deficiency, insufficiency of Kidney Yang, seminal emission, pain in the lumbar region, and weakness of the legs. *Ge Jie* is neutral in nature, and can therefore also boost the Essence and Blood. It is good for treating insufficiency of Kidney Yang and depletion and deficiency of the Essence and Blood. *Hu Tao Ren* is warm in nature as well as being moist and oily, which means that it can also moisten the Intestines and free the bowels to treat Intestinal dryness with constipation and depletion of body fluids; it is particularly suitable for the elderly or for patients with deficiency patterns and insufficiency of body fluids after illness.

Toxicity The LD_{50} for intraperitoneal injection of *Hu Tao Ren* in mice is 1583mg/kg. After intravenous injection in rabbits of 14mg/kg per day for ten days, no pathological changes were recorded in heart, liver or kidney function.

Combinations and applications

Functions	Combinations	Applications
Supplementing the Kidneys and strengthening the lumbar region and knees	*Du Zhong* (Cortex Eucommiae Ulmoidis) *Bu Gu Zhi* (Fructus Psoraleae Corylifoliae)	Limpness and aching in the lumbar region and knees and weakness of the legs due to Kidney deficiency
	Jin Qian Cao (Herba Lysimachiae) *Ji Nei Jin* (Endothelium Corneum Gigeriae Galli) *Hua Shi* (Talcum) *Hai Jin Sha* (Spora Lygodii Japonici)	Stone Lin syndrome
Astringing the Essence and stopping seminal emission	*Shu Di Huang* (Radix Rehmanniae Glutinosae Conquita) *Qian Shi* (Semen Euryales Ferocis) *Lian Zi* (Semen Nelumbinis Nuciferae)	Seminal emission and frequent urination
Moistening the Lungs, hosting Qi and stabilizing wheezing	*Ren Shen* (Radix Ginseng) *Sheng Jiang* (Rhizoma Zingiberis Officinalis Recens)	Deficiency wheezing patterns with coughing and wheezing at the slightest exertion due to failure of the Kidneys to host Qi and insufficiency of the Lungs and Kidneys
	Xing Ren (Semen Pruni Armeniacae) *Sheng Jiang* (Rhizoma Zingiberis Officinalis Recens)	Coughing and wheezing in elderly patients
Moistening the Intestines and freeing the bowels	*Huo Ma Ren* (Semen Cannabis Sativae) *Rou Cong Rong* (Herba Cistanches Deserticolae) *Dang Gui* (Radix Angelicae Sinensis)	Intestinal dryness with constipation in elderly and weak patients

Hu Lu Ba 胡芦巴 (Fenugreek seed, Semen Trigonellae Foeni-graeci)

Hu Lu Ba is the dried ripe seed of *Trigonella foenum-graecum* L., family Leguminosae.

Main ingredients *Hu Lu Ba* contains trigonelline, choline, saponins (including diosgenin, yamogenin, tigogenin, gitogenin and sitogenin), vitexin, orientin, carpaine, fatty oils, proteins, stachyose and vitamin B_1.

Properties Taste: bitter; nature: warm.

Channels entered Liver and Kidney.

Functions and indications Warms the Kidneys and reinforces Yang, dissipates cold and alleviates pain. It is indicated for cold Shan disorders, cold-damp leg Qi, cold and pain in the legs and knees or lumbar region, impotence, and seminal cold.

Common dosage 3-10g, decocted or used in pills and powders.

Precautions and contraindications *Hu Lu Ba* is contraindicated for patients with effulgent Yin deficiency-fire or damp-heat.

Modern research Lowers the blood sugar level, promotes urination and inhibits inflammation.[125]

Combinations and applications

Functions	Combinations	Applications
Warming the Kidneys and reinforcing Yang, dissipating cold and alleviating pain	*Bu Gu Zhi* (Fructus Psoraleae Corylifoliae) *Mu Gua* (Fructus Chaenomelis) *Ji Xue Teng* (Caulis Spatholobi) *Niu Xi* (Radix Achyranthis Bidentatae)	Cold-damp leg Qi and cold and pain in the legs and knees due to cold-damp pouring down and impairment of Qi transformation as a result of Yang deficiency
	Wu Zhu Yu (Fructus Evodiae Rutaecarpae) *Ba Ji Tian* (Radix Morindae Officinalis) *Chuan Lian Zi* (Fructus Meliae Toosendan)	Cold Shan disorders manifesting as pain in the lower abdomen radiating to the testicles
	Fu Pen Zi (Fructus Rubi Chingii) *Huang Jing* (Rhizoma Polygonati) *Bu Gu Zhi* (Fructus Psoraleae Corylifoliae)	Cold and pain in the lumbar region, impotence and seminal emission
	Xiao Hui Xiang (Fructus Foeniculi Vulgaris) *Ai Ye* (Folium Artemisiae Argyi)	Painful menstruation, cold and pain in the lower abdomen
	Fu Zi (Radix Lateralis Aconiti Carmichaeli Praeparata) (see notes on legal status) *Ba Ji Tian* (Radix Morindae Officinalis)	Impotence, seminal cold and dizziness due to insufficiency of Kidney Yang and debilitation of fire at the gate of vitality

Zi He Che 紫河车
(Human placenta, Placenta Hominis)

Zi He Che is dried human placenta.

Main ingredients *Zi He Che* contains ovarian hormones, interferon, progesterone, urokinase, prostaglandin E_1, lysozyme, kininase, histaminase, oxytocinase and lecithin.

Properties Taste: sweet and salty; nature: warm.

Channels entered Lung, Liver and Kidney.

Functions and indications Supplements the Kidneys and boosts the Essence, nourishes the Blood and boosts Qi, supplements the Lungs and calms wheezing. It is indicated for insufficiency of Qi and Blood, emaciation, coughing and wheezing due to Lung deficiency, tidal fever due to steaming bone disorder, night sweating, seminal emission and impotence, and infertility.

Common dosage 1.5-3g, prepared into powder, pills or capsules for oral use.

Precautions and contraindications *Zi He Che* is contraindicated in cases of internal heat due to Yin deficiency.

Modern research

1. Contains antibodies to the influenza and measles viruses.[126]
2. Has a hormone-like function.[126]
3. In powder form, it strengthens the immune function, inhibits allergies and slows the effects of ageing.[127]

Combinations and applications

Functions	Combinations	Applications
Supplementing the Kidneys and boosting the Essence	*Yin Yang Huo* (Herba Epimedii) *Lu Jiao Jiao* (Gelatinum Cornu Cervi) *Shu Di Huang* (Radix Rehmanniae Glutinosae Conquita)	Sterility, impotence, seminal emission, headache and tinnitus due to deficiency of Kidney Qi
	Huang Bai (Cortex Phellodendri) *Tian Men Dong* (Radix Asparagi Cochinchinensis) *Shu Di Huang* (Radix Rehmanniae Glutinosae Conquita) *Gui Ban* (Plastrum Testudinis) (see notes on legal status) *Du Zhong* (Cortex Eucommiae Ulmoidis) *Niu Xi* (Radix Achyranthis Bidentatae)	Steaming bone disorder, night sweating, seminal emission, limpness and aching in the lumbar region and knees and blurred vision due to Liver and Kidney deficiency
Nourishing the Blood and boosting Qi	*Dang Shen* (Radix Codonopsitis Pilosulae) *Huang Qi* (Radix Astragali seu Hedysari) *Dang Gui* (Radix Angelicae Sinensis)	Fatigued body and emaciation, a haggard complexion and stoppage of breast milk due to insufficiency of Qi and Blood deficiency
Supplementing the Lungs and calming wheezing	*Dang Shen* (Radix Codonopsitis Pilosulae) *Wu Wei Zi* (Fructus Schisandrae) *Mai Men Dong* (Radix Ophiopogonis Japonici) *Xing Ren* (Semen Pruni Armeniacae)	Enduring coughing and wheezing due to Lung deficiency

HERBS FOR SUPPLEMENTING THE BLOOD

Herbs for supplementing the Blood include herbs which can nourish and boost the Blood. They are mainly used for Blood deficiency patterns, which are essentially divided into Heart-Blood deficiency and Liver-Blood deficiency patterns.

Heart-Blood deficiency mainly manifests as a lustreless facial complexion, pale lips and tongue, palpitations and fearful throbbing, insomnia and profuse dreaming, forgetfulness, and a weak and fine pulse. Manifestations of Liver-Blood deficiency include a sallow yellow facial complexion, dizziness, tinnitus and pale nails; or delayed menstruation with scant and pale discharge, menstrual block, and a pale tongue and fine pulse.

In addition to strongly supplementing the Blood, these herbs have the concurrent functions of nourishing the Heart and fortifying the Spleen, and enriching and nourishing the Liver and Kidneys. In clinical practice, they can also be used for limpness and aching in the lumbar region and knees, and premature greying due to depletion of the Liver, Kidneys, Essence and Blood.

Generally, herbs for supplementing the Blood have limited effectiveness when used on their own, so they should be combined with other herbs depending on the nature of the pattern involved:

- add herbs for supplementing Qi in cases with Qi deficiency in order to strengthen the effect, since boosting Qi can generate Blood;
- add small dosages of herbs for quickening the Blood in cases of Blood stasis;
- add herbs for enriching Yin in cases of Yin deficiency, since Blood deficiency is frequently accompanied by Yin deficiency;
- add herbs for supplementing Qi and fortifying the Spleen in cases with Spleen and Stomach deficiency. This is because the Spleen is the root of later heaven, the source of the generation and transformation of Qi and Blood. Only when the Spleen can transport and transform normally can generation and transformation have the source required to allow herbs for supplementing the Blood to function effectively. If the Spleen fails in its function of transportation and transformation, herbs for supplementing the Blood cannot function properly.

Although herbs for supplementing the Blood can treat Blood deficiency, they are generally greasy in nature and tend to inhibit the flow of Stomach Qi, thus affecting digestion and absorption. As a result, they should not be applied in cases of damp turbidity obstructing the Middle Jiao, distension and fullness in the stomach and abdomen, loose stool and reduced appetite.

Tab. 17.3 Herbs for supplementing the Blood

Herb	Functions	Indications
Dang Gui (Radix Angelicae Sinensis)	Supplementing the Blood, quickening the Blood and alleviating pain, moistening the Intestines and freeing the bowels, dispersing swelling	Blood deficiency patterns, dizziness, menstrual irregularities, menstrual block, painful menstruation, abdominal masses, pain in the abdomen due to cold pathogenic factors, knocks and falls, pain due to Blood stasis, numbness and wind-damp Bi syndrome pain, constipation due to dryness in the Large Intestine, abscesses and sores

Shu Di Huang (Radix Rehmanniae Glutinosae Conquita)	Nourishing the Blood, enriching Yin, supplementing the Essence and replenishing the Marrow	A sallow yellow facial complexion due to Blood deficiency, dizziness, palpitations, insomnia, menstrual irregularities, limpness and aching in the lumbar region and knees, tinnitus and deafness, steaming bone disorder, night sweating, wasting and thirsting, seminal emission
Bai Shao (Radix Paeoniae Lactiflorae)	Nourishing the Blood and adjusting menstruation, constraining Yin and stopping sweating, calming and repressing Liver Yang and alleviating pain	Menstrual irregularities, uterine bleeding, spontaneous sweating, night sweating, ascendant hyperactivity of Liver Yang, headache, dizziness, pain in the chest, abdomen and hypochondrium, diarrhoea, dysentery with pain in the abdomen
He Shou Wu (Radix Polygoni Multiflori)	Supplementing and boosting the Essence and Blood, interrupting malaria, relieving toxicity, moistening the Intestines and freeing the bowels	Depletion and deficiency of the Essence and Blood, dizziness, premature greying, limpness and aching in the lumbar region and knees, seminal emission, enduring malaria, enduring dysentery, scrofula, abscesses and sores, Intestinal dryness with constipation
Sang Shen (Fructus Mori Albae)	Enriching Yin and supplementing the Blood, generating body fluids and allaying thirst, moistening the Intestines and freeing the bowels	Dizziness, tinnitus, insomnia, premature greying, wasting and thirsting, constipation
E Jiao (Gelatinum Corii Asini)	Supplementing the Blood, stopping bleeding, quieting the foetus, enriching Yin and moistening the Lungs	Palpitations due to Blood deficiency, dizziness, vomiting of blood, bleeding, uterine bleeding, vexation due to Yin deficiency, insomnia, pain in the abdomen during pregnancy, dry cough due to Yin deficiency
Long Yan Rou (Arillus Euphoriae Longanae)	Supplementing and boosting the Heart and Spleen, nourishing the Blood and quieting the Spirit	Fatigue and reduced appetite, lack of strength, emaciation, insomnia, palpitations and fearful throbbing, dizziness

Dang Gui 当归 (Chinese angelica root, Radix Angelicae Sinensis)

Dang Gui is the root of *Angelica sinensis* (Oliv.) Diels., family Umbelliferae.

Main ingredients *Dang Gui* contains volatile oils (including α-pinene, β-pinene, camphene, p-cymene, myrcene and ligustilide), p-methylbenzoalcohol, vanillin, phthalic anhydride, sucrose, fructose and vitamin B_{12}.

Properties Taste: sweet and acrid; nature: warm.

Channels entered Liver, Heart and Spleen.

Functions and indications Supplements the Blood, quickens the Blood and alleviates pain, moistens the Intestines and frees the bowels, and disperses swelling. It is indicated for Blood deficiency patterns, dizziness, menstrual irregularities, menstrual block, painful menstruation, abdominal masses, pain in the abdomen due to cold pathogenic factors, knocks and falls, pain due to Blood stasis, numbness and wind-damp Bi syndrome pain, constipation due to dryness in the Large Intestine, and abscesses and sores.

Common dosage 5-15g.

Precautions and contraindications *Dang Gui* is contraindicated in cases of obstruction of dampness in the Middle Jiao with loose stool or diarrhoea.

Remarks Use *Dang Gui Shen* (Corpus Radicis Angelicae Sinensis), the main root, for supplementing the Blood; *Dang Gui Wei* (Extremitas Radicis Angelicae Sinensis), the branches or tail of the root, for quickening the Blood; and the whole herb, *Quan Dang Gui* (Radix Angelicae Sinensis), for harmonizing the Blood. *Dang Gui* is generally used raw, but mix-frying the herb with alcohol can strengthen its function in quickening the Blood.

Comparison of functions Both *Dang Gui* (Radix Angelicae Sinensis) and *Shu Di Huang* (Radix Rehmanniae Glutinosae Conquita) are key herbs for supplementing the Blood and are frequently used together to accentuate each other's effect. However, *Dang Gui* can also quicken the Blood and performs its supplementing function without causing any side-effects of stagnation. It can also break up Blood stasis and adjust menstruation. *Shu Di Huang* has strong supplementing properties and is an important herb for enriching Yin and nourishing the Blood, but it is very cloying and may cause indigestion.

For additional comparisons, see *Bai Shao* (Radix Paeoniae Lactiflorae), *Sang Shen* (Fructus Mori Albae), *E Jiao* (Gelatinum Corii Asini) and *Ji Xue Teng* (Caulis Spatholobi).

Toxicity The LD_{50} for intraperitoneal injection in mice of an aqueous extract of *Dang Gui* is 65.8g/kg.

Modern research

1. Inhibits haematoblastic concentration, arrhythmia and cardiac ischaemia, improves microcirculation.[128, 129]
2. Promotes the production of blood, inhibits anaemia.[129-132]
3. Has a benign regulating function in the uterus; uterine contractions are inhibited by the volatile oils contained in *Dang Gui* and stimulated by the non-volatile substances it contains.[128]
4. Protects the functions of the liver, soothes the gallbladder.[133, 134]
5. Reduces the level of blood lipids.[128]
6. The polysaccharides contained in *Dang Gui* inhibit carcinoma.[132, 135]

Combinations and applications

Functions	Combinations	Applications
Supplementing the Blood	*Huang Qi* (Radix Astragali seu Hedysari)	Qi and Blood deficiency patterns, accompanied by a surging, large and deficient pulse, forceless under heavy pressure
	Shu Di Huang (Radix Rehmanniae Glutinosae Conquita) *Chuan Xiong* (Rhizoma Ligustici Chuanxiong)	A bright, white facial complexion, pale lips and nails, tinnitus, dizziness and palpitations due to Blood deficiency of the Heart and Liver
Quickening the Blood and alleviating pain	*Shu Di Huang* (Radix Rehmanniae Glutinosae Conquita) *Bai Shao* (Radix Paeoniae Lactiflorae) *Chuan Xiong* (Rhizoma Ligustici Chuanxiong)	Menstrual irregularities, painful menstruation or menstrual block due to disharmony of the Chong and Ren vessels, disharmony between Qi and Blood, Blood stagnation and Blood deficiency
	Tao Ren (Semen Persicae) *Hong Hua* (Flos Carthami Tinctorii)	Painful menstruation and menstrual block due to obstruction by Blood stasis
	Bai Shao (Radix Paeoniae Lactiflorae) *Chai Hu* (Radix Bupleuri) *Bai Zhu* (Rhizoma Atractylodis Macrocephalae)	Menstrual irregularities and painful menstruation due to disorderly counterflow of Qi and Blood with Liver depression and Qi stagnation
	Mu Dan Pi (Cortex Moutan Radicis) *Zhi Zi* (Fructus Gardeniae Jasminoidis)	Advanced menstruation or pain in the abdomen during menstruation due to heat causing the movement of Blood and Liver depression transforming into fire
	Shu Di Huang (Radix Rehmanniae Glutinosae Conquita) *Yan Hu Suo* (Rhizoma Corydalis Yanhusuo) *Xiang Fu* (Rhizoma Cyperi Rotundi)	Blood deficiency and Blood stasis, deficiency-cold in the Chong and Ren vessels, pain in the abdomen during menstruation
	Chai Hu (Radix Bupleuri) *Da Huang* (Radix et Rhizoma Rhei) *Tao Ren* (Semen Persicae) *Hong Hua* (Flos Carthami Tinctorii)	Pain, stasis and swelling in the chest and hypochondrium, knocks and falls
	Qin Jiao (Radix Gentianae Macrophyllae) *Gui Zhi* (Ramulus Cinnamomi Cassiae) *Qiang Huo* (Rhizoma et Radix Notopterygii)	Bi syndrome pain and numbness of the limbs due to an invasion of wind-cold-damp pathogenic factors
Moistening the Intestines and freeing the bowels	*Huo Ma Ren* (Semen Cannabis Sativae) *He Shou Wu* (Radix Polygoni Multiflori) *Rou Cong Rong* (Herba Cistanches Deserticolae)	Intestinal dryness with constipation due to Qi and Blood deficiency

Dispersing swelling	*Zhi Chuan Shan Jia* (Squama Manitis Pentadactylae Praeparata) (see notes on legal status) *Chi Shao* (Radix Paeoniae Rubra) *Jin Yin Hua* (Flos Lonicerae) *Chuan Bei Mu* (Bulbus Fritillariae Cirrhosae)	The initial stage of abscesses and sores with red and painful swelling, accompanied by fever and a slight aversion to cold and a forceful, rapid pulse
	Huang Qi (Radix Astragali seu Hedysari) *Shu Di Huang* (Radix Rehmanniae Glutinosae Conquita) *Rou Gui* (Cortex Cinnamomi Cassiae) *Ren Shen* (Radix Ginseng)	Non-closure of open sores due to Qi and Blood deficiency

Shu Di Huang 熟地黄 (Processed rehmannia root, Radix Rehmanniae Glutinosae Conquita)

Shu Di Huang is the root of *Rehmannia glutinosa* (Gaertn.) Libosch., family Scrophulariaceae, prepared by steaming in yellow rice wine.

Main ingredients *Shu Di Huang* contains rehmannin, catalpol, danmelittoside, leonuride, rehmanniosides, daucosterol, stachyose and glucose.

Properties Taste: sweet; nature: slightly warm.

Channels entered Liver and Kidney.

Functions and indications Nourishes the Blood, enriches Yin, and supplements the Essence and replenishes the Marrow. It is indicated for a sallow yellow facial complexion due to Blood deficiency, dizziness, palpitations, insomnia, menstrual irregularities, limpness and aching in the lumbar region and knees, tinnitus and deafness, steaming bone disorder, night sweating, wasting and thirsting, and seminal emission.

Common dosage 10-30g.

Precautions and contraindications *Shu Di Huang* is oilier in nature than its raw form, *Sheng Di Huang* (Radix Rehmanniae Glutinosae), so it is more difficult to digest. It is contraindicated for copious sputum due to Qi stagnation, fullness and distension in the stomach and abdomen, reduced appetite and loose stool.

Remarks *Shu Di Huang* should be used in combination with herbs for fortifying the Spleen and Stomach such as *Chen Pi* (Pericarpium Citri Reticulatae) or *Sha Ren* (Fructus Amomi). The herb can be used in its charred form to stop bleeding.

Comparison of functions *Di Huang*, or *Rehmannia glutinosa* (Gaertn.) Libosch., is classified into the fresh herb, *Xian Di Huang* (Radix Rehmanniae Glutinosae Recens), the dried herb, *Gan Di Huang* (Radix Rehmanniae Glutinosae Exsiccata), and the prepared herb, *Shu Di Huang* (Radix Rehmanniae Glutinosae Conquita). *Xian Di Huang* and *Gan Di Huang* are generally known as *Sheng Di Huang* (Radix Rehmanniae Glutinosae). All three varieties can enrich Yin and generate body fluids to treat depletion and deficiency of Yin, Blood and body fluids.

Xian Di Huang, sweet, bitter and very cold, is weak in enriching Yin, but is more effective in clearing heat, cooling the Blood, allaying thirst and eliminating vexation. It is often used for exuberant pathogenic heat due to Blood-heat and Yin depletion. *Gan Di Huang* is sweet, cold and moistening; it is an important herb for enriching Yin, but is not as effective as *Xian Di Huang* for clearing heat and cooling the Blood. It can be used for patterns of depletion of body fluids and Blood-heat or patterns of depletion and deficiency of the Essence, Blood, Yin and body fluids with heat. As *Shu Di Huang* is sweet and slightly warm, it specifically nourishes the Blood and enriches Yin, supplements the Essence and replenishes the Marrow; it is used to treat deficiency of Essence, Blood, Yin and body fluids accompanied by slight heat or slight cold. Since *Shu Di Huang* is relatively cloying, it is often combined with *Sha Ren* (Fructus Amomi) or *Chen Pi* (Pericarpium Citri Reticulatae) to safeguard Stomach Qi and promote the absorption of medicinals.

For additional comparisons, see *He Shou Wu* (Radix Polygoni Multiflori), *Dang Gui* (Radix Angelicae Sinensis) and *E Jiao* (Gelatinum Corii Asini).

Toxicity Rats fed a condensed decoction of 18g/kg of *Shu Di Huang* were observed for two weeks. No significant change was recorded in behaviour, weight or transaminase, and the liver and kidney continued to function without any significant pathological change.

Modern research

1. Promotes the production of blood, strengthens the immune function, lowers the blood sugar level, inhibits lipid catabolism, inhibits haematoblastic concentration, and has a clear inhibitory effect on embolisms.[136]
2. Inhibits carcinoma.[136]
3. Inhibits such fungi as Tinea barbae and Microsporum gypseum.[137]

Combinations and applications

Functions	Combinations	Applications
Nourishing the Blood	*Dang Gui* (Radix Angelicae Sinensis) *Chuan Xiong* (Rhizoma Ligustici Chuanxiong) *Bai Shao* (Radix Paeoniae Lactiflorae)	Symptoms associated with Blood deficiency such as a sallow yellow facial complexion, dizziness, palpitations, insomnia, scant menstrual flow or menstrual block
	Dang Gui (Radix Angelicae Sinensis) *Bai Shao* (Radix Paeoniae Lactiflorae) *E Jiao* (Gelatinum Corii Asini) *Ai Ye* (Folium Artemisiae Argyi)	Insufficiency of the Chong and Ren vessels due to Blood deficiency, stirring foetus, persistent uterine bleeding during pregnancy
	Xiang Fu (Rhizoma Cyperi Rotundi) *Yan Hu Suo* (Rhizoma Corydalis Yanhusuo) *Bai Shao* (Radix Paeoniae Lactiflorae) *Chuan Xiong* (Rhizoma Ligustici Chuanxiong)	Painful menstruation due to Blood deficiency or Blood stagnation, light-coloured discharge during menstruation, inhibited menstruation, pain in the lower abdomen
Enriching Yin	*Shan Zhu Yu* (Fructus Corni Officinalis) *Shan Yao* (Rhizoma Dioscoreae Oppositae) *Fu Ling* (Sclerotium Poriae Cocos) *Ze Xie* (Rhizoma Alismatis Orientalis)	Wasting and thirsting, or limpness and aching in the lumbar region and knees, dizziness, tinnitus and deafness, a red tongue with thin fur and a fine, rapid pulse due to depletion and deficiency of Kidney Yin
	Gou Qi Zi (Fructus Lycii) *Ju Hua* (Flos Chrysanthemi Morifolii) *Shan Zhu Yu* (Fructus Corni Officinalis) *Fu Ling* (Sclerotium Poriae Cocos)	Blurred vision or dry and sore eyes due to Kidney Yin deficiency

	Mai Men Dong (Radix Ophiopogonis Japonici) *Wu Wei Zi* (Fructus Schisandrae) *Shan Yao* (Rhizoma Dioscoreae Oppositae) *Dang Gui* (Radix Angelicae Sinensis) *Shan Zhu Yu* (Fructus Corni Officinalis)	Coughing and wheezing due to Yin deficiency of the Lungs and Kidneys, tidal fever, night sweating, dream emission, seminal emission
	Di Gu Pi (Cortex Lycii Radicis) *Zhi Ke* (Fructus Citri Aurantii) *Chai Hu* (Radix Bupleuri) *Zhi Mu* (Rhizoma Anemarrhenae Asphodeloidis) *Qin Jiao* (Radix Gentianae Macrophyllae) *Bie Jia* (Carapax Amydae Sinensis) (see notes on legal status)	Steaming bone disorder, fever and fatigued body resulting from insufficiency of Kidney Yin and hyperactivity of Yang due to Yin deficiency
Supplementing the Essence and replenishing the Marrow	*Shi Hu* (Herba Dendrobii) (see notes on legal status) *Rou Cong Rong* (Herba Cistanches Deserticolae) *Mai Men Dong* (Radix Ophiopogonis Japonici) *Rou Gui* (Cortex Cinnamomi Cassiae) *Shi Chang Pu* (Rhizoma Acori Graminei) *Yuan Zhi* (Radix Polygalae)	Loss of voice, lack of strength in the legs with a sunken, slow, fine and weak pulse due to deficiency of the Essence and Blood

Bai Shao 白芍 (White peony root, Radix Paeoniae Lactiflorae)

Bai Shao is the root of *Paeonia lactiflora* Pall., family Ranunculaceae.

Main ingredients *Bai Shao* contains paeoniflorin, paeonol, paeonin, albiflorin, benzoic acid, β-sitosterol, gallotannin, volatile oils, resin, starch, proteins and triterpenes.

Properties Taste: bitter and sour; nature: slightly cold.

Channels entered Liver and Spleen.

Functions and indications Nourishes the Blood and adjusts menstruation, constrains Yin and stops sweating, calms and represses Liver Yang and alleviates pain. It is indicated for menstrual irregularities, uterine bleeding, spontaneous sweating, night sweating, ascendant hyperactivity of Liver Yang, headache, dizziness, pain in the chest, abdomen and hypochondrium, diarrhoea, and dysentery with pain in the abdomen.

Common dosage 5-10g, or 15-30g to alleviate pain by calming the Liver.

Precautions and contraindications

1. *Bai Shao* should not be used on its own for deficiency-cold patterns due to Yang debilitation.
2. *Bai Shao* is incompatible with *Li Lu* (Radix et Rhizoma Veratri).

Remarks Use raw *Bai Shao* for calming the Liver, constraining Yin and stopping sweating; use *Bai Shao* stir-fried on its own or with alcohol for nourishing the Blood and adjusting menstruation.

Comparison of functions

1. Both *Bai Shao* (Radix Paeoniae Lactiflorae) and *Dang Gui* (Radix Angelicae Sinensis) can nourish the Blood. *Dang Gui* is warm and more suitable for patients with Blood deficiency accompanied by cold. *Bai Shao* is slightly cold and more suitable for patients with Blood deficiency accompanied by heat.
2. *Bai Shao* (Radix Paeoniae Lactiflorae), *Dang Gui* (Radix Angelicae Sinensis) and *Chi Shao* (Radix Paeoniae Rubra) can all alleviate pain, although their mechanism is different. *Dang Gui* supplements and quickens the Blood and moves Qi to alleviate pain; it is suitable for pain due to Blood deficiency with Blood stasis. *Chi Shao* is good for dissipating stasis to alleviate pain. Since it is slightly cold, it can also clear heat and cool the Blood, and so is particularly suitable for pain due to Blood stasis with exuberant heat. *Bai Shao* is good for nourishing the Blood and constraining Yin, and for calming the Liver and relaxing tension to alleviate pain; it is used particularly for insufficiency of Liver Yin, dull pain in the hypochondrium, and spasms and pain in the limbs due to improper nourishment of the sinews and vessels. For further details, see also *Chi Shao* (Radix Paeoniae Rubra).

Toxicity *Bai Shao* has a low level of toxicity. The LD_{50} for intraperitoneal injection in mice of the glucosides contained in *Bai Shao* is 230mg/kg. In a long-term toxicity test on dogs, 3g/kg per day of *Bai Shao* was given via intragastric administration; there was no significant difference in terms of liver and kidney function and histology in comparison with a control group.

Modern research

1. Has a tranquillizing function, alleviates pain and relieves convulsions.[138, 139]
2. Strengthens the immune function, adjusts the immune balance.[140, 141]
3. Inhibits inflammation.[138]
4. Relieves spasm of the intestinal smooth muscle.[142]
5. Inhibits gastric ulcers.[138]
6. Protects the functions of the liver.[143, 144]
7. Decoctions of *Bai Shao* inhibited various Shigella bacteria and staphylococci *in vitro*.[145]

Combinations and applications

Functions	Combinations	Applications
Nourishing the Blood and adjusting menstruation	*Dang Gui* (Radix Angelicae Sinensis) *Shu Di Huang* (Radix Rehmanniae Glutinosae Conquita) *Chuan Xiong* (Rhizoma Ligustici Chuanxiong)	Disorders associated with Blood deficiency such as dizziness, tinnitus, pale lips and nails, and scant menstrual flow with light-coloured discharge and a fine, rough pulse
	Shu Di Huang (Radix Rehmanniae Glutinosae Conquita) *Dang Gui* (Radix Angelicae Sinensis) *E Jiao* (Gelatinum Corii Asini) *Ai Ye* (Folium Artemisiae Argyi)	Menstrual irregularities or uterine bleeding with a pale tongue and a sunken and fine pulse due to Blood deficiency and insecurity of the Chong and Ren vessels
Constraining Yin and stopping sweating	*Gui Zhi* (Ramulus Cinnamomi Cassiae) *Gan Cao* (Radix Glycyrrhizae) *Sheng Jiang* (Rhizoma Zingiberis Officinalis Recens) *Da Zao* (Fructus Ziziphi Jujubae)	Externally-contracted wind-cold pathogenic factors, and disharmony between the Ying and Wei levels manifesting as spontaneous sweating due to exterior deficiency, aversion to wind, and a floating, moderate pulse

	Shu Di Huang (Radix Rehmanniae Glutinosae Conquita) *Mu Li* (Concha Ostreae) *Ma Huang Gen* (Radix Ephedrae) *Long Gu* (Os Draconis)	Palpitations and fright, night sweating due to insufficiency of Yin and Blood
Calming and repressing Liver Yang and alleviating pain	*Chai Hu* (Radix Bupleuri) *Dang Gui* (Radix Angelicae Sinensis) *Fu Ling* (Sclerotium Poriae Cocos) *Bai Zhu* (Rhizoma Atractylodis Macrocephalae) *Gan Cao* (Radix Glycyrrhizae)	Pain in the hypochondrium, distension and pain in the breasts, a pale red tongue and a string-like, deficient pulse due to Liver depression caused by Blood deficiency
	Gan Cao (Radix Glycyrrhizae)	Spasms and pain in the abdomen with a string-like and tight pulse due to Liver-Spleen disharmony, or spasms and pain in the limbs due to Liver-Blood deficiency and improper nourishment of the sinews and vessels
	Bai Zhu (Rhizoma Atractylodis Macrocephalae) *Fang Feng* (Radix Ledebouriellae Divaricatae) *Chen Pi* (Pericarpium Citri Reticulatae)	Effulgent Liver Qi due to Spleen deficiency, pain in the abdomen and rumbling intestines, diarrhoea, a thin tongue with white fur and a string-like, moderate pulse due to wood depression overwhelming earth
	Fu Ling (Sclerotium Poriae Cocos) *Bai Zhu* (Rhizoma Atractylodis Macrocephalae) *Ze Xie* (Rhizoma Alismatis Orientalis) *Dang Gui* (Radix Angelicae Sinensis)	Stirring foetus due to fright, pain in the abdomen during pregnancy
	Huang Lian (Rhizoma Coptidis) *Dang Gui* (Radix Angelicae Sinensis) *Mu Xiang* (Radix Aucklandiae Lappae) (see notes on legal status) *Gan Cao* (Radix Glycyrrhizae) *Rou Gui* (Cortex Cinnamomi Cassiae)	Damp-heat dysentery with blood in the stool, pain in the abdomen, abdominal urgency and tenesmus
	Dai Zhe Shi (Haematitum) *Niu Xi* (Radix Achyranthis Bidentatae) *Sheng Di Huang* (Radix Rehmanniae Glutinosae) *Mu Li* (Concha Ostreae)	Headache, dizziness, tinnitus, profuse dreaming and insomnia with a string-like, firm and long pulse due to ascendant hyperactivity of Liver Yang

He Shou Wu 何首乌 (Fleece-flower root, Radix Polygoni Multiflori)

He Shou Wu is the root tuber of *Polygonum multiflorum* Thunb., family Polygonaceae.

Main ingredients *He Shou Wu* contains anthraquinone derivatives, mainly chrysophanol and emodin, as well as rhein, physcion, questin, lecithin, β-sitosterol and starch.

Properties Taste: bitter, sweet and astringent; nature: slightly warm.

Channels entered Liver and Kidney.

Functions and indications Supplements and boosts the Essence and Blood, interrupts malaria, relieves toxicity, and moistens the Intestines and frees the bowels. It is indicated for depletion and deficiency of the Essence and Blood, dizziness, premature greying, limpness and aching in the lumbar region and knees, seminal emission, enduring malaria, enduring dysentery, scrofula, abscesses and sores, and Intestinal dryness with constipation.

Common dosage 10-30g; not to be decocted in an iron vessel.

Precautions and contraindications *He Shou Wu* is contraindicated in cases of loose stool and severe Phlegm-damp.

Remarks Processed *He Shou Wu* is employed to supplement and boost the Essence and Blood, secure the Kidneys and darken the hair; use raw *He Shou Wu* for interrupting malaria, relieving toxicity and moistening the Intestines. Fresh *He Shou Wu* is more effective than the raw herb for moistening the Intestines.

Comparison of functions Both *He Shou Wu* (Radix Polygoni Multiflori) and *Shu Di Huang* (Radix Rehmanniae Glutinosae Conquita) are important herbs for supplementing and boosting the Essence and Blood of the Liver and Kidneys. *Shu Di Huang* is strong and relatively greasy and may be harmful to the stomach, whereas *He Shou Wu* has more moderate properties and does not have this side-effect. *Shu Di Huang* is used for rapid and powerful supplementation, whereas *He Shou Wu* works more slowly. In addition, *He Shou Wu* has a greater range of indications than *Shu Di Huang*, also being used to interrupt malaria, relieve toxicity and moisten the Intestines.

Toxicity The toxicity of *He Shou Wu* is closely related to the way it is prepared; the processed herb is less toxic than the raw herb. The LD_{50} for the alcoholic percolate of raw *He Shou Wu* is 50g/kg, but even at amounts of 1000g/kg for the processed herb, no deaths occurred. The LD_{50} for intragastric administration of raw *He Shou Wu* is 2.7g/kg, whereas for the processed herb it is 169.4g/kg.

Modern research

1. Reduces the level of blood lipids, inhibits atherosclerosis.[146]
2. Promotes the production of blood.[147]
3. Protects the functions of the liver.[148]
4. The patent medicine derived from *He Shou Wu* – *Shou Wu Yan Shou Dan* (*He Shou Wu* Life-Extending Elixir) – slows the effects of ageing.[149]

Combinations and applications

Functions	Combinations	Applications
Supplementing and boosting the Essence and Blood	*Gou Qi Zi* (Fructus Lycii) *Tu Si Zi* (Semen Cuscutae) *Dang Gui* (Radix Angelicae Sinensis) *Niu Xi* (Radix Achyranthis Bidentatae) *Fu Ling* (Sclerotium Poriae Cocos)	Limpness and aching in the lumbar region and knees, premature greying, dizziness and blurred vision with a sunken and fine pulse due to depletion and deficiency of the Essence and Blood and insufficiency of the Liver and Kidneys
	Sha Yuan Zi (Semen Astragali Complanati) *Bai Ji Li* (Fructus Tribuli Terrestris) *Qian Shi* (Semen Euryales Ferocis) *Shu Di Huang* (Radix Rehmanniae Glutinosae Conquita) *Shan Zhu Yu* (Fructus Corni Officinalis) *Shan Yao* (Rhizoma Dioscoreae Oppositae) *Fu Ling* (Sclerotium Poriae Cocos)	Seminal emission, severe diarrhoea, limpness in the lumbar region, tinnitus, a pale tongue with white fur and a fine, weak pulse due to deficiency of the Kidneys, which thus fail to secure the Essence

Interrupting malaria	*Dang Gui* (Radix Angelicae Sinensis) *Ren Shen* (Radix Ginseng) *Chen Pi* (Pericarpium Citri Reticulatae) *Wei Jiang* (Rhizoma Zingiberis Officinalis Usta)	Non-responsive malaria due to Qi and Blood deficiency
Relieving toxicity	*Ku Shen* (Radix Sophorae Flavescentis) *Bo He* (Herba Menthae Haplocalycis) *Fang Feng* (Radix Ledebouriellae Divaricatae)	Swollen, itchy and painful sores all over the body due to externally-contracted wind toxins
	Chuan Bei Mu (Bulbus Fritillariae Cirrhosae) *Xia Ku Cao* (Spica Prunellae Vulgaris) *Dang Gui* (Radix Angelicae Sinensis) *Xiang Fu* (Rhizoma Cyperi Rotundi) *Chuan Xiong* (Rhizoma Ligustici Chuanxiong)	Non-healing scrofula, alternating chills and fever, emaciation
Moistening the Intestines and freeing the bowels	*Huo Ma Ren* (Semen Cannabis Sativae) *Hei Zhi Ma* (Semen Sesami Indici) *Dang Gui* (Radix Angelicae Sinensis)	Intestinal dryness with constipation due to Blood deficiency and depletion of body fluids in the elderly and weak, postpartum and in enduring illnesses

Appendix

Ye Jiao Teng 夜交藤 (Fleece-flower stem, Caulis Polygoni Multiflori)

Ye Jiao Teng is the vine of *He Shou Wu,* so is also known as *Shou Wu Teng*. The functions, indications, combinations and applications of *Ye Jiao Teng* are described in Chapter 14.

Sang Shen 桑椹 (Mulberry fruit, Fructus Mori Albae)

Sang Shen is the dried fruit-spike of *Morus alba* L., family Moraceae.

Main ingredients *Sang Shen* contains rutin, carotene, vitamins B_1, B_2 and C, cyanidin, linoleic acid, oleic acid, palmitic acid and proteins.

Properties Taste: sweet; nature: cold.

Channels entered Heart, Liver and Kidney.

Functions and indications Enriches Yin and supplements the Blood, generates body fluids and allays thirst, moistens the Intestines and frees the bowels. It is indicated for dizziness, tinnitus, insomnia, premature greying, wasting and thirsting, and constipation.

Common dosage 10-15g; or 30-60g when used alone.

Precautions and contraindications Since *Sang Shen* is cold in nature, it is contraindicated for patients with diarrhoea due to Spleen and Stomach deficiency-cold.

Comparison of functions *Sang Shen* (Fructus Mori Albae) and *Dang Gui* (Radix Angelicae Sinensis) are key herbs for supplementing the Blood; both can also moisten the Intestines and free the bowels. *Sang Shen* is sweet in taste and cold in nature and is effective for enriching Yin and supplementing the Blood; it is often used for dry mouth and wasting and thirsting due to Yin deficiency and Blood depletion, for dizziness, insomnia and blurred vision due to insufficiency of Liver Yin and ascendant hyperactivity of Liver Yang, and for premature greying due to insufficiency of the Liver and Kidneys. *Dang Gui* is sweet and acrid in taste, and warm in nature. It is good for warming the Blood and freeing the vessels to supplement and quicken the Blood and is suitable for treating Blood deficiency patterns with cold.

For an additional comparison, see *Sang Bai Pi* (Cortex Mori Albae Radicis).

Combinations and applications

Functions	Combinations	Applications
Enriching Yin and supplementing the Blood	*He Shou Wu* (Radix Polygoni Multiflori) *Nü Zhen Zi* (Fructus Ligustri Lucidi) *Han Lian Cao* (Herba Ecliptae Prostratae) *Du Zhong* (Cortex Eucommiae Ulmoidis)	Limpness and aching in the lumbar region and knees, dizziness, tinnitus and insomnia and premature greying due to depletion and deficiency of Yin and Blood and insufficiency of the Liver and Kidneys
Generating body fluids and allaying thirst	*Sheng Di Huang* (Radix Rehmanniae Glutinosae) *Shu Di Huang* (Radix Rehmanniae Glutinosae Conquita) *Shi Hu* (Herba Dendrobii) (see notes on legal status) *Mai Men Dong* (Radix Ophiopogonis Japonici) *Yu Zhu* (Rhizoma Polygonati Odorati) *Sha Shen* (Radix Glehniae seu Adenophorae)	Damage to body fluids, dry mouth and wasting and thirsting due to internal heat
	Tian Hua Fen (Radix Trichosanthis) *Sheng Shi Gao* (Gypsum Fibrosum Crudum) *Zhi Mu* (Rhizoma Anemarrhenae Asphodeloidis) *Tian Men Dong* (Radix Asparagi Cochinchinensis)	Add these herbs to the *Sheng Di Huang* combination for the same symptoms when internal heat is severe
	Xi Yang Shen (Radix Panacis Quinquefolii) (see notes on legal status) *Tai Zi Shen* (Radix Pseudostellariae Heterophyllae) *Huang Qi* (Radix Astragali seu Hedysari)	Add these herbs to the *Sheng Di Huang* combination for the same symptoms due to severe internal heat accompanied by Qi deficiency
Moistening the Intestines and freeing the bowels	*He Shou Wu* (Radix Polygoni Multiflori) *Hei Zhi Ma* (Semen Sesami Indici) *Huo Ma Ren* (Semen Cannabis Sativae) *Rou Cong Rong* (Herba Cistanches Deserticolae)	Intestinal dryness with constipation due to Yin depletion and Blood deficiency

E Jiao 阿胶 (Donkey-hide gelatin, Gelatinum Corii Asini)

E Jiao is the glue or gelatin prepared from skin of the donkey *Equus asinus* L., family Equidae.

Main ingredients *E Jiao* contains collagen that can generate many types of amino acid when hydrolysed, including lysine, arginine, histidine, cystine, aspartic acid and serine. It also contains calcium and sulphur.

Properties Taste: sweet; nature: neutral.

Channels entered Lung, Liver and Kidney.

Functions and indications Supplements the Blood, stops bleeding, quiets the foetus, enriches Yin and moistens the Lungs. It is indicated for palpitations due to Blood deficiency, dizziness, vomiting of blood, bleeding, uterine bleeding, vexation due to Yin deficiency, insomnia, pain in the abdomen during pregnancy, and dry cough due to Yin deficiency.

Common dosage 5-10g, dissolved by boiling in water or yellow wine or melted in a decoction.

Precautions and contraindications Since *E Jiao* is rather greasy and cloying, it can hinder digestion; it is therefore contraindicated in cases of Spleen and Stomach deficiency with reduced appetite, and for patients with vomiting and diarrhoea due to Phlegm-damp or with indigestion.

Remarks *E Jiao* fried with *Pu Huang* (Pollen Typhae) should be used to stop bleeding; for enriching Yin and moistening the Lungs, use *E Jiao* fried with *Hai Ge Ke* (Concha Meretricis seu Cyclinae).

Comparison of functions

1. *E Jiao* (Gelatinum Corii Asini) and *Dang Gui* (Radix Angelicae Sinensis) are both important materia medica for supplementing the Blood. *Dang Gui* is acrid in taste and tends to move and dissipate. It supplements the Middle Jiao with movement and is effective for supplementing and quickening the Blood while concurrently transforming stasis and alleviating pain. *E Jiao* is sweet in taste and neutral in nature. It has a preserving function in supplementing the Middle Jiao and is good for supplementing the Blood and stopping bleeding while concurrently enriching Yin and moistening the Lungs.
2. Both *E Jiao* (Gelatinum Corii Asini) and *Shu Di Huang* (Radix Rehmanniae Glutinosae Conquita) can enrich Yin and nourish the Blood. *Shu Di Huang* is sweet in taste and slightly warm in nature. Since it can supplement the Essence and replenish the Marrow, it tends to be used for patterns with deficiency and depletion of the Essence and Blood. *E Jiao* enriches Yin and moistens the Lungs and is an important medicinal for Blood and Yin deficiency patterns and for stopping bleeding.
3. For an additional comparison, see *Long Yan Rou* (Arillus Euphoriae Longanae).

Modern research

1. The collagen contained in *E Jiao* has an obvious effect on blood oxygenation.[150]
2. Strengthens the immune function.[151]

Combinations and applications

Functions	Combinations	Applications
Supplementing the Blood	*Huang Qi* (Radix Astragali seu Hedysari) *Dang Shen* (Radix Codonopsitis Pilosulae) *Dang Gui* (Radix Angelicae Sinensis)	Palpitations, dizziness, insomnia and forgetfulness with a bright white or sallow yellow facial complexion due to Blood deficiency of the Heart and Liver

Stopping bleeding	*Sheng Di Huang* (Radix Rehmanniae Glutinosae) *Bai Shao* (Radix Paeoniae Lactiflorae) *Ai Ye* (Folium Artemisiae Argyi) *Dang Gui* (Radix Angelicae Sinensis)	Profuse menstruation, uterine bleeding and pain in the lower abdomen due to cold stagnation and Blood deficiency; or bleeding during pregnancy and stirring foetus or persistent postpartum bleeding
	Pu Huang (Pollen Typhae) *Sheng Di Huang* (Radix Rehmanniae Glutinosae)	Vomiting of blood and bleeding due to Blood-heat
	Huang Qi (Radix Astragali seu Hedysari) *Sheng Di Huang* (Radix Rehmanniae Glutinosae) *Fu Zi* (Radix Lateralis Aconiti Carmichaeli Praeparata) (see notes on legal status)	Bleeding, vomiting of blood, blood in the stool and uterine bleeding due to deficiency of the Spleen, which thus fails to secure and contain the Blood
Quieting the foetus	*Ai Ye* (Folium Artemisiae Argyi)	Pain in the abdomen and stirring foetus due to fright
	Huang Lian (Rhizoma Coptidis) *Shi Liu Pi* (Pericarpium Punicae Granati) *Dang Gui* (Radix Angelicae Sinensis)	Pain in the abdomen and diarrhoea during pregnancy
Enriching Yin and moistening the Lungs	*Ma Dou Ling* (Fructus Aristolochiae) (see notes on legal status) *Xing Ren* (Semen Pruni Armeniacae) *Niu Bang Zi* (Fructus Arctii Lappae) *Gan Cao* (Radix Glycyrrhizae)	Enduring cough, hasty wheezing, dry mouth and throat, blood-streaked sputum
	Shi Gao (Gypsum Fibrosum) *Sang Ye* (Folium Mori Albae) *Xing Ren* (Semen Pruni Armeniacae) *Mai Men Dong* (Radix Ophiopogonis Japonici) *Gan Cao* (Radix Glycyrrhizae)	Dry cough without sputum or with scant, sticky sputum, vexation and thirst, dry nose and throat and a dry tongue with no fur due to dry-heat damaging the Lungs
	Huang Lian (Rhizoma Coptidis) *Bai Shao* (Radix Paeoniae Lactiflorae) *Ji Zi Huang* (raw egg yolk)	Generalized fever, vexation and insomnia, a red tongue with dry fur and a rapid pulse due to damage to Yin in febrile diseases and hyperactivity of Yang due to Yin deficiency
	Cong Bai (Bulbus Allii Fistulosi) *Feng Mi* (Mel)	Constipation due to Yin deficiency and dryness of the Intestines in the elderly

Long Yan Rou 龙眼肉 (Flesh of longan fruit, Arillus Euphoriae Longanae)

Long Yan Rou is the dried aril of *Euphoria longan* (Lour.) Steud., family Sapindaceae.

Main ingredients *Long Yan Rou* contains glucose, sucrose, adenine, choline, tartaric acid, proteins and vitamins B_1, B_2 and C.

Properties Taste: sweet; nature: warm.
Channels entered Heart and Spleen.
Functions and indications Supplements and boosts the Heart and Spleen, nourishes the Blood and quiets the Spirit. It is indicated for fatigue and reduced appetite, lack of strength, emaciation, insomnia, palpitations and fearful throbbing, and dizziness.
Common dosage 10-15g, or up to 60g when used on its own.
Precautions and contraindications *Long Yan Rou* is contraindicated in cases of dampness obstructing the Middle Jiao or externally-contracted pathogenic factors that have not yet been cleared.
Comparison of functions Both *Long Yan Rou* (Arillus Euphoriae Longanae) and *E Jiao* (Gelatinum Corii Asini) can supplement and nourish the Blood. *E Jiao* is an important materia medica for treating Yin and Blood deficiency. It is effective for stopping bleeding to treat a variety of bleeding patterns and can also enrich Yin, clear the Lungs and moisten dryness. It can be used alone or in compound prescriptions. *Long Yan Rou* is good for supplementing Qi and nourishing the Blood, but its effect is relatively weak, so it is generally used as a supporting herb in prescriptions. Unlike *E Jiao*, it also supplements and boosts the Heart and Spleen and quiets the Spirit.
Toxicity Intragastric administration to mice of a 25ml/kg solution of *Long Yan Rou* and *Ge Jie* (in a proportion of 2:1) did not result in any deaths or adverse effects within seven days.
Modern research Has a tranquillizing function and strengthens the stomach.[152]

Combinations and applications

Functions	Combinations	Applications
Supplementing and boosting the Heart and Spleen, nourishing the Blood and quieting the Spirit	*Ren Shen* (Radix Ginseng) *Dang Gui* (Radix Angelicae Sinensis) *Fu Shen* (Sclerotium Poriae Cocos cum Ligno Hospite) *Suan Zao Ren* (Semen Ziziphi Spinosae)	Palpitations and fearful throbbing, insomnia and forgetfulness, reduced appetite and fatigue due to taxation damage to the Heart and Spleen and excessive thought and preoccupation
	Huang Qi (Radix Astragali seu Hedysari) *Dang Shen* (Radix Codonopsitis Pilosulae) *Bai Zhu* (Rhizoma Atractylodis Macrocephalae) *Dang Gui* (Radix Angelicae Sinensis)	Fatigue, dizziness, spontaneous sweating, a haggard complexion, and a weak, wiry pulse

Note: To treat fatigue and lack of strength due to insufficiency of Qi and Blood, or generalized weakness in the elderly or in an enduring illness due to a weak constitution, cook 30g of *Long Yang Rou* with 3g of white sugar in a double-boiler.

HERBS FOR SUPPLEMENTING YIN

Herbs for supplementing Yin can enrich Yin, generate body fluids and moisten dryness. They are mainly used for Yin deficiency during certain chronic diseases or in the final stage of febrile diseases, as well as to treat diseases due to Yin deficiency and depletion of body fluids.

Yin deficiency patterns can be divided into deficiency of Lung, Stomach, Liver or Kidney Yin:

1. Lung Yin deficiency is characterized by dry cough, coughing of blood, vexation and thirst, dry skin, cough in Lung Wei syndrome with sticky sputum or white foam, or cough with blood-streaked sputum due to impairment of the Lungs in taxation patterns;
2. Stomach Yin deficiency manifests as red lips, a dry, red tongue with peeling fur, dry mouth, reduced appetite, vexation, or discomfort in the stomach with acid vomiting, dry retching and hiccups;
3. Liver Yin deficiency is characterized by dizziness and headache, dry eyes, vertigo, or numbness of the limbs;
4. Kidney Yin deficiency manifests as dizziness and headache, aching in the lumbar region and knees, steaming bone disorder, night sweating, a dry, red tongue without fur, seminal emission or premature ejaculation.

Each herb for supplementing Yin has its own particular strong point and should be chosen according to the principal Yin deficiency pattern. In clinical practice, herbs for supplementing Yin must be selected carefully according to their function and the presenting symptoms:

i. in cases of pathogenic heat damaging Yin in febrile diseases, they should be combined with herbs for clearing heat;
ii. in cases of Yin deficiency with internal heat, they should be combined with herbs for clearing deficiency-heat;
iii. for hyperactivity of Yang due to Yin deficiency, they should be used with herbs for subduing Yang;
iv. in cases of Yin deficiency stirring wind, they should be used with herbs for extinguishing wind;
v. in cases of Yin deficiency combined with Blood deficiency, they should be used together with herbs for supplementing the Blood.

Most herbs for supplementing Yin are sweet, cold, enriching and cloying. They should therefore not be used for disorders involving deficiency of the Spleen and Stomach, internal obstruction of Phlegm-damp, fullness in the abdomen, or loose stool.

Tab. 17.4 Herbs for supplementing Yin

Herb	Functions	Indications
Bei Sha Shen (Radix Glehniae Littoralis)	Clearing the Lungs and nourishing Yin, boosting the Stomach and generating body fluids	Dry cough or coughing of blood due to Lung-heat caused by Yin deficiency, dry mouth and throat, pain in the stomach, thirst due to damage to Yin in warm-febrile diseases
Mai Men Dong (Radix Ophiopogonis Japonici)	Nourishing Yin and moistening the Lungs, boosting the Stomach and generating body fluids, clearing the Heart and eliminating vexation, moistening the Intestines and freeing the bowels	Dry cough due to dryness of the Lungs, coughing of blood, vomiting of blood due to pulmonary consumption, Lung Wei syndrome, damage to body fluids in febrile diseases, thirst and dry mouth, dry throat, vexation and insomnia, Intestinal dryness with constipation

Bie Jia (Carapax Amydae Sinensis)	Nourishing Yin and clearing heat, subduing Yang and extinguishing wind, softening hardness and dissipating lumps	Fever due to Yin deficiency, steaming bone disorder, night sweating, damage to Yin in febrile diseases, deficiency-wind stirring internally, malaria, menstrual block, abdominal masses, child fright epilepsy
Gui Ban (Plastrum Testudinis)	Enriching Yin and subduing Yang, boosting the Kidneys and strengthening the bones, supplementing the Blood and nourishing the Heart, securing the menses and stopping uterine bleeding	Damage to Yin in seasonal febrile diseases, deficiency-wind stirring internally, ascendant hyperactivity of Liver Yang manifesting as dizziness and tinnitus, steaming bone disorder, pain in the lumbar region due to Kidney deficiency, vomiting of blood, spitting of blood, uterine bleeding, palpitations, insomnia, forgetfulness
Gou Qi Zi (Fructus Lycii)	Enriching the Kidneys and supplementing the Liver, brightening the eyes, moistening the Lungs	Limpness and aching in the lumbar region and knees due to Yin deficiency of the Liver and Kidneys, dizziness, blurred vision, consumption cough, wasting and thirsting, seminal emission
Tian Men Dong (Radix Asparagi Cochinchinensis)	Nourishing Yin and clearing heat, moistening dryness and generating body fluids	Lung-heat due to Yin deficiency, cough with or without blood, sore throat, wasting and thirsting, constipation
Bai He (Bulbus Lilii)	Moistening the Lungs and stopping coughing, clearing the Heart and quieting the Spirit	Cough due to dryness in the Lungs, damage to Yin in febrile diseases, insomnia, palpitations
Shi Hu (Herba Dendrobii)	Enriching Yin and abating fever, nourishing the Stomach and generating body fluids, brightening the eyes	Vexation and thirst due to damage to body fluids in febrile diseases, fever due to Yin deficiency, weakness in the lumbar region and legs, pain in the stomach, blurred vision due to Yin deficiency
Yu Zhu (Rhizoma Polygonati Odorati)	Enriching Yin and moistening dryness, generating body fluids and allaying thirst	Cough, dry throat and thirst, fever, headache, externally-contracted pathogenic factors in Yin deficiency patterns
Huang Jing (Rhizoma Polygonati)	Enriching Yin and moistening the Lungs, supplementing the Spleen and boosting Qi	Dry cough due to Lung Yin deficiency, limpness and aching in the lumbar region and knees, tidal fever, fatigue and poor appetite due to Qi deficiency of the Spleen and Stomach, wasting and thirsting
Han Lian Cao (Herba Ecliptae Prostratae)	Enriching and supplementing the Liver and Kidneys, cooling the Blood and stopping bleeding	Dizziness, loose teeth and premature greying due to Yin deficiency of the Liver and Kidneys; coughing of blood, nosebleed, blood in the stool, uterine bleeding, vaginal discharge

Nü Zhen Zi (Fructus Ligustri Lucidi)	Enriching and supplementing the Liver and Kidneys, supplementing the Blood and brightening the eyes	Dizziness, tinnitus, blurred vision and limpness and aching in the lumbar region and knees due to Yin deficiency of the Liver and Kidneys
Hei Zhi Ma (Semen Sesami Indici)	Supplementing and boosting the Essence and Blood, moistening dryness and lubricating the Intestines	Premature greying, dizziness and blurred vision due to insufficiency of the Essence and Blood, constipation due to Blood deficiency and depletion of body fluids

Bei Sha Shen 北沙参 (Glehnia root, Radix Glehniae Littoralis)

Bei Sha Shen is the root of *Glehnia littoralis* F. Schmidt ex Miq., family Umbelliferae.

Main ingredients *Bei Sha Shen* contains psoralen, bergapten, xanthotoxol, xanthotoxin, imperatorin, cnidilin, marmesin, scopoletin, β-sitosterol, volatile oils, alkaloids, triterpenic acids and polysaccharides.

Properties Taste: sweet and slightly bitter; nature: cool.

Channels entered Lung and Stomach.

Functions and indications Clears the Lungs and nourishes Yin, boosts the Stomach and generates body fluids. It is indicated for dry cough or coughing of blood due to Lung-heat caused by Yin deficiency, dry mouth and throat, pain in the stomach, and thirst due to damage to Yin in warm-febrile diseases.

Common dosage 10-15g, or 15-30g of the fresh herb.

Precautions and contraindications

1. *Bei Sha Shen* is contraindicated in cases of deficiency-cold in the Lungs and Stomach, or cough due to externally-contracted wind-cold.
2. *Bei Sha Shen* antagonizes *Fang Ji* (Radix Stephaniae Tetrandrae) and is incompatible with *Li Lu* (Radix et Rhizoma Veratri).

Comparison of functions See *Nan Sha Shen* (Radix Adenophorae), *Shi Hu* (Herba Dendrobii) and *Mai Men Dong* (Radix Ophiopogonis Japonici).

Modern research

1. Acetic extracts from the peel and root of *Bei Sha Shen* are effective in expelling sputum and calming wheezing.[153, 154]
2. Inhibits gastric ulcers.[155]
3. The volatile oils contained in *Bei Sha Shen* clear heat and alleviate pain.[156]

Combinations and applications

Functions	Combinations	Applications
Clearing the Lungs and nourishing Yin	*Sang Ye* (Folium Mori Albae) *Yu Zhu* (Rhizoma Polygonati Odorati) *Mai Men Dong* (Radix Ophiopogonis Japonici) *Tian Hua Fen* (Radix Trichosanthis)	Dry mouth and thirst, dry cough with scant sputum, or coughing of blood, and a red tongue with scant fur due to dry-heat damaging Lung Yin or depletion of the Essence and body fluids
	Bie Jia (Carapax Amydae Sinensis) (see notes on legal status) *Chuan Bei Mu* (Bulbus Fritillariae Cirrhosae) *Zhi Mu* (Rhizoma Anemarrhenae Asphodeloidis) *Shu Di Huang* (Radix Rehmanniae Glutinosae Conquita) *Di Gu Pi* (Cortex Lycii Radicis)	Taxation fever due to Yin deficiency of the Lungs and Kidneys, dry cough without sputum, dry skin, a bitter taste in the mouth, vexation and thirst
Boosting the Stomach and generating body fluids	*Mai Men Dong* (Radix Ophiopogonis Japonici) *Sheng Di Huang* (Radix Rehmanniae Glutinosae) *Yu Zhu* (Rhizoma Polygonati Odorati) *Shi Hu* (Herba Dendrobii) (see notes on legal status)	Pain in the stomach, reduced appetite, lack of strength, thirst and dry mouth and throat due to heat pathogenic factors damaging Yin in warm-febrile diseases

	Xing Ren (Semen Pruni Armeniacae) *Sang Ye* (Folium Mori Albae) *Zhe Bei Mu* (Bulbus Fritillariae Thunbergii) *Pi Pa Ye* (Folium Eriobotryae Japonicae)	Fever and headache, thirst, sputum that is difficult to expectorate, a red tongue with thin, white fur and a floating and rapid pulse due to invasion by externally-contracted warm-dry pathogenic factors

Appendix

Nan Sha Shen 南沙参 (Adenophora root, Radix Adenophorae)

Nan Sha Shen is the root of *Adenophora tetraphylla* (Thunb.) Fisch., *A. stricta* Miq. or related species, family Campanulaceae. Its main ingredients include taraxerone, carotene, daucosterol, β-sitosterol, octacosanoic acid and phospholipids. It is sweet and bland in taste and cool in nature and enters the Lung and Stomach channels. It is incompatible with *Li Lu* (Radix et Rhizoma Veratri).

Both *Bei Sha Shen* and *Nan Sha Shen* have the function of clearing Lung-heat and nourishing Lung Yin and can be used to treat damage to Yin in warm-febrile diseases, fever due to generalized deficiency and cough due to Yin deficiency. *Nan Sha Shen* is comparatively stronger than *Bei Sha Shen* in clearing the Lungs and dispelling Phlegm; it is frequently used for cough due to Lung-heat with sputum that is difficult to expectorate. *Bei Sha Shen* is more effective for moistening the Lungs and is used for dry cough without sputum due to insufficiency of Lung Yin and for deficiency taxation cough with Lung deficiency and expectoration of blood. Fresh *Nan Sha Shen* is moist in quality and is very good for clearing heat and generating body fluids; it is used for thirst due to damage to Yin in febrile diseases.

Mai Men Dong 麦门冬 (Ophiopogon root, Radix Ophiopogonis Japonici)

Mai Men Dong is the tuberous root of *Ophiopogon japonicus* (Thunb.) Ker-Gawl., family Liliaceae.

Main ingredients *Mai Men Dong* contains ophiopogonin, β-sitosterol, amino acids, glucose and glucosides.

Properties Taste: sweet and slightly bitter; nature: slightly cold.

Channels entered Lung, Heart and Stomach.

Functions and indications Nourishes Yin and moistens the Lungs, boosts the Stomach and generates body fluids, clears the Heart and eliminates vexation, moistens the Intestines and frees the bowels. It is indicated for dry cough due to dryness of the Lungs, coughing of blood, vomiting of blood due to pulmonary consumption, Lung Wei syndrome, damage to body fluids in febrile diseases, thirst and dry mouth, dry throat, vexation and insomnia, and Intestinal dryness with constipation.

Common dosage 10-15g.

Precautions and contraindications *Mai Men Dong* is contraindicated in cases of Phlegm-fluids and damp turbidity in the Lungs and Stomach, cough due to externally-contracted wind-cold, and diarrhoea due to Spleen deficiency.

Remarks Use *Mai Men Dong* without its core for nourishing Lung Yin and Stomach Yin; use the whole herb for clearing the Heart and eliminating vexation.

Comparison of functions Both *Mai Men Dong* (Radix Ophiopogonis Japonici) and *Sha Shen* (Radix Glehniae seu Adenophorae) can clear Lung-heat, nourish Lung Yin, moisten Lung dryness, and boost the Stomach, generate body fluids and allay thirst. They are often used in combination to treat dry cough with scant sputum due to Lung-heat and Yin deficiency, and for taxation cough with expectoration of blood; they are also used together for insufficiency of Stomach Yin, thirst due to damage to body fluids, reduced appetite, and retching. *Mai Men Dong* can also clear the Heart to eliminate vexation and quiet the Spirit; it is used for vexation, insomnia, palpitations and forgetfulness due to Yin deficiency with heat signs, and for night fever due to pathogenic heat invading the Ying level. *Nan Sha Shen* (Radix Adenophorae) can also dispel Phlegm and is used for dry cough with sticky sputum due to damage to body fluids.

For an additional comparison, see *Tian Men Dong* (Radix Asparagi Cochinchinensis).

Toxicity Mice fed an alcoholic extract of 0.45g of *Mai Men Dong* initially exhibited a reduction in activity but recovered to a normal state after half an hour. No deaths or adverse effects were reported after mice were given an intravenous injection in the tail of 1ml of *Mai Men Dong* (the equivalent of 100 times the normal dosage for humans).

Modern research

1. Inhibits the central nervous system to act as a tranquillizer; decoctions of *Mai Men Dong* inhibit convulsions [157]
2. Increases the nutritional blood supply in the cardiac muscle, inhibits arrhythmia.[157]
3. Raises the white blood cell count, inhibits inflammation, and expands the smooth muscle in the bronchus.[157]

Combinations and applications

Functions	Combinations	Applications
Nourishing Yin and moistening the Lungs	*Sang Ye* (Folium Mori Albae) *Shi Gao* (Gypsum Fibrosum) *Xing Ren* (Semen Pruni Armeniacae) *E Jiao* (Gelatinum Corii Asini) *Ren Shen* (Radix Ginseng)	Damage to Lung Qi and Lung Yin by warm-dry pathogenic factors, manifesting as fever and headache, dry cough without sputum, wheezing due to counterflow Qi, thirst and dry throat, and a dry tongue with no fur
	Sheng Di Huang (Radix Rehmanniae Glutinosae) *Xuan Shen* (Radix Scrophulariae Ningpoensis) *Mu Dan Pi* (Cortex Moutan Radicis) *Bo He* (Herba Menthae Haplocalycis) *Chuan Bei Mu* (Bulbus Fritillariae Cirrhosae)	Diphtheria with spots on the tonsils, sore throat, fever, dry nose and lips, rapid pulse
	Sheng Di Huang (Radix Rehmanniae Glutinosae) *Shu Di Huang* (Radix Rehmanniae Glutinosae Conquita) *Bai He* (Bulbus Lilii) *Bai Shao* (Radix Paeoniae Lactiflorae) *Dang Gui* (Radix Angelicae Sinensis) *Bai Bu* (Radix Stemonae)	Sore and dry throat, coughing and wheezing, blood-streaked sputum, taxation cough, heat in the palms and soles, a red tongue with sparse fur and a fine, rapid pulse due to deficiency-fire flaming upwards caused by Yin deficiency of the Lungs and Kidneys
	Tian Men Dong (Radix Asparagi Cochinchinensis) *Feng Mi* (Mel)	Vomiting of blood due to pulmonary consumption, or dry cough with blood-streaked sputum

Boosting the Stomach and generating body fluids	*Ren Shen* (Radix Ginseng) *Ban Xia* (Rhizoma Pinelliae Ternatae) *Gan Cao* (Radix Glycyrrhizae)	Lung Wei syndrome, coughing and wheezing, shortness of breath, dry mouth and throat and a deficient and rapid pulse due to insufficiency of Stomach Yin and deficiency-fire flaming upwards and damaging Lung Yin
	Yu Zhu (Rhizoma Polygonati Odorati) *Sheng Di Huang* (Radix Rehmanniae Glutinosae) *Bei Sha Shen* (Radix Glehniae Littoralis)	Damage to Yin after seasonal febrile diseases, manifesting as thirst and dry throat, fatigued body and lack of strength, vexation in the Heart and a deficient and rapid pulse
	Ze Xie (Rhizoma Alismatis Orientalis) *Che Qian Zi* (Semen Plantaginis) *Huang Lian* (Rhizoma Coptidis) *Mu Li* (Concha Ostreae) *Sang Piao Xiao* (Oötheca Mantidis)	Incessant wasting and thirsting, vexation and thirst drawing fluid intake, frequent urination and lack of strength in the limbs
Clearing the Heart and eliminating vexation	*Sheng Di Huang* (Radix Rehmanniae Glutinosae) *Dan Zhu Ye* (Herba Lophatheri Gracilis) *Huang Lian* (Rhizoma Coptidis) *Xuan Shen* (Radix Scrophulariae Ningpoensis) *Mu Dan Pi* (Cortex Moutan Radicis)	Pathogenic heat invading the Ying level in seasonal febrile diseases, night fever, vexation and agitation, a red tongue and a fine, rapid pulse
	Suan Zao Ren (Semen Ziziphi Spinosae) *Sheng Di Huang* (Radix Rehmanniae Glutinosae) *Zhi Mu* (Rhizoma Anemarrhenae Asphodeloidis) *Tian Men Dong* (Radix Asparagi Cochinchinensis) *Dang Gui* (Radix Angelicae Sinensis)	Fever due to Yin deficiency, palpitations, vexation and insomnia, profuse dreaming
	Ren Shen (Radix Ginseng) *Wu Wei Zi* (Fructus Schisandrae)	Depletion of Qi and Yin, manifesting as fatigued limbs, shortness of breath, palpitations and insomnia, profuse sweating and thirst, dry mouth with a desire to drink, accompanied by a bound or regularly interrupted pulse and a pale red tongue
Moistening the Intestines and freeing the bowels	*Sheng Di Huang* (Radix Rehmanniae Glutinosae) *Xuan Shen* (Radix Scrophulariae Ningpoensis)	Yangming-type seasonal febrile diseases, insufficiency of the Essence and body fluids, constipation, thirst, a dry and red tongue and a fine, rapid pulse

Bie Jia 鳖甲 (Chinese soft-shelled turtle shell, Carapax Amydae Sinensis)

Bie Jia is the shell of *Amyda sinensis* (Wiegmann), also known as *Trionyx sinensis* (Wiegmann), family Trionychidae.

Legal status *Bie Jia* is a restricted substance listed in Appendix I of the Convention on International Trade in Endangered Species of Wild Fauna and Flora (CITES). All trade in this materia medica is presently banned.

Main ingredients *Bie Jia* contains collagen, keratin, iodine, vitamin D, calcium phosphate and calcium carbonate.

Properties Taste: salty; nature: cold.

Channels entered Liver, Spleen and Kidney.

Functions and indications Nourishes Yin and clears heat, subdues Yang and extinguishes wind, softens hardness and dissipates lumps. It is indicated for fever due to Yin deficiency, steaming bone disorder, night sweating, damage to Yin in febrile diseases, deficiency-wind stirring internally, malaria, menstrual block, abdominal masses, and child fright epilepsy.

Common dosage 10-30g; decocted for 30 minutes before adding other substances.

Precautions and contraindications *Bie Jia* is contraindicated in cases of Spleen and Stomach deficiency-cold, loose stool and reduced appetite, and during pregnancy.

Remarks Raw *Bie Jia* is used for nourishing Yin and subduing Yang, whereas *Bie Jia* mix-fried with vinegar is effective for softening hardness and dissipating lumps.

Comparison of functions See *Gui Ban* (Plastrum Testudinis).

Modern research

1. Inhibits the generation of connective tissue, thus dissipating masses.[158]
2. Increases plasma protein, thus inhibiting anaemia in hepatic diseases.[159]

Combinations and applications

Functions	Combinations	Applications
Nourishing Yin and clearing heat	*Qing Hao* (Herba Artemisiae Chinghao) *Sheng Di Huang* (Radix Rehmanniae Glutinosae) *Zhi Mu* (Rhizoma Anemarrhenae Asphodeloidis) *Mu Dan Pi* (Cortex Moutan Radicis)	Final stage of febrile diseases with damage to Yin, manifesting as night fever abating at dawn, emaciation despite intake of food, a red tongue with sparse fur, and a rapid pulse
	Gui Ban (Plastrum Testudinis) (see notes on legal status) *Mu Li* (Concha Ostreae) *Bai Wei* (Radix Cynanchi Atrati)	Non-abating slight fever and vexing heat in the five hearts due to Qi and Yin deficiency in the final stage of warm diseases
	Yin Chai Hu (Radix Stellariae Dichotomae) *Zhi Mu* (Rhizoma Anemarrhenae Asphodeloidis) *Hu Huang Lian* (Rhizoma Picrorhizae Scrophulariiflorae) *Di Gu Pi* (Cortex Lycii Radicis) *Qin Jiao* (Radix Gentianae Macrophyllae)	Non-abating slight fever due to Yin deficiency of the Liver and Kidneys; or night sweating, steaming bone disorder and emaciation due to intense heat pathogenic factors with red lips and a red face, and a fine, rapid pulse

	Ren Shen (Radix Ginseng) *Huang Qi* (Radix Astragali seu Hedysari) *Sang Bai Pi* (Cortex Mori Albae Radicis) *Zi Wan* (Radix Asteris Tatarici) *Jie Geng* (Radix Platycodi Grandiflori) *Zhi Mu* (Rhizoma Anemarrhenae Asphodeloidis)	Steaming bone disorder, taxation fever and deficiency taxation cough due to deficiency-heat in the Lungs and Yin deficiency with scant Blood
Subduing Yang and extinguishing wind	*Shu Di Huang* (Radix Rehmanniae Glutinosae Conquita) *Bai Shao* (Radix Paeoniae Lactiflorae) *Mu Li* (Concha Ostreae) *E Jiao* (Gelatinum Corii Asini) *Mai Men Dong* (Radix Ophiopogonis Japonici)	Deficiency-wind stirring internally due to damage to Yin in the final stage of seasonal febrile diseases, manifesting as a dry tongue with black teeth, spasms in the fingers, or fright epilepsy, with a sunken and rapid pulse
	Feng Mi (Mel)	Child fright epilepsy
Softening hardness and dissipating lumps	*Mu Dan Pi* (Cortex Moutan Radicis) *Chai Hu* (Radix Bupleuri) *Bai Shao* (Radix Paeoniae Lactiflorae) *Tao Ren* (Semen Persicae)	Malaria with an enlarged liver and spleen and a soot-black facial complexion
	Zhi Mu (Rhizoma Anemarrhenae Asphodeloidis) *Chang Shan* (Radix Dichroae Febrifugae) *Dan Zhu Ye* (Herba Lophatheri Gracilis) *Di Gu Pi* (Cortex Lycii Radicis) *Shi Gao* (Gypsum Fibrosum)	Lingering malarial conditions
	Da Huang (Radix et Rhizoma Rhei) *Hu Po* (Succinum)	Abdominal masses due to Qi stagnation and Blood stasis, menstrual block, pain in the abdomen

Gui Ban 龟板
(Freshwater turtle plastron, Plastrum Testudinis)

Gui Ban is the plastron of *Chinemys reevesii* (Gray), family Testudinidae.

Legal status *Gui Ban* is a restricted substance listed in Appendix II of the Convention on International Trade in Endangered Species of Wild Fauna and Flora (CITES). Appropriate import and export permits are required for trade in this materia medica.

Main ingredients *Gui Ban* contains collagen, keratin, proteins, amino acids and calcium salts.

Properties Taste: sweet and salty; nature: cold.

Channels entered Liver, Kidney and Heart.

Functions and indications Enriches Yin and subdues Yang, boosts the Kidneys and strengthens the bones, supplements the Blood and nourishes the Heart, secures the menses and stops uterine bleeding. It is indicated for damage to Yin in seasonal febrile diseases, deficiency-wind stirring internally, ascendant hyperactivity of Liver Yang manifesting as dizziness and tinnitus, steaming bone disorder, pain in the lumbar region due to Kidney deficiency, vomiting of blood, spitting of blood, uterine bleeding, palpitations, insomnia, and forgetfulness.

Common dosage 10-30g, broken up and decocted for 30 minutes before adding other substances.

Precautions and contraindications

1. *Gui Ban* is contraindicated in cases of damp-cold in the Stomach.
2. According to the ancient canons, *Gui Ban* can soften hardness and dissipate masses to aid in difficult labour; it is therefore also contraindicated during pregnancy.

Comparison of functions Both *Gui Ban* (Plastrum Testudinis) and *Bie Jia* (Carapax Amydae Sinensis) are important substances for enriching Yin and subduing Yang; they are often used in combination for Yin deficiency with Yang hyperactivity. *Gui Ban* is stronger in enriching Yin and can also boost the Kidneys and strengthen the bones, and supplement the Blood and nourish the Heart. *Bie Jia* is more effective for abating fever, and is also better than *Gui Ban* for softening hardness and dissipating stasis. In addition, it can be used for abdominal masses, enduring malaria and menstrual block.

Toxicity The LD_{50} for *Gui Ban* cannot be tested, since its toxicity is too low.

Modern research

1. Inhibits Mycobacterium tuberculosis.[160]
2. Strengthens the immune function.[160]
3. Regulates the synthesis of nucleic acid in the liver and spleen.[161]

Combinations and applications

Functions	Combinations	Applications
Enriching Yin and subduing Yang	*E Jiao* (Gelatinum Corii Asini) *Sheng Di Huang* (Radix Rehmanniae Glutinosae) *Mu Li* (Concha Ostreae) *Bai Shao* (Radix Paeoniae Lactiflorae) *Ji Zi Huang* (raw egg yolk)	Damage to Yin in seasonal febrile diseases and deficiency-wind stirring internally, manifesting as dizziness, fatigued body, vexation or fright epilepsy, with a deficient and weak pulse and a crimson tongue with sparse fur
	Sheng Di Huang (Radix Rehmanniae Glutinosae) *Shi Jue Ming* (Concha Haliotidis) *Ju Hua* (Flos Chrysanthemi Morifolii) *Gou Teng* (Ramulus Uncariae cum Uncis)	Ascendant hyperactivity of Liver Yang, manifesting as dizziness and tinnitus, and a string-like and rapid pulse
	Niu Xi (Radix Achyranthis Bidentatae) *Dai Zhe Shi* (Haematitum) *Long Gu* (Os Draconis) *Xuan Shen* (Radix Scrophulariae Ningpoensis) *Bai Shao* (Radix Paeoniae Lactiflorae) *Tian Men Dong* (Radix Asparagi Cochinchinensis)	Liver-wind stirring internally due to Yin deficiency, manifesting as gradual disablement of the limbs, facial spasms, or dizziness with possible falls or unconsciousness, and a string-like, long and forceful pulse
	Huang Bai (Cortex Phellodendri) *Zhi Mu* (Rhizoma Anemarrhenae Asphodeloidis) *Shu Di Huang* (Radix Rehmanniae Glutinosae Conquita)	Yin deficiency of the Liver and Kidneys and deficiency-fire flaming upwards, manifesting as steaming bone disorder, night sweating, seminal emission, cough with or without blood, pain and heat in the feet and knees

	Bie Jia (Carapax Amydae Sinensis) (see notes on legal status) *Mu Li* (Concha Ostreae) *Bai Shao* (Radix Paeoniae Lactiflorae) *Sheng Di Huang* (Radix Rehmanniae Glutinosae) *E Jiao* (Gelatinum Corii Asini)	Spasms of the hands and feet due to improper nourishment of the sinews and vessels, depletion of body fluids and Yin deficiency
	Gou Qi Zi (Fructus Lycii) *Ren Shen* (Radix Ginseng) *Lu Jiao* (Cornu Cervi)	Dream emission, seminal emission, emaciation and blurred vision due to effulgent Yin deficiency-fire
Boosting the Kidneys and strengthening the bones	*Shu Di Huang* (Radix Rehmanniae Glutinosae Conquita) *Niu Xi* (Radix Achyranthis Bidentatae) *Suo Yang* (Herba Cynomorii Songarici) *Bai Shao* (Radix Paeoniae Lactiflorae) *Huang Bai* (Cortex Phellodendri)	Limpness and aching in the lumbar region and knees, Wei syndrome of the sinews and bones, lack of strength in the legs and feet, difficulty in walking, and a red tongue with sparse fur due to effulgent Yin deficiency-fire and failure to nourish the sinews and bones
Supplementing the Blood and nourishing the Heart	*Shi Chang Pu* (Rhizoma Acori Graminei) *Yuan Zhi* (Radix Polygalae) *Long Gu* (Os Draconis)	Palpitations, insomnia and forgetfulness due to improper nourishment of the Heart as a result of Blood deficiency
Securing the menses and stopping uterine bleeding	*Mu Li* (Concha Ostreae)	Profuse menstruation and uterine bleeding due to Blood-heat caused by Yin deficiency

Appendix

Gui Ban Jiao **龟板胶 (Freshwater turtle plastron glue, Gelatinum Plastri Testudinis)**

Gui Ban Jiao is the concentrated glue obtained by boiling the plastron of *Gui Ban*. As with *Gui Ban*, *Gui Ban Jiao* requires appropriate permits for trade. *Gui Ban Jiao* is sweet and salty in taste and neutral in nature. It can enrich Yin and supplement the Blood, and stop bleeding. It is used for Blood depletion and Yin deficiency, steaming bone disorder, coughing of blood, bleeding, palpitations and vexation, pain in the lumbar region due to Kidney deficiency, weakness of the feet and knees, and uterine bleeding. It is contraindicated for damp-cold in the Stomach.

Gou Qi Zi 枸杞子 (Wolfberry fruit, Fructus Lycii)

Gou Qi Zi is the fruit of *Lycium barbarum* L. or *L. chinense* Mill., family Solanaceae.

Main ingredients *Gou Qi Zi* contains betaine, carotene, thiamine, riboflavin, nicotinic acid, ascorbic acid, β-sitosterol, linoleic acid, physalien, atropine and scopoletin.

Properties Taste: sweet; nature: neutral.

Channels entered Liver, Kidney and Lung.

Functions and indications Enriches the Kidneys and supplements the Liver, brightens the eyes, and moistens the Lungs. It is indicated for limpness and aching in the lumbar region and knees due to

Yin deficiency of the Liver and Kidneys, dizziness, blurred vision, consumption cough, wasting and thirsting, and seminal emission.

Common dosage 5-10g.

Precautions and contraindications *Gou Qi Zi* is contraindicated in cases of full-heat due to external pathogenic factors, dampness due to Spleen deficiency, and diarrhoea.

Remarks *Gou Qi Zi* is an important herb for enriching the Kidneys and supplementing the Liver since it can moderately supplement Yin and Yang of the Liver and Kidneys. It is used for disorders due to Essence depletion, deficiency and overwork.

Toxicity *Gou Qi Zi* has a very low level of toxicity. The LD_{50} for subcutaneous injection in mice of aqueous extracts of the herb is 8.32g/kg.

Modern research

1. Strengthens the immune function and inhibits carcinoma.[162, 163]
2. Increases the testosterone level to strengthen the body and slow the ageing process.[164]
3. Lowers blood pressure, reduces the level of blood lipids, lowers the blood sugar level and stimulates respiration.[165]
4. Decoctions of *Gou Qi Zi* strengthen uterine contractions.[166]

Combinations and applications

Functions	Combinations	Applications
Enriching the Kidneys and supplementing the Liver, brightening the eyes	*Sheng Di Huang* (Radix Rehmanniae Glutinosae) *Tian Men Dong* (Radix Asparagi Cochinchinensis)	Limpness and aching in the lumbar region and knees, seminal emission and a sunken, fine and rapid pulse due to Yin deficiency of the Liver and Kidneys
	Sheng Di Huang (Radix Rehmanniae Glutinosae) *Gui Ban* (Plastrum Testudinis) (see notes on legal status) *Xu Duan* (Radix Dipsaci) *Niu Xi* (Radix Achyranthis Bidentatae)	Wei syndrome of the bones due to Kidney deficiency, aching in the lumbar region and knees
	Huang Qi (Radix Astragali seu Hedysari) *Ren Shen* (Radix Ginseng) *Dang Gui* (Radix Angelicae Sinensis) *Bai Shao* (Radix Paeoniae Lactiflorae)	Frequent urination and thirst due to depletion of Kidney Qi
	Tu Si Zi (Semen Cuscutae) *Wu Wei Zi* (Fructus Schisandrae) *Fu Pen Zi* (Fructus Rubi Chingii) *Che Qian Zi* (Semen Plantaginis)	Kidney deficiency with such manifestations as scant semen, impotence, premature ejaculation, seminal emission, seminal cold or infertility
	Ju Hua (Flos Chrysanthemi Morifolii) *Shu Di Huang* (Radix Rehmanniae Glutinosae Conquita) *Shan Zhu Yu* (Fructus Corni Officinalis) *Fu Ling* (Sclerotium Poriae Cocos) *Ze Xie* (Rhizoma Alismatis Orientalis)	Dizziness and blurred vision with a sunken and fine pulse due to Yin deficiency of the Liver and Kidneys

	Shu Di Huang (Radix Rehmanniae Glutinosae Conquita) *Tu Si Zi* (Semen Cuscutae) *Gui Ban Jiao* (Gelatinum Plastri Testudinis) (see notes on legal status) *Niu Xi* (Radix Achyranthis Bidentatae)	Dizziness, deafness, spontaneous sweating, night sweating and internal heat due to insufficiency of the Liver and Kidneys
	Bei Sha Shen (Radix Glehniae Littoralis) *Mai Men Dong* (Radix Ophiopogonis Japonici) *Dang Gui* (Radix Angelicae Sinensis) *Sheng Di Huang* (Radix Rehmanniae Glutinosae) *Chuan Lian Zi* (Fructus Meliae Toosendan)	Pain in the stomach and hypochondrium, acid regurgitation and dry mouth and throat due to Yin deficiency of the Liver and Kidneys with constrained Liver Qi, reduced body fluids, a red tongue, and a deficient, string-like pulse
Moistening the Lungs	*Chuan Bei Mu* (Bulbus Fritillariae Cirrhosae) *Zhi Mu* (Rhizoma Anemarrhenae Asphodeloidis) *Mai Men Dong* (Radix Ophiopogonis Japonici)	Enduring cough with scant sputum or blood in the sputum, and tidal fever due to Lung Yin deficiency in enduring diseases

Tian Men Dong 天门冬
(Lucid asparagus root, Radix Asparagi Cochinchinensis)

Tian Men Dong is the dried tuberous root of *Asparagus cochinchinensis* (Lour.) Merr., family Liliaceae.

Main ingredients *Tian Men Dong* contains asparagine, citrulline, serine, threonine, proline, glycine, amino acids, β-sitosterol, smilagenin, glucose, pectin and oligosaccharides.

Properties Taste: sweet and bitter; nature: very cold.

Channels entered Lung and Kidney.

Functions and indications Nourishes Yin and clears heat, moistens dryness and generates body fluids. It is indicated for Lung-heat due to Yin deficiency, cough with or without blood, sore throat, wasting and thirsting, and constipation.

Common dosage 6-15g.

Precautions and contraindications *Tian Men Dong* is contraindicated in cases of Spleen and Stomach deficiency-cold with reduced appetite and loose stool.

Comparison of functions *Tian Men Dong* (Radix Asparagi Cochinchinensis), *Mai Men Dong* (Radix Ophiopogonis Japonici) and *Bai He* (Bulbus Lilii) can all nourish Yin, moisten dryness and generate body fluids, and are effective in supplementing Lung Yin to clear heat. They can be used to treat dry cough and coughing of blood due to insufficiency of Lung Yin, dry throat and thirst due to damage to body fluids in febrile diseases, Intestinal dryness with constipation, and wasting and thirsting due to internal heat. They are often used in combination.

Mai Men Dong can also boost the Stomach to stop vomiting and clear the Heart to eliminate vexation in order to treat dry mouth and thirst due to insufficiency of Stomach Yin, night fever due to pathogenic heat invading the Ying level in warm-febrile diseases, vexation and agitation, and palpitations and insomnia due to Yin deficiency with heat signs. *Tian Men Dong* has a stronger effect in clearing heat and moistening dryness and can also enrich and nourish Kidney Yin to treat tidal fever and night sweating due to insufficiency of Kidney Yin. *Bai He* can clear the Heart and quiet the Spirit and is often used for damage to Yin in febrile diseases, deficiency vexation and palpitations due to insufficiency of Qi and body fluids, and insomnia and profuse dreaming.

Modern research

1. A decoction of *Tian Men Dong* inhibited such pathogenic micro-organisms as Bacillus anthracis, α- and β-haemolytic streptococci, Corynebacterium diphtheriae and Staphylococcus aureus *in vitro*.[167]
2. Inhibits carcinoma.[168]
3. Dilates external blood vessels, lowers blood pressure, strengthens heart contractions, slows the heart rate and reduces the amount of urine produced.[169]

Combinations and applications

Functions	Combinations	Applications
Nourishing Yin and clearing heat	*Mai Men Dong* (Radix Ophiopogonis Japonici) *Bai Bu* (Radix Stemonae)	Dry cough, sore throat and coughing of blood due to Lung-heat caused by Yin deficiency
	Bai He (Bulbus Lilii) *Chuan Bei Mu* (Bulbus Fritillariae Cirrhosae) *Jie Geng* (Radix Platycodi Grandiflori) *Sang Bai Pi* (Cortex Mori Albae Radicis)	Cough with sticky sputum that is difficult to expectorate due to Phlegm-heat congesting the Lungs and damage to body fluids
	Sheng Di Huang (Radix Rehmanniae Glutinosae) *Nan Sha Shen* (Radix Adenophorae) *Bai Bu* (Radix Stemonae) *Tian Hua Fen* (Radix Trichosanthis)	Wasting and thirsting due to body fluids being consumed by internal heat
	Jie Geng (Radix Platycodi Grandiflori) *Shan Dou Gen* (Radix Sophorae Tonkinensis) *Ban Lan Gen* (Radix Isatidis seu Baphicacanthi) *Niu Bang Zi* (Fructus Arctii Lappae)	Sore throat due to heat toxins
	Dong Gua Ren (Semen Benincasae Hispidae) *Tao Ren* (Semen Persicae) *Yi Yi Ren* (Semen Coicis Lachrymajobi) *Yu Xing Cao* (Herba Houttuyniae Cordatae) *Jie Geng* (Radix Platycodi Grandiflori)	Lung abscess
Moistening dryness and generating body fluids	*Xuan Shen* (Radix Scrophulariae Ningpoensis) *Mai Men Dong* (Radix Ophiopogonis Japonici) *Sheng Di Huang* (Radix Rehmanniae Glutinosae) *Huo Ma Ren* (Semen Cannabis Sativae)	Constipation due to Yin deficiency and dryness of the Large Intestine

Bai He 百合
(Lily bulb, Bulbus Lilii)

Bai He is the dried bulb of *Lilium lancifolium* Thunb., *L. brownii* F. E. Brown var. *viridulum* Baker or *L. pumilum* DC., family Liliaceae.

Main ingredients *Bai He* contains regalosides, lilioside, brownioside, alkaloids, starch, proteins, fats and colchiceine.

Properties Taste: sweet and bland; nature: slightly cold.

Channels entered Heart and Lung.

Functions and indications Moistens the Lungs and stops coughing, clears the Heart and quiets the Spirit. It is indicated for cough due to dryness in the Lungs, damage to Yin in febrile diseases, insomnia, and palpitations.

Common dosage 10-30g.

Precautions and contraindications *Bai He* is contraindicated in cases of cough due to wind-cold or loose stool due to cold in the Middle Jiao.

Comparison of functions Both *Bai He* (Bulbus Lilii) and *Yu Zhu* (Rhizoma Polygonati Odorati) enter the Lung channel; they can moisten the Lungs and enrich Yin and clear heat and generate body fluids. *Bai He* also enters the Heart channel and can clear heat from the Heart and quiet the Spirit. It is used for deficiency vexation and fright palpitations, insomnia and profuse dreaming. It is a key herb for treating lily disease (Yin deficiency of the Heart and Lungs due to depression binding of the seven emotions or during convalescence after a severe illness). *Yu Zhu* concurrently enters the Stomach channel and is good at enriching Stomach Yin, moistening Stomach dryness and generating body fluids to allay thirst. It is often used for damage to Yin in febrile diseases, depletion of body fluids, and thirst due to vexation heat.

For additional comparisons, see *Tian Men Dong* (Radix Asparagi Cochinchinensis) and *Bai Bu* (Radix Stemonae).

Modern research

1. Stops coughing, expels sputum, has a tranquilizing function, and strengthens the body.[170]
2. The colchiceine contained in *Bai He* inhibits the degeneration of carcinoma cells.[171]

Combinations and applications

Functions	Combinations	Applications
Moistening the Lungs and stopping coughing	*Sheng Di Huang* (Radix Rehmanniae Glutinosae) *Xuan Shen* (Radix Scrophulariae Ningpoensis) *Zhe Bei Mu* (Bulbus Fritillariae Thunbergii) *Mai Men Dong* (Radix Ophiopogonis Japonici)	Enduring, dry cough or coughing of blood with fever and night sweating due to dryness in the Lungs damaging Yin
	Kuan Dong Hua (Flos Tussilaginis Farfarae)	Lung-heat manifesting as enduring cough damaging Yin accompanied by blood-streaked sputum
Clearing the Heart and quieting the Spirit	*Sheng Di Huang* (Radix Rehmanniae Glutinosae) *Zhi Mu* (Rhizoma Anemarrhenae Asphodeloidis)	Febrile diseases damaging Yin with insufficiency of Qi and body fluids, manifesting as vexation and thirst, deficiency vexation and fright palpitations, insomnia and profuse dreaming

Shi Hu 石斛
(Dendrobium, Herba Dendrobii)

Shi Hu is the fresh or dried stem of *Dendrobium loddigesii* Rolfe., *D. chrysanthum* Wall., *D. fimbriatum* Hook. var. *oculatum* Hook., *D. nobile* Lindl. or *D. candidum* Wall. ex Lindl., family Orchidaceae.

Legal status *Shi Hu* is a restricted substance listed in Appendix II of the Convention on International Trade in Endangered Species of Wild Fauna and Flora (CITES). Appropriate import and export permits are required for trade in this materia medica.

Main ingredients *Shi Hu* contains alkaloids (including dendrobine, nobiline, dendroxine and dendramine), starch and dendrin.

Properties Taste: sweet and bland; nature: slightly cold.

Channels entered Stomach and Kidney.

Functions and indications Enriches Yin and abates fever, nourishes the Stomach and generates body fluids, and brightens the eyes. It is indicated for vexation and thirst due to damage to body fluids in febrile diseases, fever due to Yin deficiency, weakness in the lumbar region and legs, pain in the stomach, and blurred vision due to Yin deficiency.

Common dosage 6-15g, or 15-30g of the fresh herb, decocted before other herbs.

Precautions and contraindications

1. Since *Shi Hu* can constrain pathogenic factors, it should not be used in the initial stage of warm-febrile diseases.
2. Since *Shi Hu* can also reinforce dampness, it is contraindicated for warm-damp patterns before warm-damp transforms to dryness, and in cases of thin, loose stool and thick, slimy tongue fur.

Comparison of functions *Shi Hu* (Herba Dendrobii), *Sha Shen* (Radix Glehniae seu Adenophorae) and *Yu Zhu* (Rhizoma Polygonati Odorati) all enter the Stomach channel. They can clear heat, enrich Yin and generate body fluids to treat damage to body fluids in febrile diseases or insufficiency of Stomach Yin, dry mouth and thirst. *Sha Shen* and *Yu Zhu* also enter the Lung channel; they can nourish Lung Yin and moisten Lung dryness to treat dry cough due to Yin deficiency.

Sha Shen is good at clearing the Lungs and moistening dryness to stop coughing in order to treat patterns of heat damaging Lung Yin with such manifestations as dry cough with scant sputum, enduring cough and hoarse voice, and blood-streaked sputum. *Yu Zhu* is better for enriching and moistening to nourish Yin without cloying. It is used for Yin deficiency patterns, externally-contracted wind-heat, fever and headache, cough, sore throat and thirst. *Shi Hu* is very effective for clearing heat and is frequently employed for damage to Yin and body fluids in febrile diseases. It can also enrich Kidney Yin and abate deficiency fever and is often used for depletion of body fluids due to Yin deficiency and non-abating of deficiency fever.

Modern research

1. Helps prevent cataracts.[172-174]
2. Strengthens the immune function.[175]

Combinations and applications

Functions	Combinations	Applications
Enriching Yin and abating fever	*Sheng Di Huang* (Radix Rehmanniae Glutinosae) *Mai Men Dong* (Radix Ophiopogonis Japonici) *Tian Hua Fen* (Radix Trichosanthis) *Yu Zhu* (Rhizoma Polygonati Odorati)	Slight fever with vexation and thirst, dry mouth and throat, and a red tongue with scant fur due to damage to body fluids in febrile diseases

	Mai Men Dong (Radix Ophiopogonis Japonici) *Sheng Di Huang* (Radix Rehmanniae Glutinosae) *Xuan Shen* (Radix Scrophulariae Ningpoensis)	Yin deficiency and depletion of body fluids associated with insufficiency of Kidney Yin, manifesting as non-abating deficiency fever, dry and sore throat, a red tongue and scant body fluids
	Niu Xi (Radix Achyranthis Bidentatae) *Sheng Di Huang* (Radix Rehmanniae Glutinosae) *Gou Qi Zi* (Fructus Lycii) *Mu Gua* (Fructus Chaenomelis) *Bai Shao* (Radix Paeoniae Lactiflorae) *Suan Zao Ren* (Semen Ziziphi Spinosae)	Aching in the lumbar region and pain in the legs due to depletion and deficiency of Yin and Blood and insufficiency of the Liver and Kidneys
Nourishing the Stomach and generating body fluids	*Huo Xiang* (Herba Agastaches seu Pogostemi) *Mu Dan Pi* (Cortex Moutan Radicis) *Chen Pi* (Pericarpium Citri Reticulatae)	Pain in the stomach
	Sha Shen (Radix Glehniae seu Adenophorae) *Bai Bian Dou* (Semen Dolichoris Lablab) *Mai Men Dong* (Radix Ophiopogonis Japonici) *Bai Shao* (Radix Paeoniae Lactiflorae) *Zhu Ru* (Caulis Bambusae in Taeniis)	No desire for food and drink, abdominal discomfort, dull or scorching pain in the stomach, dry retching or belching, with a smooth tongue and scant fur due to insufficiency of Stomach Yin in a variety of diseases
Brightening the eyes	*Gou Qi Zi* (Fructus Lycii) *Ju Hua* (Flos Chrysanthemi Morifolii) *Shu Di Huang* (Radix Rehmanniae Glutinosae Conquita) *Sheng Di Huang* (Radix Rehmanniae Glutinosae) *Tu Si Zi* (Semen Cuscutae) *Mai Men Dong* (Radix Ophiopogonis Japonici) *Jue Ming Zi* (Semen Cassiae)	Blurred vision due to improper nourishment of the eyes caused by Yin deficiency of the Liver and Kidneys

Yu Zhu 玉竹
(Fragrant Solomon seal rhizome, Rhizoma Polygonati Odorati)

Yu Zhu is the dried rhizome of *Polygonatum odoratum* (Mill.) Druce (also known as *Polygonatum officinale* All.), family Liliaceae.

Main ingredients *Yu Zhu* contains convallamarin, convallarin, quercitol, holosides and vitamin A.

Properties Taste: sweet; nature: slightly cold.

Channels entered Lung and Stomach.

Functions and indications Enriches Yin and moistens dryness, generates body fluids and allays thirst. It is indicated for cough, dry throat and thirst, fever, headache, and externally-contracted pathogenic factors in Yin deficiency patterns.

Common dosage 10-15g.

Precautions and contraindications Since *Yu Zhu* is moistening and slightly cold, it is contraindicated in cases of Spleen and Stomach deficiency, Phlegm-damp brewing internally, or loose stool due to cold in the Middle Jiao.

Remarks Use raw *Yu Zhu* for clearing heat; use the herb processed with wine for enriching Yin and moistening the Lungs and Stomach.

Comparison of functions Both *Yu Zhu* (Rhizoma Polygonati Odorati) and *Huang Jing* (Rhizoma Polygonati) are sweet and can enrich Yin and moisten the Lungs to treat dry cough due to Lung deficiency; they can also boost the Stomach and nourish Yin to treat Yin damage of the Spleen and Stomach, dry mouth and reduced appetite, dry stool, and red tongue with scant fur. *Yu Zhu* is slightly cold and tends to enrich Yin to generate body fluids; it is often used for dry cough and dry mouth with scant body fluids. It nourishes Yin without cloying to treat cough with fever, sore throat and thirst. *Huang Jing* is neutral but cloying. It can boost Qi and enrich Yin and is an important herb for supplementing the Lungs, Spleen and Kidneys to treat reduced appetite and fatigue due to Qi deficiency of the Spleen and Stomach, limpness and aching in the lumbar region and knees, dizziness, and premature greying due to Kidney deficiency and Essence depletion.

For additional comparisons, see *Bai He* (Bulbus Lilii) and *Shi Hu* (Herba Dendrobii).

Modern research

1. Lowers blood pressure and strengthens the heart, protects the heart against acute cardiac ischaemia.[176]
2. Relieves arteriosclerosis.[176]
3. Strengthens the immune function and lowers the blood sugar level.[176]

Combinations and applications

Functions	Combinations	Applications
Enriching Yin and moistening dryness, generating body fluids and allaying thirst	*Nan Sha Shen* (Radix Adenophorae) *Mai Men Dong* (Radix Ophiopogonis Japonici)	Dry cough with scant sputum, dry throat and thirst and a red tongue due to dry-heat damaging the Lungs
	Sha Shen (Radix Glehniae seu Adenophorae) *Sheng Di Huang* (Radix Rehmanniae Glutinosae) *Mai Men Dong* (Radix Ophiopogonis Japonici) *Bing Tang* (Saccharon Crystallinum)	Vexation heat and thirst, dry mouth and tongue due to depletion and consumption of body fluids and damage to Stomach Yin in febrile diseases
	Bai Wei (Radix Cynanchi Atrati) *Jie Geng* (Radix Platycodi Grandiflori) *Bo He* (Herba Menthae Haplocalycis) *Cong Bai* (Bulbus Allii Fistulosi)	Externally-contracted wind-heat, fever, headache, slight aversion to cold, vexation and thirst with a dry tongue and a floating and rapid pulse in patients with Yin deficiency patterns

Huang Jing 黄精
(Siberian Solomon seal rhizome, Rhizoma Polygonati)

Huang Jing is the dried rhizome of *Polygonatum sibiricum* Red., *P. kingianum* Coll. et Hemsl. or *P. cyrtonema* Hua, family Liliaceae.

Main ingredients *Huang Jing* contains alkaloids, nicotinic acid, aspartic acid, homoserine, digitalis glycoside, starch and sugars.

Properties Taste: sweet; nature: neutral.
Channels entered Spleen, Lung and Kidney.
Functions and indications Enriches Yin and moistens the Lungs, supplements the Spleen and boosts Qi. It is indicated for dry cough due to Lung Yin deficiency, limpness and aching in the lumbar region and knees, tidal fever, fatigue and poor appetite due to Qi deficiency of the Spleen and Stomach, and wasting and thirsting.
Common dosage 10-20g, or 30-60g of the fresh herb.
Precautions and contraindications The enriching and cloying properties of *Huang Jing* mean that it can reinforce dampness and obstruct the Stomach; it is therefore contraindicated in cases of congestion and stagnation of Phlegm-damp, loose stool due to cold in the Middle Jiao, or distension of the abdomen due to Qi stagnation.
Comparison of functions Both *Huang Jing* (Rhizoma Polygonati) and *Shan Yao* (Rhizoma Dioscoreae Oppositae) are sweet and neutral and enter the Spleen, Lung and Kidney channels. They can neutrally supplement these three channels, boost Qi and nourish Yin to treat dry cough due to Lung deficiency, reduced appetite and fatigue due to Spleen deficiency, pain in the lumbar region due to Kidney deficiency, and wasting and thirsting. *Shan Yao* is also suitable for loose stool due to Spleen deficiency and coughing and wheezing due to Lung deficiency; in addition, as it has an astringent function, it can secure the Essence, reduce urine and stop vaginal discharge. *Huang Jing* is better than *Shan Yao* in terms of enriching Yin and moistening dryness. It is often used for dry cough due to Yin deficiency, dry mouth and reduced appetite, and dry stool and a red tongue without fur due to Yin damage of the Spleen and Stomach.

For an additional comparison, see *Yu Zhu* (Rhizoma Polygonati Odorati).

Modern research

1. Restores the blood-producing function inhibited by cobalt-60.[177]
2. Inhibits the adrenocortical function.[178]
3. Strengthens the immune function.[179, 180]
4. Aqueous extracts of *Huang Jing* inhibited Salmonella typhi, Staphylococcus aureus and acid-fast bacteria *in vitro*.[181]
5. Reduces the level of blood lipids, lowers the blood sugar level, and inhibits the effects of ageing.[182-184]

Combinations and applications

Functions	Combinations	Applications
Enriching Yin and moistening the Lungs	*Sha Shen* (Radix Glehniae seu Adenophorae) *Mai Men Dong* (Radix Ophiopogonis Japonici) *Zhi Mu* (Rhizoma Anemarrhenae Asphodeloidis) *Chuan Bei Mu* (Bulbus Fritillariae Cirrhosae) *Sheng Di Huang* (Radix Rehmanniae Glutinosae)	Dry cough with scant sputum, a red tongue and scant fur due to Lung Yin deficiency
	Sheng Di Huang (Radix Rehmanniae Glutinosae) *E Jiao* (Gelatinum Corii Asini) *San Qi* (Radix Notoginseng) *Tian Men Dong* (Radix Asparagi Cochinchinensis) *Bai Bu* (Radix Stemonae)	Tidal fever, night sweating, taxation cough with expectoration of blood, and deficiency and weakness due to Yin deficiency of the Lungs and Kidneys

	Gou Qi Zi (Fructus Lycii) *Dang Gui* (Radix Angelicae Sinensis) *Shu Di Huang* (Radix Rehmanniae Glutinosae Conquita)	Dizziness, palpitations, premature greying, and limpness and aching in the lumbar region and knees due to depletion and deficiency of the Essence and Blood in the aftermath of a prolonged illness
	Huang Qi (Radix Astragali seu Hedysari) *Shan Yao* (Rhizoma Dioscoreae Oppositae) *Tian Hua Fen* (Radix Trichosanthis) *Wu Wei Zi* (Fructus Schisandrae) *Sheng Di Huang* (Radix Rehmanniae Glutinosae) *Mai Men Dong* (Radix Ophiopogonis Japonici)	Wasting and thirsting with excessive fluid intake due to Yin deficiency with internal heat
Supplementing the Spleen and boosting Qi	*Dang Shen* (Radix Codonopsitis Pilosulae) *Bai Zhu* (Rhizoma Atractylodis Macrocephalae) *Fu Ling* (Sclerotium Poriae Cocos)	Fatigue and lack of strength, poor appetite and a weak and deficient pulse due to Qi deficiency of the Spleen and Stomach
	Sheng Di Huang (Radix Rehmanniae Glutinosae) *Mai Men Dong* (Radix Ophiopogonis Japonici) *Nan Sha Shen* (Radix Adenophorae)	Vexation and thirst, reduced appetite and a red tongue due to heat consuming Qi and Yin in the final stage of febrile diseases
	Yu Zhu (Rhizoma Polygonati Odorati) *Mai Men Dong* (Radix Ophiopogonis Japonici) *Shi Hu* (Herba Dendrobii) (see notes on legal status) *Shan Yao* (Rhizoma Dioscoreae Oppositae) *Wu Mei* (Fructus Pruni Mume) *Wu Wei Zi* (Fructus Schisandrae)	Yin deficiency of the Spleen and Stomach, manifesting as dry mouth, reduced appetite, inability to taste food, and dry stool, with a red tongue without fur

Han Lian Cao 旱莲草 (Eclipta, Herba Ecliptae Prostratae)

Han Lian Cao (also known as *Mo Han Lian*) is the dried aerial parts of *Eclipta prostrata* L., family Compositae.

Main ingredients *Han Lian Cao* contains thiophene compounds (including A-terthienyl, A-terthienyl methanol and α-formyl-α-terthienyl), stigmasterol, wedelolactone, saponins, nicotine, tannin, vitamin A, ecliptine, proteins and flavones.

Properties Taste: sweet and sour; nature: cold.

Channels entered Liver and Kidney.

Functions and indications Enriches and supplements the Liver and Kidneys, cools the Blood and stops bleeding. It is indicated for dizziness, loose teeth and premature greying due to Yin deficiency of the Liver and Kidneys; and for coughing of blood, nosebleed, blood in the stool, uterine bleeding, and vaginal discharge.

Common dosage 10-15g, or double this dosage for the fresh herb; appropriate dosage for external application.

Precautions and contraindications *Han Lian Cao* is contraindicated for diarrhoea due to Yang deficiency of the Spleen and Stomach.

Comparison of functions Both *Han Lian Cao* (Herba Ecliptae Prostratae) and *Nü Zhen Zi* (Fructus Ligustri Lucidi) can supplement Liver and Kidney Yin to treat Yin deficiency of the Liver and Kidneys, manifesting as dizziness, limpness and aching in the lumbar region and knees and premature greying. *Han Lian Cao* is cold in nature and can also cool the Blood and stop bleeding to treat a variety of bleeding patterns caused by Blood-heat due to Yin deficiency. *Nü Zhen Zi* is cool in nature and supplements without cloying. It can also brighten the eyes and is often used for blurred vision due to depletion and deficiency of the Liver and Kidneys.

Modern research

1. The powder and steep of *Han Lian Cao* can stop bleeding.[185]
2. Protects the liver and has a detoxifying function.[186, 187]
3. Strengthens the immune function.[188]
4. A tincture of *Han Lian Cao* had a certain inhibitory effect on Staphylococcus aureus and Shigella flexneri *in vitro*.[185]

Combinations and applications

Functions	Combinations	Applications
Enriching and supplementing the Liver and Kidneys	*Nü Zhen Zi* (Fructus Ligustri Lucidi) *Sang Shen* (Fructus Mori Albae)	Dizziness, blurred vision and premature greying due to Yin deficiency of the Liver and Kidneys
Cooling the Blood and stopping bleeding	*Sheng Di Huang* (Radix Rehmanniae Glutinosae)	Coughing of blood due to Lung deficiency
	Che Qian Cao (Herba Plantaginis)	Blood in the urine
	Xian He Cao (Herba Agrimoniae Pilosae)	Blood in the stool, uterine bleeding

Notes:

1. The powder or paste of fresh *Han Lian Cao* can be applied externally for bleeding due to knocks and falls.
2. A decoction of 30g of *Han Lian Cao* can be added to chicken soup to treat red and white vaginal discharge.

Nü Zhen Zi 女贞子
(Glossy privet fruit, Fructus Ligustri Lucidi)

Nü Zhen Zi is the dried fruit of *Ligustrum lucidum* Ait., family Oleaceae.

Main ingredients *Nü Zhen Zi* contains glucose, oleanolic acid, mannitol, palmitic acid, stearic acid, phospholipids and microelements.

Properties Taste: sweet and bitter; nature: cool.

Channels entered Liver and Kidney.

Functions and indications Enriches and supplements the Liver and Kidneys, supplements the Blood and brightens the eyes. It is indicated for dizziness, tinnitus, blurred vision and limpness and aching in the lumbar region and knees due to Yin deficiency of the Liver and Kidneys.

Common dosage 10-15g.

Precautions and contraindications *Nü Zhen Zi* is contraindicated in cases of Yang deficiency, or diarrhoea due to Spleen and Stomach deficiency-cold.

Remarks *Nü Zhen Zi* has supplementing and clearing functions and is effective for enriching Liver and Kidney Yin, darkening the hair and brightening the eyes. It is commonly used for patients with Yin deficiency of the Liver and Kidneys.

Comparison of functions See *Han Lian Cao* (Herba Ecliptae Prostratae).

Modern research

1. Raises the white blood cell count.[189]
2. The steep of *Nü Zhen Zi* and the amylose contained in the herb strengthen the immune function.[190, 191]
3. Increases the volume of blood supply to the coronary artery.[192]
4. Inhibits carcinoma.[193]
5. Inhibits inflammation.[194]
6. Reduces the level of blood lipids.[195]

Combinations and applications

Functions	Combinations	Applications
Enriching and supplementing the Liver and Kidneys, supplementing the Blood and brightening the eyes	*Han Lian Cao* (Herba Ecliptae Prostratae) *Sang Shen* (Fructus Mori Albae)	Dizziness, premature greying and limpness in the lumbar region and knees due to Yin deficiency of the Liver and Kidneys
	Sheng Di Huang (Radix Rehmanniae Glutinosae) *Gou Qi Zi* (Fructus Lycii) *Ju Hua* (Flos Chrysanthemi Morifolii) *Sha Yuan Zi* (Semen Astragali Complanati)	Blurred vision, tinnitus and forgetfulness due to Yin deficiency of the Liver and Kidneys
	Di Gu Pi (Cortex Lycii Radicis) *Sheng Di Huang* (Radix Rehmanniae Glutinosae) *Mu Dan Pi* (Cortex Moutan Radicis)	Insufficiency of the Liver and Kidneys and fever due to Yin deficiency, manifesting as steaming bone disorder with taxation fever, night sweating and seminal emission

Hei Zhi Ma 黑芝麻
(Black sesame seed, Semen Sesami Indici)

Hei Zhi Ma is the dried ripe seed of *Sesamum indicum* DC., family Pedaliaceae.

Main ingredients *Hei Zhi Ma* contains fatty oils (including oleic, linoleic, palmitic, arachidic and stearic acids), α- and β-globulin, albumin, histidine, sesamin, sesamol, sesamolin, sitosterol, stigmasterol, glucose, galactose, fructose, sucrose, sesamose, vitamins B_6 and E, and calcium.

Properties Taste: sweet; nature: neutral.

Channels entered Liver and Kidney.

Functions and indications Supplements and boosts the Essence and Blood, moistens dryness and lubricates the Intestines. It is indicated for premature greying, dizziness and blurred vision due to insufficiency of the Essence and Blood, and for constipation due to Blood deficiency and depletion of body fluids.

Common dosage 10-30g; generally stir-fried for internal use.

Precautions and contraindications *Hei Zhi Ma* is contraindicated for patients with loose stool and diarrhoea due to Spleen deficiency.

Toxicity The seeds of *Hei Zhi Ma* can cause diarrhoea. This herb should be stir-fried before internal use; it has been reported that intake of large dosages of raw *Hei Zhi Ma* resulted in partial obstruction of the intestines.

Combinations and applications

Functions	Combinations	Applications
Supplementing and boosting the Essence and Blood	*He Shou Wu* (Radix Polygoni Multiflori) *Tu Si Zi* (Semen Cuscutae) *Sheng Di Huang* (Radix Rehmanniae Glutinosae) *Du Zhong* (Cortex Eucommiae Ulmoidis) *Niu Xi* (Radix Achyranthis Bidentatae) *Nü Zhen Zi* (Fructus Ligustri Lucidi)	Premature greying, dizziness and blurred vision, lack of strength in lumbar region and knees and frequent urination at night due to Liver and Kidney deficiency and insufficiency of the Essence and Blood
	Yi Yi Ren (Semen Coicis Lachrymajobi) *Sheng Di Huang* (Radix Rehmanniae Glutinosae) (steep in wine and drink the liquid)	Wind Bi syndrome and weakness in the elderly, lack of strength in the limbs and aching in the lumbar region and knees
	Bai Zhu (Rhizoma Atractylodis Macrocephalae) *Wei Ling Xian* (Radix Clematidis)	Wind-damp patterns, pain in the lumbar region and legs, wandering wind that sometimes moves and sometimes stops
Moistening dryness and lubricating the Intestines	*Dang Gui* (Radix Angelicae Sinensis) *Rou Cong Rong* (Herba Cistanches Deserticolae) *Sheng He Shou Wu* (Radix Polygoni Multiflori Cruda) *Huo Ma Ren* (Semen Cannabis Sativae)	Intestinal dryness with constipation due to Blood deficiency and depletion of body fluids

Notes:

1. After being ground to a powder, *Hei Zhi Ma* can be taken on its own or boiled with rice in a congee to treat premature greying due to insufficiency of the Essence and Blood, dizziness and blurred vision.
2. Raw *Hei Zhi Ma* can be mashed to a pulp and applied to clove sores to disperse swelling and close sores; it can also be used in this form to treat insect bites.
3. The juice from a decoction of *Hei Zhi Ma* can be used as a mouth wash to treat toothache.

Modern research references

1. H. Saito et al., 'The effect of ginseng and its saponins on experimental amnesia in mice and on the cell culture of neurons' (Proceedings of the Fifth International Ginseng Symposium, Seoul, 1988), 92.
2. Zhang Juntian et al., *Yao Xue Xue Bao* [Pharmacology Journal] 23, 1 (1988): 12.
3. M. Liu et al., 'The effect of ginsenoside R_{b1} and R_{gi} on synaptosomal AT phase and calmodulin in rat hippocampus' (Programme and Abstracts of the Third China-Japan Joint Meeting on Pharmacology, Beijing, 1993) 008, 12.
4. Jin Ruomin et al., *Zhong Yao Tong Bao* [Bulletin of Chinese Materia Medica] 8, 1 (1983): 34.

5. Pei Yinquan et al., *Bei Jing Yi Ke Da Xue Xue Bao* [Journal of Beijing Medical University] 18, 2 (1986): 124.
6. Fang Yunxiang et al., *Zhong Xi Yi Jie He Za Zhi* [Journal of Integrated TCM and Western Medicine] 7, 6 (1987): 354.
7. Chen Changxun et al., *Yao Xue Tong Bao* [Pharmacology Bulletin] 20, 12 (1985): 713.
8. Xun Yanjun et al., *Yao Xue Tong Bao* 23, 5 (1988): 284.
9. Wang Benxiang, *Ren Shen De Yan Jiu* [Ginseng Research] (Tianjin: Tianjin Science and Technology Publishing House, 1985), 124–127.
10. Wang Benxiang et al., 'Study on the hypoglycaemic mechanism of ginseng glycopeptides' (Symposia Proceedings of the 5th Japan-China Symposium on Medical and Pharmaceutical Research into Chinese and Japanese Traditional Medicines, Fourth International Symposium on Traditional Medicine, Toyoma, 1995), 101.
11. Wang Benxiang et al., *Ren Shen Yan Jiu* [Ginseng Research] 2 (1991): 22.
12. M. Katano et al., 'A tumour growth inhibitory substance isolated from *Panax ginseng*' (Proceedings of the Fifth International Ginseng Symposium, Seoul, 1988), 33.
13. M. Kimura et al., 'Further purified ginseng extract fraction (D-O-ANA) of insulin release and its mode of action compared with the isolated residual components' (Proceedings of the Fourth International Ginseng Symposium, Korea Ginseng and Tobacco Research Institute, Korea, 1984), 191.
14. J. Liu et al., 'The effect of ginseng on the β-adrenoreceptor-cAMP system and the endocranium of aged rats' (Programme and Abstracts of the Third China-Japan Joint Meeting on Pharmacology, Beijing, 1993), 96.
15. Liu Ping et al., *Chang Bai Shan Zhong Yi Yao Yan Jiu Yu Fa Zhan* [Changbaishan Research and Development of Traditional Chinese Medicine and Materia Medica] 2, 3 (1993): 43 and 2, 4 (1993): 34.
16. Tian Yuwang et al., *Zhong Yao Yao Li Yu Lin Chuang* [Pharmacology and Clinical Application of Chinese Materia Medica] 10, 1 (1994): 27.
17. Chen Yuchun et al., *Fu Jian Yi Yao Za Zhi* [Fujian Journal of Medicine and Pharmacology] 14, 3 (1992): 33.
18. Zhang Congyun et al., *Zhong Yi Yao Xue Bao* [Journal of Traditional Chinese Medicine and Materia Medica] 6 (1995): 45.
19. Wang Kaizhen et al., *Zhong Yao Tong Bao* [Bulletin of Chinese Materia Medica] 11, 8 (1986): 53.
20. Pang Laixiang et al., *Xi Bei Yao Xue Za Zhi* [Northwest Journal of Pharmacology] 3, 3 (1988): 45.
21. Zhou Ran et al., *Bei Jing Zhong Yi Xue Yuan Xue Bao* [Journal of Beijing College of Traditional Chinese Medicine] 14, 5 (1991): 47.
22. Wang Zhong et al., *Jiang Su Zhong Yi Za Zhi* [Jiangsu Journal of Traditional Chinese Medicine] 4, 3 (1983): 58.
23. Han Pusheng et al., *Zhong Yao Yao Li Yu Lin Chuang* [Pharmacology and Clinical Application of Chinese Materia Medica] 6, 1 (1990): 19.
24. He Xingdong et al., *Lin Chuang Zhong Yao Shou Ce* [Clinical Handbook of Chinese Materia Medica] (Beijing: People's Medical Publishing House, 1998), 289.
25. Pan Siyuan et al., *Zhong Yao Yao Li Yu Lin Chuang* [Pharmacology and Clinical Application of Chinese Materia Medica] 8, 5 (1992): 22.
26. Huang Chengcai, *Zhong Yao Xin Yao Yu Lin Chuang Yao Li* [New Drugs of Chinese Materia Medica and Clinical Pharmacology] 4, 4 (1993): 50.
27. Yang Yingzhen et al., *Shanghai Yi Ke Da Xue Xue Bao* [Journal of Shanghai Medical University] 16, 2 (1989): 87.
28. Guo Zhaogui et al., *Zhong Yi Za Zhi* [Journal of Traditional Chinese Medicine] 21, 5 (1980): 73.
29. Zhou Honghao et al., *Hu Nan Yi Xue Yuan Xue Bao* [Journal of Hunan Medical College] 6, 4 (1981): 277.
30. Ma Lanfang et al., *Zhong Hua Xue Ye Xue Za Zhi* [Chinese Journal of Haematology] 9, 3 (1988): 148.
31. Lin Peiying et al., *Guang Zhou Yi Yao* [Guangzhou Journal of Medicine and Pharmacology] 14, 3 (1983): 27.
32. Xu Xihong et al., *Zhe Jiang Zhong Yi Yao Za Zhi* [Zhejiang Journal of Traditional Chinese Medicine and Materia Medica] 1 (1991): 39.
33. Yang Dezhi et al., *Zhong Xi Yi Jie He Za Zhi* [Journal of Integrated TCM and Western Medicine] 13, 10 (1993): 616.
34. Zhang Yindi et al., *Yao Xue Xue Bao* [Pharmacology Journal] 5 (1984): 333.
35. Liang Xiaochun et al., *Zhong Xi Yi Jie He Za Zhi* [Journal of Integrated TCM and Western Medicine] 13, 10 (1993): 587.
36. Meng Xianyi, *Zhong Cheng Yao Yan Jiu* [Chinese Medicinal Preparation Research] 10 (1982): 40.
37. Dai Yuru et al., *Nan Jing Zhong Yi Xue Yuan Xue Bao* [Journal of Nanjing College of Traditional Chinese Medicine] 4 (1988): 40.
38. Le Zhaosheng et al., *Zhong Yao Tong Bao* [Bulletin of Chinese Materia Medica] 10, 1 (1985): 44.
39. Liu Guosheng et al., *Yao Xue Lun Wen Zhai Yao* [Digest of Pharmacology Dissertations] (1978): 269.
40. Sun Xicai et al., *Shan Xi Zhong Yi* [Shaanxi Journal of Traditional Chinese Medicine] 6 (1988): 282.
41. Zhang Luoxiu et al., *Shang Hai Yi Ke Da Xue Xue Bao* [Journal of Shanghai Medical University] 15, 2 (1988): 101.

42. Wang Wenjuan, *Zhong Yi Yao Nian Jian* [Year Book of Traditional Chinese Medicine] (Beijing: Chinese TCM Publishing House, 1991), 430.
43. Zhang Qingbo, *Shang Hai Yi Xue* [Shanghai Medical Journal] 10 (1989): 613.
44. Yang Xu (translator), *Guo Wai Yi Xue – Zhong Yi Zhong Yao Fen Ce* [Foreign Medicine – TCM Fascicule] 9, 5 (1987): 54.
45. He Yuzhuo (translator), *Guo Wai Yi Xue – Zhong Yi Zhong Yao Fen Ce* 11, 6 (1989): 32.
46. Bian Ruqian et al., *Zhe Jiang Yi Ke Da Xue Xue Bao* [Journal of Zhejiang Medical University] 1 (1982): 273.
47. Zhu Yan, *Zhong Yao Yao Li Yu Ying Yong* [Pharmacology and Application of Chinese Materia Medica] (Beijing: People's Medical Publishing House, 1954), 231.
48. Xiong Gulang, *Biomedicine and Therapeutics* 14 (1985): 134.
49. Hu Zhihou, *Yao Xue Xue Bao* [Pharmacology Journal] 23, 7 (1988): 553.
50. Wang Shanyuan, *Ke Xue Tong Bao* [Science Bulletin] 12 (1958): 379.
51. Yang Guang (translator), *Guo Wai Yi Xue – Zhong Yi Zhong Yao Fen Ce* [Foreign Medicine – TCM Fascicule] 10, 5 (1988): 20.
52. He Xingdong et al., *Lin Chuang Zhong Yao Shou Ce*, 294.
53. Lei Zaiquan and Zhang Tingmo, *Zhong Hua Lin Chuang Zhong Yao Xue* [Chinese Clinical Materia Medica] (Beijing: People's Medical Publishing House, 1998), 1622.
54. S.C. Chou et al., *Med Pharmacol Exp* 16, 5 (1967): 407.
55. Ma Zhenya et al., *Shan Xi Zhong Yi Xue Yuan Xue Bao* [Journal of Shaanxi College of Traditional Chinese Medicine] 2 (1979): 1.
56. Li Xianggao, *Te Chan Ke Xue Shi Yan* [Scientific Experiments on Special Herb Production] (1980): 56.
57. Jiang Mengliang et al., *Research on Special Products* 4 (1993): 13.
58. Li Minzhen et al., *Guang Xi Zhong Yi Yao* [Guangxi Journal of Traditional Chinese Medicine and Materia Medica] 12, 5 (1989): 45.
59. Ba Tu et al., *Bai Qiu En Yi Ke Da Xue Xue Bao* [Journal of Bethune Medical University] 17, 6 (1991): 566.
60. Li Jingbo et al., *Bai Qiu En Yi Ke Da Xue Xue Bao* 18, 1 (1992): 24.
61. He Xingdong et al., *Lin Chuang Zhong Yao Shou Ce*, 290.
62. Lei Zaiquan and Zhang Tingmo, *Zhong Hua Lin Chuang Zhong Yao Xue*, 1643.
63. He Xingdong et al., *Lin Chuang Zhong Yao Shou Ce*, 297.
64. Fan Yuling et al., *Zhong Cao Yao Tong Xun* [Chinese Herbs Newsletter] 8 (1979): 4.
65. Pan Linshi (translator), *Fu Jian Yi Yao Za Zhi* [Fujian Journal of Medicine and Pharmacology] 2 (1980): 64.
66. Ding Yuxiong et al., *Zhong Cao Yao* [Journal of Chinese Herbs] 17, 5 (1986): 44.
67. Ding Yuxiong et al., *Zhong Cheng Yao* [Journal of Chinese Medicinal Preparations] 13, 1 (1991): 27.
68. Lin Peiying et al., *Zhong Cheng Yao Yan Jiu* [Chinese Medicinal Preparation Research] 12 (1984): 28.
69. Lian Yushu, *Zhong Yi Yao Xue Bao* [Journal of Traditional Chinese Medicine and Materia Medica] 6 (1988): 41.
70. Ding Yan, *Zhong Guo Mian Yi Xue Za Zhi* [Chinese Journal of Immunology] 9, 3 (1993): 185.
71. Zhao Peng, *Bei Jing Zhong Yi Xue Yuan Xue Bao* [Journal of Beijing College of Traditional Chinese Medicine] 11, 6 (1988): 41.
72. Liu Baoqing, *Zhong Cao Yao* [Journal of Chinese Herbs] 11, 5 (1980): 201.
73. Liu Chongming, *Shen Yang Yao Xue Yuan Xue Bao* [Journal of Shenyang Pharmacology College] 13 (1981): 9.
74. Gong Lansheng, *Liao Ning Zhong Yi Za Zhi* [Liaoning Journal of Traditional Chinese Medicine] 10 (1981): 45.
75. Yuan Bingxiang, *Xi Bei Yao Xue Za Zhi* [Northwest Journal of Pharmacology] 7, 3 (1992): 15.
76. Liu Huibo, *Zhong Yao Yao Li Yu Lin Chuang* [Pharmacology and Clinical Application of Chinese Materia Medica] 6, 2 (1990): 18.
77. Zeng Yi, *Zhong Hua Yi Xue Za Zhi* [Chinese Journal of Medicine] 50, 8 (1964): 521.
78. Hubei Province Bronchitis Group, *Collection of Traditional Chinese Medicine Research Documents* 6 (1976): 44.
79. Shenyang Pharmacology College No. 42 Yin Yang Huo Research Group, *Shen Yang Yao Xue Yuan Xue Bao* [Journal of Shenyang Pharmacology College] 8 (1977): 90.
80. Xiao Jinsong et al., *Zhong Guo Zhong Yao Za Zhi* [Journal of Chinese Materia Medica] 15, 9 (1990): 45.
81. Huang Guifang et al., *Zhong Cheng Yao* [Journal of Chinese Medicinal Preparations] 12, 6 (1990): 27.
82. Zhang Lanling et al., *Shi Yong Zhong Liu Xue Za Zhi* [Journal of Practical Oncology] 1, 3 (1987): 3.
83. He Xingdong et al., *Lin Chuang Zhong Yao Shou Ce*, 314.
84. Lei Zaiquan and Zhang Tingmo, *Zhong Hua Lin Chuang Zhong Yao Xue*, 1713.
85. He Xingdong et al., *Lin Chuang Zhong Yao Shou Ce*, 305.
86. Ibid., 306.
87. Lei Zaiquan and Zhang Tingmo, *Zhong Hua Lin Chuang Zhong Yao Xue*, 1716.
88. Li Bingru et al., *Zhong Yi Za Zhi* [Journal of Traditional Chinese Medicine] 7 (1984): 63.
89. Shen Daoxiu et al., *Shang Hai Zhong Yi Yao Za Zhi* [Shanghai Journal of Traditional Chinese Medicine and Materia Medica] 11 (1985): 46.

90. Qiao Zhisheng et al., *Zhong Xi Yi Jie He Za Zhi* [Journal of Integrated TCM and Western Medicine] 11, 7 (1991): 415.
91. Qian Zengnian et al., *Zhong Cheng Yao Yan Jiu* [Chinese Medicinal Preparation Research] 11 (1986): 32.
92. Chen Quansheng et al., *Zhong Guo Zhong Yao Za Zhi* [Journal of Chinese Materia Medica] 14, 10 (1989): 42.
93. Maternity Hospital Affiliated to Tianjin Medical College, *Tian Jin Yi Yao* [Tianjin Journal of Medicine and Pharmacology] 1 (1973): 36.
94. Yang Yican et al., *Zhong Xi Yi Jie He Za Zhi* [Journal of Integrated TCM and Western Medicine] 7, 12 (1987): 736.
95. Yang Yican et al., *Shan Xi Xin Yi Yao* [Shaanxi New Medical Journal] 10 (1983): 49.
96. Zhao Jianbin et al., *Shan Xi Zhong Yi* [Shaanxi Journal of Traditional Chinese Medicine] 11, 9 (1990): 427.
97. Lu Zehua et al., *Zhong Xi Yi Jie He Za Zhi* [Journal of Integrated TCM and Western Medicine] 10, 6 (1990): 370.
98. Zhu Dayuan et al., *Yao Xue Xue Bao* [Pharmacology Journal] 14, 10 (1979): 605.
99. Sun Yan et al., *Zhong Hua Yi Xue Za Zhi* [Chinese Journal of Medicine] 61, 2 (1981): 97.
100. Ma Rou et al., *Zhong Xi Yi Jie He Za Zhi* [Journal of Integrated TCM and Western Medicine] 9 (1984): 533.
101. He Xingdong et al., *Lin Chuang Zhong Yao Shou Ce*, 309.
102. Ibid., 302.
103. Tang Chenkang et al., *Xi Bei Yao Xue Za Zhi* [Northwest Journal of Pharmacology] 2, 1 (1987): 57.
104. Yin Zhongzhu et al., *Zhong Yao Yao Li Yu Lin Chuang* [Pharmacology and Clinical Application of Chinese Materia Medica] 4, 4 (1988): 26.
105. Xu Qingyuan, *Shan Xi Yi Xue Za Zhi* [Shaanxi Journal of Medicine] 16, 5 (1987): 61.
106. Zhou Peifang et al., *Zhong Cheng Yao Yan Jiu* [Chinese Medicinal Preparation Research] 12 (1984): 44.
107. Chen Guangjuan et al., *Zhong Cao Yao* [Journal of Chinese Herbs] 24, 2 (1993): 81.
108. Lei Zaiquan and Zhang Tingmo, *Zhong Hua Lin Chuang Zhong Yao Xue*, 1687.
109. He Xingdong et al., *Lin Chuang Zhong Yao Shou Ce*, 310.
110. Bao Tiantong et al., *Zhong Xi Yi Jie He Za Zhi* [Journal of Integrated TCM and Western Medicine] 8, 6 (1988): 352.
111. Wang Qin et al., *Zhong Yao Tong Bao* [Bulletin of Chinese Materia Medica] 12, 11 (1987): 42.
112. Lou Yaqing et al., *Zhong Cao Yao* [Journal of Chinese Herbs] 17, 5 (1986): 209.
113. Tang Rongjiang et al., *Zhong Cao Yao* 16, 6 (1985): 489.
114. Zhang Shishan et al., *Yao Xue Xue Bao* [Pharmacology Journal] 16, 3 (1981): 139.
115. Wang Meiying, *Shang Hai Yi Ke Da Xue Xue Bao* [Journal of Shanghai Medical University] 16, 5 (1989): 386.
116. Deng Qingqing et al., *Zhong Guo Zhong Yao Za Zhi* [Journal of Chinese Materia Medica] 18, 2 (1993): 115.
117. Liu Chao et al., *Zhong Xi Yi Jie He Za Zhi* [Journal of Integrated TCM and Western Medicine] 12, 5 (1992): 267.
118. Dong Rui et al., *Bei Jing Yi Xue* [Beijing Journal of Medicine] 6 (1981): 364.
119. Pan Qingqing et al., *Ji Sheng Chong Xue He Ji Sheng Chong Bing Za Zhi* [Journal of Parasitology and Parasitic Diseases] 4, 4 (1985): 303.
120. Li Changchun et al., *Fu Jian Yi Yao Za Zhi* [Fujian Journal of Medicine and Pharmacology] 5 (1983): 311.
121. Wang Junmo, *Zhong Cheng Yao Yan Jiu* [Chinese Medicinal Preparation Research] 11 (1985): 27.
122. Chen Yi et al., *Zhong Cao Yao* [Journal of Chinese Herbs] 16, 5 (1985): 33.
123. Wang Junmo et al., *Xian Dai Ying Yong Yao Xue* [Current Applied Pharmacology] 4, 3 (1987): 4.
124. Wang Benxian, *Xin Bian Zhong Yao Xue Ci Dian* [New Dictionary of Chinese Materia Medica] (Tianjin: Tianjin Science and Technology Publishing House, 1996), 1226.
125. Wang Benxian, *Xin Bian Zhong Yao Xue Ci Dian*, 865.
126. He Xingdong et al., *Lin Chuang Zhong Yao Shou Ce*, 313.
127. Lei Zaiquan and Zhang Tingmo, *Zhong Hua Lin Chuang Zhong Yao Xue*, 1690.
128. Xiao Lin, *Zhong Cheng Yao* [Journal of Chinese Medicinal Preparations] 11, 2 (1989): 35.
129. Xu Lina et al., *Zhong Guo Yao Li Xue Bao* [Chinese Journal of Pharmacology] 2, 1 (1981): 35.
130. Wu Jianxin et al., *Jiang Su Zhong Yi Za Zhi* [Jiangsu Journal of Traditional Chinese Medicine] 8, 1 (1992): 16.
131. Wu Jianxin et al., *Zhong Yao Yao Li Yu Lin Chuang* [Pharmacology and Clinical Application of Chinese Materia Medica] 9, 6 (1993): 22.
132. Wang Yaping et al., *Zhong Xi Yi Jie He Za Zhi* [Journal of Integrated TCM and Western Medicine] 11, 1 (1991): 61.
133. Cheng Bin et al., *Zhong Guo Xin Yao Za Zhi* [Chinese Journal of New Drugs] 1, 4 (1992): 31.
134. Huang Ziping et al., *Lin Chuang Gan Dan Bing Za Zhi* [Journal of Clinical Hepatology] 9, 1 (1993): 32.
135. Mei Qibing et al., *Zhong Guo Yao Li Xue Bao* [Chinese Journal of Pharmacology] 9, 3 (1988): 279.

136. He Xingdong et al., *Lin Chuang Zhong Yao Shou Ce*, 319.
137. Lei Zaiquan and Zhang Tingmo, *Zhong Hua Lin Chuang Zhong Yao Xue*, 1759.
138. Deng Wenlong, *Zhong Yi Fang Ji Yao Li Yu Ying Yong* [Pharmacology and Application of TCM Prescriptions] (Chongqing: Chongqing Publishing House, 1990), 290.
139. Zhang Yan et al., *Zhong Guo Yao Li Tong Bao* [Chinese Bulletin of Pharmacology] 10, 5 (1994): 372.
140. Sun Xiumei et al., *Zhong Guo Zhong Yao Za Zhi* [Journal of Chinese Materia Medica] 15, 6 (1990): 344.
141. Zhang Hong et al., *Zhong Guo Yao Li Xue Yu Du Li Xue Za Zhi* [Chinese Journal of Pharmacology and Toxicology] 4, 3 (1990): 190.
142. Chinese Herbal Research Office of Shanghai Medical Materials Company, *Zhong Cheng Yao Yan Jiu* [Chinese Medicinal Preparation Research] 1 (1978): 28.
143. Chen Minzhu et al., *Mian Yi Yao Li Jin Zhan Ji Chu Yu Lin Chuang* [Developments in Immune Pharmacology Basics and Clinical Application] (Beijing: China Science and Technology Publishing House, 1993), 133.
144. Dai Liming et al., *Zhong Guo Yao Li Tong Bao* [Chinese Bulletin of Pharmacology] 9, 6 (1993): 449.
145. Xiao Shangxi et al., *An Hui Yi Ke Da Xue Xue Bao* [Journal of Anhui Medical University] 26, 4 (1991): 250.
146. Zhao Bin et al., *Zhong Cheng Yao Yan Jiu* [Chinese Medicinal Preparation Research] 10 (1984): 6.
147. Zhou Zhiwen et al., *Zhong Yao Yao Li Yu Lin Chuang* [Pharmacology and Clinical Application of Chinese Materia Medica] 7, 5 (1991): 19.
148. Yoshiyuki Kimura et al., *Planta Med* 49, 1 (1983): 51.
149. Zou Xian, *Lao Nian Xue Za Zhi* [Journal of Geriatrics] 4, 1 (1986): 53.
150. Wang Zhihai et al., *Shan Dong Zhong Yi Za Zhi* [Shandong Journal of Traditional Chinese Medicine] 11, 1 (1992): 35.
151. Lu Chengbiao et al., *Zhong Yao Yao Li Yu Lin Chuang* [Pharmacology and Clinical Application of Chinese Materia Medica] 7, 4 (1991): 329.
152. He Xingdong et al., *Lin Chuang Zhong Yao Shou Ce*, 324.
153. Wang Jian, *Zhong Yao Tong Bao* [Bulletin of Chinese Materia Medica] 12, 12 (1987): 38.
154. Deng Shixian et al., *Zhong Cao Yao* [Journal of Chinese Herbs] 12, 2 (1981): 20.
155. Cui Jingchao et al., *Zhong Xi Yi Jie He Za Zhi* [Journal of Integrated TCM and Western Medicine] special volume (1988): 45.
156. Wang Yusheng et al., *Zhong Yao Yao Li Yu Ying Yong* [Pharmacology and Application of Chinese Materia Medica] (Beijing: People's Medical Publishing House, 1988), 302.
157. He Xingdong et al., *Lin Chuang Zhong Yao Shou Ce*, 326.
158. Lei Zaiquan and Zhang Tingmo, *Zhong Hua Lin Chuang Zhong Yao Xue*, 1831.
159. He Xingdong et al., *Lin Chuang Zhong Yao Shou Ce*, 334.
160. Lei Zaiquan and Zhang Tingmo, *Zhong Hua Lin Chuang Zhong Yao Xue*, 1828.
161. He Xingdong et al., *Lin Chuang Zhong Yao Shou Ce*, 333.
162. Zhu Chengwei et al., *Zhong Cheng Yao Yan Jiu* [Chinese Medicinal Preparation Research] 5 (1979): 46.
163. Du Shouying et al., *Zhong Guo Mian Yi Xue Za Zhi* [Chinese Journal of Immunology] 10, 6 (1994): 356.
164. Dai Shouzhi et al., *Lao Nian Xue Za Zhi* [Journal of Geriatrics] 10, 2 (1990): 94.
165. Li Hongguang et al., *Shen Yang Yao Xue Yuan Xue Bao* [Journal of Shenyang Pharmacology College] 8, 3 (1991): 233.
166. Hou Lingling et al., *Shan Xi Zhong Yi* [Shaanxi Journal of Traditional Chinese Medicine] 3 (1985): 141.
167. Jiangsu New Medical College, *Zhong Yao Da Ci Dian* [Dictionary of Chinese Materia Medica] volume 1 (Shanghai: Shanghai People's Publishing House, 1977), 318.
168. Du Xuhua et al., *Shen Yang Yao Xue Yuan Xue Bao* [Journal of Shenyang Pharmacology College] 7, 3 (1990): 197.
169. Chinese Herbal Medicine Information Centre of the State Administrative Bureau of Medicine and Pharmacology, *Zhi Wu Yao You Xiao Cheng Fen Shou Ce* [Handbook of Effective Ingredients of Herbal Medicine] (Beijing: People's Medical Publishing House, 1986), 93.
170. He Xingdong et al., *Lin Chuang Zhong Yao Shou Ce*, 329.
171. Lei Zaiquan and Zhang Tingmo, *Zhong Hua Lin Chuang Zhong Yao Xue*, 1807.
172. Yang Tao et al., *Bei Jing Yi Ke Da Xue Xue Bao* [Journal of Beijing Medical University] 23, 2 (1991): 97.
173. Yang Tao et al., *Journal of Biological Chemistry* 7, 6 (1991): 731.
174. Ibid., 8, 1 (1992): 21.
175. Shi Zili et al., *He Nan Zhong Yi* [Henan Journal of Traditional Chinese Medicine] 9, 2 (1989): 35.
176. He Xingdong et al., *Lin Chuang Zhong Yao Shou Ce*, 328.
177. Xu Xiangyu, *Yi Xue Zi Liao* [Medical Documents] 2 (1981): 81.
178. Xue Fang, *Xin Zhong Yi* [New Journal of Traditional Chinese Medicine] 10 (1983): 21.

179. Ling Shusen, *Jiang Su Yi Yao* [Jiangsu Journal of Medicine and Pharmacology] 5 (1982): 5.
180. Tan Hengshan, *Zhong Cao Yao* [Journal of Chinese Herbs] 20, 11 (1989): 36.
181. Wang Yusheng et al., *Zhong Yao Yao Li Yu Ying Yong*, 1032.
182. Zhang Rongrui, *Jiang Su Zhong Yi Za Zhi* [Jiangsu Journal of Traditional Chinese Medicine] 7 (1988): 41.
183. Lin Yiping, *Fu Jian Yi Yao Za Zhi* [Fujian Journal of Medicine and Pharmacology] 1 (1992): 29.
184. Liu Zhongshen, *Zhong Yi Yao Xue Bao* [Journal of Traditional Chinese Medicine and Materia Medica] 3 (1990): 44.
185. Hubei Provincial Drug Testing Institute, *Hu Bei Zhong Yao Zhi* [Hubei Records of Chinese Materia Medica] volume 1 (Wuhan: Hubei People's Publishing House, 1985), 506.
186. B. Singh et al., *Phytotherapy Res* 7 (1993): 154.
187. H. Wager et al., *Planta Med* 5 (1986): 372.
188. Hu Huijuan et al., *Zhong Guo Yao Ke Da Xue Xue Bao* [Journal of Chinese Pharmacology University] 23, 1 (1992): 55.
189. Sun Yan et al., *Zhong Guo Lin Chuang Yao Li Xue Za Zhi* [Chinese Journal of Clinical Pharmacology] 6, 2 (1990): 72.
190. Qian Tuisheng, *Zhong Yi Za Zhi* [Journal of Traditional Chinese Medicine] 2, 3 (1980): 75.
191. Dai Yue et al., *Zhong Guo Yao Ke Da Xue Xue Bao* [Journal of Chinese Pharmacology University] 18, 4 (1987): 301.
192. Peng Rui et al., *Zhong Yao Tong Bao* [Bulletin of Chinese Materia Medica] 8, 3 (1983): 32.
193. Zhao Ying et al., *Zhong Yi Yao Xue Bao* [Journal of Traditional Chinese Medicine and Materia Medica] 6 (1990): 47.
194. Dai Yue et al., *Zhong Guo Zhong Yao Za Zhi* [Journal of Chinese Materia Medica] 14, 7 (1989): 47.
195. Hao Zhiqi et al., *Zhong Guo Zhong Yao Za Zhi* 17, 7 (1992): 429.

Chapter 18

Herbs for promoting astriction

收涩药

Herbs for promoting astriction

Most herbs for promoting astriction are warm or neutral in nature and sour or astringent in taste. They can be used for profuse sweating, diarrhoea, vaginal discharge and seminal emission, and can stop bleeding and coughing. These herbs are used for patterns of Qi, Blood, Essence and body fluid desertion or patterns due to vital Qi deficiency with failure of the ability to control certain body functions.

These patterns manifest as spontaneous sweating, night sweating, enduring diarrhoea and dysentery, prolapse of the rectum, seminal emission, premature ejaculation, frequent urination, urinary incontinence, incessant uterine bleeding or chronic bleeding patterns. In such cases, significant depletion of original Qi or other disorders may occur if herbs for promoting astriction are not applied immediately.

It must be borne in mind that herbs for promoting astriction are only able to treat temporary manifestations of symptoms; they cannot treat the root cause of the disease. Hence, these herbs must be used in combination with other herbs, the choice of which is determined by the nature of the symptoms involved:

1. for patients with spontaneous sweating due to Qi deficiency or night sweating due to Yin deficiency, herbs for promoting astriction should be combined with herbs for supplementing Qi or herbs for supplementing Yin;
2. for patients with enduring diarrhoea and dysentery or incessant vaginal discharge due to Yang deficiency of the Spleen and Kidneys, herbs for promoting astriction should be combined with herbs for supplementing the Spleen and boosting Qi, and herbs for warming the Kidneys and supplementing Yang;
3. for patients with incessant seminal emission, enuresis and frequent urination due to insecurity of the Essence gate caused by Kidney deficiency, herbs for supplementing the Kidneys should be added;
4. for patients with incessant uterine bleeding due to deficiency and depletion of the Liver and Kidneys and insecurity of the Chong and Ren vessels, herbs for supplementing the Liver and Kidneys and securing the Chong and Ren vessels should be added;
5. for patients with enduring cough and deficiency wheezing due to Lung and Kidney deficiency, herbs for promoting astriction should be combined with herbs for supplementing and boosting the Lungs and Kidneys and herbs for hosting Qi and calming wheezing.

In all these instances, combining these herbs enables both the root and manifestation of the condition to be treated simultaneously.

Herbs for promoting astriction should not be applied in cases of unreleased exterior patterns or in the initial stage of diarrhoea and cough.

Herbs for promoting astriction can be divided into four types:

- herbs for securing the exterior and stopping sweating;
- herbs for constraining the Lungs and stopping coughing;
- herbs for astringing the Intestines and stopping diarrhoea; and
- herbs for securing the Essence, reducing urination and stopping vaginal discharge.

HERBS FOR SECURING THE EXTERIOR AND STOPPING SWEATING

Herbs for securing the exterior and stopping sweating can regulate the Wei level to secure the exterior and constrain sweating. They are mainly used for spontaneous sweating due to Qi deficiency, night sweating caused by Yin deficiency resulting in failure to control body fluids, and Yang heat forcing the discharge of body fluids.

These herbs should be added to other herbs depending on the nature of the cause of the sweating. For spontaneous sweating due to Qi deficiency, they should be used in combination with herbs for boosting Qi and securing the exterior, whereas for night sweating due to Yin deficiency, they should be combined with herbs for enriching Yin and eliminating steam (from steaming bone disorder).

Since 'sweat is the fluid of the Heart', diseases of the Heart will also result in sweating. For diseases due to Heart Yin deficiency, herbs for securing the exterior and stopping sweating should be used together with herbs for enriching Heart Yin, whereas for disorders caused by Heart-fire flaming upwards, they should be added to herbs for clearing heat from the Heart and draining fire.

In cases of profuse sweating or symptoms such as Yang collapse accompanied by a weak pulse, apply herbs such as *Ren Shen* (Radix Ginseng) to supplement depleted Yang in order to cure the root symptoms; it is not sufficient just to use herbs for securing the exterior and stopping sweating.

Tab. 18.1 Herbs for securing the exterior and stopping sweating

Herb	Functions	Indications
Ma Huang Gen (Radix Ephedrae)	Constraining the Lungs and stopping sweating	Spontaneous sweating and night sweating
Fu Xiao Mai (Fructus Tritici Aestivi Levis)	Constraining sweating, abating taxation fever	Spontaneous sweating due to Qi deficiency, night sweating due to Yin deficiency, taxation fever, steaming bone disorder

Ma Huang Gen 麻黄根 (Ephedra root, Radix Ephedrae)

Ma Huang Gen is the dried root of *Ephedra sinica* Stapf., *E. intermedia* Schrenk et C. A. Mey. or *E. equisetina* Bge., family Ephedraceae.

Main ingredients *Ma Huang Gen* contains mao-konine, ephedradines A, B, C and D, mahuannins A, B, C and D, and ephedrannin.

Properties Taste: sweet; nature: neutral.

Channel entered Lung.

Functions and indications Constrains the Lungs and stops sweating. It is indicated for spontaneous sweating and night sweating.

Common dosage 3-10g; appropriate dosage of the powder for external application.

Precautions and contraindications As a result of its action in stopping sweating, *Ma Huang Gen* is contraindicated in cases with exterior patterns.

Remarks *Ma Huang Gen* has a strong astringent effect in stopping sweating and can be used for all types of sweating due to deficiency patterns.

Modern research

1. The ephedradines A, B, C and D contained in *Ma Huang Gen* reduce blood pressure and block neuroganglions.[1-3]
2. Slows the heart rate.[4]
3. Inhibits sweating.[4]

Combinations and applications

Functions	Combinations	Applications
Constraining the Lungs and stopping sweating	*Huang Qi* (Radix Astragali seu Hedysari) *Bai Zhu* (Rhizoma Atractylodis Macrocephalae)	Spontaneous sweating due to Qi deficiency
	Ren Shen (Radix Ginseng) *Fu Zi* (Radix Lateralis Aconiti Carmichaeli Praeparata) (see notes on legal status)	Spontaneous sweating due to Yang deficiency
	Sheng Di Huang (Radix Rehmanniae Glutinosae) *Huang Lian* (Rhizoma Coptidis)	Tidal fever and night sweating due to Yin deficiency with heat signs forcing the discharge of body fluids
	Shu Di Huang (Radix Rehmanniae Glutinosae Conquita) *Shan Zhu Yu* (Fructus Corni Officinalis) *Long Gu* (Os Draconis) *Mu Li* (Concha Ostreae)	Night sweating due to Yin deficiency
	Dang Gui (Radix Angelicae Sinensis) *Huang Qi* (Radix Astragali seu Hedysari)	Persistent sweating postpartum due to Qi deserting with the Blood

Note: *Ma Huang Gen* can be ground to a fine powder with *Mu Li* (Concha Ostreae) for external application to stop sweating due to deficiency.

Fu Xiao Mai 浮小麦 (Light wheat grain, Fructus Tritici Aestivi Levis)

Fu Xiao Mai is the dried unripe caryopsis of *Triticum aestivum* L., family Gramineae.

Main ingredients *Fu Xiao Mai* contains starch, proteins, sugars, fatty oils, coarse fibres, dextrin, lecithin and allantoin.

Properties Taste: sweet and salty; nature: cool.

Channel entered Heart.

Functions and indications Constrains sweating and abates taxation fever. It is indicated for spontaneous sweating due to Qi deficiency, night sweating due to Yin deficiency, taxation fever, and steaming bone disorder.

Common dosage 15-30g in decoction; or 3-5g baked and ground into powder for oral use.

Remarks

1. With its sweet taste and cool nature, *Fu Xiao Mai* is able to boost Qi and clear heat. It can be used to treat all types of sweating due to deficiency.
2. The herb can be used alone in decoction or prepared as a powder for oral intake with rice congee.

Modern research

1. Inhibits sweat gland secretion.[5]
2. Has a tranquillizing effect.[6]

Combinations and applications

Functions	Combinations	Applications
Constraining sweating, abating taxation fever	*Huang Qi* (Radix Astragali seu Hedysari) *Mu Li* (Concha Ostreae) *Ma Huang Gen* (Radix Ephedrae)	Spontaneous sweating due to Qi deficiency
	Wu Wei Zi (Fructus Schisandrae) *Di Gu Pi* (Cortex Lycii Radicis) *Mai Men Dong* (Radix Ophiopogonis Japonici)	Vexation and agitation and night sweating due to heat harassing in Yin deficiency
	Di Gu Pi (Cortex Lycii Radicis) *Sheng Di Huang* (Radix Rehmanniae Glutinosae) *Mai Men Dong* (Radix Ophiopogonis Japonici)	Steaming bone disorder and taxation fever due to Yin deficiency with heat signs

HERBS FOR CONSTRAINING THE LUNGS AND STOPPING COUGHING

Most of the herbs in this section are sour and astringent and enter the Lung channel. They have the functions of constraining Lung Qi, stopping coughing and calming wheezing, and are used principally for enduring coughing and wheezing that does not respond to treatment, coughing and wheezing due to Lung deficiency and hasty breathing on exertion, or for Lung and Kidney deficiency with impairment of the ability to contain and host, or for wheezing due to Lung and Kidney deficiency with exhalation exceeding inhalation.

Some herbs for constraining the Lungs and stopping coughing can also clear the Lungs and bear fire downwards or enrich Yin and moisten dryness to treat Phlegm-fire depressing the Lungs, coughing and wheezing due to counterflow Qi and taxation cough due to Yin deficiency.

In addition, some of these herbs enter the Large Intestine channel and can astringe the Intestines and stop diarrhoea to treat enduring diarrhoea and dysentery with slippery intestines.

As these herbs are sour and constraining and promote astriction, they are contraindicated for the initial stage of cough and in cases of damp-heat dysentery and food accumulation with diarrhoea.

Tab. 18.2 Herbs for constraining the Lungs and stopping coughing

Herb	Functions	Indications
Wu Wei Zi (Fructus Schisandrae)	Constraining the Lungs and enriching the Kidneys, generating body fluids and constraining sweating, astringing the Essence and stopping diarrhoea, quieting the Heart and Spirit	Enduring cough and deficiency wheezing, thirst due to damage to body fluids, spontaneous sweating and night sweating, emaciation, wasting and thirsting, dream emission, seminal emission, enduring diarrhoea and dysentery, palpitations, insomnia, profuse dreaming
Wu Mei (Fructus Pruni Mume)	Constraining the Lungs and stopping coughing, astringing the Intestines and stopping diarrhoea, generating body fluids and allaying thirst, expelling roundworm and alleviating pain, stopping bleeding	Enduring cough due to Lung deficiency, enduring diarrhoea and dysentery, wasting and thirsting, pain in the abdomen and vomiting due to roundworm, uterine bleeding, sore throat
Wu Bei Zi (Galla Rhois Chinensis)	Internal use for constraining the Lungs and bearing fire downwards, astringing the Intestines and stopping diarrhoea, securing the Essence and stopping seminal emission, stopping bleeding	Enduring cough due to Lung deficiency, enduring diarrhoea and dysentery, spontaneous sweating and night sweating, seminal emission, blood in the stool, uterine bleeding
	External use for absorbing dampness and closing sores	Abscesses and sores, prolapse of the rectum, haemorrhoids
He Zi (Fructus Terminaliae Chebulae)	Astringing the Intestines and stopping diarrhoea, constraining the Lungs and stopping coughing, benefiting the throat and restoring the voice	Enduring diarrhoea and dysentery, prolapse of the rectum, enduring cough, loss of voice, blood in the stool, haemorrhoidal bleeding, vaginal discharge

Wu Wei Zi 五味子
(Schisandra fruit, Fructus Schisandrae)

Wu Wei Zi is the mature fruit of *Schisandra chinensis* (Turcz.) Baill. or *S. sphenanthera* Rehd. et Wils., family Magnoliaceae.

Main ingredients *Wu Wei Zi* contains volatile oils (including α- and β-pinene, camphene, myrcene, α-terpinene, limonene, bornyl acetate, linalool and benzoic acid), saccharides, arginine, schisandrin, schisandrol, gomisins, carbohydrates, resin, tannin, and vitamins C and E.

Properties Taste: sour; nature: warm.

Channels entered Lung, Kidney and Heart.

Functions and indications Constrains the Lungs and enriches the Kidneys, generates body fluids and constrains sweating, astringes the Essence and stops diarrhoea, and quiets the Heart and Spirit. It is indicated for enduring cough and deficiency wheezing, thirst due to damage to body fluids, spontaneous sweating and night sweating, emaciation, wasting and thirsting, dream emission, seminal emission, enduring diarrhoea and dysentery, palpitations, insomnia, and profuse dreaming.

Common dosage 2-6g; or 1-3g of powder for oral use.

Precautions and contraindications As *Wu Wei Zi* is sour and has an astringent function, it is contraindicated in cases of internal full-heat combined with unreleased exterior patterns, and in the initial stage of cough or measles.

Comparison of functions See *Wu Mei* (Fructus Pruni Mume) and *Wu Bei Zi* (Galla Rhois Chinensis).

Toxicity Oral administration to mice of 10-15g/kg of the fatty oils contained in the seeds of *Schisandra chinensis* or 0.28g/kg of the volatile oils contained in these seeds resulted in restricted activity, respiratory difficulties, loss of balance and death. A few cases have been reported of a burning sensation in the stomach, acid regurgitation and pain in the abdomen after administration of the herb to humans.

Modern research

1. Strengthens the process of inhibition and stimulation of the central nervous system.[7]
2. Regulates blood circulation in the cardiovascular system, dilates blood vessels and lowers blood pressure.[7]
3. Stimulates breathing, expels sputum and stops coughing.[8]
4. Strongly inhibits Mycobacterium tuberculosis and staphylococci.[8, 9]
5. Oral intake of a powder of *Wu Wei Zi* prepared with *Suan Zao Ren* (Semen Ziziphi Spinosae) can lower the transaminase of patients suffering from chronic hepatitis.[10]

Combinations and applications

Functions	Combinations	Applications
Constraining the Lungs and enriching the Kidneys	*Shu Di Huang* (Radix Rehmanniae Glutinosae Conquita) *Shan Zhu Yu* (Fructus Corni Officinalis) *Fu Ling* (Sclerotium Poriae Cocos) *Mu Dan Pi* (Cortex Moutan Radicis)	Wheezing, red face and hiccups due to Kidney Yin deficiency
	Ren Shen (Radix Ginseng) *Gan Jiang* (Rhizoma Zingiberis Officinalis) *Zi Wan* (Radix Asteris Tatarici) *Kuan Dong Hua* (Flos Tussilaginis Farfarae)	Coughing and wheezing due to Lung deficiency

	Fu Ling (Sclerotium Poriae Cocos) *Gan Cao* (Radix Glycyrrhizae) *Xi Xin* (Herba cum Radice Asari) *Gan Jiang* (Rhizoma Zingiberis Officinalis)	Cough with copious, thin sputum due to cold invading the Lung channel
	Sheng Di Huang (Radix Rehmanniae Glutinosae) *Xu Duan* (Radix Dipsaci) *Lu Rong* (Cornu Cervi Parvum)	Emaciation, shortness of breath, profuse dreaming, back pain and wheezing during movement due to Yin deficiency of the Lungs and Kidneys
Generating body fluids and constraining sweating	*Ren Shen* (Radix Ginseng) *Mai Men Dong* (Radix Ophiopogonis Japonici)	Shortness of breath, fatigue and lack of strength, thirst, profuse sweating, dry mouth and dry cough due to heat damaging Qi and Yin
	Mu Li (Concha Ostreae) *Ma Huang Gen* (Radix Ephedrae) *Bai Zi Ren* (Semen Biotae Orientalis) *Ren Shen* (Radix Ginseng)	Night sweating due to Yin deficiency or spontaneous sweating due to Yang deficiency
	Huang Qi (Radix Astragali seu Hedysari) *Mai Men Dong* (Radix Ophiopogonis Japonici) *Tian Hua Fen* (Radix Trichosanthis) *Sheng Di Huang* (Radix Rehmanniae Glutinosae)	Wasting and thirsting with thirst and a large fluid intake due to Yin deficiency with internal heat
Astringing the Essence and stopping diarrhoea	*Duan Long Gu* (Os Draconis Calcinatum) *Sang Piao Xiao* (Oötheca Mantidis)	Seminal emission and diarrhoea due to Kidney deficiency
	Rou Dou Kou (Semen Myristicae Fragrantis) *Wu Zhu Yu* (Fructus Evodiae Rutaecarpae) *Bu Gu Zhi* (Fructus Psoraleae Corylifoliae)	Early-morning diarrhoea, reduced appetite and reduced food intake, aching and cold in the lumbar region and fatigue due to deficiency-cold of the Spleen and Kidneys
	Wu Zhu Yu (Fructus Evodiae Rutaecarpae)	Seminal emission and urinary turbidity due to deficiency of the Kidneys, which thus fail to secure the Essence
Quieting the Heart and Spirit	*Suan Zao Ren* (Semen Ziziphi Spinosae) *Dan Shen* (Radix Salviae Miltiorrhizae) *Mai Men Dong* (Radix Ophiopogonis Japonici) *Sheng Di Huang* (Radix Rehmanniae Glutinosae) *Dang Gui* (Radix Angelicae Sinensis)	Deficiency vexation, palpitations, insomnia, forgetfulness and profuse dreaming due to non-interaction of the Heart and Kidneys or improper nourishment of the Heart and Spirit due to depletion damage to Yin and Blood

Wu Mei 乌梅
(Black plum, Fructus Pruni Mume)

Wu Mei is the fruit of *Prunus mume* (Sieb.) Sieb. et Zucc., family Rosaceae.

Main ingredients *Wu Mei* contains citric, malic, succinic, tartaric and oleanolic acids, sitosterol, amygdalin and benzaldehyde.

Properties Taste: sour and astringent; nature: neutral.

Channels entered Liver, Spleen, Lung and Large Intestine.

Functions and indications Constrains the Lungs and stops coughing, astringes the Intestines and stops diarrhoea, generates body fluids and allays thirst, expels roundworm and alleviates pain, and stops bleeding. It is indicated for enduring cough due to Lung deficiency, enduring diarrhoea and dysentery, wasting and thirsting, pain in the abdomen and vomiting due to roundworm, uterine bleeding, and sore throat.

Common dosage 3-10g, the maximum dosage is about 30g; appropriate dosage of the fresh herb as a paste or charred and ground into a powder for external application.

Precautions and contraindications As *Wu Mei* is sour and has an astringent function, it is contraindicated in cases of exterior patterns or stagnation of full-heat internally.

Remarks Use char-fried *Wu Mei* to stop bleeding.

Comparison of functions Both *Wu Mei* (Fructus Pruni Mume) and *Wu Wei Zi* (Fructus Schisandrae) are sour in taste and can constrain the Lungs to stop coughing, astringe the Intestines to stop diarrhoea, and generate body fluids to allay thirst. They can be used for enduring cough due to Lung deficiency, enduring diarrhoea and dysentery, wasting and thirsting due to deficiency-heat, and thirst due to damage to body fluids. *Wu Wei Zi* is an important herb for securing Kidney Essence and boosting Qi; it can constrain the Lungs to stop coughing in the Upper Jiao, enrich the Kidneys to secure Kidney Essence in the Lower Jiao, constrain sweating in the exterior, and generate body fluids and quiet the Heart and Spirit in the interior. *Wu Mei* is extremely sour and can also expel roundworm to alleviate pain, promote contraction to stop bleeding, and disperse the toxins of sores. It is used for pain in the abdomen due to roundworm and for bleeding patterns in the lower body, such as uterine bleeding and blood in the stool and urine.

Modern research Contracts the gallbladder and increases bile secretion, promotes the discharge of bile, inhibits contraction of the intestinal smooth muscle.[11, 12]

Combinations and applications

Functions	Combinations	Applications
Constraining the Lungs and stopping coughing	*E Jiao* (Gelatinum Corii Asini) *Xing Ren* (Semen Pruni Armeniacae) *Ban Xia* (Rhizoma Pinelliae Ternatae)	Enduring cough with scant sputum or dry cough without sputum due to Lung deficiency
Astringing the Intestines and stopping diarrhoea	*He Zi* (Fructus Terminaliae Chebulae) *Rou Dou Kou* (Semen Myristicae Fragrantis)	Enduring diarrhoea and dysentery
	Huang Lian (Rhizoma Coptidis) *Feng Mi* (Mel)	Dysentery accompanied by no desire for food and drink

Generating body fluids and allaying thirst	*Dan Dou Chi* (Semen Sojae Praeparatum) *Mai Men Dong* (Radix Ophiopogonis Japonici)	Wasting and thirsting, vexation in the Heart, oppression in the chest
	Mai Men Dong (Radix Ophiopogonis Japonici) *Tian Hua Fen* (Radix Trichosanthis) *Ge Gen* (Radix Puerariae) *Ren Shen* (Radix Ginseng)	Slight fever, vexation and thirst due to Yin deficiency
	Jin Yin Hua (Flos Lonicerae) *Xiong Huang* (Realgar) (see notes on legal status) *Feng Mi* (Mel)	Sore and swollen throat
Expelling roundworm and alleviating pain	*Xi Xin* (Herba cum Radice Asari) *Hua Jiao* (Pericarpium Zanthoxyli) *Huang Lian* (Rhizoma Coptidis) *Gan Jiang* (Rhizoma Zingiberis Officinalis)	Pain in the abdomen and vomiting due to roundworm
Stopping bleeding	*Huai Hua* (Flos Sophorae Japonicae) *Ce Bai Ye* (Cacumen Biotae Orientalis) *Xiao Ji* (Herba Cephalanoploris seu Cirsii) *Ou Jie* (Nodus Nelumbinis Nuciferae Rhizomatis)	Uterine bleeding, blood in the stool, blood in the urine

Note: In addition, *Wu Mei* can also be applied externally as a plaster to treat sores with pus.

Wu Bei Zi 五倍子
(Chinese gall, Galla Rhois Chinensis)

Wu Bei Zi is the gall produced mainly by the parasitic aphids, *Melaphis chinensis* (Bell) Baker, on the leaf of *Rhus chinensis* Mill., *R. potaninii* Maxim. or *R. punjabensis* Stew. var. *sinica* Diels (Rehd. et Wils.), family Anacardiaceae.

Legal status *Wu Bei Zi* was listed in a document entitled *A Review of Restricted Herbal Ingredients* issued by the Medicines Control Agency (MCA) in the UK in September 2001 with a view to the possible imposition of restrictions on its use at a future date. The MCA is concerned that a related plant, *Rhus radicans*, is restricted to external use only in Schedule II of the Medicines (Retail Sale or Supply of Herbal Remedies) Order 1977 and that other species may present a risk to public health.

Main ingredients *Wu Bei Zi* contains gallotannin, resin, fats and starch.

Properties Taste: sour and salty; nature: cold.

Channels entered Lung, Large Intestine and Kidney.

Functions and indications

Internal use: Constrains the Lungs and bears fire downwards, astringes the Intestines and stops diarrhoea, secures the Essence and stops seminal emission, and stops bleeding; it is indicated for enduring cough due to Lung deficiency, enduring diarrhoea and dysentery, spontaneous sweating and night sweating, seminal emission, blood in the stool, and uterine bleeding.

External use: Absorbs dampness and closes sores; it is indicated for abscesses and sores, prolapse of the rectum, and haemorrhoids.

Common dosage 1.5-6g, prepared in pills or powder for oral use; or appropriate dosage for external application as a powder or wash.

Precautions and contraindications *Wu Bei Zi* is contraindicated in cases of cough due to external pathogenic factors or diarrhoea due to damp-heat.

Comparison of functions Both *Wu Bei Zi* (Galla Rhois Chinensis) and *Wu Wei Zi* (Fructus Schisandrae) are sour in taste and can constrain the Lungs to stop coughing, constrain sweating to stop sweating, secure the Essence to stop seminal emission, and astringe the Intestines to stop diarrhoea. They can be used for enduring cough due to Lung deficiency, spontaneous sweating and night sweating, seminal emission, and enduring diarrhoea and dysentery. *Wu Bei Zi* also has the functions of clearing the Lungs and bearing fire downwards, and promoting contraction to stop bleeding; it is therefore used to treat cough due to Lung-heat, uterine bleeding, blood in the stool and urine, and bleeding due to external injury. *Wu Wei Zi* can also enrich the Kidneys, boost Qi and quiet the Heart and Spirit to treat wheezing due to Lung and Kidney deficiency, thirst due to damage to body fluids, wasting and thirsting, and palpitations and insomnia.

Toxicity Intraperitoneal injection in mice of 0.25ml of a pure *Wu Wei Zi* solution resulted in all the animals dying within 12 hours; when the dose was reduced to 1/10 of this quantity, no changes were observed in the animals. Very large dosages of the herb can cause focal necrosis of liver cells.

Modern research

1. Stops diarrhoea and bleeding.[13]
2. Inhibits ulcers, shortens bleeding time and decreases the amount of bleeding, clearly reduces the amount of gastric acid.[13]
3. *Wu Bei Zi* inhibited Staphylococcus aureus, Streptococcus pneumoniae, Salmonella typhi and Pseudomonas aeruginosa *in vitro*.[13, 14]
4. Inhibits contraction of the intestinal smooth muscle.[13]

Combinations and applications

Functions	Combinations	Applications
Constraining the Lungs and bearing fire downwards	*Wu Wei Zi* (Fructus Schisandrae) *Ying Su Ke* (Pericarpium Papaveris Somniferi) (see notes on legal status)	Enduring cough due to Lung deficiency
	Gua Lou (Fructus Trichosanthis) *Huang Qin* (Radix Scutellariae Baicalensis) *Bei Mu* (Bulbus Fritillariae)	Cough due to Lung-heat
Astringing the Intestines and stopping diarrhoea	*He Zi* (Fructus Terminaliae Chebulae) *Wu Wei Zi* (Fructus Schisandrae)	Enduring diarrhoea and dysentery, blood in the stool, prolapse of the rectum
Securing the Essence and stopping seminal emission	*Fu Ling* (Sclerotium Poriae Cocos) *Long Gu* (Os Draconis)	Seminal emission and urinary incontinence due to Kidney deficiency
Stopping bleeding	*Zong Lü Tan* (Fibra Carbonisata Trachycarpi Stipulae) *Xue Yu Tan* (Crinis Carbonisatus Hominis) *Lian Fang Tan* (Receptaculum Nelumbinis Nuciferae Carbonisatum)	Uterine bleeding
	Huai Hua (Flos Sophorae Japonicae) *Di Yu* (Radix Sanguisorbae Officinalis) (decocted for use as a steam wash)	Haemorrhoids, blood in the stool

Other applications:

1. *Wu Bei Zi* can be used alone externally ground into a powder or as a decoction for steam-washing to relieve toxicity, disperse swelling and close sores; it is indicated for the swelling and toxins of sores and boils, damp sores with flow of water, non-closure of ulcerating sores, and prolapse of the rectum and uterus.
2. Mixing powdered *Wu Bei Zi* with water and applying the paste to the navel before sleeping can stop spontaneous sweating and night sweating.

He Zi 诃子 (Chebula fruit, Fructus Terminaliae Chebulae)

He Zi is the dried fruit of *Terminalia chebula* Retz., or *T. chebula* Retz. var. *tomentella* Kurt., family Combretacae.

Main ingredients *He Zi* contains 30–40% of tannins, as well as chebulinic acid, chebulagic acid, corilagin, terchebin, glucogallin, ellagic acid, shikimic acid, quinic acid, sennoside A, chebulin, tannase, arabinose, fructose, dextrose and sucrose.

Properties Taste: bitter, sour and astringent; nature: neutral.

Channels entered Lung, Stomach and Large Intestine.

Functions and indications Astringes the Intestines and stops diarrhoea, constrains the Lungs and stops coughing, benefits the throat and restores the voice. It is indicated for enduring diarrhoea and dysentery, prolapse of the rectum, enduring cough, loss of voice, blood in the stool, haemorrhoidal bleeding, and vaginal discharge.

Common dosage 3-10g.

Precautions and contraindications

1. *He Zi* is contraindicated in cases with exterior patterns or accumulation and stagnation of damp-heat in the interior.
2. This herb is also contraindicated in the initial stage of cough or dysentery.
3. Dosage should be reduced for patients with Qi deficiency.

Remarks Use raw *He Zi* for constraining the Lungs, benefiting the throat and treating loss of voice; use the roasted herb for astringing the Intestines and stopping diarrhoea.

Modern research

1. A decoction of *He Zi* had a strong inhibitory effect *in vitro* on Shigella shigae, Pseudomonas aeruginosa and Corynebacterium diphtheriae.[14, 15]
2. Has a papaverine-like function in relaxing the intestinal smooth muscle.[15]

Combinations and applications

Functions	Combinations	Applications
Astringing the Intestines and stopping diarrhoea	*Mu Xiang* (Radix Aucklandiae Lappae) (see notes on legal status) *Huang Lian* (Rhizoma Coptidis)	Enduring diarrhoea and dysentery and pain in the abdomen with residual damp-heat
	Gan Jiang (Rhizoma Zingiberis Officinalis) *Ying Su Ke* (Pericarpium Papaveris Somniferi) (see notes on legal status) *Chen Pi* (Pericarpium Citri Reticulatae)	Enduring diarrhoea and prolapse of the rectum due to deficiency-cold

Constraining the Lungs and stopping coughing, benefiting the throat and restoring the voice	*Ren Shen* (Radix Ginseng) *Wu Wei Zi* (Fructus Schisandrae)	Enduring cough, shortness of breath and a weak pulse due to Lung Qi deficiency
	Jie Geng (Radix Platycodi Grandiflori) *Gan Cao* (Radix Glycyrrhizae)	Loss of voice due to Lung deficiency
	Xing Ren (Semen Pruni Armeniacae) *Tong Cao* (Medulla Tetrapanacis Papyriferi)	Enduring cough and loss of voice due to Phlegm-fire congesting the Lungs
	Bo He (Herba Menthae Haplocalycis) *Niu Bang Zi* (Fructus Arctii Lappae) *Chan Tui* (Periostracum Cicadae)	Sore throat and loss of voice due to repeated external contraction of pathogenic factors, incessant and enduring cough

Note: *He Zi* can also be used to treat uterine bleeding, vaginal discharge and urinary incontinence due to depletion and deficiency of the Liver and Kidneys.

HERBS FOR ASTRINGING THE INTESTINES AND STOPPING DIARRHOEA

Most of the herbs in this section are sweet and astringent or sour and astringent and enter the Large Intestine channel. They have the functions of astringing the Intestines and stopping diarrhoea and dysentery and are mainly used to treat deficiency-cold of the Spleen and Kidneys, manifesting as enduring diarrhoea and dysentery, slippery intestines, and pain in the abdomen that likes pressure or warmth, accompanied by a pale tongue with white fur. These herbs can be combined with herbs for fortifying the Spleen and boosting Qi and with herbs for warming the Kidneys and moving the Spleen, thus treating the root and manifestation of the condition simultaneously.

Herbs for astringing the Intestines and stopping diarrhoea are contraindicated in the initial stage of diarrhoea and dysentery and in cases of accumulation and stagnation of damp-heat in the Large Intestine.

Some of the herbs in this section can also stem profuse uterine bleeding, stop vaginal discharge, astringe the Essence and stop emission; they are used for uterine bleeding, vaginal discharge, seminal emission and enuresis.

Tab. 18.3 Herbs for astringing the Intestines and stopping diarrhoea

Herb	Functions	Indications
Yu Yu Liang (Limonitum)	Astringing the Intestines and stopping diarrhoea, promoting contraction and stopping bleeding	Enduring diarrhoea and dysentery, uterine bleeding and incessant vaginal discharge
Chi Shi Zhi (Halloysitum Rubrum)	Astringing the Intestines and stopping diarrhoea, promoting contraction and stopping bleeding, generating flesh and closing sores	Enduring diarrhoea and dysentery, prolapse of the rectum, uterine bleeding, blood in the stool, vaginal discharge, non-healing sores
Rou Dou Kou (Semen Myristicae Fragrantis)	Astringing the Intestines and stopping diarrhoea, warming the Middle Jiao and moving Qi	Enduring diarrhoea due to Spleen and Stomach deficiency-cold, early-morning diarrhoea due to deficiency-cold of the Spleen and Kidneys, reduced appetite, distension and pain in the stomach and abdomen
Shi Liu Pi (Pericarpium Punicae Granati)	Astringing the Intestines and stopping diarrhoea, killing worms and alleviating pain, stemming profuse uterine bleeding and stopping vaginal discharge	Enduring diarrhoea and dysentery, prolapse of the rectum, pain in the abdomen due to worms, seminal emission, uterine bleeding, vaginal discharge
Chun Pi (Cortex Ailanthi Altissimae)	Clearing heat and drying dampness, astringing the Intestines and stopping diarrhoea, stopping vaginal discharge and stopping bleeding, killing worms and alleviating itching	Enduring diarrhoea and dysentery, blood in the stool, uterine bleeding and profuse menstruation, vaginal discharge, roundworm, sores and tinea
Lian Zi (Semen Nelumbinis Nuciferae)	Nourishing the Heart and quieting the Spirit, boosting the Kidneys and securing the Essence, supplementing the Spleen and stopping diarrhoea	Palpitations, profuse dreaming, dream emission, seminal emission, enduring diarrhoea and dysentery, uterine bleeding, vaginal discharge

Qian Shi (Semen Euryales Ferocis)	Fortifying the Spleen and stopping diarrhoea, securing the Kidneys and astringing the Essence, dispelling dampness and stopping vaginal discharge	Diarrhoea due to Spleen deficiency; seminal emission, urinary turbidity and urinary incontinence due to Kidney deficiency; vaginal discharge

Yu Yu Liang 禹余粮 (Limonite, Limonitum)

Yu Yu Liang is the powder made from the naturally-occurring hydrous iron oxide limonite.

Main ingredients *Yu Yu Liang* contains ferric oxide FeO(OH), phosphates, aluminium, manganese, potassium and sodium.

Properties Taste: sweet and astringent; nature: neutral.

Channels entered Large Intestine and Stomach.

Functions and indications Astringes the Intestines and stops diarrhoea, promotes contraction and stops bleeding. It is indicated for enduring diarrhoea and dysentery, uterine bleeding and incessant vaginal discharge.

Common dosage 10–15g.

Precautions and contraindications

1. As *Yu Yu Liang* is astringent, it is contraindicated for full patterns.
2. *Yu Yu Liang* should used with caution during pregnancy; according to *Ben Cao Gang Mu* [The Materia Medica Compendium], this substance has a 'midwifery function'.

Comparison of functions Both *Yu Yu Liang* (Limonitum) and *Chi Shi Zhi* (Halloysitum Rubrum) have the functions of astringing the Intestines and stopping diarrhoea. They are frequently used in combination to treat enduring diarrhoea and dysentery, blood in the stool, prolapse of the rectum, and uterine bleeding and incessant vaginal discharge due to insecurity of the Lower Jiao. Although *Yu Yu Liang* is heavier than *Chi Shi Zhi*, the latter substance is warmer. As a result, *Chi Shi Zhi* is also used externally for closing sores and generating flesh to treat the non-closure of open sores, water flowing from damp sores and bleeding due to external injury. *Yu Yu Liang* is used specifically for astringing the Lower Jiao, as it is more effective than *Chi Shi Zhi* in stopping bleeding and vaginal discharge.

Modern research

1. Stops diarrhoea.[16]
2. Stops bleeding.[16]

Combinations and applications

Functions	Combinations	Applications
Astringing the Intestines and stopping diarrhoea	*Chi Shi Zhi* (Halloysitum Rubrum)	Enduring diarrhoea and dysentery due to insecurity of the Lower Jiao and slipperiness of the Intestines
	Bu Gu Zhi (Fructus Psoraleae Corylifoliae) *Bai Zhu* (Rhizoma Atractylodis Macrocephalae) *Gan Cao* (Radix Glycyrrhizae)	Diarrhoea due to Yang deficiency of the Spleen and Kidneys or weak constitution in the elderly
Promoting contraction and stopping bleeding	*Ren Shen* (Radix Ginseng) *Dang Gui* (Radix Angelicae Sinensis) *Shu Di Huang* (Radix Rehmanniae Glutinosae Conquita) *Chi Shi Zhi* (Halloysitum Rubrum)	Uterine bleeding due to the Chong and Ren vessels failing to contain
	Hai Piao Xiao (Os Sepiae seu Sepiellae) *Duan Mu Li* (Concha Ostreae, calcined) *Bai Guo* (Semen Ginkgo Bilobae)	Incessant vaginal discharge due to insufficiency of the lower origin and insecurity of the Dai vessel

Chi Shi Zhi 赤石脂 (Red halloysite, Halloysitum Rubrum)

Chi Shi Zhi is a silicate salt mineral of the polyhydrate kaolinate group; it owes its red colour to the presence of iron oxide.

Main ingredients *Chi Shi Zhi* contains hydrated aluminium silicate $[Al_4(Si_4O_{10})(OH)_8].4H_2O$, as well as ferric oxide, manganese, magnesium and calcium.

Properties Taste: sweet, sour and astringent; nature: warm.

Channels entered Spleen, Stomach and Large Intestine.

Functions and indications Astringes the Intestines and stops diarrhoea, promotes contraction and stops bleeding, generates flesh and closes sores. It is indicated for enduring diarrhoea and dysentery, prolapse of the rectum, uterine bleeding, blood in the stool, vaginal discharge, and non-healing sores.

Common dosage 10-20g in oral decoction, or prepared into pills and powder; appropriate dosage of the powder for external application.

Precautions and contraindications

1. *Chi Shi Zhi* is contraindicated in cases of enduring diarrhoea with accumulation and stagnation of damp-heat.
2. This substance should be used with caution during pregnancy.
3. *Chi Shi Zhi* antagonizes *Guan Gui* (Cortex Tubiformis Cinnamomi Cassiae).

Comparison of functions See *Yu Yu Liang* (Limonitum).

Modern research Stops gastrointestinal bleeding, absorbs toxic materials in the digestive tract and protects the mucous membrane.[8]

Combinations and applications

Functions	Combinations	Applications
Astringing the Intestines and stopping diarrhoea	*Yu Yu Liang* (Limonitum)	Enduring diarrhoea or dysentery with thin stool
	Gan Jiang (Rhizoma Zingiberis Officinalis) *Jing Mi* (Oryza Sativa)	Dysentery with blood and pus in the stool due to deficiency-cold
Promoting contraction and stopping bleeding	*Ren Shen* (Radix Ginseng) *Huang Qi* (Radix Astragali seu Hedysari) *Sheng Ma* (Rhizoma Cimicifugae)	Prolapse of the rectum due to Qi deficiency fall and insufficiency of middle Qi
	Ce Bai Ye (Cacumen Biotae Orientalis) *Hai Piao Xiao* (Os Sepiae seu Sepiellae) (roasted together and ground into a powder for oral use)	Uterine bleeding
	Huai Hua (Flos Sophorae Japonicae) *Di Yu* (Radix Sanguisorbae Officinalis)	Blood in the stool
	Bai Shao (Radix Paeoniae Lactiflorae) *Gan Jiang* (Rhizoma Zingiberis Officinalis)	Clear and thin or persistent red and white vaginal discharge due to insufficiency of Kidney Qi
Generating flesh and closing sores	*Long Gu* (Os Draconis) *Lu Gan Shi* (Calamina) *Xue Jie* (Resina Draconis) *Ru Xiang* (Gummi Olibanum) (prepared into a powder for external application)	Non-closure of ulcerating sores

Note: Used externally, *Chi Shi Zhi* is also effective for damp sores and bleeding due to knocks and falls.

Rou Dou Kou 肉豆蔻 (Nutmeg, Semen Myristicae Fragrantis)

Rou Dou Kou is the dried seed of *Myristica fragrans* Houtt., family Myristicaceae.

Main ingredients *Rou Dou Kou* contains volatile oils (including α-pinene, d-camphene, myristicin, d-borneol, dl-terpineol, geraniol, eugenol and safrole), fatty oils, starch and proteins.

Properties Taste: acrid; nature: warm.

Channels entered Spleen, Stomach and Large Intestine.

Functions and indications Astringes the Intestines and stops diarrhoea, warms the Middle Jiao and moves Qi. It is indicated for enduring diarrhoea due to Spleen and Stomach deficiency-cold, early-morning diarrhoea due to deficiency-cold of the Spleen and Kidneys, reduced appetite, and distension and pain in the stomach and abdomen.

Common dosage 3-10g; or 1.5-3g prepared into pills or powder for oral use.

Precautions and contraindications *Rou Dou Kou* is contraindicated in cases of damp-heat dysentery.

Remarks

1. Roasted *Rou Dou Kou* can strengthen the effect of warming the Middle Jiao and stopping diarrhoea.
2. *Rou Dou Kou* astringes without causing stagnation and moves without dispersing.

Toxicity Powdered *Rou Dou Kou* given orally to cats can lead to a semi-comatose state; after death, changes in liver fats were found. Oral administration to cats of 0.5-1.0ml/kg of myristicin caused death (with incomplete absorption of the substance in the gastrointestinal tract); subcutaneous injection of 0.12ml resulted in extensive changes to the liver. Slight overdoses of *Rou Dou Kou* manifest as hallucinations or nausea and dizziness; in severe cases, symptoms may include delirium, unconsciousness, dilated pupils, areflexia or even death.

Modern research

1. Regulates contractions of the smooth muscle in the digestive tract.[17]
2. Increases the secretion of gastric liquids; promotes digestion in small dosages, while inhibiting it in large dosages.[17]
3. Has an obvious sedative function.[18]

Combinations and applications

Functions	Combinations	Applications
Astringing the Intestines and stopping diarrhoea	*He Zi* (Fructus Terminaliae Chebulae) *Ying Su Ke* (Pericarpium Papaveris Somniferi) (see notes on legal status) *Dang Shen* (Radix Codonopsitis Pilosulae) *Bai Zhu* (Rhizoma Atractylodis Macrocephalae) *Rou Gui* (Cortex Cinnamomi Cassiae)	Enduring diarrhoea due to Spleen and Stomach deficiency-cold
	Bu Gu Zhi (Fructus Psoraleae Corylifoliae) *Wu Wei Zi* (Fructus Schisandrae) *Wu Zhu Yu* (Fructus Evodiae Rutaecarpae)	Early-morning diarrhoea due to deficiency-cold of the Spleen and Kidneys (in severe cases, with non-transformation of food)
Warming the Middle Jiao and moving Qi	*Mu Xiang* (Radix Aucklandiae Lappae) (see notes on legal status) *Jiang Ban Xia* (Rhizoma Pinelliae Ternatae, processed with ginger)	Distension and pain in the stomach and abdomen, reduced appetite and vomiting due to Stomach-cold

Shi Liu Pi 石榴皮 (Pomegranate rind, Pericarpium Punicae Granati)

Shi Liu Pi is the dried pericarp of *Punica granatum* L., family Punicaceae.

Main ingredients *Shi Liu Pi* contains gallic acid, malic acid, ursolic acid, isoquercitrin, granatin B, punicalagin, punicalin, tannin, resin and mannitol.

Properties Taste: sour and astringent; nature: warm.

Channels entered Stomach and Large Intestine.

Functions and indications Astringes the Intestines and stops diarrhoea, kills worms and alleviates pain, stems profuse uterine bleeding and stops vaginal discharge. It is indicated for enduring diarrhoea and dysentery, prolapse of the rectum, pain in the abdomen due to worms, seminal emission, uterine bleeding, and vaginal discharge.

Common dosage 3-10g as a decoction or prepared as pills and powders; for external application, it can also be ground into a powder for topical use or decocted for a steam wash.

Precautions and contraindications *Shi Liu Pi* is contraindicated for full patterns and for the initial stage of diarrhoea and dysentery due to damp-heat.

Remarks Char-fried *Shi Liu Pi* is used to stop bleeding.

Modern research

1. A decoction of *Shi Liu Pi* inhibited Shigella shigae, Bacterium coli, Salmonella typhi and Pseudomonas aeruginosa *in vitro*.[19]
2. Expels worms.[20]

Combinations and applications

Functions	Combinations	Applications
Astringing the Intestines and stopping diarrhoea	*Huang Lian* (Rhizoma Coptidis) *Huang Bai* (Cortex Phellodendri) *Dang Gui* (Radix Angelicae Sinensis)	Enduring dysentery due to damp-heat
	Dang Shen (Radix Codonopsitis Pilosulae) *Huang Qi* (Radix Astragali seu Hedysari) *Sheng Ma* (Rhizoma Cimicifugae)	Prolapse of the rectum caused by middle Qi fall due to enduring diarrhoea and dysentery
Killing worms and alleviating pain	*Bing Lang* (Semen Arecae Catechu) *Shi Jun Zi* (Fructus Quisqualis Indicae)	Roundworm, tapeworm, and pain in the abdomen due to worm accumulation
Stemming profuse uterine bleeding and stopping vaginal discharge	*Dang Gui* (Radix Angelicae Sinensis) *E Jiao* (Gelatinum Corii Asini) *Ai Ye Tan* (Folium Artemisiae Argyi Carbonisatum)	Uterine bleeding and incessant bleeding during pregnancy
	Hai Piao Xiao (Os Sepiae seu Sepiellae) *Chun Pi* (Cortex Ailanthi Altissimae)	Red and white vaginal discharge

Notes:

1. *Shi Liu Pi* can be char-fried, ground and mixed with oil for external application to treat psoriasis.
2. This herb can also be used in a concentrated decoction with *Ming Fan* (Alumen) in a steam wash to treat prolapse of the rectum.

Chun Pi 椿皮 (Ailanthus bark, Cortex Ailanthi Altissimae)

Chun Pi is the dried bark of the root or stem of *Ailanthus altissima* (Mill.) Swingle, family Simaroubaceae.

Main ingredients The root bark of *Chun Pi* contains mersosin and tannin; the stem bark contains ailanthone, amarolide, acetyl amarolide, quassin and neoquassin.

Properties Taste: bitter and astringent; nature: cold.

Channels entered Large Intestine and Liver.

Functions and indications Clears heat and dries dampness, astringes the Intestines and stops diarrhoea, stops vaginal discharge and stops bleeding, kills worms and alleviates itching. It is indicated for enduring diarrhoea and dysentery, blood in the stool, uterine bleeding and profuse menstruation, vaginal discharge, roundworm, sores and tinea.

Common dosage 3-5g in decoctions; appropriate dosage for external application, either as a decoction for a wash or boiled to a paste for topical use.

Precautions and contraindications *Chun Pi* is contraindicated for patients with Spleen and Stomach deficiency-cold because of its bitter taste and cold nature.

Comparison of functions Both *Chun Pi* (Cortex Ailanthi Altissimae) and *Huang Bai* (Cortex Phellodendri) can clear heat and dry dampness and are often used together to accentuate each other's effect in treating vaginal discharge and diarrhoea and dysentery due to damp-heat. *Chun Pi* has the function of promoting contraction and securing astriction and is often used for uterine bleeding and blood in the stool due to Blood-heat and for enduring diarrhoea and dysentery. *Huang Bai* is more effective in clearing heat and drying dampness. It has the ability to drain ministerial fire at the gate of vitality and is also often used for effulgent Yin deficiency-fire patterns.

Combinations and applications

Functions	Combinations	Applications
Clearing heat and drying dampness, astringing the Intestines and stopping diarrhoea, stopping vaginal discharge and stopping bleeding	*He Zi* (Fructus Terminaliae Chebulae) *Ding Xiang* (Flos Caryophylli)	Enduring dysentery
	Di Yu (Radix Sanguisorbae Officinalis)	Diarrhoea and dysentery due to damp-heat
	Hua Shi (Talcum)	Dysentery due to damp-heat, blood in the stool, white vaginal discharge
	Gui Ban (Plastrum Testudinis) (see notes on legal status) *Bai Shao* (Radix Paeoniae Lactiflorae) *Huang Bai* (Cortex Phellodendri)	Uterine bleeding and profuse menstruation due to Blood-heat
	Huang Bai (Cortex Phellodendri) *Bai Shao* (Radix Paeoniae Lactiflorae) *Gao Liang Jiang* (Rhizoma Alpiniae Officinari) or, as an alternative combination, *Ku Shen* (Radix Sophorae Flavescentis) *Huang Bai* (Cortex Phellodendri) *Zhi Zi* (Fructus Gardeniae Jasminoidis)	Red and white vaginal discharge due to damp-heat pouring down

	Cang Zhu (Rhizoma Atractylodis) *Chen Pi* (Pericarpium Citri Reticulatae) *Ban Xia* (Rhizoma Pinelliae Ternatae)	Vaginal discharge with a slippery pulse due to Phlegm-damp pouring down

Notes:

1. *Chun Pi* also has the function of drying dampness, killing worms and alleviating itching and can therefore be used as an external wash to treat sores and tinea.
2. *Chun Pi* can be used on its own or in combination with *Ce Bai Ye* (Cacumen Biotae Orientalis), *Sheng Ma* (Rhizoma Cimicifugae) and *Chi Shao* (Radix Paeoniae Rubra) for blood in the stool and haemorrhoidal bleeding.

Lian Zi 莲子 (Lotus seed, Semen Nelumbinis Nuciferae)

Lian Zi is the mature seed of *Nelumbo nucifera* Gaertn., family Nymphaeaceae.

Main ingredients *Lian Zi* contains raffinose, starch, proteins, fats, carbohydrates, calcium and phosphorus; the seed pod contains oxoushinsunine and n-norarmepavine.

Properties Taste: sweet and astringent; nature: neutral.

Channels entered Spleen, Kidney and Heart.

Functions and indications Nourishes the Heart and quiets the Spirit, boosts the Kidneys and secures the Essence, supplements the Spleen and stops diarrhoea. It is indicated for palpitations, profuse dreaming, dream emission, seminal emission, enduring diarrhoea and dysentery, uterine bleeding, and vaginal discharge.

Common dosage 6–10g.

Precautions and contraindications *Lian Zi* is contraindicated in cases of constipation.

Comparison of functions See *Qian Shi* (Semen Euryales Ferocis).

Modern research

1. Inhibits rhinopharyngoceles.[21]
2. Possesses astringing, tranquillizing and slightly supplementing functions.[22]

Combinations and applications

Functions	Combinations	Applications
Nourishing the Heart and quieting the Spirit	*Mai Men Dong* (Radix Ophiopogonis Japonici) *Bai Zi Ren* (Semen Biotae Orientalis) *Fu Shen* (Sclerotium Poriae Cocos cum Ligno Hospite)	Deficiency vexation, palpitations, profuse dreaming and insomnia due to non-interaction of the Heart and Kidneys
Boosting the Kidneys and securing the Essence	*Sha Yuan* Zi (Semen Astragali Complanati) *Long Gu* (Os Draconis) *Mu Li* (Concha Ostreae) *Qian Shi* (Semen Euryales Ferocis)	Premature ejaculation, seminal emission, fatigue and lack of strength, pain in the lumbar region, tinnitus, and limp and aching limbs due to deficiency of the Kidneys, which therefore fail to secure the Essence
	Yi Zhi Ren (Fructus Alpiniae Oxyphyllae) *Long Gu* (Os Draconis)	White urinary turbidity, dream emission and seminal emission due to insufficiency of the Heart and Kidneys

	Bai Zhu (Rhizoma Atractylodis Macrocephalae) *Fu Ling* (Sclerotium Poriae Cocos)	Deficiency of the Spleen with failure of its transportation function, manifesting as profuse white vaginal discharge due to water and dampness pouring down, fatigue and reduced food intake
Supplementing the Spleen and stopping diarrhoea	*Ren Shen* (Radix Ginseng) *Bai Zhu* (Rhizoma Atractylodis Macrocephalae) *Yi Yi Ren* (Semen Coicis Lachrymajobi) *Shan Yao* (Rhizoma Dioscoreae Oppositae)	Spleen deficiency with exuberance of dampness, manifesting as diarrhoea, poor appetite, fullness and oppression in the chest and stomach, and lack of strength in the limbs
	Huang Lian (Rhizoma Coptidis) *Ren Shen* (Radix Ginseng)	Enduring dysentery, reduced appetite and reduced food intake
	Fu Ling (Sclerotium Poriae Cocos) *Jing Mi* (Oryza Sativa)	Indigestion due to Spleen and Stomach deficiency
	Fu Ling (Sclerotium Poriae Cocos) *Ding Xiang* (Flos Caryophylli) *Sheng Jiang* (Rhizoma Zingiberis Officinalis Recens)	Cough and hiccups, vomiting, distension and fullness in the stomach and abdomen due to postpartum cold in the Stomach

Appendix

Lian Zi Xin 莲子心 (Lotus plumule, Plumula Nelumbinis Nuciferae)

Lian Zi Xin is the plumule and radicle of *Nelumbo nucifera* Gaertn.

Lian Zi Xin is bitter in taste and cold in nature. Entering the Heart and Pericardium channels, it has the functions of clearing the Heart, stopping bleeding and astringing the Essence. *Lian Zi Xin* can be used with *Xuan Shen* (Radix Scrophulariae Ningpoensis), *Mai Men Dong* (Radix Ophiopogonis Japonici) and *Dan Zhu Ye* (Herba Lophatheri Gracilis) to treat vexation heat and clouded Spirit in febrile diseases. Oral intake of *Lian Zi Xin* in powder form is effective against vomiting of blood or seminal emission. The common dosage is 1.5-3g.

Lian Xu 莲须 (Lotus stamen, Stamen Nelumbinis Nuciferae)

Lian Xu is the stamen of *Nelumbo nucifera* Gaertn.

Lian Xu is sweet and astringent in taste and neutral in nature. Entering the Spleen, Kidney and Heart channels, *Lian Xu* is used to clear the Heart and secure the Kidneys, astringe the Essence, and stop bleeding. It is often combined with *Sha Yuan Zi* (Semen Astragali Complanati), *Qian Shi* (Semen Euryales Ferocis), *Long Gu* (Os Draconis) and *Mu Li* (Concha Ostreae) to treat seminal emission, frequent urination and urinary incontinence due to Kidney deficiency. *Lian Xu* can also be employed for vomiting of blood and uterine bleeding. The common dosage is 1.5-5g.

Lian Fang 莲房 (Lotus receptacle, Receptaculum Nelumbinis Nuciferae)

Lian Fang is the receptacle of *Nelumbo nucifera* Gaertn.

Lian Fang is bitter and astringent in taste and warm in nature. Entering the Liver, Spleen and Kidney channels, it is used to disperse Blood stasis and stop bleeding. It is most effective in stopping bleeding in its charred form. *Lian Fang* is used for uterine bleeding, blood in the urine and stool, and persistent flow of lochia. The common dosage is 5-10g.

He Ye 荷叶 (Lotus leaf, Folium Nelumbinis Nuciferae)

He Ye is the leaf of *Nelumbo nucifera* Gaertn.

He Ye is bitter and astringent in taste and neutral in nature. Entering the Heart, Liver and Spleen channels, it is used to clear summerheat, bear Yang upwards, and stop bleeding. *He Ye* is often combined with *Jin Yin Hua* (Flos Lonicerae), *Bian Dou Hua* (Flos Dolichoris Lablab) and *Xi Gua Cui Yi* (Epicarpium Citrulli Vulgaris) to clear summerheat, and with *Sheng Di Huang* (Radix Rehmanniae Glutinosae) and *Ce Bai Ye* (Cacumen Biotae Orientalis) to stop bleeding. The common dosage is 3-10g.

Qian Shi 芡实
(Euryale seed, Semen Euryales Ferocis)

Qian Shi is the dried seed of *Euryale ferox* Salisb., family Nymphaeaceae.

Main ingredients *Qian Shi* contains pyrano-glucosides, starch, proteins, fatty oils, calcium, phosphorus, iron, and vitamins B_2 and C.

Properties Taste: sweet and astringent; nature: neutral.

Channels entered Spleen and Kidney.

Functions and indications Fortifies the Spleen and stops diarrhoea, secures the Kidneys and astringes the Essence, dispels dampness and stops vaginal discharge. It is indicated for diarrhoea due to Spleen deficiency; seminal emission, urinary turbidity and urinary incontinence due to Kidney deficiency; and vaginal discharge.

Common dosage 10-15g.

Precautions and contraindications *Qian Shi* is contraindicated in cases of inhibited urination and defecation.

Comparison of functions Both *Qian Shi* (Semen Euryales Ferocis) and *Lian Zi* (Semen Nelumbinis Nuciferae) can fortify the Spleen to stop diarrhoea and secure the Kidneys to astringe the Essence. However, *Qian Shi* has a stronger effect in securing the Kidneys and is used for seminal emission, urinary incontinence and uterine bleeding due to Kidney deficiency. *Lian Zi* is better for supplementing the Spleen and nourishing the Heart and is often used for diarrhoea due to Spleen deficiency and for disorders due to non-interaction of the Heart and Kidneys.

Modern research *Qian Shi* has a nourishing, moisturizing and astringent function.[23]

Combinations and applications

Functions	Combinations	Applications
Fortifying the Spleen and stopping diarrhoea	*Dang Shen* (Radix Codonopsitis Pilosulae) *Bai Zhu* (Rhizoma Atractylodis Macrocephalae) *Shan Yao* (Rhizoma Dioscoreae Oppositae) *Fu Ling* (Sclerotium Poriae Cocos) *Lian Zi* (Semen Nelumbinis Nuciferae)	Enduring diarrhoea due to Spleen deficiency, a sallow yellow facial complexion, oppression in the stomach and poor appetite
Securing the Kidneys and astringing the Essence	*Jin Ying Zi* (Fructus Rosae Laevigatae)	Seminal emission, urinary incontinence and limpness and aching in the lumbar region and knees due to insecurity of Kidney Qi

	Fu Ling (Sclerotium Poriae Cocos)	White turbidity due to insufficiency of Kidney Qi
Dispelling dampness and stopping vaginal discharge	*Shan Yao* (Rhizoma Dioscoreae Oppositae) *Huang Bai* (Cortex Phellodendri) *Bai Guo* (Semen Ginkgo Bilobae) *Che Qian Zi* (Semen Plantaginis)	Thick, yellow, fishy-smelling vaginal discharge due to damp-heat in Spleen deficiency patterns
	Shan Zhu Yu (Fructus Corni Officinalis) *Tu Si Zi* (Semen Cuscutae) *Jin Ying Zi* (Fructus Rosae Laevigatae)	Thin, clear, flowing vaginal discharge due to Spleen and Kidney deficiency, deficiency-cold of the lower origin, impairment of the retaining function of the Dai vessel and failure of the securing function of the Ren vessel

Note: *Qian Shi* can be prepared as pills with an equal dosage of *Fu Ling* (Sclerotium Poriae Cocos) for oral intake with salty water to treat vaginal discharge.

HERBS FOR SECURING THE ESSENCE, REDUCING URINATION AND STOPPING VAGINAL DISCHARGE

Most of the herbs in this section are sour in nature and enter the Liver and Kidney channels. Herbs for securing the Essence, reducing urination and stopping vaginal discharge have the functions of supplementing the Kidneys and securing the Essence in order to reduce urination and stop other discharge from the Lower Jiao.

These herbs are mainly indicated for premature ejaculation, seminal emission or urinary turbidity due to the Kidneys failing to perform their storage function as a result of Kidney Qi deficiency; for frequent urination and urinary incontinence due to deficiency-cold in the Lower Jiao and failure of the Bladder to transform Qi; and for vaginal discharge caused by failure of the transportation and transformation function due to Spleen deficiency and dampness attacking the Lower Jiao. They are often used in combination with herbs for supplementing the Spleen and Kidneys.

Tab. 18.4 Herbs for securing the Essence, reducing urination and stopping vaginal discharge

Herb	Functions	Indications
Shan Zhu Yu (Fructus Corni Officinalis)	Supplementing and boosting the Liver and Kidneys, astringing the Essence and reducing urine, securing the menses and stopping bleeding, constraining sweating and curtailing desertion	Limpness and aching in the lumbar region and knees, dizziness, impotence, seminal emission, frequent urination, sweating, profuse menstruation
Sang Piao Xiao (Oötheca Mantidis)	Supplementing the Kidneys and reinforcing Yang, securing the Essence and reducing urine	Seminal emission, white turbidity, frequent urination, urinary incontinence, vaginal discharge, impotence
Hai Piao Xiao (Os Sepiae seu Sepiellae)	Promoting contraction and stopping bleeding, securing the Essence and stopping vaginal discharge, controlling acidity and alleviating pain, absorbing dampness and closing sores	Uterine bleeding, bleeding in the Lungs and Stomach, bleeding due to external injury, seminal emission, vaginal discharge, pain in the stomach and acid vomiting, damp sores, eczema, ulcerating sores
Fu Pen Zi (Fructus Rubi Chingii)	Boosting the Kidneys, securing the Essence and reducing urine, brightening the eyes	Seminal emission and urinary incontinence, frequent urination, impotence, sterility, cold uterus and infertility, blurred vision due to insufficiency of the Liver and Kidneys
Jin Ying Zi (Fructus Rosae Laevigatae)	Securing the Essence and reducing urine, astringing the Intestines and stopping diarrhoea	Seminal emission, urinary incontinence and frequent urination, clear and thin vaginal discharge, enduring diarrhoea and dysentery, prolapse of the rectum or uterus, uterine bleeding

Shan Zhu Yu 山茱萸
(Asiatic Cornelian cherry fruit, Fructus Corni Officinalis)

Shan Zhu Yu is the pulp of the ripe fruit of *Cornus officinalis* Sieb. et Zucc., family Cornaceae.

Main ingredients *Shan Zhu Yu* contains cornin, verbenalin, ursolic acid, loganin, morroniside, sweroside, saponins, tannin, malic acid and vitamin A.

Properties Taste: sour and astringent; nature: slightly warm.

Channels entered Liver and Kidney.

Functions and indications Supplements and boosts the Liver and Kidneys, astringes the Essence and reduces urine, secures the menses and stops bleeding, constrains sweating and curtails desertion. It is indicated for limpness and aching in the lumbar region and knees, dizziness, impotence, seminal emission, frequent urination, sweating, and profuse menstruation.

Common dosage 5-10g, decocted with water or prepared as pills; the maximum dosage is about 30g for curtailing desertion in emergencies.

Precautions and contraindications As *Shan Zhu Yu* is warm and astringent, it is contraindicated in cases of damp-heat or painful or difficult urination.

Remarks *Shan Zhu Yu* is a strongly astringent herb, but has a mild function in supplementing and boosting the Liver and Kidneys. It can be used for all patterns with incessant and excessive loss of body fluids due to Liver and Kidney deficiency.

Modern research

1. Has an anti-diabetic function.[24]
2. Raises the white blood cell count and strengthens the immune function.[24]
3. Lowers blood pressure and promotes urination.[24]
4. A decoction of the fruit of *Shan Zhu Yu* inhibited Staphylococcus aureus and Shigella shigae *in vitro*.[25]

Combinations and applications

Functions	Combinations	Applications
Supplementing and boosting the Liver and Kidneys	*Shu Di Huang* (Radix Rehmanniae Glutinosae Conquita) *Shan Yao* (Rhizoma Dioscoreae Oppositae)	Limpness and aching in the lumbar region and knees, dizziness and tinnitus due to depletion and deficiency of the Essence and Blood and insufficiency of the Liver and Kidneys
	Rou Gui (Cortex Cinnamomi Cassiae) *Fu Zi* (Radix Lateralis Aconiti Carmichaeli Praeparata) (see notes on legal status) *Lu Jiao Jiao* (Gelatinum Cornu Cervi) *Shu Di Huang* (Radix Rehmanniae Glutinosae Conquita)	Fear of cold, cold limbs and impotence due to insufficiency of Kidney Yang
	Shu Di Huang (Radix Rehmanniae Glutinosae Conquita) *Shan Yao* (Rhizoma Dioscoreae Oppositae) *Ze Xie* (Rhizoma Alismatis Orientalis) *Fu Ling* (Sclerotium Poriae Cocos) *Zhi Mu* (Rhizoma Anemarrhenae Asphodeloidis) *Huang Bai* (Cortex Phellodendri)	Tidal fever and steaming bone disorder, night sweating, dream emission and dizziness with a fine and rapid pulse due to insufficiency of Kidney Yin and flaming upwards of deficiency-fire

Astringing the Essence and reducing urine	*Bu Gu Zhi* (Fructus Psoraleae Corylifoliae) *Dang Gui* (Radix Angelicae Sinensis) *She Xiang* (Secretio Moschi) (see notes on legal status)	Impotence or seminal emission due to insufficiency of Kidney Yang
	Shu Di Huang (Radix Rehmanniae Glutinosae Conquita) *Gou Qi Zi* (Fructus Lycii) *Tu Si Zi* (Semen Cuscutae)	Seminal emission and dream emission due to depletion of true Yin and failure of the storage function of the Kidneys
	Yi Zhi Ren (Fructus Alpiniae Oxyphyllae) *Sha Yuan Zi* (Semen Astragali Complanati) *Fu Pen Zi* (Fructus Rubi Chingii) *Sang Piao Xiao* (Oötheca Mantidis)	Frequent urination and urinary incontinence in the elderly due to insufficiency of Qi in the Kidneys, which thus fail to secure and contain
Securing the menses and stopping bleeding	*Hai Piao Xiao* (Os Sepiae seu Sepiellae) *Qian Cao Tan* (Radix Rubiae Cordifoliae Carbonisata) *Zong Lü Tan* (Fibra Carbonisata Trachycarpi Stipulae) *Huang Qi* (Radix Astragali seu Hedysari) *Duan Long Gu* (Os Draconis Calcinatum)	Profuse menstruation, uterine bleeding, palpitations and shortness of breath due to insecurity of the Chong and Ren vessels
Constraining sweating and curtailing desertion	*Sheng Long Gu* (Os Draconis Crudum) *Mu Li* (Concha Ostreae) *Bai Shao* (Radix Paeoniae Lactiflorae) *Ren Shen* (Radix Ginseng) *Fu Zi* (Radix Lateralis Aconiti Carmichaeli Praeparata) (see notes on legal status)	Deficiency desertion in enduring diseases or profuse sweating, cold limbs and a faint pulse with Yang Qi verging on desertion

Sang Piao Xiao 桑螵蛸
(Mantis egg-case, Oötheca Mantidis)

Sang Piao Xiao is the egg-case of *Tenodera sinensis* Saussure, *Statilia maculata* (Thunb.) or *Hierodula patellifera* (Serville), family Mantidae.

Main ingredients *Sang Piao Xiao* contains proteins, fats, coarse fibres, iron, calcium and carotene pigment.

Properties Taste: sweet and salty; nature: neutral.

Channels entered Liver and Kidney.

Functions and indications Supplements the Kidneys and reinforces Yang, secures the Essence and reduces urine. It is indicated for seminal emission, white turbidity, frequent urination, urinary incontinence, vaginal discharge, and impotence.

Common dosage 3-10g.

Precautions and contraindications *Sang Piao Xiao* is contraindicated in cases of effulgent Yin deficiency-fire, or frequent urination due to heat in the Bladder.

Comparison of functions See *Hai Piao Xiao* (Os Sepiae seu Sepiellae).

Modern research

1. Has a slight effect in inhibiting urination.[26, 27]
2. Reduces sweating.[26, 27]

Combinations and applications

Functions	Combinations	Applications
Supplementing the Kidneys and reinforcing Yang, securing the Essence and reducing urine	*Long Gu* (Os Draconis) *Shi Chang Pu* (Rhizoma Acori Graminei) *Yuan Zhi* (Radix Polygalae) *Dang Shen* (Radix Codonopsitis Pilosulae) *Gui Ban* (Plastrum Testudinis) (see notes on legal status)	Frequent urination, urinary incontinence, seminal emission, fatigue and forgetfulness due to Heart and Kidney deficiency
	Shan Zhu Yu (Fructus Corni Officinalis) *Tu Si Zi* (Semen Cuscutae)	Frequent urination or urinary incontinence in the elderly due to impairment of the containment function as a result of insufficiency of Kidney Yang
	Shan Zhu Yu (Fructus Corni Officinalis) *Tu Si Zi* (Semen Cuscutae) *Sha Yuan Zi* (Semen Astragali Complanati) *Fu Pen Zi* (Fructus Rubi Chingii)	Seminal emission and white turbidity due to insecurity of the Essence gate and insufficiency of the lower origin
	Rou Cong Rong (Herba Cistanches Deserticolae) *Tu Si Zi* (Semen Cuscutae) *Lu Rong* (Cornu Cervi Parvum)	Impotence, seminal emission or white vaginal discharge due to Yang deficiency of the Spleen and Kidneys
	Long Gu (Os Draconis) *Mu Li* (Concha Ostreae) *Shan Yao* (Rhizoma Dioscoreae Oppositae) *Qian Cao Gen* (Radix Rubiae Cordifoliae)	Profuse, thin and continuous or bloody vaginal discharge with limpness and aching in the lumbar region, a haggard complexion and a sunken pulse due to Yang deficiency of the Spleen and Kidneys
	Xiao Hui Xiang (Fructus Foeniculi Vulgaris) *Hua Jiao* (Pericarpium Zanthoxyli)	Cold Shan disorders due to invasion of cold, and pain in the lower abdomen due to deficiency-cold in the Lower Jiao

Hai Piao Xiao 海螵蛸
(Cuttlefish bone, Os Sepiae seu Sepiellae)

Hai Piao Xiao (also known as *Wu Zei Gu*) is the internal calcareous shell of *Sepia esculenta* Hoyle or *Sepiella maindroni* de Rochebrune, family Sepiidae.
Main ingredients *Hai Piao Xiao* contains calcium carbonate, calcium phosphate, sodium chloride and magnesium chloride.
Properties Taste: salty and astringent; nature: slightly warm.
Channels entered Liver, Kidney and Stomach.
Functions and indications Promotes contraction and stops bleeding, secures the Essence and stops vaginal discharge, controls acidity and alleviates pain, absorbs dampness and closes sores. It is indicated for uterine bleeding, bleeding in the Lungs and Stomach, bleeding due to external injury, seminal emission, vaginal discharge, pain in the stomach

and acid vomiting, damp sores, eczema, and ulcerating sores.

Common dosage 6-12g; where ground to a powder for oral intake, 1.5-3g each time; appropriate dosage as a powder for external application.

Precautions and contraindications *Hai Piao Xiao* should not be taken over a long period or it may cause constipation; it should not be given in large dosages to patients with Yin deficiency and excessive heat.

Comparison of functions Both *Hai Piao Xiao* (Os Sepiae seu Sepiellae) and *Sang Piao Xiao* (Oötheca Mantidis) can secure the Essence and stop vaginal discharge; they are used to treat seminal emission, white turbidity and vaginal discharge. *Sang Piao Xiao* can also supplement the Kidneys and reinforce Yang to treat impotence due to Kidney deficiency; it is particularly effective in the treatment of urinary incontinence, frequent urination, seminal emission and vaginal discharge caused by insufficiency of Kidney Yang. *Hai Piao Xiao* has a stronger effect in securing astriction, while concurrently promoting contraction, stopping bleeding, closing damp sores and controlling acidity to alleviate pain.

Modern research

1. Effective in treating ulcers in the digestive tract.[28]
2. Promotes the repair of bone defects.[29]

Combinations and applications

Functions	Combinations	Applications
Promoting contraction and stopping bleeding	*Qian Cao Gen* (Radix Rubiae Cordifoliae) *Zong Lü Tan* (Fibra Carbonisata Trachycarpi Stipulae) *Wu Bei Zi* (Galla Rhois Chinensis) *Huang Qi* (Radix Astragali seu Hedysari) *Shan Zhu Yu* (Fructus Corni Officinalis)	Uterine bleeding due to insecurity of the Chong and Ren vessels
	Bai Ji (Rhizoma Bletillae Striatae) (see notes on legal status)	Bleeding in the Lungs and Stomach
Securing the Essence and stopping vaginal discharge	*Shan Zhu Yu* (Fructus Corni Officinalis) *Tu Si Zi* (Semen Cuscutae) *Sha Yuan Zi* (Semen Astragali Complanati) *Long Gu* (Os Draconis)	Seminal emission due to the Kidneys failing to secure and store the Essence
	Shan Yao (Rhizoma Dioscoreae Oppositae) *Mu Li* (Concha Ostreae) *Xu Duan* (Radix Dipsaci)	Clear, thin vaginal discharge with limpness and aching in the lumbar region and knees due to damage to the Ren and Dai vessels and insufficiency of the Liver and Kidneys
	Bai Zhi (Radix Angelicae Dahuricae) *Xue Yu Tan* (Crinis Carbonisatus Hominis)	Red and white vaginal discharge due to damp turbidity pouring down
Controlling acidity and alleviating pain	*Zhe Bei Mu* (Bulbus Fritillariae Thunbergii)	Pain in the stomach and acid vomiting due to Spleen and Stomach deficiency-cold

Absorbing dampness and closing sores	*Huang Bai* (Cortex Phellodendri) *Huang Lian* (Rhizoma Coptidis) *Qing Dai* (Indigo Naturalis) *Duan Shi Gao* (Gypsum Fibrosum Calcinatum) (ground into a powder for external application)	Damp sores and eczema
	Duan Shi Gao (Gypsum Fibrosum Calcinatum) *Ming Fan* (Alumen) *Bai Zhi* (Radix Angelicae Dahuricae) *Hong Shen* (Radix Ginseng Rubra) *Bing Pian* (Borneolum) (ground to a fine powder and applied topically)	Ulcerating sores with large amounts of pus

Note: *Hai Piao Xiao* can be used on its own as a powder for external application to stop bleeding due to external injury.

Fu Pen Zi 覆盆子 (Chinese raspberry, Fructus Rubi Chingii)

Fu Pen Zi is the dried fruit of *Rubus chingii* Hu, family Rosaceae.

Main ingredients *Fu Pen Zi* contains citric acid, malic acid, salicylic acid, naphtha, pectin, glucose, vitamin C and ellagic acid.

Properties Taste: sweet and sour; nature: slightly warm.

Channels entered Liver and Kidney.

Functions and indications Boosts the Kidneys, secures the Essence and reduces urine, and brightens the eyes. It is indicated for seminal emission and urinary incontinence, frequent urination, impotence, sterility, cold uterus and infertility, and blurred vision due to insufficiency of the Liver and Kidneys.

Common dosage 3-10g.

Precautions and contraindications *Fu Pen Zi* is contraindicated for patients with difficult and painful urination and in cases of scant urine due to Kidney deficiency with fire.

Comparison of functions See *Jin Ying Zi* (Fructus Rosae Laevigatae).

Modern research

1. Has an oestrogen-like function.[30]
2. Inhibits Vibrio cholerae.[30]

Combinations and applications

Functions	Combinations	Applications
Boosting the Kidneys, securing the Essence and reducing urine	*Sha Yuan Zi* (Semen Astragali Complanati) *Shan Zhu Yu* (Fructus Corni Officinalis) *Qian Shi* (Semen Euryales Ferocis)	Dream emission, seminal emission, impotence and sterility due to insufficiency of the Kidneys
	Sang Piao Xiao (Oötheca Mantidis) *Yi Zhi Ren* (Fructus Alpiniae Oxyphyllae) *Jin Ying Zi* (Fructus Rosae Laevigatae)	Urinary incontinence, dribbling after urination and frequent urination with the Bladder failing to retain the urine due to deficiency-cold of the lower origin

	Gou Qi Zi (Fructus Lycii) *Tu Si Zi* (Semen Cuscutae) *Wu Wei Zi* (Fructus Schisandrae)	Infertility and cold uterus or seminal emission, sterility, impotence and seminal cold due to insufficiency of Kidney Yang
Brightening the eyes	*Gou Qi Zi* (Fructus Lycii) *Sha Yuan Zi* (Semen Astragali Complanati) *Tu Si Zi* (Semen Cuscutae) *Shu Di Huang* (Radix Rehmanniae Glutinosae Conquita)	Blurred vision due to insufficiency of the Liver and Kidneys

Jin Ying Zi 金樱子 (Cherokee rose fruit, Fructus Rosae Laevigatae)

Jin Ying Zi is the ripe fruit of *Rosa laevigata* Michx., family Rosaceae.

Main ingredients *Jin Ying Zi* contains citric acid, malic acid, digallic acid, tannin, resin, vitamin C, saponins, fructose, sucrose and starch.

Properties Taste: sour and astringent; nature: neutral.

Channels entered Kidney, Bladder and Large Intestine.

Functions and indications Secures the Essence and reduces urine, astringes the Intestines and stops diarrhoea. It is indicated for seminal emission, urinary incontinence and frequent urination, clear and thin vaginal discharge, enduring diarrhoea and dysentery, prolapse of the rectum or uterus, and uterine bleeding.

Common dosage 6-12g; decocted, boiled to a paste or used in pills.

Precautions and contraindications Since *Jin Ying Zi* is astringent, it is contraindicated in cases of full-fire or full pathogenic factors.

Comparison of functions Both *Jin Ying Zi* (Fructus Rosae Laevigatae) and *Fu Pen Zi* (Fructus Rubi Chingii) can secure the Essence and reduce urine to treat seminal emission, urinary incontinence, frequent urination and vaginal discharge. *Fu Pen Zi* can also boost the Liver and Kidneys and brighten the eyes while securing the Essence; it is frequently used for patterns of Kidney deficiency or insufficiency of the Liver and Kidneys to treat impotence and sterility due to Kidney deficiency and blurred vision due to insufficiency of the Liver and Kidneys. *Jin Ying Zi* is effective in promoting astriction to astringe the Intestines and stop diarrhoea and is often used for enduring diarrhoea and dysentery.

Modern research

1. Decoctions of *Jin Ying Zi* have an inhibitory effect on Staphylococcus aureus, Escherichia coli, Pseudomonas aeruginosa and Clostridium tetani.[31]
2. Promotes the secretion of gastric juices and reduces intestinal mucous membrane secretions.[31]

Combinations and applications

Functions	Combinations	Applications
Securing the Essence and reducing urine	*Tu Si Zi* (Semen Cuscutae) *Bu Gu Zhi* (Fructus Psoraleae Corylifoliae)	Seminal emission due to insufficiency of Kidney Qi and insecurity of the Essence gate

	Sang Piao Xiao (Oötheca Mantidis) *Yi Zhi Ren* (Fructus Alpiniae Oxyphyllae) *Shan Yao* (Rhizoma Dioscoreae Oppositae)	Urinary incontinence and frequent urination due to the Bladder failing to retain the urine and insufficiency of Kidney Qi
	Qian Shi (Semen Euryales Ferocis)	Turbid urine and non-separation of the clear and the turbid due to insecurity of Kidney Qi
	Chun Pi (Cortex Ailanthi Altissimae) *Ji Guan Hua* (Flos Celosiae Cristatae) *Qian Shi* (Semen Euryales Ferocis)	Clear, thin vaginal discharge due to the Dai vessel failing in its retaining function and depletion and deficiency of Kidney Qi
Astringing the Intestines and stopping diarrhoea	*Dang Shen* (Radix Codonopsitis Pilosulae) *Qian Shi* (Semen Euryales Ferocis) *Wu Wei Zi* (Fructus Schisandrae) *Bai Zhu* (Rhizoma Atractylodis Macrocephalae) *Shan Yao* (Rhizoma Dioscoreae Oppositae)	Enduring diarrhoea and dysentery due to Spleen deficiency
	Lian Zi (Semen Nelumbinis Nuciferae) *Qian Shi* (Semen Euryales Ferocis) *Ying Su Ke* (Pericarpium Papaveris Somniferi) (see notes on legal status)	Enduring dysentery

Note: *Jin Ying Zi* is also used in combination with *Dang Shen* (Radix Codonopsitis Pilosulae), *Huang Qi* (Radix Astragali seu Hedysari) and *Sheng Ma* (Rhizoma Cimicifugae) to treat prolapse of the rectum and uterus.

Modern research references

1. H. Hikino et al., *CA* 99 (1983): 136830.
2. Suntory Ltd., *CA* 99 (1983): 119549.
3. Y. Kasahara et al., *CA* 99 (1983): 181328.
4. Liu Zhi (translator), *Guo Wai Yi Xue – Zhong Yi Zhong Yao Fen Ce* [Foreign Medicine – TCM Fascicule] 4 (1981): 12.
5. He Xingdong et al., *Lin Chuang Zhong Yao Shou Ce* [Clinical Handbook of Chinese Materia Medica] (Beijing: People's Medical Publishing House, 1998), 341.
6. Ding Xuemin et al., *Chang Yong Zhong Yi Fang Yao Shou Ce* [Handbook of Commonly-Used Chinese Herbs and Prescriptions] (Changsha: Hunan Science and Technology Publishing House, 1982), 107.
7. Lei Zaiquan and Zhang Tingmo, *Zhong Hua Lin Chuang Zhong Yao Xue* [Chinese Clinical Materia Medica] (Beijing: People's Medical Publishing House, 1998), 1626.
8. He Xingdong et al., *Lin Chuang Zhong Yao Shou Ce*, 337.
9. Ding Xuemin et al., *Chang Yong Zhong Yi Fang Yao Shou Ce*, 108.
10. Ling Yikui et al., *Zhong Yao Xue* [Chinese Materia Medica] (Shanghai: Shanghai Science and Technology Publishing House, 1998), 246.
11. Su Jingtang, *Zhong Cao Yao* [Journal of Chinese Herbs] 18, 4 (1987): 28.
12. Zhou Zi, *Zhong Yi Yao Xin Xi* [Traditional Chinese Medicine and Materia Medica News] 1 (1986): 29.
13. He Xingdong et al., *Lin Chuang Zhong Yao Shou Ce*, 340.
14. Ding Xuemin et al., *Chang Yong Zhong Yi Fang Yao Shou Ce*, 104.
15. He Xingdong et al., *Lin Chuang Zhong Yao Shou Ce*, 344.
16. Wang Benxian, *Xin Bian Zhong Yao Xue Ci Dian* [New Dictionary of Chinese Materia Medica] (Tianjin: Tianjin Science and Technology Publishing House, 1996), 911.
17. He Xingdong et al., *Lin Chuang Zhong Yao Shou Ce*, 345.
18. Lei Zaiquan and Zhang Tingmo, *Zhong Hua Lin Chuang Zhong Yao Xue*, 1861.
19. Wu Zongrong, *Jiang Xi Yi Yao* [Jiangxi Journal of Medicine and Pharmacology] 7 (1965): 906.
20. J.P. Wibaut et al., *Arch Biochem Biophys* 69 (1957): 27.
21. He Xingdong et al., *Lin Chuang Zhong Yao Shou Ce*, 348.
22. Ding Xuemin et al., *Chang Yong Zhong Yi Fang Yao Shou Ce*, 105.
23. Lei Zaiquan and Zhang Tingmo, *Zhong Hua Lin Chuang Zhong Yao Xue*, 1889.

24. He Xingdong et al., *Lin Chuang Zhong Yao Shou Ce*, 350.
25. Lei Zaiquan and Zhang Tingmo, *Zhong Hua Lin Chuang Zhong Yao Xue*, 1879.
26. He Xingdong et al., *Lin Chuang Zhong Yao Shou Ce*, 351.
27. Ding Xuemin et al., *Chang Yong Zhong Yi Fang Yao Shou Ce*, 106.
28. Huang Zheyuan, *Hai Yang Yao Wu Xue Gai Lun* [An Introduction to Marine Materia Medica] (Fuzhou: Fujian Science and Technology Publishing House, 1987), 33.
29. Liu Yi et al., *Fu Jian Zhong Yi Yao* [Fujian Journal of Traditional Chinese Medicine and Materia Medica] 19, 3 (1988): 49.
30. He Xingdong et al., *Lin Chuang Zhong Yao Shou Ce*, 352.
31. Pharmaceutical Institute of the Chinese Academy of Medical Science, *Zhong Yao Zhi* [Chinese Materia Medica Records] (Beijing: People's Medical Publishing House, 1993), 461.

Chapter 19

Herbs for inducing vomiting

涌吐药

Herbs for inducing vomiting

Herbs for inducing vomiting are bitter and cold and can cause the vomiting of toxic substances, abiding food and Phlegm-fluids. They are used for toxins from harmful food substances collecting and lingering in the Stomach without being absorbed; for the stagnation and non-transformation of abiding food that has not yet entered the Intestines, accompanied by distension and pain in the stomach and abdomen; for congestion of Phlegm-fluids obstructed in the chest and diaphragm or throat with difficulty in breathing; and for Phlegm turbidity clouding the clear orifices, and epilepsy, mania and withdrawal.

These herbs have a very strong effect and are generally toxic. This drastic vomiting-inducing characteristic may affect the normal functioning of the Zang-Fu organs. Improper use of these herbs will cause serious problems. This means that herbs for inducing vomiting must only be used for patients with a strong constitution. Consequently, they are contraindicated for weak and elderly patients, children, women during pregnancy and postpartum, and for patients suffering from loss of blood, dizziness, palpitations, and coughing and wheezing.

When applying these herbs, attention must be paid to their dosage, administration and antidotes. Generally, a small dosage should be given at first; the dosage can then be increased gradually, thus avoiding toxic side-effects or excessive vomiting. After taking these herbs, patients should drink some warm boiled water to strengthen the effect, or use supplementary methods to reinforce the vomiting function. If vomiting cannot be stopped, an antidote should be applied immediately. After vomiting, the patient should rest, and not eat for a certain time. After restoration of the gastrointestinal function, a liquid diet and easily-digestible food can be taken to nourish Stomach Qi.

The harsh nature of these herbs and their after-effects mean that they are rarely used in the clinic nowadays.

Tab. 19 Herbs for inducing vomiting

Herb	Functions	Indications
Chang Shan (Radix Dichroae Febrifugae)	Inducing vomiting to expel Phlegm-fluids, killing worms and interrupting malaria	Phlegm-fluids congesting the chest, malaria
Gua Di (Pedicellus Cucumeris)	Internal use for inducing vomiting to expel Phlegm or food	Congestion of Phlegm-heat and food accumulation
	External use for dispelling damp-heat and abating jaundice	Damp-heat jaundice, headache due to dampness

Chang Shan 常山 (Dichroa root, Radix Dichroae Febrifugae)

Chang Shan is the dried root of *Dichroa febrifuga* Lour., family Saxifragaceae.

Main ingredients *Chang Shan* contains α-, β- and γ-dichroines, febrifugine, isofebrifugine, dichroidine and umbelliferone.

Properties Taste: bitter and acrid; nature: cold; toxic.

Channels entered Lung, Heart and Liver.

Functions and indications Induces vomiting to expel Phlegm-fluids, kills worms and interrupts malaria. It is indicated for Phlegm-fluids congesting the chest and for malaria.

Common dosage 5-10g.

Precautions and contraindications

1. *Chang Shan* should be used with caution for patients with a weak constitution because its strong function in inducing vomiting may damage vital Qi.
2. *Chang Shan* is contraindicated during pregnancy.

Remarks Raw *Chang Shan* is better for inducing vomiting; stir-fry the herb with wine when used for its anti-malarial function.

Comparison of functions According to *Ben Cao Gang Mu* [The Materia Medica Compendium], *Chang Shan* (Radix Dichroae Febrifugae) induces vomiting to expel Phlegm-fluids in malarial disorders, *Gua Di* (Pedicellus Cucumeris) induces vomiting to expel congestion of Phlegm-heat, *Lai Fu Zi* (Semen Raphani Sativi) induces vomiting to expel Phlegm-fluids due to Qi stagnation, and *Li Lu* (Radix et Rhizoma Veratri) induces vomiting to expel wind-Phlegm.

Toxicity The LD_{50} for oral administration to mice of the alkaloids contained in *Chang Shan* is 7.79mg/kg, with the LD_{50} for both β-dichroine and γ-dichroine being around 6.5mg/kg. The dichroines in *Chang Shan* stimulate the vagus and sympathetic nerve endings in the gastrointestinal tract, thus causing vomiting. Symptoms of overdose include nausea and vomiting, pain in the abdomen and diarrhoea, and blood in the stool; in severe cases, the blood capillary vessels may be destroyed, leading to gastrointestinal hyperaemia or haemorrhage.

Modern research

1. Decoctions of *Chang Shan* have an effect on malaria which is clearly stronger than that of quinine.[1]
2. Decoctions of *Chang Shan* can relieve fever.[1]
3. Lowers blood pressure.[2]
4. Excites the smooth muscle in the uterus.[2]
5. Inhibits arrhythmia.[2]

Combinations and applications

Functions	Combinations	Applications
Inducing vomiting to expel Phlegm-fluids, killing worms and interrupting malaria	*Gan Cao* (Radix Glycyrrhizae) *Feng Mi* (Mel)	Phlegm-fluids congesting the chest and diaphragm, desire to vomit without vomiting
	Bing Lang (Semen Arecae Catechu) *Cao Guo* (Fructus Amomi Tsaoko) *Qing Pi* (Pericarpium Citri Reticulatae Viride)	Warm-febrile diseases and malaria due to damp pathogenic factors

Gua Di 瓜蒂 (Muskmelon pedicle, Pedicellus Cucumeris)

Gua Di is the dried pedicle of *Cucumis melo* L., family Cucurbitaceae.

Main ingredients *Gua Di* contains cucurbitacins, saponins and amino acids.

Properties Taste: bitter; nature: cold; toxic.

Channel entered Stomach.

Functions and indications

1. Internal use: induces vomiting to expel Phlegm or food. It is indicated for congestion of Phlegm-heat and food accumulation.
2. External use: dispels damp-heat and abates jaundice. It is indicated for damp-heat jaundice and headache due to dampness.

Common dosage 2.5-5g; or 0.10-0.15g prepared as pills or powder for oral use; appropriate dosage for external application.

Precautions and contraindications *Gua Di* is contraindicated for patients with a weak constitution or with vomiting or expectoration of blood or in the absence of full pathogenic factors in the upper body.

Remarks *Gua Di* can be used in a decoction or as pills and powder. Ingesting a lump of sugar after oral intake of the herb can strengthen the emetic effect. If the vomiting is too strong, oral ingestion of 0.10-0.15g of *She Xiang* (Secretio Moschi) with water traditionally acts as an antidote (see notes on legal status for the availability of *She Xiang*).

Comparison of functions See *Chang Shan* (Radix Dichroae Febrifugae).

Toxicity The LD_{50} for oral administration to mice of cucurbitacin B is 14.0 ± 3.0mg/kg, that of subcutaneous injection is 1.0 ± 0.07mg/kg. The melotoxin contained in *Gua Di* can stimulate the mucous membrane of the stomach, resulting in severe vomiting. Overdosage can result in a burning pain in the stomach, severe vomiting (the vomitus may contain blood or bile) and diarrhoea; in more serious cases, symptoms of overdose may include a reduction in blood pressure, respiratory difficulty, convulsions and coma, or even death.

Modern research Oral intake excites the vomiting centre and induces vomiting and diarrhoea.[3]

Combinations and applications

1. Inducing vomiting to expel Phlegm or food:
   - *Gua Di* can be prepared into a powder in equal quantities with *Yu Jin* (Radix Curcumae) to treat epilepsy, diphtheria and throat Bi syndrome due to congestion of Phlegm-heat; take orally with warm water, 3g each time.
   - to treat food collecting and stagnating in the stomach with focal distension and pain in the chest and below the heart, or for food poisoning, *Gua Di* can be used in a powder in equal quantities with *Chi Xiao Dou* (Semen Phaseoli Calcarati), or decocted with *Dan Dou Chi* (Semen Sojae Praeparatum); 3g each time. Stop using the powder when vomiting occurs.
2. Dispelling damp-heat and abating jaundice:
   - To treat damp-heat jaundice, inhale a little of the powder into the nostrils two to three times a day until a yellow discharge is obtained. The same procedure can be used for headache, dizziness and nasal congestion in patients susceptible to dampness.

Modern research references

1. Lei Zaiquan and Zhang Tingmo, *Zhong Hua Lin Chuang Zhong Yao Xue* [Chinese Clinical Materia Medica] (Beijing: People's Medical Publishing House, 1998), 1908.
2. He Xingdong et al., *Lin Chuang Zhong Yao Shou Ce* [Clinical Handbook of Chinese Materia Medica] (Beijing: People's Medical Publishing House, 1998), 357.
3. Ibid., 356.

Chapter 20

Substances for external application 外用药

Substances for external application

Substances for external application refer to herbs and other substances applied to the surface of the body to treat local conditions and disorders. The substances included in this chapter are commonly used externally. Although some of them may be used with caution internally, their toxicity means that such application is mainly restricted to the clinic.

Substances for external application achieve their effect through contact with the skin. They have the functions of relieving toxicity and killing worms, drying dampness and alleviating itching, transforming putrefaction and generating flesh, expelling pus and dispersing swelling, and stopping bleeding by astriction. They are used to treat abscesses, sores, toxic swellings, scabies, external injuries, and ENT and eye diseases. Since these disorders occur in different areas of the body and manifest in different ways, substances for external application can be used in a variety of topical treatments as powders, pastes mixed with sesame oil or tea infusions, ointments, rubs, dressings, mouth washes, eye drops, herbal baths, steam-washes and suppositories.

In clinical practice, substances for external application should be used in combination with other herbs as appropriate according to the nature of the condition:

1. for local bleeding, use them with herbs for stopping bleeding;
2. for inflammation with local swelling and redness, use them with herbs for clearing heat and relieving toxicity, and herbs for dispersing swelling and alleviating pain;
3. for excessive secretion in sores, use them with herbs for promoting astriction;
4. for local ulceration, combine them with herbs for generating flesh.

When applying these substances, attention should be paid to the following aspects:

i. Many of these substances have drastic toxicity. Improper usage (especially improper internal usage) will result in poisoning, so the dosage must be strictly controlled. Even when used externally, the dosage should also be controlled when a substance is applied to a large wound, thus avoiding the absorption of toxins.
ii. For internal use, these substances are generally prepared as pills or powders so they can be absorbed slowly and the dosage can be controlled.
iii. For highly toxic substances, pharmaceutical regulations must be followed to ensure safe use (note should also be taken of legal status).

Tab. 20 Substances for external application

Herb	Functions	Indications
Xiong Huang (Realgar)	Relieving toxicity and killing worms, drying dampness and dispelling Phlegm, settling fright	Swollen and painful abscesses, throat wind, alopecia areata (glossy scalp wind), sores, poisonous snake bites, tetanus, convulsions, epilepsy, scabies and tinea, herpes zoster
Liu Huang (Sulphur)	Internal use for supplementing fire, invigorating Yang and freeing the bowels; external use for relieving toxicity, killing worms and alleviating itching	Cold wheezing due to Kidney deficiency, impotence and seminal cold, cold and limpness in the lumbar region and knees, constipation, frequent urination, cold and pain in the abdomen, eczema, scabies and tinea, itchy skin
Ming Fan (Alumen)	Internal use for stopping bleeding and stopping diarrhoea, dispelling Phlegm and opening the orifices	Wind-stroke Phlegm collapse, epilepsy, enduring diarrhoea, blood in the stool, uterine bleeding
	External use for drying dampness and alleviating itching, relieving toxicity and killing worms	Scabies, eczema, itching, mouth and tongue sores, vaginal discharge
She Chuang Zi (Fructus Cnidii Monnieri)	Warming the Kidneys and invigorating Yang, dispelling wind and dissipating cold, drying dampness, killing worms and alleviating itching	Internal use for impotence due to Kidney Yang deficiency, infertility due to cold uterus, lumbar and limb joint pain or vaginal discharge due to damp-cold; external use for pudendal itch, scabies, eczema
Er Cha (Pasta Acaciae seu Uncariae)	External use for absorbing dampness, closing sores and generating flesh, stopping bleeding	Damp sores and weeping ulcers, Gan of the teeth and gums, mouth sores, lower body Gan, bleeding due to external injury
Chan Su (Venenum Bufonis)	Relieving toxicity and dispersing swelling, alleviating pain, opening the orifices and arousing the brain	Swelling and toxins of abscesses and sores, swollen and painful throat, toothache, vomiting and diarrhoea, pain in the abdomen
Feng Fang (Nidus Vespae)	Dispelling wind-damp, invigorating Kidney Yang, relieving toxicity	Abscesses and sores, breast abscess, scrofula, scabies, toothache, wind-damp Bi syndrome pain, urticaria (dormant papules)
Xue Jie (Resina Draconis)	Stopping bleeding, dispelling Blood stasis and alleviating pain, closing sores and generating flesh	Pain in the heart and abdomen due to Blood stasis, postpartum pain in the abdomen, knocks and falls, bleeding due to external injury, non-healing abscesses and sores

Qing Fen (Calomelas)	Internal use for promoting the movement of water and freeing the bowels	Distension in the abdomen, oedema, difficult urination, constipation
	External use for killing worms and relieving toxicity	Abscesses, boils, sores, stubborn tinea, syphilis
Lu Gan Shi (Calamina)	External use for brightening the eyes and removing eye screen, absorbing dampness, closing sores and generating flesh	Red, sore and swollen eyes, wind eye with ulceration of the eyelid rim, eye screen, profuse lacrimation and fear of light, non-healing abscesses and sores
Peng Sha (Borax)	Internal use for clearing heat and transforming Phlegm	Hoarse voice and sore throat due to congestion of Phlegm-heat, difficult expectoration of sputum
	External use for relieving toxicity and preventing putrefaction	Mouth and tongue sores, sore and swollen throat, red eyes and eye screen

Xiong Huang 雄黄 (Realgar, Realgar)

Xiong Huang is a red mineral ore mainly composed of arsenic (II) sulphide.

Legal status The use of this materia medica is illegal in the UK as a result of its toxic nature.

Main ingredients *Xiong Huang* contains arsenic (II) sulphide (As_2S_2) and small quantities of salts of other heavy metals.

Properties Taste: acrid and bitter; nature: warm; toxic.

Channels entered Heart, Liver and Stomach.

Functions and indications Relieves toxicity and kills worms, dries dampness and dispels Phlegm, and settles fright. It is indicated for swollen and painful abscesses, throat wind, alopecia areata (glossy scalp wind), sores, poisonous snake bites, tetanus, convulsions, epilepsy, scabies and tinea, and herpes zoster.

Common dosage Appropriate dosage prepared as a powder for external application; 0.3-0.9g for oral use in pills.

Precautions and contraindications

1. *Xiong Huang* is contraindicated in cases of Yin deficiency and depletion of Blood, and during pregnancy.
2. Since it is easy for this substance to be absorbed through the skin, it must not be applied to a large area or for a long time.
3. *Xiong Huang* should not be calcined, as this process causes it to decompose into As_2O_3, which is extremely toxic.

Comparison of functions See *Liu Huang* (Sulphur).

Toxicity *Xiong Huang* is extremely toxic. Administration by intravenous drip to laboratory animals resulted in immediate death. The LD_{50} for intravenous injection of arsenic sulphide in rabbits is 80mg/kg. The toxicity of *Xiong Huang* is attributable to As_2O_3, which damages a number of organs in the body. Arsenic compounds are accumulative poisons, and for this reason the use of *Xiong Huang* is prohibited in the UK.

Modern research

1. Liquid preparations of *Xiong Huang* inhibited the growth of Mycobacterium tuberculosis hominis and Mycobacterium tuberculosis bovis on culture media.[1]
2. Solutions of *Xiong Huang* inhibited many types of dermatophytes *in vitro*.[2]
3. Inhibits schistosomes.[3]

Combinations and applications

Functions	Combinations	Applications
Relieving toxicity and killing worms, drying dampness and dispelling Phlegm	*Ru Xiang* (Gummi Olibanum) *Mo Yao* (Myrrha) *She Xiang* (Secretio Moschi) (see notes on legal status) *Feng Mi* (Mel) (prepared as pills for oral use)	Hard, swollen and painful abscesses and sores
	Ming Fan (Alumen)	Red and swollen itchy abscesses, and itchy scabies and tinea due to wind-damp
	Ba Dou Shuang (Pulvis Crotonis Semenis) *Yu Jin* (Radix Curcumae)	Throat wind, throat Bi syndrome, tonsillitis and Phlegm-saliva congestion

	Xiong Zhu Dan Zhi (Bilis Suis, male pig bile) (external application as a powder)	Alopecia areata (glossy scalp wind)
	Bing Lang (Semen Arecae Catechu) *Qian Niu Zi* (Semen Pharbitidis) (decoction for internal use)	Worms, and pain in the abdomen due to worm accumulation
	Fang Feng (Radix Ledebouriellae Divaricatae) *Cao Wu* (Radix Aconiti Kusnezoffii) (see notes on legal status)	Tetanus, opisthotonos or convulsions due to Liver-wind stirring internally
	Wu Bei Zi (Galla Rhois Chinensis) *Ming Fan* (Alumen) *Wu Mei* (Fructus Pruni Mume) (decoction for internal use)	Haemorrhoidal bleeding
Settling fright	*Dan Nan Xing* (Pulvis Arisaematis cum Felle Bovis)	Frequent epilepsy

Note: *Xiong Huang* can be ground to a powder and mixed with vinegar to treat poisonous snake and insect bites and wasp stings.

Liu Huang 硫黄 (Sulphur, Sulphur)

Liu Huang is processed natural sulphur.

Main ingredients *Liu Huang* contains sulphur and certain impurities (including lime, iron, tellurium and selenium).

Properties Taste: sour; nature: warm; toxic.

Channels entered Kidney and Large Intestine.

Functions and indications Internal use for supplementing fire, invigorating Yang and freeing the bowels; external use for relieving toxicity, killing worms and alleviating itching. It is indicated for cold wheezing due to Kidney deficiency, impotence and seminal cold, cold and limpness in the lumbar region and knees, constipation, frequent urination, cold and pain in the abdomen, eczema, scabies and tinea, and itchy skin.

Common dosage 1-3g for oral use in pills or powder; appropriate dosage of the powder mixed with *Ma You* (Oleum Sesami) for external application.

Precautions and contraindications

1. *Liu Huang* is contraindicated in cases of effulgent Yin deficiency-fire and during pregnancy.
2. *Liu Huang* antagonizes *Po Xiao* (Mirabilitum Non-Purum).

Comparison of functions Both *Liu Huang* (Sulphur) and *Xiong Huang* (Realgar) are toxic; they relieve toxicity and kill worms by attacking toxin with toxin and are often used for scabies and tinea (for *Xiong Huang*, see notes on legal status). However, *Xiong Huang* has a stronger effect in relieving toxicity and treating swollen abscesses and clove sores; it is better for killing intestinal worms, drying dampness and settling fright. *Liu Huang* has a stronger effect externally in killing worms and alleviating itching and is often used for scabies and tinea, eczema, and itchy skin; used internally, it can invigorate Yang and free the bowels.

Toxicity The LD_{50} for *Liu Huang* given to mice via intragastric administration is 20g/kg. *Liu Huang* is transformed in the intestinal tract into hydrogen sulphide, which controls the activity of certain enzymes and can impede oxidation reactions. Overdosage can lead to nausea and vomiting, distension in the abdomen and diarrhoea, blood in the stool, dizziness and headache, general lack of strength, tinnitus, palpitations, high temperature and in extreme cases, coma. *Liu Huang* is generally used externally nowadays, with the result that reports of toxic side-effects are infrequent.

Modern research

1. Kills scabies mites in external application.[4]
2. Inhibits inflammation and stops coughing.[5]
3. Strengthens the inhibitory function of chlorpromazine and sodium pentothal.[6]
4. Internal use results in diarrhoea.[7]

Combinations and applications

Functions	Combinations	Applications
Supplementing fire, invigorating Yang and freeing the bowels (internal use)	*Rou Gui* (Cortex Cinnamomi Cassiae) *Fu Zi* (Radix Lateralis Aconiti Carmichaeli Praeparata) (see notes on legal status)	Deficiency wheezing and shortness of breath due to Kidney Yang deficiency resulting in failure of the Kidneys to host Qi
	Bu Gu Zhi (Fructus Psoraleae Corylifoliae) *Lu Rong* (Cornu Cervi Parvum)	Impotence, seminal emission, frequent urination, and cold and limpness in the lumbar region and knees due to depletion of Kidney Yang and exhaustion of fire at the gate of vitality
	Ban Xia (Rhizoma Pinelliae Ternatae) *Sheng Jiang* (Rhizoma Zingiberis Officinalis Recens)	Constipation and cold limbs due to insufficiency of Kidney Yang in the elderly
	Yan Hu Suo (Rhizoma Corydalis Yanhusuo) *Wu Ling Zhi* (Excrementum Trogopteri) *Hu Jiao* (Fructus Piperis Nigri) *Bai Dou Kou* (Fructus Amomi Kravanh)	Cold and pain in the stomach and abdomen due to Yang deficiency of the Middle Jiao
Relieving toxicity, killing worms and alleviating itching (external use)	*Qian Dan* (Minium) (ground into a powder and mixed with sesame oil)	Scabies, wet- and dry-type tinea
	She Chuang Zi (Fructus Cnidii Monnieri) *Ku Fan* (Alumen Praeparatum) (ground into a powder)	Damp sores and itching in the genital region
	Ku Fan (Alumen Praeparatum) *Duan Shi Gao* (Gypsum Fibrosum Calcinatum) *Qing Dai* (Indigo Naturalis) *Bing Pian* (Borneolum) (ground into a powder and mixed with sesame oil)	Eczema and itchy skin
	Bing Lang (Semen Arecae Catechu) *Bing Pian* (Borneolum) (ground into a powder and mixed with sesame oil)	Rosacea

Ming Fan 明矾 (Alum, Alumen)

Ming Fan (otherwise known as *Bai Fan*) is a white or colourless crystalline compound of aluminium potassium sulphate.

Main ingredients *Ming Fan* is aluminium potassium sulphate $KAl(SO_4)_2.12H_2O$.

Properties Taste: sour and astringent; nature: cold.

Channels entered Lung, Liver, Spleen and Large Intestine.

Functions and indications

Internal use: stops bleeding and stops diarrhoea, dispels Phlegm and opens the orifices. It is indicated for wind-stroke Phlegm collapse, epilepsy, enduring diarrhoea, blood in the stool, and uterine bleeding.

External use: dries dampness and alleviates itching, relieves toxicity and kills worms. It is indicated for scabies, eczema, itching, mouth and tongue sores, and vaginal discharge.

Common dosage 1-3g in pills or powder for oral use; appropriate dosage for external application as a powder or paste.

Precautions and contraindications

1. *Ming Fan* is contraindicated for patients with a deficient constitution and weak stomach or in cases without damp-heat and Phlegm-fire.
2. Overuse can easily lead to vomiting.

Remarks In its crude form, *Ming Fan* used internally can eliminate wind-Phlegm, stop diarrhoea and stop bleeding; in its calcined form for external application, *Ku Fan* (Alumen Praeparatum), the substance is effective for drying dampness and alleviating itching.

Toxicity The LD_{50} for *Ming Fan* in acute toxicity tests on mice was 2.15g/kg. Large dosages had a strong stimulatory effect, burnt the oral cavity and throat, and caused vomiting and diarrhoea. Other experiments indicated that long-term use or overdosage impaired the renal function. Symptoms of overdose include ulceration of the gums, nausea and vomiting, pain in the abdomen and diarrhoea, blood in the urine or deficiency desertion. Internal use of *Ming Fan* is very rare these days; if the substance is used internally, dosage should be strictly controlled.

Modern research

1. Effective *in vitro* against staphylococci, Streptococcus pneumoniae, Trichomonas vaginalis and many other pathogenic micro-organisms.[8-10]
2. Promotes biliary secretion.[11]
3. Stimulates the gastric mucous membrane to induce reflex vomiting and secrete sputum.[12]

Combinations and applications

Functions	Combinations	Applications
Stopping bleeding and stopping diarrhoea (internal use)	*Wu Wei Zi* (Fructus Schisandrae) *He Zi* (Fructus Terminaliae Chebulae)	Enduring diarrhoea with rumbling intestines and a sensation of prolapsed rectum due to weak constitution in the elderly and Spleen and Kidney depletion
	Di Yu (Radix Sanguisorbae Officinalis) *Xue Yu Tan* (Crinis Carbonisatus Hominis) *Wu Bei Zi* (Galla Rhois Chinensis)	Blood in the stool, uterine bleeding, bleeding due to external injury
Dispelling Phlegm and opening the orifices (internal use)	*Ban Xia* (Rhizoma Pinelliae Ternatae) *Zao Jiao Ci* (Spina Gleditsiae Sinensis)	Wind-stroke manifesting as Phlegm collapse, clouded Spirit and inability to speak, Phlegm-saliva congestion, and a gurgling sound in the throat

	Yu Jin (Radix Curcumae)	Epilepsy due to Phlegm-heat congesting the orifices of the Heart
Drying dampness and alleviating itching, relieving toxicity and killing worms (external use)	*Liu Huang* (Sulphur) *Qing Fen* (Calomelas) (see notes on legal status) (ground into a powder)	Itchy skin due to scabies sores
	Huang Bai (Cortex Phellodendri) *Ku Shen* (Radix Sophorae Flavescentis) *She Chuang Zi* (Fructus Cnidii Monnieri) (grind *Ming Fan* into a powder for use on its own or with these herbs)	Profuse vaginal discharge with pudendal itch due to damp-heat pouring down
	Xiong Huang (Realgar) (see notes on legal status) (ground into a powder)	Itchy eczema due to wind-damp-heat toxins with dribbling discharge of yellow water after scratching
	Qing Dai (Indigo Naturalis) *Bing Pian* (Borneolum) (ground into a powder)	Mouth and tongue sores
	Huang Lian (Rhizoma Coptidis) *Xue Jie* (Resina Draconis) (for use as an external wash)	Non-healing, foul-smelling ulcerating sores

She Chuang Zi 蛇床子 (Cnidium fruit, Fructus Cnidii Monnieri)

She Chuang Zi is the dried fruit of *Cnidium monnieri* (L.) Cusson, family Umbelliferae.

Main ingredients *She Chuang Zi* contains l-pinene, l-camphene, bornyl isovalerate, isoborneol, osthole, cnidimine, isopimpinelline, bergapten, columbianetin, columbianadin, cnidiadin, xanthotoxol, xanthotoxin, imperatorin, palmitic acid and β-sitosterol.

Properties Taste: acrid and bitter; nature: warm.

Channel entered Kidney.

Functions and indications Warms the Kidneys and invigorates Yang, dispels wind and dissipates cold, dries dampness, kills worms and alleviates itching. It is indicated for internal use to treat impotence due to Kidney Yang deficiency, infertility due to cold uterus, and lumbar and limb joint pain or vaginal discharge due to damp-cold; and for external use to treat pudendal itch, scabies and eczema.

Common dosage 3-10g; 15-30g for use as an external wash.

Precautions and contraindications Internal use of *She Chuang Zi* is contraindicated in cases of vaginal discharge due to damp-heat, insufficiency of Kidney Yin or easily-stirred ministerial fire.

Comparison of functions Both *She Chuang Zi* (Fructus Cnidii Monnieri) and *Ku Shen* (Radix Sophorae Flavescentis) are very effective in drying dampness and dispelling wind, and in killing worms to alleviate itching. They can be used in combination to treat pudendal itch, vaginal discharge, generalized itchy skin, and scabies, sores and stubborn tinea. *She Chuang Zi* warms the Kidneys and invigorates Yang and is suitable for internal use to treat impotence and infertility. *Ku Shen* is effective in clearing heat and drying dampness, while concurrently promoting urination; it can be used for damp-heat dysentery, inhibited urination due to retention of damp-heat, and damp-heat jaundice.

Toxicity The LD_{50} for oral administration to mice of the coumarins contained in *She Chuang Zi* is 2.44g/kg. Rats given up to 60mg/kg of the coumarins in *She Chuang Zi* via intragastric administration once a day for 31 days did not exhibit any clear difference when compared against a control group in terms of weight, plasma or the main organs. *She Chuang Zi* has a low level of toxicity and there have been no reports to date of overdose.

Modern research

1. Preparations of *She Chuang Zi* inhibited Staphylococcus aureus, Pseudomonas aeruginosa, Trichomonas vaginalis and other pathogenic micro-organisms *in vitro*.[13]
2. Has a sex hormone-like function.[14]

Combinations and applications

Functions	Combinations	Applications
Warming the Kidneys and invigorating Yang (internal use)	*Wu Wei Zi* (Fructus Schisandrae) *Tu Si Zi* (Semen Cuscutae)	Impotence due to Kidney Yang deficiency, infertility due to cold uterus
Dispelling wind and dissipating cold (internal use)	*Sang Ji Sheng* (Ramulus Loranthi) *Du Zhong* (Cortex Eucommiae Ulmoidis) *Gou Ji* (Rhizoma Cibotii Barometz) (see notes on legal status) *Du Huo* (Radix Angelicae Pubescentis)	Lumbar and limb joint pain due to damp-cold Bi syndrome
	Shan Zhu Yu (Fructus Corni Officinalis) *Shan Yao* (Rhizoma Dioscoreae Oppositae) *Lu Jiao Jiao* (Gelatinum Cornu Cervi) *Wu Wei Zi* (Fructus Schisandrae)	Cold-damp vaginal discharge patterns with clear and thin discharge and cold and pain in the lumbar region and knees due to insufficiency of Kidney Yang
Drying dampness, killing worms and alleviating itching (external use)	*Bai Bu* (Radix Stemonae) *Ku Shen* (Radix Sophorae Flavescentis) *Hua Jiao* (Pericarpium Zanthoxyli) (prepared as a decoction for use as an external wash)	Eczema of the scrotum, scabies
	Ming Fan (Alumen) (prepared as a decoction for use as an external wash)	Pudendal itch due to an invasion of wind toxins and cold-damp pouring down
	Huang Bai (Cortex Phellodendri) *Ku Shen* (Radix Sophorae Flavescentis) *Hua Jiao* (Pericarpium Zanthoxyli) *Ku Fan* (Alumen Praeparatum) (prepared as a vaginal suppository)	Itching in the vagina

Note: Use 30g of *She Chuang Zi* mixed with 9g of *Huang Bai* (Cortex Phellodendri) and glycerin gelatin as a vaginal suppository (2g once a day) to treat trichomoniasis or unbearable itching in the vagina.

Er Cha 儿茶 (Catechu, Pasta Acaciae seu Uncariae)

Er Cha is the dried concentrated decoction prepared from the peeled branch and heartwood of *Acacia catechu* (L.) Willd., family Leguminosae, or *Uncaria gambier* Roxb., family Rubiaceae (also known as *Er Cha Gou Teng*).

Main ingredients *Er Cha* contains catechuic acid, catechu tannic acid, l- and dl-catechin, l- and dl-epicatechin, phlobatannin, fisetin, quercetin and quercetagetin; *Er Cha Gou Teng* contains catechin, catechu tannic acid, quercetin, gambirine and roxburghines A-E.

Properties Taste: bitter and astringent; nature: cool.

Channel entered Lung.

Functions and indications External use: absorbs dampness, closes sores and generates flesh, and stops bleeding. It is indicated for damp sores and weeping ulcers, Gan of the teeth and gums, mouth sores, lower body Gan, and bleeding due to external injury.

Common dosage 0.1-1g in pills and powders for oral use (see *Remarks* below); appropriate dosage for external application, ground into a powder and sprinkled on wounds or applied directly as a paste.

Remarks When taken orally, *Er Cha* also has the functions of clearing the Lungs and transforming Phlegm, generating body fluids, stopping bleeding and stopping diarrhoea. It is indicated for cough due to Lung-heat, thirst due to summerheat damaging body fluids, bleeding due to internal injury, and enduring diarrhoea and dysentery. However, this herb is seldom administered by this method nowadays.

Toxicity Laboratory mice died after intravenous injection of 200-300mg/kg of *Er Cha*. Oral administration to cats and rats of 50mg/kg per day of the pyrocatechol contained in *Er Cha* resulted in loss of consciousness, paralysis and death within 48 hours due to respiratory and circulatory failure.

Modern research

1. Inhibited Staphylococcus aureus, Staphylococcus albus, β-haemolytic streptococci and Candida albicans *in vitro*.[15]
2. Stops diarrhoea.[15]
3. Relieves toxicity.[15]

Combinations and applications

Function	Combinations	Applications
Absorbing dampness, closing sores and generating flesh (external use)	*Ru Xiang* (Gummi Olibanum) *Mo Yao* (Myrrha) *Bing Pian* (Borneolum) *Xue Jie* (Resina Draconis) *Duan Long Gu* (Os Draconis Calcinatum) (ground into a powder for external application)	Damp sores and weeping ulcers
	Qing Fen (Calomelas) (see notes on legal status) *Xue Jie* (Resina Draconis) (ground into a powder for external application)	Non-closure of ulcerating sores
	Peng Sha (Borax) (ground into a powder for topical application)	Gan of the teeth and gums, mouth sores
	Zhen Zhu (Margarita) *Bing Pian* (Borneolum) (ground into a powder for external application)	Lower body Gan, genital sores

Stopping bleeding (external use)	*Duan Long Gu* (Os Draconis Calcinatum) *Xue Jie* (Resina Draconis) *Bai Ji* (Rhizoma Bletillae Striatae) (see notes on legal status) *Jiang Xiang* (Lignum Dalbergiae Odoriferae)	Bleeding due to external injury

Chan Su 蟾酥 (Toad venom, Venenum Bufonis)

Chan Su is the dried secretion of the skin glands of the toad, *Bufo bufo gargarizans* Cantor or *B. melanostictus* Schneider, family Bufonidae.

Main ingredients *Chan Su* contains bufotalin, cinobufagin, cinobufotalin, telocinobufagin, bufalin, gamabufotalin, resibufogenin, cinobufotalidin, bufotalinin, cinobufaginol, arenobufagin, bufarenogin, bufotenine, bufotenidine and arginine.

Properties Taste: acrid and sweet; nature: warm; toxic.

Channels entered Stomach and Heart.

Functions and indications Relieves toxicity and disperses swelling, alleviates pain, opens the orifices and arouses the brain. It is indicated for swelling and toxins of abscesses and sores, swollen and painful throat, toothache, vomiting and diarrhoea, and pain in the abdomen.

Common dosage 0.015-0.03g for internal use in pills or powder; appropriate dosage for external application as a powder or paste.

Precautions and contraindications

1. *Chan Su* is contraindicated during pregnancy because it can induce contraction of the uterus.
2. As *Chan Su* is toxic, overdosage must be avoided.
3. During external application, care should be taken to ensure that the substance is kept out of the eyes.

Remarks The toxic nature of *Chan Su* enables it to relieve toxicity by attacking toxin with toxin. It is commonly used externally to treat swollen and painful sores and is also effective for throat conditions.

Toxicity The liposoluble constituents of *Chan Su* are more toxic than the water-soluble constituents. Mice injected with 625 times the normal dosage for humans of the water-soluble constituents of *Chan Su* did not exhibit signs of overdose. The LD_{50} for intravenous injection in mice of an alcoholic extract of *Chan Su* is 208mg/kg. The toxicity of the substance is reduced considerably by boiling. Many cases of overdose are due to over-consumption of *Liu Shen Wan* (Six Spirits Pill), which contains *Chan Su*.

Modern research

1. Strengthens the heart, raises blood pressure and stimulates respiration.[16, 17]
2. Inhibits inflammation.[18]
3. Has a local anaesthetic function.[19]
4. Stops coughing and calms wheezing, but is not effective in expelling sputum.[20]

Combinations and applications

Functions	Combinations	Applications
Relieving toxicity and dispersing swelling	*Ru Xiang* (Gummi Olibanum) *Zhu Sha* (Cinnabaris) (see notes on legal status)	Swelling and toxins of abscesses and sores

	Xiong Huang (Realgar) (see notes on legal status) *Zhen Zhu* (Margarita) *Niu Huang* (Calculus Bovis) *She Xiang* (Secretio Moschi) (see notes on legal status) *Bing Pian* (Borneolum)	Sore and swollen throat, throat wind, tonsillitis
Alleviating pain, opening the orifices and arousing the brain	*Ding Xiang* (Flos Caryophylli) *Cang Zhu* (Rhizoma Atractylodis) *She Xiang* (Secretio Moschi) (see notes on legal status)	Acute vomiting and diarrhoea, pain in the abdomen and sudden collapse due to summerheat and damp-turbid pathogenic factors
	Chuan Wu (Radix Aconiti Carmichaeli) (see notes on legal status) *Cao Wu* (Radix Aconiti Kusnezoffii) (see notes on legal status) *Tian Nan Xing* (Rhizoma Arisaematis) *Ban Xia* (Rhizoma Pinelliae Ternatae)	Prepared as a powder for external application with a local anaesthetic effect

Feng Fang 蜂房
(Hornet nest, Nidus Vespae)

Feng Fang is the honeycomb built by hornets, especially *Polistes olivaceus* (Degeer), *P. japonicus* Saussure or *Parapolybia varia* Fabr., family Vespidae.

Main ingredients *Feng Fang* contains beeswax and resin.

Properties Taste: sweet; nature: neutral; toxic.

Channels entered Lung and Stomach.

Functions and indications Dispels wind-damp, invigorates Kidney Yang, and relieves toxicity. It is indicated for abscesses and sores, breast abscess, scrofula, scabies, toothache, wind-damp Bi syndrome pain, and urticaria (dormant papules).

Common dosage 6-12g in decoctions; or 1.5-3g as a powder for oral use; appropriate dosage for external application.

Precautions and contraindications

1. *Feng Fang* should be used with caution in cases of Qi and Blood deficiency.
2. *Feng Fang* is contraindicated in cases of impairment of the Kidney function and ulcerated abscesses.

Toxicity The LD_{50} for intravenous injection in mice of an aqueous extract of *Feng Fang* is 12g/kg. The minimum toxic dosage is 30g for decoctions, 10g for powders. After the oils contained in *Feng Fang* have been absorbed by the body, they are excreted by the kidneys; the metabolized products stimulate the glomerulus blood capillaries resulting in acute nephritis. The toxic nature of *Feng Fang* means that it is no longer used for expelling worms.

Modern research

1. Inhibits inflammation, alleviates pain and lowers body temperature.[21]
2. Stops bleeding, strengthens myocardial contraction, lowers blood pressure and promotes urination.[22]
3. Inhibits carcinoma.[23]
4. The volatile oils contained in *Feng Fang* expel tapeworm.[23]
5. Overdosage inhibited respiration and induced acute nephritis in animals (see also *Toxicity*).[22]

Combinations and applications

Functions	Combinations	Applications
Dispelling wind-damp	*Tu Bie Chong* (Eupolyphaga seu Steleophaga) *Quan Xie* (Buthus Martensi) *Wu Gong* (Scolopendra Subspinipes)	Red, swollen, painful and stiff joints due to wind-damp
	Chan Tui (Periostracum Cicadae) *Fu Ping* (Herba Spirodelae Polyrrhizae) *Di Fu Zi* (Fructus Kochiae Scopariae)	Itchy skin and urticaria (dormant papules)
	Ru Xiang (Gummi Olibanum) *Xi Xin* (Herba cum Radice Asari) (prepared as a decoction for gargling)	'Wind worm' toothache
Invigorating Kidney Yang	*Sang Piao Xiao* (Oötheca Mantidis)	Urinary incontinence
Relieving toxicity	Oral intake of 1.5-3g of the powder prepared by mixing yellow-baked *Feng Fang* with rice wine (a large amount of water should be drunk when taking the mixture)	Initial stage of breast abscess before pus appears in the abscess
	Local application of the paste made from a powder of yellow-baked *Feng Fang* mixed with *Mi Cu* (Acetum Oryzae, rice vinegar)	Sloughing abscess
	Local application of the paste made by mixing powdered *Feng Fang* with pork fat	Scrofula
	Tian Nan Xing (Rhizoma Arisaematis) *Chi Xiao Dou* (Semen Phaseoli Calcarati) *Sheng Cao Wu* (Radix Aconiti Kusnezoffii Cruda) *Ming Fan* (Alumen) (prepared as a powder and mixed with *Mi Cu*, rice vinegar)	Hard and painful swelling and local redness in the initial stage of abscesses

Xue Jie 血竭
(Dragon's blood, Resina Draconis)

Xue Jie is the resinous secretion from the fruits of *Daemonorops draco* (Bl.) and related species, family Palmae.

Main ingredients *Xue Jie* contains dracoalban, dracorubin, nordracoalban, nordracorubin, flavonols, chalcone, resin, gum, benzoic acid and cinnamic acid.

Properties Taste: sweet and salty; nature: neutral.

Channels entered Heart and Liver.

Functions and indications Stops bleeding, dispels Blood stasis and alleviates pain, closes sores and generates flesh. It is indicated for pain in the heart and abdomen due to Blood stasis, postpartum pain in the abdomen, knocks and falls, bleeding due to external injury, and non-healing abscesses and sores.

Common dosage 1-1.5g, prepared as pills or powder; appropriate dosage for external application as a powder or plaster.

Precautions and contraindications *Xue Jie* is contraindicated for internal use in cases without Blood stasis and during pregnancy.

Modern research

1. Promotes urination in small dosages, whereas large dosages lead to toxic side-effects.[24]
2. Stops bleeding.[25]
3. Inhibits coagulation, and decreases the viscosity of blood and plasma.[25]

Combinations and applications

Functions	Combinations	Applications
Stopping bleeding, dispelling Blood stasis and alleviating pain (internal use)	*Ru Xiang* (Gummi Olibanum) *Mo Yao* (Myrrha) *Hong Hua* (Flos Carthami Tinctorii) *Bing Pian* (Borneolum)	Stabbing pain in the heart and abdomen due to Blood stasis, postpartum pain in the abdomen and menstrual block due to Blood stasis
Stopping bleeding, closing sores and generating flesh (external use)	*Ru Xiang* (Gummi Olibanum) *Er Cha* (Pasta Acaciae seu Uncariae) *Mo Yao* (Myrrha)	Knocks and falls, pain in the sinews and bones, or bleeding due to external injury
	Qian Dan (Minium) (apply as a powder to the opening of the sores)	Chronic, non-healing sores

Qing Fen 轻粉 (Calomel, Calomelas)

Qing Fen is a crystalline mercurous chloride (Hg_2Cl_2).

Legal status The use of this materia medica is illegal in the UK as a result of its toxic nature.

Main ingredients *Qing Fen* contains mercurous chloride (Hg_2Cl_2).

Properties Taste: acrid; nature: cold; extremely toxic.

Channels entered Large Intestine and Small Intestine.

Functions and indications

Internal use: promotes the movement of water and frees the bowels; it is indicated for distension in the abdomen, oedema, difficult urination, and constipation.

External use: kills worms and relieves toxicity; it is indicated for abscesses, boils, sores, stubborn tinea, and syphilis.

Common dosage Appropriate dosage for external application; or 0.1-0.2g prepared as pills or powder for oral use.

Precautions and contraindications

1. *Qing Fen* should be used with extreme caution internally as a result of its highly toxic nature (see *Legal status* above); even externally, the substance must not be used long-term and the dosage must not be exceeded.
2. *Qing Fen* is contraindicated during pregnancy.

Toxicity The LD_{50} for *Qing Fen* given via intragastric administration is 410mg/kg for mice and 1740mg/kg for rats. Mercury builds up within the body and damages the central and autonomic nervous systems. Symptoms of acute poisoning include enlargement of the kidneys, acute corrosive gastroenteritis and circulation problems. Chronic poisoning results in nervous exhaustion, a metallic taste in the mouth, swollen gums, bleeding, loose teeth, nausea and vomiting, lack of appetite, pain in the abdomen and diarrhoea.

Modern research

1. Inhibited dermatophytes *in vitro*.[26]
2. Inhibits carcinoma.[27]

Combinations and applications

Functions	Combinations	Applications
Promoting the movement of water and freeing the bowels (internal use)	*Da Huang* (Radix et Rhizoma Rhei) *Jing Da Ji* (Radix Euphorbiae Pekinensis) *Gan Sui* (Radix Euphorbiae Kansui)	Full patterns of swelling and constipation, manifesting as distension in the abdomen with oedema and difficult urination and defecation due to the collection of water and dampness
Killing worms and relieving toxicity (external use)	*Xue Jie* (Resina Draconis) *Zi Cao* (Radix Arnebiae seu Lithospermi) (prepared as a powder)	Non-closure of open sores
	Ru Xiang (Gummi Olibanum) *Xue Jie* (Resina Draconis) *Hai Piao Xiao* (Os Sepiae seu Sepiellae) *Duan Long Gu* (Os Draconis Calcinatum) (prepared as a powder)	Frostbite
	Feng Xiang Zhi (Resina Liquidambaris) *Song Xiang* (Resina Pini) (make a powder from equal amounts of *Qing Fen* and these substances and mix with sesame oil)	Stubborn tinea

Lu Gan Shi 炉甘石 (Calamine, Calamina)

Lu Gan Shi is a natural ore, smithsonite, of the calcite group.

Main ingredients *Lu Gan Shi* contains zinc carbonate ($ZnCO_3$). Calcined *Lu Gan Shi* contains zinc oxide.

Properties Taste: sweet; nature: neutral.

Channels entered Liver and Stomach.

Functions and indications External use: brightens the eyes and removes eye screen, absorbs dampness, closes sores and generates flesh. It is indicated for external use to treat red, sore and swollen eyes, wind eye with ulceration of the eyelid rim, eye screen, profuse lacrimation and fear of light, and non-healing abscesses and sores.

Common dosage As *Lu Gan Shi* is only used externally, the appropriate dosage should be chosen depending on the condition involved.

Precautions and contraindications Not to be used internally.

Comparison of functions See *Peng Sha* (Borax).

Modern research

1. Has an astringent function.[28]
2. External application relieves itching and inhibits certain bacteria.[28]

Combinations and applications

Functions	Combinations	Applications
Brightening the eyes and removing eye screen, absorbing dampness, closing sores and generating flesh (external use)	*Huang Lian* (Rhizoma Coptidis) *Bing Pian* (Borneolum) *Peng Sha* (Borax) (prepared as eye drops)	Wind eye with ulceration of the eyelid rim, eye screen outcrop (pterygium), red eyes and profuse lacrimation
	Huang Bai (Cortex Phellodendri) *Qing Dai* (Indigo Naturalis) *Duan Shi Gao* (Gypsum Fibrosum Calcinatum)	Itchy eczema, damp skin sores with constant drainage of water and pus

Peng Sha 硼砂
(Borax, Borax)

Peng Sha is a crystalline mineral salt refined from borax ores.

Main ingredients *Peng Sha* contains hydrated disodium tetraborate ($Na_2B_4O_7.10H_2O$).

Properties Taste: sweet and salty; nature: cool.

Channels entered Lung and Stomach.

Functions and indications

Internal use: clears heat and transforms Phlegm. It is indicated for hoarse voice and sore throat due to congestion of Phlegm-heat, and for difficult expectoration of sputum.

External use: relieves toxicity and prevents putrefaction. It is indicated for mouth and tongue sores, sore and swollen throat, and red eyes and eye screen.

Common dosage 1.5-3g; appropriate dosage for external application as a paste or fine powder.

Precautions and contraindications *Peng Sha* is mainly used externally; oral administration calls for great caution.

Remarks Use crude *Peng Sha* for transforming Phlegm; use the calcined substance for external applications.

Comparison of functions Both *Peng Sha* (Borax) and *Lu Gan Shi* (Calamina) are mild, relatively non-toxic materia medica used frequently in the treatment of eye, mouth and throat conditions. *Peng Sha* is cool in nature and is better for clearing heat and relieving toxicity; it acts as an antiseptic when used externally. *Peng Sha* can also be used for clearing the Lungs to transform Phlegm. *Lu Gan Shi* is neutral in nature and functions better in absorbing dampness and closing sores; it is used externally for non-healing abscesses and sores.

Modern research

1. Solutions of *Peng Sha* inhibited many bacteria *in vitro*, including Streptococcus pneumoniae and Pseudomonas aeruginosa.[29]
2. Relieves toxicity and attenuates hyperthyroidism due to fluorosis.[12]

Combinations and applications

Functions	Combinations	Applications
Clearing heat and transforming Phlegm (internal use)	*Tian Hua Fen* (Radix Trichosanthis) *Qing Dai* (Indigo Naturalis) *Zhu Li* (Succus Bambusae)	Chronic cough and hoarse voice with thick, sticky, yellow sputum due to congestion of Phlegm-heat
Relieving toxicity and preventing putrefaction (external use)	*Bing Pian* (Borneolum) *Xuan Ming Fen* (Mirabilitum Depuratum) (prepared as a powder)	Sore and swollen throat, mouth and tongue sores
	Bing Pian (Borneolum) (used as eye drops)	Red, sore and swollen eyes, eye screen outcrop (pterygium)

Modern research references

1. Cao Zhaobo et al., *Zhong Cao Yao* [Journal of Chinese Herbs] 17, 12 (1986): 35.
2. He Xingdong et al., *Lin Chuang Zhong Yao Shou Ce* [Clinical Handbook of Chinese Materia Medica] (Beijing: People's Medical Publishing House, 1998), 362.
3. Lei Zaiquan and Zhang Tingmo, *Zhong Hua Lin Chuang Zhong Yao Xue* [Chinese Clinical Materia Medica] (Beijing: People's Medical Publishing House, 1998), 1908.
4. Shandong Provincial Hospital, *Shi Yong Yao Wu Shou Ce* [Practical Handbook of Medicines] (Jinan: Shandong Science and Technology Publishing House, 1987), 940.
5. Ye Xianchun, *Zhong Yao Xue* [Chinese Materia Medica] (Shanghai: Shanghai College of TCM Press, 1988), 758.
6. Yan Zhenghua, *Zhong Yao Xue* [Chinese Materia Medica] (Beijing: People's Medical Publishing House, 1991), 908.
7. Wang Yusheng et al., *Zhong Yao Yao Li Yu Ying Yong* [Pharmacology and Application of Chinese Materia Medica] (Beijing: People's Medical Publishing House, 1988), 1154.
8. Jiangsu New Medical College, *Zhong Yao Da Ci Dian* [Dictionary of Chinese Materia Medica] (Shanghai: Shanghai Science and Technology Publishing House, 1986), 680.
9. Yu Jianwen et al., *Yun Nan Zhong Yi Za Zhi* [Yunnan Journal of Traditional Chinese Medicine] 11, 3 (1990): 26.
10. Wu Jingpu, *Nan Jing Zhong Yi Xue Yuan Xue Bao* [Journal of Nanjing College of Traditional Chinese Medicine] 1 (1985): 46.
11. Chen Xiangming et al., *Zhong Yao Tong Bao* [Bulletin of Chinese Materia Medica] 13, 12 (1988): 48.
12. He Xingdong et al., *Lin Chuang Zhong Yao Shou Ce*, 367.
13. Lei Zaiquan and Zhang Tingmo, *Zhong Hua Lin Chuang Zhong Yao Xue*, 1685.
14. Pharmacology Faculty of Shandong Medical College, *Zhong Cao Yao Yao Li Xue* [Pharmacology of Chinese Herbs] (Jinan: Shandong Science and Technology Publishing House, 1976), 188.
15. Wang Benxian, *Xin Bian Zhong Yao Xue Ci Dian* [New Dictionary of Chinese Materia Medica] (Tianjin: Tianjin Science and Technology Publishing House, 1996), 29.
16. Xie Jingtian, *Zhong Guo Yao Li Xue Bao* [Chinese Journal of Pharmacology] 6, 4 (1985): 254.
17. Ibid., 6, 3 (1985): 169.
18. Tian Jiatai, *Jia Mu Si Yi Xue Yuan Xue Bao* [Journal of Jiamusi Medical College] 3 (1977): 49.
19. Liu Zhongyu, *Jiang Xi Yi Yao* [Jiangxi Journal of Medicine and Pharmacology] 5, 3 (1965): 665.
20. Xue Kaixian, *Xin Yi Yao Xue Za Zhi* [New Medicine and Pharmacology Journal] 1 (1974): 39.
21. Meng Yingqin et al., *Zhong Cao Yao* [Journal of Chinese Herbs] 14, 9 (1983): 21.
22. Lei Zaiquan and Zhang Tingmo, *Zhong Hua Lin Chuang Zhong Yao Xue*, 1952.
23. Wang Zheng, *Shan Xi Xin Yi Yao* [Shaanxi New Medical Journal] 8, 11 (1979): 51.
24. He Xingdong et al., *Lin Chuang Zhong Yao Shou Ce*, 378.
25. Wang Benxian, *Xin Bian Zhong Yao Xue Ci Dian*, 498.
26. Yang Zhenyu et al., *Zhong Cao Yao* [Journal of Chinese Herbs] 21, 8 (1990): 26.
27. Zhang Tingdong et al., *Collected Papers of the Second Conference of the Chinese Academy of Integrated TCM and Western Medicine* (1985), 18-19.
28. He Xingdong et al., *Lin Chuang Zhong Yao Shou Ce*, 366.
29. Lei Zaiquan and Zhang Tingmo, *Zhong Hua Lin Chuang Zhong Yao Xue*, 1350.

Appendices

LIST OF APPENDICES

Appendix 1 Index of materia medica covered by individual monographs

The materia medica in this index are listed in four-column tabular format with each sub-index beginning with a different column – pinyin, pharmaceutical name or English name. All materia medica are indexed to the pages containing the relevant monograph. Please note that Appendix 6 provides a listing of individual materia medica (by pinyin and pharmaceutical name) cross-referenced to the main herb of the combinations in which they appear.

Appendix 1a Index of materia medica by pinyin name

(listed alphabetically without any distinction made between tones)

Pinyin	Simplified Chinese characters	Pharmaceutical name	English name	Page
Bai Shen	白参	Radix Ginseng Alba	White ginseng	514
Bai Tou Weng	白头翁	Radix Pulsatillae Chinensis	Chinese pulsatilla root	107
Bai Wei	白薇	Radix Cynanchi Atrati	Black-end swallowwort root	142
Bai Xian Pi	白鲜皮	Cortex Dictamni Dasycarpi Radicis	Dittany root bark	90
Bai Zhi	白芷	Radix Angelicae Dahuricae	White angelica root	33
Bai Zhu	白术	Rhizoma Atractylodis Macrocephalae	White atractylodes rhizome	521
Bai Zi Ren	柏子仁	Semen Biotae Orientalis	Chinese arborvitae seed	462
Ban Bian Lian	半边莲	Herba Lobeliae Chinensis cum Radice	Chinese lobelia	111
Ban Lan Gen	板蓝根	Radix Isatidis seu Baphicacanthi	Isatis root	101
Ban Xia	半夏	Rhizoma Pinelliae Ternatae	Pinellia tuber	399
Bei Mu	贝母	Bulbus Fritillariae	Fritillary bulb	413
Bei Sha Shen	北沙参	Radix Glehniae Littoralis	Glehnia root	579
Bi Xie	萆薢	Rhizoma Dioscoreae (Hypoglaucae seu Septemlobae)	Yam rhizome	236
Bian Xu	扁蓄	Herba Polygoni Avicularis	Prostrate knotweed	233
Bie Jia	鳖甲	Carapax Amydae Sinensis	Chinese soft-shelled turtle shell	583
Bing Lang	槟榔	Semen Arecae Catechu	Areca seed	311
Bing Pian	冰片	Borneolum (Syntheticum)	Borneol	503
Bo He	薄荷	Herba Menthae Haplocalycis	Peppermint	45
Bu Gu Zhi	补骨脂	Fructus Psoraleae Corylifoliae	Psoralea fruit	548
Cang Er Zi	苍耳子	Fructus Xanthii Sibirici	Cocklebur fruit	36
Cang Zhu	苍术	Rhizoma Atractylodis	Atractylodes rhizome	201
Cao Dou Kou	草豆蔻	Semen Alpiniae Katsumadai	Katsumada galangal seed	206
Cao Guo	草果	Fructus Amomi Tsaoko	Tsaoko fruit	208
Cao Wu	草乌	Radix Aconiti Kusnezoffii	Wild aconite root	253
Ce Bai Ye	侧柏叶	Cacumen Biotae Orientalis	Chinese arborvitae twig and leaf	328
Chai Hu	柴胡	Radix Bupleuri	Chinese thorowax root	51
Chan Su	蟾酥	Venenum Bufonis	Toad venom	657
Chan Tui	蝉蜕	Periostracum Cicadae	Cicada slough	55
Chang Shan	常山	Radix Dichroae Febrifugae	Dichroa root	642
Che Qian Cao	车前草	Herba Plantaginis	Plantain herb	227
Che Qian Zi	车前子	Semen Plantaginis	Plantain seed	226
Chen Pi	陈皮	Pericarpium Citri Reticulatae	Tangerine peel	272
Chen Xiang	沉香	Lignum Aquilariae Resinatum	Chinese eaglewood	279
Chi Fu Ling	赤茯苓	Sclerotium Poriae Cocos Rubrae	Red poria	219
Chi Shao	赤芍	Radix Paeoniae Rubra	Red peony root	133
Chi Shi Zhi	赤石脂	Halloysitum Rubrum	Red halloysite	622

Pinyin	Simplified Chinese characters	Pharmaceutical name	English name	Page
Di Yu Tan	地榆炭	Radix Sanguisorbae Officinalis Carbonisata	Charred sanguisorba root	327
Ding Xiang	丁香	Flos Caryophylli	Cloves	262
Dong Chong Xia Cao	冬虫夏草	Cordyceps Sinensis	Chinese caterpillar fungus	554
Dong Gua Pi	冬瓜皮	Epicarpium Benincasae Hispidae	Wax gourd peel	223
Dong Gua Ren	冬瓜仁	Semen Benincasae Hispidae	Wax gourd seed	224
Du Huo	独活	Radix Angelicae Pubescentis	Pubescent angelica root	174
Du Zhong	杜仲	Cortex Eucommiae Ulmoidis	Eucommia bark	542
Duan Long Gu	煅龙骨	Os Draconis Calcinatum	Calcined dragon bone	455
Duan Shi Gao	煅石膏	Gypsum Fibrosum Calcinatum	Calcined gypsum	69
E Jiao	阿胶	Gelatinum Corii Asini	Donkey-hide gelatin	573
E Zhu	莪术	Rhizoma Curcumae	Zedoary rhizome	385
Er Cha	儿茶	Pasta Acaciae seu Uncariae	Catechu	656
Fa Ban Xia	法半夏	Rhizoma Pinelliae Ternatae Praeparata	Prepared pinellia tuber	399
Fan Xie Ye	番泻叶	Folium Sennae	Senna leaf	159
Fang Feng	防风	Radix Ledebouriellae Divaricatae (Radix Saposhnikoviae Divaricatae)	Ledebouriella root (Saposhnikovia root)	30
Fang Ji	防己	Radix Stephaniae Tetrandrae	Stephania root	183
Fei Zi	榧子	Semen Torreyae Grandis	Torreya nut	316
Fen Bi Xie	粉萆薢	Rhizoma Dioscoreae Hypoglaucae	Collett yam rhizome	236
Feng Fang	蜂房	Nidus Vespae	Hornet nest	658
Fo Shou	佛手	Fructus Citri Sarcodactylis	Finger citron fruit or Buddha's hand	282
Fo Shou Hua	佛手花	Flos Citri Sarcodactylis	Finger citron flower	283
Fu Hai Shi	浮海石	Os Costaziae seu Pumex	Costazia bone or pumice	422
Fu Ling	茯苓	Sclerotium Poriae Cocos	Poria	217
Fu Ling Pi	茯苓皮	Cortex Poriae Cocos	Poria skin	219
Fu Pen Zi	覆盆子	Fructus Rubi Chingii	Chinese raspberry	635
Fu Ping	浮萍	Herba Spirodelae Polyrrhizae	Common ducksmeat herb	59
Fu Shen	茯神	Sclerotium Poriae Cocos cum Ligno Hospite	Poria with hostwood	219
Fu Xiao Mai	浮小麦	Fructus Tritici Aestivi Levis	Light wheat grain	610
Fu Zi	附子	Radix Lateralis Aconiti Carmichaeli Praeparata	Prepared Sichuan aconite daughter root	250
Gan Cao	甘草	Radix Glycyrrhizae	Liquorice root	523
Gan Di Huang	干地黄	Radix Rehmanniae Glutinosae Exsiccata	Dried rehmannia root	129
Gan Jiang	干姜	Rhizoma Zingiberis Officinalis	Dried ginger	253
Gan Sui	甘遂	Radix Euphorbiae Kansui	Kansui root	162
Gao Ben	藁本	Rhizoma et Radix Ligustici	Chinese lovage root	35

Pinyin	Simplified Chinese characters	Pharmaceutical name	English name	Page
Hu Lu Ba	胡芦巴	Semen Trigonellae Foeni-graeci	Fenugreek seed	558
Hu Po	琥珀	Succinum	Amber	457
Hu Tao Ren/ Hu Tao Rou	胡桃仁/胡桃肉	Semen Juglandis Regiae	Walnut kernel	557
Hu Zhang	虎杖	Radix et Rhizoma Polygoni Cuspidati	Giant knotweed root and rhizome	241
Hua Jiao	花椒	Pericarpium Zanthoxyli	Chinese prickly ash	259
Hua Rui Shi	花蕊石	Ophicalcitum	Ophicalcite	337
Hua Shi	滑石	Talcum	Talc	227
Huai Hua	槐花	Flos Sophorae Japonicae	Pagoda tree flower	329
Huai Jiao	槐角	Fructus Sophorae Japonicae	Pagoda tree fruit	330
Huai Niu Xi	怀牛膝	Radix Achyranthis Bidentatae	Achyranthes root	375
Huang Bai	黄柏	Cortex Phellodendri	Amur cork tree bark	84
Huang Bai Tan	黄柏炭	Cortex Phellodendri Carbonisatus	Charred amur cork tree bark	85
Huang Jing	黄精	Rhizoma Polygonati	Siberian Solomon seal rhizome	593
Huang Ju Hua	黄菊花	Flos Aureus Chrysanthemi Morifolii	Yellow chrysanthemum flower	50
Huang Lian	黄连	Rhizoma Coptidis	Golden thread rhizome	82
Huang Qi	黄芪	Radix Astragali seu Hedysari	Milk vetch or sweet vetch root	518
Huang Qin	黄芩	Radix Scutellariae Baicalensis	Baical skullcap root	81
Huang Qin Tan	黄芩炭	Radix Scutellariae Baicalensis Carbonisata	Charred baical skullcap root	81
Huang Yao Zi	黄药子	Rhizoma Dioscoreae Bulbiferae	Air potato yam	427
Huo Ma Ren	火麻仁	Semen Cannabis Sativae	Hemp seed	151
Huo Xiang	藿香	Herba Agastaches seu Pogostemi	Agastache or patchouli	199
Ji Nei Jin	鸡内金	Endothelium Corneum Gigeriae Galli	Internal lining of chicken gizzard	302
Ji Xue Teng	鸡血藤	Caulis Spatholobi	Spatholobus stem	378
Jiang Can	僵蚕	Bombyx Batryticatus	Stiff silkworm	493
Jiang Huang	姜黄	Rhizoma Curcumae Longae	Turmeric rhizome	364
Jiang Xiang	降香	Lignum Dalbergiae Odoriferae	Dalbergia heartwood	338
Jiao Mu	椒目	Semen Zanthoxyli	Chinese prickly ash seed	260
Jie Geng	桔梗	Radix Platycodi Grandiflori	Platycodon root	406
Jin Qian Cao	金钱草	Herba Lysimachiae	Lysimachia	240
Jin Yin Hua	金银花	Flos Lonicerae	Honeysuckle flower	95
Jin Ying Zi	金樱子	Fructus Rosae Laevigatae	Cherokee rose fruit	636
Jing Da Ji	京大戟	Radix Euphorbiae Pekinensis	Peking spurge root	163
Jing Jie	荆芥	Herba Schizonepetae Tenuifoliae	Schizonepeta herb	28

Pinyin	Simplified Chinese characters	Pharmaceutical name	English name	Page
Lu Jiao Shuang	鹿角霜	Cornu Cervi Degelatinatum	Degelatined mature deer antler	540
Lu Lu Tong	路路通	Fructus Liquidambaris	Sweetgum fruit	180
Lu Rong	鹿茸	Cornu Cervi Parvum	Pilose antler of young deer	538
Lü Dou	绿豆	Semen Phaseoli Radiati	Mung bean	125
Lü Dou Yi	绿豆衣	Testa Phaseoli Radiati	Mung bean skin	126
Luo Shi Teng	络石藤	Caulis Trachelospermi Jasminoidis	Chinese star jasmine stem	187
Ma Bo	马勃	Sclerotium Lasiosphaerae seu Calvatiae	Puff-ball	116
Ma Chi Xian	马齿苋	Herba Portulacae Oleraceae	Purslane	117
Ma Dou Ling	马兜铃	Fructus Aristolochiae	Aristolochia fruit	439
Ma Huang	麻黄	Herba Ephedrae	Ephedra	20
Ma Huang Gen	麻黄根	Radix Ephedrae	Ephedra root	609
Mai Men Dong	麦门冬	Radix Ophiopogonis Japonici	Ophiopogon root	580
Mai Ya	麦芽	Fructus Hordei Vulgaris Germinatus	Barley sprout	299
Man Jing Zi	蔓荆子	Fructus Viticis	Chaste-tree fruit	56
Mang Xiao	芒硝	Mirabilitum	Mirabilite	157
Mei Gui Hua	玫瑰花	Flos Rosae Rugosae	Chinese rose flower	289
Mian Bi Xie	绵萆薢	Rhizoma Dioscoreae Septemlobae	Seven-lobed yam rhizome	236
Ming Fan	明矾	Alumen	Alum	653
Mo Han Lian	墨旱莲	Herba Ecliptae Prostratae	Eclipta	595
Mo Yao	没药	Myrrha	Myrrh	366
Mu Dan Pi	牡丹皮	Cortex Moutan Radicis	Tree peony root bark	132
Mu Gua	木瓜	Fructus Chaenomelis	Chinese quince fruit	175
Mu Hu Die	木蝴蝶	Semen Oroxyli Indici	Oroxylum seed	120
Mu Li	牡蛎	Concha Ostreae	Oyster shell	473
Mu Tong	木通	Caulis Mutong	Mutong stem	229
Mu Xiang	木香	Radix Aucklandiae Lappae	Aucklandia root	276
Mu Zei	木贼	Herba Equiseti Hiemalis	Scouring rush herb	60
Nan Gua Zi	南瓜子	Semen Cucurbitae Moschatae	Pumpkin seed	313
Nan Sha Shen	南沙参	Radix Adenophorae	Adenophora root	580
Niu Bang Zi	牛蒡子	Fructus Arctii Lappae	Great burdock fruit	46
Niu Huang	牛黄	Calculus Bovis	Cow bezoar	482
Niu Xi	牛膝	Radix Achyranthis Bidentatae	Achyranthes root	375
Nü Zhen Zi	女贞子	Fructus Ligustri Lucidi	Glossy privet fruit	596
Ou Jie	藕节	Nodus Nelumbinis Nuciferae Rhizomatis	Node of lotus rhizome	344
Pang Da Hai	胖大海	Semen Sterculiae Lychnophorae	Boat-fruited sterculia seed	426
Pao Jiang	炮姜	Rhizoma Zingiberis Officinalis Praeparata	Prepared dried ginger	346

Pinyin	Simplified Chinese characters	Pharmaceutical name	English name	Page
Shan Dou Gen	山豆根	Radix Sophorae Tonkinensis	Subprostrate sophora root	115
Shan Yang Jiao	山羊角	Cornu Naemorhedi	Goat horn	481
Shan Yao	山药	Rhizoma Dioscoreae Oppositae	Chinese yam	526
Shan Zha	山楂	Fructus Crataegi	Hawthorn fruit	297
Shan Zhu Yu	山茱萸	Fructus Corni Officinalis	Asiatic Cornelian cherry fruit	631
She Chuang Zi	蛇床子	Fructus Cnidii Monnieri	Cnidium fruit	654
She Gan	射干	Rhizoma Belamcandae Chinensis	Belamcanda rhizome	106
She Xiang	麝香	Secretio Moschi	Musk	501
Shen Jin Cao	伸筋草	Herba Lycopodii Japonici	Club moss	178
Shen Qu	神曲	Massa Fermentata	Medicated leaven	298
Sheng Di Huang	生地黄	Radix Rehmanniae Glutinosae	Rehmannia root	129
Sheng Di Huang Tan	生地黄炭	Radix Rehmanniae Glutinosae Carbonisata	Charred rehmannia root	129
Sheng Jiang	生姜	Rhizoma Zingiberis Officinalis Recens	Fresh ginger	39
Sheng Jiang Pi	生姜皮	Cortex Zingiberis Officinalis Recens	Ginger rhizome skin	39
Sheng Ma	升麻	Rhizoma Cimicifugae	Bugbane rhizome	57
Sheng Shi Gao	生石膏	Gypsum Fibrosum Crudum	Crude gypsum	69
Shi Chang Pu	石菖蒲	Rhizoma Acori Graminei	Grass-leaf sweetflag rhizome	505
Shi Gao	石膏	Gypsum Fibrosum	Gypsum	69
Shi Hu	石斛	Herba Dendrobii	Dendrobium	591
Shi Jue Ming	石决明	Concha Haliotidis	Abalone shell	472
Shi Jun Zi	使君子	Fructus Quisqualis Indicae	Rangoon creeper fruit	309
Shi Liu Pi	石榴皮	Pericarpium Punicae Granati	Pomegranate rind	624
Shi Wei	石韦	Folium Pyrrosiae	Pyrrosia leaf	235
Shu Di Huang	熟地黄	Radix Rehmanniae Glutinosae Conquita	Processed rehmannia root	565
Shui Niu Jiao	水牛角	Cornu Bubali	Water buffalo horn	136
Shui Zhi	水蛭	Hirudo seu Whitmania	Leech	387
Su Geng	苏梗	Caulis Perillae Frutescentis	Perilla stem	28
Su He Xiang	苏合香	Styrax Liquidus	Liquid storax	503
Su Mu	苏木	Lignum Sappan	Sappan wood	382
Su Zi	苏子	Fructus Perillae Frutescentis	Perilla fruit	432
Suan Zao Ren	酸枣仁	Semen Ziziphi Spinosae	Spiny jujube seed	460
Suo Yang	锁阳	Herba Cynomorii Songarici	Cynomorium stem	551
Tai Zi Shen	太子参	Radix Pseudostellariae Heterophyllae	Pseudostellaria root	531
Tao Ren	桃仁	Semen Persicae	Peach kernel	372
Tian Hua Fen	天花粉	Radix Trichosanthis	Trichosanthes root	71
Tian Ma	天麻	Rhizoma Gastrodiae Elatae	Gastrodia tuber	486

Pinyin	Simplified Chinese characters	Pharmaceutical name	English name	Page
Xin Yi Hua	辛夷花	Flos Magnoliae	Magnolia flower	38
Xing Ren	杏仁	Semen Pruni Armeniacae	Apricot kernel	431
Xiong Huang	雄黄	Realgar	Realgar	650
Xu Chang Qing	徐长卿	Radix Cynanchi Paniculati	Paniculate swallowwort root	188
Xu Duan	续断	Radix Dipsaci	Dipsacus root	544
Xuan Fu Hua	旋复花	Flos Inulae	Inula flower	410
Xuan Ming Fen	玄明粉	Mirabilitum Depuratum	Refined mirabilite	158
Xuan Shen	玄参	Radix Scrophulariae Ningpoensis	Figwort root	130
Xue Jie	血竭	Resina Draconis	Dragon's blood	659
Ya Dan Zi	鸦胆子	Fructus Bruceae Javanicae	Brucea fruit	118
Yan Hu Suo	延胡索	Rhizoma Corydalis Yanhusuo	Corydalis tuber	361
Yang Jin Hua	洋金花	Flos Daturae	Datura flower	444
Ye Jiao Teng	夜交藤	Caulis Polygoni Multiflori	Fleece-flower stem	464
Ye Ju Hua	野菊花	Flos Chrysanthemi Indici	Wild chrysanthemum flower	108
Yi Mu Cao	益母草	Herba Leonuri Heterophylli	Motherwort	374
Yi Tang	饴糖	Saccharum Granorum	Malt sugar	533
Yi Yi Ren	薏苡仁	Semen Coicis Lachrymajobi	Coix seed	219
Yi Zhi Ren	益智仁	Fructus Alpiniae Oxyphyllae	Bitter cardamom	549
Yin Chai Hu	银柴胡	Radix Stellariae Dichotomae	Stellaria root	140
Yin Chen Hao	茵陈蒿	Herba Artemisiae Scopariae	Oriental wormwood	239
Yin Yang Huo	淫羊藿	Herba Epimedii	Epimedium	540
Yu Jin	郁金	Radix Curcumae	Turmeric root tuber	362
Yu Li Ren	郁李仁	Semen Pruni	Bush cherry stone	152
Yu Mi Xu	玉米须	Stylus Zeae Mays	Corn silk	238
Yu Xing Cao	鱼腥草	Herba Houttuyniae Cordatae	Houttuynia	104
Yu Yu Liang	禹余粮	Limonitum	Limonite	621
Yu Zhu	玉竹	Rhizoma Polygonati Odorati	Fragrant Solomon seal rhizome	592
Yuan Hua	芫花	Flos Daphnes Genkwa	Genkwa flower	165
Yuan Zhi	远志	Radix Polygalae	Polygala root	461
Zao Jiao	皂角	Fructus Gleditsiae Sinensis	Chinese honey locust fruit	408
Zao Jiao Ci	皂角刺	Spina Gleditsiae Sinensis	Spine of Chinese honey locust fruit	409
Zao Xin Tu	灶心土	Terra Flava Usta	Oven earth	348
Ze Lan	泽兰	Herba Lycopi Lucidi	Bugleweed	380
Ze Xie	泽泻	Rhizoma Alismatis Orientalis	Water plantain rhizome	221
Zhe Bei Mu	浙贝母	Bulbus Fritillariae Thunbergii	Zhejiang fritillary bulb	414
Zhen Zhu	珍珠	Margarita	Pearl	477
Zhen Zhu Mu	珍珠母	Concha Margaritifera	Mother-of-pearl	478
Zhi Gan Cao	炙甘草	Radix Glycyrrhizae Praeparata	Prepared liquorice root	524
Zhi Ke (Zhi Qiao)	枳壳	Fructus Citri Aurantii	Ripe bitter orange fruit	275

Appendix 1b Index of materia medica by pharmaceutical name

Pharmaceutical name	English name	Pinyin	Simplified Chinese characters	Page
Acaciae seu Uncariae, Pasta	Catechu	*Er Cha*	儿茶	656
Acanthopanacis Gracilistyli Radicis, Cortex	Acanthopanax root bark	*Wu Jia Pi*	五加皮	191
Achyranthis Bidentatae, Radix	Achyranthes root	*Niu Xi (Huai Niu Xi)*	牛膝 (怀牛膝)	375
Aconiti, Radix	Aconite mother root	*Wu Tou*	乌头	252
Aconiti Carmichaeli, Radix	Sichuan aconite mother root	*Chuan Wu*	川乌	252
Aconiti Carmichaeli Praeparata, Radix Lateralis	Prepared Sichuan aconite daughter root	*Fu Zi*	附子	250
Aconiti Kusnezoffii, Radix	Wild aconite root	*Cao Wu*	草乌	253
Acori Graminei, Rhizoma	Grass-leaf sweetflag rhizome	*Shi Chang Pu*	石菖蒲	505
Adenophorae, Radix	Adenophora root	*Nan Sha Shen*	南沙参	580
Agastaches seu Pogostemi, Herba	Agastache or patchouli	*Huo Xiang*	藿香	199
Agkistrodon	Long-noded pit viper	*Qi She (Bai Hua She)*	蕲蛇 (白花蛇)	176
Agrimoniae Pilosae, Gemma	Agrimony bud	*He Cao Ya*	鹤草芽	314
Agrimoniae Pilosae, Herba	Hairy vein agrimony	*Xian He Cao*	仙鹤草	341
Ailanthi Altissimae, Cortex	Ailanthus bark	*Chun Pi*	椿皮	625
Albizziae Julibrissin, Cortex	Albizzia bark	*He Huan Pi*	合欢皮	463
Alismatis Orientalis, Rhizoma	Water plantain rhizome	*Ze Xie*	泽泻	221
Allii Fistulosi, Bulbus	Chinese green onion	*Cong Bai*	葱白	42
Allii Macrostemi, Bulbus	Chinese chive	*Xie Bai*	薤白	287
Allii Tuberosi, Semen	Chinese leek seed	*Jiu Cai Zi*	韭菜子	554
Aloes, Herba	Aloe	*Lu Hui*	芦荟	159
Alpiniae Katsumadai, Semen	Katsumada galangal seed	*Cao Dou Kou*	草豆蔻	206
Alpiniae Officinari, Rhizoma	Lesser galangal rhizome	*Gao Liang Jiang*	高良姜	263
Alpiniae Oxyphyllae, Fructus	Bitter cardamom	*Yi Zhi Ren*	益智仁	549
Alumen	Alum	*Ming Fan*	明矾	653
Alumen Praeparatum	Prepared alum	*Ku Fan*	枯矾	653
Amomi, Fructus	Amomum fruit	*Sha Ren*	砂仁	204
Amomi Kravanh, Fructus	Round cardamom fruit	*Bai Dou Kou*	白豆蔻	205
Amomi Tsaoko, Fructus	Tsaoko fruit	*Cao Guo*	草果	208
Ampelopsis Japonicae, Radix	Japanese peppervine root	*Bai Lian*	白蔹	124
Amydae Sinensis, Carapax	Chinese soft-shelled turtle shell	*Bie Jia*	鳖甲	583
Andrographitis Paniculatae, Herba	Green chiretta	*Chuan Xin Lian*	穿心莲	109
Anemarrhenae Asphodeloidis, Rhizoma	Anemarrhena rhizome	*Zhi Mu*	知母	70

Pharmaceutical name	English name	Pinyin	Simplified Chinese characters	Page
Biotae Orientalis, Cacumen	Chinese arborvitae twig and leaf	*Ce Bai Ye*	侧柏叶	328
Biotae Orientalis, Semen	Chinese arborvitae seed	*Bai Zi Ren*	柏子仁	462
Bletillae Striatae, Rhizoma	Bletilla rhizome	*Bai Ji*	白及	340
Boehmeriae Niveae, Radix	Ragon grass root	*Zhu Ma Gen*	苎麻根	332
Bombyx Batryticatus	Stiff silkworm	*Jiang Can*	僵蚕	493
Borax	Borax	*Peng Sha*	硼砂	662
Borneolum (Syntheticum)	Borneol	*Bing Pian*	冰片	503
Bovis, Calculus	Cow bezoar	*Niu Huang*	牛黄	482
Bruceae Javanicae, Fructus	Brucea fruit	*Ya Dan Zi*	鸦胆子	118
Bubali, Cornu	Water buffalo horn	*Shui Niu Jiao*	水牛角	136
Bufonis, Venenum	Toad venom	*Chan Su*	蟾酥	657
Bupleuri, Radix	Chinese thorowax root	*Chai Hu*	柴胡	51
Buthus Martensi	Scorpion	*Quan Xie*	全蝎	489
Calamina	Calamine	*Lu Gan Shi*	炉甘石	661
Callicarpae, Folium	Callicarpa leaf	*Zi Zhu*	紫珠	343
Calomelas	Calomel	*Qing Fen*	轻粉	660
Cannabis Sativae, Semen	Hemp seed	*Huo Ma Ren*	火麻仁	151
Carthami Tinctorii, Flos	Safflower	*Hong Hua*	红花	370
Caryophylli, Flos	Cloves	*Ding Xiang*	丁香	262
Cassiae, Semen	Cassia seed	*Jue Ming Zi*	决明子	77
Cephalanoploris seu Cirsii, Herba	Field thistle	*Xiao Ji*	小蓟	326
Cervi, Cornu	Mature deer antler	*Lu Jiao*	鹿角	539
Cervi Degelatinatum, Cornu	Degelatined mature deer antler	*Lu Jiao Shuang*	鹿角霜	540
Cervi Parvum, Cornu	Pilose antler of young deer	*Lu Rong*	鹿茸	538
Chaenomelis, Fructus	Chinese quince fruit	*Mu Gua*	木瓜	175
Chrysanthemi Indici, Flos	Wild chrysanthemum flower	*Ye Ju Hua*	野菊花	108
Chrysanthemi Morifolii, Flos	Chrysanthemum flower	*Ju Hua*	菊花	49
Chrysanthemi Morifolii, Flos Albus	White chrysanthemum flower	*Bai Ju Hua*	白菊花	50
Chrysanthemi Morifolii, Flos Aureus	Yellow chrysanthemum flower	*Huang Ju Hua*	黄菊花	50
Cibotii Barometz, Rhizoma	Cibot rhizome	*Gou Ji*	狗脊	192
Cicadae, Periostracum	Cicada slough	*Chan Tui*	蝉蜕	55
Cimicifugae, Rhizoma	Bugbane rhizome	*Sheng Ma*	升麻	57
Cinnabaris	Cinnabar	*Zhu Sha*	朱砂	453
Cinnamomi Cassiae, Cortex	Cassia bark	*Rou Gui*	肉桂	254
Cinnamomi Cassiae, Ramulus	Cinnamon twig	*Gui Zhi*	桂枝	22
Cirsii Japonici, Herba seu Radix	Japanese thistle	*Da Ji*	大蓟	325
Cistanches Deserticolae, Herba	Desert-living cistanche	*Rou Cong Rong*	肉苁蓉	550

Pharmaceutical name	English name	Pinyin	Simplified Chinese characters	Page
Cynanchi Paniculati, Radix	Paniculate swallowwort root	*Xu Chang Qing*	徐长卿	188
Cynanchi Stauntonii, Radix et Rhizoma	Willow-leaf swallowwort rhizome	*Bai Qian*	白前	411
Cynomorii Songarici, Herba	Cynomorium stem	*Suo Yang*	锁阳	551
Cyperi Rotundi, Rhizoma	Nut-grass rhizome	*Xiang Fu*	香附	277
Dalbergiae Odoriferae, Lignum	Dalbergia heartwood	*Jiang Xiang*	降香	338
Daphnes Genkwa, Flos	Genkwa flower	*Yuan Hua*	芫花	165
Daturae, Flos	Datura flower	*Yang Jin Hua*	洋金花	444
Dendrobii, Herba	Dendrobium	*Shi Hu*	石斛	591
Dianthi, Herba	Chinese pink herb	*Qu Mai*	瞿麦	232
Dichroae Febrifugae, Radix	Dichroa root	*Chang Shan*	常山	642
Dictamni Dasycarpi Radicis, Cortex	Dittany root bark	*Bai Xian Pi*	白鲜皮	90
Dioscoreae, Rhizoma	Yam rhizome	*Bi Xie*	萆薢	236
Dioscoreae Bulbiferae, Rhizoma	Air potato yam	*Huang Yao Zi*	黄药子	427
Dioscoreae Hypoglaucae, Rhizoma	Collett yam rhizome	*Fen Bi Xie*	粉萆薢	236
Dioscoreae Oppositae, Rhizoma	Chinese yam	*Shan Yao*	山药	526
Dioscoreae Septemlobae, Rhizoma	Seven-lobed yam rhizome	*Mian Bi Xie*	绵萆薢	236
Dipsaci, Radix	Dipsacus root	*Xu Duan*	续断	544
Dolichoris Lablab, Semen	White hyacinth bean	*Bai Bian Dou*	白扁豆	528
Draconis, Os	Dragon bone	*Long Gu*	龙骨	455
Draconis Calcinatum, Os	Calcined dragon bone	*Duan Long Gu*	煅龙骨	455
Draconis, Resina	Dragon's blood	*Xue Jie*	血竭	659
Drynariae, Rhizoma	Drynaria rhizome	*Gu Sui Bu*	骨碎补	382
Dryopteris Crassirhizomae, Rhizoma	Basket fern	*Guan Zhong*	贯众	113
Ecliptae Prostratae, Herba	Eclipta	*Han Lian Cao (Mo Han Lian)*	旱莲草 (墨旱莲)	595
Elsholtziae seu Moslae, Herba	Aromatic madder	*Xiang Ru*	香薷	40
Ephedrae, Herba	Ephedra	*Ma Huang*	麻黄	20
Ephedrae, Radix	Ephedra root	*Ma Huang Gen*	麻黄根	609
Epimedii, Herba	Epimedium	*Yin Yang Huo*	淫羊藿	540
Equiseti Hiemalis, Herba	Scouring rush herb	*Mu Zei*	木贼	60
Eriobotryae Japonicae, Folium	Loquat leaf	*Pi Pa Ye*	枇杷叶	441
Erythrinae, Cortex	Erythrina bark	*Hai Tong Pi*	海桐皮	186
Eucommiae Ulmoidis, Cortex	Eucommia bark	*Du Zhong*	杜仲	542
Eupatorii Fortunei, Herba	Eupatorium	*Pei Lan*	佩兰	203
Euphorbiae Kansui, Radix	Kansui root	*Gan Sui*	甘遂	162

Pharmaceutical name	English name	Pinyin	Simplified Chinese characters	Page
Imperatae Cylindricae, Rhizoma	Cogon grass rhizome	*Bai Mao Gen*	白茅根	331
Indigo Naturalis	Natural indigo	*Qing Dai*	青黛	103
Inulae, Flos	Inula flower	*Xuan Fu Hua*	旋复花	410
Isatidis seu Baphicacanthi, Folium	Woad leaf	*Da Qing Ye*	大青叶	102
Isatidis seu Baphicacanthi, Radix	Isatis root	*Ban Lan Gen*	板蓝根	101
Juglandis Regiae, Semen	Walnut kernel	*He Tao Ren/ Hu Tao Ren/ Hu Tao Rou*	核桃仁/ 胡桃仁/ 胡桃肉	557
Junci Effusi, Medulla	Rush pith	*Deng Xin Cao*	灯心草	237
Kochiae Scopariae, Fructus	Broom cypress fruit	*Di Fu Zi*	地肤子	234
Laminariae seu Eckloniae, Thallus	Laminaria	*Kun Bu*	昆布	426
Lasiosphaerae seu Calvatiae, Sclerotium	Puff-ball	*Ma Bo*	马勃	116
Ledebouriellae Divaricatae, Radix	Ledebouriella root	*Fang Feng*	防风	30
Leonuri Heterophylli, Herba	Motherwort	*Yi Mu Cao*	益母草	374
Lepidii seu Descurainiae, Semen	Lepidium or descurainia seed	*Ting Li Zi*	葶苈子	436
Ligustici, Rhizoma et Radix	Chinese lovage root	*Gao Ben*	藁本	35
Ligustici Chuanxiong, Rhizoma	Sichuan lovage rhizome	*Chuan Xiong*	川芎	359
Ligustri Lucidi, Fructus	Glossy privet fruit	*Nü Zhen Zi*	女贞子	596
Lilii, Bulbus	Lily bulb	*Bai He*	百合	590
Limonitum	Limonite	*Yu Yu Liang*	禹余粮	621
Linderae Strychnifoliae, Radix	Lindera root	*Wu Yao*	乌药	285
Liquidambaris, Fructus	Sweetgum fruit	*Lu Lu Tong*	路路通	180
Litchi Chinensis, Semen	Lychee seed	*Li Zhi He*	荔枝核	289
Lobeliae Chinensis, Herba cum Radice	Chinese lobelia	*Ban Bian Lian*	半边莲	111
Lonicerae, Flos	Honeysuckle flower	*Jin Yin Hua*	金银花	95
Lonicerae Japonicae, Caulis	Honeysuckle stem	*Ren Dong Teng*	忍冬藤	96
Lophatheri Gracilis, Herba	Lophatherum herb	*Dan Zhu Ye*	淡竹叶	76
Loranthi, Ramulus	Mulberry mistletoe	*Sang Ji Sheng*	桑寄生	190
Lumbricus	Earthworm	*Di Long*	地龙	488
Lycii, Fructus	Wolfberry fruit	*Gou Qi Zi*	枸杞子	586
Lycii Radicis, Cortex	Wolfberry root bark	*Di Gu Pi*	地骨皮	139
Lycopi Lucidi, Herba	Bugleweed	*Ze Lan*	泽兰	380
Lycopodii Japonici, Herba	Club moss	*Shen Jin Cao*	伸筋草	178
Lygodii Japonici, Herba	Climbing fern	*Hai Jin Sha Teng*	海金沙藤	231
Lygodii Japonici, Spora	Climbing fern spore	*Hai Jin Sha*	海金沙	230
Lysimachiae, Herba	Lysimachia	*Jin Qian Cao*	金钱草	240

Pharmaceutical name	English name	Pinyin	Simplified Chinese characters	Page
Oroxyli Indici, Semen	Oroxylum seed	*Mu Hu Die*	木蝴蝶	120
Oryzae Sativae Germinatus, Fructus	Rice sprout	*Dao Ya*	稻芽	300
Ostreae, Concha	Oyster shell	*Mu Li*	牡蛎	473
Paeoniae Lactiflorae, Radix	White peony root	*Bai Shao*	白芍	567
Paeoniae Rubra, Radix	Red peony root	*Chi Shao*	赤芍	133
Panacis Quinquefolii, Radix	American ginseng root	*Xi Yang Shen*	西洋参	529
Paridis, Rhizoma	Paris root	*Chong Lou*	重楼	110
Patriniae cum Radice, Herba	Patrinia	*Bai Jiang Cao*	败酱草	122
Perillae Frutescentis, Caulis	Perilla stem	*Su Geng*	苏梗	28
Perillae Frutescentis, Folium	Perilla leaf	*Zi Su Ye*	紫苏叶	27
Perillae Frutescentis, Fructus	Perilla fruit	*Su Zi*	苏子	432
Persicae, Semen	Peach kernel	*Tao Ren*	桃仁	372
Peucedani, Radix	Hogfennel root	*Qian Hu*	前胡	417
Pharbitidis, Semen	Morning glory seed	*Qian Niu Zi*	牵牛子	164
Phaseoli Calcarati, Semen	Aduki bean	*Chi Xiao Dou*	赤小豆	224
Phaseoli Radiati, Semen	Mung bean	*Lü Dou*	绿豆	125
Phaseoli Radiati, Testa	Mung bean skin	*Lü Dou Yi*	绿豆衣	126
Phellodendri, Cortex	Amur cork tree bark	*Huang Bai*	黄柏	84
Phellodendri Carbonisatus, Cortex	Charred amur cork tree bark	*Huang Bai Tan*	黄柏炭	85
Phragmitis Communis, Rhizoma	Reed rhizome	*Lu Gen*	芦根	75
Phragmitis Communis Recens, Rhizoma	Fresh reed rhizome	*Xian Lu Gen*	鲜芦根	75
Picrorhizae Scrophularii-florae, Rhizoma	Picrorhiza rhizome	*Hu Huang Lian*	胡黄连	141
Pinelliae Ternatae, Rhizoma	Pinellia tuber	*Ban Xia*	半夏	399
Pinelliae Ternatae Depurata, Rhizoma	Purified pinellia tuber	*Qing Ban Xia*	清半夏	399
Pinelliae Ternatae Praeparata, Rhizoma	Prepared pinellia tuber	*Fa Ban Xia*	法半夏	399
Piperis Kadsurae, Caulis	Kadsura pepper stem	*Hai Feng Teng*	海风藤	179
Plantaginis, Herba	Plantain herb	*Che Qian Cao*	车前草	227
Plantaginis, Semen	Plantain seed	*Che Qian Zi*	车前子	226
Plastri Testudinis, Gelatinum	Freshwater turtle plastron glue	*Gui Ban Jiao*	龟板胶	586
Platycodi Grandiflori, Radix	Platycodon root	*Jie Geng*	桔梗	406
Pogostemi, Herba	Patchouli	*Guang Huo Xiang*	广藿香	199
Polygalae, Radix	Polygala root	*Yuan Zhi*	远志	461
Polygonati, Rhizoma	Siberian Solomon seal rhizome	*Huang Jing*	黄精	593
Polygonati Odorati, Rhizoma	Fragrant Solomon seal rhizome	*Yu Zhu*	玉竹	592
Polygoni Avicularis, Herba	Prostrate knotweed	*Bian Xu*	扁蓄	233
Polygoni Cuspidati, Radix et Rhizoma	Giant knotweed root and rhizome	*Hu Zhang*	虎杖	241

Pharmaceutical name	English name	Pinyin	Simplified Chinese characters	Page
Rosae Laevigatae, Fructus	Cherokee rose fruit	*Jin Ying Zi*	金樱子	636
Rosae Rugosae, Flos	Chinese rose flower	*Mei Gui Hua*	玫瑰花	289
Rubi Chingii, Fructus	Chinese raspberry	*Fu Pen Zi*	覆盆子	635
Rubiae Cordifoliae, Radix	Madder root	*Qian Cao Gen*	茜草根	334
Rubiae Cordifoliae Carbonisata, Radix	Charred madder root	*Qian Cao Tan*	茜草炭	335
Saccharum Granorum	Malt sugar	*Yi Tang*	饴糖	533
Salviae Miltiorrhizae, Radix	Red sage root	*Dan Shen*	丹参	369
Sanguisorbae Officinalis, Radix	Sanguisorba root	*Di Yu*	地榆	327
Sanguisorbae Officinalis Carbonisata, Radix	Charred sanguisorba root	*Di Yu Tan*	地榆炭	327
Saposhnikoviae Divaricatae, Radix	Saposhnikovia root	*Fang Feng*	防风	30
Sappan, Lignum	Sappan wood	*Su Mu*	苏木	382
Sargassi, Herba	Seaweed	*Hai Zao*	海藻	425
Sargentodoxae Cuneatae, Caulis	Sargentodoxa vine	*Hong Teng*	红藤	123
Schisandrae, Fructus	Schisandra fruit	*Wu Wei Zi*	五味子	612
Schizonepetae Tenuifoliae, Herba	Schizonepeta herb	*Jing Jie*	荆芥	28
Schizonepetae Tenuifoliae, Spica	Schizonepeta spike	*Jing Jie Sui*	荆芥穗	29
Schizonepetae Tenuifoliae Carbonisata, Herba	Charred schizonepeta herb	*Jing Jie Tan*	荆芥炭	29
Scolopendra Subspinipes	Centipede	*Wu Gong*	蜈蚣	491
Scrophulariae Ningpoensis, Radix	Figwort root	*Xuan Shen*	玄参	130
Scutellariae Baicalensis, Radix	Baical skullcap root	*Huang Qin*	黄芩	81
Scutellariae Baicalensis Carbonisata, Radix	Charred baical skullcap root	*Huang Qin Tan*	黄芩炭	81
Sennae, Folium	Senna leaf	*Fan Xie Ye*	番泻叶	159
Sepiae seu Sepiellae, Os	Cuttlefish bone	*Hai Piao Xiao/ Wu Zei Gu*	海螵蛸/乌贼骨	633
Sesami Indici, Semen	Black sesame seed	*Hei Zhi Ma*	黑芝麻	597
Setariae Italicae Germinatus, Fructus	Millet sprout	*Gu Ya*	谷芽	301
Siegesbeckiae, Herba	Siegesbeckia herb	*Xi Xian Cao*	豨莶草	185
Sinapis Albae, Semen	White mustard seed	*Bai Jie Zi*	白芥子	407
Smilacis Glabrae, Rhizoma	Glabrous green briar rhizome	*Tu Fu Ling*	土茯苓	112
Sojae Praeparatum, Semen	Prepared soybean	*Dan Dou Chi*	淡豆豉	54
Sophorae Flavescentis, Radix	Flavescent sophora root	*Ku Shen*	苦参	86
Sophorae Japonicae, Flos	Pagoda tree flower	*Huai Hua*	槐花	329
Sophorae Japonicae, Fructus	Pagoda tree fruit	*Huai Jiao*	槐角	330
Sophorae Tonkinensis, Radix	Subprostrate sophora root	*Shan Dou Gen*	山豆根	115
Sparganii Stoloniferi, Rhizoma	Burreed tuber	*San Leng*	三棱	386

Pharmaceutical name	English name	Pinyin	Simplified Chinese characters	Page
Zanthoxyli, Semen	Chinese prickly ash seed	*Jiao Mu*	椒目	260
Zeae Mays, Stylus	Corn silk	*Yu Mi Xu*	玉米须	238
Zingiberis Officinalis, Rhizoma	Dried ginger	*Gan Jiang*	干姜	253
Zingiberis Officinalis Praeparata, Rhizoma	Prepared dried ginger	*Pao Jiang*	炮姜	346
Zingiberis Officinalis Recens, Cortex	Ginger rhizome skin	*Sheng Jiang Pi*	生姜皮	39
Zingiberis Officinalis Recens, Rhizoma	Fresh ginger	*Sheng Jiang*	生姜	39
Zingiberis Officinalis Usta, Rhizoma	Roasted ginger	*Wei Jiang*	煨姜	39
Ziziphi Jujubae, Fructus	Chinese date	*Da Zao*	大枣	532
Ziziphi Spinosae, Semen	Spiny jujube seed	*Suan Zao Ren*	酸枣仁	460

Appendix 1c Index of materia medica by English name

English name	Pharmaceutical name	Pinyin	Simplified Chinese characters	Page
Baical skullcap root	Radix Scutellariae Baicalensis	*Huang Qin*	黄芩	81
Baical skullcap root, charred	Radix Scutellariae Baicalensis Carbonisata	*Huang Qin Tan*	黄芩炭	81
Bamboo sap, dried	Succus Bambusae	*Zhu Li*	竹沥	421
Bamboo shavings	Caulis Bambusae in Taeniis	*Zhu Ru*	竹茹	418
Barley sprout	Fructus Hordei Vulgaris Germinatus	*Mai Ya*	麦芽	299
Basket fern	Rhizoma Dryopteris Crassirhizomae	*Guan Zhong*	贯众	113
Belamcanda rhizome	Rhizoma Belamcandae Chinensis	*She Gan*	射干	106
Bitter apricot kernel	Semen Pruni Armeniacae Amarum	*Ku Xing Ren*	苦杏仁	431
Bitter cardamom	Fructus Alpiniae Oxyphyllae	*Yi Zhi Ren*	益智仁	549
Bitter orange fruit, immature	Fructus Immaturus Citri Aurantii	*Zhi Shi*	枳实	274
Bitter orange fruit, ripe	Fructus Citri Aurantii	*Zhi Ke (Zhi Qiao)*	枳壳	275
Black-end swallowwort root	Radix Cynanchi Atrati	*Bai Wei*	白薇	142
Black plum	Fructus Pruni Mume	*Wu Mei*	乌梅	614
Black sesame seed	Semen Sesami Indici	*Hei Zhi Ma*	黑芝麻	597
Bletilla rhizome	Rhizoma Bletillae Striatae	*Bai Ji*	白及	340
Boat-fruited sterculia seed	Semen Sterculiae Lychnophorae	*Pang Da Hai*	胖大海	426
Borax	Borax	*Peng Sha*	硼砂	662
Borneol	Borneolum (Syntheticum)	*Bing Pian*	冰片	503
Broom cypress fruit	Fructus Kochiae Scopariae	*Di Fu Zi*	地肤子	234
Brucea fruit	Fructus Bruceae Javanicae	*Ya Dan Zi*	鸦胆子	118
Buddha's hand	Fructus Citri Sarcodactylis	*Fo Shou*	佛手	282
Bugbane rhizome	Rhizoma Cimicifugae	*Sheng Ma*	升麻	57
Bugleweed	Herba Lycopi Lucidi	*Ze Lan*	泽兰	380
Burreed tuber	Rhizoma Sparganii Stoloniferi	*San Leng*	三棱	386
Bush cherry stone	Semen Pruni	*Yu Li Ren*	郁李仁	152
Calamine	Calamina	*Lu Gan Shi*	炉甘石	661
Callicarpa leaf	Folium Callicarpae	*Zi Zhu*	紫珠	343
Calomel	Calomelas	*Qing Fen*	轻粉	660
Carbonized palm petiole fibre	Fibra Carbonisata Trachycarpi Stipulae	*Zong Lü Tan*	棕榈炭	343
Cassia bark	Cortex Cinnamomi Cassiae	*Rou Gui*	肉桂	254
Cassia seed	Semen Cassiae	*Jue Ming Zi*	决明子	77
Catechu	Pasta Acaciae seu Uncariae	*Er Cha*	儿茶	656
Cat-tail pollen	Pollen Typhae	*Pu Huang*	蒲黄	336
Centipede	Scolopendra Subspinipes	*Wu Gong*	蜈蚣	491
Chaste-tree fruit	Fructus Viticis	*Man Jing Zi*	蔓荆子	56
Chebula fruit	Fructus Terminaliae Chebulae	*He Zi*	诃子	617
Cherokee rose fruit	Fructus Rosae Laevigatae	*Jin Ying Zi*	金樱子	636

English name	Pharmaceutical name	Pinyin	Simplified Chinese characters	Page
Cinnamon twig	Ramulus Cinnamomi Cassiae	*Gui Zhi*	桂枝	22
Citron fruit	Fructus Citri Medicae seu Wilsonii	*Xiang Yuan*	香橼	283
Clam shell	Concha Meretricis seu Cyclinae	*Hai Ge Ke*	海蛤壳	423
Climbing fern	Herba Lygodii Japonici	*Hai Jin Sha Teng*	海金沙藤	231
Climbing fern spore	Spora Lygodii Japonici	*Hai Jin Sha*	海金沙	230
Cloves	Flos Caryophylli	*Ding Xiang*	丁香	262
Club moss	Herba Lycopodii Japonici	*Shen Jin Cao*	伸筋草	178
Cnidium fruit	Fructus Cnidii Monnieri	*She Chuang Zi*	蛇床子	654
Cocklebur fruit	Fructus Xanthii Sibirici	*Cang Er Zi*	苍耳子	36
Cockroach, wingless	Eupolyphaga seu Steleophaga	*Tu Bie Chong*	土鳖虫	388
Codonopsis root	Radix Codonopsitis Pilosulae	*Dang Shen*	党参	517
Cogon grass rhizome	Rhizoma Imperatae Cylindricae	*Bai Mao Gen*	白茅根	331
Coix seed	Semen Coicis Lachrymajobi	*Yi Yi Ren*	薏苡仁	219
Collett yam rhizome	Rhizoma Dioscoreae Hypoglaucae	*Fen Bi Xie*	粉萆薢	236
Coltsfoot flower	Flos Tussilaginis Farfarae	*Kuan Dong Hua*	款冬花	438
Common ducksmeat herb	Herba Spirodelae Polyrrhizae	*Fu Ping*	浮萍	59
Common fennel seed	Fructus Foeniculi Vulgaris	*Xiao Hui Xiang*	小茴香	260
Corn silk	Stylus Zeae Mays	*Yu Mi Xu*	玉米须	238
Corydalis tuber	Rhizoma Corydalis Yanhusuo	*Yan Hu Suo*	延胡索	361
Costazia bone	Os Costaziae	*Fu Hai Shi*	浮海石	422
Cow bezoar	Calculus Bovis	*Niu Huang*	牛黄	482
Croton frost	Pulvis Crotonis Semenis	*Ba Dou Shuang*	巴豆霜	166
Croton seed	Semen Crotonis Tiglii	*Ba Dou*	巴豆	166
Curculigo rhizome	Rhizoma Curculiginis Orchioidis	*Xian Mao*	仙茅	547
Cuttlefish bone	Os Sepiae seu Sepiellae	*Hai Piao Xiao/ Wu Zei Gu*	海螵蛸/ 乌贼骨	633
Cyathula root	Radix Cyathulae Officinalis	*Chuan Niu Xi*	川牛膝	375
Cynomorium stem	Herba Cynomorii Songarici	*Suo Yang*	锁阳	551
Dalbergia heartwood	Lignum Dalbergiae Odoriferae	*Jiang Xiang*	降香	338
Dandelion	Herba Taraxaci cum Radice	*Pu Gong Ying*	蒲公英	98
Datura flower	Flos Daturae	*Yang Jin Hua*	洋金花	444
Degelatined mature deer antler	Cornu Cervi Degelatinatum	*Lu Jiao Shuang*	鹿角霜	540
Dendrobium	Herba Dendrobii	*Shi Hu*	石斛	591
Desert-living cistanche	Herba Cistanches Deserticolae	*Rou Cong Rong*	肉苁蓉	550
Dichroa root	Radix Dichroae Febrifugae	*Chang Shan*	常山	642
Dipsacus root	Radix Dipsaci	*Xu Duan*	续断	544
Dittany root bark	Cortex Dictamni Dasycarpi Radicis	*Bai Xian Pi*	白鲜皮	90
Dodder seed	Semen Cuscutae	*Tu Si Zi*	菟丝子	541

English name	Pharmaceutical name	Pinyin	Simplified Chinese characters	Page
Gecko	Gekko	*Ge Jie*	蛤蚧	556
Genkwa flower	Flos Daphnes Genkwa	*Yuan Hua*	芫花	165
Giant knotweed root and rhizome	Radix et Rhizoma Polygoni Cuspidati	*Hu Zhang*	虎杖	241
Ginger, dried	Rhizoma Zingiberis Officinalis	*Gan Jiang*	干姜	253
Ginger, fresh	Rhizoma Zingiberis Officinalis Recens	*Sheng Jiang*	生姜	39
Ginger, prepared dried	Rhizoma Zingiberis Officinalis Praeparata	*Pao Jiang*	炮姜	346
Ginger, roasted	Rhizoma Zingiberis Officinalis Usta	*Wei Jiang*	煨姜	39
Ginger rhizome skin	Cortex Zingiberis Officinalis Recens	*Sheng Jiang Pi*	生姜皮	39
Ginkgo nut	Semen Ginkgo Bilobae	*Bai Guo*	白果	443
Ginseng	Radix Ginseng	*Ren Shen*	人参	514
Ginseng, red	Radix Ginseng Rubra	*Hong Shen*	红参	514
Ginseng, white	Radix Ginseng Alba	*Bai Shen*	白参	514
Glabrous green briar rhizome	Rhizoma Smilacis Glabrae	*Tu Fu Ling*	土茯苓	112
Glehnia root	Radix Glehniae Littoralis	*Bei Sha Shen*	北沙参	579
Globethistle root	Radix Rhapontici seu Echinopsis	*Lou Lu*	漏芦	121
Glossy privet fruit	Fructus Ligustri Lucidi	*Nü Zhen Zi*	女贞子	596
Goat horn	Cornu Naemorhedi	*Shan Yang Jiao*	山羊角	481
Golden thread rhizome	Rhizoma Coptidis	*Huang Lian*	黄连	82
Grass-leaf sweetflag rhizome	Rhizoma Acori Graminei	*Shi Chang Pu*	石菖蒲	505
Great burdock fruit	Fructus Arctii Lappae	*Niu Bang Zi*	牛蒡子	46
Green chiretta	Herba Andrographitis Paniculatae	*Chuan Xin Lian*	穿心莲	109
Green tangerine peel	Pericarpium Citri Reticulatae Viride	*Qing Pi*	青皮	280
Gypsum	Gypsum Fibrosum	*Shi Gao*	石膏	69
Gypsum, calcined	Gypsum Fibrosum Calcinatum	*Duan Shi Gao*	煅石膏	69
Gypsum, crude	Gypsum Fibrosum Crudum	*Sheng Shi Gao*	生石膏	69
Haematite	Haematitum	*Dai Zhe Shi*	代赭石	475
Hairy vein agrimony	Herba Agrimoniae Pilosae	*Xian He Cao*	仙鹤草	341
Hawthorn fruit	Fructus Crataegi	*Shan Zha*	山楂	297
Hemp seed	Semen Cannabis Sativae	*Huo Ma Ren*	火麻仁	151
Hogfennel root	Radix Peucedani	*Qian Hu*	前胡	417
Honeysuckle flower	Flos Lonicerae	*Jin Yin Hua*	金银花	95
Honeysuckle stem	Caulis Lonicerae Japonicae	*Ren Dong Teng*	忍冬藤	96
Hornet nest	Nidus Vespae	*Feng Fang*	蜂房	658
Houttuynia	Herba Houttuyniae Cordatae	*Yu Xing Cao*	鱼腥草	104
Human placenta	Placenta Hominis	*Zi He Che*	紫河车	559

English name	Pharmaceutical name	Pinyin	Simplified Chinese characters	Page
Lotus receptacle	Receptaculum Nelumbinis Nuciferae	*Lian Fang*	莲房	627
Lotus rhizome node	Nodus Nelumbinis Nuciferae Rhizomatis	*Ou Jie*	藕节	344
Lotus seed	Semen Nelumbinis Nuciferae	*Lian Zi*	莲子	626
Lotus stamen	Stamen Nelumbinis Nuciferae	*Lian Xu*	莲须	627
Lucid asparagus root	Radix Asparagi Cochinchinensis	*Tian Men Dong*	天门冬	588
Lychee seed	Semen Litchi Chinensis	*Li Zhi He*	荔枝核	289
Lysimachia	Herba Lysimachiae	*Jin Qian Cao*	金钱草	240
Madder root	Radix Rubiae Cordifoliae	*Qian Cao Gen*	茜草根	334
Madder root, charred	Radix Rubiae Cordifoliae Carbonisata	*Qian Cao Tan*	茜草炭	335
Magnetite	Magnetitum	*Ci Shi*	磁石	454
Magnolia bark	Cortex Magnoliae Officinalis	*Hou Po*	厚朴	200
Magnolia flower	Flos Magnoliae	*Xin Yi Hua*	辛夷花	38
Malt sugar	Saccharum Granorum	*Yi Tang*	饴糖	533
Mantis egg-case	Oötheca Mantidis	*Sang Piao Xiao*	桑螵蛸	632
Mature deer antler	Cornu Cervi	*Lu Jiao*	鹿角	539
Mature deer antler, degelatined	Cornu Cervi Degelatinatum	*Lu Jiao Shuang*	鹿角霜	540
Mature deer antler glue	Gelatinum Cornu Cervi	*Lu Jiao Jiao*	鹿角胶	539
Medicated leaven	Massa Fermentata	*Shen Qu*	神曲	298
Milk vetch or sweet vetch root	Radix Astragali seu Hedysari	*Huang Qi*	黄芪	518
Millet sprout	Fructus Setariae Italicae Germinatus	*Gu Ya*	谷芽	301
Mirabilite	Mirabilitum	*Mang Xiao*	芒硝	157
Mirabilite, impure	Mirabilitum Non-Purum	*Po Xiao*	朴硝	157
Mirabilite, refined	Mirabilitum Depuratum	*Xuan Ming Fen*	玄明粉	158
Morinda root	Radix Morindae Officinalis	*Ba Ji Tian*	巴戟天	545
Morning glory seed	Semen Pharbitidis	*Qian Niu Zi*	牵牛子	164
Mother-of-pearl	Concha Margaritifera	*Zhen Zhu Mu*	珍珠母	478
Motherwort	Herba Leonuri Heterophylli	*Yi Mu Cao*	益母草	374
Mugwort leaf	Folium Artemisiae Argyi	*Ai Ye*	艾叶	347
Mulberry fruit	Fructus Mori Albae	*Sang Shen*	桑椹	571
Mulberry mistletoe	Ramulus Loranthi	*Sang Ji Sheng*	桑寄生	190
Mulberry twig	Ramulus Mori Albae	*Sang Zhi*	桑枝	184
Mung bean	Semen Phaseoli Radiati	*Lü Dou*	绿豆	125
Mung bean skin	Testa Phaseoli Radiati	*Lü Dou Yi*	绿豆衣	126
Musk	Secretio Moschi	*She Xiang*	麝香	501
Muskmelon pedicle	Pedicellus Cucumeris	*Gua Di*	瓜蒂	643
Mutong stem	Caulis Mutong	*Mu Tong*	木通	229
Myrrh	Myrrha	*Mo Yao*	没药	366
Natural indigo	Indigo Naturalis	*Qing Dai*	青黛	103
Notoginseng root	Radix Notoginseng	*San Qi*	三七	333

English name	Pharmaceutical name	Pinyin	Simplified Chinese characters	Page
Poria with hostwood	Sclerotium Poriae Cocos cum Ligno Hospite	*Fu Shen*	茯神	219
Prepared alum	Alumen Praeparatum	*Ku Fan*	枯矾	653
Prepared dried ginger	Rhizoma Zingiberis Officinalis Praeparata	*Pao Jiang*	炮姜	346
Prepared jack-in-the-pulpit tuber	Rhizoma Arisaematis Praeparata	*Zhi Nan Xing*	制南星	402
Prepared liquorice root	Radix Glycyrrhizae Praeparata	*Zhi Gan Cao*	炙甘草	524
Prepared pinellia tuber	Rhizoma Pinelliae Ternatae Praeparata	*Fa Ban Xia*	法半夏	399
Prepared Sichuan aconite daughter root	Radix Lateralis Aconiti Carmichaeli Praeparata	*Fu Zi*	附子	250
Prepared soybean	Semen Sojae Praeparatum	*Dan Dou Chi*	淡豆豉	54
Processed rehmannia root	Radix Rehmanniae Glutinosae Conquita	*Shu Di Huang*	熟地黄	565
Prostrate knotweed	Herba Polygoni Avicularis	*Bian Xu*	扁蓄	233
Prunella spike	Spica Prunellae Vulgaris	*Xia Ku Cao*	夏枯草	74
Pseudostellaria root	Radix Pseudostellariae Heterophyllae	*Tai Zi Shen*	太子参	531
Psoralea fruit	Fructus Psoraleae Corylifoliae	*Bu Gu Zhi*	补骨脂	548
Pubescent angelica root	Radix Angelicae Pubescentis	*Du Huo*	独活	174
Puff-ball	Sclerotium Lasiosphaerae seu Calvatiae	*Ma Bo*	马勃	116
Pumice	Pumex	*Fu Hai Shi*	浮海石	422
Pumpkin seed	Semen Cucurbitae Moschatae	*Nan Gua Zi*	南瓜子	313
Purple aster root	Radix Asteris Tatarici	*Zi Wan*	紫菀	437
Purslane	Herba Portulacae Oleraceae	*Ma Chi Xian*	马齿苋	117
Pyrrosia leaf	Folium Pyrrosiae	*Shi Wei*	石韦	235
Radish seed	Semen Raphani Sativi	*Lai Fu Zi*	莱菔子	301
Ragon grass root	Radix Boehmeriae Niveae	*Zhu Ma Gen*	苎麻根	332
Rangoon creeper fruit	Fructus Quisqualis Indicae	*Shi Jun Zi*	使君子	309
Realgar	Realgar	*Xiong Huang*	雄黄	650
Red ginseng	Radix Ginseng Rubra	*Hong Shen*	红参	514
Red halloysite	Halloysitum Rubrum	*Chi Shi Zhi*	赤石脂	622
Red peony root	Radix Paeoniae Rubra	*Chi Shao*	赤芍	133
Red poria	Sclerotium Poriae Cocos Rubrae	*Chi Fu Ling*	赤茯苓	219
Red sage root	Radix Salviae Miltiorrhizae	*Dan Shen*	丹参	369
Reed rhizome	Rhizoma Phragmitis Communis	*Lu Gen*	芦根	75
Reed rhizome, fresh	Rhizoma Phragmitis Communis Recens	*Xian Lu Gen*	鲜芦根	75
Rehmannia root	Radix Rehmanniae Glutinosae	*Sheng Di Huang*	生地黄	129
Rehmannia root, charred	Radix Rehmanniae Glutinosae Carbonisata	*Sheng Di Huang Tan*	生地黄炭	129

English name	Pharmaceutical name	Pinyin	Simplified Chinese characters	Page
Sichuan aconite mother root	Radix Aconiti Carmichaeli	*Chuan Wu*	川乌	252
Sichuan chinaberry	Fructus Meliae Toosendan	*Chuan Lian Zi*	川楝子	284
Sichuan fritillary bulb	Bulbus Fritillariae Cirrhosae	*Chuan Bei Mu*	川贝母	413
Sichuan lovage rhizome	Rhizoma Ligustici Chuanxiong	*Chuan Xiong*	川芎	359
Siegesbeckia herb	Herba Siegesbeckiae	*Xi Xian Cao*	豨莶草	185
Soybean, prepared	Semen Sojae Praeparatum	*Dan Dou Chi*	淡豆豉	54
Spatholobus stem	Caulis Spatholobi	*Ji Xue Teng*	鸡血藤	378
Spiny jujube seed	Semen Ziziphi Spinosae	*Suan Zao Ren*	酸枣仁	460
Stellaria root	Radix Stellariae Dichotomae	*Yin Chai Hu*	银柴胡	140
Stemona root	Radix Stemonae	*Bai Bu*	百部	433
Stephania root	Radix Stephaniae Tetrandrae	*(Han) Fang Ji*	(汉)防己	183
Stiff silkworm	Bombyx Batryticatus	*Jiang Can*	僵蚕	493
Storax, liquid	Styrax Liquidus	*Su He Xiang*	苏合香	503
Subprostrate sophora root	Radix Sophorae Tonkinensis	*Shan Dou Gen*	山豆根	115
Sulphur	Sulphur	*Liu Huang*	硫黄	651
Sweet wormwood	Herba Artemisiae Chinghao	*Qing Hao*	青蒿	138
Sweetgum fruit	Fructus Liquidambaris	*Lu Lu Tong*	路路通	180
Tabasheer	Concretio Silicea Bambusae	*Tian Zhu Huang*	天竺黄	420
Talc	Talcum	*Hua Shi*	滑石	227
Tangerine leaf	Folium Citri Reticulatae	*Ju Ye*	橘叶	274
Tangerine peel	Pericarpium Citri Reticulatae	*Chen Pi*	陈皮	272
Tangerine peel, red part	Pars Rubra Epicarpii Citri Erythrocarpae	*Ju Hong*	橘红	274
Tangerine pip	Semen Citri Reticulatae	*Ju He*	橘核	273
Tangerine pith	Retinervus Fructus Citri Reticulatae	*Ju Luo*	橘络	274
Toad venom	Venenum Bufonis	*Chan Su*	蟾酥	657
Torreya nut	Semen Torreyae Grandis	*Fei Zi*	榧子	316
Tree peony root bark	Cortex Moutan Radicis	*Mu Dan Pi*	牡丹皮	132
Tribulus fruit	Fructus Tribuli Terrestris	*Bai Ji Li*	白蒺藜	479
Trichosanthes fruit	Fructus Trichosanthis	*Gua Lou*	栝蒌	415
Trichosanthes husk	Pericarpium Trichosanthis	*Gua Lou Pi*	栝蒌皮	416
Trichosanthes root	Radix Trichosanthis	*Tian Hua Fen*	天花粉	71
Trichosanthes seed	Semen Trichosanthis	*Gua Lou Ren*	栝蒌仁	416
Tsaoko fruit	Fructus Amomi Tsaoko	*Cao Guo*	草果	208
Turmeric rhizome	Rhizoma Curcumae Longae	*Jiang Huang*	姜黄	364
Turmeric root tuber	Radix Curcumae	*Yu Jin*	郁金	362
Typhoneum rhizome	Rhizoma Typhonii Gigantei	*Bai Fu Zi*	白附子	404
Umbellate pore	Sclerotium Polypori Umbellati	*Zhu Ling*	猪苓	222
Uncaria stem and thorns	Ramulus Uncariae cum Uncis	*Gou Teng*	钩藤	484
Vaccaria seed	Semen Vaccariae Segetalis	*Wang Bu Liu Xing*	王不留行	379

Appendix 2 Index of other materia medica

The materia medica in this index are not covered by individual monographs within this book. They are listed in four-column tabular format with each sub-index beginning with a different column – pinyin, pharmaceutical name or English name. Please note that Appendix 6 provides a listing of individual materia medica (by pinyin and pharmaceutical name) cross-referenced to the main herb of the combinations in which they appear.

Appendix 2a Index of materia medica by pinyin name

(listed alphabetically without any distinction made between tones)

Pinyin	Simplified Chinese characters	Pharmaceutical name	English name
Ai Ye Tan	艾叶炭	Folium Artemisiae Argyi Carbonisatum	Charred mugwort leaf
An Xi Xiang	安息香	Benzoinum	Benzoin
Bai Jiu	白酒	Granorum Spiritus Incolor	White alcohol
Ban Mao	斑蝥	Mylabris	Blister beetle
Ban Xia Qu	半夏曲	Massa Fermentata Pinelliae	Pinellia tuber leaven
Ban Zhi Lian	半枝莲	Herba Scutellariae Barbatae	Barbated skullcap herb
Bi Ba	荜茇	Fructus Piperis Longi	Long pepper fruit
Bian Dou Hua	扁豆花	Flos Dolichoris Lablab	White hyacinth bean flower
Bing Tang	冰糖	Saccharon Crystallinum	Sugar candy
Can Sha	蚕砂	Excrementum Bombycis Mori	Silkworm droppings
Chen Hu Lu	陈葫芦	Fructus Lagenariae Depressae	Bottle gourd
Chong Wei Zi	茺蔚子	Semen Leonuri Heterophylli	Motherwort seed
Da Suan	大蒜	Bulbus Allii Sativi	Garlic bulb
Dai Mao	玳瑁	Carapax Eretmochelydis	Hawksbill turtle shell
Dong Gua Zi	冬瓜子	Semen Benincasae Hispidae	Wax gourd seed
Dong Kui Zi	冬葵子	Semen Malvae Verticillatae	Musk mallow seed
E Bu Shi Cao	鹅不食草	Herba Centipedae	Centipeda herb
Feng Mi	蜂蜜	Mel	Honey
Feng Xiang Zhi	枫香脂	Resina Liquidambaris	Sweetgum resin
Gan Song	甘松	Radix Nardostachydis	Nardostachys root
Gu Jing Cao	谷精草	Scapus et Flos Eriocaulonis Buergeriani	Pipewort flower
Gua Lou Gen	栝蒌根	Radix Trichosanthis	Trichosanthes root
Guan Gui	官桂	Cortex Tubiformis Cinnamomi Cassiae	Cinnamon inner bark
Guan Mu Tong	关木通	Caulis Aristolochiae Manshuriensis	Aristolochia stem

Pinyin	Simplified Chinese characters	Pharmaceutical name	English name
Han Shui Shi	寒水石	Calcitum	Calcite
He Huan Hua	合欢花	Flos Albizziae Julibrissin	Albizzia flower
Hou Po Hua	厚朴花	Flos Magnoliae Officinalis	Magnolia flower
Hu Jiao	胡椒	Fructus Piperis Nigri	Pepper fruit
Huai Hua Mi	槐花米	Flos Sophorae Japonicae Immaturus	Immature pagoda tree flower
Huai Hua Tan	槐花炭	Flos Sophorae Japonicae Carbonisatus	Charred pagoda tree flower
Huang Jiu	黄酒	Vinum Aureum	Yellow wine
Ji Guan Hua	鸡冠花	Flos Celosiae Cristatae	Cockscomb flower
Jiao San Xian	焦三仙	Scorch-fried combination of Fructus Crataegi, Massa Fermentata and Fructus Hordei Vulgaris Germinatus	Scorch-fried combination of hawthorn fruit, medicated leaven and barley sprout
Jing Mi	粳米	Oryza Sativa	Polished round grain rice
Jiu Xiang Chong	九香虫	Aspongopus	Stink bug
Ku Shi Lian Zi	苦石莲子	Semen Caesalpiniae Minax	Lotus fruit
Lang Du	狼毒	Radix Euphorbiae Fischerianae	Euphorbia
Li Lu	藜芦	Radix et Rhizoma Veratri	Veratrum root
Lian Fang Tan	莲房炭	Receptaculum Nelumbinis Nuciferae Carbonisatum	Charred lotus receptacle
Long Chi	龙齿	Dens Draconis	Fossilized teeth
Ma You	麻油	Oleum Sesami	Sesame oil
Meng Chong	虻虫	Tabanus	Gadfly
Mi Tuo Seng	密陀僧	Lithargyrum	Litharge
Pi Shuang	砒霜	Arsenicum	Arsenic
Qian Dan	铅丹	Minium	Lead oxide
Qian Li Guang	千里光	Herba Senecionis Scandentis	Climbing groundsel
Qian Nian Jian	千年健	Rhizoma Homalomenae Occultae	Homalomena rhizome
Qing Guo	青果	Fructus Canarii Albi	Chinese white olive
Qing Ma Zi	苘麻子	Semen Abutilonis Theophrasti	Indian mallow seed
Qing Meng Shi	青礞石	Lapis Chloriti	Chlorite schist
Qing Xiang Zi	清湘子	Semen Celosiae Argenteae	Celosia seed
San Qi Hua	三七花	Flos Notoginseng	Notoginseng flower
Shan Ci Gu	山慈菇	Pseudobulbus Shancigu	Cremastra or common pleione pseudobulb
Shang Lu	商陆	Radix Phytolaccae	Pokeberry root
Sheng Cao Wu	生草乌	Radix Aconiti Kusnezoffii Cruda	Raw wild aconite root
Sheng Chuan Wu	生川乌	Radix Aconiti Carmichaeli Cruda	Raw Sichuan aconite mother root
Sheng He Shou Wu	生何首乌	Radix Polygoni Multiflori Cruda	Raw fleece-flower root
Sheng Jiang Zhi	生姜汁	Succus Rhizomatis Zingiberis Officinalis Recens	Fresh ginger juice

Pinyin	Simplified Chinese characters	Pharmaceutical name	English name
Sheng Long Gu	生龙骨	Os Draconis Crudum	Crude dragon bone
Shi Bing	柿饼	Fructus Kaki Exsiccatus	Dried persimmon
Shi Da Gong Lao Ye	十大功劳叶	Folium Mahoniae	Chinese mahonia leaf
Shi Di	柿蒂	Calyx Diospyri Kaki	Persimmon calyx
Shui Yin	水银	Hydrargyrum	Mercury
Si Gua Luo	丝瓜络	Fasciculus Vascularis Luffae	Dried vegetable sponge skeleton
Song Xiang	松香	Resina Pini	Rosin
Song Zi Ren	松子仁	Semen Pini	Pine nut
Tan Xiang	檀香	Lignum Santali Albi	Sandalwood heartwood
Teng Li Gen	藤梨根	Radix Actinidiae Chinensis	Chinese actinidia root
Tu Bei Mu	土贝母	Tuber Bolbostemmatis	Bolbostemma tuber
Tu Gua Ren	土瓜仁	Semen Trichosanthis Cucumeroidis	Cucumber gourd seed
Wa Leng Zi	瓦楞子	Concha Arcae	Ark shell
Wu Shao She	乌梢蛇	Zaocys Dhumnades	Black-tail snake
Xi Gua Cui Yi	西瓜翠衣	Epicarpium Citrulli Vulgaris	Watermelon skin
Xi Gua Shuang	西瓜霜	Pulvis Fructus Citrulli Vulgaris	Watermelon powder
Xi He Liu	西河柳	Cacumen Tamaricis	Tamarisk twig
Xi Jiao	犀角	Cornu Rhinoceri	Rhinoceros horn
Xiang Fu Zi	香附子	Semen Cyperi Rotundi	Nut-grass seed
Xiong Zhu Dan Zhi	雄猪胆汁	Bilis Suis	Male pig bile
Xue Yu Tan	血余炭	Crinis Carbonisatus Hominis	Charred human hair
Ya Xiao	牙消	Mirabilitum Equidens	Horse-tooth mirabilite
Yang Qi Shi	阳起石	Actinolitum	Actinolite
Ying Su Ke	罂粟壳	Pericarpium Papaveris Somniferi	Opium poppy husk
Zao Jiao Zi	皂角子	Semen Gleditsiae Sinensis	Chinese honey locust seed
Zhi Chuan Shan Jia	炙穿山甲	Squama Manitis Pentadactylae Praeparata	Prepared pangolin scales
Zhi Pa Ye	炙杷叶	Folium Eriobotryae Japonicae Praeparatum	Prepared loquat leaf
Zi Ran Tong	自然铜	Pyritum	Pyrite

Appendix 2b Index of materia medica by pharmaceutical name

Pharmaceutical name	English name	Pinyin	Simplified Chinese characters
Abutilonis Theophrasti, Semen	Indian mallow seed	*Qing Ma Zi*	苘麻子
Aconiti Carmichaeli Cruda, Radix	Raw Sichuan aconite mother root	*Sheng Chuan Wu*	生川乌
Aconiti Kusnezoffii Cruda, Radix	Raw wild aconite root	*Sheng Cao Wu*	生草乌
Actinidiae Chinensis, Radix	Chinese actinidia root	*Teng Li Gen*	藤梨根
Actinolitum	Actinolite	*Yang Qi Shi*	阳起石
Albizziae Julibrissin, Flos	Albizzia flower	*He Huan Hua*	合欢花
Allii Sativi, Bulbus	Garlic bulb	*Da Suan*	大蒜
Arcae, Concha	Ark shell	*Wa Leng Zi*	瓦楞子
Aristolochiae Manshuriensis, Caulis	Aristolochia stem	*Guan Mu Tong*	关木通
Arsenicum	Arsenic	*Pi Shuang*	砒霜
Artemisiae Argyi Carbonisatum, Folium	Charred mugwort leaf	*Ai Ye Tan*	艾叶炭
Aspongopus	Stink bug	*Jiu Xiang Chong*	九香虫
Benincasae Hispidae, Semen	Wax gourd seed	*Dong Gua Zi*	冬瓜子
Benzoinum	Benzoin	*An Xi Xiang*	安息香
Bolbostemmatis, Tuber	Bolbostemma tuber	*Tu Bei Mu*	土贝母
Bombycis Mori, Excrementum	Silkworm droppings	*Can Sha*	蚕砂
Caesalpiniae Minax, Semen	Lotus fruit	*Ku Shi Lian Zi*	苦石莲子
Calcitum	Calcite	*Han Shui Shi*	寒水石
Canarii Albi, Fructus	Chinese white olive	*Qing Guo*	青果
Celosiae Argenteae, Semen	Celosia seed	*Qing Xiang Zi*	清湘子
Celosiae Cristatae, Flos	Cockscomb flower	*Ji Guan Hua*	鸡冠花
Centipedae, Herba	Centipeda herb	*E Bu Shi Cao*	鹅不食草
Chloriti, Lapis	Chlorite schist	*Qing Meng Shi*	青礞石
Cinnamomi Cassiae, Cortex Tubiformis	Cinnamon inner bark	*Guan Gui*	官桂
Citrulli Vulgaris, Epicarpium	Watermelon skin	*Xi Gua Cui Yi*	西瓜翠衣
Citrulli Vulgaris, Pulvis Fructus	Watermelon powder	*Xi Gua Shuang*	西瓜霜
Cyperi Rotundi, Semen	Nut-grass seed	*Xiang Fu Zi*	香附子
Diospyri Kaki, Calyx	Persimmon calyx	*Shi Di*	柿蒂
Dolichoris Lablab, Flos	White hyacinth bean flower	*Bian Dou Hua*	扁豆花
Draconis, Dens	Fossilized teeth	*Long Chi*	龙齿
Draconis Crudum, Os	Crude dragon bone	*Sheng Long Gu*	生龙骨
Eretmochelydis, Carapax	Hawksbill turtle shell	*Dai Mao*	玳瑁
Eriobotryae Japonicae Praeparatum, Folium	Prepared loquat leaf	*Zhi Pa Ye*	炙杷叶
Eriocaulonis Buergeriani, Scapus et Flos	Pipewort flower	*Gu Jing Cao*	谷精草
Euphorbiae Fischerianae, Radix	Euphorbia	*Lang Du*	狼毒
Gleditsiae Sinensis, Semen	Chinese honey locust seed	*Zao Jiao Zi*	皂角子
Granorum Spiritus Incolor	White alcohol	*Bai Jiu*	白酒

Pharmaceutical name	English name	Pinyin	Simplified Chinese characters
Homalomenae Occultae, Rhizoma	Homalomena rhizome	*Qian Nian Jian*	千年健
Hominis, Crinis Carbonisatus	Charred human hair	*Xue Yu Tan*	血余炭
Hydrargyrum	Mercury	*Shui Yin*	水银
Kaki Exsiccatus, Fructus	Dried persimmon	*Shi Bing*	柿饼
Lagenariae Depressae, Fructus	Bottle gourd	*Chen Hu Lu*	陈葫芦
Leonuri Heterophylli, Semen	Motherwort seed	*Chong Wei Zi*	茺蔚子
Liquidambaris, Resina	Sweetgum resin	*Feng Xiang Zhi*	枫香脂
Lithargyrum	Litharge	*Mi Tuo Seng*	密陀僧
Luffae, Fasciculus Vascularis	Dried vegetable sponge skeleton	*Si Gua Luo*	丝瓜络
Magnoliae Officinalis, Flos	Magnolia flower	*Hou Po Hua*	厚朴花
Mahoniae, Folium	Chinese mahonia leaf	*Shi Da Gong Lao Ye*	十大功劳叶
Malvae Verticillatae, Semen	Musk mallow seed	*Dong Kui Zi*	冬葵子
Manitis Pentadactylae Praeparata, Squama	Prepared pangolin scales	*Zhi Chuan Shan Jia*	炙穿山甲
Mel	Honey	*Feng Mi*	蜂蜜
Minium	Lead oxide	*Qian Dan*	铅丹
Mirabilitum Equidens	Horse-tooth mirabilite	*Ya Xiao*	牙消
Mylabris	Blister beetle	*Ban Mao*	斑蝥
Nardostachydis, Radix	Nardostachys root	*Gan Song*	甘松
Nelumbinis Nuciferae Carbonisatum, Receptaculum	Charred lotus receptacle	*Lian Fang Tan*	莲房炭
Notoginseng, Flos	Notoginseng flower	*San Qi Hua*	三七花
Oryza Sativa	Polished round grain rice	*Jing Mi*	粳米
Papaveris Somniferi, Pericarpium	Opium poppy husk	*Ying Su Ke*	罂粟壳
Phytolaccae, Radix	Pokeberry root	*Shang Lu*	商陆
Pinelliae, Massa Fermentata	Pinellia tuber leaven	*Ban Xia Qu*	半夏曲
Pini, Resina	Rosin	*Song Xiang*	松香
Pini, Semen	Pine nut	*Song Zi Ren*	松子仁
Piperis Longi, Fructus	Long pepper fruit	*Bi Ba*	荜茇
Piperis Nigri, Fructus	Pepper fruit	*Hu Jiao*	胡椒
Polygoni Multiflori Cruda, Radix	Raw fleece-flower root	*Sheng He Shou Wu*	生何首乌
Pyritum	Pyrite	*Zi Ran Tong*	自然铜
Rhinoceri, Cornu	Rhinoceros horn	*Xi Jiao*	犀角
Saccharon Crystallinum	Sugar candy	*Bing Tang*	冰糖
Santali Albi, Lignum	Sandalwood heartwood	*Tan Xiang*	檀香
Scutellariae Barbatae, Herba	Barbated skullcap herb	*Ban Zhi Lian*	半枝莲
Senecionis Scandentis, Herba	Climbing groundsel	*Qian Li Guang*	千里光
Sesami, Oleum	Sesame oil	*Ma You*	麻油
Shancigu, Pseudobulbus	Cremastra or common pleione pseudobulb	*Shan Ci Gu*	山慈菇

Pharmaceutical name	English name	Pinyin	Simplified Chinese characters
Sophorae Japonicae Carbonisatus, Flos	Charred pagoda tree flower	*Huai Hua Tan*	槐花炭
Sophorae Japonicae Immaturus, Flos	Immature pagoda tree flower	*Huai Hua Mi*	槐花米
Suis, Bilis	Male pig bile	*Xiong Zhu Dan Zhi*	雄猪胆汁
Tabanus	Gadfly	*Meng Chong*	虻虫
Tamaricis, Cacumen	Tamarisk twig	*Xi He Liu*	西河柳
Trichosanthis, Radix	Trichosanthes root	*Gua Lou Gen*	栝蒌根
Trichosanthis Cucumeroidis, Semen	Cucumber gourd seed	*Tu Gua Ren*	土瓜仁
Veratri, Radix et Rhizoma	Veratrum root	*Li Lu*	藜芦
Vinum Aureum	Yellow wine	*Huang Jiu*	黄酒
Zaocys Dhumnades	Black-tail snake	*Wu Shao She*	乌梢蛇
Zingiberis Officinalis Recens, Succus Rhizomatis	Fresh ginger juice	*Sheng Jiang Zhi*	生姜汁

Appendix 2c Index of materia medica by English name

English name	Pharmaceutical name	Pinyin	Simplified Chinese characters
Actinolite	Actinolitum	*Yang Qi Shi*	阳起石
Albizzia flower	Flos Albizziae Julibrissin	*He Huan Hua*	合欢花
Aristolochia stem	Caulis Aristolochiae Manshuriensis	*Guan Mu Tong*	关木通
Ark shell	Concha Arcae	*Wa Leng Zi*	瓦楞子
Arsenic	Arsenicum	*Pi Shuang*	砒霜
Barbated skullcap herb	Herba Scutellariae Barbatae	*Ban Zhi Lian*	半枝莲
Benzoin	Benzoinum	*An Xi Xiang*	安息香
Black-tail snake	Zaocys Dhumnades	*Wu Shao She*	乌梢蛇
Blister beetle	Mylabris	*Ban Mao*	斑蝥
Bolbostemma tuber	Tuber Bolbostemmatis	*Tu Bei Mu*	土贝母
Bottle gourd	Fructus Lagenariae Depressae	*Chen Hu Lu*	陈葫芦
Calcite	Calcitum	*Han Shui Shi*	寒水石
Celosia seed	Semen Celosiae Argenteae	*Qing Xiang Zi*	清湘子
Centipeda herb	Herba Centipedae	*E Bu Shi Cao*	鹅不食草
Charred human hair	Crinis Carbonisatus Hominis	*Xue Yu Tan*	血余炭
Chinese actinidia root	Radix Actinidiae Chinensis	*Teng Li Gen*	藤梨根
Chinese honey locust seed	Semen Gleditsiae Sinensis	*Zao Jiao Zi*	皂角子
Chinese mahonia leaf	Folium Mahoniae	*Shi Da Gong Lao Ye*	十大功劳叶
Chinese white olive	Fructus Canarii Albi	*Qing Guo*	青果
Chlorite schist	Lapis Chloriti	*Qing Meng Shi*	青礞石
Cinnamon inner bark	Cortex Tubiformis Cinnamomi Cassiae	*Guan Gui*	官桂
Climbing groundsel	Herba Senecionis Scandentis	*Qian Li Guang*	千里光
Cockscomb flower	Flos Celosiae Cristatae	*Ji Guan Hua*	鸡冠花
Cremastra or common pleione pseudobulb	Pseudobulbus Shancigu	*Shan Ci Gu*	山慈菇
Cucumber gourd seed	Semen Trichosanthis Cucumeroidis	*Tu Gua Ren*	土瓜仁
Dragon bone, crude	Os Draconis Crudum	*Sheng Long Gu*	生龙骨
Dried vegetable sponge skeleton	Fasciculus Vascularis Luffae	*Si Gua Luo*	丝瓜络
Euphorbia	Radix Euphorbiae Fischerianae	*Lang Du*	狼毒
Fleece-flower root, raw	Radix Polygoni Multiflori Cruda	*Sheng He Shou Wu*	生何首乌
Fossilized teeth	Dens Draconis	*Long Chi*	龙齿
Gadfly	Tabanus	*Meng Chong*	虻虫
Garlic bulb	Bulbus Allii Sativi	*Da Suan*	大蒜
Ginger juice, fresh	Succus Rhizoma Zingiberis Officinalis Recens	*Sheng Jiang Zhi*	生姜汁
Hawksbill turtle shell	Carapax Eretmochelydis	*Dai Mao*	玳瑁
Homalomena rhizome	Rhizoma Homalomenae Occultae	*Qian Nian Jian*	千年健

English name	Pharmaceutical name	Pinyin	Simplified Chinese characters
Honey	Mel	*Feng Mi*	蜂蜜
Horse-tooth mirabilite	Mirabilitum Equidens	*Ya Xiao*	牙消
Human hair, charred	Crinis Carbonisatus Hominis	*Xue Yu Tan*	血余炭
Indian mallow seed	Semen Abutilonis Theophrasti	*Qing Ma Zi*	苘麻子
Lead oxide	Minium	*Qian Dan*	铅丹
Litharge	Lithargyrum	*Mi Tuo Seng*	密陀僧
Long pepper fruit	Fructus Piperis Longi	*Bi Ba*	荜茇
Loquat leaf, prepared	Folium Eriobotryae Japonicae Praeparatum	*Zhi Pa Ye*	炙杷叶
Lotus fruit	Semen Caesalpiniae Minax	*Ku Shi Lian Zi*	苦石莲子
Lotus receptacle, charred	Receptaculum Nelumbinis Nuciferae Carbonisatum	*Lian Fang Tan*	莲房炭
Magnolia flower	Flos Magnoliae Officinalis	*Hou Po Hua*	厚朴花
Male pig bile	Bilis Suis	*Xiong Zhu Dan Zhi*	雄猪胆汁
Mercury	Hydrargyrum	*Shui Yin*	水银
Motherwort seed	Semen Leonuri Heterophylli	*Chong Wei Zi*	茺蔚子
Mugwort leaf, charred	Folium Artemisiae Argyi Carbonisatum	*Ai Ye Tan*	艾叶炭
Musk mallow seed	Semen Malvae Verticillatae	*Dong Kui Zi*	冬葵子
Nardostachys root	Radix Nardostachydis	*Gan Song*	甘松
Notoginseng flower	Flos Notoginseng	*San Qi Hua*	三七花
Nut-grass seed	Semen Cyperi Rotundi	*Xiang Fu Zi*	香附子
Opium poppy husk	Pericarpium Papaveris Somniferi	*Ying Su Ke*	罂粟壳
Pagoda tree flower, charred	Flos Sophorae Japonicae Carbonisatus	*Huai Hua Tan*	槐花炭
Pagoda tree flower, immature	Flos Sophorae Japonicae Immaturus	*Huai Hua Mi*	槐花米
Pangolin scales, prepared	Squama Manitis Pentadactylae Praeparata	*Zhi Chuan Shan Jia*	炙穿山甲
Pepper fruit	Fructus Piperis Nigri	*Hu Jiao*	胡椒
Persimmon, dried	Fructus Kaki Exsiccatus	*Shi Bing*	柿饼
Persimmon calyx	Calyx Diospyri Kaki	*Shi Di*	柿蒂
Pine nut	Semen Pini	*Song Zi Ren*	松子仁
Pinellia tuber leaven	Massa Fermentata Pinelliae	*Ban Xia Qu*	半夏曲
Pipewort flower	Scapus et Flos Eriocaulonis Buergeriani	*Gu Jing Cao*	谷精草
Pokeberry root	Radix Phytolaccae	*Shang Lu*	商陆
Pyrite	Pyritum	*Zi Ran Tong*	自然铜
Rhinoceros horn	Cornu Rhinoceri	*Xi Jiao*	犀角
Rice, polished round-grain	Oryza Sativa	*Jing Mi*	粳米
Rosin	Resina Pini	*Song Xiang*	松香
Sandalwood heartwood	Lignum Santali Albi	*Tan Xiang*	檀香
Sesame oil	Oleum Sesami	*Ma You*	麻油

English name	Pharmaceutical name	Pinyin	Simplified Chinese characters
Sichuan aconite mother root, raw	Radix Aconiti Carmichaeli Cruda	*Sheng Chuan Wu*	生川乌
Silkworm droppings	Excrementum Bombycis Mori	*Can Sha*	蚕砂
Stink bug	Aspongopus	*Jiu Xiang Chong*	九香虫
Sugar candy	Saccharon Crystallinum	*Bing Tang*	冰糖
Sweetgum resin	Resina Liquidambaris	*Feng Xiang Zhi*	枫香脂
Tamarisk twig	Cacumen Tamaricis	*Xi He Liu*	西河柳
Trichosanthes root	Radix Trichosanthis	*Gua Lou Gen*	栝蒌根
Veratrum root	Radix et Rhizoma Veratri	*Li Lu*	藜芦
Watermelon powder	Pulvis Fructus Citrulli Vulgaris	*Xi Gua Shuang*	西瓜霜
Watermelon skin	Epicarpium Citrulli Vulgaris	*Xi Gua Cui Yi*	西瓜翠衣
Wax gourd seed	Semen Benincasae Hispidae	*Dong Gua Zi*	冬瓜子
White alcohol	Granorum Spiritus Incolor	*Bai Jiu*	白酒
White hyacinth bean flower	Flos Dolichoris Lablab	*Bian Dou Hua*	扁豆花
Wild aconite root, raw	Radix Aconiti Kusnezoffii Cruda	*Sheng Cao Wu*	生草乌
Yellow wine	Vinum Aureum	*Huang Jiu*	黄酒

Appendix 3 Selective glossary of TCM terms used

It is beyond the scope of this book to explain all the terminology used. We have assumed that readers will already be familiar with the most common terms used in TCM. The purpose of this glossary is twofold: to explain terms that may not have been encountered regularly and to provide some background to other terms that may have been translated differently in other books, thus enabling the concept to be recognized and confusion between terms circumvented.

Abdominal masses

zhēng jiǎ 癥瘕

Abdominal masses refer to disorders due to lumps binding and accumulating in the abdomen. They are divided into immovable masses (*zhēng*) and movable masses (*jiǎ*). Masses that are immovable, possess a definite form, and give rise to pain in a fixed location (*zhēng*) are related to the Zang organs and belong to the Xue level; masses that are movable (sometimes forming, sometimes dissipating), possess no definite form and give rise to pain without a fixed location (*jiǎ*) are related to the Fu organs and belong to the Qi level. According to *Zhu Bing Yuan Hou Lun · Zheng Jia Bing Zhu Hou* [General Treatise on Causes and Symptoms · Causes and Symptoms of Diseases Due to Abdominal Masses]: '*Zhēng* are gradually formed due to cold or warmth causing Qi deficiency in the Zang-Fu organs, with non-dispersion of food, which accumulates in the interior. They are often caused by dietary irregularities, debilitation of Stomach Qi, depletion of Spleen Qi, Qi stagnation and Blood stasis in the abdomen.' According to *Zhu Bing Yuan Hou Lun · Jia Bing Hou* [General Treatise on Causes and Symptoms · Diseases Due to *Jiǎ* Masses]: '*Jiǎ* diseases are caused by excessive cold or warmth and non-dispersion of food contending with Zang Qi to accumulate in the abdomen and bind into masses with pain; these masses move with Qi.' The *Yi Xue Ru Men* [Entry to Medicine], published in 1575, states that abdominal masses are mostly seen in women and accumulations (*jī jù*) in men.

Abscesses

yōng jū 痈疽

A collective term for acute suppurative disorders. *Yōng* abscesses can be classified into internal and external types. Internal *yōng* abscesses appear in the Zang-Fu organs, whereas external *yōng* abscesses appear on the external surface of the body. These abscesses have a large, shallow surface, do not have a head, and are characterized by redness, swelling, heat and pain. External *yōng* abscesses do not normally penetrate into the sinews and bones. They are generally caused by external contraction of the six excesses, improper diet, external injury and pathogenic toxins causing disharmony between the Ying and Wei levels, the congealing and gathering of pathogenic heat, and Qi stagnation and Blood stasis. *Jū* abscesses are deep-rooted. Caused by the obstruction and stagnation of Qi and Blood due to pathogenic toxins, they occur in the space between the flesh, sinews and bones. They are now divided into *jū* abscesses with heads and *jū* abscesses without heads, although the latter type was not recognized before the Song Dynasty. In the initial stage, *jū* abscesses with heads are the size of millet grains, itchy and painful and with hard roots; they subsequently expand in size with an increase in the amount of pus, turning red and giving a sensation of scorching heat. *Jū* abscesses without heads appear deep in the sinews and bones with diffuse swelling and no alteration in the colour of the skin; pain can penetrate to the bones. These abscesses are difficult to disperse, ulcerate or close, and may damage the sinews and bones after ulceration.

Accumulations
jī jù 积聚
A general term for disorders involving lumps, distension or pain in the abdomen generally caused by binding depression of the seven emotions with Qi stagnation and Blood stasis, by internal damage due to improper diet with Phlegm stagnation, or by an imbalance of cold and heat with vital Qi deficiency and stagnation of pathogenic factors. Accumulated masses (*jī*) are characterized by obvious lumps with distension and pain in a fixed location and are a disorder of the Zang organs, whereas shapeless masses (*jù*) are characterized by a vague migratory mass with no fixed location and some distension and are a disorder of the Fu organs.

Binding in the chest
jié xiōng 结胸
This term refers to the internal binding of pathogenic Qi resulting in distension, fullness and pain in the chest, diaphragm and abdomen. The condition results from the inward fall of exterior heat or full pathogenic factors invading the interior to bind together with water in the chest.

Blood in the stool
biàn xuè 便血
Refers to bleeding from the anus. Bleeding can be before the passage of stool, in the stool or after the passage of stool. The blood can be clear or turbid, bright or dark. Blood in the stool is mainly caused by accumulation of damp-heat in the Intestines, Spleen and Stomach deficiency-cold, insufficiency of Qi in the Middle Jiao, toxins invading the Intestines and Stomach, or wind-heat invading the Lower Jiao and injuring the Blood vessels.

Clouded Spirit and delirious speech
shén hūn zhān yǔ 神昏谵语
Clouded Spirit refers to coma and loss of consciousness, whereas delirious speech refers to a severe disorder manifesting as unclear Spirit and Mind and nonsensical talk due to full-heat in the Yangming channel or warm pathogenic factors invading the Ying and Xue levels resulting in pathogenic heat harassing the Spirit.

Clove sore
dīng chuāng 疔疮
Clove sores get their name from the shape of the sore, which resembles a clove or nail; these sores are small in shape with a deep root and are hard like a nail. They are caused by improper diet, unclean food or externally-contracted wind pathogenic factors and fire toxins; they may also erupt due to external injury with contraction of toxins. Clove sores often occur on the face and less frequently on the limbs and trunk. They change quickly in appearance; at the initial stage, they are the size of rice grains with hard roots and white tops. They subsequently warm up and turn red, gradually swelling in size and becoming painful. Once the sore ulcerates and the root is ejected, the swelling disperses and the pain disappears.

Cold congealing and Qi stagnation
hán níng qì zhì 寒凝气滞
A disorder of pathogenic cold congealing to cause obstruction and stagnation of Qi, manifesting as distension and pain in the abdomen, swelling of the shins, limpness or paralysis, and cold limbs.

Collapse
jué zhèng 厥证
Collapse includes conditions of sudden falling over or fainting and loss of consciousness; in most cases, the collapse is of short duration and is followed by gradual recovery. It is generally caused by sudden chaotic counterflow of Qi, abnormal upward-bearing and downward-bearing of Qi, and the inability of Qi and Blood to move properly. The condition was mentioned in ancient works and was classified as cold collapse (*hán jué*), heat collapse (*rè jué*), roundworm collapse (*huí jué*), Phlegm collapse (*tán jué*), food collapse (*shí jué*), Qi collapse (*qì jué*) and Blood collapse (*xuè jué*). *Jué* can also be taken to include disorders manifesting as counterflow cold of the limbs with cold hands and feet.

Deep-source nasal congestion
bí yuān 鼻渊
This condition manifests as profuse and constant running of turbid discharge from the nose, often accompanied by headache, nasal congestion and a reduced sense of smell. It is classified into two types – deficiency and full. The deficiency type is mostly caused by Qi deficiency of the Spleen and Lungs due to vital Qi failing to overcome pathogenic factors. The full type is generally caused by wind-heat in the Lung channel, heat depression in the Gallbladder, and damp-heat in the Spleen and Stomach that ascends to invade and scorch the nasal sinuses.

Deficiency patterns
xū zhèng 虚证
Deficiency refers to diminished functional activity in the body due to insufficiency of Qi, Blood, body fluids or Essence. It manifests as listlessness of Essence-Spirit, a dull facial complexion, fatigue and lack of strength, emaciation, palpitations and shortness of breath, spontaneous sweating and night sweating, loose stool and diarrhoea, frequent urination or urinary incontinence, a pale and enlarged tongue with crimson fur, and a deficient, fine and forceless pulse.

Depression (or depression patterns)
yù zhèng 郁证
The term depression is used to describe disorders caused by an inability to diffuse and disperse stagnation. Depression can originate from external contraction of one or more of the six excesses that cannot be immediately resolved and dissipated, or from internal damage by the seven emotions that cannot be dispersed immediately, thus obstructing the Qi dynamic. Depression may also be caused by other factors such as overeating and overwork.

The ancient classic *Simple Questions* (*Su Wen*) classified depression into wood depression (*mù yù*), fire depression (*huǒ yù*), earth depression (*tǔ yù*), metal depression (*jīn yù*) and water depression (*shuǐ yù*). In *Dan Xi Xin Fa*, written by Zhu Zhen-feng in the Yuan dynasty, depression is categorized into Qi depression (*qì yù*), Blood depression (*xuè yù*), damp depression (*shī yù*), heat depression (*rè yù*), Phlegm depression (*tán yù*), and food depression (*shí yù*).

The full type of depression pattern often includes depression binding of Liver Qi, depression Qi transforming into fire and depression binding of Phlegm and Qi; the deficiency type of depression pattern often includes damage to the Mind due to prolonged depression and effulgent Yin deficiency-fire.

Desertion pattern
tuō zhèng 脱证
A critical pathological disorder caused by a sudden worsening of the patient's condition, severe exhaustion of Yin, Yang, Qi and Blood, and the departure of Yin and Yang. It manifests as continuous sweating with pearls of sweat, extremely cold limbs, open mouth and closed eyes, limp hands and enuresis, and a faint and fine pulse verging on expiry. Clinically, exhaustion of Essence and Qi due to wind-stroke, profuse sweating, profuse diarrhoea, major bleeding or large amounts of seminal discharge leading to the departure of Yin and Yang are referred to as fulminant desertion. Deficiency desertion manifests as deficiency of original Qi due to chronic diseases and gradual consumption of Essence and Qi. In Western medicine, this category includes heart, lung, liver or kidney failure.

Early-morning diarrhoea
wǔ gēng xiè 五更泻
In the past in China, the night was divided into five periods or watches. The fifth watch (*wǔ gēng*) lasted from 4 a.m. to 6 a.m. Early-morning diarrhoea refers to diarrhoea that habitually starts during the fifth watch. It has a number of causes such as deficiency of Kidney Yang, insufficiency of fire at the gate of vitality, failure to warm and nourish the Spleen and Stomach, and alcohol, food or cold accumulation. Apart from diarrhoea, it manifests as abdominal pain, rumbling intestines, and cold body and limbs.

Effulgent Yin deficiency-fire
yīn xū huǒ wàng 阴虚火旺
This term refers to deficiency-fire exuberance due to depletion of Yin-Essence. It manifests as vexation and agitation, bad temper, tidal reddening of the face, and dry mouth and sore throat.

Fearful throbbing
zhēng chōng 怔忡
A condition characterized by severe palpitations with a sensation of fright or uncontrollable palpitations with agitation.

Five taxations
wǔ láo 五劳
The five taxations refer to the causes of five types of taxation disease as originally summarized in the ancient classic *Simple Questions* (*Su Wen*): prolonged use of the eyes damages the Blood, prolonged lying damages Qi, prolonged sitting damages the flesh, prolonged standing damages the bones, and prolonged walking damages the sinews. Later they were also taken to refer to five types of overstrain as the cause of disease: excessive ambition, mental strain, sorrow, anxiety, and fatigue. In addition, the five taxations can also refer to taxation of the five organs – Lungs, Liver, Heart, Spleen and Kidneys.

Focal distension
pǐ 痞
A term referring to disorders with a subjective sensation of blockage and fullness in the chest and abdomen, but with no sensation of pain under pressure. *Shang Han Lun · Bian Taiyang Bing Mai Zheng Bing Zhi* [On Cold Damage · Identification of Taiyang Diseases: Pulse, Signs and Treatment] states: 'Where disease erupts from Yang but descends and heat enters, this is binding in the chest (*jié xiōng*); where disease erupts from Yin but descends, this is focal distension (*pǐ*) .... If patients experience a sensation of fullness and hardness and there is pain below the heart, this is binding in the chest; if patients experience a sensation of fullness without pain, this is focal distension.' According to the Ming dynasty work *Chi Shui Xuan Zhu · Pi Qi Men* [Red Water and Suspended Pearl · On Focal Distension and Qi]: '*Pǐ* is a disorder caused by deep-lying Yin and amassment of Yang and is formed by Qi ascending but not transporting; it is located below the heart and in the middle .... *Pǐ* can only be felt as an internal sensation of blockage and oppression, with no sign of external distension and can therefore be distinguished from distension and fullness, which have external signs and can be felt by touching.' Focal distension can be caused by deficiency of middle Qi, which thus fails to transport and transform, by accumulation of food and Phlegm inhibiting transformation, and by over-exuberance of damp-heat causing earth to overwhelm below the heart.

Focal distension and fullness
pǐ mǎn 痞满
This term refers to focal distension (*pǐ*), fullness (*mǎn*) and oppression (*mèn*) in the chest and stomach without pain. *Jing Yue Quan Shu · Shang Han Dian* [Jing Yue's Complete Compendium · On Cold Damage] states: 'If patients experience fullness without pain, this is focal distension and fullness (*pǐ mǎn*), but not binding in the chest (*jié xiōng*).' *Shou Shi Bao Yuan · Pi Man* [Achieving Longevity by Guarding the Source · Focal Distension and Fullness] states: 'Focal distension and fullness (*pǐ mǎn*) is different from distension and fullness (*zhàng mǎn*), which is not only internal distension but also has an externally tangible form; *pǐ* is an internal sensation of focal distension and oppression but has no external form.' *Za Bing Yuan Liu Xi Zhu · Zhong Zhang Yuan Liu* [Discourse on the Origin and Development of Miscellaneous Diseases · Origin and Development of Swelling and Distension] states: 'Focal distension and fullness is a disease of the Spleen and is caused by deficiency of Spleen Qi and Qi depression, thus inhibiting movement and transportation.' Focal distension and fullness can therefore be caused by insufficiency of middle Qi, which thus fails to perform its transportation and transformation function, as well as by food accumulation, Phlegm binding, and exuberant damp-heat.

Full patterns

shí zhèng 实证

Full patterns result from obstruction and stagnation due to external pathogenic factors attacking the body, Phlegm-fire, Blood stasis, water-damp, food accumulation or worm accumulation. They are characterized by high fever, distension and pain in the abdomen, oppression in the chest, vexation and agitation, clouded Spirit and delirious speech, congestion of Phlegm or saliva, constipation, inhibited urination, thick and slimy tongue fur, and a full pulse.

Gan

gān 疳

Gan is a general term including Gan patterns, Gan accumulation and Gan diseases. It refers to disorders of chronic nutritional impairment caused by abnormality of the transportation and transformation functions of the Spleen and Stomach. It often occurs in children under five due to improper feeding and dietary imbalance damaging the Spleen and Stomach, or can result from infection by the six excesses, infectious toxins, worms, or febrile or chronic diseases causing Spleen and Stomach deficiency. Although there are a number of causes, the key site of the disorder is located in the Spleen and Stomach.

Gan accumulation

gān jī 疳积

A general syndrome of accumulation and stagnation generally occurring in children under five and caused by a desire for cold, raw, sweet, fatty, sticky or greasy food leading to food stagnating in the stomach and resulting in the Spleen and Stomach failing to digest. Clinically, it manifests initially as a yellow facial complexion and a thin body, dry or loose stool, unquiet sleep, profuse sweating, grinding of teeth during sleep and a propensity to lie on the abdomen. More serious cases are characterized by emaciation, lack of energy, a swollen abdomen, and dry and thin hair.

Hyperactivity of Liver Yang

gān yáng shàng kàng 肝阳上亢

Refers to symptoms caused by depletion of Kidney-water failing to enrich and nourish Liver-wood, or by insufficiency of Liver Yin resulting in Yin failing to subdue Yang. It manifests as dizziness, headache, red face, tinnitus, a bitter taste in the mouth, red tongue, and a string-like, fine and rapid pulse.

Lin syndrome

lín zhèng 淋证

This syndrome is characterized by urinary urgency, difficult and painful urination (often with scorching heat and a stinging pain), constant dribbling, and frequent urination with short voidings. It generally results from damp-heat accumulating in the Bladder accompanied by Qi stagnation, or from weak constitution with advancing age, middle Qi fall and poor Qi transformation due to Kidney deficiency. Depending on the cause of the disorder and the nature of other conditions, Lin syndrome can be classified into stone, blood, heat, Qi and turbid Lin (the five syndromes referred to in this book); other texts also refer to taxation, Phlegm and summer-heat Lin syndromes.

Liver-fire flaming upwards

gān huǒ shàng yán 肝火上炎

Liver-fire flaming upwards refers to a state in which Liver depression and Qi stagnation transform fire, which flames upwards along the Liver channel. It may result from damage to the Liver from excessive anger, ascending counterflow of exuberant Liver Qi, extremes of the seven emotions, or retention of heat in the Liver channel. Liver-fire manifests in the upper part of the body and tends to ascend.

Lung Wei syndrome

fèi wěi 肺痿

A disorder caused by desiccated lobes of the Lungs due to deficiency-heat or deficiency-cold. Lung Wei syndrome due to deficiency-heat manifests as a low cough, spitting of sticky sputum, dry mouth and throat, shortness of breath, hasty wheezing, emaciation or tidal fever, dry hair, a dry and red tongue, and a deficient and rapid pulse. Lung Wei syndrome due to deficiency-cold manifests as cough with thin and frothy sputum, a cold body, fatigued Spirit, absence of thirst, frequent urination, pale tongue, and a weak and deficient pulse.

Mania and withdrawal
diān kuáng 癫狂
This term refers to disorders in the category of mental confusion (possibly even as serious as madness). Withdrawal (*diān*) belongs to Yin and tends to be a deficiency pattern, manifesting as tranquil depression; mania (*kuáng*) belongs to Yang and tends to be a full pattern, manifesting as agitation. However, a prolonged withdrawal disorder can cause Phlegm depression transforming into fire, which leads to mania, and prolonged mania can result in insufficiency of vital Qi and lead to withdrawal. The two conditions are therefore always related to one another.

Phlegm-fluids
tán yǐn 痰饮
Phlegm-fluid patterns are caused by the retention of body fluids in the Stomach and Intestines due to blockage of Qi and the vessels, with water and Qi collecting in the chest to form Phlegm. They are characterized by emaciation, reduced appetite, rumbling intestines and loose stool.

Phlegm-fluid patterns are one of the four types of disorders due to the collection and accumulation of water, the others being suspended fluids (*xuán yǐn*), manifesting as distension and fullness in the hypochondrium, and cough or dragging pain in the hypochondrium when swallowing saliva; spillage fluids (*yì yǐn*), manifesting as fluid congestion in the muscles and flesh due to Spleen deficiency; and propping fluids (*zhī yǐn*), manifesting as an excess of fluid accumulating in the chest due to impairment of the purifying and downward-bearing functions of the Lungs.

In more detailed terms, fluids in the Heart manifest as fearful throbbing and dizziness, fluids in the Lungs as hasty wheezing and cough, fluids in the Spleen as shortness of breath, focal distension and fullness, fluids in the Liver as pain and fullness in the hypochondrium, fluids in the Kidneys as palpitations, fluids in the Stomach as fullness in the stomach and thirst and immediate vomiting after drinking, fluids in the Intestines as a gurgling sound and diarrhoea, fluids in the channels and network vessels as paralysis moving from one side to another, and fluids in the upper part of the body as oedema of the face.

Phlegm nodes
tán hé 痰核
This term refers to local lumps caused by Phlegm-damp accumulation due to deficiency of the Spleen, which fails to perform its transportation function. Phlegm nodes manifest as lumps under the skin and local redness without any sensation of heat. The lumps are of varying sizes, neither painful nor hard, and move when pushed. Phlegm nodes frequently occur in the neck, jaw, limbs and back. They are often accompanied by wind-heat in the upper part of the body and by damp-heat in the lower part.

Plum-pit Qi
méi hé qì 梅核气
This condition refers to the sensation of a foreign object being stuck in the throat. It is often caused by depression binding of the emotions and Mind, and Phlegm and Qi congealing and stagnating.

Qi dynamic
qì jī 气机
Refers to the four basic types of Qi movement – upward-bearing, downward-bearing, inward and outward – with which the physiological functions and pathological activities of the Zang-Fu organs and the channels and network vessels can be summarized.

Qi stagnation
qì zhì 气滞
Qi stagnation occurs when the Qi of the Zang-Fu organs and the channels and network vessels is obstructed and blocked. It can be caused by pathogenic Qi or depression binding of the seven emotions, or by a weak constitution and Qi deficiency resulting in failure to move Qi. A variety of symptoms are manifested depending on which organs or channels and vessels are affected. Qi stagnation in the Spleen manifests as reduced appetite and distension, fullness and pain in the stomach; symptoms of Qi stagnation in the Liver include transverse counterflow of Liver Qi, pain in the hypochondrium and anger; and Qi stagnation in the Lungs manifests as turbid Lung Qi, copious sputum, and coughing and wheezing. Severe Qi stagnation can cause Blood stasis.

Severe pain in the Heart
jué xīn tōng 厥心痛
This refers to pain in the Heart due to Qi ascending counterflow overwhelming the Heart; it is caused by disorders of the Kidneys, Stomach, Spleen, Liver and Heart.

Shan disorders
shàn 疝 ***(or shàn qì*** 疝气***)***
This term has three meanings in traditional Chinese medicine: 1) a collective term for disorders relating to the protrusion of part of an organ from a body cavity, which is often accompanied by symptoms of Qi pain. Such disorders include protrusions through the abdominal wall or into the groin or projection downwards from the abdominal cavity into the intestinal section of the scrotum; 2) disorders of the external genitalia, testicles and scrotum, such as ulcers and swelling with pus; 3) severe abdominal pain around the navel accompanied by difficult urination and constipation.

Taxation (or deficiency taxation)
láo 劳 ***(or xū láo*** 虚劳***)***
This is a general term referring to a variety of chronic debilitating diseases resulting mainly from depletion of and damage to the Zang-Fu organs and insufficiency of Qi, Blood, Yin and Yang. Taxation results from deficiency patterns caused by damage to vital Qi; some infectious diseases and disorders also manifest as deficiency patterns. Taxation may also be caused by an improper lifestyle, overwork or extreme deficiency.

Taxation cough
láo ké 劳咳
Taxation cough indicates a prolonged cough caused by an externally-contracted pathogenic factor and internal damage to the seven emotions.

Vexation and agitation
fán zào 烦躁
Vexation and agitation indicate patterns manifesting as agitation and irritability due to heat depression and occurring in many types of disorders caused by internal damage or external pathogenic factors. These patterns can be divided into deficiency, full, hot and cold types. Where external pathogenic factors are involved, vexation and agitation without sweating generally belong to deficiency patterns, whereas vexation and agitation after sweating are full patterns. In disorders due to internal damage, vexation is generally more pronounced than agitation; this is often the case with effulgent Yin deficiency-fire patterns.

Wei syndrome
wěi zhèng 痿证
A term referring to weakness of the limbs and lack of strength, particularly in the lower limbs, which may even result in muscular atrophy (with impairment of the motor function). It is mainly caused by heat in the Zang organs, particularly heat in the Lungs, which results in damage to body fluids with an invasion of damp-heat, or by insufficiency of Qi and Blood, and depletion and deficiency of the Liver and Kidneys.

Appendix 4 Listing of functions in English, pinyin and simplified Chinese characters

abating deficiency-heat	*tuì xū rè*	退虚热
abating fever	*tuì rè*	退热
abating jaundice	*tuì huáng (dǎn)*	退黄(疸)
abating taxation fever	*tuì láo rè*	退劳热
absorbing dampness	*shōu shī*	收湿
adjusting and harmonizing the nature of herbs	*tiáo hé yào xìng*	调和药性
adjusting and harmonizing the Ying and Wei levels	*tiáo hé yíng wèi*	调和营卫
adjusting menstruation	*tiáo jīng*	调经
allaying thirst	*zhǐ kě*	止渴
alleviating Bi syndrome pain	*zhǐ bì tòng*	止痹痛
alleviating itching	*zhǐ yǎng*	止痒
alleviating pain	*zhǐ tòng*	止痛
alleviating tetany	*zhǐ jìng*	止痉
allowing constrained Liver Qi to flow freely	*shū gān jiě yù*	疏肝解郁
aromatically opening the orifices	*fāng xiāng kāi qiào*	芳香开窍
arousing the brain	*xǐng nǎo*	醒脑
arousing the Spirit	*xǐng shén*	醒神
arousing the Spleen	*xǐng pí*	醒脾
astringing the Essence	*sè jīng*	涩精
astringing the Intestines	*sè cháng*	涩肠
attacking accumulation	*gōng jī*	攻积
attacking toxins	*gōng dú*	攻毒
bearing counterflow Qi downwards	*jiàng nì xià qì*	降逆下气
bearing fire downwards	*jiàng huǒ*	降火
bearing Qi downwards	*jiàng qì*	降气
bearing Yang upwards	*shēng yáng*	升阳
benefiting the diaphragm	*lì gé*	利膈
benefiting the Gallbladder	*lì dǎn*	利胆
benefiting the joints	*lì guān jié*	利关节
benefiting the orifices	*lì qiào*	利窍
benefiting the throat	*lì yān*	利咽
boosting defensive Qi	*yì wèi*	益卫
boosting Kidney Yin	*yì shèn yīn*	益肾阴
boosting Qi	*yì qì*	益气
boosting the Essence and Blood	*yì jīng xuè*	益精血
boosting the Kidneys	*yì shèn*	益肾
boosting the Liver	*yì gān*	益肝
boosting the Lungs	*yì fèi*	益肺
boosting the Stomach	*yì wèi*	益胃
breaking up (Blood) stasis	*pò yū*	破瘀
breaking up Qi (stagnation)	*pò qì*	破气
brightening the eyes	*míng mù*	明目
calming and repressing Liver Yang	*píng yì gān yáng*	平抑肝阳
calming the Liver	*píng gān*	平肝

calming wheezing	*píng chuǎn*	平喘
causing milk to descend	*xià rǔ*	下乳
causing Qi to descend	*xià qì*	下气
clearing and benefiting the head and eyes	*qīng lì tóu mù*	清利头目
clearing damp-heat	*qīng shī rè*	清湿热
clearing deficiency-heat	*qīng xū rè*	清虚热
clearing fire	*qīng huǒ*	清火
clearing Heart-fire	*qīng xīn huǒ*	清心火
clearing heat	*qīng rè*	清热
clearing Liver-fire	*qīng gān huǒ*	清肝火
clearing summerheat	*qīng shǔ*	清暑
clearing the Heart	*qīng xīn*	清心
clearing the Intestines	*qīng cháng*	清肠
clearing the Liver	*qīng gān*	清肝
clearing the Lungs	*qīng fèi*	清肺
closing sores	*liǎn chuāng*	敛疮
constraining sweating	*liǎn hàn*	敛汗
constraining the Lungs	*liǎn fèi*	敛肺
constraining Yin	*liǎn yīn*	敛阴
controlling acidity	*zhì suān*	制酸
cooling the Blood	*liàng xuè*	凉血
curtailing desertion	*gù tuō*	固脱
diffusing and dissipating wind-heat	*xuān sàn fēng rè*	宣散风热
diffusing Lung Qi	*xuān fèi* *(xuān tōng fèi qì)*	宣肺 (宣通肺气)
dislodging Phlegm	*huò tán*	豁痰
dispelling cold	*qū hán*	祛寒
dispelling damp-heat	*qū shī rè*	祛湿热
dispelling dampness	*qū shī*	祛湿
dispelling Phlegm	*qū tán*	祛痰
dispelling (Blood) stasis	*qū yū*	祛瘀
dispelling wind	*qū fēng*	祛风
dispelling wind-cold	*qū fēng hán*	祛风寒
dispelling wind-damp	*qū fēng shī*	祛风湿
dispelling wind-heat	*qū fēng rè*	祛风热
dispersing abdominal masses	*xiāo zhēng*	消癥
dispersing abscesses	*xiāo yōng*	消痈
dispersing accumulation	*xiāo jī*	消积
dispersing fluids	*xiāo yǐn*	消饮
dispersing focal distension	*xiāo pǐ*	消痞
dispersing food (accumulation)	*xiāo shí*	消食
dispersing Gan	*xiāo gān*	消疳
dispersing goitre	*xiāo yǐng*	消瘿
dispersing haemorrhoids	*xiāo zhì*	消痔
dispersing Phlegm	*xiāo tán*	消痰
dispersing stagnation	*xiāo zhì*	消滞
dispersing (Blood) stasis	*xiāo yū*	消瘀
dispersing stones	*xiāo shí*	消石
dispersing swelling	*xiāo zhǒng*	消肿
dissipating cold	*sàn hán*	散寒
dissipating externally-contracted wind-heat	*sàn fēng rè xié*	散风热邪

dissipating lumps	*sàn jié*	散结
dissipating (Blood) stasis	*sàn yū*	散瘀
dissipating swelling	*sàn zhǒng*	散肿
dissipating wind	*sàn fēng*	散风
dissipating wind-cold	*fā sàn fēng hán*	发散风寒
dissipating wind-heat	*shū sàn fēng rè*	疏散风热
draining cold accumulation downwards	*xiè xià lěng jī*	泻下冷积
draining downwards	*xiè xià*	泻下
draining fire	*xiè huǒ*	泻火
draining the Lungs	*xiè fèi*	泻肺
draining water	*xiè shuǐ*	泻水
drawing out toxins	*tuō dú*	托毒
drying dampness	*zào shī*	燥湿
eliminating Bi syndrome	*chú bì*	除痹
eliminating Bi syndrome pain	*chú bì zhǐ tòng*	除痹止痛
eliminating dampness	*chú shī*	除湿
eliminating eye screen	*qù yì*	去翳
eliminating focal distension	*chú pǐ*	除痞
eliminating Gan fever	*chú gān rè*	除疳热
eliminating steam (in steaming bone disorder or, more broadly, fever due to Yin deficiency)	*chú zhēng*	除蒸
eliminating vexation	*chú fán*	除烦
emolliating the Liver	*róu gān*	柔肝
enriching and supplementing the Liver and Kidneys	*zī bǔ gān shèn*	滋补肝肾
enriching the Kidneys	*zī shèn*	滋肾
enriching Yin	*zī yīn*	滋阴
expelling (Blood) stasis	*zhú yū*	逐瘀
expelling damp-cold	*zhú shī hán*	逐湿寒
expelling fluids	*zhú yǐn*	逐饮
expelling pus	*pái nóng*	排脓
expelling roundworm	*qū huí*	驱蛔
expelling stones	*pái shí*	排石
expelling water	*zhú shuǐ*	逐水
expelling wind	*qū fēng*	驱风
expelling worms	*zhú chóng*	逐虫
exterminating lice	*miè shī*	灭虱
extinguishing wind	*xī fēng*	熄风
fortifying the Spleen	*jiàn pí*	健脾
freeing Bi syndrome	*tōng bì*	通痹
freeing Lin syndrome	*tōng lín*	通淋
freeing menstruation	*tōng jīng*	通经
freeing milk	*tōng rǔ*	通乳
freeing obstructions	*tōng bì*	通闭
freeing Phlegm	*tōng tán*	通痰
freeing Qi	*tōng qì*	通气
freeing the Blood vessels	*xuān tōng xuè mài*	宣通血脉
freeing the bowels	*tōng biàn*	通便
freeing the channels	*tōng jīng*	通经
freeing the network vessels	*tōng luò*	通络

freeing the orifices	*tōng qiào*	通窍
freeing the vessels	*tōng mài*	通脉
freeing Yang	*tōng yáng*	通阳
generating body fluids	*shēng jīn*	生津
generating flesh	*shēng jī*	生肌
guiding out stagnation	*dǎo zhì*	导滞
guiding the downward movement of Blood	*yǐn xuè xià xíng*	引血下行
harmonizing Shaoyang	*hé jiě shào yáng*	和解少阳
harmonizing the Blood	*hé xuè*	和血
harmonizing the Middle (Jiao)	*hé zhōng*	和中
harmonizing the Stomach	*hé wèi*	和胃
hastening delivery	*cuī shēng*	催生
hosting Qi	*nà qì*	纳气
increasing the appetite (opening the Stomach)	*kāi wèi*	开胃
increasing wisdom	*zēng zhì*	增智
inducing sweating	*fā hàn*	发汗
inducing vomiting	*yǒng tù*	涌吐
interrupting malaria	*jié nüè*	截疟
invigorating Yang	*zhuàng yáng*	壮阳
joining fractures	*xù zhé*	续折
joining the sinews and bones	*xù jīn jiē gǔ*	续筋接骨
killing worms	*shā chóng*	杀虫
loosening the chest	*kuān xiōng*	宽胸
loosening the Middle (Jiao)	*kuān zhōng*	宽中
lowering blood pressure	*jiàng (xuè) yā*	降(血)压
lubricating the Intestines	*huá cháng*	滑肠
moderating and harmonizing the nature of herbs	*huǎn hé yào xìng*	缓和药性
moistening dryness	*rùn zào*	润燥
moistening the Intestines	*rùn cháng*	润肠
moistening the Lungs	*rùn fèi*	润肺
moving Qi	*xíng qì*	行气
moving water	*xíng shuǐ*	行水
nourishing the Blood	*yǎng xuè*	养血
nourishing the Heart	*yǎng xīn*	养心
nourishing the Liver	*yǎng gān*	养肝
nourishing the Stomach	*yǎng wèi*	养胃
nourishing Yin	*yǎng yīn*	养阴
opening depression	*kāi yù*	开郁
opening the orifices	*kāi qiào*	开窍
opening up and diffusing Lung Qi	*kāi xuān fèi qì*	开宣肺气
overcoming dampness	*shèng shī*	胜湿
percolating dampness	*shèn shī*	渗湿
preventing putrefaction	*fáng fǔ*	防腐

promoting astriction	*shōu sè*	收涩
promoting contraction	*shōu liǎn*	收敛
promoting the elimination of dampness	*lì shī*	利湿
promoting the movement of Qi	*lì qì*	利气
promoting the movement of water	*lì shuǐ*	利水
promoting urination	*lì niào*	利尿
putrefying and consuming warts	*fǔ shí zhuì yóu*	腐蚀赘疣
quickening the Blood	*huó xuè*	活血
quickening the network vessels	*huó luò*	活络
quieting the foetus	*ān tāi*	安胎
quieting the Heart	*níng xīn*	宁心
quieting the Spirit	*ān shén*	安神
raising the fall	*jǔ xiàn*	举陷
reducing swelling	*tuì zhǒng*	退肿
reducing urination	*suō xiǎo biàn*	缩小便
reducing urine	*suō niào*	缩尿
regulating Qi	*lǐ qì*	理气
regulating the Blood	*lǐ xuè*	理血
regulating the Chong and Ren vessels	*tiáo lǐ chōng rèn*	调理冲任
reinforcing Yang	*zhù yáng*	助阳
relaxing tension	*huǎn jí*	缓急
releasing flesh	*jiě jī*	解肌
releasing the exterior	*jiě biǎo*	解表
relieving depression	*jiě yù*	解郁
relieving summerheat	*jiě shǔ*	解暑
relieving tetany	*jiě jìng*	解痉
relieving the toxicity of sores	*jiě chuāng dú*	解疮毒
relieving toxicity	*jiě dú*	解毒
removing eye screen	*tuì yì*	退翳
repelling foulness	*bì huì*	避秽
repelling turbidity	*bì zhuó*	避浊
replenishing the Marrow	*tián suǐ*	填髓
restoring the voice	*kāi yīn*	开音
returning Yang	*huí yáng*	回阳
securing astriction	*gù sè*	固涩
securing the Essence	*gù jīng*	固精
securing the exterior	*gù biǎo*	固表
securing the Kidneys	*gù shèn*	固肾
securing the menses	*gù jīng*	固经
separating the clear and the turbid	*fēn bié qīng zhuó*	分别清浊
settling fright	*zhèn jīng*	镇惊
settling tetany	*zhèn jìng*	镇痉
settling the Heart	*zhèn xīn*	镇心
sharpening the hearing	*cōng ěr*	聪耳
sharpening the wits	*yì zhì*	益智
softening hardness	*ruǎn jiān*	软坚
soothing the Liver	*shū gān*	舒肝
soothing the sinews	*shū jīn*	舒筋
stabilizing wheezing	*dìng chuǎn*	定喘

stemming counterflow	*jiù nì*	救逆
stemming profuse uterine bleeding	*jiù bēng*	救崩
stopping bleeding	*zhǐ xuè*	止血
stopping coughing	*zhǐ ké*	止咳
stopping diarrhoea	*zhǐ xiè*	止泻
stopping dysentery	*zhǐ lì*	止痢
stopping seminal emission	*zhǐ yí*	止遗
stopping sweating	*zhǐ hàn*	止汗
stopping uterine bleeding	*zhǐ bēng*	止崩
stopping vaginal discharge	*zhǐ dài*	止带
stopping vomiting	*zhǐ ǒu*	止呕
strengthening the bones	*jiàn gǔ*	健骨
strengthening the lumbar region and knees	*qiáng yāo xī*	强腰膝
strengthening the sinews and bones	*qiáng jiàn jīn gǔ*	强健筋骨
strongly supplementing original Qi	*dà bǔ yuán qì*	大补元气
subduing Yang	*qián yáng*	潜阳
supplementing and boosting the Essence and Blood	*bǔ yì jīng xuè*	补益精血
supplementing and boosting the Heart and Spleen	*bǔ yì xīn pí*	补益心脾
supplementing and boosting the Liver and Kidneys	*bǔ yì gān shèn*	补益肝肾
supplementing deficiency	*bǔ xū*	补虚
supplementing fire	*bǔ huǒ*	补火
supplementing Kidney Yang	*bǔ shèn yáng*	补肾阳
supplementing Qi	*bǔ qì*	补气
supplementing the Blood	*bǔ xuè*	补血
supplementing the Essence	*bǔ jīng*	补精
supplementing the Kidneys	*bǔ shèn*	补肾
supplementing the Liver	*bǔ gān*	补肝
supplementing the Liver and Kidneys	*bǔ gān shèn*	补肝肾
supplementing the Lungs	*bǔ fèi*	补肺
supplementing the Middle (Jiao)	*bǔ zhōng*	补中
supplementing the Spleen	*bǔ pí*	补脾
supplementing Yang	*bǔ yáng*	补阳
supplementing Yin	*bǔ yīn*	补阴
supporting vital Qi	*fú zhù zhèng qì*	扶助正气
terminating lactation	*huí rǔ*	回乳
transforming accumulation	*huà jī*	化积
transforming dampness	*huà shī*	化湿
transforming fluids	*huà yǐn*	化饮
transforming Phlegm	*huà tán*	化痰
transforming Qi	*huà qì*	化气
transforming stagnation	*huà zhì*	化滞
transforming (Blood) stasis	*huà yū*	化瘀
treating injuries	*liáo shāng*	疗伤
treating seafood poisoning	*jiě yú xiè dú*	解鱼蟹毒
treating sores	*liáo chuāng*	疗疮
treating tinea	*liáo xuǎn*	疗癣
uplifting Yang Qi	*shēng jǔ yáng qì*	升举阳气
venting macules and papules	*tòu fā bān zhěn*	透发斑疹
venting papules	*tòu zhěn*	透疹

warming and freeing the channels and vessels	*wēn tōng jīng mài*	温通经脉
warming and transforming water-fluids	*wēn huà shuǐ yǐn*	温化水饮
warming the channels	*wēn jīng*	温经
warming the interior	*wēn lǐ*	温里
warming the Kidneys	*nuǎn shèn/wēn shèn*	暖肾/温肾
warming the Lungs	*wēn fèi*	温肺
warming the Middle (Jiao)	*wēn zhōng*	温中
warming the Spleen	*wēn pí*	温脾
warming the Spleen and Kidneys	*wēn xù pí shèn*	温煦脾肾
warming the Stomach	*wēn wèi*	温胃
warming Yang	*wēn yáng*	温阳

Appendix 5 Cross-reference of functions to individual materia medica

Appendix 6 Cross-reference of individual materia medica to the combinations in which they appear

This appendix indicates the main herb for each combination in which the materia medica listed appear. For space reasons, the corresponding pharmaceutical names of the herbs in the combinations have not been listed; they can be found in Appendix 1.

Appendix 7 Cross-reference of applications to materia medica combinations

Appendix 8 Classification of materia medica according to commonly-seen patterns and symptoms

In contrast to the chapters in this book, which are compiled according to function, this appendix is classified on the basis of a selection of commonly-seen patterns and symptoms with the aim of enabling readers to gain an idea of which materia medica are suitable for treating the symptoms in question. Reference can then be made to the main herb and its combinations for further information (the page numbers stated relate to the start of the monograph concerned). The legal status of some of these materia medica must also be borne in mind (see the note at the end of the introduction, pages 11 to 13).

1. Abdominal distension patterns

a. Damp obstruction damaging the Middle Jiao

Bai Dou Kou (Fructus Amomi Kravanh), 205; *Cang Zhu* (Rhizoma Atractylodis), 201; *Cao Guo* (Fructus Amomi Tsaoko), 208; *Chen Pi* (Pericarpium Citri Reticulatae), 272; *Da Fu Pi* (Pericarpium Arecae Catechu), 288; *Hou Po* (Cortex Magnoliae Officinalis), 200; *Pei Lan* (Herba Eupatorii Fortunei), 203; *Sha Ren* (Fructus Amomi), 204

b. Qi stagnation in the Spleen and Stomach

Bai Dou Kou (Fructus Amomi Kravanh), 205; *Bing Lang* (Semen Arecae Catechu), 311; *Chen Pi* (Pericarpium Citri Reticulatae), 272; *Chen Xiang* (Lignum Aquilariae Resinatum), 279; *Da Fu Pi* (Pericarpium Arecae Catechu), 288; *Hou Po* (Cortex Magnoliae Officinalis), 200; *Lai Fu Zi* (Semen Raphani Sativi), 301; *Mu Xiang* (Radix Aucklandiae Lappae), 276; *Sha Ren* (Fructus Amomi), 204; *Su Geng* (Caulis Perillae Frutescentis), 28; *Wu Yao* (Radix Linderae Strychnifoliae), 285; *Zhi Ke* (Fructus Citri Aurantii), 275; *Zhi Shi* (Fructus Immaturus Citri Aurantii), 274

2. Abdominal masses and accumulations

Bie Jia (Carapax Amydae Sinensis), 583; *Chuan Shan Jia* (Squama Manitis Pentadactylae), 389; *Da Huang* (Radix et Rhizoma Rhei), 155; *E Zhu* (Rhizoma Curcumae), 385; *Hong Hua* (Flos Carthami Tinctorii), 370; *Mang Xiao* (Mirabilitum), 157; *Mo Yao* (Myrrha), 366; *Mu Li* (Concha Ostreae), 473; *Ru Xiang* (Gummi Olibanum), 365; *San Leng* (Rhizoma Sparganii Stoloniferi), 386; *Shan Zha* (Fructus Crataegi), 297; *She Gan* (Rhizoma Belamcandae Chinensis), 106; *She Xiang* (Secretio Moschi), 501; *Shui Zhi* (Hirudo seu Whitmania), 387; *Tao Ren* (Semen Persicae), 372; *Tu Bie Chong* (Eupolyphaga seu Steleophaga), 388; *Yu Jin* (Radix Curcumae), 362

3. Bi syndrome

a. Bi syndrome due to insufficiency of the Liver and Kidneys

Ba Ji Tian (Radix Morindae Officinalis), 545; *Gou Ji* (Rhizoma Cibotii Barometz), 192; *Niu Xi* (Radix Achyranthis Bidentatae), 375; *Rou Gui* (Cortex Cinnamomi Cassiae), 254; *Sang Ji Sheng* (Ramulus Loranthi), 190; *Suo Yang* (Herba Cynomorii Songarici), 551; *Wu Jia Pi* (Cortex Acanthopanacis Gracilistyli Radicis), 191; *Xian Mao* (Rhizoma Curculiginis Orchioidis), 547; *Xu Duan* (Radix Dipsaci), 544

b. Stubborn Bi syndrome due to wind-damp

Chuan Shan Jia (Squama Manitis Pentadactylae), 389; *Di Long* (Lumbricus), 488; *Quan Xie* (Buthus Martensi), 489; *Ru Xiang* (Gummi Olibanum), 365; *Wei Ling Xian* (Radix Clematidis), 177; *Wu Gong* (Scolopendra Subspinipes), 491

c. Wind-cold-damp Bi syndrome

Ba Ji Tian (Radix Morindae Officinalis), 545; *Bi Xie* (Rhizoma Dioscoreae Hypoglaucae seu Septemlobae), 236; *Cang Zhu* (Rhizoma Atractylodis), 201; *Chuan Xiong* (Rhizoma Ligustici Chuanxiong), 359; *Dang Gui* (Radix Angelicae Sinensis), 563; *Du Huo* (Radix Angelicae Pubescentis), 174; *Fang Feng* (Radix Ledebouriellae Divaricatae), 30; *Fang Ji* (Radix Stephaniae Tetrandrae), 183; *Fu Zi* (Radix Lateralis Aconiti

Carmichaeli Praeparata), 250; *Gao Ben* (Rhizoma et Radix Ligustici), 35; *Gou Ji* (Rhizoma Cibotii Barometz), 192; *Gui Zhi* (Ramulus Cinnamomi Cassiae), 22; *Hai Feng Teng* (Caulis Piperis Kadsurae), 179; *Jiang Huang* (Rhizoma Curcumae Longae), 364; *Lu Lu Tong* (Fructus Liquidambaris), 180; *Ma Huang* (Herba Ephedrae), 20; *Mu Gua* (Fructus Chaenomelis), 175; *Qi She* (Agkistrodon), 176; *Qiang Huo* (Rhizoma et Radix Notopterygii), 32; *Qin Jiao* (Radix Gentianae Macrophyllae), 181; *Rou Gui* (Cortex Cinnamomi Cassiae), 254; *Ru Xiang* (Gummi Olibanum), 365; *Sang Ji Sheng* (Ramulus Loranthi), 190; *Shen Jin Cao* (Herba Lycopodii Japonici), 178; *Wei Ling Xian* (Radix Clematidis), 177; *Wu Gong* (Scolopendra Subspinipes), 491; *Wu Jia Pi* (Cortex Acanthopanacis Gracilistyli Radicis), 191; *Xi Xin* (Herba cum Radice Asari), 24; *Xu Chang Qing* (Radix Cynanchi Paniculati), 188

d. Wind-damp-heat Bi syndrome

Bai Xian Pi (Cortex Dictamni Dasycarpi Radicis), 90; *Bi Xie* (Rhizoma Dioscoreae Hypoglaucae seu Septemlobae), 236; *Di Long* (Lumbricus), 488; *Fang Ji* (Radix Stephaniae Tetrandrae), 183; *Luo Shi Teng* (Caulis Trachelospermi Jasminoidis), 187; *Mu Gua* (Fructus Chaenomelis), 175; *Mu Tong* (Caulis Mutong), 229; *Niu Xi* (Radix Achyranthis Bidentatae), 375; *Qin Jiao* (Radix Gentianae Macrophyllae), 181; *Ren Dong Teng* (Caulis Lonicerae Japonicae), 96; *Sang Zhi* (Ramulus Mori Albae), 184; *Xi Xian Cao* (Herba Siegesbeckiae), 185; *Yi Yi Ren* (Semen Coicis Lachrymajobi), 219

4. Bleeding patterns

a. Bleeding due to external injury

Bai Ji (Rhizoma Bletillae Striatae), 340; *Duan Long Gu* (Os Draconis Calcinatum), 455; *Er Cha* (Pasta Acaciae seu Uncariae), 656; *Hua Rui Shi* (Ophicalcitum), 337; *Ming Fan* (Alumen), 653; *Pu Huang* (Pollen Typhae), 336; *San Qi* (Radix Notoginseng), 333; *Xue Jie* (Resina Draconis), 659

b. Blood-heat patterns

Da Huang Tan (Radix et Rhizoma Rhei Carbonisatae), 155; *Di Yu* (Radix Sanguisorbae Officinalis), 327; *E Jiao* (Gelatinum Corii Asini), 573; *Huai Hua* (Flos Sophorae Japonicae), 329; *Huai Jiao* (Fructus Sophorae Japonicae), 330; *Yu Jin* (Radix Curcumae), 362; *Zhu Ma Gen* (Radix Boehmeriae Niveae), 332

c. Frenetic movement of hot Blood

Ai Ye (Folium Artemisiae Argyi), 347; *Bai Mao Gen* (Rhizoma Imperatae Cylindricae), 331; *Ce Bai Ye* (Cacumen Biotae Orientalis), 328; *Da Huang Tan* (Radix et Rhizoma Rhei Carbonisatae), 155; *Da Ji* (Herba seu Radix Cirsii Japonici), 325; *Dai Zhe Shi* (Haematitum), 475; *Di Gu Pi* (Cortex Lycii Radicis), 139; *Han Lian Cao* (Herba Ecliptae Prostratae), 595; *Huang Qin Tan* (Radix Scutellariae Baicalensis Carbonisata), 81; *Ma Chi Xian* (Herba Portulacae Oleraceae), 117; *Mu Dan Pi* (Cortex Moutan Radicis), 132; *Qian Cao Gen* (Radix Rubiae Cordifoliae), 334; *Qing Dai* (Indigo Naturalis), 103; *San Qi* (Radix Notoginseng), 333; *Sheng Di Huang* (Radix Rehmanniae Glutinosae), 129; *Shui Niu Jiao* (Cornu Bubali), 136; *Xiao Ji* (Herba Cephalanoploris seu Cirsii), 326; *Yu Jin* (Radix Curcumae), 362; *Zhi Zi* (Fructus Gardeniae Jasminoidis), 72; *Zong Lü Tan* (Fibra Carbonisata Trachycarpi Stipulae), 343

d. Incessant bleeding

Chi Shi Zhi (Halloysitum Rubrum), 622; *Ming Fan* (Alumen), 653; *Mu Li* (Concha Ostreae), 473; *Ou Jie* (Nodus Nelumbinis Nuciferae Rhizomatis), 344; *Xian He Cao* (Herba Agrimoniae Pilosae), 341; *Xu Duan* (Radix Dipsaci), 544; *Yu Yu Liang* (Limonitum), 621; *Zong Lü Tan* (Fibra Carbonisata Trachycarpi Stipulae), 343

e. Obstruction due to Blood stasis

Hua Rui Shi (Ophicalcitum), 337; *Jiang Xiang* (Lignum Dalbergiae Odoriferae), 338; *Pu Huang* (Pollen Typhae), 336; *San Qi* (Radix Notoginseng), 333

f. Qi failing to contain the Blood

Duan Long Gu (Os Draconis Calcinatum), 455; *E Jiao* (Gelatinum Corii Asini), 573; *Huang Qi* (Radix Astragali seu Hedysari), 518; *Lu Jiao Jiao* (Gelatinum Cornu Cervi), 539; *Pao Jiang* (Rhizoma Zingiberis Officinalis Praeparata), 346; *Qian Cao Gen* (Radix Rubiae Cordifoliae), 334; *San Qi* (Radix Notoginseng), 333; *Zao Xin Tu* (Terra Flava Usta), 348

5. Block patterns

a. Clouded Spirit due to cold block

She Xiang (Secretio Moschi), 501; *Shi Chang Pu* (Rhizoma Acori Graminei), 505; *Su He Xiang* (Styrax Liquidus), 503; *Zao Jiao* (Fructus Gleditsiae Sinensis), 408

b. Clouded Spirit due to heat block
Bing Pian (Borneolum), 503; *Ling Yang Jiao* (Cornu Antelopis), 481; *Ming Fan* (Alumen), 653; *Niu Huang* (Calculus Bovis), 482; *She Xiang* (Secretio Moschi), 501

6. Blurred vision
Bo He (Herba Menthae Haplocalycis), 45; *Che Qian Zi* (Semen Plantaginis), 226; *Ci Shi* (Magnetitum), 454; *Fu Pen Zi* (Fructus Rubi Chingii), 635; *Gou Qi Zi* (Fructus Lycii), 586; *Gui Ban* (Plastrum Testudinis), 584; *Han Lian Cao* (Herba Ecliptae Prostratae), 595; *He Shou Wu* (Radix Polygoni Multiflori), 569; *Hei Zhi Ma* (Semen Sesami Indici), 597; *Ju Hua* (Flos Chrysanthemi Morifolii), 49; *Jue Ming Zi* (Semen Cassiae), 77; *Mu Zei* (Herba Equiseti Hiemalis), 60; *Nü Zhen Zi* (Fructus Ligustri Lucidi), 596; *Sang Ye* (Folium Mori Albae), 48; *Sha Yuan Zi* (Semen Astragali Complanati), 552; *Shi Hu* (Herba Dendrobii), 591; *Shi Jue Ming* (Concha Haliotidis), 472; *Shu Di Huang* (Radix Rehmanniae Glutinosae Conquita), 565; *Tu Si Zi* (Semen Cuscutae), 541; *Zhen Zhu Mu* (Concha Margaritifera), 478; *Zhu Sha* (Cinnabaris), 453; *Zi He Che* (Placenta Hominis), 559

7. Breast abscess
Bai Zhi (Radix Angelicae Dahuricae), 33; *Ban Bian Lian* (Herba Lobeliae Chinensis cum Radice), 111; *Ban Xia* (Rhizoma Pinelliae Ternatae), 399; *Chi Shao* (Radix Paeoniae Rubra), 133; *Dan Shen* (Radix Salviae Miltiorrhizae), 369; *Gan Cao* (Radix Glycyrrhizae), 523; *Gua Lou* (Fructus Trichosanthis), 415; *Jin Yin Hua* (Flos Lonicerae), 95; *Ju Ye* (Folium Citri Reticulatae), 274; *Lian Qiao* (Fructus Forsythiae Suspensae), 97; *Lou Lu* (Radix Rhapontici seu Echinopsis), 121; *Lu Jiao* (Cornu Cervi), 539; *Mang Xiao* (Mirabilitum), 157; *Niu Huang* (Calculus Bovis), 482; *Pu Gong Ying* (Herba Taraxaci cum Radice), 98; *Qing Pi* (Pericarpium Citri Reticulatae Viride), 280; *Tian Hua Fen* (Radix Trichosanthis), 71; *Wang Bu Liu Xing* (Semen Vaccariae Segetalis), 379; *Xia Ku Cao* (Spica Prunellae Vulgaris), 74; *Xu Duan* (Radix Dipsaci), 544; *Yi Mu Cao* (Herba Leonuri Heterophylli), 374; *Yuan Zhi* (Radix Polygalae), 461; *Zhe Bei Mu* (Bulbus Fritillariae Thunbergii), 414; *Zi Hua Di Ding* (Herba Violae Yedoensitis), 100

8. Burns and scalds
Bai Lian (Radix Ampelopsis Japonicae), 124; *Ce Bai Ye* (Cacumen Biotae Orientalis), 328; *Di Yu* (Radix Sanguisorbae Officinalis), 327; *Duan Shi Gao* (Gypsum Fibrosum Calcinatum), 69; *Zi Zhu* (Folium Callicarpae), 343

9. Chest Bi syndrome
a. Bi syndrome obstruction due to Blood stasis
Chuan Xiong (Rhizoma Ligustici Chuanxiong), 359; *Hong Hua* (Flos Carthami Tinctorii), 370; *Hu Po* (Succinum), 457; *Jiang Xiang* (Lignum Dalbergiae Odoriferae), 338; *Pu Huang* (Pollen Typhae), 336; *She Xiang* (Secretio Moschi), 501; *Tao Ren* (Semen Persicae), 372; *Wu Ling Zhi* (Excrementum Trogopteri), 367; *Xie Bai* (Bulbus Allii Macrostemi), 287; *Yu Jin* (Radix Curcumae), 362

b. Bi syndrome obstruction due to Phlegm turbidity
Chen Pi (Pericarpium Citri Reticulatae), 272; *Gua Lou* (Fructus Trichosanthis), 415; *Gui Zhi* (Ramulus Cinnamomi Cassiae), 22; *Zhi Shi* (Fructus Immaturus Citri Aurantii), 274

c. Yang deficiency
Fu Zi (Radix Lateralis Aconiti Carmichaeli Praeparata), 250; *Xi Xin* (Herba cum Radice Asari), 24

10. Common cold
a. Initial stage of damp-warm diseases
Bai Dou Kou (Fructus Amomi Kravanh), 205; *Hua Shi* (Talcum), 227; *Huang Lian* (Rhizoma Coptidis), 82; *Huang Qin* (Radix Scutellariae Baicalensis), 81; *Huo Xiang* (Herba Agastaches seu Pogostemi), 199; *Jin Yin Hua* (Flos Lonicerae), 95; *Pei Lan* (Herba Eupatorii Fortunei), 203; *Tong Cao* (Medulla Tetrapanacis Papyriferi), 232; *Yin Chen Hao* (Herba Artemisiae Scopariae), 239

b. Summerheat-damp exterior patterns
Bai Bian Dou (Semen Dolichoris Lablab), 528; *Huo Xiang* (Herba Agastaches seu Pogostemi), 199; *Jin Yin Hua* (Flos Lonicerae), 95; *Pei Lan* (Herba Eupatorii Fortunei), 203; *Qing Hao* (Herba Artemisiae Chinghao), 138; *Xiang Ru* (Herba Elsholtziae seu Moslae), 40

c. Summerheat-heat exterior patterns
He Ye (Folium Nelumbinis Nuciferae), 628; *Hua Shi* (Talcum), 227; *Lü Dou* (Semen Phaseoli Radiati), 125; *Qing Hao* (Herba Artemisiae Chinghao), 138; *Xiang Ru* (Herba Elsholtziae seu Moslae), 40

d. Wind-cold-type common cold

Bai Zhi (Radix Angelicae Dahuricae), 33; *Cang Er Zi* (Fructus Xanthii Sibirici), 36; *Chai Hu* (Radix Bupleuri), 51; *Cong Bai* (Bulbus Allii Fistulosi), 42; *Dan Dou Chi* (Semen Sojae Praeparatum), 54; *Fang Feng* (Radix Ledebouriellae Divaricatae), 30; *Gao Ben* (Rhizoma et Radix Ligustici), 35; *Ge Gen* (Radix Puerariae), 53; *Gui Zhi* (Ramulus Cinnamomi Cassiae), 22; *Jing Jie* (Herba Schizonepetae Tenuifoliae), 28; *Ma Huang* (Herba Ephedrae), 20; *Qiang Huo* (Rhizoma et Radix Notopterygii), 32; *Sheng Jiang* (Rhizoma Zingiberis Officinalis Recens), 39; *Xi Xin* (Herba cum Radice Asari), 24; *Xiang Ru* (Herba Elsholtziae seu Moslae), 40; *Xin Yi Hua* (Flos Magnoliae), 38; *Zi Su Ye* (Folium Perillae Frutescentis), 27

e. Wind-heat-type common cold

Bo He (Herba Menthae Haplocalycis), 45; *Chai Hu* (Radix Bupleuri), 51; *Chan Tui* (Periostracum Cicadae), 55; *Dan Dou Chi* (Semen Sojae Praeparatum), 54; *Fang Feng* (Radix Ledebouriellae Divaricatae), 30; *Fu Ping* (Herba Spirodelae Polyrrhizae), 59; *Ge Gen* (Radix Puerariae), 53; *Jin Yin Hua* (Flos Lonicerae), 95; *Jing Jie* (Herba Schizonepetae Tenuifoliae), 28; *Ju Hua* (Flos Chrysanthemi Morifolii), 49; *Lian Qiao* (Fructus Forsythiae Suspensae), 97; *Man Jing Zi* (Fructus Viticis), 56; *Niu Bang Zi* (Fructus Arctii Lappae), 46; *Sang Ye* (Folium Mori Albae), 48

11. Constipation

a. Constipation due to binding of heat

Da Huang (Radix et Rhizoma Rhei), 155; *Fan Xie Ye* (Folium Sennae), 159; *Lu Hui* (Herba Aloes), 159; *Mang Xiao* (Mirabilitum), 157; *Qian Niu Zi* (Semen Pharbitidis), 164; *Zhi Shi* (Fructus Immaturus Citri Aurantii), 274

b. Constipation due to cold accumulation

Ba Dou (Semen Crotonis Tiglii), 166; *Liu Huang* (Sulphur), 651

c. Intestinal dryness with constipation

Bai Zi Ren (Semen Biotae Orientalis), 462; *Dang Gui* (Radix Angelicae Sinensis), 563; *E Jiao* (Gelatinum Corii Asini), 573; *Gua Lou Ren* (Semen Trichosanthis), 416; *He Shou Wu* (Radix Polygoni Multiflori), 569; *Hei Zhi Ma* (Semen Sesami Indici), 597; *Hu Tao Ren* (Semen Juglandis Regiae), 557; *Huo Ma Ren* (Semen Cannabis Sativae), 151; *Jue Ming Zi* (Semen Cassiae), 77; *Mai Men Dong* (Radix Ophiopogonis Japonici), 580; *Niu Bang Zi* (Fructus Arctii Lappae), 46; *Rou Cong Rong* (Herba Cistanches Deserticolae), 550; *Sang Shen* (Fructus Mori Albae), 571; *Su Zi* (Fructus Perillae Frutescentis), 432; *Suo Yang* (Herba Cynomorii Songarici), 551; *Tao Ren* (Semen Persicae), 372; *Tian Men Dong* (Radix Asparagi Cochinchinensis), 588; *Xing Ren* (Semen Pruni Armeniacae), 431; *Yu Li Ren* (Semen Pruni), 152; *Zhi Mu* (Rhizoma Anemarrhenae Asphodeloidis), 70

12. Cough

a. Cough due to cold-Phlegm

Ai Di Cha (Herba Ardisiae Japonicae), 442; *Bai Jie Zi* (Semen Sinapis Albae), 407; *Gan Cao* (Radix Glycyrrhizae), 523; *Ju Hong* (Pars Rubra Epicarpii Citri Erythrocarpae), 274; *Sheng Jiang* (Rhizoma Zingiberis Officinalis Recens), 39; *Su Zi* (Fructus Perillae Frutescentis), 432; *Tian Nan Xing* (Rhizoma Arisaematis), 401; *Xuan Fu Hua* (Flos Inulae), 410

b. Cough due to dry Phlegm

Bai He (Bulbus Lilii), 590; *Bei Sha Shen* (Radix Glehniae Littoralis), 579; *E Jiao* (Gelatinum Corii Asini), 573; *Kuan Dong Hua* (Flos Tussilaginis Farfarae), 438; *Mai Men Dong* (Radix Ophiopogonis Japonici), 580; *Sang Ye* (Folium Mori Albae), 48; *Tian Hua Fen* (Radix Trichosanthis), 71; *Xing Ren* (Semen Pruni Armeniacae), 431; *Yu Zhu* (Rhizoma Polygonati Odorati), 592; *Zhi Mu* (Rhizoma Anemarrhenae Asphodeloidis), 70

c. Cough due to Lung-cold

Gan Jiang (Rhizoma Zingiberis Officinalis), 253; *Wu Wei Zi* (Fructus Schisandrae), 612; *Zi Wan* (Radix Asteris Tatarici), 437

d. Cough due to Lung-heat

Ai Di Cha (Herba Ardisiae Japonicae), 442; *Bai Guo* (Semen Ginkgo Bilobae), 443; *Bai Hua She She Cao* (Herba Hedyotidis Diffusae), 119; *Bai Jiang Cao* (Herba Patriniae cum Radice), 122; *Bai Mao Gen* (Rhizoma Imperatae Cylindricae), 331; *Bai Wei* (Radix Cynanchi Atrati), 142; *Ce Bai Ye* (Cacumen Biotae Orientalis), 328; *Che Qian Zi* (Semen Plantaginis), 226; *Chuan Xin Lian* (Herba Andrographitis Paniculatae), 109; *Di Gu Pi* (Cortex Lycii Radicis), 139; *Dong Gua Ren* (Semen Benincasae Hispidae), 224; *Gan Cao* (Radix Glycyrrhizae), 523; *Gua Lou* (Fructus

Trichosanthis), 415; *Hu Zhang* (Radix et Rhizoma Polygoni Cuspidati), 241; *Huang Qin* (Radix Scutellariae Baicalensis), 81; *Lu Gen* (Rhizoma Phragmitis Communis), 75; *Ma Bo* (Sclerotium Lasiosphaerae seu Calvatiae), 116; *Ma Dou Ling* (Fructus Aristolochiae), 439; *Ma Huang* (Herba Ephedrae), 20; *Mu Hu Die* (Semen Oroxyli Indici), 120; *Nan Sha Shen* (Radix Adenophorae), 580; *Niu Bang Zi* (Fructus Arctii Lappae), 46; *Pi Pa* Ye (Folium Eriobotryae Japonicae), 441; *Pu Gong Ying* (Herba Taraxaci cum Radice), 98; *Qian Hu* (Radix Peucedani), 417; *Qing Dai* (Indigo Naturalis), 103; *Shan Dou Gen* (Radix Sophorae Tonkinensis), 115; *She Gan* (Rhizoma Belamcandae Chinensis), 106; *Shi Gao* (Gypsum Fibrosum), 69; *Shi Wei* (Folium Pyrrosiae), 235; *Tian Hua Fen* (Radix Trichosanthis), 71; *Tian Men Dong* (Radix Asparagi Cochinchinensis), 588; *Tian Nan Xing* (Rhizoma Arisaematis), 401; *Wu Bei Zi* (Galla Rhois Chinensis), 615; *Yu Xing Cao* (Herba Houttuyniae Cordatae), 104; *Zhi Mu* (Rhizoma Anemarrhenae Asphodeloidis), 70; *Zi Wan* (Radix Asteris Tatarici), 437

e. Cough due to Phlegm-damp

Bai Qian (Radix et Rhizoma Cynanchi Stauntonii), 411; *Ban Xia* (Rhizoma Pinelliae Ternatae), 399; *Bing Lang* (Semen Arecae Catechu), 311; *Chen Pi* (Pericarpium Citri Reticulatae), 272; *Fo Shou* (Fructus Citri Sarcodactylis), 282; *Hou Po* (Cortex Magnoliae Officinalis), 200; *Ju Hong* (Pars Rubra Epicarpii Citri Erythrocarpae), 274; *Qian Hu* (Radix Peucedani), 417; *Tian Nan Xing* (Rhizoma Arisaematis), 401; *Xiang Yuan* (Fructus Citri Medicae seu Wilsonii), 283

f. Cough due to Phlegm-heat

Dan Nan Xing (Pulvis Arisaematis cum Felle Bovis), 403; *Fu Hai Shi* (Os Costaziae seu Pumex), 422; *Gan Cao* (Radix Glycyrrhizae), 523; *Gua Lou* (Fructus Trichosanthis), 415; *Hai Ge Ke* (Concha Meretricis seu Cyclinae), 423; *Pang Da Hai* (Semen Sterculiae Lychnophorae), 426; *Tian Men Dong* (Radix Asparagi Cochinchinensis), 588; *Xuan Fu Hua* (Flos Inulae), 410; *Zhe Bei Mu* (Bulbus Fritillariae Thunbergii), 414; *Zhu Li* (Succus Bambusae), 421; *Zhu Ru* (Caulis Bambusae in Taeniis), 418

g. Cough due to wind-cold

Bai Bu (Radix Stemonae), 433; *Bai Qian* (Radix et Rhizoma Cynanchi Stauntonii), 411; *Gan Cao* (Radix Glycyrrhizae), 523; *Jie Geng* (Radix Platycodi Grandiflori), 406; *Ma Huang* (Herba Ephedrae), 20; *Zi Wan* (Radix Asteris Tatarici), 437

h. Cough due to wind-heat

Gan Cao (Radix Glycyrrhizae), 523; *Jie Geng* (Radix Platycodi Grandiflori), 406; *Niu Bang Zi* (Fructus Arctii Lappae), 46; *Pi Pa* Ye (Folium Eriobotryae Japonicae), 441; *Qian Hu* (Radix Peucedani), 417; *Xing Ren* (Semen Pruni Armeniacae), 431; *Zhe Bei Mu* (Bulbus Fritillariae Thunbergii), 414

i. Taxation cough with coughing of blood

Ai Di Cha (Herba Ardisiae Japonicae), 442; *Bai Bu* (Radix Stemonae), 433; *Bai He* (Bulbus Lilii), 590; *Bai Ji* (Rhizoma Bletillae Striatae), 340; *Bai Qian* (Radix et Rhizoma Cynanchi Stauntonii), 411; *Bei Sha Shen* (Radix Glehniae Littoralis), 579; *Bie Jia* (Carapax Amydae Sinensis), 583; *Dong Chong Xia Cao* (Cordyceps Sinensis), 554; *E Jiao* (Gelatinum Corii Asini), 573; *Ge Jie* (Gekko), 556; *Gou Qi Zi* (Fructus Lycii), 586; *Gua Lou* (Fructus Trichosanthis), 415; *Gui Ban* (Plastrum Testudinis), 584; *Hua Rui Shi* (Ophicalcitum), 337; *Huang Jing* (Rhizoma Polygonati), 593; *Kuan Dong Hua* (Flos Tussilaginis Farfarae), 438; *Mai Men Dong* (Radix Ophiopogonis Japonici), 580; *Tian Men Dong* (Radix Asparagi Cochinchinensis), 588; *Xi Yang Shen* (Radix Panacis Quinquefolii), 529; *Xian He Cao* (Herba Agrimoniae Pilosae), 341; *Zi Wan* (Radix Asteris Tatarici), 437

13. Damage to the sinews, knocks and falls

Chuan Xiong (Rhizoma Ligustici Chuanxiong), 359; *Da Huang* (Radix et Rhizoma Rhei), 155; *Dang Gui Wei* (Extremitas Radicis Angelicae Sinensis), 563; *Du Zhong* (Cortex Eucommiae Ulmoidis), 542; *Gu Sui Bu* (Rhizoma Drynariae), 382; *Hong Hua* (Flos Carthami Tinctorii), 370; *Hu Zhang* (Radix et Rhizoma Polygoni Cuspidati), 241; *Liu Ji Nu* (Herba Artemisiae Anomalae), 383; *Mo Yao* (Myrrha), 366; *Niu Xi* (Radix Achyranthis Bidentatae), 375; *Ru Xiang* (Gummi Olibanum), 365; *San Qi* (Radix Notoginseng), 333; *She Xiang* (Secretio Moschi), 501; *Shen Jin Cao* (Herba Lycopodii Japonici), 178; *Su Mu* (Lignum Sappan), 382; *Tao Ren* (Semen Persicae), 372; *Tu Bie Chong* (Eupolyphaga seu Steleophaga), 388; *Wei Ling Xian* (Radix Clematidis), 177; *Wu Ling Zhi* (Excrementum Trogopteri), 367; *Xu Duan* (Radix Dipsaci), 544; *Xue Jie* (Resina Draconis), 659; *Yan Hu Suo* (Rhizoma Corydalis Yanhusuo), 361

14. Deficiency (or deficiency taxation) patterns

a. Depletion and deficiency of the Essence and Blood

Dong Chong Xia Cao (Cordyceps Sinensis), 554; *Ge Jie* (Gekko), 556; *He Shou Wu* (Radix Polygoni Multiflori), 569; *Hei Zhi Ma* (Semen Sesami Indici), 597; *Huang Jing* (Rhizoma Polygonati), 593; *Lu Jiao Jiao* (Gelatinum Cornu Cervi), 539; *Lu Rong* (Cornu Cervi Parvum), 538; *Rou Cong Rong* (Herba Cistanches Deserticolae), 550; *Shan Zhu Yu* (Fructus Corni Officinalis), 631; *Shu Di Huang* (Radix Rehmanniae Glutinosae Conquita), 565; *Zi He Che* (Placenta Hominis), 559

b. Heart and/or Liver Blood deficiency patterns

Bai Shao (Radix Paeoniae Lactiflorae), 567; *Da Zao* (Fructus Ziziphi Jujubae), 532; *Dang Gui* (Radix Angelicae Sinensis), 563; *Dang Shen* (Radix Codonopsitis Pilosulae), 517; *E Jiao* (Gelatinum Corii Asini), 573; *He Shou Wu* (Radix Polygoni Multiflori), 569; *Hei Zhi Ma* (Semen Sesami Indici), 597; *Huang Qi* (Radix Astragali seu Hedysari), 518; *Ren Shen* (Radix Ginseng), 514; *Sang Shen* (Fructus Mori Albae), 571; *Shu Di Huang* (Radix Rehmanniae Glutinosae Conquita), 565; *Zi He Che* (Placenta Hominis), 559

c. Kidney Yang deficiency patterns

Ba Ji Tian (Radix Morindae Officinalis), 545; *Bu Gu Zhi* (Fructus Psoraleae Corylifoliae), 548; *Dong Chong Xia Cao* (Cordyceps Sinensis), 554; *Du Zhong* (Cortex Eucommiae Ulmoidis), 542; *Fu Pen Zi* (Fructus Rubi Chingii), 635; *Fu Zi* (Radix Lateralis Aconiti Carmichaeli Praeparata), 250; *Ge Jie* (Gekko), 556; *Hu Lu Ba* (Semen Trigonellae Foeni-graeci), 558; *Hu Tao Ren* (Semen Juglandis Regiae), 557; *Jiu Cai Zi* (Semen Allii Tuberosi), 554; *Lu Jiao Jiao* (Gelatinum Cornu Cervi), 539; *Lu Jiao Shuang* (Cornu Cervi Degelatinatum), 540; *Lu Rong* (Cornu Cervi Parvum), 538; *Rou Cong Rong* (Herba Cistanches Deserticolae), 550; *Rou Gui* (Cortex Cinnamomi Cassiae), 254; *Sha Yuan Zi* (Semen Astragali Complanati), 552; *Shan Zhu Yu* (Fructus Corni Officinalis), 631; *Suo Yang* (Herba Cynomorii Songarici), 551; *Tu Si Zi* (Semen Cuscutae), 541; *Xian Mao* (Rhizoma Curculiginis Orchioidis), 547; *Yi Zhi Ren* (Fructus Alpiniae Oxyphyllae), 549; *Yin Yang Huo* (Herba Epimedii), 540; *Zi He Che* (Placenta Hominis), 559

d. Liver and/or Kidney Yin deficiency patterns

Bie Jia (Carapax Amydae Sinensis), 583; *Du Zhong* (Cortex Eucommiae Ulmoidis), 542; *E Jiao* (Gelatinum Corii Asini), 573; *Gou Ji* (Rhizoma Cibotii Barometz), 192; *Gou Qi Zi* (Fructus Lycii), 586; *Gui Ban* (Plastrum Testudinis), 584; *Han Lian Cao* (Herba Ecliptae Prostratae), 595; *He Shou Wu* (Radix Polygoni Multiflori), 569; *Nü Zhen Zi* (Fructus Ligustri Lucidi), 596; *Sang Ji Sheng* (Ramulus Loranthi), 190; *Sang Shen* (Fructus Mori Albae), 571; *Sang Ye* (Folium Mori Albae), 48; *Sha Yuan Zi* (Semen Astragali Complanati), 552; *Shan Yao* (Rhizoma Dioscoreae Oppositae), 526; *Shan Zhu Yu* (Fructus Corni Officinalis), 631; *Shi Hu* (Herba Dendrobii), 591; *Shu Di Huang* (Radix Rehmanniae Glutinosae Conquita), 565; *Tu Si Zi* (Semen Cuscutae), 541; *Wu Jia Pi* (Cortex Acanthopanacis Gracilistyli Radicis), 191; *Wu Wei Zi* (Fructus Schisandrae), 612; *Xu Duan* (Radix Dipsaci), 544

e. Lung and/or Stomach Yin deficiency patterns

Bei Sha Shen (Radix Glehniae Littoralis), 579; *Gan Cao* (Radix Glycyrrhizae), 523; *Gou Qi Zi* (Fructus Lycii), 586; *Huang Jing* (Rhizoma Polygonati), 593; *Mai Men Dong* (Radix Ophiopogonis Japonici), 580; *Nan Sha Shen* (Radix Adenophorae), 580; *Shi Hu* (Herba Dendrobii), 591; *Tai Zi Shen* (Radix Pseudostellariae Heterophyllae), 531; *Tian Men Dong* (Radix Asparagi Cochinchinensis), 588; *Wu Wei Zi* (Fructus Schisandrae), 612; *Xi Yang Shen* (Radix Panacis Quinquefolii), 529; *Yu Zhu* (Rhizoma Polygonati Odorati), 592; *Zhi Mu* (Rhizoma Anemarrhenae Asphodeloidis), 70

f. Lung Qi deficiency patterns

Dang Shen (Radix Codonopsitis Pilosulae), 517; *Huang Qi* (Radix Astragali seu Hedysari), 518; *Ren Shen* (Radix Ginseng), 514; *Shan Yao* (Rhizoma Dioscoreae Oppositae), 526; *Tai Zi Shen* (Radix Pseudostellariae Heterophyllae), 531; *Xi Yang Shen* (Radix Panacis Quinquefolii), 529

g. Middle Qi fall

Chai Hu (Radix Bupleuri), 51; *Dang Shen* (Radix Codonopsitis Pilosulae), 517; *Huang Qi* (Radix Astragali seu Hedysari), 518; *Ren Shen* (Radix Ginseng), 514; *Sheng Ma* (Rhizoma Cimicifugae), 57; *Shi Liu Pi* (Pericarpium Punicae Granati), 624

h. Spleen Qi deficiency patterns

Bai Bian Dou (Semen Dolichoris Lablab), 528; *Bai Zhu* (Rhizoma Atractylodis Macrocephalae), 521; *Da Zao* (Fructus Ziziphi Jujubae), 532; *Dang Shen* (Radix Codonopsitis Pilosulae), 517; *Gan Cao*

(Radix Glycyrrhizae), 523; *Huang Jing* (Rhizoma Polygonati), 593; *Huang Qi* (Radix Astragali seu Hedysari), 518; *Lian Zi* (Semen Nelumbinis Nuciferae), 626; *Long Yan Rou* (Arillus Euphoriae Longanae), 574; *Ren Shen* (Radix Ginseng), 514; *Shan Yao* (Rhizoma Dioscoreae Oppositae), 526; *Tai Zi Shen* (Radix Pseudostellariae Heterophyllae), 531; *Yi Tang* (Saccharum Granorum), 533; *Yi Yi Ren* (Semen Coicis Lachrymajobi), 219

15. Desertion patterns

Fu Zi (Radix Lateralis Aconiti Carmichaeli Praeparata), 250; *Gan Jiang* (Rhizoma Zingiberis Officinalis), 253; *Ren Shen* (Radix Ginseng), 514; *Rou Gui* (Cortex Cinnamomi Cassiae), 254; *Shan Zhu Yu* (Fructus Corni Officinalis), 631

16. Diarrhoea and dysentery

a. Bloody dysentery due to heat toxins

Bai Tou Weng (Radix Pulsatillae Chinensis), 107; *Di Yu* (Radix Sanguisorbae Officinalis), 327; *Jin Yin Hua* (Flos Lonicerae), 95; *Ma Chi Xian* (Herba Portulacae Oleraceae), 117; *Qin Pi* (Cortex Fraxini), 89; *Ya Dan Zi* (Fructus Bruceae Javanicae), 118

b. Damp-heat dysentery

Bai Shao (Radix Paeoniae Lactiflorae), 567; *Chuan Xin Lian* (Herba Andrographitis Paniculatae), 109; *Chun Pi* (Cortex Ailanthi Altissimae), 625; *Da Huang* (Radix et Rhizoma Rhei), 155; *Ge Gen* (Radix Puerariae), 53; *Hu Huang Lian* (Rhizoma Picrorhizae Scrophulariiflorae), 141; *Huang Bai* (Cortex Phellodendri), 84; *Huang Lian* (Rhizoma Coptidis), 82; *Huang Qin* (Radix Scutellariae Baicalensis), 81; *Ku Shen* (Radix Sophorae Flavescentis), 86; *Ma Chi Xian* (Herba Portulacae Oleraceae), 117; *Mu Gua* (Fructus Chaenomelis), 175; *San Qi* (Radix Notoginseng), 333; *Xie Bai* (Bulbus Allii Macrostemi), 287; *Yu Xing Cao* (Herba Houttuyniae Cordatae), 104

c. Diarrhoea due to cold-damp

Cao Dou Kou (Semen Alpiniae Katsumadai), 206; *Cao Guo* (Fructus Amomi Tsaoko), 208; *Hou Po* (Cortex Magnoliae Officinalis), 200; *Zhu Ling* (Sclerotium Polypori Umbellati), 222

d. Diarrhoea due to Spleen deficiency

Bai Bian Dou (Semen Dolichoris Lablab), 528; *Bai Zhi* (Radix Angelicae Dahuricae), 33; *Bai Zhu* (Rhizoma Atractylodis Macrocephalae), 521; *Cang Zhu* (Rhizoma Atractylodis), 201; *Chai Hu* (Radix Bupleuri), 51; *Che Qian Zi* (Semen Plantaginis), 226; *Dang Shen* (Radix Codonopsitis Pilosulae), 517; *Dao Ya* (Fructus Oryzae Sativae Germinatus), 300; *Fang Feng* (Radix Ledebouriellae Divaricatae), 30; *Fu Ling* (Sclerotium Poriae Cocos), 217; *Ge Gen* (Radix Puerariae), 53; *Lian Zi* (Semen Nelumbinis Nuciferae), 626; *Long Gu* (Os Draconis), 455; *Qian Shi* (Semen Euryales Ferocis), 628; *Shan Yao* (Rhizoma Dioscoreae Oppositae), 526; *Tu Si Zi* (Semen Cuscutae), 541; *Yi Yi Ren* (Semen Coicis Lachrymajobi), 219; *Zhu Ling* (Sclerotium Polypori Umbellati), 222

e. Early-morning diarrhoea

Bu Gu Zhi (Fructus Psoraleae Corylifoliae), 548; *Rou Dou Kou* (Semen Myristicae Fragrantis), 623; *Wu Wei Zi* (Fructus Schisandrae), 612; *Wu Zhu Yu* (Fructus Evodiae Rutaecarpae), 257

f. Enduring diarrhoea and dysentery

Cang Zhu (Rhizoma Atractylodis), 201; *Chi Shi Zhi* (Halloysitum Rubrum), 622; *Chun Pi* (Cortex Ailanthi Altissimae), 625; *Dang Shen* (Radix Codonopsitis Pilosulae), 517; *He Zi* (Fructus Terminaliae Chebulae), 617; *Huang Qi* (Radix Astragali seu Hedysari), 518; *Jin Ying Zi* (Fructus Rosae Laevigatae), 636; *Qian Shi* (Semen Euryales Ferocis), 628; *Rou Dou Kou* (Semen Myristicae Fragrantis), 623; *Sheng Ma* (Rhizoma Cimicifugae), 57; *Shi Liu Pi* (Pericarpium Punicae Granati), 624; *Wu Bei Zi* (Galla Rhois Chinensis), 615; *Wu Mei* (Fructus Pruni Mume), 614; *Wu Wei Zi* (Fructus Schisandrae), 612. *Xian He Cao* (Herba Agrimoniae Pilosae), 341; *Yu Yu Liang* (Limonitum), 621; *Zao Xin Tu* (Terra Flava Usta), 348

g. Summerheat-damp diarrhoea

Bai Bian Dou (Semen Dolichoris Lablab), 528; *Che Qian Zi* (Semen Plantaginis), 226; *Huo Xiang* (Herba Agastaches seu Pogostemi), 199; *Xiang Ru* (Herba Elsholtziae seu Moslae), 40

17. Dizziness

a. Dizziness due to Blood deficiency

Bai Shao (Radix Paeoniae Lactiflorae), 567; *Bai Zhu* (Rhizoma Atractylodis Macrocephalae), 521; *Da Zao* (Fructus Ziziphi Jujubae), 532; *Dang Gui* (Radix Angelicae Sinensis), 563; *Dang Shen* (Radix Codonopsitis Pilosulae), 517; *E Jiao* (Gelatinum Corii Asini), 573; *He Shou Wu* (Radix Polygoni Multiflori), 569; *Shu Di Huang* (Radix Rehmanniae Glutinosae Conquita), 565

b. Dizziness due to Liver and Kidney deficiency
Gou Qi Zi (Fructus Lycii), 586; *He Shou Wu* (Radix Polygoni Multiflori), 569; *Hei Zhi Ma* (Semen Sesami Indici), 597; *Sang Shen* (Fructus Mori Albae), 571; *Sha Yuan Zi* (Semen Astragali Complanati), 552; *Shan Zhu Yu* (Fructus Corni Officinalis), 631; *Sheng Di Huang* (Radix Rehmanniae Glutinosae), 129

c. Dizziness due to Phlegm-fluids
Gui Zhi (Ramulus Cinnamomi Cassiae), 22; *Xuan Fu Hua* (Flos Inulae), 410; *Ze Xie* (Rhizoma Alismatis Orientalis), 221

d. Dizziness due to wind-Phlegm
Bai Fu Zi (Rhizoma Typhonii Gigantei), 404; *Ban Xia* (Rhizoma Pinelliae Ternatae), 399; *Tian Ma* (Rhizoma Gastrodiae Elatae), 486; *Tian Nan Xing* (Rhizoma Arisaematis), 401

e. Dizziness due to Yin deficiency of the Liver and/or Kidneys
Du Zhong (Cortex Eucommiae Ulmoidis), 542; *Gou Qi Zi* (Fructus Lycii), 586; *Han Lian Cao* (Herba Ecliptae Prostratae), 595; *Nü Zhen Zi* (Fructus Ligustri Lucidi), 596; *Shan Yao* (Rhizoma Dioscoreae Oppositae), 526; *Shan Zhu Yu* (Fructus Corni Officinalis), 631; *Shu Di Huang* (Radix Rehmanniae Glutinosae Conquita), 565; *Yin Yang Huo* (Herba Epimedii), 540

f. Liver Yang dizziness
Bai Ji Li (Fructus Tribuli Terrestris), 479; *Bai Shao* (Radix Paeoniae Lactiflorae), 567; *Chuan Xiong* (Rhizoma Ligustici Chuanxiong), 359; *Ci Shi* (Magnetitum), 454; *Dai Zhe Shi* (Haematitum), 475; *Du Zhong* (Cortex Eucommiae Ulmoidis), 542; *Gou Teng* (Ramulus Uncariae cum Uncis), 484; *Gui Ban* (Plastrum Testudinis), 584; *Ju Hua* (Flos Chrysanthemi Morifolii), 49; *Jue Ming Zi* (Semen Cassiae), 77; *Ling Yang Jiao* (Cornu Antelopis), 481; *Long Gu* (Os Draconis), 455; *Mu Li* (Concha Ostreae), 473; *Niu Xi* (Radix Achyranthis Bidentatae), 375; *Sang Ye* (Folium Mori Albae), 48; *Shi Jue Ming* (Concha Haliotidis), 472; *Tian Ma* (Rhizoma Gastrodiae Elatae), 486; *Xia Ku Cao* (Spica Prunellae Vulgaris), 74; *Yu Mi Xu* (Stylus Zeae Mays), 238; *Zhen Zhu Mu* (Concha Margaritifera), 478

18. Eczema
Ai Ye (Folium Artemisiae Argyi), 347; *Bai Xian Pi* (Cortex Dictamni Dasycarpi Radicis), 90; *Bai Zhi* (Radix Angelicae Dahuricae), 33; *Bian Xu* (Herba Polygoni Avicularis), 233; *Cang Er Zi* (Fructus Xanthii Sibirici), 36; *Chuan Xin Lian* (Herba Andrographitis Paniculatae), 109; *Di Fu Zi* (Fructus Kochiae Scopariae), 234; *Di Yu* (Radix Sanguisorbae Officinalis), 327; *Fang Ji* (Radix Stephaniae Tetrandrae), 183; *Hai Ge Ke* (Concha Meretricis seu Cyclinae), 423; *Hai Piao Xiao* (Os Sepiae seu Sepiellae), 633; *Hai Tong Pi* (Cortex Erythrinae), 186; *Hua Shi* (Talcum), 227; *Huang Bai* (Cortex Phellodendri), 84; *Jing Jie* (Herba Schizonepetae Tenuifoliae), 28; *Ku Lian Pi* (Cortex Meliae Radicis), 310; *Ku Shen* (Radix Sophorae Flavescentis), 86; *Liu Huang* (Sulphur), 651; *Long Dan Cao* (Radix Gentianae Scabrae), 88; *Lu Gan Shi* (Calamina), 661; *Ming Fan* (Alumen), 653; *She Chuang Zi* (Fructus Cnidii Monnieri), 654; *Shi Gao* (Gypsum Fibrosum), 69; *Tu Fu Ling* (Rhizoma Smilacis Glabrae), 112; *Wu Zhu Yu* (Fructus Evodiae Rutaecarpae), 257; *Xi Xian Cao* (Herba Siegesbeckiae), 185; *Xu Chang Qing* (Radix Cynanchi Paniculati), 188; *Yin Chen Hao* (Herba Artemisiae Scopariae), 239; *Zi Cao* (Radix Arnebiae seu Lithospermi), 135

19. Focal distension
Ba Dou (Semen Crotonis Tiglii), 166; *Bai Qian* (Radix et Rhizoma Cynanchi Stauntonii), 411; *Bai Zhu* (Rhizoma Atractylodis Macrocephalae), 521; *Ban Xia* (Rhizoma Pinelliae Ternatae), 399; *Dan Shen* (Radix Salviae Miltiorrhizae), 369; *Fo Shou* (Fructus Citri Sarcodactylis), 282; *Gua Lou* (Fructus Trichosanthis), 415; *Huo Xiang* (Herba Agastaches seu Pogostemi), 199; *Jie Geng* (Radix Platycodi Grandiflori), 406; *Mu Xiang* (Radix Aucklandiae Lappae), 276; *Qing Hao* (Herba Artemisiae Chinghao), 138; *Tian Ma* (Rhizoma Gastrodiae Elatae), 486; *Tian Nan Xing* (Rhizoma Arisaematis), 401; *Xiang Fu* (Rhizoma Cyperi Rotundi), 277; *Xuan Fu Hua* (Flos Inulae), 410; *Yu Jin* (Radix Curcumae), 362; *Zhi Ke* (Fructus Citri Aurantii), 275; *Zhi Shi* (Fructus Immaturus Citri Aurantii), 274

20. Food accumulation
Bing Lang (Semen Arecae Catechu), 311; *Da Huang* (Radix et Rhizoma Rhei), 155; *Dao Ya* (Fructus Oryzae Sativae Germinatus), 300; *E Zhu* (Rhizoma Curcumae), 385; *Gu Ya* (Fructus Setariae Italicae Germinatus), 301; *Hou Po* (Cortex Magnoliae Officinalis), 200; *Ji Nei Jin* (Endothelium Corneum Gigeriae Galli), 302; *Ju Hong* (Pars Rubra Epicarpii Citri Erythrocarpae),

274; *Lai Fu Zi* (Semen Raphani Sativi), 301; *Mai Ya* (Fructus Hordei Vulgaris Germinatus), 299; *Qian Niu Zi* (Semen Pharbitidis), 164; *Qing Pi* (Pericarpium Citri Reticulatae Viride), 280; *San Leng* (Rhizoma Sparganii Stoloniferi), 386; *Sha Ren* (Fructus Amomi), 204; *Shan Yao* (Rhizoma Dioscoreae Oppositae), 526; *Shan Zha* (Fructus Crataegi), 297; *Shen Qu* (Massa Fermentata), 298; *Zhi Shi* (Fructus Immaturus Citri Aurantii), 274

21. Fractures
Gu Sui Bu (Rhizoma Drynariae), 382; *He Huan Pi* (Cortex Albizziae Julibrissin), 463; *Liu Ji Nu* (Herba Artemisiae Anomalae), 383; *Su Mu* (Lignum Sappan), 382; *Tu Bie Chong* (Eupolyphaga seu Steleophaga), 388; *Xu Duan* (Radix Dipsaci), 544

22. Fright wind and fright epilepsy
Bie Jia (Carapax Amydae Sinensis), 583; *Chong Lou* (Rhizoma Paridis), 110; *Dan Nan Xing* (Pulvis Arisaematis cum Felle Bovis), 403; *Di Long* (Lumbricus), 488; *Gou Teng* (Ramulus Uncariae cum Uncis), 484; *Gui Ban* (Plastrum Testudinis), 584; *Hu Po* (Succinum), 457; *Jiang Can* (Bombyx Batryticatus), 493; *Ling Yang Jiao* (Cornu Antelopis), 481; *Lu Hui* (Herba Aloes), 159; *Niu Huang* (Calculus Bovis), 482; *Qi She* (Agkistrodon), 176; *Qing Dai* (Indigo Naturalis), 103; *Quan Xie* (Buthus Martensi), 489; *Tian Ma* (Rhizoma Gastrodiae Elatae), 486; *Tian Zhu Huang* (Concretio Silicea Bambusae), 420; *Wu Gong* (Scolopendra Subspinipes), 491; *Yang Jin Hua* (Flos Daturae), 444; *Zhen Zhu* (Margarita), 477; *Zhen Zhu Mu* (Concha Margaritifera), 478; *Zhu Li* (Succus Bambusae), 421

23. Full-heat patterns in the Qi level
Dan Zhu Ye (Herba Lophatheri Gracilis), 76; *Huang Bai* (Cortex Phellodendri), 84; *Huang Lian* (Rhizoma Coptidis), 82; *Huang Qin* (Radix Scutellariae Baicalensis), 81; *Lu Gen* (Rhizoma Phragmitis Communis), 75; *Shi Gao* (Gypsum Fibrosum), 69; *Tian Hua Fen* (Radix Trichosanthis), 71; *Zhi Mu* (Rhizoma Anemarrhenae Asphodeloidis), 70; *Zhi Zi* (Fructus Gardeniae Jasminoidis), 72

24. Full-heat patterns in the Ying and Xue levels (including patterns of heat entering the Pericardium)
Chi Shao (Radix Paeoniae Rubra), 133; *Dan Shen* (Radix Salviae Miltiorrhizae), 369; *Huang Lian* (Rhizoma Coptidis), 82; *Jin Yin Hua* (Flos Lonicerae), 95; *Lian Qiao* (Fructus Forsythiae Suspensae), 97; *Lian Zi Xin* (Plumula Nelumbinis Nuciferae), 627; *Mu Dan Pi* (Cortex Moutan Radicis), 132; *Sheng Di Huang* (Radix Rehmanniae Glutinosae), 129; *Shui Niu Jiao* (Cornu Bubali), 136; *Xuan Shen* (Radix Scrophulariae Ningpoensis), 130; *Zi Cao* (Radix Arnebiae seu Lithospermi), 135

25. Gan accumulation
Hu Huang Lian (Rhizoma Picrorhizae Scrophulariiflorae), 141; *Ji Nei Jin* (Endothelium Corneum Gigeriae Galli), 302; *Lei Wan* (Sclerotium Omphaliae Lapidescens), 315; *Lu Hui* (Herba Aloes), 159; *Shi Jun Zi* (Fructus Quisqualis Indicae), 309; *Yin Chai Hu* (Radix Stellariae Dichotomae), 140

26. Haemorrhoids
Bai Lian (Radix Ampelopsis Japonicae), 124; *Bai Tou Weng* (Radix Pulsatillae Chinensis), 107; *Di Yu* (Radix Sanguisorbae Officinalis), 327; *Hu Huang Lian* (Rhizoma Picrorhizae Scrophulariiflorae), 141; *Huai Hua* (Flos Sophorae Japonicae), 329; *Huang Bai* (Cortex Phellodendri), 84; *Jing Jie Tan* (Herba Schizonepetae Tenuifoliae Carbonisata), 28; *Ku Shen* (Radix Sophorae Flavescentis), 86; *Lu Hui* (Herba Aloes), 159; *Ma Chi Xian* (Herba Portulacae Oleraceae), 117; *Ma Dou Ling* (Fructus Aristolochiae), 439; *Mu Zei* (Herba Equiseti Hiemalis), 60; *Wu Bei Zi* (Galla Rhois Chinensis), 615; *Xiong Huang* (Realgar), 650; *Yu Jin* (Radix Curcumae), 362; *Yu Xing Cao* (Herba Houttuyniae Cordatae), 104

27. Headache

a. Ascendant hyperactivity of Liver Yang
Bai Shao (Radix Paeoniae Lactiflorae), 567; *Chuan Xiong* (Rhizoma Ligustici Chuanxiong), 359; *Du Zhong* (Cortex Eucommiae Ulmoidis), 542; *Ju Hua* (Flos Chrysanthemi Morifolii), 49; *Niu Xi* (Radix Achyranthis Bidentatae), 375; *Sang Ye* (Folium Mori Albae), 48; *Shi Jue Ming* (Concha Haliotidis), 472; *Tian Ma* (Rhizoma Gastrodiae Elatae), 486; *Xia Ku Cao* (Spica Prunellae Vulgaris), 74

b. Blood stasis headache
Chuan Xiong (Rhizoma Ligustici Chuanxiong), 359; *She Xiang* (Secretio Moschi), 501

c. Channel conductors

i. for Taiyang headache
Gao Ben (Rhizoma et Radix Ligustici), 35; *Qiang Huo* (Rhizoma et Radix Notopterygii), 32

ii. for Yangming headache
Bai Zhi (Radix Angelicae Dahuricae), 33; *Sheng Ma* (Rhizoma Cimicifugae), 57

iii. for Shaoyang headache
Chai Hu (Radix Bupleuri), 51; *Huang Qin* (Radix Scutellariae Baicalensis), 81

iv. for Jueyin (reverting Yin) headache
Wu Zhu Yu (Fructus Evodiae Rutaecarpae), 257

v. for Shaoyin headache
Xi Xin (Herba cum Radice Asari), 24

d. Liver-fire headache

Gou Teng (Ramulus Uncariae cum Uncis), 484; *Huai Hua* (Flos Sophorae Japonicae), 329; *Huai Jiao* (Fructus Sophorae Japonicae), 330; *Huang Qin* (Radix Scutellariae Baicalensis), 81; *Jue Ming Zi* (Semen Cassiae), 77; *Ling Yang Jiao* (Cornu Antelopis), 481; *Long Dan Cao* (Radix Gentianae Scabrae), 88; *Lu Hui* (Herba Aloes), 159

e. Liver-wind headache

Di Long (Lumbricus), 488; *Ju Hua* (Flos Chrysanthemi Morifolii), 49; *Niu Xi* (Radix Achyranthis Bidentatae), 375; *Quan Xie* (Buthus Martensi), 489; *Shi Jue Ming* (Concha Haliotidis), 472; *Tian Ma* (Rhizoma Gastrodiae Elatae), 486

f. Wind-cold headache

Bai Zhi (Radix Angelicae Dahuricae), 33; *Cang Er Zi* (Fructus Xanthii Sibirici), 36; *Chuan Wu* (Radix Aconiti Carmichaeli), 252; *Chuan Xiong* (Rhizoma Ligustici Chuanxiong), 359; *Fang Feng* (Radix Ledebouriellae Divaricatae), 30; *Gao Ben* (Rhizoma et Radix Ligustici), 35; *Jing Jie* (Herba Schizonepetae Tenuifoliae), 28; *Qiang Huo* (Rhizoma et Radix Notopterygii), 32; *Xi Xin* (Herba cum Radice Asari), 24; *Xin Yi Hua* (Flos Magnoliae), 38; *Zi Su Ye* (Folium Perillae Frutescentis), 27

g. Wind-cold-damp headache

Cang Zhu (Rhizoma Atractylodis), 201; *Du Huo* (Radix Angelicae Pubescentis), 174

h. Wind-heat headache

Ban Lan Gen (Radix Isatidis seu Baphicacanthi), 101; *Bo He* (Herba Menthae Haplocalycis), 45; *Chuan Xiong* (Rhizoma Ligustici Chuanxiong), 359; *Ge Gen* (Radix Puerariae), 53; *Gou Teng* (Ramulus Uncariae cum Uncis), 484; *Jiang Can* (Bombyx Batryticatus), 493; *Jie Geng* (Radix Platycodi Grandiflori), 406; *Jin Yin Hua* (Flos Lonicerae), 95; *Ju Hua* (Flos Chrysanthemi Morifolii), 49; *Lian Qiao* (Fructus Forsythiae Suspensae), 97; *Man Jing Zi* (Fructus Viticis), 56; *Sheng Ma* (Rhizoma Cimicifugae), 57; *Yu Zhu* (Rhizoma Polygonati Odorati), 592

i. Wind-Phlegm headache

Bai Fu Zi (Rhizoma Typhonii Gigantei), 404; *Ban Xia* (Rhizoma Pinelliae Ternatae), 399; *Tian Ma* (Rhizoma Gastrodiae Elatae), 486; *Tian Nan Xing* (Rhizoma Arisaematis), 401

28. Hiccups

Chen Pi (Pericarpium Citri Reticulatae), 272; *Chen Xiang* (Lignum Aquilariae Resinatum), 279; *Dai Zhe Shi* (Haematitum), 475; *Ding Xiang* (Flos Caryophylli), 262; *Wu Wei Zi* (Fructus Schisandrae), 612; *Zhu Ru* (Caulis Bambusae in Taeniis), 418

29. Impotence

Ba Ji Tian (Radix Morindae Officinalis), 545; *Bu Gu Zhi* (Fructus Psoraleae Corylifoliae), 548; *Ding Xiang* (Flos Caryophylli), 262; *Dong Chong Xia Cao* (Cordyceps Sinensis), 554; *Du Zhong* (Cortex Eucommiae Ulmoidis), 542; *Fu Pen Zi* (Fructus Rubi Chingii), 635; *Fu Zi* (Radix Lateralis Aconiti Carmichaeli Praeparata), 250; *Ge Jie* (Gekko), 556; *Gou Qi Zi* (Fructus Lycii), 586; *Hu Lu Ba* (Semen Trigonellae Foeni-graeci), 558; *Jiu Cai Zi* (Semen Allii Tuberosi), 554; *Liu Huang* (Sulphur), 651; *Lu Rong* (Cornu Cervi Parvum), 538; *Ren Shen* (Radix Ginseng), 514; *Rou Cong Rong* (Herba Cistanches Deserticolae), 550; *Rou Gui* (Cortex Cinnamomi Cassiae), 254; *Sang Piao Xiao* (Oötheca Mantidis), 632; *Shan Zhu Yu* (Fructus Corni Officinalis), 631; *She Chuang Zi* (Fructus Cnidii Monnieri), 654; *Suo Yang* (Herba Cynomorii Songarici), 551; *Tu Si Zi* (Semen Cuscutae), 541; *Xian Mao* (Rhizoma Curculiginis Orchioidis), 547; *Yin Yang Huo* (Herba Epimedii), 540; *Zi He Che* (Placenta Hominis), 559

30. Infertility

Ba Ji Tian (Radix Morindae Officinalis), 545; *Fu Pen Zi* (Fructus Rubi Chingii), 635; *Fu Zi* (Radix Lateralis Aconiti Carmichaeli Praeparata), 250; *Gou Qi Zi* (Fructus Lycii), 586; *Ling Yang Jiao* (Cornu Antelopis), 481; *Lu Rong* (Cornu

Cervi Parvum), 538; *Rou Cong Rong* (Herba Cistanches Deserticolae), 550; *Rou Gui* (Cortex Cinnamomi Cassiae), 254; *She Chuang Zi* (Fructus Cnidii Monnieri), 654; *Zi He Che* (Placenta Hominis), 559

31. Intestinal abscess

Bai Hua She She Cao (Herba Hedyotidis Diffusae), 119; *Bai Jiang Cao* (Herba Patriniae cum Radice), 122; *Bai Zhi* (Radix Angelicae Dahuricae), 33; *Da Huang* (Radix et Rhizoma Rhei), 155; *Dong Gua Ren* (Semen Benincasae Hispidae), 224; *Gua Lou Ren* (Semen Trichosanthis), 416; *Hong Teng* (Caulis Sargentodoxae Cuneatae), 123; *Jin Yin Hua* (Flos Lonicerae), 95; *Mu Dan Pi* (Cortex Moutan Radicis), 132; *Pu Gong Ying* (Herba Taraxaci cum Radice), 98; *Tao Ren* (Semen Persicae), 372; *Yi Yi Ren* (Semen Coicis Lachrymajobi), 219; *Zi Hua Di Ding* (Herba Violae Yedoensitis), 100

32. Jaundice

a. Damp-heat jaundice (Yang-type jaundice)

Ai Di Cha (Herba Ardisiae Japonicae), 442; *Bai Hua She She Cao* (Herba Hedyotidis Diffusae), 119; *Bai Mao Gen* (Rhizoma Imperatae Cylindricae), 331; *Bai Xian Pi* (Cortex Dictamni Dasycarpi Radicis), 90; *Ban Bian Lian* (Herba Lobeliae Chinensis cum Radice), 111; *Che Qian Zi* (Semen Plantaginis), 226; *Chi Xiao Dou* (Semen Phaseoli Calcarati), 224; *Da Huang* (Radix et Rhizoma Rhei), 155; *Da Qing Ye* (Folium Isatidis seu Baphicacanthi), 102; *Gua Di* (Pedicellus Cucumeris), 643; *Hai Jin Sha Teng* (Herba Lygodii Japonici), 231; *Hu Zhang* (Radix et Rhizoma Polygoni Cuspidati), 241; *Huang Bai* (Cortex Phellodendri), 84; *Huang Lian* (Rhizoma Coptidis), 82; *Huang Qin* (Radix Scutellariae Baicalensis), 81; *Jin Qian Cao* (Herba Lysimachiae), 240; *Ku Shen* (Radix Sophorae Flavescentis), 86; *Long Dan Cao* (Radix Gentianae Scabrae), 88; *Mu Xiang* (Radix Aucklandiae Lappae), 276; *Pu Gong Ying* (Herba Taraxaci cum Radice), 98; *Qin Jiao* (Radix Gentianae Macrophyllae), 181; *Yin Chen Hao* (Herba Artemisiae Scopariae), 239; *Yu Jin* (Radix Curcumae), 362; *Zhi Zi* (Fructus Gardeniae Jasminoidis), 72

b. Jaundice due to cold-damp obstruction (Yin-type jaundice)

Fu Zi (Radix Lateralis Aconiti Carmichaeli Praeparata), 250; *Yin Chen Hao* (Herba Artemisiae Scopariae), 239

33. Leg Qi

a. Leg Qi due to cold-damp pouring down

Bing Lang (Semen Arecae Catechu), 311; *Chi Xiao Dou* (Semen Phaseoli Calcarati), 224; *Hu Lu Ba* (Semen Trigonellae Foeni-graeci), 558; *Mu Gua* (Fructus Chaenomelis), 175; *Wu Zhu Yu* (Fructus Evodiae Rutaecarpae), 257; *Yi Yi Ren* (Semen Coicis Lachrymajobi), 219

b. Leg Qi due to damp-heat pouring down

Fang Ji (Radix Stephaniae Tetrandrae), 183; *Huang Bai* (Cortex Phellodendri), 84; *Long Dan Cao* (Radix Gentianae Scabrae), 88; *Mu Gua* (Fructus Chaenomelis), 175; *Mu Tong* (Caulis Mutong), 229; *Niu Xi* (Radix Achyranthis Bidentatae), 375; *Yi Yi Ren* (Semen Coicis Lachrymajobi), 219

34. Limpness and aching in the lumbar region and knees

Ba Ji Tian (Radix Morindae Officinalis), 545; *Bi Xie* (Rhizoma Dioscoreae Hypoglaucae seu Septemlobae), 236; *Du Zhong* (Cortex Eucommiae Ulmoidis), 542; *Gou Ji* (Rhizoma Cibotii Barometz), 192; *Gou Qi Zi* (Fructus Lycii), 586; *Gui Ban* (Plastrum Testudinis), 584; *He Shou Wu* (Radix Polygoni Multiflori), 569; *Hei Zhi Ma* (Semen Sesami Indici), 597; *Hu Tao Ren* (Semen Juglandis Regiae), 557; *Huang Jing* (Rhizoma Polygonati), 593; *Liu Huang* (Sulphur), 651; *Lu Rong* (Cornu Cervi Parvum), 538; *Mu Li* (Concha Ostreae), 473; *Niu Xi* (Radix Achyranthis Bidentatae), 375; *Nü Zhen Zi* (Fructus Ligustri Lucidi), 596; *Qian Shi* (Semen Euryales Ferocis), 628; *Sang Ji Sheng* (Ramulus Loranthi), 190; *Sang Shen* (Fructus Mori Albae), 571; *Sha Yuan Zi* (Semen Astragali Complanati), 552; *Shan Yao* (Rhizoma Dioscoreae Oppositae), 526; *Shan Zhu Yu* (Fructus Corni Officinalis), 631; *Sheng Di Huang* (Radix Rehmanniae Glutinosae), 129; *Shi Hu* (Herba Dendrobii), 591; *Shu Di Huang* (Radix Rehmanniae Glutinosae Conquita), 565; *Suo Yang* (Herba Cynomorii Songarici), 551; *Tu Si Zi* (Semen Cuscutae), 541; *Wu Jia Pi* (Cortex Acanthopanacis Gracilistyli Radicis), 191; *Yin Yang Huo* (Herba Epimedii), 540

35. Lin syndrome

a. Blood Lin syndrome

Bai Mao Gen (Rhizoma Imperatae Cylindricae), 331; *Bai Wei* (Radix Cynanchi Atrati), 142; *Ce Bai Ye* (Cacumen Biotae Orientalis), 328; *Da Ji* (Herba seu Radix Cirsii Japonici), 325; *Fu Hai Shi* (Os Costaziae seu Pumex), 422; *Hai Jin Sha* (Spora Lygodii Japonici), 230; *Hu Po* (Succinum), 457; *Jin Yin Hua* (Flos Lonicerae), 95; *Niu Xi* (Radix Achyranthis Bidentatae), 375; *Pu Huang* (Pollen Typhae), 336; *Shi Wei* (Folium Pyrrosiae), 235; *Xiao Ji* (Herba Cephalanoploris seu Cirsii), 326; *Zhu Ma Gen* (Radix Boehmeriae Niveae), 332

b. *Heat Lin syndrome*
Bai Hua She She Cao (Herba Hedyotidis Diffusae), 119; *Bai Mao Gen* (Rhizoma Imperatae Cylindricae), 331; *Bai Wei* (Radix Cynanchi Atrati), 142; *Bian Xu* (Herba Polygoni Avicularis), 233; *Che Qian Zi* (Semen Plantaginis), 226; *Chuan Xin Lian* (Herba Andrographitis Paniculatae), 109; *Da Huang* (Radix et Rhizoma Rhei), 155; *Dan Zhu Ye* (Herba Lophatheri Gracilis), 76; *Deng Xin Cao* (Medulla Junci Effusi), 237; *Di Fu Zi* (Fructus Kochiae Scopariae), 234; *Hai Jin Sha* (Spora Lygodii Japonici), 230; *Hu Po* (Succinum), 457; *Hua Shi* (Talcum), 227; *Huang Bai* (Cortex Phellodendri), 84; *Huang Qin* (Radix Scutellariae Baicalensis), 81; *Jin Qian Cao* (Herba Lysimachiae), 240; *Ku Shen* (Radix Sophorae Flavescentis), 86; *Lian Qiao* (Fructus Forsythiae Suspensae), 97; *Long Dan Cao* (Radix Gentianae Scabrae), 88; *Mu Tong* (Caulis Mutong), 229; *Pu Gong Ying* (Herba Taraxaci cum Radice), 98; *Qu Mai* (Herba Dianthi), 232; *Shi Wei* (Folium Pyrrosiae), 235; *Tong Cao* (Medulla Tetrapanacis Papyriferi), 232; *Tu Fu Ling* (Rhizoma Smilacis Glabrae), 112; *Yu Xing Cao* (Herba Houttuyniae Cordatae), 104; *Zhi Zi* (Fructus Gardeniae Jasminoidis), 72; *Zhu Ling* (Sclerotium Polypori Umbellati), 222; *Zhu Ma Gen* (Radix Boehmeriae Niveae), 332

c. *Stone Lin syndrome*
Che Qian Zi (Semen Plantaginis), 226; *Fu Hai Shi* (Os Costaziae seu Pumex), 422; *Hai Jin Sha* (Spora Lygodii Japonici), 230; *Hu Po* (Succinum), 457; *Hu Tao Ren* (Semen Juglandis Regiae), 557; *Hua Shi* (Talcum), 227; *Ji Nei Jin* (Endothelium Corneum Gigeriae Galli), 302; *Jin Qian Cao* (Herba Lysimachiae), 240; *Jin Yin Hua* (Flos Lonicerae), 95; *Qu Mai* (Herba Dianthi), 232; *Shi Wei* (Folium Pyrrosiae), 235

d. *Turbid Lin syndrome*
Bi Xie (Rhizoma Dioscoreae Hypoglaucae seu Septemlobae), 236; *Hu Zhang* (Radix et Rhizoma Polygoni Cuspidati), 241; *Zhu Ling* (Sclerotium Polypori Umbellati), 222

36. Lung abscess
Bai Ji (Rhizoma Bletillae Striatae), 340; *Bai Jiang Cao* (Herba Patriniae cum Radice), 122; *Chuan Bei Mu* (Bulbus Fritillariae Cirrhosae), 413; *Chuan Xin Lian* (Herba Andrographitis Paniculatae), 109; *Dong Gua Ren* (Semen Benincasae Hispidae), 224; *He Huan Pi* (Cortex Albizziae Julibrissin), 463; *Jie Geng* (Radix Platycodi Grandiflori), 406; *Jin Yin Hua* (Flos Lonicerae), 95; *Kuan Dong Hua* (Flos Tussilaginis Farfarae), 438; *Lu Gen* (Rhizoma Phragmitis Communis), 75; *Pu Gong Ying* (Herba Taraxaci cum Radice), 98; *Tao Ren* (Semen Persicae), 372; *Tian Men Dong* (Radix Asparagi Cochinchinensis), 588; *Yi Yi Ren* (Semen Coicis Lachrymajobi), 219; *Yu Xing Cao* (Herba Houttuyniae Cordatae), 104; *Zhe Bei Mu* (Bulbus Fritillariae Thunbergii), 414

37. Macular or maculopapular eruptions due to warm or heat toxins
Ban Lan Gen (Radix Isatidis seu Baphicacanthi), 101; *Chi Shao* (Radix Paeoniae Rubra), 133; *Da Qing Ye* (Folium Isatidis seu Baphicacanthi), 102; *Hong Hua* (Flos Carthami Tinctorii), 370; *Mu Dan Pi* (Cortex Moutan Radicis), 132; *Qing Dai* (Indigo Naturalis), 103; *Xuan Shen* (Radix Scrophulariae Ningpoensis), 130; *Zi Cao* (Radix Arnebiae seu Lithospermi), 135

38. Malaria

a. *Cold malaria*
Bing Lang (Semen Arecae Catechu), 311; *Cao Guo* (Fructus Amomi Tsaoko), 208; *Chang Shan* (Radix Dichroae Febrifugae), 642; *Xian He Cao* (Herba Agrimoniae Pilosae), 341; *Ya Dan Zi* (Fructus Bruceae Javanicae), 118

b. *Heat malaria*
Bing Lang (Semen Arecae Catechu), 311; *Chai Hu* (Radix Bupleuri), 51; *Chang Shan* (Radix Dichroae Febrifugae), 642; *He Shou Wu* (Radix Polygoni Multiflori), 569; *Qing Hao* (Herba Artemisiae Chinghao), 138; *Xian He Cao* (Herba Agrimoniae Pilosae), 341; *Ya Dan Zi* (Fructus Bruceae Javanicae), 118

39. Measles

a. *Initial stage of measles*
Bo He (Herba Menthae Haplocalycis), 45; *Ge Gen* (Radix Puerariae), 53; *Jing Jie* (Herba Schizonepetae Tenuifoliae), 28

b. Measles rash

Lu Gen (Rhizoma Phragmitis Communis), 75; *Zhu Ma Gen* (Radix Boehmeriae Niveae), 332

c. Non-eruption of measles rash

Chan Tui (Periostracum Cicadae), 55; *Fu Ping* (Herba Spirodelae Polyrrhizae), 59; *Niu Bang Zi* (Fructus Arctii Lappae), 46; *Sheng Ma* (Rhizoma Cimicifugae), 57; *Zi Cao* (Radix Arnebiae seu Lithospermi), 135

40. Menstrual block

Ai Di Cha (Herba Ardisiae Japonicae), 442; *Chi Shao* (Radix Paeoniae Rubra), 133; *Chuan Shan Jia* (Squama Manitis Pentadactylae), 389; *Chuan Xiong* (Rhizoma Ligustici Chuanxiong), 359; *Da Huang* (Radix et Rhizoma Rhei), 155; *Da Zao* (Fructus Ziziphi Jujubae), 532; *Dan Shen* (Radix Salviae Miltiorrhizae), 369; *Dang Gui* (Radix Angelicae Sinensis), 563; *E Zhu* (Rhizoma Curcumae), 385; *Gui Zhi* (Ramulus Cinnamomi Cassiae), 22; *Hong Hua* (Flos Carthami Tinctorii), 370; *Hong Teng* (Caulis Sargentodoxae Cuneatae), 123; *Hu Po* (Succinum), 457; *Hu Zhang* (Radix et Rhizoma Polygoni Cuspidati), 241; *Ji Xue Teng* (Caulis Spatholobi), 378; *Jiang Huang* (Rhizoma Curcumae Longae), 364; *Liu Ji Nu* (Herba Artemisiae Anomalae), 383; *Lu Lu Tong* (Fructus Liquidambaris), 180; *Mang Xiao* (Mirabilitum), 157; *Mo Yao* (Myrrha), 366; *Mu Dan Pi* (Cortex Moutan Radicis), 132; *Mu Tong* (Caulis Mutong), 229; *Niu Xi* (Radix Achyranthis Bidentatae), 375; *Qian Cao Gen* (Radix Rubiae Cordifoliae), 334; *Qu Mai* (Herba Dianthi), 232; *Rou Gui* (Cortex Cinnamomi Cassiae), 254; *Ru Xiang* (Gummi Olibanum), 365; *San Leng* (Rhizoma Sparganii Stoloniferi), 386; *She Xiang* (Secretio Moschi), 501; *Shui Zhi* (Hirudo seu Whitmania), 387; *Su Mu* (Lignum Sappan), 382; *Tao Ren* (Semen Persicae), 372; *Tu Bie Chong* (Eupolyphaga seu Steleophaga), 388; *Wang Bu Liu Xing* (Semen Vaccariae Segetalis), 379; *Wu Ling Zhi* (Excrementum Trogopteri), 367; *Xiang Fu* (Rhizoma Cyperi Rotundi), 277; *Ze Lan* (Herba Lycopi Lucidi), 380

41. Menstrual irregularities

a. Insufficiency of Liver-Blood

Bai Shao (Radix Paeoniae Lactiflorae), 567; *Chai Hu* (Radix Bupleuri), 51; *Dang Gui* (Radix Angelicae Sinensis), 563; *Ji Xue Teng* (Caulis Spatholobi), 378; *Shu Di Huang* (Radix Rehmanniae Glutinosae Conquita), 565

b. Lower Jiao deficiency-cold or deficiency-cold in the Chong and Ren vessels

Ai Ye (Folium Artemisiae Argyi), 347; *Bai Shao* (Radix Paeoniae Lactiflorae), 567; *Chuan Xiong* (Rhizoma Ligustici Chuanxiong), 359; *Dang Gui* (Radix Angelicae Sinensis), 563; *Rou Gui* (Cortex Cinnamomi Cassiae), 254; *Wu Zhu Yu* (Fructus Evodiae Rutaecarpae), 257

c. Qi stagnation and Blood stasis

Chi Shao (Radix Paeoniae Rubra), 133; *Chuan Xiong* (Rhizoma Ligustici Chuanxiong), 359; *Dan Shen* (Radix Salviae Miltiorrhizae), 369; *Dang Gui* (Radix Angelicae Sinensis), 563; *E Zhu* (Rhizoma Curcumae), 385; *Hong Hua* (Flos Carthami Tinctorii), 370; *Ji Xue Teng* (Caulis Spatholobi), 378; *Jiang Huang* (Rhizoma Curcumae Longae), 364; *Liu Ji Nu* (Herba Artemisiae Anomalae), 383; *Lu Lu Tong* (Fructus Liquidambaris), 180; *Mei Gui Hua* (Flos Rosae Rugosae), 289; *Niu Xi* (Radix Achyranthis Bidentatae), 375; *Pu Huang* (Pollen Typhae), 336; *Qian Cao Gen* (Radix Rubiae Cordifoliae), 334; *Qu Mai* (Herba Dianthi), 232; *San Leng* (Rhizoma Sparganii Stoloniferi), 386; *Shan Zha* (Fructus Crataegi), 297; *Shui Zhi* (Hirudo seu Whitmania), 387; *Su Mu* (Lignum Sappan), 382; *Tao Ren* (Semen Persicae), 372; *Tu Bie Chong* (Eupolyphaga seu Steleophaga), 388; *Wang Bu Liu Xing* (Semen Vaccariae Segetalis), 379; *Wu Ling Zhi* (Excrementum Trogopteri), 367; *Wu Yao* (Radix Linderae Strychnifoliae), 285; *Xiang Fu* (Rhizoma Cyperi Rotundi), 277; *Yan Hu Suo* (Rhizoma Corydalis Yanhusuo), 361; *Yi Mu Cao* (Herba Leonuri Heterophylli), 374; *Ze Lan* (Herba Lycopi Lucidi), 380

42. Nasal congestion and deep-source nasal congestion

Bai Zhi (Radix Angelicae Dahuricae), 33; *Cang Er Zi* (Fructus Xanthii Sibirici), 36; *Xi Xin* (Herba cum Radice Asari), 24; *Xin Yi Hua* (Flos Magnoliae), 38

43. Non-closure of sores

Bai Lian (Radix Ampelopsis Japonicae), 124; *Bing Pian* (Borneolum), 503; *Chi Shi Zhi* (Halloysitum Rubrum), 622; *Dan Shen* (Radix Salviae Miltiorrhizae), 369; *Dang Gui* (Radix Angelicae Sinensis), 563; *Duan Shi Gao* (Gypsum Fibrosum Calcinatum), 69; *Er Cha* (Pasta Acaciae seu Uncariae), 656; *Hai Piao Xiao* (Os Sepiae seu Sepiellae), 633; *Huang Qi* (Radix Astragali seu

Hedysari), 518; *Lu Gan Shi* (Calamina), 661; *Mo Yao* (Myrrha), 366; *Qing Fen* (Calomelas), 660; *Ru Xiang* (Gummi Olibanum), 365; *Wu Bei Zi* (Galla Rhois Chinensis), 615; *Xue Jie* (Resina Draconis), 659; *Zhen Zhu* (Margarita), 477

44. Non-ulcerating sores with discharge of pus
Chuan Shan Jia (Squama Manitis Pentadactylae), 389; *Lu Rong* (Cornu Cervi Parvum), 538

45. Oedema

a. Oedema due to damp-heat congestion and obstruction
Bai Mao Gen (Rhizoma Imperatae Cylindricae), 331; *Che Qian Zi* (Semen Plantaginis), 226; *Fang Ji* (Radix Stephaniae Tetrandrae), 183; *Mu Tong* (Caulis Mutong), 229; *Ting Li Zi* (Semen Lepidii seu Descurainiae), 436; *Tong Cao* (Medulla Tetrapanacis Papyriferi), 232

b. Oedema due to failure of the Lungs to diffuse and bear downwards
Bing Lang (Semen Arecae Catechu), 311; *Fang Ji* (Radix Stephaniae Tetrandrae), 183; *Fu Ping* (Herba Spirodelae Polyrrhizae), 59; *Ma Huang* (Herba Ephedrae), 20; *Sang Bai Pi* (Cortex Mori Albae Radicis), 435; *Sheng Jiang Pi* (Cortex Zingiberis Officinalis Recens), 39; *Ting Li Zi* (Semen Lepidii seu Descurainiae), 436

c. Oedema due to Spleen deficiency with exuberant dampness
Bai Zhu (Rhizoma Atractylodis Macrocephalae), 521; *Da Fu Pi* (Pericarpium Arecae Catechu), 288; *Fu Ling* (Sclerotium Poriae Cocos), 217; *Huang Qi* (Radix Astragali seu Hedysari), 518; *Yi Yi Ren* (Semen Coicis Lachrymajobi), 219; *Yu Mi Xu* (Stylus Zeae Mays), 238; *Ze Xie* (Rhizoma Alismatis Orientalis), 221; *Zhu Ling* (Sclerotium Polypori Umbellati), 222

d. Oedema due to Yang deficiency of the Spleen and Kidneys
Che Qian Zi (Semen Plantaginis), 226; *Fu Ling* (Sclerotium Poriae Cocos), 217; *Fu Zi* (Radix Lateralis Aconiti Carmichaeli Praeparata), 250; *Gan Jiang* (Rhizoma Zingiberis Officinalis), 253; *Rou Gui* (Cortex Cinnamomi Cassiae), 254

e. Oedema in full Yang patterns
Gan Sui (Radix Euphorbiae Kansui), 162; *Jing Da Ji* (Radix Euphorbiae Pekinensis), 163; *Yuan Hua* (Flos Daphnes Genkwa), 165

46. Pain in the abdomen

a. Pain due to cold in the Middle Jiao
Ba Dou (Semen Crotonis Tiglii), 166; *Bai Zhi* (Radix Angelicae Dahuricae), 33; *Cao Dou Kou* (Semen Alpiniae Katsumadai), 206; *Ding Xiang* (Flos Caryophylli), 262; *Fu Zi* (Radix Lateralis Aconiti Carmichaeli Praeparata), 250; *Gan Jiang* (Rhizoma Zingiberis Officinalis), 253; *Gao Liang Jiang* (Rhizoma Alpiniae Officinari), 263; *Gui Zhi* (Ramulus Cinnamomi Cassiae), 22; *Hua Jiao* (Pericarpium Zanthoxyli), 259; *Rou Gui* (Cortex Cinnamomi Cassiae), 254; *Wu Zhu Yu* (Fructus Evodiae Rutaecarpae), 257; *Xiao Hui Xiang* (Fructus Foeniculi Vulgaris), 260; *Yi Zhi Ren* (Fructus Alpiniae Oxyphyllae), 549

b. Pain due to worm accumulation
Chuan Lian Zi (Fructus Meliae Toosendan), 284; *Guan Zhong* (Rhizoma Dryopteris Crassirhizomae), 113; *Hua Jiao* (Pericarpium Zanthoxyli), 259; *Qian Niu Zi* (Semen Pharbitidis), 164; *Shi Jun Zi* (Fructus Quisqualis Indicae), 309; *Shi Liu Pi* (Pericarpium Punicae Granati), 624; *Xiong Huang* (Realgar), 650

c. Postpartum pain due to Blood stasis
Bai Jiang Cao (Herba Patriniae cum Radice), 122; *Chi Shao* (Radix Paeoniae Rubra), 133; *Da Huang* (Radix et Rhizoma Rhei), 155; *Dan Shen* (Radix Salviae Miltiorrhizae), 369; *Li Zhi He* (Semen Litchi Chinensis), 289; *Pu Huang* (Pollen Typhae), 336; *Shan Zha* (Fructus Crataegi), 297; *Su Mu* (Lignum Sappan), 382; *Tao Ren* (Semen Persicae), 372; *Tu Bie Chong* (Eupolyphaga seu Steleophaga), 388; *Xue Jie* (Resina Draconis), 659; *Ze Lan* (Herba Lycopi Lucidi), 380

47. Pain in the hypochondrium
Bai Ji Li (Fructus Tribuli Terrestris), 479; *Bai Shao* (Radix Paeoniae Lactiflorae), 567; *Chai Hu* (Radix Bupleuri), 51; *Chi Shao* (Radix Paeoniae Rubra), 133; *Chuan Lian Zi* (Fructus Meliae Toosendan), 284; *Chuan Xiong* (Rhizoma Ligustici Chuanxiong), 359; *Fo Shou* (Fructus Citri Sarcodactylis), 282; *Jiang Huang* (Rhizoma Curcumae Longae), 364; *Ju Ye* (Folium Citri Reticulatae), 274; *Long Dan Cao* (Radix Gentianae Scabrae), 88; *Mai Ya* (Fructus Hordei Vulgaris Germinatus), 299; *Mu Dan Pi* (Cortex Moutan Radicis), 132; *Mu Xiang* (Radix Aucklandiae Lappae), 276; *Qing Pi* (Pericarpium Citri Reticulatae Viride), 280; *Wu Yao* (Radix Linderae Strychnifoliae), 285; *Wu Zhu Yu* (Fructus Evodiae

Rutaecarpae), 257; *Xiang Fu* (Rhizoma Cyperi Rotundi), 277; *Xiang Yuan* (Fructus Citri Medicae seu Wilsonii), 283; *Xiao Hui Xiang* (Fructus Foeniculi Vulgaris), 260; *Yu Jin* (Radix Curcumae), 362; *Zhi Ke* (Fructus Citri Aurantii), 275

48. Pain in the stomach

a. *Cold pathogenic factors settling in the Stomach*
Bai Dou Kou (Fructus Amomi Kravanh), 205; *Cao Dou Kou* (Semen Alpiniae Katsumadai), 206; *Ding Xiang* (Flos Caryophylli), 262; *Gao Liang Jiang* (Rhizoma Alpiniae Officinari), 263; *Sheng Jiang* (Rhizoma Zingiberis Officinalis Recens), 39; *Xiao Hui Xiang* (Fructus Foeniculi Vulgaris), 260

b. *Qi stagnation in the Spleen and Stomach*
Mu Xiang (Radix Aucklandiae Lappae), 276; *Wu Yao* (Radix Linderae Strychnifoliae), 285; *Xiang Fu* (Rhizoma Cyperi Rotundi), 277; *Xiang Yuan* (Fructus Citri Medicae seu Wilsonii), 283

c. *Spleen and Stomach deficiency-cold*
Bai Zhu (Rhizoma Atractylodis Macrocephalae), 521; *Gan Cao* (Radix Glycyrrhizae), 523; *Gan Jiang* (Rhizoma Zingiberis Officinalis), 253; *Hai Piao Xiao* (Os Sepiae seu Sepiellae), 633; *Wu Zhu Yu* (Fructus Evodiae Rutaecarpae), 257

49. Painful menstruation

Ai Ye (Folium Artemisiae Argyi), 347; *Chai Hu* (Radix Bupleuri), 51; *Chuan Xiong* (Rhizoma Ligustici Chuanxiong), 359; *Da Huang* (Radix et Rhizoma Rhei), 155; *Dan Shen* (Radix Salviae Miltiorrhizae), 369; *Dang Gui* (Radix Angelicae Sinensis), 563; *Gui Zhi* (Ramulus Cinnamomi Cassiae), 22; *Hong Hua* (Flos Carthami Tinctorii), 370; *Hu Lu Ba* (Semen Trigonellae Foeni-graeci), 558; *Hu Zhang* (Radix et Rhizoma Polygoni Cuspidati), 241; *Ji Xue Teng* (Caulis Spatholobi), 378; *Mang Xiao* (Mirabilitum), 157; *Mu Dan Pi* (Cortex Moutan Radicis), 132; *Niu Xi* (Radix Achyranthis Bidentatae), 375; *Pu Huang* (Pollen Typhae), 336; *Rou Gui* (Cortex Cinnamomi Cassiae), 254; *Ru Xiang* (Gummi Olibanum), 365; *Shan Zha* (Fructus Crataegi), 297; *Shu Di Huang* (Radix Rehmanniae Glutinosae Conquita), 565; *Su Mu* (Lignum Sappan), 382; *Tao Ren* (Semen Persicae), 372; *Wang Bu Liu Xing* (Semen Vaccariae Segetalis), 379; *Wu Ling Zhi* (Excrementum Trogopteri), 367; *Wu Zhu Yu* (Fructus Evodiae Rutaecarpae), 257; *Xiang Fu* (Rhizoma Cyperi Rotundi), 277; *Xiao Hui Xiang* (Fructus Foeniculi Vulgaris), 260; *Yan Hu Suo* (Rhizoma Corydalis Yanhusuo), 361; *Yi Mu Cao* (Herba Leonuri Heterophylli), 374; *Yu Jin* (Radix Curcumae), 362; *Ze Lan* (Herba Lycopi Lucidi), 380

50. Palpitations and insomnia

a. *Deficiency patterns*
Bai Zi Ren (Semen Biotae Orientalis), 462; *Dan Shen* (Radix Salviae Miltiorrhizae), 369; *E Jiao* (Gelatinum Corii Asini), 573; *Fu Ling* (Sclerotium Poriae Cocos), 217; *Gui Ban* (Plastrum Testudinis), 584; *He Huan Pi* (Cortex Albizziae Julibrissin), 463; *Long Gu* (Os Draconis), 455; *Long Yan Rou* (Arillus Euphoriae Longanae), 574; *Mai Men Dong* (Radix Ophiopogonis Japonici), 580; *Ren Shen* (Radix Ginseng), 514; *Suan Zao Ren* (Semen Ziziphi Spinosae), 460; *Wu Wei Zi* (Fructus Schisandrae), 612; *Ye Jiao Teng* (Caulis Polygoni Multiflori), 464; *Yuan Zhi* (Radix Polygalae), 461

b. *Full patterns*
Ci Shi (Magnetitum), 454; *Hu Po* (Succinum), 457; *Long Gu* (Os Draconis), 455; *Mu Li* (Concha Ostreae), 473; *Zhen Zhu* (Margarita), 477; *Zhen Zhu Mu* (Concha Margaritifera), 478; *Zhu Sha* (Cinnabaris), 453

51. Papules

a. *Dormant papules*
Fang Feng (Radix Ledebouriellae Divaricatae), 30; *Feng Fang* (Nidus Vespae), 658; *Fu Ping* (Herba Spirodelae Polyrrhizae), 59; *Sheng Di Huang* (Radix Rehmanniae Glutinosae), 129; *Xu Chang Qing* (Radix Cynanchi Paniculati), 188

b. *Wind papules*
Bai Ji Li (Fructus Tribuli Terrestris), 479; *Bai Xian Pi* (Cortex Dictamni Dasycarpi Radicis), 90; *Bo He* (Herba Menthae Haplocalycis), 45; *Chan Tui* (Periostracum Cicadae), 55; *Jiang Can* (Bombyx Batryticatus), 493; *Lu Lu Tong* (Fructus Liquidambaris), 180; *Qi She* (Agkistrodon), 176; *Ye Jiao Teng* (Caulis Polygoni Multiflori), 464

52. Plum-pit Qi (globus hystericus)

Ban Xia (Rhizoma Pinelliae Ternatae), 399; *Hou Po* (Cortex Magnoliae Officinalis), 200

53. Postpartum stasis and obstruction

Chi Shao (Radix Paeoniae Rubra), 133; *Chuan Xiong* (Rhizoma Ligustici Chuanxiong), 359; *Dan Shen* (Radix Salviae Miltiorrhizae), 369; *Hong Hua* (Flos Carthami Tinctorii), 370; *Jiang Huang*

(Rhizoma Curcumae Longae), 364; *Liu Ji Nu* (Herba Artemisiae Anomalae), 383; *Niu Xi* (Radix Achyranthis Bidentatae), 375; *Pu Huang* (Pollen Typhae), 336; *San Leng* (Rhizoma Sparganii Stoloniferi), 386; *Su Mu* (Lignum Sappan), 382; *Tao Ren* (Semen Persicae), 372; *Wu Ling Zhi* (Excrementum Trogopteri), 367; *Xue Jie* (Resina Draconis), 659; *Yi Mu Cao* (Herba Leonuri Heterophylli), 374; *Ze Lan* (Herba Lycopi Lucidi), 380

54. Red eyes

a. Liver-fire flaming upwards

Chan Tui (Periostracum Cicadae), 55; *Huai Hua* (Flos Sophorae Japonicae), 329; *Huai Jiao* (Fructus Sophorae Japonicae), 330; *Jue Ming Zi* (Semen Cassiae), 77; *Ling Yang Jiao* (Cornu Antelopis), 481; *Long Dan Cao* (Radix Gentianae Scabrae), 88; *Pu Gong Ying* (Herba Taraxaci cum Radice), 98; *Qin Pi* (Cortex Fraxini), 89; *Sang Ye* (Folium Mori Albae), 48; *Shi Jue Ming* (Concha Haliotidis), 472; *Xia Ku Cao* (Spica Prunellae Vulgaris), 74; *Zhen Zhu Mu* (Concha Margaritifera), 478; *Zhi Zi* (Fructus Gardeniae Jasminoidis), 72

b. Liver-heat attacking upwards

Che Qian Zi (Semen Plantaginis), 226; *Huang Lian* (Rhizoma Coptidis), 82; *Lu Gan Shi* (Calamina), 661; *Peng Sha* (Borax), 662; *Ye Ju Hua* (Flos Chrysanthemi Indici), 108; *Zhen Zhu* (Margarita), 477

c. Wind-heat disturbing upwards

Bai Ji Li (Fructus Tribuli Terrestris), 479; *Bo He* (Herba Menthae Haplocalycis), 45; *Chan Tui* (Periostracum Cicadae), 55; *Fang Feng* (Radix Ledebouriellae Divaricatae), 30; *Gou Teng* (Ramulus Uncariae cum Uncis), 484; *Jiang Can* (Bombyx Batryticatus), 493; *Jin Yin Hua* (Flos Lonicerae), 95; *Ju Hua* (Flos Chrysanthemi Morifolii), 49; *Jue Ming Zi* (Semen Cassiae), 77; *Man Jing Zi* (Fructus Viticis), 56; *Mu Zei* (Herba Equiseti Hiemalis), 60; *Qiang Huo* (Rhizoma et Radix Notopterygii), 32; *Zhen Zhu* (Margarita), 477

55. Scabies and tinea

Ba Dou (Semen Crotonis Tiglii), 166; *Bai Xian Pi* (Cortex Dictamni Dasycarpi Radicis), 90; *Feng Fang* (Nidus Vespae), 658; *Ku Lian Pi* (Cortex Meliae Radicis), 310; *Ku Shen* (Radix Sophorae Flavescentis), 86; *Liu Huang* (Sulphur), 651; *Lou Lu* (Radix Rhapontici seu Echinopsis), 121; *Lu Hui* (Herba Aloes), 159; *Lu Lu Tong* (Fructus Liquidambaris), 180; *Ming Fan* (Alumen), 653; *Qing Fen* (Calomelas), 660; *She Chuang Zi* (Fructus Cnidii Monnieri), 654; *Xiong Huang* (Realgar), 650; *Ye Jiao Teng* (Caulis Polygoni Multiflori), 464; *Zao Jiao Ci* (Spina Gleditsiae Sinensis), 409; *Zi Cao* (Radix Arnebiae seu Lithospermi), 135

56. Scrofula, Phlegm nodes and goitre

Bai Fu Zi (Rhizoma Typhonii Gigantei), 404; *Bai Ji* (Rhizoma Bletillae Striatae), 340; *Bai Wei* (Radix Cynanchi Atrati), 142; *Ban Xia* (Rhizoma Pinelliae Ternatae), 399; *Chuan Bei Mu* (Bulbus Fritillariae Cirrhosae), 413; *Chuan Shan Jia* (Squama Manitis Pentadactylae), 389; *Feng Fang* (Nidus Vespae), 658; *Fu Hai Shi* (Os Costaziae seu Pumex), 422; *Hai Ge Ke* (Concha Meretricis seu Cyclinae), 423; *Hai Tong Pi* (Cortex Erythrinae), 186; *Hai Zao* (Herba Sargassi), 425; *He Shou Wu* (Radix Polygoni Multiflori), 569; *Huang Yao Zi* (Rhizoma Dioscoreae Bulbiferae), 427; *Jiang Can* (Bombyx Batryticatus), 493; *Jing Da Ji* (Radix Euphorbiae Pekinensis), 163; *Kun Bu* (Thallus Laminariae seu Eckloniae), 426; *Lian Qiao* (Fructus Forsythiae Suspensae), 97; *Lou Lu* (Radix Rhapontici seu Echinopsis), 121; *Mu Li* (Concha Ostreae), 473; *Niu Huang* (Calculus Bovis), 482; *Pu Gong Ying* (Herba Taraxaci cum Radice), 98; *Quan Xie* (Buthus Martensi), 489; *Ru Xiang* (Gummi Olibanum), 365; *She Gan* (Rhizoma Belamcandae Chinensis), 106; *Tu Fu Ling* (Rhizoma Smilacis Glabrae), 112; *Wu Gong* (Scolopendra Subspinipes), 491; *Xia Ku Cao* (Spica Prunellae Vulgaris), 74; *Xuan Shen* (Radix Scrophulariae Ningpoensis), 130; *Zhe Bei Mu* (Bulbus Fritillariae Thunbergii), 414

57. Seminal emission

Ba Ji Tian (Radix Morindae Officinalis), 545; *Bu Gu Zhi* (Fructus Psoraleae Corylifoliae), 548; *Dong Chong Xia Cao* (Cordyceps Sinensis), 554; *Fu Pen Zi* (Fructus Rubi Chingii), 635; *Ge Jie* (Gekko), 556; *Gou Qi Zi* (Fructus Lycii), 586; *Gui Ban* (Plastrum Testudinis), 584; *Hai Piao Xiao* (Os Sepiae seu Sepiellae), 633; *He Shou Wu* (Radix Polygoni Multiflori), 569; *Hu Tao Ren* (Semen Juglandis Regiae), 557; *Huang Bai* (Cortex Phellodendri), 84; *Ji Nei Jin* (Endothelium Corneum Gigeriae Galli), 302; *Jin Ying Zi* (Fructus Rosae Laevigatae), 636; *Jiu Cai Zi* (Semen Allii Tuberosi), 554; *Lian Xu* (Stamen Nelumbinis Nuciferae), 627; *Lian Zi* (Semen Nelumbinis Nuciferae), 626; *Lian Zi Xin* (Plumula Nelumbinis

Nuciferae), 627; *Liu Huang* (Sulphur), 651; *Long Gu* (Os Draconis), 455; *Mu Li* (Concha Ostreae), 473; *Qian Shi* (Semen Euryales Ferocis), 628; *Rou Cong Rong* (Herba Cistanches Deserticolae), 550; *Sang Piao Xiao* (Oötheca Mantidis), 632; *Sha Yuan Zi* (Semen Astragali Complanati), 552; *Shan Yao* (Rhizoma Dioscoreae Oppositae), 526; *Sheng Di Huang* (Radix Rehmanniae Glutinosae), 129; *Suo Yang* (Herba Cynomorii Songarici), 551; *Tu Si Zi* (Semen Cuscutae), 541; *Wu Bei Zi* (Galla Rhois Chinensis), 615; *Wu Wei Zi* (Fructus Schisandrae), 612; *Yi Zhi Ren* (Fructus Alpiniae Oxyphyllae), 549; *Ze Xie* (Rhizoma Alismatis Orientalis), 221; *Zi He Che* (Placenta Hominis), 559

58. Shan disorders

Bing Lang (Semen Arecae Catechu), 311; *Chuan Lian Zi* (Fructus Meliae Toosendan), 284; *Chuan Wu* (Radix Aconiti Carmichaeli), 252; *Ding Xiang* (Flos Caryophylli), 262; *Fu Zi* (Radix Lateralis Aconiti Carmichaeli Praeparata), 250; *Gao Liang Jiang* (Rhizoma Alpiniae Officinari), 263; *Hai Zao* (Herba Sargassi), 425; *Hu Lu Ba* (Semen Trigonellae Foeni-graeci), 558; *Ju He* (Semen Citri Reticulatae), 273; *Li Zhi He* (Semen Litchi Chinensis), 289; *Mu Xiang* (Radix Aucklandiae Lappae), 276; *Qing Pi* (Pericarpium Citri Reticulatae Viride), 280; *Sang Piao Xiao* (Oötheca Mantidis), 632; *Shan Zha* (Fructus Crataegi), 297; *Wu Yao* (Radix Linderae Strychnifoliae), 285; *Wu Zhu Yu* (Fructus Evodiae Rutaecarpae), 257; *Xiang Fu* (Rhizoma Cyperi Rotundi), 277; *Xiao Hui Xiang* (Fructus Foeniculi Vulgaris), 260; *Yan Hu Suo* (Rhizoma Corydalis Yanhusuo), 361

59. Snake and insect bites

Bai Fu Zi (Rhizoma Typhonii Gigantei), 404; *Bai Hua She She Cao* (Herba Hedyotidis Diffusae), 119; *Bai Wei* (Radix Cynanchi Atrati), 142; *Ban Bian Lian* (Herba Lobeliae Chinensis cum Radice), 111; *Chong Lou* (Rhizoma Paridis), 110; *Chuan Xin Lian* (Herba Andrographitis Paniculatae), 109; *Hu Zhang* (Radix et Rhizoma Polygoni Cuspidati), 241; *Huang Yao Zi* (Rhizoma Dioscoreae Bulbiferae), 427; *Jin Qian Cao* (Herba Lysimachiae), 240; *Ma Chi Xian* (Herba Portulacae Oleraceae), 117; *Wu Gong* (Scolopendra Subspinipes), 491; *Wu Ling Zhi* (Excrementum Trogopteri), 367; *Xi Xian Cao* (Herba Siegesbeckiae), 185; *Xiong Huang* (Realgar), 650; *Xu Chang Qing* (Radix Cynanchi Paniculati), 188; *Zi Hua Di Ding* (Herba Violae Yedoensitis), 100

60. Steaming bone disorder

Gui Ban (Plastrum Testudinis), 584; *Mu Dan Pi* (Cortex Moutan Radicis), 132; *Shu Di Huang* (Radix Rehmanniae Glutinosae Conquita), 565; *Ze Xie* (Rhizoma Alismatis Orientalis), 221; *Zhi Mu* (Rhizoma Anemarrhenae Asphodeloidis), 70

a. with taxation fever

Bie Jia (Carapax Amydae Sinensis), 583; *Fu Xiao Mai* (Fructus Tritici Aestivi Levis), 610; *Nü Zhen Zi* (Fructus Ligustri Lucidi), 596; *Qing Hao* (Herba Artemisiae Chinghao), 138;

b. with tidal fever

Di Gu Pi (Cortex Lycii Radicis), 139; *Hu Huang Lian* (Rhizoma Picrorhizae Scrophulariiflorae), 141; *Huang Bai* (Cortex Phellodendri), 84; *Qin Jiao* (Radix Gentianae Macrophyllae), 181; *Shan Zhu Yu* (Fructus Corni Officinalis), 631; *Yin Chai Hu* (Radix Stellariae Dichotomae), 140

61. Stirring foetus

Ai Ye (Folium Artemisiae Argyi), 347; *Bai Shao* (Radix Paeoniae Lactiflorae), 567; *Bai Zhu* (Rhizoma Atractylodis Macrocephalae), 521; *Du Zhong* (Cortex Eucommiae Ulmoidis), 542; *E Jiao* (Gelatinum Corii Asini), 573; *Huang Qin* (Radix Scutellariae Baicalensis), 81; *Sang Ji Sheng* (Ramulus Loranthi), 190; *Sha Ren* (Fructus Amomi), 204; *Tu Si Zi* (Semen Cuscutae), 541; *Xu Duan* (Radix Dipsaci), 544; *Zhu Ma Gen* (Radix Boehmeriae Niveae), 332; *Zi Su Ye* (Folium Perillae Frutescentis), 27

62. Stoppage of breast milk

Bai Ji Li (Fructus Tribuli Terrestris), 479; *Chuan Shan Jia* (Squama Manitis Pentadactylae), 389; *Lou Lu* (Radix Rhapontici seu Echinopsis), 121; *Lu Lu Tong* (Fructus Liquidambaris), 180; *Mu Tong* (Caulis Mutong), 229; *Tong Cao* (Medulla Tetrapanacis Papyriferi), 232; *Wang Bu Liu Xing* (Semen Vaccariae Segetalis), 379; *Xu Duan* (Radix Dipsaci), 544

63. Sweating

a. Night sweating

Bai He (Bulbus Lilii), 590; *Bai Shao* (Radix Paeoniae Lactiflorae), 567; *Bai Zi Ren* (Semen Biotae Orientalis), 462; *Bie Jia* (Carapax Amydae Sinensis), 583; *Di Gu Pi* (Cortex Lycii Radicis), 139; *Fu Xiao Mai* (Fructus Tritici Aestivi Levis), 610; *Gui Ban* (Plastrum Testudinis), 584; *Hu Huang Lian* (Rhizoma Picrorhizae Scrophulariiflorae),

141; *Huang Bai* (Cortex Phellodendri), 84; *Huang Jing* (Rhizoma Polygonati), 593; *Huang Qi* (Radix Astragali seu Hedysari), 518; *Long Gu* (Os Draconis), 455; *Ma Huang Gen* (Radix Ephedrae), 609; *Mu Li* (Concha Ostreae), 473; *Nü Zhen Zi* (Fructus Ligustri Lucidi), 596; *Qing Hao* (Herba Artemisiae Chinghao), 138; *Shan Zhu Yu* (Fructus Corni Officinalis), 631; *Sheng Di Huang* (Radix Rehmanniae Glutinosae), 129; *Shu Di Huang* (Radix Rehmanniae Glutinosae Conquita), 565; *Suan Zao Ren* (Semen Ziziphi Spinosae), 460; *Wu Bei Zi* (Galla Rhois Chinensis), 615; *Wu Wei Zi* (Fructus Schisandrae), 612; *Yin Chai Hu* (Radix Stellariae Dichotomae), 140; *Zhi Mu* (Rhizoma Anemarrhenae Asphodeloidis), 70; *Zi He Che* (Placenta Hominis), 559

b. Spontaneous sweating

Bai Shao (Radix Paeoniae Lactiflorae), 567; *Bai Zhu* (Rhizoma Atractylodis Macrocephalae), 521; *Dong Chong Xia Cao* (Cordyceps Sinensis), 554; *Fu Xiao Mai* (Fructus Tritici Aestivi Levis), 610; *Gan Cao* (Radix Glycyrrhizae), 523; *Huang Qi* (Radix Astragali seu Hedysari), 518; *Long Gu* (Os Draconis), 455; *Ma Huang Gen* (Radix Ephedrae), 609; *Mu Li* (Concha Ostreae), 473; *Ren Shen* (Radix Ginseng), 514; *Suan Zao Ren* (Semen Ziziphi Spinosae), 460; *Tai Zi Shen* (Radix Pseudostellariae Heterophyllae), 531; *Wu Bei Zi* (Galla Rhois Chinensis), 615; *Wu Wei Zi* (Fructus Schisandrae), 612

64. Swollen abscesses and sores

Bai Hua She She Cao (Herba Hedyotidis Diffusae), 119; *Bai Ji* (Rhizoma Bletillae Striatae), 340; *Bai Jiang Cao* (Herba Patriniae cum Radice), 122; *Bai Lian* (Radix Ampelopsis Japonicae), 124; *Bai Zhi* (Radix Angelicae Dahuricae), 33; *Ban Bian Lian* (Herba Lobeliae Chinensis cum Radice), 111; *Chan Su* (Venenum Bufonis), 657; *Chong Lou* (Rhizoma Paridis), 110; *Da Huang* (Radix et Rhizoma Rhei), 155; *He Huan Pi* (Cortex Albizziae Julibrissin), 463; *He Shou Wu* (Radix Polygoni Multiflori), 569; *Hong Teng* (Caulis Sargentodoxae Cuneatae), 123; *Hu Zhang* (Radix et Rhizoma Polygoni Cuspidati), 241; *Huang Bai* (Cortex Phellodendri), 84; *Huang Qin* (Radix Scutellariae Baicalensis), 81; *Jiang Can* (Bombyx Batryticatus), 493; *Jin Yin Hua* (Flos Lonicerae), 95; *Jing Da Ji* (Radix Euphorbiae Pekinensis), 163; *Lian Qiao* (Fructus Forsythiae Suspensae), 97; *Lü Dou* (Semen Phaseoli Radiati), 125; *Luo Shi Teng* (Caulis Trachelospermi Jasminoidis), 187; *Ma Chi Xian* (Herba Portulacae Oleraceae), 117; *Mang Xiao* (Mirabilitum), 157; *Mo Yao* (Myrrha), 366; *Mu Dan Pi* (Cortex Moutan Radicis), 132; *Niu Bang Zi* (Fructus Arctii Lappae), 46; *Niu Huang* (Calculus Bovis), 482; *Pu Gong Ying* (Herba Taraxaci cum Radice), 98; *Quan Xie* (Buthus Martensi), 489; *Ru Xiang* (Gummi Olibanum), 365; *San Qi* (Radix Notoginseng), 333; *Shan Dou Gen* (Radix Sophorae Tonkinensis), 115; *Sheng Ma* (Rhizoma Cimicifugae), 57; *Tian Hua Fen* (Radix Trichosanthis), 71; *Wu Bei Zi* (Galla Rhois Chinensis), 615; *Wu Gong* (Scolopendra Subspinipes), 491; *Xiao Ji* (Herba Cephalanoploris seu Cirsii), 326; *Xiong Huang* (Realgar), 650; *Ye Ju Hua* (Flos Chrysanthemi Indici), 108; *Yi Mu Cao* (Herba Leonuri Heterophylli), 374; *Yu Xing Cao* (Herba Houttuyniae Cordatae), 104; *Zao Jiao* (Fructus Gleditsiae Sinensis), 408; *Zhi Zi* (Fructus Gardeniae Jasminoidis), 72; *Zhu Ma Gen* (Radix Boehmeriae Niveae), 332; *Zi Hua Di Ding* (Herba Violae Yedoensitis), 100

65. Syphilis

Qing Fen (Calomelas), 660; *Tu Fu Ling* (Rhizoma Smilacis Glabrae), 112

66. Tetanus

Bai Fu Zi (Rhizoma Typhonii Gigantei), 404; *Fang Feng* (Radix Ledebouriellae Divaricatae), 30; *Jiang Can* (Bombyx Batryticatus), 493; *Qi She* (Agkistrodon), 176; *Quan Xie* (Buthus Martensi), 489; *Tian Ma* (Rhizoma Gastrodiae Elatae), 486; *Tian Nan Xing* (Rhizoma Arisaematis), 401; *Wu Gong* (Scolopendra Subspinipes), 491; *Xiong Huang* (Realgar), 650

67. Tetany

a. Deficiency Liver-wind patterns

Bie Jia (Carapax Amydae Sinensis), 583; *Gui Ban* (Plastrum Testudinis), 584; *Mu Li* (Concha Ostreae), 473; *Tian Ma* (Rhizoma Gastrodiae Elatae), 486

b. Full Liver-wind patterns

Di Long (Lumbricus), 488; *Gou Teng* (Ramulus Uncariae cum Uncis), 484; *Jiang Can* (Bombyx Batryticatus), 493; *Ling Yang Jiao* (Cornu Antelopis), 481; *Niu Huang* (Calculus Bovis), 482; *Quan Xie* (Buthus Martensi), 489; *Tian Ma* (Rhizoma Gastrodiae Elatae), 486; *Wu Gong* (Scolopendra Subspinipes), 491

68. Throat Bi syndrome and tonsillitis

a. Exuberant fire in the Lungs and Stomach
Chan Su (Venenum Bufonis), 657; *Huang Qin* (Radix Scutellariae Baicalensis), 81; *Mai Men Dong* (Radix Ophiopogonis Japonici), 580; *Peng Sha* (Borax), 662; *Shan Dou Gen* (Radix Sophorae Tonkinensis), 115; *Xuan Shen* (Radix Scrophulariae Ningpoensis), 130

b. Wind-heat invading upwards
Bing Pian (Borneolum), 503; *Bo He* (Herba Menthae Haplocalycis), 45; *Chan Su* (Venenum Bufonis), 657; *Jiang Can* (Bombyx Batryticatus), 493; *Jie Geng* (Radix Platycodi Grandiflori), 406; *Jin Yin Hua* (Flos Lonicerae), 95; *Lian Qiao* (Fructus Forsythiae Suspensae), 97; *Ma Bo* (Sclerotium Lasiosphaerae seu Calvatiae), 116; *Mu Hu Die* (Semen Oroxyli Indici), 120; *Niu Bang Zi* (Fructus Arctii Lappae), 46; *Xuan Ming Fen* (Mirabilitum Depuratum), 157

69. Tinnitus and deafness

a. Ascendant hyperactivity of Liver Yang
Gui Ban (Plastrum Testudinis), 584; *Long Gu* (Os Draconis), 455; *Mu Li* (Concha Ostreae), 473; *Niu Xi* (Radix Achyranthis Bidentatae), 375; *Shi Jue Ming* (Concha Haliotidis), 472; *Zhen Zhu Mu* (Concha Margaritifera), 478

b. Blood deficiency
Bai Shao (Radix Paeoniae Lactiflorae), 567; *Dang Gui* (Radix Angelicae Sinensis), 563

c. Kidney deficiency
Ci Shi (Magnetitum), 454; *Gu Sui Bu* (Rhizoma Drynariae), 382; *He Shou Wu* (Radix Polygoni Multiflori), 569; *Lian Zi* (Semen Nelumbinis Nuciferae), 626; *Nü Zhen Zi* (Fructus Ligustri Lucidi), 596; *Sang Shen* (Fructus Mori Albae), 571; *Sha Yuan Zi* (Semen Astragali Complanati), 552; *Shan Zhu Yu* (Fructus Corni Officinalis), 631; *Sheng Di Huang* (Radix Rehmanniae Glutinosae), 129; *Shi Chang Pu* (Rhizoma Acori Graminei), 505; *Shu Di Huang* (Radix Rehmanniae Glutinosae Conquita), 565; *Ze Xie* (Rhizoma Alismatis Orientalis), 221

70. Toothache

a. Toothache due to Stomach-fire
Huang Qin (Radix Scutellariae Baicalensis), 81; *Shan Dou Gen* (Radix Sophorae Tonkinensis), 115; *Sheng Ma* (Rhizoma Cimicifugae), 57; *Shi Gao* (Gypsum Fibrosum), 69

b. Toothache due to wind-cold
Bai Zhi (Radix Angelicae Dahuricae), 33; *Feng Fang* (Nidus Vespae), 658; *Xi Xin* (Herba cum Radice Asari), 24; *Xu Chang Qing* (Radix Cynanchi Paniculati), 188

71. Urinary incontinence
Ba Ji Tian (Radix Morindae Officinalis), 545; *Bu Gu Zhi* (Fructus Psoraleae Corylifoliae), 548; *Feng Fang* (Nidus Vespae), 658; *Fu Pen Zi* (Fructus Rubi Chingii), 635; *He Zi* (Fructus Terminaliae Chebulae), 617; *Ji Nei Jin* (Endothelium Corneum Gigeriae Galli), 302; *Jin Ying Zi* (Fructus Rosae Laevigatae), 636; *Lian Xu* (Stamen Nelumbinis Nuciferae), 627; *Long Gu* (Os Draconis), 455; *Mu Li* (Concha Ostreae), 473; *Qian Shi* (Semen Euryales Ferocis), 628; *Sang Piao Xiao* (Oötheca Mantidis), 632; *Shan Zhu Yu* (Fructus Corni Officinalis), 631; *Tu Si Zi* (Semen Cuscutae), 541; *Wu Yao* (Radix Linderae Strychnifoliae), 285; *Xian Mao* (Rhizoma Curculiginis Orchioidis), 547; *Yi Zhi Ren* (Fructus Alpiniae Oxyphyllae), 549

72. Urinary turbidity
Bai Guo (Semen Ginkgo Bilobae), 443; *Bi Xie* (Rhizoma Dioscoreae Hypoglaucae seu Septemlobae), 236; *Qian Shi* (Semen Euryales Ferocis), 628; *Sang Piao Xiao* (Oötheca Mantidis), 632; *Tu Si Zi* (Semen Cuscutae), 541; *Wu Wei Zi* (Fructus Schisandrae), 612; *Yi Zhi Ren* (Fructus Alpiniae Oxyphyllae), 549; *Ze Xie* (Rhizoma Alismatis Orientalis), 221

73. Vaginal discharge

a. Vaginal discharge due to cold-damp
Bai Bian Dou (Semen Dolichoris Lablab), 528; *Bai Lian* (Radix Ampelopsis Japonicae), 124; *Bai Zhi* (Radix Angelicae Dahuricae), 33; *Gou Ji* (Rhizoma Cibotii Barometz), 192; *Hai Piao Xiao* (Os Sepiae seu Sepiellae), 633; *Jin Ying Zi* (Fructus Rosae Laevigatae), 636; *Lian Zi* (Semen Nelumbinis Nuciferae), 626; *Long Gu* (Os Draconis), 455; *Lu Rong* (Cornu Cervi Parvum), 538; *Mu Li* (Concha Ostreae), 473; *Sha Yuan Zi* (Semen Astragali Complanati), 552; *She Chuang Zi* (Fructus Cnidii Monnieri), 654; *Tu Si Zi* (Semen Cuscutae), 541

b. Vaginal discharge due to damp-heat
Bai Bian Dou (Semen Dolichoris Lablab), 528; *Bai Guo* (Semen Ginkgo Bilobae), 443; *Bai Lian* (Radix Ampelopsis Japonicae), 124; *Bai Tou Weng*

(Radix Pulsatillae Chinensis), 107; *Bai Zhi* (Radix Angelicae Dahuricae), 33; *Cang Zhu* (Rhizoma Atractylodis), 201; *Chun Pi* (Cortex Ailanthi Altissimae), 625; *Da Huang* (Radix et Rhizoma Rhei), 155; *Dong Gua Ren* (Semen Benincasae Hispidae), 224; *Fu Ling* (Sclerotium Poriae Cocos), 217; *Hu Zhang* (Radix et Rhizoma Polygoni Cuspidati), 241; *Huang Bai* (Cortex Phellodendri), 84; *Jin Qian Cao* (Herba Lysimachiae), 240; *Ku Shen* (Radix Sophorae Flavescentis), 86; *Long Dan Cao* (Radix Gentianae Scabrae), 88; *Ming Fan* (Alumen), 653; *Qian Shi* (Semen Euryales Ferocis), 628; *Qin Pi* (Cortex Fraxini), 89; *Shan Yao* (Rhizoma Dioscoreae Oppositae), 526; *Tu Fu Ling* (Rhizoma Smilacis Glabrae), 112; *Yi Yi Ren* (Semen Coicis Lachrymajobi), 219

74. Vomiting

a. Vomiting due to damp obstruction in the Middle Jiao

Cang Zhu (Rhizoma Atractylodis), 201; *Cao Dou Kou* (Semen Alpiniae Katsumadai), 206; *Cao Guo* (Fructus Amomi Tsaoko), 208; *Gan Jiang* (Rhizoma Zingiberis Officinalis), 253; *Huo Xiang* (Herba Agastaches seu Pogostemi), 199; *Sha Ren* (Fructus Amomi), 204

b. Vomiting due to Qi stagnation in the Spleen and Stomach

Xiang Yuan (Fructus Citri Medicae seu Wilsonii), 283; *Zi Su Ye* (Folium Perillae Frutescentis), 27

c. Vomiting due to Spleen and Stomach deficiency-cold

Chen Pi (Pericarpium Citri Reticulatae), 272; *Chen Xiang* (Lignum Aquilariae Resinatum), 279; *Ding Xiang* (Flos Caryophylli), 262; *Huo Xiang* (Herba Agastaches seu Pogostemi), 199; *Pao Jiang* (Rhizoma Zingiberis Officinalis Praeparata), 346; *Wu Zhu Yu* (Fructus Evodiae Rutaecarpae), 257; *Zao Xin Tu* (Terra Flava Usta), 348

d. Vomiting due to Stomach-cold

Bai Dou Kou (Fructus Amomi Kravanh), 205; *Ding Xiang* (Flos Caryophylli), 262; *Gan Jiang* (Rhizoma Zingiberis Officinalis), 253; *Gao Liang Jiang* (Rhizoma Alpiniae Officinari), 263; *Huo Xiang* (Herba Agastaches seu Pogostemi), 199; *Rou Dou Kou* (Semen Myristicae Fragrantis), 623; *Sheng Jiang* (Rhizoma Zingiberis Officinalis Recens), 39; *Wu Zhu Yu* (Fructus Evodiae Rutaecarpae), 257

e. Vomiting due to Stomach-heat

Ban Xia (Rhizoma Pinelliae Ternatae), 399; *Huang Lian* (Rhizoma Coptidis), 82; *Lu Gen* (Rhizoma Phragmitis Communis), 75; *Pi Pa* Ye (Folium Eriobotryae Japonicae), 441; *Sheng Jiang* (Rhizoma Zingiberis Officinalis Recens), 39; *Zhi Zi* (Fructus Gardeniae Jasminoidis), 72; *Zhu Ru* (Caulis Bambusae in Taeniis), 418

75. Wasting and thirsting

Di Gu Pi (Cortex Lycii Radicis), 139; *Fu Ping* (Herba Spirodelae Polyrrhizae), 59; *Ge Gen* (Radix Puerariae), 53; *Gou Qi Zi* (Fructus Lycii), 586; *Gua Lou* (Fructus Trichosanthis), 415; *Huang Jing* (Rhizoma Polygonati), 593; *Huang Qi* (Radix Astragali seu Hedysari), 518; *Mai Men Dong* (Radix Ophiopogonis Japonici), 580; *Qin Jiao* (Radix Gentianae Macrophyllae), 181; *Ren Shen* (Radix Ginseng), 514; *Sang Bai Pi* (Cortex Mori Albae Radicis), 435; *Sang Shen* (Fructus Mori Albae), 571; *Shan Yao* (Rhizoma Dioscoreae Oppositae), 526; *Sheng Di Huang* (Radix Rehmanniae Glutinosae), 129; *Shu Di Huang* (Radix Rehmanniae Glutinosae Conquita), 565; *Tian Hua Fen* (Radix Trichosanthis), 71; *Tian Men Dong* (Radix Asparagi Cochinchinensis), 588; *Tu Si Zi* (Semen Cuscutae), 541; *Wu Mei* (Fructus Pruni Mume), 614; *Wu Wei Zi* (Fructus Schisandrae), 612; *Xuan Shen* (Radix Scrophulariae Ningpoensis), 130; *Zhi Mu* (Rhizoma Anemarrhenae Asphodeloidis), 70

76. Wei syndrome

a. Lung Wei syndrome

Bai Ji (Rhizoma Bletillae Striatae), 340; *Chuan Bei Mu* (Bulbus Fritillariae Cirrhosae), 413; *Gua Lou* (Fructus Trichosanthis), 415; *Mai Men Dong* (Radix Ophiopogonis Japonici), 580

b. Wei syndrome of the lower limbs

Hai Zao (Herba Sargassi), 425; *Huang Bai* (Cortex Phellodendri), 84; *Huang Qi* (Radix Astragali seu Hedysari), 518; *Kun Bu* (Thallus Laminariae seu Eckloniae), 426; *Niu Xi* (Radix Achyranthis Bidentatae), 375

c. Wei syndrome of the sinews and bones

Gou Qi Zi (Fructus Lycii), 586; *Gui Ban* (Plastrum Testudinis), 584; *Sang Ji Sheng* (Ramulus Loranthi), 190; *Wu Jia Pi* (Cortex Acanthopanacis Gracilistyli Radicis), 191; *Xian Mao* (Rhizoma Curculiginis Orchioidis), 547

77. Wheezing patterns

a. *Cold fluids collecting internally involving the Lungs*

Ban Xia (Rhizoma Pinelliae Ternatae), 399; *Gan Jiang* (Rhizoma Zingiberis Officinalis), 253; *Gui Zhi* (Ramulus Cinnamomi Cassiae), 22; *Hou Po* (Cortex Magnoliae Officinalis), 200; *Ma Huang* (Herba Ephedrae), 20; *Su Zi* (Fructus Perillae Frutescentis), 432; *Xi Xin* (Herba cum Radice Asari), 24

b. *Lung and Kidney deficiency*

Bu Gu Zhi (Fructus Psoraleae Corylifoliae), 548; *Chen Xiang* (Lignum Aquilariae Resinatum), 279; *Ci Shi* (Magnetitum), 454; *Dai Zhe Shi* (Haematitum), 475; *Dong Chong Xia Cao* (Cordyceps Sinensis), 554; *Ge Jie* (Gekko), 556; *Hu Tao Ren* (Semen Juglandis Regiae), 557; *Liu Huang* (Sulphur), 651; *Ren Shen* (Radix Ginseng), 514; *Shan Yao* (Rhizoma Dioscoreae Oppositae), 526; *Wu Wei Zi* (Fructus Schisandrae), 612; *Zi He Che* (Placenta Hominis), 559

c. *Lung-heat congestion*

Ce Bai Ye (Cacumen Biotae Orientalis), 328; *Chuan Xin Lian* (Herba Andrographitis Paniculatae), 109; *Di Long* (Lumbricus), 488; *Gan Cao* (Radix Glycyrrhizae), 523; *Gua Lou* (Fructus Trichosanthis), 415; *Ma Dou Ling* (Fructus Aristolochiae), 439; *Niu Bang Zi* (Fructus Arctii Lappae), 46; *Pi Pa* Ye (Folium Eriobotryae Japonicae), 441; *Qian Hu* (Radix Peucedani), 417; *Ren Shen* (Radix Ginseng), 514; *Sang Bai Pi* (Cortex Mori Albae Radicis), 435; *Shi Gao* (Gypsum Fibrosum), 69; *Xing Ren* (Semen Pruni Armeniacae), 431

78. Wind-stroke

a. *Sequelae of wind-stroke*

Bing Pian (Borneolum), 503; *Di Long* (Lumbricus), 488; *Du Zhong* (Cortex Eucommiae Ulmoidis), 542; *Qi She* (Agkistrodon), 176; *Qin Jiao* (Radix Gentianae Macrophyllae), 181; *Quan Xie* (Buthus Martensi), 489; *Tian Zhu Huang* (Concretio Silicea Bambusae), 420

b. *Wind-stroke due to Phlegm-heat*

Dan Nan Xing (Pulvis Arisaematis cum Felle Bovis), 403; *Niu Huang* (Calculus Bovis), 482; *Zhu Li* (Succus Bambusae), 421

c. *Wind-stroke due to Phlegm obstruction or congestion*

She Xiang (Secretio Moschi), 501; *Tian Nan Xing* (Rhizoma Arisaematis), 401; *Zao Jiao* (Fructus Gleditsiae Sinensis), 408

d. *Wind-stroke with Phlegm collapse*

Bing Pian (Borneolum), 503; *Ming Fan* (Alumen), 653; *Su He Xiang* (Styrax Liquidus), 503; *Zao Jiao* (Fructus Gleditsiae Sinensis), 408

79. Worms

a. *Hookworm*

Bian Xu (Herba Polygoni Avicularis), 233; *Bing Lang* (Semen Arecae Catechu), 311; *Fei Zi* (Semen Torreyae Grandis), 316; *Guan Zhong* (Rhizoma Dryopteris Crassirhizomae), 113; *Ku Lian Pi* (Cortex Meliae Radicis), 310; *Lei Wan* (Sclerotium Omphaliae Lapidescens), 315; *Shi Jun Zi* (Fructus Quisqualis Indicae), 309

b. *Roundworm and pinworm*

Bian Xu (Herba Polygoni Avicularis), 233; *Bing Lang* (Semen Arecae Catechu), 311; *Chuan Lian Zi* (Fructus Meliae Toosendan), 284; *Fei Zi* (Semen Torreyae Grandis), 316; *Guan Zhong* (Rhizoma Dryopteris Crassirhizomae), 113; *Hua Jiao* (Pericarpium Zanthoxyli), 259; *Ku Lian Pi* (Cortex Meliae Radicis), 310; *Lei Wan* (Sclerotium Omphaliae Lapidescens), 315; *Lu Hui* (Herba Aloes), 159; *Nan Gua Zi* (Semen Cucurbitae Moschatae), 313; *Qian Niu Zi* (Semen Pharbitidis), 164; *Shi Jun Zi* (Fructus Quisqualis Indicae), 309; *Shi Liu Pi* (Pericarpium Punicae Granati), 624; *Wu Mei* (Fructus Pruni Mume), 614

c. *Tapeworm*

Bing Lang (Semen Arecae Catechu), 311; *Fei Zi* (Semen Torreyae Grandis), 316; *Guan Zhong* (Rhizoma Dryopteris Crassirhizomae), 113; *He Cao Ya* (Gemma Agrimoniae Pilosae), 314; *Lei Wan* (Sclerotium Omphaliae Lapidescens), 315; *Nan Gua Zi* (Semen Cucurbitae Moschatae), 313; *Qian Niu Zi* (Semen Pharbitidis), 164; *Shi Liu Pi* (Pericarpium Punicae Granati), 624; *Xiong Huang* (Realgar), 650

d. *Threadworm*

Bai Bu (Radix Stemonae), 433; *Bing Lang* (Semen Arecae Catechu), 311; *Qian Niu Zi* (Semen Pharbitidis), 164

80. Yin abscesses and streaming sores

Bai Jie Zi (Semen Sinapis Albae), 407; *Lu Jiao Jiao* (Gelatinum Cornu Cervi), 539; *Lu Rong* (Cornu Cervi Parvum), 538; *Ma Huang* (Herba Ephedrae), 20; *Rou Gui* (Cortex Cinnamomi Cassiae), 254

Appendix 9 Index of channels entered

Lung

Large Intestine

Stomach

Spleen

Heart

Bai Zi Ren (Semen Biotae Orientalis), 462
Ban Bian Lian (Herba Lobeliae Chinensis cum Radice), 111
Ban Lan Gen (Radix Isatidis seu Baphicacanthi), 101
Bing Pian (Borneolum), 504
Cao Wu (Radix Aconiti Kusnezoffii), 253
Chan Su (Venenum Bufonis), 657
Chang Shan (Radix Dichroae Febrifugae), 642
Chi Xiao Dou (Semen Phaseoli Calcarati), 224
Chuan Bei Mu (Bulbus Fritillariae Cirrhosae), 413
Chuan Wu (Radix Aconiti Carmichaeli), 252
Ci Shi (Magnetitum), 454
Da Huang (Radix et Rhizoma Rhei), 155
Da Ji (Herba seu Radix Cirsii Japonici), 325
Da Qing Ye (Folium Isatidis seu Baphicacanthi), 102
Dai Zhe Shi (Haematitum), 475
Dan Shen (Radix Salviae Miltiorrhizae), 369
Dan Zhu Ye (Herba Lophatheri Gracilis), 76
Dang Gui (Radix Angelicae Sinensis), 563
Deng Xin Cao (Medulla Junci Effusi), 237
Fu Ling (Sclerotium Poriae Cocos), 217
Fu Shen (Sclerotium Poriae Cocos cum Ligno Hospite), 219
Fu Xiao Mai (Fructus Tritici Aestivi Levis), 610
Fu Zi (Radix Lateralis Aconiti Carmichaeli Praeparata), 250
Gan Cao (Radix Glycyrrhizae), 524
Gan Jiang (Rhizoma Zingiberis Officinalis), 253
Gui Ban (Plastrum Testudinis), 584
Gui Zhi (Ramulus Cinnamomi Cassiae), 22
He Huan Pi (Cortex Albizziae Julibrissin), 463
He Ye (Folium Nelumbinis Nuciferae), 628
Hong Hua (Flos Carthami Tinctorii), 370
Hu Po (Succinum), 457
Huang Lian (Rhizoma Coptidis), 82
Ji Xue Teng (Caulis Spatholobi), 378
Jin Yin Hua (Flos Lonicerae), 95
Ku Shen (Radix Sophorae Flavescentis), 86
Lian Qiao (Fructus Forsythiae Suspensae), 97
Lian Xu (Stamen Nelumbinis Nuciferae), 627
Lian Zi (Semen Nelumbinis Nuciferae), 626
Lian Zi Xin (Plumula Nelumbinis Nuciferae), 627
Ling Yang Jiao (Cornu Antelopis), 481
Liu Ji Nu (Herba Artemisiae Anomalae), 383
Long Gu (Os Draconis), 455
Long Yan Rou (Arillus Euphoriae Longanae), 575
Lü Dou (Semen Phaseoli Radiati), 125
Lü Dou Yi (Testa Phaseoli Radiati), 126
Luo Shi Teng (Caulis Trachelospermi Jasminoidis), 187
Mai Men Dong (Radix Ophiopogonis Japonici), 580
Mo Yao (Myrrha), 366
Mu Dan Pi (Cortex Moutan Radicis), 132
Mu Tong (Caulis Mutong), 229
Niu Huang (Calculus Bovis), 482
Pu Huang (Pollen Typhae), 336
Qu Mai (Herba Dianthi), 233
Ren Dong Teng (Caulis Lonicerae Japonicae), 96
Rou Gui (Cortex Cinnamomi Cassiae), 255
Ru Xiang (Gummi Olibanum), 365
Sang Shen (Fructus Mori Albae), 571
She Xiang (Secretio Moschi), 501
Sheng Di Huang (Radix Rehmanniae Glutinosae), 129
Shi Chang Pu (Rhizoma Acori Graminei), 505
Shui Niu Jiao (Cornu Bubali), 136
Su He Xiang (Styrax Liquidus), 503
Su Mu (Lignum Sappan), 382
Suan Zao Ren (Semen Ziziphi Spinosae), 460
Tao Ren (Semen Persicae), 372
Tian Zhu Huang (Concretio Silicea Bambusae), 420
Wu Wei Zi (Fructus Schisandrae), 612
Xi Yang Shen (Radix Panacis Quinquefolii), 529
Xiao Ji (Herba Cephalanoploris seu Cirsii), 326
Xiong Huang (Realgar), 650
Xue Jie (Resina Draconis), 659
Yan Hu Suo (Rhizoma Corydalis Yanhusuo), 361
Yang Jin Hua (Flos Daturae), 444
Ye Jiao Teng (Caulis Polygoni Multiflori), 464
Yi Mu Cao (Herba Leonuri Heterophylli), 374
Yu Jin (Radix Curcumae), 362
Yuan Zhi (Radix Polygalae), 461
Zhe Bei Mu (Bulbus Fritillariae Thunbergii), 414
Zhen Zhu (Margarita), 477
Zhen Zhu Mu (Concha Margaritifera), 478
Zhi Zi (Fructus Gardeniae Jasminoidis), 72
Zhu Li (Succus Bambusae), 421
Zhu Ma Gen (Radix Boehmeriae Niveae), 332
Zhu Sha (Cinnabaris), 453
Zi Cao (Radix Arnebiae seu Lithospermi), 135
Zi Hua Di Ding (Herba Violae Yedoensitis), 100

Small Intestine

Bai Hua She She Cao (Herba Hedyotidis Diffusae), 119
Ban Bian Lian (Herba Lobeliae Chinensis cum Radice), 111
Che Qian Cao (Herba Plantaginis), 227
Che Qian Zi (Semen Plantaginis), 226
Chi Xiao Dou (Semen Phaseoli Calcarati), 224
Chuan Lian Zi (Fructus Meliae Toosendan), 284
Chuan Xin Lian (Herba Andrographitis Paniculatae), 109
Da Fu Pi (Pericarpium Arecae Catechu), 288
Dan Zhu Ye (Herba Lophatheri Gracilis), 76
Deng Xin Cao (Medulla Junci Effusi), 237
Dong Gua Pi (Epicarpium Benincasae Hispidae), 224

Bladder

Kidney

Pericardium

San Jiao

Gallbladder

Liver

Appendix 10 Index of comparisons of functions

Hai Jin Sha (Spora Lygodii Japonici),
Bi Xie (Rhizoma Dioscoreae Hypoglaucae seu Septemlobae), *Jin Qian Cao* (Herba Lysimachiae) and *Shi Wei* (Folium Pyrrosiae), 240; *Shi Wei* (Folium Pyrrosiae), 230
Hai Piao Xiao (Os Sepiae seu Sepiellae),
Sang Piao Xiao (Oötheca Mantidis), 634
Hai Zao (Herba Sargassi),
Fu Hai Shi (Os Costaziae seu Pumex), *Hai Ge Ke* (Concha Meretricis seu Cyclinae) and *Kun Bu* (Thallus Laminariae seu Eckloniae), 423
Han Lian Cao (Herba Ecliptae Prostratae),
Nü Zhen Zi (Fructus Ligustri Lucidi), 596
He Cao Ya (Gemma Agrimoniae Pilosae),
Bing Lang (Semen Arecae Catechu) and *Nan Gua Zi* (Semen Cucurbitae Moschatae), 314
He Shou Wu (Radix Polygoni Multiflori),
Shu Di Huang (Radix Rehmanniae Glutinosae Conquita), 570
Hong Hua (Flos Carthami Tinctorii),
Tao Ren (Semen Persicae), 372
Hong Teng (Caulis Sargentodoxae Cuneatae),
Bai Jiang Cao (Herba Patriniae cum Radice) and *Yu Xing Cao* (Herba Houttuyniae Cordatae), 122
Hou Po (Cortex Magnoliae Officinalis),
Cang Zhu (Rhizoma Atractylodis), 202
Hu Huang Lian (Rhizoma Picrorhizae Scrophulariiflorae),
Huang Lian (Rhizoma Coptidis), 141
Hu Po (Succinum),
Zhu Sha (Cinnabaris), 457
Hu Tao Ren (Semen Juglandis Regiae),
Ge Jie (Gekko), 557
Hua Shi (Talcum),
Che Qian Zi (Semen Plantaginis), 226; *Shi Gao* (Gypsum Fibrosum), 228
Huai Hua (Flos Sophorae Japonicae),
Di Yu (Radix Sanguisorbae Officinalis), 330
Huang Bai (Cortex Phellodendri),
Chun Pi (Cortex Ailanthi Altissimae), 625; *Huang Lian* (Rhizoma Coptidis) and *Huang Qin* (Radix Scutellariae Baicalensis), 85; *Ku Shen* (Radix Sophorae Flavescentis), 86; *Long Dan Cao* (Radix Gentianae Scabrae), 88
Huang Jing (Rhizoma Polygonati),
Shan Yao (Rhizoma Dioscoreae Oppositae), 594; *Yu Zhu* (Rhizoma Polygonati Odorati), 593
Huang Lian (Rhizoma Coptidis),
Hu Huang Lian (Rhizoma Picrorhizae Scrophulariiflorae), 141; *Huang Bai* (Cortex Phellodendri) and *Huang Qin* (Radix Scutellariae Baicalensis), 85
Huang Qi (Radix Astragali seu Hedysari),
Ren Shen (Radix Ginseng), 519
Huang Qin (Radix Scutellariae Baicalensis),
Huang Bai (Cortex Phellodendri) and *Huang Lian* (Rhizoma Coptidis), 85
Huo Ma Ren (Semen Cannabis Sativae),
Yu Li Ren (Semen Pruni), 152
Huo Xiang (Herba Agastaches seu Pogostemi),
Pei Lan (Herba Eupatorii Fortunei) and *Xiang Ru* (Herba Elsholtziae seu Moslae), 203; *Zi Su Ye* (Folium Perillae Frutescentis), 199

Ji Xue Teng (Caulis Spatholobi),
Dang Gui (Radix Angelicae Sinensis), 378
Jiang Can (Bombyx Batryticatus),
Quan Xie (Buthus Martensi) and *Wu Gong* (Scolopendra Subspinipes), 493
Jiang Huang (Rhizoma Curcumae Longae),
Yu Jin (Radix Curcumae), 364
Jie Geng (Radix Platycodi Grandiflori),
Bai Qian (Radix et Rhizoma Cynanchi Stauntonii), 411; *Xing Ren* (Semen Pruni Armeniacae), 431
Jin Qian Cao (Herba Lysimachiae),
Bi Xie (Rhizoma Dioscoreae Hypoglaucae seu Septemlobae), *Hai Jin Sha* (Spora Lygodii Japonici) and *Shi Wei* (Folium Pyrrosiae), 240
Jin Yin Hua (Flos Lonicerae),
Lian Qiao (Fructus Forsythiae Suspensae), 97
Jin Ying Zi (Fructus Rosae Laevigatae),
Fu Pen Zi (Fructus Rubi Chingii), 636
Jing Da Ji (Radix Euphorbiae Pekinensis),
Gan Sui (Radix Euphorbiae Kansui) and *Yuan Hua* (Flos Daphnes Genkwa), 165
Jing Jie (Herba Schizonepetae Tenuifoliae),
Bo He (Herba Menthae Haplocalycis), 45; *Fang Feng* (Radix Ledebouriellae Divaricatae), 30
Ju Hua (Flos Chrysanthemi Morifolii),
Gou Teng (Ramulus Uncariae cum Uncis), 485; *Qin Pi* (Cortex Fraxini), 89; *Sang Ye* (Folium Mori Albae), 50; *Ye Ju Hua* (Flos Chrysanthemi Indici), 108
Jue Ming Zi (Semen Cassiae),
Shi Jue Ming (Concha Haliotidis), 472; *Xia Ku Cao* (Spica Prunellae Vulgaris), 77

Ku Lian Pi (Cortex Meliae Radicis),
Chuan Lian Zi (Fructus Meliae Toosendan), 310; *Shi Jun Zi* (Fructus Quisqualis Indicae), 309
Ku Shen (Radix Sophorae Flavescentis),
Bai Xian Pi (Cortex Dictamni Dasycarpi Radicis), 90; *Huang Bai* (Cortex Phellodendri), 86; *She Chuang Zi* (Fructus Cnidii Monnieri), 654

Appendix 11 Chinese titles of books and journals cited in modern research references

1. Books

Chang Yong Zhong Yao Yao Li Yu Ying Yong	常用中药药理与应用	Pharmacology and Application of Commonly-Used Chinese Materia Medica
Chang Yong Zhong Yao Xian Dai Yan Jiu Yu Lin Chuang	常用中药现代研究与临床	Current Research and Clinical Application of Commonly-Used Chinese Materia Medica
Chang Yong Zhong Yi Fang Yao Shou Ce	常用中医方药手册	Handbook of Commonly-Used Chinese Herbs and Prescriptions
Hai Yang Yao Wu Xue Gai Lun	海洋药物学概论	An Introduction to Marine Materia Medica
Hu Bei Zhong Yao Zhi	湖北中药志	Hubei Records of Chinese Materia Medica
Lin Chuang Zhong Yao Shou Ce	临床中药手册	Clinical Handbook of Chinese Materia Medica
Mian Yi Yao Li Jin Zhan-Ji Chu Yu Lin Chuang	免疫药理进展-基础与临床	Developments in Immune Pharmacology – Basics and Clinical Application
Quan Guo Qing Re Jie Du Yao Hui Yi Lun Wen Ji	全国清热解毒药会议论文集	Collection of Papers from the National Conference on Materia Medica for Clearing Heat and Relieving Toxicity
Quan Guo Zhong Cao Yao Hui Bian	全国中草药汇编	National Collection of Chinese Herbs
Ren Shen De Yan Jiu	人参的研究	Ginseng Research
Shi Yong Yao Wu Shou Ce	实用药物手册	Practical Handbook of Medicines
Xin Bian Zhong Yao Xue Ci Dian	新编中药学辞典	New Dictionary of Chinese Materia Medica
Yao Li Xue Jin Zhan	药理学进展	Development of Pharmacology
Zhi Wu Yao You Xiao Cheng Fen Shou Ce	植物药有效成分手册	Handbook of Active Ingredients of Herbal Medicine
Zhong Cao Yao Yao Li Xue	中草药药理学	Pharmacology of Chinese Herbs
Zhong Cao Yao You Xiao Cheng Fen Shou Ce	中草药有效成分手册	Handbook of Effective Ingredients of Chinese Medicinal Herbs
Zhong Hua Lin Chuang Zhong Yao Xue	中华临床中药学	Chinese Clinical Materia Medica
Zhong Yao Cai Zhi Yan Jiu	中药材之研究	Research on Chinese Materia Medica
Zhong Yao Da Ci Dian	中药大辞典	Dictionary of Chinese Materia Medica
Zhong Yao Xue	中药学	Chinese Materia Medica
Zhong Yao Yao Li Yu Ying Yong	中药药理与应用	Pharmacology and Application of Chinese Materia Medica
Zhong Yao Zhi	中药志	Chinese Materia Medica Records
Zhong Yi Fang Ji Yao Li Yu Ying Yong	中医方剂药理与应用	Pharmacology and Application of TCM Prescriptions
Zhong Yi Yao Nian Jian	中医药年鉴	Year Book of Traditional Chinese Medicine

2. Journals

Ai Zheng	癌症	Journal of Cancer
An Hui Yi Ke Da Xue Xue Bao	安徽医科大学学报	Journal of Anhui Medical University
An Hui Yi Xue Yuan Xue Bao	安徽医学院学报	Journal of Anhui Medical College
An Hui Zhong Yi Xue Yuan Xue Bao	安徽中医学院学报	Journal of Anhui College of Traditional Chinese Medicine
Bai Qiu En Yi Ke Da Xue Xue Bao	白求恩医科大学学报	Journal of Bethune Medical University
Bao Tou Yi Xue	包头医学	Baotou Journal of Medicine
Bei Jing Da Xue Yi Xue Yuan Xue Bao	北京大学医学院学报	Journal of Beijing University Medical College
Bei Jing Yi Ke Da Xue Xue Bao	北京医科大学学报	Journal of Beijing Medical University
Bei Jing Yi Xue	北京医学	Beijing Journal of Medicine
Bei Jing Yi Xue Yuan Xue Bao	北京医学院学报	Journal of Beijing Medical College
Bei Jing Yi Yao Gong Ye	北京医药工业	Beijing Medical and Pharmacology Industry
Bei Jing Zhong Yi Xue Yuan Xue Bao	北京中医学院学报	Journal of Beijing College of Traditional Chinese Medicine
Bei Jing Zhong Yi Za Zhi	北京中医杂志	Beijing Journal of Traditional Chinese Medicine
Chang Bai Shan Zhong Yi Yao Yan Jiu Yu Fa Zhan	长白山中医药研究与发展	Changbaishan Research and Development of Traditional Chinese Medicine and Materia Medica
Chang Yong Zhong Yao De Yao Li Yu Ying Yong	常用中药的药理与应用	Pharmacology and Application of Commonly-Used Chinese Materia Medica
Cheng Du Zhong Yi Xue Yuan Xue Bao	成都中医学院学报	Journal of Chengdu College of TCM
Da Lian Yi Xue Yuan Xue Bao	大连医学院学报	Journal of Dalian College of Medicine
Di Er Jun Yi Da Xue Xue Bao	第二军医大学学报	Journal of Second Military Medical University
Di San Jun Yi Da Xue Xue Bao	第三军医大学学报	Journal of Third Military Medical University
Di Yi Jun Yi Da Xue Xue Bao	第一军医大学学报	Journal of First Military Medical University
Dong Wu Xue Za Zhi	动物学杂志	Zoology Journal
Fu Jian Yi Yao Za Zhi	福建医药杂志	Fujian Journal of Medicine and Pharmacology
Fu Jian Zhong Yi Yao	福建中医药	Fujian Journal of Traditional Chinese Medicine and Materia Medica
Gan Su Zhong Yi Xue Yuan Xue Bao	甘肃中医学院学报	Journal of Gansu College of TCM
Guang Xi Yi Xue	广西医学	Guangxi Journal of Medicine
Guang Xi Yi Yao Tong Xun	广西医药通讯	Guangxi Medicine and Pharmacology Newsletter
Guang Xi Zhong Yi Yao	广西中医药	Guangxi Journal of Traditional Chinese Medicine and Materia Medica
Guang Zhou Yi Yao	广州医药	Guangzhou Journal of Medicine and Pharmacology
Guo Wai Yao Xun	国外药讯	Foreign Pharmacology Newsletter
Guo Wai Yi Xue – Yao Xue Fen Ce	国外医学 - 药学分册	Foreign Medicine – Pharmacology Fascicule

Guo Wai Yi Xue – Zhi Wu Yao Fen Ce	国外医学 - 植物药分册	Foreign Medicine – Herbs Fascicule
Guo Wai Yi Xue – Zhong Yi Zhong Yao Fen Ce	国外医学 - 中医中药分册	Foreign Medicine – TCM Fascicule
Ha Er Bin Yi Ke Da Xue Xue Bao	哈尔滨医科大学学报	Journal of Harbin Medical University
He Bei Zhong Yi	河北中医	Hebei Journal of Traditional Chinese Medicine
He Nan Yi Xue Yuan Xue Bao	河南医学院学报	Journal of Henan Medical College
He Nan Zhong Yi	河南中医	Henan Journal of Traditional Chinese Medicine
Hu Bei Yi Xue Yuan Xue Bao	湖北医学院学报	Journal of Hubei Medical College
Hu Nan Yi Xue Qing Bao	湖南医学情报	Hunan Medical Information
Hu Nan Yi Xue Yuan Xue Bao	湖南医学院学报	Journal of Hunan Medical College
Hu Nan Yi Yao Za Zhi	湖南医药杂志	Hunan Journal of Medicine and Pharmacology
Hu Nan Zhong Yi Za Zhi	湖南中医杂志	Hunan Journal of Traditional Chinese Medicine
Hua Xi Yao Xue Za Zhi	华西药学杂志	Huaxi Pharmacology Journal
Hua Xi Yi Ke Da Xue Xue Bao	华西医科大学学报	Journal of Huaxi Medical University
Hua Xue Xue Bao	化学学报	Chemistry Journal
Ji Chu Yi Xue Yu Lin Chuang	基础医学与临床	Foundations of Medicine and Clinical Application
Ji Sheng Chong Xue He Ji Sheng Chong Bing Za Zhi	寄生虫学和寄生虫病杂志	Journal of Parasitology and Parasitic Diseases
Jia Mu Si Yi Xue Yuan Xue Bao	佳木斯医学院学报	Journal of Jiamusi Medical College
Jiang Su Sheng Zhong Yao Yan Jiu Suo Suo Kan	江苏省中药研究所所刊	Internal Journal of Jiangsu Chinese Materia Medica Research Institute
Jiang Su Yi Yao	江苏医药	Jiangsu Journal of Medicine and Pharmacology
Jiang Su Zhong Yi Za Zhi	江苏中医杂志	Jiangsu Journal of Traditional Chinese Medicine
Jiang Xi Yi Xue Yuan Xue Bao	江西医学院学报	Journal of Jiangxi Medical College
Jiang Xi Yi Yao	江西医药	Jiangxi Journal of Medicine and Pharmacology
Jiang Xi Zhong Yi Yao	江西中医药	Jiangxi Journal of Traditional Chinese Medicine and Materia Medica
Ke Ji Zi Liao Hui Bian	科技资料汇编	Collection of Scientific Papers
Ke Xue Tong Bao	科学通报	Science Bulletin
Lan Zhou Yi Xue Yuan Xue Bao	兰州医学院学报	Journal of Lanzhou Medical College
Lao Nian Xue Za Zhi	老年学杂志	Journal of Geriatrics
Liao Ning Zhong Yi Za Zhi	辽宁中医杂志	Liaoning Journal of Traditional Chinese Medicine
Lin Chuang Gan Dan Bing Za Zhi	临床肝胆病杂志	Journal of Clinical Hepatology
Nan Jing Tie Dao Yi Xue Yuan Xue Bao	南京铁道医学院学报	Journal of Nanjing Railway Medical College
Nan Jing Yao Xue Yuan Xue Bao	南京药学院学报	Journal of Nanjing Pharmacology College
Nan Jing Yi Xue Yuan Xue Bao	南京医学院学报	Journal of Nanjing Medical College
Nan Jing Zhong Yi Xue Yuan Xue Bao	南京中医学院学报	Journal of Nanjing College of Traditional Chinese Medicine
Qing Hai Yi Xue Yuan Xue Bao	青海医学院学报	Journal of Qinghai Medical College
Ren Shen Yan Jiu	人参研究	Ginseng Research
Ri Ben Yao Li Xue Za Zhi	日本药理学杂志	Japanese Journal of Pharmacology

Shan Dong Yi Ke Da Xue Xue Bao	山东医科大学学报	Journal of Shandong Medical University
Shan Dong Yi Xue Yuan Xue Bao	山东医学院学报	Journal of Shandong College of Medicine
Shan Dong Yi Yao	山东医药	Shandong Medical Journal
Shan Dong Zhong Yi Xue Yuan Xue Bao	山东中医学院学报	Journal of Shandong College of Traditional Chinese Medicine
Shan Dong Zhong Yi Za Zhi	山东中医杂志	Shandong Journal of Traditional Chinese Medicine
Shan Xi Yi Xue Yuan Xue Bao	山西医学院学报	Journal of Shanxi College of Medicine
Shan Xi Yi Yao	山西医药	Shanxi Medical Journal
Shan Xi Yi Yao Za Zhi	山西医药杂志	Shanxi Journal of Medicine and Pharmacology
Shan Xi Xin Yi Yao	陕西新医药	Shaanxi New Medical Journal
Shan Xi Yi Xue Za Zhi	陕西医学杂志	Shaanxi Journal of Medicine
Shan Xi Zhong Yi	陕西中医	Shaanxi Journal of Traditional Chinese Medicine
Shan Xi Zhong Yi Xue Yuan Xue Bao	陕西中医学院学报	Journal of Shaanxi College of Traditional Chinese Medicine
Shang Hai Di Yi Yi Xue Yuan Xue Bao	上海第一医学院学报	Journal of Shanghai No. 1 Medical College
Shang Hai Yi Ke Da Xue Xue Bao	上海医科大学学报	Journal of Shanghai Medical University
Shang Hai Yi Xue	上海医学	Shanghai Medical Journal
Shang Hai Zhong Yi Yao Za Zhi	上海中医药杂志	Shanghai Journal of Traditional Chinese Medicine and Materia Medica
Shen Yang Yao Xue Yuan Xue Bao	沈阳药学院学报	Journal of Shenyang Pharmacology College
Sheng Li Ke Xue	生理科学	Physiological Science
Sheng Li Ke Xue Jin Zhan	生理科学进展	Developments in Physiological Science
Sheng Li Xue Bao	生理学报	Physiology Journal
Sheng Yao Xue Za Zhi	生药学杂志	Journal of Raw Herbs
Sheng Zhi Yu Bi Yun	生殖与避孕	Reproduction and Contraception
Shi Yan Sheng Wu Xue Bao	实验生物学报	Journal of Experimental Biology
Shi Yong Zhong Liu Xue Za Zhi	实用肿瘤学杂志	Journal of Practical Oncology
Shou Yi Ke Ji Za Zhi	兽医科技杂志	Journal of Veterinary Medicine Science and Technology
Si Chuan Da Xue Xue Bao	四川大学学报	Journal of Sichuan University
Si Chuan Yi Xue	四川医学	Sichuan Journal of Medicine
Tai Wan Yi Xue Hui Za Zhi	台湾医学会杂志	Journal of Taiwan Medical Association
Te Chan Ke Xue Shi Yan	特产科学实验	Scientific Experiments on Special Herb Production
Tian Jin Yi Ke Da Xue Xue Bao	天津医科大学学报	Journal of Tianjin Medical University
Tian Jin Yi Xue Tong Xun	天津医学通讯	Tianjin Medical Newsletter
Tian Jin Yi Xue Za Zhi	天津医学杂志	Tianjin Journal of Medicine
Tian Jin Yi Yao	天津医药	Tianjin Journal of Medicine and Pharmacology
Tong Ji Yi Ke Da Xue Xue Bao	同济医科大学学报	Journal of Tongji Medical University

Wei Liang Yuan Su	微量元素	Trace Elements
Wei Sheng Fang Yi Tong Xun	卫生防疫通讯	Health and Epidemic Prevention Newsletter
Wei Sheng Wu Xue Bao	微生物学报	Micro-organism Journal
Wei Sheng Wu Xue Tong Bao	微生物学通报	Micro-organism Bulletin
Wen Zhou Yi Xue Yuan Xue Bao	温州医学院学报	Journal of Wenzhou Medical College
Xi An Yi Xue Yuan Xue Bao	西安医学院学报	Journal of Xi'an Medical College
Xi Bei Yao Xue Za Zhi	西北药学杂志	Northwest Journal of Pharmacology
Xian Dai Ying Yong Yao Xue	现代应用药学	Current Applied Pharmacology
Xin Jiang Zhong Yi Yao	新疆中医药	Xinjiang Journal of Traditional Chinese Medicine and Materia Medica
Xin Yao Yu Lin Chuang	新药与临床	New Drugs and Clinical Applications
Xin Yi Xue	新医学	New Journal of Medicine
Xin Yi Xue Bao	新医学报	New Medical Journal
Xin Yi Xue Zi Liao	新医学资料	New Medical Documents
Xin Yi Yao Xue Za Zhi	新医药学杂志	New Medicine and Pharmacology Journal
Xin Yi Yao Yan Jiu	新医药研究	New Medicine and Materia Medica Research Journal
Xin Zhong Yi	新中医	New Journal of Traditional Chinese Medicine
Yao Jian Gong Ye Tong Xun	药检工业通讯	Medicine Inspection Industry Newsletter
Yao Wu Fen Xi Za Zhi	药物分析杂志	Chinese Journal of Pharmacological Analysis
Yao Xue Lun Wen Zhai Yao	药学论文摘要	Digest of Pharmacology Dissertations
Yao Xue Tong Bao	药学通报	Pharmacology Bulletin
Yao Xue Xue Bao	药学学报	Pharmacology Journal
Yao Xue Za Zhi	药学杂志	Journal of Pharmacology
Yi Xue Zhong Yang Za Zhi	医学中央杂志	Medical Centre Journal
Yi Xue Zi Liao	医学资料	Medical Documents
Yi Yao Gong Ye	医药工业	Medical and Pharmaceutical Industry Journal
Yun Nan Yi Yao	云南医药	Yunnan Journal of Medicine and Pharmacology
Yun Nan Zhong Yi Za Zhi	云南中医杂志	Yunnan Journal of Traditional Chinese Medicine
Zhe Jiang Tong Xun	浙江通讯	Zhejiang Newsletter
Zhe Jiang Yi Ke Da Xue Xue Bao	浙江医科大学学报	Journal of Zhejiang Medical University
Zhe Jiang Yi Xue	浙江医学	Zhejiang Journal of Medicine
Zhe Jiang Zhong Liu Tong Xun	浙江肿瘤通讯	Zhejiang Tumour Newsletter
Zhe Jiang Zhong Yi Yao Za Zhi	浙江中医药杂志	Zhejiang Journal of Traditional Chinese Medicine and Materia Medica
Zhe Jiang Zhong Yi Za Zhi	浙江中医杂志	Zhejiang Journal of Traditional Chinese Medicine
Zhong Cao Yao	中草药	Journal of Chinese Herbs
Zhong Cao Yao Tong Bao	中草药通报	Bulletin of Chinese Herbs
Zhong Cao Yao Tong Xun	中草药通讯	Chinese Herbs Newsletter

Zhong Cao Yao Yan Jiu Zi Liao	中草药研究资料	Chinese Medicinal Herbs Research Documentation
Zhong Cheng Yao	中成药	Journal of Chinese Medicinal Preparations
Zhong Cheng Yao Yan Jiu	中成药研究	Chinese Medicinal Preparation Research
Zhong Guo Hai Yang Yao Wu	中国海洋药物	Chinese Marine Materia Medica
Zhong Guo Lin Chuang Yao Li Xue Za Zhi	中国临床药理学杂志	Chinese Journal of Clinical Pharmacology
Zhong Guo Mian Yi Xue Za Zhi	中国免疫学杂志	Chinese Journal of Immunology
Zhong Guo Nong Cun Yi Xue	中国农村医学	Chinese Rural Medicine
Zhong Guo Sheng Li Ke Xue Za Zhi	中国生理科学杂志	Chinese Journal of Physiological Science
Zhong Guo Xin Yao Za Zhi	中国新药杂志	Chinese Journal of New Drugs
Zhong Guo Yao Ke Da Xue Xue Bao	中国药科大学学报	Journal of Chinese Pharmacology University
Zhong Guo Yao Li Tong Bao	中国药理通报	Chinese Bulletin of Pharmacology
Zhong Guo Yao Li Tong Xun	中国药理通讯	Chinese Pharmacology Newsletter
Zhong Guo Yao Li Xue Bao	中国药理学报	Chinese Journal of Pharmacology
Zhong Guo Yao Li Xue Tong Bao	中国药理学通报	Chinese Pharmacology Bulletin
Zhong Guo Yao Li Xue Yu Du Li Xue Za Zhi	中国药理学与毒理学杂志	Chinese Journal of Pharmacology and Toxicology
Zhong Guo Yao Xue Za Zhi	中国药学杂志	Journal of Chinese Pharmacology
Zhong Guo Yi Ke Da Xue Xue Bao	中国医科大学学报	Journal of Chinese Medical University
Zhong Guo Yi Xue Ke Xue Yuan Xue Bao	中国医学科学院学报	Journal of the Chinese Academy of Medical Science
Zhong Guo Yi Xue Ke Xue Yuan Lun Wen Zhai Yao	中国医学科学院论文摘要	Digest of the Chinese Academy of Medical Science Discussion Papers
Zhong Guo Yi Xue Za Zhi	中华医学杂志	China Medical Journal
Zhong Guo Yi Yao Xue Bao	中国医药学报	Chinese Journal of Medicine and Pharmacology
Zhong Guo Yi Yuan Yao Xue Za Zhi	中国医院药学杂志	Chinese Journal of Hospital Pharmacology
Zhong Guo Zhong Yao Za Zhi	中国中药杂志	Journal of Chinese Materia Medica
Zhong Hua Fang She Xue Za Zhi	中华放射学杂志	Chinese Radiology Journal
Zhong Hua Hu Li Za Zhi	中华护理杂志	Chinese Journal of Nursing
Zhong Hua Lao Nian Bing Xue Za Zhi	中华老年病学杂志	Chinese Journal of Geriatrics
Zhong Hua Nei Ke Za Zhi	中华内科杂志	Chinese Journal of Internal Medicine
Zhong Hua Pi Fu Ke Za Zhi	中华皮肤科杂志	Chinese Dermatology Journal
Zhong Hua Wai Ke Za Zhi	中华外科杂志	Chinese Journal of Surgery
Zhong Hua Wei Sheng Wu He Mian Yi Za Zhi	中华微生物和免疫杂志	Chinese Micro-organism and Immunization Journal
Zhong Hua Xin Xue Guan Bing Za Zhi	中华心血管病杂志	Chinese Journal of Cardiology
Zhong Hua Xin Yi Xue Bao	中华新医学报	Chinese Journal of New Medicine
Zhong Hua Xue Ye Xue Za Zhi	中华血液学杂志	Chinese Journal of Haematology
Zhong Hua Yi Xue Za Zhi	中华医学杂志	Chinese Journal of Medicine
Zhong Ma Tong Xun	中麻通讯	Chinese Anaesthetics Newsletter
Zhong Xi Yi Jie He Za Zhi	中西医结合杂志	Journal of Integrated TCM and Western Medicine

Zhong Xi Yi Jie He Zi Liao Hui Bian	中西医结合资料汇编	Collection of Scientific Papers on Integrated TCM and Western Medicine
Zhong Yao Cai	中药材	Chinese Materia Medica
Zhong Yao Ke Yan Jian Bao	中药科研简报	Chinese Materia Medica Scientific Research Briefing
Zhong Yao Tong Bao	中药通报	Bulletin of Chinese Materia Medica
Zhong Yao Xin Yao Yu Lin Chuang Yao Li	中药新药与临床药理	New Drugs of Chinese Materia Medica and Clinical Pharmacology
Zhong Yao Yao Li Yu Lin Chuang	中药药理与临床	Pharmacology and Clinical Application of Chinese Materia Medica
Zhong Yi Xue Yan Jiu Can Kao	中医学研究参考	Journal of Chinese Medicine Research
Zhong Yi Yan Jiu	中医研究	Traditional Chinese Medicine Research
Zhong Yi Yao Xin Xi	中医药信息	Traditional Chinese Medicine and Materia Medica News
Zhong Yi Yao Xue Bao	中医药学报	Journal of Traditional Chinese Medicine and Materia Medica
Zhong Yi Yao Yan Jiu	中医药研究	Traditional Chinese Medicine and Materia Medica Research
Zhong Yi Za Zhi	中医杂志	Journal of Traditional Chinese Medicine

Bibliography

Academy of Traditional Chinese Medicine and Guangzhou College of Traditional Chinese Medicine, *Jian Ming Zhong Yi Ci Dian* 简明中医辞典 [Concise Dictionary of Traditional Chinese Medicine], Beijing: People's Medical Publishing House, 1979.

Bao Xiangao, *Yan Fang Xin Bian* 验方新编 [New Compilation of Classical Formulae], Beijing: People's Medical Publishing House, 1998.

Ding Xuemin et al., *Chang Yong Zhong Yi Fang Yao Shou Ce* 常用中医方药手册 [Handbook of Commonly-Used Chinese Herbs and Prescriptions], Changsha: Hunan Science and Technology Publishing House, 1982.

Ding Zhaomeng, *Zhong Yao Yao Xiao Yu Lin Chuang* 中药药效与临床 [Pharmacodynamics and Clinical Application of Chinese Materia Medica], Beijing: Chinese Medical and Pharmaceutical Science and Technology Publishing House, 1999.

Editorial Committee of Chinese-English, Chinese-French, Chinese-German, Chinese-Japanese and Chinese-Russian Medical Dictionary, *Han Ying Yi Xue Da Ci Dian* 汉英医学大词典 [The Chinese-English Medical Dictionary], Beijing: People's Medical Publishing House, 1994.

Foreign Language Teaching and Research Section of Beijing Medical College, *Han Ying Chang Yong Yi Xue Ci Hui* 汉英常用医学词汇 [Chinese-English Glossary of Commonly Used Medical Terminology], Beijing: People's Medical Publishing House, 1982.

Gao Xuemei et al., *Zhong Yao Xue* 中药学 [Chinese Materia Medica], Beijing: People's Medical Publishing House, 2000.

Gong Shideng, *Lin Zheng Yong Yao Jing Yan* 临证用药经验 [Clinical Experience of Application of Materia Medica Based on Pattern Identification], Beijing: People's Medical Publishing House, 1999.

He Xingdong et al., *Lin Chuang Zhong Yao Shou Ce* 临床中药手册 [Clinical Handbook of Chinese Materia Medica], Beijing: People's Medical Publishing House, 1998.

Hu Zhijian, *Zhong Yao Lin Zheng Ying Yong* 中药临证应用 [Clinical Application of Chinese Materia Medica], Hohhot: Inner Mongolia People's Publishing House, 1980.

Jiangsu New Medical College, *Zhong Yao Da Ci Dian* 中药大词典 [Dictionary of Chinese Materia Medica], revised edition, Shanghai: Shanghai Science and Technology Publishing House, 1986.

Lei Zaiquan and Zhang Tingmo, *Zhong Hua Lin Chuang Zhong Yao Xue* 中华临床中药学 [Chinese Clinical Materia Medica], Beijing: People's Medical Publishing House, 1998.

Li Shizhen (Ming dynasty), *Ben Cao Gang Mu* 本草纲目 [Materia Medica Compendium], Beijing: People's Medical Publishing House, 1982 (modern re-edition).

Ling Yiduo, *Zhong Yao Xue* 中药学 [Chinese Materia Medica], Shanghai: Shanghai Science and Technology Publishing House, 1998.

Liu Chinian, *Gu Jin Yao Fang Zong Heng* 古今药方纵横 [Discussion on Ancient and Modern Formulae, third volume], Beijing: People's Medical Publishing House, 1998.

Liu Shengsi, *Jing Yue Xin Fang Ba Zhen Qian Jie Yu Ying Yong* 景岳新方八阵浅解与应用 [Brief Explanation and Application of Jing Yue's Formulae], Beijing: People's Medical Publishing House, 1999.

Ou Ming, *Han Ying Zhong Yi Ci Dian* 汉英中医辞典 [Chinese-English Dictionary of Traditional Chinese Medicine], Guangzhou: Guangdong Science and Technology Publishing House, 1993.

Pharmacopoeia Commission of the PRC, *Pharmacopoeia of the People's Republic of China (English Edition)*, Beijing: Chemical Industry Press, 2000.

Xie Pangen, *Shi Er Jing Lin Chuang Yong Yao Shou Ce* 十二经临床用药手册 [Clinical and Pharmaceutical Manual of the Twelve Channels], Beijing: Chinese Medical and Pharmaceutical Science and Technology Publishing House, 1992.

Xie Zongwan et al., *Quan Guo Zhong Cao Yao Hui Bian* 全国中草药汇编 [National Collection of Chinese Herbs], 2nd edition, Beijing: People's Medical Publishing House, 1996.

Wang Benxian, *Xin Bian Zhong Yao Xue Ci Dian* 新编中药学辞典 [New Dictionary of Chinese Materia Medica], Tianjin: Tianjin Science and Technology Publishing House, 1996.

Wang Yusheng et al., *Zhong Yao Yao Li Yu Ying Yong* 中药药理与应用 [Pharmacology and Application of Chinese Materia Medica], Beijing: People's Medical Publishing House, 1998.

Wiseman, Nigel, *English-Chinese Chinese-English Dictionary of Chinese Medicine*, Changsha: Hubei Science and Technology Publishing House, 1996.

Yang Baifo, *Shi Yong Jing Fang Ji Cheng* 实用精方集成 [Practical Collection of Classical Formulae], Beijing: People's Medical Publishing House, 1997.

Yang Yiya, *Zhong Yao* 中药 [Chinese Materia Medica], Shijiazhuang: Hebei Science and Technology Publishing House, 1994.

Yuan Yixiang, Ren Jixue and Huang Long, *Han Ying Shuang Jie Zhong Yi Da Ci Dian* 汉英双解中医大辞典 [Chinese-English Dictionary of Traditional Chinese Medicine], Beijing: People's Medical Publishing House, 1997.

Zhang Xianchen et al., *Zhong Yao Jing Hua* 中药精华 [Essentials of Chinese Materia Medica], Hefei: Anhui Science and Technology Publishing House, 1988.

Zou Jilong, *Gu Jin Yao Fang Zong Heng* 古今药方纵横 [Discussions on Ancient and Modern Formulae, second volume], Beijing: People's Medical Publishing House, 1998.